Clinical Evaluation and Diagnostic Tests for Neuromuscular Disorders

Clinical Evaluation and Diagnostic Tests for Neuromuscular Disorders

Tulio E. Bertorini, M.D.

Professor, Departments of Neurology and Pathology, University of Tennessee Health Science Center, Memphis; Co-Director, Neurology Training Program; Director, Clinical Neurophysiology Training Program, University of Tennessee Health Science Center; Director, Neurology and Electromyography Laboratory, Methodist University Hospital, Wesley Neurology Clinic, Wesley Neuromuscular Laboratory, and Midsouth Muscular Dystrophy Association Clinic, Memphis

With 32 Contributing Authors

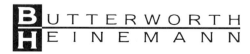

An Imprint of Elsevier Science

Amsterdam • Boston • London • Oxford • New York • Paris
San Diego • San Francisco • Singapore • Sydney • Tokyo

MT

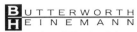

An Imprint of Elsevier Science

225 Wildwood Avenue
Woburn, MA 01801

Notice

Neurology is an ever-changing field. Standard safety precautions must be followed, but as new research and clinical experience broaden our knowledge, changes in treatment and drug therapy may become necessary or appropriate. Readers are advised to check the most current product information provided by the manufacturer of each drug to be administered to verify the recommended dose, the method and duration of administration, and contraindications. It is the responsibility of the treating physician, relying on experience and knowledge of the patient, to determine dosages and the best treatment for each individual patient. Neither the Publisher nor the author assume any liability for any injury and/or damage to persons or property arising from this publication.

The Publisher

Library of Congress Cataloging-in-Publication Data

Clinical evaluation and diagnostic tests for neuromuscular disorders / edited by Tulio E.
Bertorini ; with 32 contributing authors. – 1st ed.
        p. ; cm.
    Includes bibliographical references and index.
    ISBN 0-7506-7290-0
      1. Neuromuscular diseases—Diagnosis. I. Bertorini, Tulio E.
    [DNLM: 1. Neuromuscular Diseases—diagnosis. 2. Diagnostic Techniques,
  Neurological. 3. Electromyography. WE 550 C6403 2002]
  RC925.7.C56 2002
  616.7'44075—dc21

                                                            2002017678

Publisher: Susan F. Pioli
Editorial Assistant: Joan Ryan

SSC/MVY

Printed in the United States of America
Last digit is the print number: 9 8 7 6 5 4 3 2 1

7/12/04

Contents

Color Plates A1–A10 follow page 24.

Color Plates B1–B54 follow page 624.

Contributing Authors

Paul E. Barkhaus, M.D.
Associate Professor, Department of Neurology, Medical College of Wisconsin, Milwaukee; Attending Staff and Director, Neuromuscular Diseases, Neurology Service, Milwaukee Veterans Administration Medical Center

Tulio E. Bertorini, M.D.
Professor, Departments of Neurology and Pathology, University of Tennessee Health Science Center, Memphis; Co-Director, Neurology Training Program; Director, Clinical Neurophysiology Training Program, University of Tennessee Health Science Center; Director, Neurology and Electromyography Laboratory, Methodist University Hospital, Wesley Neurology Clinic, Wesley Neuromuscular Laboratory, and Midsouth Muscular Dystrophy Association Clinic, Memphis

Emma Ciafaloni, M.D.
Assistant Professor, Department of Medicine, Division of Neurology, Duke University Medical Center, Durham, North Carolina

Salvatore DiMauro, M.D.
Lucy G. Moses Professor of Neurology, Columbia University College of Physicians and Surgeons, New York

Alberto L. Dubrovsky, M.D.
Associate Professor of Neurology, University of Buenos Aires School of Medicine, Buenos Aires, Argentina; Director, Neuromuscular Unit, Hospital Frances, Buenos Aires

J. Rafael Gorospe, M.D., Ph.D.
Assistant Professor of Pediatrics, Research Center for Genetic Medicine, Children's National Medical Center, George Washington University School of Medicine, Washington, D.C.

Alan Graves, M.D.
Radiologist, Department of Radiology, Methodist Hospitals of Memphis, Memphis, Tennessee

Judy W. Griffin, M.S., P.T.
Clinical Professor, Department of Physical Therapy, University of Tennessee Health Science Center, Memphis

Hollis Halford, M.D.
Radiologist, Department of Radiology, Methodist Hospitals of Memphis, Memphis, Tennessee

Eric P. Hoffman, Ph.D.
A. James Clark Chair of Molecular Medicine, Professor of Pediatrics, Biochemistry, and Molecular Biology, and Director, Research Center for Genetic Medicine, Children's National Medical Center, George Washington University School of Medicine, Washington, D.C.

Linda H. Horner, H.T. (A.S.C.P.), E.M.T. (M.S.A.)
Research Coordinator, Department of Neurology, University of Tennessee Health Science Center, Memphis

Horacio Kaufmann, M.D.
Associate Professor, Department of Neurology, Mount Sinai School of Medicine, New York; Attending Physician, Department of Neurology, Mount Sinai Medical Center, New York

Jun Kimura, M.D.
Professor of Neurology and Director, Electromyography Laboratory, University of Iowa College of Medicine, University of Iowa Hospitals and Clinics, Iowa City

Sindu Krishna, Ph.D.
Staff Associate, Department of Neurology, Columbia University College of Physicians and Surgeons, New York

Raffaele Lodi, M.D., Ph.D.
Associate Professor, Department of Medicine, Clinical Magnetic Resonance Spectroscopy Unit, Clinica e Biotecnologia Applicata D. Campanacci, Università di Bologna, Bologna, Italy

Catherine Lomen-Hoerth, M.D., Ph.D.
Assistant Professor in Residence, Department of Neurology, University of California, San Francisco

Carlos A. Luciano, M.D.
Associate Professor of Neurology and Assistant Director, RCMI-Clinical Research Center, Department of Medicine, Division of Neurology, University of Puerto Rico School of Medicine, San Juan; Staff Neurologist, University District Hospital, San Juan

Ricardo A. Maselli, M.D.
Professor, Department of Neurology, University of California, Davis; University of California Davis Medical Center, Sacramento

Janice M. Massey, M.D.
Professor, Department of Medicine, Division of Neurology, Duke University Medical Center, Durham, North Carolina

Daniel L. Menkes, M.D.
Associate Professor, Department of Neurology, University of Tennessee Health Science Center, Memphis; Director of Clinical Neurophysiology, The Regional Medical Center, Memphis

Ali Naini, Ph.D.
Research Scientist and Director, Molecular Neurogenetics, Department of Neurology, Columbia University College of Physicians and Surgeons, New York

Sanjeev D. Nandedkar, Ph.D.
Clinical Applications Manager, Oxford Instruments Medical Systems, Hawthorne, New York

Pushpa Narayanaswami, M.D.
Clinical Assistant Professor, Department of Neurology, University of Tennessee Health Science Center, Memphis; Neurologist, Wesley Neurology Clinic, Methodist University Hospital, Memphis

Shin J. Oh, M.D.
Professor, Department of Neurology, University of Alabama at Birmingham; Medical Director, Department of Clinical Neurophysiology, Electromyography Laboratory, Muscle/Nerve Histopathology Laboratory, University of Alabama Hospital, Birmingham

Mary L. O'Toole, Ph.D.
Professor, Department of Obstetrics, Gynecology and Women's Health, Saint Louis University, St. Louis

Kandasami Senthilkumar, M.D.
Fellow, Department of Neurology, Clinical Neurophysiology Program, University of Tennessee Health Science Center, Methodist University Hospital, Memphis; Neurologist, Christus Saint Elizabeth Hospital, Memorial Herman Baptist Hospital, Beaumont, Texas

Sara Shanske, Ph.D.
Research Scientist, Department of Neurology, Columbia University College of Physicians and Surgeons, New York

Erik Stålberg, M.D., Ph.D., F.R.C.P.
Professor Emeritus, Uppsala University, Uppsala, Sweden; Chairman, Department of Clinical Neurophysiology, Uppsala University Hospital, Uppsala

Tanja Taivassalo, Ph.D.
Research Associate, Neuromuscular Center, Institute for Exercise and Environmental Medicine, University of Texas Southwestern Medical Center, Dallas

Jože V. Trontelj, M.D., D.Sc.
Professor of Neurology, Medical Faculty, University of Ljubljana, Slovenia; Neurologist and Clinical Neurophysiologist, Department of Neurology, Institute of Clinical Neurophysiology, University Medical Center, Ljubljana

Renato J. Verdugo, M.D.
Associate Professor, Faculty of Medicine, Universidad de Chile, Santiago

Annabel K. Wang, M.D.
Assistant Professor, Department of Neurology, Mount Sinai School of Medicine, New York; Attending Physician, Department of Neurology, Mount Sinai Medical Center, New York

Preface

The field of neuromuscular disorders has expanded rapidly in the last 20 years, providing the clinician with multiple areas of knowledge to explore and understand. The purpose of this book is to present clinicians and trainees with overviews of the clinical approaches and the applications of the different diagnostic tests for these conditions, incorporating not only those used routinely but also new methodologies. This book, however, is not intended to be a treatise on neuromuscular disorders and their treatment.

The standard diagnostic tests are explained in a didactic way that we expect will help those new in the field, whereas newer techniques are covered in enough detail to be useful as a reference source. Also, to provide the reader the opportunity to review each chapter independently, I have taken the liberty of allowing some information to be repeated. Should there be a need to seek more in-depth coverage of the various areas, excellent textbooks—some of which are works by our collaborators—are available.

The book has one problem—that I am the editor—and for that I have no excuse. But I believe that I have been able to seek the expert and enthusiastic help of an exceptional group of collaborators, including prestigious authorities and young investigators, who have contributed to this endeavor. I hope that the product of our efforts will be valuable to those who care for patients with neuromuscular disorders.

Tulio E. Bertorini

Acknowledgments

I want to thank the Methodist University Hospital and Wesley Neurology Clinic in Memphis for their support, particularly Judy DeFranco for reviewing our manuscripts and Drs. Paul Deaton and Amado Freire for their suggestions.

I also want to thank those who helped in preparing various chapters, including Julie Carter, Cindy Culver, and Helen Hamm for their hard work and dedication, and John Conner, Lisa Everhardt, and Sue Maccarino. I particularly would like to thank Jason Peck for his excellent artwork and Nancy Smith, Librarian at the Methodist University Hospital, for her assistance. Thanks also to Susan Pioli and Andrea Sherman from Butterworth–Heinemann for their encouragement and valuable help, and to Holly Hoe for her meticulous and outstanding work.

I am particularly thankful for the authors and collaborators of the various chapters of this book for their unselfish hard work, dedication, and kindness.

I want to express my appreciation and dedicate my work to my wife, Emma, and our children, Tulio, Paola, Francisco, and Jason; to my father, Nicolas (Nico); and to the memory of my mother, Enriqueta (Queta).

1

Overview and Classification of Neuromuscular Disorders

Tulio E. Bertorini

Neuromuscular diseases are those that involve the peripheral nervous system, which includes the anterior horn cells (motor neuron diseases), roots (radiculopathies), plexi (plexopathies), peripheral nerves (neuropathies), neuromuscular junctions (myasthenia gravis [MG]), and muscle fiber (myopathies) (Figure 1.1). These disorders affect the motor unit, an anatomic and physiologic structure formed by the anterior horn, its axon, and the number of muscle fibers innervated by that neuron. Because peripheral nerve roots and plexi carry not only axons from the motor unit, but also those of the autonomic nervous system and sensory neurons, neuropathies, radiculopathies, and plexopathies also manifest symptoms and signs caused by dysfunction of these fibers, such as numbness, pain, and dysautonomia.

Neuromuscular diseases can be caused by diverse pathologic processes. For example, the lower motor neurons might be affected by infections (poliomyelitis) or genetic defects (spinal muscular atrophy), whereas both the lower and upper motor neurons are involved in amyotrophic lateral sclerosis (ALS). In radiculopathies, the motor or sensory roots, or both, can be damaged by focal compression, as in disk disease, causing a localized radiculopathy with motor or sensory symptoms restricted to the involved root. Simultaneous dysfunction of multiple roots occurs in some disorders that also involve the peripheral nerve, such as Guillain-Barré syndrome (polyradiculoneuropathy) (see Figure 1.1).

The cervical, brachial, or lumbosacral plexus are affected by compression due to aneurysms or tumors, radiation injury, or, in some cases, an infectious or autoimmune process, such as neuralgic amyotrophy. In these, the symptoms and signs correspond to the degree and extent of the damage. The posterior root ganglia may be the target of different processes, such as infection by the herpes zoster virus or a more generalized autoimmune disorder, such as Sjögren's syndrome or paraneoplastic ganglioneuritis.

The neuropathies include an extensive group of disorders that can be either focal (carpal tunnel syndrome) or diffuse (polyneuropathy). Their signs and symptoms depend on the type of nerve fiber affected (motor or sensory), whether small or large fibers are involved, and whether the damage is predominantly of myelin (demyelina-

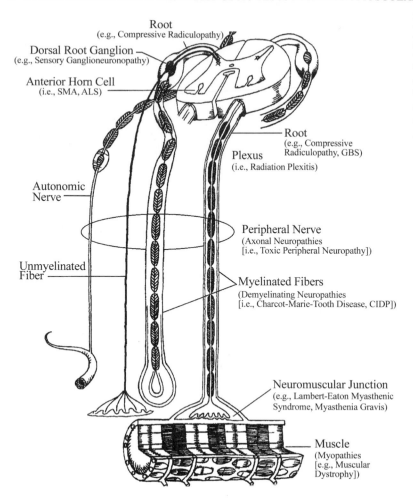

Root
(e.g., Compressive Radiculopathy)

Dorsal Root Ganglion
(e.g., Sensory Ganglioneuronopathy)

Anterior Horn Cell
(i.e., SMA, ALS)

Root
(e.g., Compressive Radiculopathy, GBS)

Plexus
(i.e., Radiation Plexitis)

Autonomic Nerve

Peripheral Nerve
(Axonal Neuropathies
[i.e., Toxic Peripheral Neuropathy])

Unmyelinated Fiber

Myelinated Fibers
(Demyelinating Neuropathies
[i.e., Charcot-Marie-Tooth Disease, CIDP])

Neuromuscular Junction
(e.g., Lambert-Eaton Myasthenic
Syndrome, Myasthenia Gravis)

Muscle
(Myopathies
[e.g., Muscular
Dystrophy])

Figure 1.1 The components of the peripheral nervous system and location of the various types of neuromuscular diseases. (ALS = amyotrophic lateral sclerosis; CIDP = chronic inflammatory demyelinating polyradiculopathy; GBS = Guillain-Barré syndrome; SMA = spinal muscular atrophy.)

tion) or axons (axonal degeneration). The clinical picture varies with single-nerve involvement (mononeuritis), simultaneous involvement of several individual nerves (mononeuritis multiplex), or involvement of most nerves in a symmetric fashion (distal symmetrical polyneuropathies).

Diseases of the neuromuscular junction include presynaptic processes, such as botulism and Lambert-Eaton myasthenic syndrome (LEMS), and postsynaptic disorders, such as autoimmune MG or the slow channel syndrome.

Primary muscle disorders, or myopathies, are those that affect the muscle fiber itself, either by alteration of its structural components (dystrophinopathies), autoimmune damage (polymyositis), or metabolic derangement (glycogen storage disease). They can also be caused by genetic disorders of the ionic channels, as in the myotonias, or infectious, toxic, or endocrine disease.

MAJOR SYMPTOMS AND SIGNS OF NEUROMUSCULAR DISORDERS

The following are the major symptoms and signs of neuromuscular disorders; Table 1.1 lists their characteristics according to location of the disease.

Table 1.1 Neuromuscular Diseases: Clinical Evaluation

Clinical Parameter	Motor Neuron Disease	Polyneuropathy	Diseases of Neuromuscular Junction	Myopathy
Pattern of weakness	Variable, symmetric in most, often asymmetric in ALS	Distal > proximal	Proximal > distal, fluctuates, often involves extraocular muscles	Proximal > distal
Fasciculations	Yes	Sometimes	No	No
Deep tendon reflexes	Variable, decreased in most, increased in ALS	Decreased or absent	Normal in postsynaptic disorders (myasthenia gravis), decreased in presynaptic disorders (Lambert-Eaton myasthenic syndrome and botulism)	Normal initially, may be decreased in later stages (ankle reflexes often preserved until very late)
Sensory loss	No	Usually present	No	No

ALS = amyotrophic lateral sclerosis.

Weakness and Atrophy

The most common symptom of neuromuscular disorders is weakness, which is frequently accompanied by atrophy. In motor neuron diseases, the weakness can be generalized, but an asymmetric presentation may occur initially in ALS. In most myopathies, weakness is symmetrical and proximal, whereas it is predominantly distal in polyneuropathies.[1] In mononeuropathies, radiculopathies, or plexopathies, it involves only muscles innervated by the affected nerve, root, or plexus. Disorders of the neuromuscular junction usually manifest with fluctuating weakness. This is especially true in MG, in which extraocular, eyelid, and bulbar muscle involvement is common, whereas atrophy is rare.

Tone

Tone, the normal resistance of muscle to passive movement, is often decreased (*hypotonia*) in neuromuscular diseases, owing to damage or atrophy of muscle fibers or from impaired proprioceptive input. Hypotonia may be the main manifestation of neuromuscular disease in newborns and infants. Spasticity with the characteristic "clasp-knife" increase in muscle tone occurs in conditions that affect the upper motor neuron, as in ALS.

Fasciculations

Fasciculations are spontaneous depolarizations of motor units and are characteristically seen in motor neuron disorders, but they can also be observed less conspicuously in neuropathies and radiculopathies. Fasciculations without weakness and atrophy may occur in healthy individuals.

Myotonia

Myotonia, or muscle stiffness and difficulty relaxing after contraction, is caused by continuous muscle fiber depolarization. This is a feature of some myopathies (channelopathies).

Reflexes

Muscle stretch reflexes, particularly the distal reflexes, are classically decreased or absent early in neuropathies. They are usually normal in myopathies until later in the course of the disease. Most anterior horn cell diseases demonstrate hyporeflexia, although some, such as ALS, are characterized by hyper-reflexia. Reflexes are normal in MG but are usually diminished in the presynaptic disorders of neuromuscular transmission. Reflexes are usually absent in neuromuscular disorders presenting as floppy infants. In radiculopathies, plexopathies, or mononeuropathies, only the reflexes whose pathways involve the affected root, nerve, or plexus are diminished or absent.

Sensation

Abnormalities of sensation occur only in disorders involving sensory nerve fibers. In neuropathies, sensation is decreased distally; in radiculopathies, plexopathies, and mononeuropathies, the deficit follows their designated dermatomes. In these conditions, there may also be so-called positive symptoms, such as painful paresthesias, and autonomic symptoms, such as decreased sweating or tearing and impotence.

Muscle Pain, Exercise Intolerance, and Myoglobinuria

Exercise intolerance with pain occurs in metabolic myopathies.[2] Intense exercise in these conditions may result in muscle necrosis with secondary release of myoglobin in quantities above the renal threshold for this protein, resulting in myoglobinuria. This can also be induced by other causes, such as toxins and trauma.

LABORATORY EVALUATION

The findings in laboratory studies of neuromuscular disease are summarized in Table 1.2.

Serum Muscle Enzymes

Serum enzymes, especially creatine kinase, but also aldolase, alanine aminotransferase (ALT), aspartate aminotransferase (AST) and lactate dehydrogenase (LDH), are characteristically elevated in myopathies[2,3]; for this reason, measurements of serum enzymes are helpful in the diagnoses of myopathies, in which they are elevated from muscle necrosis, although mild elevations may also occur in anterior horn cell diseases.

Nerve Conduction Studies

Nerve conduction velocity studies evaluate mainly large, myelinated motor and sensory axons. In demyelinating diseases, there is slowing of conduction and conduction block or dispersion of the compound muscle action potentials. Focal slowing of con-

Table 1.2 Neuromuscular Diseases: Laboratory Evaluation

Test	Motor Neuron Disease	Polyneuropathy	Myopathy	Diseases of Neuromuscular Junction
Serum muscle enzymes	Normal or mild elevation	Normal	Increased	Normal
Nerve conduction studies	Normal or low-amplitude CMAPs, normal SNAPs	Usually slow nerve conduction velocities or low-amplitude CMAPs and SNAPs	Normal	Normal
Electromyography	Decreased number of motor units, evidence of denervation and reinnervation (large motor units)	Decreased number of motor units, evidence of denervation and reinnervation (large motor units)	Normal number of motor units of short duration and low amplitude, and frequently polyphasic	Normal or small motor units, variability of motor unit size
Repetitive nerve stimulation test	Usually normal, decremental responses can occur	Normal	Normal	Decrement of CMAP at low rate of stimulation, increment at fast rates in presynaptic disorders
Muscle biopsy	Denervation (atrophic angular and target fibers, fiber-type grouping, group atrophy)	Denervation (atrophic angular and target fibers, fiber-type grouping)	"Myopathic" (necrosis, storage material, inflammation)	Normal or some type II muscle fiber atrophy

CMAP = compound muscle action potential; SNAP = sensory nerve action potential.

duction or conduction block is seen in entrapment neuropathies. In axonal neuropathies, nerve conduction is relatively normal with absent or diminished amplitude motor and sensory-evoked responses. In radiculopathies, nerve conduction velocities and amplitudes of the sensory nerve action potentials (SNAPs) are normal, even in the presence of sensory impairment clinically, because the posterior root ganglion and its axon are usually not affected.

In motor neuron diseases, the SNAPs are normal, and motor nerve conduction velocities are also usually normal, whereas the amplitude of the compound muscle action potential (CMAP) is often decreased. Nerve conduction velocities are normal in disorders of the neuromuscular junction. Measurements of the latency of the H reflexes and F responses or motor nerve conduction using root stimulation are valuable techniques in the study and diagnosis of the proximal segments of nerve in neuropathies, radiculopathies, and plexopathies, wherein responses can be slow or absent.[4]

Repetitive motor nerve stimulation with supramaximal stimuli at slow rates produces a decremental response of the CMAP in disorders of neuromuscular transmission, such as MG. In presynaptic defects, such as LEMS, there is an initial low amplitude of the CMAP, owing to decreased acetylcholine (ACh) release, and this increases during fast-frequency repetitive stimulation (20–50 Hz) or after tetanic contractions ("post-tetanic facilitation"). Those abnormalities do not occur in myopathies. Rarely, decremental responses may occur in motor neuron disorders and neuropathies.

Histologic and Electrophysiologic Evaluations in Various Neuromuscular Diseases

A motor unit innervates muscle fibers of a single type. These intermix with fibers of other motor units. This normal "checkerboard" pattern of muscle fiber distribution is demonstrated on muscle biopsy with histochemical staining.

Damage to a motor neuron or its axon results in denervation hypersensitivity to ACh, caused by increased expression of the ACh receptor over the entire surface of the muscle membrane, rather than being limited to the normal site at the neuromuscular junction. The electrophysiologic correlate of this phenomenon is spontaneous depolarization of individual muscle fibers on electromyography (EMG), called *fibrillations* or *positive sharp waves* (fibrillations that have lost their negative component). When the number of motor neurons or axons that are damaged increases, the number of motor units that can be activated with increasing force of muscle contraction diminishes. This is reflected in a reduced recruitment of motor units on EMG.

The histologic correlate of denervation of individual muscle fibers is the presence of atrophic angulated fibers. In chronic disease, axons from normal motor neurons reinnervate these fibers, causing a loss of the normal checkerboard pattern, and groups of fibers of the same type are then seen on enzyme histochemistry ("fiber-type grouping"). When the reinnervating neuron or its axons are damaged, the entire group of muscle fibers innervated by that neuron atrophies, producing "group atrophy." The EMG correlate of fiber-type grouping is the presence of large-amplitude, long-duration motor units, because a larger number of muscle fibers of the same unit is included in the recording range of the EMG needle electrode. In radiculopathies, plexopathies, or mononeuropathies, these changes occur in a restricted fashion, involving muscles innervated by the affected root, plexus, or nerve. In radiculopathies, denervation potentials are frequently seen in paraspinal muscles, because the posterior rami are usually affected. A summary of the clinical and electrophysiologic findings in focal diseases (single root, or plexus and mononeuropathy) is presented in Table 1.3.

In myopathies, the motor neurons and axons remain intact, but individual muscle fibers are damaged from necrosis or other pathologic processes. Fiber atrophy and hypertrophy, rounding of fibers, and internal nucleation with increased connective tissue are found on muscle biopsy.[3] In some myopathies, the biopsy findings may lead to a specific diagnosis—for example, inflammation in polymyositis and absent dystrophin staining in Duchenne's dystrophy, or the glycogen accumulation and lack of staining for specific glycolytic enzymes in glycogen storage diseases.

In these disorders, damage to individual muscle fibers causes the motor units on EMG to appear smaller in amplitude and shorter in duration. The number of units required to perform a certain level of contraction is increased because each unit has fewer fibers, but the number of motor units is not decreased. This causes early, full recruitment of motor units during voluntary effort.[5]

Other Studies

Magnetic resonance spectroscopy is used in the analysis of characteristics of energy use in muscle during exercise, particularly in metabolic myopathies, whereas biochemistry is used for a definitive etiologic diagnosis. Western blot studies are performed on muscle biopsies to detect specific protein deficiencies, as in the dystrophinopathies.

Table 1.3 Clinical and Laboratory Descriptions of Segmental Neurologic Disorders

	Mononeuropathy	**Plexopathy**	**Radiculopathy**
Muscle weakness and reflexes	Weakness, decreased reflexes in muscle innervated by single nerves	Weakness or decreased reflexes in muscles innervated by roots from affected plexus area (e.g., trunk) but by different nerves	Weakness in muscles innervated by the same root but different nerves
Sensory deficit	Follows a single nerve territory	Follows a plexus sensory territory	Follows territory of the involved root
Limb needle electromyography	Signs of denervation following the territory of one nerve	Signs of denervation in multiple nerves involved by affected plexus area (e.g., lower trunk = hand muscles of ulnar, median nerves)	Signs of denervation in muscles innervated by the same root but different nerves
Paraspinal needle electromyography	No paraspinal muscle denervation	No paraspinal muscle denervation	Paraspinal muscle denervation is common
Motor nerve conduction velocity	Slow in affected nerve (CMAP amplitude could be decreased when stimulating the affected nerve)	Normal (CMAP amplitude could be decreased when stimulating nerves, which axons travel through the affected plexus), slowing across Erb's point	Normal (CMAP amplitude could be decreased when stimulating nerves, which axons originate in affected roots)
Sensory-evoked responses	Low amplitude and/or prolonged latency SNAP	Low-amplitude SNAP in nerves that axons travel through the affected plexus area	Normal SNAP
Proximal responses: F response/H reflex	Could be slow or absent in affected nerves	Could be slow or absent in nerves from affected plexus area	Could be slow or absent in nerves from affected root

CMAP = compound muscle action potential; SNAP = sensory nerve action potential.

Many neuromuscular disorders can now be diagnosed by DNA studies of muscle and, most important, in lymphocytes without having to subject the patient to an invasive procedure, such as a muscle biopsy.

Nerve biopsy may be useful in the evaluation of some peripheral neuropathies to analyze axonal degeneration or demyelination and inflammation or to determine the presence of storage material, such as amyloid.

CLASSIFICATION OF NEUROMUSCULAR DISEASES

The following simple classification (Table 1.4) is not intended as a rigid demarcation between the various disease entities, but rather to provide a working sequence to be used in the book. It follows, in a simplified manner, the standard classifications used by Walton, Rowland, and McLeod,[6] and, later in the book, *Disorders of Voluntary Muscle*,[7] with some updated additions, but these, as do other classifications, have limitations, omissions, and repetitions.

Stressing the difficulties of classifying diseases, Vance made the following comment in a recent editorial regarding Charcot-Marie-Tooth disease,[8] in which alteration of the same gene causes variable phenotypes:

> It is a humbling reminder that nature does not follow or meet the human desire to recognize and classify the world around us. Rather, it seems to delight in providing twists and turns that defy our attempts at logical thought process. Yet we need to have some useful classification system so that each clinician, researcher, and patient can communicate effectively.

The difficulty in classifying these diseases is apparent when one considers, for example, that a condition such as bulbospinal muscular atrophy (Kennedy's syndrome) is classified here as a motor neuron disease, yet patients might also show evidence of peripheral nerve involvement. Limb-girdle dystrophy type 2B is classified separately from the distal muscular dystrophy of the Miyoshi type, despite the fact that they are allelic, both caused by a deficiency of the muscle membrane protein dysferlin.

There are also some redundancies in this classification, such as the inclusion of the myotonias as channelopathies as well as "diseases with excessive motor unit activity," and all the toxic myopathies, neuropathies, and entrapment neuropathies are not included. Finally, the inherited myopathies are not all classified according to their protein defect, and the classical method of separating the Duchenne's and Becker's dystrophies from limb-girdle muscular dystrophies is used. Tables of genetic defects and protein abnormalities in these and other inherited neuromuscular diseases are included in Chapter 20 on molecular genetics. This field is, however, advancing so rapidly that it is likely that when this book is published, new protein deficiencies will have been found in these diseases, making this classification obsolete.

Table 1.4 Classification of Neuromuscular Diseases

Motor neuron diseases
Predominantly upper motor neuron
Idiopathic
    Primary lateral sclerosis (usually develops lower motor
        neuron signs later, thus ALS)
Hereditary
    Familial spastic paraplegia, autosomal dominant
        (Strümpell's disease), autosomal recessive,
        X-linked recessive
Associated with other conditions
    Cervical spondylosis, spinocerebellar degeneration,
        tumors, inflammation
Infectious
    HTLV-I, HIV
Upper and lower motor neuron (ALS)
Idiopathic
    Classic ALS, Guamanian ALS
Hereditary
    Familial ALS, late onset, autosomal dominant, juvenile,
        autosomal recessive X-linked ALS with dystonia
Progressive bulbar palsy (usually develops into, or is a
    form of, classic ALS)
Predominantly anterior horn cell disease
Idiopathic
    Progressive SMA, neurogenic quadriceps amyotrophy,
        postpolio amyotrophy, benign focal amyotrophy
        (monomelic amyotrophy)

Hereditary
    Familial SMA
    Infantile (Werdnig-Hoffman disease) or SMA1
    Intermediate or SMA2
    Juvenile (Kugelberg-Welander disease) or SMA3
    Adult SMA
    Bulbospinal (spinal-bulbar) muscular atrophy (Kennedy's
        syndrome), X-linked, autosomal dominant
    Scapuloperoneal syndromes
    Distal SMA
Congenital
    Möbius' syndrome
    Fazio-Londe disease (progressive bulbar palsy of childhood)
    Arthrogryposis multiplex congenita (neurogenic)
Metabolic
    Hexosaminidase A deficiency
    Polyglycosan body disease
    Hyperparathyroidism, hyperinsulinism, others
Paraneoplastic
Autoimmune
Associated with other conditions
    Multiple system degeneration
    Huntington's disease
    Pick's disease
    Cerebellar ataxia (i.e., Machado-Joseph disease)
    Other degenerative disorders

Infections (e.g., polio, other viruses)
Traumatic, post-traumatic
Radiation injury
Others
  Tumors, vascular, spinal stenosis, lead intoxication
Diseases of peripheral nerves
Segmental neuropathy
Radiculopathy (traumatic, compressive, inflammatory,
  autoimmune, others)
Plexopathy (tumor, autoimmune and hereditary neuralgia
  amyotrophy, radiation, compressive, others)
Focal neuropathy: mononeuropathy (entrapments, trauma,
  tumors, vascular inflammatory, vasculitic, diabetic);
  mononeuritis multiplex (vascular, inflammatory,
  diabetic-ischemic), infectious (leprosy, Lyme dis-
  ease), autoimmune
Multifocal motor neuropathy (also listed under Peripheral
  polyneuropathy [autoimmune, chronic])
Peripheral polyneuropathy
Hereditary
  Motor sensory[a]
    Demyelinating
      Autosomal dominant
        CMT 1 (CMT 1A, 1B, 1C, 1D)
        Hereditary neuropathy with predisposition to
          pressure palsy (allelic to CMT 1A)
      X-linked recessive
        CMT X
    Axonal
      CMT 2 (2A, 2B, 2C, 2D, 2E)
    Autosomal dominant demyelinating, infantile
      Dejerine-Sottas disease (CMT 3A, 3B, 3C, 3D,
      3E), most with the same genetic defects as in
      CMT 1
    Autosomal recessive childhood onset (CMT 4A, 4B,
      4C, 4D, 4E, 4F)
    Others (e.g., CMT with optic neuropathy or
      ophthalmoplegia)
  Hereditary sensory and autonomic neuropathy (HSAN)
    HSAN-I
    HSAN-II (Morvan's disease)
    HSAN-III (Riley-Day syndrome)
    HSAN IV, V, VI
  Neuroaxonal atrophy
  Giant axonal neuropathy
  Chédiak-Higashi syndrome
  Spinocerebellar degeneration with neuropathy, such as
    Friedreich's ataxia, others
  Familial amyloid neuropathy due to transthyretin, apoli-
    poprotein A, gelsolin mutations
  Sphingolipidoses
    Metachromatic leukodystrophy
    Globoid cell leukodystrophy
      (Krabbe's disease)
    Fabry's disease
    Niemann-Pick disease
    Farber's disease
  Porphyrias
    Acute intermittent, variegate, coproporphyria, ami-
      nolevulinic acid dehydratase deficiencies

Peroxisomal disorders
  Refsum's disease (hereditary motor and sensory neu-
    ropathy IV)
  Adrenomyeloneuropathy
Lipoprotein disorders
  Abetalipoproteinemia (Bassen-Kornzweig syndrome),
    hypolipoproteinemia
  Tangier disease (an alphalipoproteinemia)
  Hypobetalipoproteinemia
Cerebrotendinous xanthomatosis
Defects of DNA repair
  Ataxia telangiectasia
  Xeroderma pigmentosum
  Cockayne's syndrome
Others
  Primary hyperoxaluria
  Mitochondrial diseases
  Familial vitamin E deficiency
  Familial vitamin B_{12} deficiency
Autoimmune
  Acute
    Inflammatory demyelinating polyneuropathy (classic
      Guillain-Barré syndrome)
    Motor axonal neuropathy
    Motor sensory axonal neuropathy
    Acute dysautonomic neuropathy
    Miller Fisher syndrome
    Sensory Guillain-Barré syndrome
  Chronic
    Chronic inflammatory demyelinating polyneuropathy
    Multifocal motor neuropathy, multifocal motor sen-
      sory neuropathy
    Distal autoimmune demyelinating polyneuropathy
      (with and without myelin-associated glycoprotein
      antibodies)
    Sensory chronic inflammatory demyelinating poly-
      neuropathy
    Paraneoplastic
    Vasculitic
    Cryoglobulinemia, idiopathic, with systemic diseases
    Sarcoidosis
    Ganglioneuritis, in Sjögren's syndrome, paraneoplastic
Neuropathies associated with gammopathy
  Waldenström's macroglobulinemia, primary amyloidosis
  Secondary amyloidosis, β_2-microglobulin deposition
  Monoclonal gammopathy of undetermined significance,
    associated with myeloma, POEMS syndrome
Infectious
  Herpes zoster
  Leprosy
  HTLV-I
  HIV
  Diphtheria
  Chaga's disease
  Hepatitis
  Cytomegalic virus lumbosacral polyradiculopathy
  Others
Nutritional, acquired metabolic, endocrine
  Thiamine deficiency
  Pyridoxine deficiency

Table 1.4 *Continued*

Peripheral polyneuropathy—continued
  B_{12} deficiency
  Vitamin E deficiency
  Diabetes
  Hyperinsulinemia
  Acromegaly
  Uremia
  Toxins
    Lead
    Arsenic
    Thallium
    Alcohol
    Saxitoxin
    Organophosphates
    N-hexane
    Others
  Drug-induced
    Ethambutol
    Vincristine
    Pyridoxine
    Isoniazid
    Nitrofurantoin
    Metronidazole
    Cisplatin
    Thalidomide
    Amiodarone
    Perhexiline
    Dapsone
    Cimetidine
    Phenytoin
    Allopurinol
    Others
Disorders of neuromuscular transmission, acquired
Presynaptic
Autoimmune
  Lambert-Eaton myasthenic syndrome, with and without
    cancer
  Toxic
    Botulism
    Snake bite intoxication
    Tick paralysis
    Drug-induced (e.g., aminoglycosides)
Pre- and postsynaptic
Autoimmune
  Some cases of autoimmune myasthenia
Toxic
  Organophosphate poisoning
Postsynaptic
Autoimmune
  Classic myasthenia gravis
  Autoimmune myasthenia gravis caused by penicillamine
  Acquired slow channel syndrome
Congenital myasthenic syndromes (CMSs)
Presynaptic
  Defect in ACh resynthesis (familial infantile myasthenia
    or CMS with episodic apnea)

CMS with paucity of synaptic vesicles and reduced
  quantal release
CMS resembling Lambert-Eaton myasthenic syndrome
Synaptic
  End-plate acetylcholinesterase deficiency
Postsynaptic
  With kinetic abnormalities of ACh receptor
    Slow channel myasthenic syndromes
    Fast channel myasthenic syndromes
  ACh receptor deficiency with or without minor kinetic
    abnormalities
    Due to mutations in ACh receptor genes
    Due to rapsyn gene mutations
  Others
Myopathies
Congenital myopathies[b]
Central core disease
Multicore disease
Nemaline myopathy (also an adult-onset type)
Myotubular myopathy
Centronuclear myopathy, sporadic, autosomal recessive
Congenital fiber-type disproportion
Fingerprint myopathy
Sarcotubular myopathy
Rigid spine syndrome
Reducing body myopathy
Hyaline body myopathy, spheroid body myopathy (both
    myofibrillar myopathies)
Cytoplasmic body myopathy
Zebra body myopathy
Trilaminar body myopathy
Familial myopathy with tubular aggregates
Congenital myopathy with excess of thin myofilaments
Others
Muscular dystrophies[a]
Dystrophinopathies
  Duchenne's
  Becker's
Limb-girdle muscular dystrophy
  Autosomal dominant: 1A, 1B (lamin A/C gene muta-
    tion), 1C (caveolin deficiency), 1D, 1E
  Autosomal recessive: 2A (calpain deficiency), 2B (dys-
    ferlin deficiency); sarcoglycan deficiency due to
    sarcoglycan gene mutations: 2C (γ-sarcoglycan),
    2D (α-sarcoglycan), 2E (β-sarcoglycan), 2F (δ-
    sarcoglycan), 2G (telethonin gene mutation), 2H
    (TRIM 32 gene), 2I (fukutin-related protein gene)
  Limb-girdle dystrophy with epidermolysis bullosa
Bethlem myopathy
Emery-Dreifuss muscular dystrophy: X-linked (emerin
    deficiency), autosomal dominant (lamin A/C gene
    mutation)
Facioscapulohumeral dystrophy
Scapuloperoneal syndrome
Scapulohumeral syndrome
Oculopharyngeal dystrophy

Oculopharyngeodistal dystrophy
Congenital muscular dystrophy
  Merosin deficient
  Integrin α_7 deficient
  Congenital muscular dystrophy with rigid spine
  Fukuyama type
  Muscle-eye-brain
  Walker-Warburg syndrome
Myotonic dystrophy (DM1 and DM2), Proximal myotonic
  myopathy (PROMM)
Distal muscular dystrophy
  Autosomal recessive, juvenile onset, posterior compart-
    ment of the legs (Miyoshi type)
  Autosomal recessive, juvenile onset, anterior compart-
    ment of the legs (Nonaka type or hereditary inclu-
    sion body myopathy?)
  Autosomal dominant (leg predominantly), juvenile
    myopathy (Laig type)
  Autosomal dominant late onset, predominantly in hands
    (Welander type)
  Autosomal dominant late onset, predominantly in legs
    (Markesberry-Griggs/Udd type)
Myofibrillar (desmin myopathy)
Distal myopathy with vocal cord paralysis
Metabolic myopathies
Disorders of glycogen storage
  Acid maltase deficiency (Type II)
  Debrancher enzyme deficiency (Type III)
  Branching enzyme deficiency (Type IV)
  Myophosphorylase deficiency (Type V)
  Phosphofructokinase deficiency (Type VII)
  Phosphorylase b kinase deficiency (Type VIII)
  Phosphoglycerate kinase deficiency (Type IX)
  Phosphoglycerate mutase deficiency (Type X)
  Lactate dehydrogenase deficiency (Type XI)
  Aldolase A deficiency (Type XII)
  β-Enolase deficiency (Type XIII)
Disorders of lipid metabolism
  Defects of the carnitine cycle
    Primary systemic carnitine deficiency
    Secondary carnitine deficiency
    Inborn errors of metabolism (i.e., defects of mitochon-
      drial respiratory chain, disorders of branched chain
      amino acid metabolism)
    Acquired (e.g., malnutrition, cirrhosis)
    Carnitine-acylcarnitine translocase deficiency
    CPT II deficiency (CPT I is present in liver and muscle
      but only a liver deficiency has been described.)
  Defects of β-oxidation
    Short-chain acyl-CoA dehydrogenase (SCAD)
      deficiency
    Medium-chain acyl-CoA dehydrogenase (MCAD)
      deficiency
    Very-long-chain acyl-CoA dehydrogenase (VLCAD)
      deficiency
    Trifunctional protein (TP) deficiency
    Long-chain 3-hydroxyacyl-CoA dehydrogenase
      (LCHAD) deficiency

    Short-chain 3-hydroxyacyl-CoA dehydrogenase
      (SCHAD) deficiency
    Electron-transfer flavoprotein (ETF) deficiency
    ETF CoQ_{10} oxidoreductase deficiency
    Hydroxy-acyl-CoA dehydrogenase deficiency
Defects of the mitochondrial respiratory chain
  Myopathies due to defects in mitochondrial DNA
    Mutations affecting mitochondrial protein synthesis
      (can result in multisystem disorders or encephalop-
      athy [see below] but sometimes presents only as a
      muscle disease)
    Mutations in protein coding genes (i.e., LHON, MILS,
      defects of Complex I, Complex III, or Complex IV
      or COX deficiency)
  Myopathies due to defects in nuclear DNA
    CoQ_{10} deficiency
    Complex IV (COX) deficiency (also caused by mito-
      chondrial DNA mutations)
  Encephalomyopathies
    Progressive external ophthalmoplegia (PEO)
    Isolated skeletal myopathy
    Kearns-Sayre syndrome (KSS)
    Mitochondrial encephalopathy with lactic acidosis and
      stroke-like episodes (MELAS)
    Myoclonic epilepsy with ragged red fibers (MERRF)
    Neuropathy, ataxia, retinitis pigmentosa (NARP)
    Mitochondrial DNA depletion and infantile lactic acidosis
    Mitochondrial neurogastrointestinal encephalomyopa-
      thy (MNGIE)
    Alpers' disease
    Myopathy with lipomatosis (this is usually associated
      with one of the MERRF)
    Others
Mitochondrial hypermetabolism (Luft's disease)
Myoadenylate deaminase deficiency
Myosin adenosinetriphosphatase deficiency (Brody's disease)
Muscle channelopathies
Sodium channel disease
  Hyperkalemic periodic paralysis, hyperkalemic periodic
    paralysis with cardiac arrhythmia (Andersen's
    syndrome)
  Paramyotonia congenita
  Acetazolamide-sensitive myotonia
  Myotonia fluctuans
  Myotonia permanens
Chloride channel myopathies
  Myotonia congenita, autosomal recessive
  Myotonia congenita, autosomal dominant
  Fluctuating myotonia congenita
  Myotonia levior
Calcium channel myopathies
  Malignant hyperthermia
  Hypokalemic periodic paralysis, hypokalemic paralysis
    with hypogonadism
Inflammatory myopathies
Autoimmune
  Idiopathic adult PM
  Idiopathic childhood PM

Table 1.4 *Continued*

Inflammatory myopathies—continued
  Neonatal PM
  Adult DM
  Childhood DM
  PM or DM associated with connective tissue disorders
  PM or DM associated with cancer
  PM associated with monoclonal gammopathies
  Acute myositis of children; postviral myositis of adults
  Myositis and fasciitis in the hypereosinophilic syndrome
  PM with other systemic diseases
  Inclusion body myositis
  Focal myositis
  PM with agammaglobulinemia
  Putative myositis
Infectious
  Viral myositis
  PM with acquired immunodeficiency syndrome, HTLV-I
    infection
  Toxoplasmosis, cysticercosis
  Fungi
  Bacteria
  Others
Endocrine myopathies
Hypo- and hyperthyroidism
Acromegaly
Hyperadrenalism
Hyperparathyroidism
Others
Toxic myopathies[c]
Drug-induced
  Necrotizing
    Cholesterol-lowering drugs
      Clofibrate
      Gemfibrozil
      Hydroxymethylglutaryl-CoA reductase inhibitors
      Niacin
      Others
    Cyclophilins (cyclosporine and tacrolimus), labetalol,
      propofol, epsilon aminocaproic acid, others
    Amphiphilic (drug-induced autophagic lysosomal myop-
      athy)
      Chloroquine
      Hydroxychloroquine

  Amiodarone
  Others
Antimicrotubular
  Colchicine
  Vincristine
  Others
Mitochondrial damage
  Zidovudine
  Germanium
  Others
Drug-induced inflammation: procainamide, L-tryp-
  tophan, cimetidine, L-dopa, penicillamine, pheny-
  toin, lamotrigine, toxic oil, propylthiouracil
Impaired protein synthesis
  Corticosteroids
  Finasteride
  Emetine
  Elinafide
  Others
Drug-induced hypokalemia
  Diuretics
  Amphotericin B
  Licorice
  Others
Other
  Acute quadriplegic myopathy of critical illness
  Meperidine, pentazocine (produces muscle fibrosis)
Toxins
  Alcohol
  Serotonin syndrome
  Cocaine, heroin
Diseases of motor unit hyperactivity
Stiff-man syndrome
Tetany due to hypocalcemia or hypomagnesemia, alka-
  losis
Isaacs' syndrome
Infectious, toxic: tetanus, strychnine, organophosphates
Myotonias: symptomatic and hereditary (congenital) (see
  Muscle channelopathies)
Rippling muscle disease
Schwartz-Jampel syndrome
Benign cramp fasciculations syndrome

ACh = acetylcholine; ALS = amyotrophic lateral sclerosis; CMT = Charcot-Marie-Tooth disease; CoA = coenzyme A; CoQ$_{10}$ = coenzyme Q$_{10}$; COX = cytochrome oxidase; CPT = carnitine palmitoyl transferase; DM = dermatomyositis; HIV = human immuno- deficiency virus; HTLV-I = human T-cell lymphotrophic virus type1; LHON = Leber hereditary optic neuropathy; MILS = maternally inherited Leigh syndrome; PM = polymyositis; POEMS = polyneuropathy, organomegaly, endocrinopathy, M protein, and skin changes; SMA = spinal muscular atrophy.

[a]A complete list of these with their genetic defects can be found in Chapter 20.
[b]Congenital muscular dystrophy is listed under Muscular dystrophies.
[c]Modified from Zaida OO, Ruff RL, Kaminski HJ. Endocrine and Toxic Myopathies. In AHV Shapira, RC Griggs (eds), Muscle Diseases. Boston: Butterworth–Heinemann, 1999.

REFERENCES

1. Brooke M. The Symptoms and Signs of Neuromuscular Disease. In M Brooke (ed), A Clinician's View of Neuromuscular Diseases. Baltimore: Williams & Wilkins, 1986;1–33.
2. Brooke M. Clinical Evaluation of Patients with Neuromuscular Diseases. In AHV Shapira, R Griggs (eds), Muscle Diseases. Boston: Butterworth–Heinemann, 1999; 1–24.
3. Griggs RC, Mendell JR, Miller RG. Evaluation of Patients with Myopathy. In RC Griggs, JR Mendell, RG Miller (eds), Evaluation and Treatment of Myopathies: Contemporary Neurology Series. Philadelphia: FA Davis, 1995;17–78.
4. Oh SJ. Clinical Electromyography and Nerve Conduction Studies. In SJ Oh (ed), Nerve Conduction in Polyneuropathies. Baltimore: University Park Press, 1984;419–480.
5. Bertorini TE. EMG in Polymyositis and Dermatomyositis. In MC Dalakas (ed), Polymyositis and Dermatomyositis. Boston: Butterworth, 1988.
6. Walton J, Rowland LP, McLeod JG. World Federation of Neurology Research Group on Neuromuscular Disorders. J Neurol Sci 1988;86:333–360.
7. Walton J, Rowland LP. Clinical Examination, Differential Diagnosis and Classification. In JN Walton, G Karpati, D Hilton-Jones (eds), Disorders of Voluntary Muscle. New York: Churchill Livingstone, 1994;499–552.
8. Vance JM. The many faces of Charcot-Marie-Tooth disease. Arch Neurol 2000;57(5):638–640.

Clinical Evaluation and Clinical Laboratory Tests

Tulio E. Bertorini

For proper diagnosis and management of neuromuscular diseases, it is very important to obtain a complete history, perform a thorough examination, and order the appropriate laboratory studies. We present here first the clinical approach to these patients, followed by a description of laboratory studies and specific clinical tests that are useful to arrive at the diagnosis.

THE HISTORY

A detailed medical history should include the mode of onset and progression to learn whether the disease is acute or chronic, recurrent or episodic, or has been present since birth, and whether it is hereditary or sporadic. The history should also determine whether the condition is generalized or segmental and whether it affects the motor or sensory system, or both.

In children, information should be obtained about the antenatal period and delivery, as well as the Apgar scores. It is particularly important to include details of their developmental milestones, especially motor milestones. Deviations from the following should be noted. Normally, a child rolls over by 4 months, sits by 5–6 months, sits securely while unattended by 9 months, and pulls to a standing position by 10–12 months. A child stands alone and may walk independently at 15 months (9–16 months), and at 2 years can run well. More details of developmental milestones are available in the literature.[1]

The past and concurring general medical history is also of utmost importance. For example, some inflammatory myopathies and neuropathies are associated with other disimmune conditions or preceded by infectious diseases, whereas a history of weight loss may be an indication of an underlying malignancy. There should also be an inquiry as to the work environment and possible exposure to toxins, alcohol, and medication use, because, for example, various toxins cause peripheral neuropathy, or myopathies, which could also be caused by cholesterol-lowering agents, whereas penicillamine can induce myasthenia gravis (MG).

Table 2.1 Neuromuscular Disorders That May Present with Acute Generalized Weakness

Motor neuron diseases
   Poliomyelitis
   Amyotrophic lateral sclerosis (rarely)
Neuropathies
   Guillain-Barré syndrome and variants
   Porphyria, particularly acute intermittent
   Dinoflagellate toxins
   Diphtheria
   Arsenic poisoning and other acute toxic neuropathies
Disorders of neuromuscular transmission
   Botulism and other biological toxins (black widow spider bite)
   Organophosphate poisoning
   Lambert-Eaton myasthenic syndrome
   Hypermagnesemia
   Myasthenia gravis
Myopathies
   Rhabdomyolysis (from various causes, e.g., metabolic, toxic, infectious)
   Polymyositis/dermatomyositis
   Infectious myositis (e.g., trichinosis, toxoplasmosis)
   Electrolyte imbalance (e.g., hypo- and hyperkalemia, hypermagnesemia, hypocalcemia, hypercalcemia, hypophosphatemia)
   Hyperthyroidism
   Toxins
   Intensive care myopathy

Knowledge of the family history is very useful because many neuromuscular diseases are hereditary. A detailed pedigree tree should be drawn and consanguinity among parents noted.

When obtaining the medical history, the patient should also be asked specifically about important neuromuscular symptoms, which are described in the following sections.

Muscle Weakness

Weakness is a frequent complaint in most neuromuscular disorders, except in purely sensory neuropathies, some radiculopathies, and entrapment syndromes. Knowledge of the distribution, onset, and course of muscle weakness assists in narrowing down the differential diagnosis.

Progression

Acute muscle weakness progressing up to 4 weeks occurs in Guillain-Barré syndrome (GBS) and in other diseases from which GBS should be differentiated (Table 2.1). Conditions such as the periodic paralyses, exercise-induced rhabdomyolysis, and some inflammatory neuropathies manifest with recurrent weak-

Table 2.2 Conditions That Present with Progressive Subacute or Chronic Proximal Muscle Weakness

Progressive spinal muscular atrophy
Bulbospinal muscular atrophy (Kennedy's disease)
Amyotrophic lateral sclerosis (sometimes)
Chronic inflammatory demyelinating neuropathy
Lambert-Eaton myasthenic syndrome
Myasthenia gravis
Endocrine diseases (e.g., hypothyroidism, Cushing's disease, hyperparathyroidism)
Drugs (e.g., steroids, cholesterol-lowering agents, zidovudine, colchicine, chloroquine)
Toxins (e.g., alcoholic myopathy)
Electrolyte imbalance
Congenital myopathies (usually of earlier onset)
Muscular dystrophies
Polymyositis and dermatomyositis
Inclusion body myositis
Adult "nemaline" or "rod" myopathy
Mitochondrial myopathy
Juvenile and adult forms of acid maltase deficiency
Carnitine deficiency

ness, whereas in disorders of neuromuscular transmission, particularly MG, this characteristically fluctuates during the day. Progressive weakness lasting 1–2 months is considered subacute, as it occurs in chronic inflammatory demyelinating polyneuropathy (CIDP). The progression can be chronic for months in inflammatory myopathies and in some patients with CIDP. Other conditions such as the muscular dystrophies, some metabolic myopathies, and familial neuropathies progress for years or throughout life.

Distribution

Knowledge of the distribution of weakness assists in differentiation of the various types of diseases. For example, weakness is usually proximal in spinal muscular atrophy (SMA) and in most myopathies (Table 2.2),[2,3] although in some myopathies it can be more prominent in distal muscles (Table 2.3). In neuropathies, weakness characteristically begins in the legs, but it may also manifest initially or be more prominent in the upper extremities in multifocal motor neuropathy (MMN), porphyria, and plexopathies and in some entrapment neuropathies. The presentation is variable in amyotrophic lateral sclerosis (ALS), but a distal, asymmetric weakness starting in the hands occurs frequently.

Weakness in Selected Muscle Groups

Extraocular Muscles. Weakness of the eyelids and extraocular muscles could be prominent in some myopathies. A history of droopy eyelids, particularly if intermittent and accompanied by diplopia, is suggestive of MG, whereas ptosis and acute paralysis of extraocular muscles occur in Miller Fisher syndrome and in some patients with otherwise classical GBS. In botulism, ptosis is usually accompanied by

Table 2.3 Neuromuscular Diseases That Manifest with Prominent Distal Weakness

Distal spinal muscular atrophy

Amyotrophic lateral sclerosis

Polyneuropathies, particularly axonal

Slow channel congenital and acquired myasthenic syndromes

Distal autoimmune myasthenia gravis

Debrancher enzyme deficiency

Phosphorylase B kinase deficiency

Myotubular myopathy

Facioscapulohumeral dystrophy

Myotonic dystrophy

Scapuloperoneal syndromes

Inclusion body myositis

Distal muscular dystrophies

    Adult onset, autosomal dominant upper extremity predominantly (Welander type)

    Adult onset, autosomal dominant lower extremity predominantly (Markesberry-Griggs/Udd type)

    Juvenile onset, autosomal recessive posterior compartment (Myoshi type)

    Juvenile onset, autosomal recessive anterior compartment (Nonaka type)

    Juvenile onset autosomal dominant, lower extremity predominant (Laing type)

    Distal myopathy with vocal cord paralysis

    Oculopharyngeo-distal dystrophy

    Myofibrillar or "desmin" myopathy

autonomic symptoms such as lack of tearing, pupillary paralysis, and anhidrosis. Acute diplopia from unilateral ocular nerve paralysis occurs in mononeuritis or mononeuritis multiplex, as in diabetes, sarcoidosis, or vasculitis (Table 2.4). Chronic, symmetric, progressive extraocular weakness, frequently without diplopia, can be seen in some myopathies, such as in mitochondrial disorders.

Table 2.4 Diseases That Can Present with Ptosis or Limitation of Extraocular Movements, or Both

Congenital anomalies (e.g., Möbius' syndrome)

Miller Fisher syndrome

Botulism

Lambert-Eaton myasthenic syndrome[a]

Myasthenia gravis

Congenital myasthenic syndromes (e.g., slow channel syndrome)

Mitochondrial myopathy

Oculopharyngeal dystrophy[b]

Ocular myopathy

Ophthalmoplegia from a vasculopathy, such as diabetes causing III or VI nerve palsies, sarcoidosis, and vasculitis

Myotonic dystrophy[a]

Myotubular myopathy[a]

[a]Mainly mild ptosis; ophthalmoplegia is unusual.

[b]May develop mild ophthalmoplegia.

Table 2.5 Neuromuscular Causes of Prominent Dysphagia

Amyotrophic lateral sclerosis, particularly progressive bulbar palsy
Bulbospinal muscular atrophy
Myasthenia gravis
Congenital myasthenic syndromes
Botulism
Lambert-Eaton myasthenic syndrome
Guillain-Barré syndrome and, in rare cases, chronic demyelinating inflammatory polyneuropathy
Diphtheria
Oculopharyngeal dystrophy
Polymyositis
Dermatomyositis
Inclusion body myositis
Myotonic dystrophy
Mitochondrial myopathy

Source: Adapted from Evaluation of the Patient with Myopathy. In R Griggs, JR Mendell, RG Miller (eds), Evaluation and Treatment of Myopathies. Contemporary Neurology Series. Philadelphia: FA Davis, 1995;37, with permission.

Speech and Swallowing. The clinician should investigate whether the patient's speech has changed in tone, cadence, and pitch (dysphonia), and note whether the change is intermittent or progressive. Accompanying difficulty swallowing (dysphagia) should be noted (Table 2.5). Intermittent dysphonia and dysphagia occur in patients with MG, whereas they are progressive in oculopharyngeal dystrophy (OPMD), some spinocerebellar degenerations, and inflammatory myopathies. These are also complaints of patients with motor neuron disease or with some mitochondrial myopathies. Speech difficulties from vocal cord paralysis also occur rarely in inflammatory neuropathies, in some forms of Charcot-Marie-Tooth (CMT) disease, and in a form of distal muscular dystrophy.

Respiratory Muscle Weakness and Respiratory Failure. Respiratory insufficiency may be an early manifestation of weakness in diseases that present with acute paralysis, such as GBS and in MG, or may occur in the later stages of progressive disorders, such as ALS, muscular dystrophy, inflammatory myopathies, and acid maltase deficiency, among others.[4] Respiratory failure may sometimes be the initial presentation in some progressive diseases, such as ALS, acid maltase deficiency, and MG (Table 2.6).

Facial and Neck Muscle Weakness. Acute, bilateral facial diplegia is seen in GBS, whereas unilateral facial weakness occurs in idiopathic Bell's palsy, CIDP, vasculitis, diabetes, and sarcoidosis. In sarcoidosis, the facial weakness may be recurrent or bilateral. A slowly progressive, symmetric facial weakness is seen in fascioscapulohumeral muscular dystrophy (FSHMD), myotubular and mitochondrial myopathies, myotonic dystrophy (MD*), and some familial amyloidosis.

---

*For this disease, others use the abbreviation *DM* for *dystrophic myotonia*. It will not be used here, so as to avoid confusion with *dermatomyositis* (DM)

Table 2.6 Neuromuscular Diseases Manifesting with Respiratory Insufficiency

---

Respiratory insufficiency may be initial manifestation
    Amyotrophic lateral sclerosis
    Guillain-Barré syndrome
    Botulism
    Organophosphate poisoning
    Polymyositis/dermatomyositis
    Acid maltase deficiency
    Acute rhabdomyolysis and myoglobinemia of different causes (see Table 2.18)
    Myasthenia gravis
Respiratory insufficiency could develop during disease progression
    Amyotrophic lateral sclerosis
    Guillain-Barré syndrome
    Chronic inflammatory demyelinating neuropathy
    Myasthenia gravis
    Congenital myasthenic syndromes
    Muscular dystrophies
    Polymyositis/dermatomyositis, inclusion body myositis
    Congenital myopathies
    Mitochondrial myopathies
    Acid maltase deficiency

Cervical muscles (splenius, longus colli, scalenus, sternocleidomastoid, and "strap" muscles) are important to keep the head in an upright position. Weakness of these muscles may cause patients with myopathy or motor neuron disease to have difficulty in maintaining the head erect while in a wheelchair or while accelerating or decelerating a car.[3]

Although in neuromuscular diseases neck flexors are usually more affected, some patients develop the "dropped head syndrome" in which the head falls forward due to a more prominent neck extensor muscle weakness.

Limb Weakness. Difficulties in combing their hair and placing objects in higher cabinets are common complaints in patients with shoulder girdle weakness, whereas difficulty in writing and grasping objects and a tendency to drop things from the hand indicate distal upper-extremity involvement.

Weakness of the hip extensors usually causes inability to rise from a low chair or toilet seat, whereas difficulty ascending stairs indicates mainly weakness of hip flexors but also the quadriceps. Patients with distal leg weakness and foot drop might catch the stairs with the affected foot or when negotiating curbs. Patients with quadriceps weakness, as in inclusion body myositis (IBM), have more difficulty descending stairs. This difficulty occurs because while descending the stairs, the quadricep is markedly stressed to support the body while the opposite limb is lowered.[3]

The complaint of dragging the feet while walking may occur in patients with ALS or peripheral neuropathy from a foot drop, which also causes a steppage gait.

Table 2.7 Neuromuscular Diseases Associated with Muscle Pain

Pain at rest

    Motor neuron disease, neuropathies with cramps

    Guillain-Barré syndrome

    Fibromyalgia

    Fasciitis

    Polymyalgia rheumatica

    Polymyositis/dermatomyositis

    Viral myositis

    Trichinosis and other parasites

    Sarcoidosis

    Myotubular myopathy

    Myopathy with tubular aggregates

    Familial vacuolar myopathy

    Dystrophinopathies (pain sometimes, particularly at night)

    Electrolyte imbalance (low K, Ca, Mg, Na, high Na)

    Hypothyroidism

    Toxins, alcoholic myopathy

    Medication (cholesterol-lowering drugs, zidovudine)

    Muscle pain fasciculation syndrome

    Leg muscle pain in the "painful leg, moving toes" syndrome from focal neuropathy or radiculopathy

Exercise intolerance and exercise-induced muscle pains

    Neurogenic diseases with cramps that worsen with exercise

    Myoadenylate deaminase deficiency

    Mitochondrial myopathy such as Complex I, III, and coenzyme Q_{10} deficiencies. (Pain is not as prominent as in glycogen storage diseases; exercise intolerance, fatigue, or myoglobinuria may occur.)

    Myotonias (rare)

    Glycogen storage diseases (i.e., deficiencies of phosphorylase, phosphofructokinase, phosphorylase B kinase, phosphoglycerate kinase, phosphoglycerate mutase, lactate dehydrogenase, aldolase A, B enolase)

    Carnitine palmitoyl transferase deficiency. (Pain might occur only during myoglobinuric attacks; exercise intolerance is less severe than in the glycogen storage diseases.)

    Some cases of very-long-chain acyl-CoA dehydrogenase deficiency

CoA = coenzyme A.

Muscle Pain

Muscle pain is frequent in some neuromuscular disorders and can occur at rest or during exercise (Table 2.7).

Muscle Pain at Rest

Muscle pain can occur at rest in patients with acute myopathies, such as viral myositis or rhabdomyolysis from any cause, and is also a common complaint of

Table 2.8 Muscle Cramps or Fasciculations, or Both

Motor neuron disease
Radiculopathies
Neuropathy
Electrolyte imbalance (e.g., hyponatremia or hypocalcemia)
Schwartz-Jampel syndrome
Pregnancy
Familial cramp, cramp fasciculations syndrome
Myopathy with tubular aggregates

patients with GBS. In polymyalgia rheumatica and fasciitis, the pain is more chronic and diffuse and is sometimes aggravated by exercise. In polymyositis (PM) and dermatomyositis (DM), weakness can be accompanied by pain. This complaint is rare in IBM.

Those with fibromyalgia syndrome have muscle aches throughout the day and night, and the aches are usually more prominent in "tender" points. A series of clinical criteria for the diagnosis of fibromyalgia has been published.[5,6] It is, however, frequently difficult to separate this condition from a purely psychogenic disorder.

Other diseases accompanied by pain at rest include familial myopathy with tubular aggregates[7] and cramp-fasciculation syndrome.[8] Painful cramps occur in motor neuron diseases and some neuropathies (Table 2.8). Muscle stiffness, which can be accompanied by pain, occurs in stiff-man syndrome[9] and rarely is a complaint of patients with myotonia.

Pain may be present at rest but is aggravated by exercise and is accompanied by stiffness in hypothyroidism, chronic alcoholism, inflammatory myopathies, and in patients receiving medications such as clofibrate. Young children with Duchenne's muscular dystrophy (DMD) also may complain of muscle pain at night or after exercise.

Muscle Pain during Exercise

Exercise intolerance with pain occurs frequently in patients with metabolic myopathies, such as glycogen storage diseases,[10] myoadenylate deaminase deficiency,[11] Brody's disease,[12] and carnitine palmitoyl transferase (CPT) deficiency.[13] In CPT deficiency and mitochondrial disease, pain is not as severe as in glycogen storage disease. It may only occur during an attack of myoglobinuria and, in CPT deficiency, it is usually present only after prolonged exercise or fasting, or both.

Patients with glycogen storage diseases may have exercise-induced muscle contractures that are electrically silent on electromyography. These are caused by a lack of calcium reuptake by the sarcoplasmic reticulum, thereby impairing muscle relaxation. In these patients, pain occurs with high-intensity exercise and frequently improves when exercise is continued. This phenomenon is called the "second wind." Normally, the fuel source for muscle contraction and relaxation comes from glycogenolysis, which is impaired in these diseases. With prolonged exercise, free fatty acids are mobilized to provide an alternative source of energy, causing the second wind phenomenon.

Muscle Fatigue

Patients with diseases of the neuromuscular junction such as MG and Lambert-Eaton myasthenic syndrome (LEMS)* often complain of fatigue. In MG, fatigue is brought about or worsens with prolonged exertion, whereas increased activity may temporarily improve strength in LEMS. Fatigue is also not an uncommon complaint in mitochondrial and inflammatory myopathies and also occurs in PM, DM, and neurogenic disorders, such as ALS and inflammatory neuropathies.

Chronic fatigue syndrome is another condition associated with exercise intolerance that is difficult to define because it lacks clear anatomic or physiologic findings. The Centers for Disease Control and Prevention has, however, established research criteria for the diagnosis of this disorder.[14,15]

Muscle Stiffness

Muscle stiffness or "tightness" is not unusual in disorders that affect the upper motor neuron or that cause spasticity and in extrapyramidal syndromes that cause rigidity. These are relatively easy to diagnose during the examination. Among the conditions that cause muscle stiffness is stiff-man syndrome, in which patients have persistent stiffness in axial muscles, particularly the abdominals and lumbar paraspinals.

Stiffness also occurs in other disorders associated with motor unit hyperactivity, such as Isaacs' syndrome,[16] Brody's disease,[12] and rippling muscle disease.[17] Patients with these conditions complain of stiffness or spasms which worsen during activity, whereas patients with myotonia also frequently have this symptom but, in these patients, it usually improves with exercise.

Patients with polymyalgia rheumatica and PM, DM, or both, not only complain of muscle pain but also refer to their muscles as being "stiff." This is also a symptom in hyperparathyroidism, hypothyroidism, tetany, and, more acutely, tetanus (see Table 2.9).

Numbness

Complaints of distal numbness are common in polyneuropathies. In radiculopathies, numbness is present in the territory of the affected nerve roots. In mononeuropathies, the deficit is in the territory of the affected nerve. Numbness begins in the lower extremities in most generalized neuropathies but can start in the hands in vitamin B_{12} deficiency. In some forms of amyloidosis, amyloid deposition may result in carpal tunnel syndrome, causing hand numbness.

Spontaneous Neurogenic Pain

Spontaneous limb pain is a common symptom in neuropathy. The so-called nerve trunk pain that occurs in most root compressions or with other forms of nerve trunk

---

*This disorder is also called *Lambert-Eaton syndrome* (LES) by some authors in this book.

Table 2.9 Neuromuscular Conditions Associated with Muscle Stiffness at Rest*

Stiff-man syndrome
Amyotrophic lateral sclerosis, progressive lateral sclerosis
Isaac's syndrome
Schwartz-Jampel syndrome
Myotonia (e.g., myotonic dystrophy, proximal myotonic myopathy, myotonia congenita)
Polymyositis
Rippling muscle disease
Hypothyroidism
Hyperparathyroidism, tetany
Tetanus
Drugs, toxins (e.g., clofibrate)
Myopathies with prominent contractures (e.g., pentazocine-induced)

*Painful stiffness or contractures may develop in glycogen storage diseases only during exercise.

damage is focal and intense, sometimes like a toothache or piercing knife. A sharp-shooting pain also occurs in radiculopathy from root stretching.

A pain elicited by warming and accompanied by redness of the skin, also called *angry backfiring nociceptor syndrome*,[18] corresponds to the complex regional pain syndrome I, previously termed *reflex sympathetic dystrophy*. Dysesthetic burning pain, or causalgia, occurs in traumatic nerve lesions; this and other post-traumatic neuralgias are considered as complex regional pain syndrome II and are also usually accompanied by skin changes. Some patients with nerve injury have the so-called triple cold syndrome, in which there is burning pain and mechanical hyperalgesia in a cold and pale limb that worsen with cooling of the limb. Burning pain occurs in polyneuropathies, especially those affecting the small nerve fibers. The term *allodynia* refers to pain elicited by a stimulation that is normally nonpainful, such as cold or touch. *Anesthesia dolorosa* describes a painful syndrome in areas of decreased sensitivity.

Paresthesias

Tingling paresthesias and the sensation of "prickling" or " pins and needles"—particularly in the feet and distal legs—are common complaints in neuropathies, particularly in those affecting unmyelinated nerve fibers, such as diabetic, alcoholic, and toxic neuropathies (Table 2.10). Paresthesias, however, also occur in some demyelinating neuropathies, such as CIDP.

Autonomic Symptoms

Patients with peripheral neuropathy may have symptoms of autonomic nervous system dysfunction, such as generalized or distal abnormalities of sweating (either increased or decreased), which in focal neuropathies may be seen in the territory of the affected nerve. Those with dysautonomic polyneuropathy may also complain

Color Plate A1 Retinal degeneration in a patient with spinocerebellar degeneration. (Courtesy of Dr. Richard Drewry.)

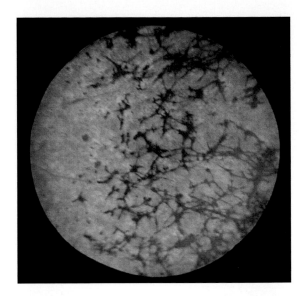

Color Plate A2 Atypical retinal degeneration in a patient with a mitochondrial myopathy (Kearns-Sayre syndrome).

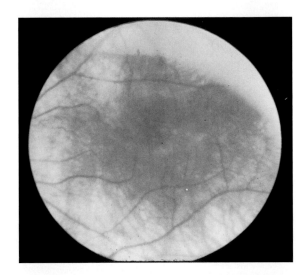

Color Plate A3 Cotton wool exudates in the retina in a patient with diabetes and peripheral neuropathy.

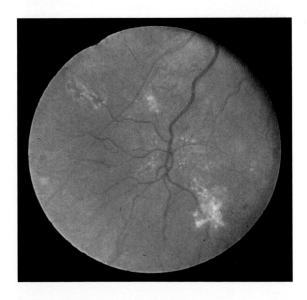

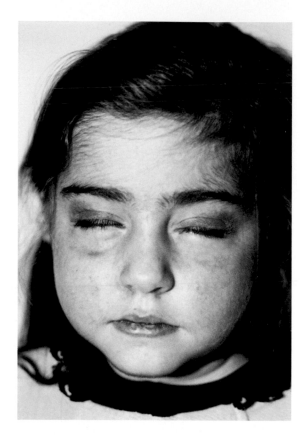

Color Plate A4 Heliotrope rash in a child with dermatomyositis.

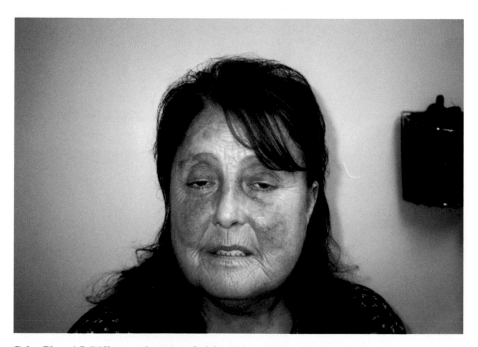

Color Plate A5 Diffuse erythematous facial rash in an adult with dermatomyositis.

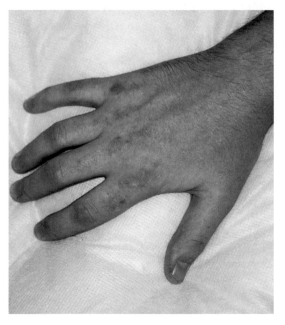

Color Plate A6 Erythema in the dorsum of the joints in the hand of a patient with dermatomyositis.

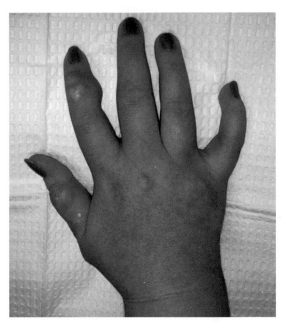

Color Plate A7 Fusiform fingers with calcifications in a patient with mixed connective tissue disease.

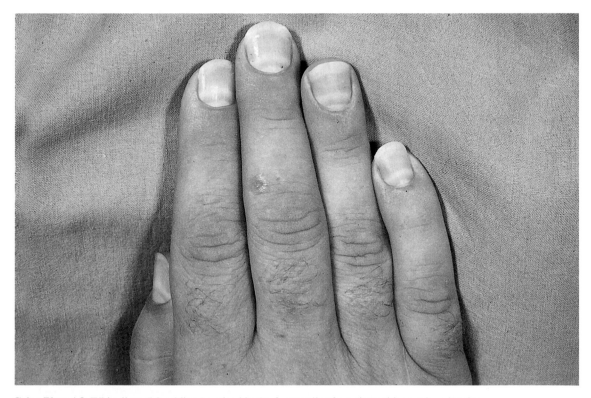

Color Plate A8 White lines (Mees' lines) noticed in the fingernails of a patient with arsenic poisoning.

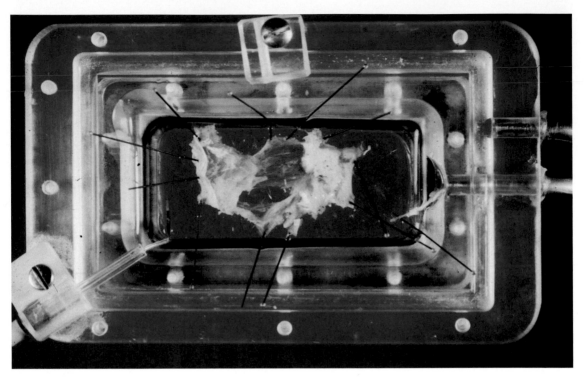

Color Plate A9 Example of muscles used for in vitro microelectrode studies. Dissected external intercostal muscle pinned down to a layer of sylgard covering the bottom of a recording chamber.

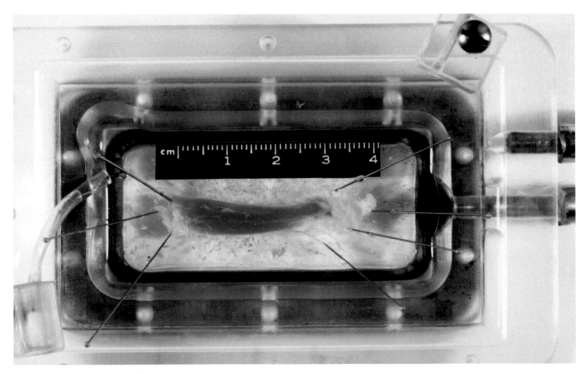

Color Plate A10 Example of muscles used for in vitro microelectrode studies. A bundle of intact muscle fibers from the anconeus muscle of an adult patient.

Table 2.10 Predominantly Sensory Neuropathy

Diabetes mellitus
Amyloidosis
Sjögren's syndrome
Paraneoplastic neuropathy
Pyridoxine intoxication
Familial sensory neuropathies
B_{12} deficiency
Hypothyroidism
Vitamin E deficiency
Neuropathy with antibodies against myelin-associated glycoprotein (sensory-motor, distal)
Sensory chronic inflammatory demyelinating polyneuropathy, sensory Guillain-Barré
   syndrome
Human immunodeficiency virus polyneuropathy
Some neurotoxins (e.g., thallium intoxication)
Medications (e.g., cisplatinum, thalidomide, metronidazole)
Cryptogenic neuropathy

---

of constipation, impotence, urinary difficulties, and lightheadedness, caused by orthostatic hypotension. Hypoglycemia may be asymptomatic in diabetics from autonomic neuropathy, because the symptoms of hypoglycemia are caused by sympathetic overactivity.

Autonomic dysfunction is common in amyloidosis, LEMS, and hereditary sensory and autonomic neuropathies. It is also seen in approximately 20% of patients with GBS and is very prominent in the acute pandysautonomic neuropathies. Thus, patients with these diseases need to be monitored carefully for hypertensive crisis and arrhythmias.

PHYSICAL EXAMINATION

General Examination

The examination of patients with neuromuscular disorders should not be limited to evaluation of muscle and nerve function but should also include careful general physical observations, because systemic manifestations may provide clues in the etiologic diagnosis. This is particularly important in mitochondrial disorders that can have multisystem manifestations, such as stroke-like episodes, retinal degeneration, hearing loss, lipomas, ataxia, and cardiac disease. Other examples include the presence of liver and spleen enlargement in patients with a neuropathy, which could be suggestive of POEMS syndrome (*p*olyneuropathy, *o*rganomegaly, *e*ndocrinopathy, *M* protein, *s*kin changes) or alcoholism, whereas visceromegaly in a floppy baby suggests a multisystem problem, such as Pompe's disease. Enlarged salivary glands with dry mouth and decreased tears occur in Sjögren's syndrome, whereas enlarged orange tonsils are characteristic of Tangier disease.

Retinal degeneration can occur in patients with mitochondrial myopathy (see Color Plates A1 and A2), Refsum's disease, and abetalipoproteinemia. A retinopathy with microaneurysms and cotton wool exudates is characteristic of diabetes (see Color Plate A3), whereas optic atrophy or hearing loss may occur in CMT disease. FSHMD may be associated with hearing loss and Coats' syndrome with retinal detachment and exudates.[19]

During the eye examination, it is helpful to look for the presence of cataracts that occurs in some diseases, such as MD, Fabry's, and Refsum's diseases. Corneal opacity occurs in gelsolin familial amyloidosis, and vitreous opacities can be observed in transthyretin amyloidosis.[20,21]

Detailed evaluation of the skin can also provide clues in the diagnosis—for example, a thick skin is seen in patients with systemic sclerosis or hypothyroidism, purpura in cryoglobulinemia, angiokeratosis in Fabry's disease, or ichthyosis in Refsum's disease. Those with lepromatous leprosy have multiple erythematous macules and a "leonine" facies, whereas patients with lupus erythematosus have a characteristic butterfly rash on the face. Skin changes in DM include a malar rash and the classic heliotrope (see Color Plates A4 and A5) as well as scaling and erythema on the extensor surfaces of the joints, including the Gottron's rash seen over the knuckles (see Color Plate A6) and in the classic shawl or cape distribution in the exposed areas of the shoulders and chest. Abnormal capillaries of the nail folds and thickening skin of the fingertips, or "carpenter's fingers," also can be seen. Subcutaneous calcification may be seen in childhood DM (Figure 2.1A).

The examiner should also look for herpetic lesions (see Figure 2.1B) in acute focal radiculopathies and for joint deformity and ulnar deviation of the wrist or fusiform appearance of the fingers that occur in connective tissue disorders (see Color Plate A7), which can be associated with carpal tunnel syndrome and PM. A clue in the diagnosis of patients with a neuropathy with intellectual impairment and ataxia is the presence of xanthomas in the Achilles' tendon, which are characteristic of cerebrotendinous xanthomatosis (see Figure 2.1C).

The presence of Mees' lines (white lines on finger nails—see Color Plate A8) is indicative of heavy metal intoxication, particularly arsenic; nails that appear whiter are also seen in the POEMS syndrome. Thallium intoxication, on the other hand, causes alopecia.

Other important observations that provide clues in the diagnosis include the presence of a high arched palate in congenital myopathies, feet with high arches and hammer toes (Figure 2.2) in hereditary neuropathies and some distal myopathies, and scoliosis in those with long-standing weakness since childhood.

The neurologic examination should be complete and not limited to the peripheral nervous system. For example, evaluation of mental function is important because retardation or regressing milestones occur in some of these disorders, such as congenital MD and metachromatic leukodystrophy (MLD). A "neuropathic" tremor is seen in some forms of CMT disease (e.g., Roussy-Lévy syndrome), CIDP, and paraproteinemic neuropathies, and sensory ataxia also occurs in some large-fiber neuropathies. This chapter, however, emphasizes only the examination of the peripheral nervous system.

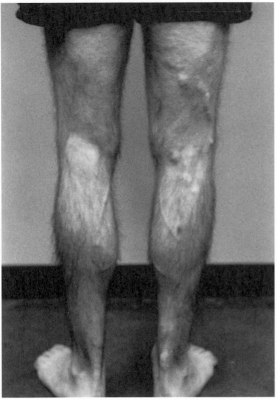

A

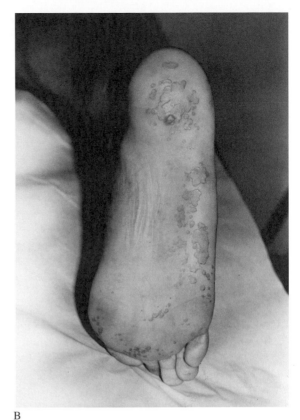

B

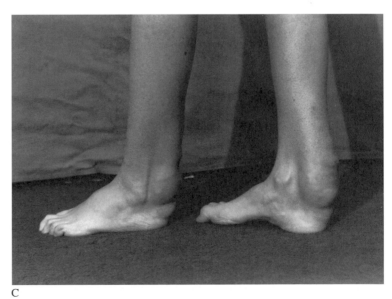

Figure 2.1 A. Subcutaneous calcifications in a young man with dermatomyositis. **B.** Herpetic vesicles in the S1 root territory. Herpes zoster infection. **C.** Xanthomas of the Achillies' tendon in a patient with cerebrotendinous xanthomatosis.

C

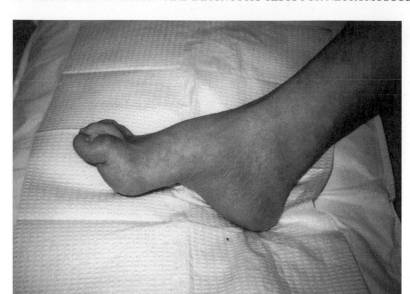

Figure 2.2 High arch and hammertoes in a patient with Charcot-Marie-Tooth disease.

Neuromuscular Evaluation

Analysis of Posture and Gait

The clinician should first observe whether the patients use their arms to push up while rising from a chair or whether there is hyperflexion of the trunk when standing because of hip extensor weakness.

After this, the patient's posture should be observed while standing for the presence of scoliosis or exaggerated lumbar lordosis. Lordosis is seen in patients with weak hip extensors and lumbar paraspinal muscles; this exaggerated posture aids in maintaining the center of gravity. A prominent lordosis is also seen in patients with the stiff-man syndrome (Figure 2.3), caused by spasms of lumbar paraspinal muscles.

The patient is then asked to raise his or her arms with the forearm supinated to a horizontal position to determine whether there is downward drift with pronation of the limb, the "pronator drift" that may be seen in diseases of the upper motor neuron, even without prominent shoulder weakness on manual muscle testing (MMT). With the eyes closed, a gradual "drift" above the horizontal is seen in those with prominent proprioceptive deficit.

A Romberg test should also be done while the patient is standing to determine whether there is a proprioceptive deficit of the legs, which occurs in large-fiber neuropathies.

During the analysis of gait, the examiner should observe for the characteristic scissoring or "circumduction" gait of spasticity. Weakness of the foot dorsiflexors produces the classical steppage gait in neuropathies, whereas the waddling gait is seen in most myopathies and some motor neuron diseases, such as juvenile SMA, owing to prominent hip flexor weakness. In these patients, the pelvis is tilted and the hip is flexed with a circular motion rather than a direct flexion.[3] A gait with hyperextension of the knee can be seen in those with prominent quadriceps muscle weakness (Figure 2.4). Patients should also be asked to walk on the heels and toes to detect mild weakness of the foot dorsiflexors and plantar flexors.

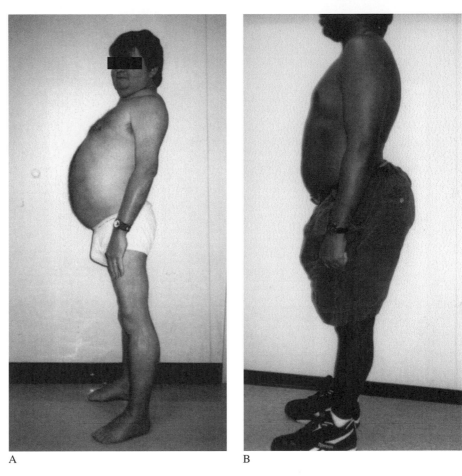

A   B

Figure 2.3 A. Lordosis, calf hypertrophy, and atrophy of the thigh muscles in a patient with Becker's muscular dystrophy. **B.** Prominent lordosis in a patient with stiff-man syndrome.

Figure 2.4 The figure demonstrates a hyperextended knee while walking in a patient with muscular dystrophy with predominant quadriceps muscle weakness.

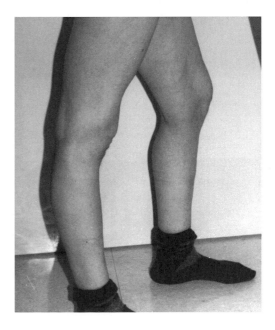

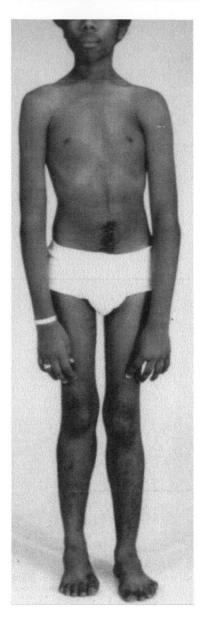

Figure 2.5 Patient with juvenile spinal muscular atrophy showing hyperpronation of the arms with atrophy of the pectoralis quadriceps muscles and mild calf hypertrophy.

Evaluation of the movements of the upper extremities while the patient stands and walks is also useful; for example, those with weakness of shoulder abduction may pronate the arms while standing or walking (Figure 2.5).

A characteristic manifestation of proximal lower-extremity weakness is the Gower's sign, which is the maneuver of "climbing over the legs" to stand to compensate for hip extensor weakness (Figure 2.6).[22,23] In less severe cases, a modification of this sign is used to rise from the floor. This was described by Dr. Michael Brooke as the "butt-first" maneuver, because the buttocks are pushed up before the trunk.[22]

Figure 2.6 Patient with late infantile acid maltase deficiency showing the Gower's sign. Also notice the hyperextension of the elbow while sitting.

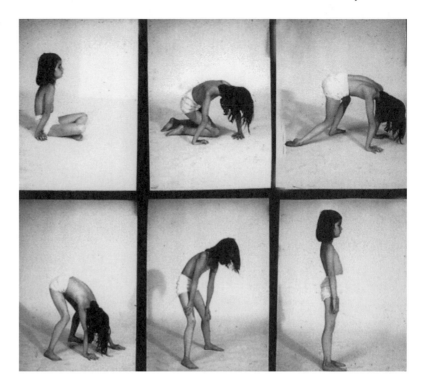

Knee extensor and hip flexor function can be assessed by asking the patient to step on a stool. Difficulty in performing this task is caused by the iliopsoas or quadriceps weakness.

Comprehensive assessment of neuromuscular function and functional ability scores, with disease-specific evaluations used for follow-up, are available. Protocols for these are included in Appendix III.

Examination of the Eyelids and Extraocular Muscles

The eye examination should determine the presence of ptosis that, when unilateral and accompanied by a small pupil, is characteristic of the Horner's syndrome (Figure 2.7), seen in some lesions of the lower trunk of the brachial plexus. Chronic,

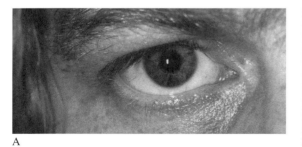
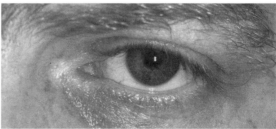

A   B

Figure 2.7 Horner's syndrome on the left eye (**B**) in a patient with lymphoma of the lower brachial plexus. Notice ptosis and a smaller pupil and compare with normal eye (**A**).

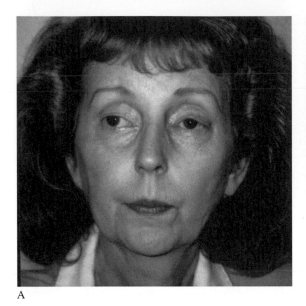 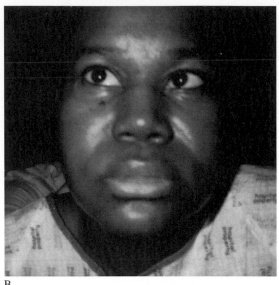

A   B

Figure 2.8 A. Ptosis and symmetrical limitation of gaze in a patient with mitochondrial myopathy. **B.** Patient with sarcoidosis showing abducens palsy with spontaneous adduction of the left eye.

bilateral, and symmetric ptosis occurs in several myopathies, such as MD, myotubular myopathy, and some mitochondrial disorders (Figure 2.8A). A mild, bilateral ptosis could be seen in LEMS. In OPMD (Figure 2.9), patients have the characteristic "astronomist posture" of overcontracting the frontalis muscle and tilting the head backward to overcome the ptosis.[24] The astronomist posture can also be seen in patients with other diseases, such as mitochondrial myopathy.

The examiner should also evaluate for eyelid fatigue during sustained upward gaze, which is typical of MG. During the examination, it is important to distinguish true ptosis from pseudo-ptosis and from blepharospasm. In these conditions, there is contraction of the orbicularis oculi, and the lower eyelid of the "ptotic" eye is contracted and thus raised.

Extraocular muscle evaluation should determine whether there is limitation of eye movements, diplopia, or both. For isolation of the weak muscle, the red glass test and the Lancaster red-green rod test are useful.

Bilateral and symmetric limitation of eye movements can occur in mitochondrial myopathy, the so-called ocular myopathies, slow channel syndrome, and advanced cases of OPMD. Limitation of eye movement is frequently associated with exophthalmos in thyroid eye disease. Ophthalmoplegia occurs acutely in Miller Fisher syndrome (Figure 2.10), whereas paralysis of an individual ocular muscle suggests a condition such as sarcoidosis (see Figure 2.8B) or a vasculopathy like diabetic ophthalmoplegia (Figure 2.11), in which the third nerve involvement usually spares the pupil.

Careful evaluation of eye movements is important in MG, a disease that can present with several types of abnormality, from isolated muscle weakness to a complete external ophthalmoplegia (Table 2.11). Ptosis, however, is the most common finding in MG, is frequently asymmetric, and worsens during repetitive eye opening or during saccadic tests[24] and sustained upward gaze (Figure 2.12). To observe for levator fatigue during sustained upward gaze, it is helpful to press the patient's forehead to avoid his or her use of the frontalis muscle to elevate the lid.

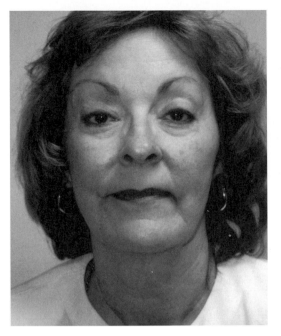

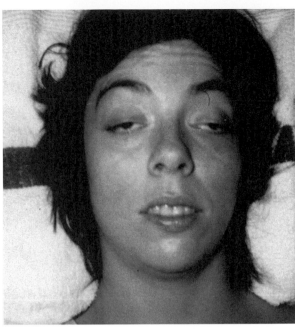

Figure 2.9 The astronomist posture in a patient with oculopharyngeal dystrophy.

Figure 2.10 Ophthalmoplegia and ptosis in a patient with Miller Fisher syndrome.

Some myasthenic patients may also have "paradoxical" reversal of ptosis, in which the ptosis switches from one eye to the other during the day.[24] Eyelid "hopping" or twitching during lateral gaze accompanied by extraocular muscle fatigue can be seen. In MG, it is also useful to observe for ptosis that develops in the apparently normal eye when the examiner raises the patient's affected ptotic eyelid. This happens because normally there is bilateral central innervation of the levators; when this bilateral central innervation is suppressed by passively lifting the ptotic eyelid, there is unmasking of the mild weakness and ptosis in the apparently normal eye (Hering's law) (Figure 2.13).[25]

A very important finding in MG is "Cogan's lid-twitch" sign.[26] This is observed when the patient is asked to look down for a brief moment, then to return his or her

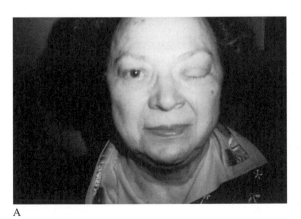

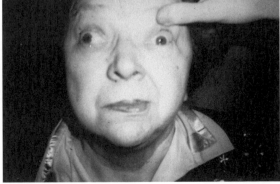

A

B

Figure 2.11 A. Patient with diabetic third nerve palsy with ptosis of the left eye. **B.** Limitation of adduction of the same eye.

Table 2.11 Ocular Signs in Myasthenia Gravis

Levator palpebrae weakness
   Ptosis with sustained upward gaze
   Lid twitch and lid nystagmus of sustained upward gaze
   Lid retraction
   Cogan's lid-twitch sign
   Lid hopping
   Lid retraction of the contralateral eye and enhancement of contralateral ptosis on manual
      lifting of the ptotic eye
Weakness of orbicularis oculi
   Afternoon ectropion
   Peek sign
Weakness of extraocular movements
   Diplopia and ocular paresis
   Gaze paretic nystagmus
   Fatiguing saccades

Source: Adapted from JS Barton, M Fouladvand. Ocular Aspects of Myasthenia Gravis. In J Corbett (ed), Neuroophthalmology for the General Neurologist. New York: Thieme, 2000;7–20.

gaze to the primary position. In the Cogan's sign, the eyelid elevates excessively and then returns to the neutral position, appearing as a brief "twitch," after which it becomes ptotic again. This overshoot is caused by the temporary resting of the elevator during downward gaze.

Myasthenics may also show eyelid retraction during vertical gaze, although this is most characteristic of thyroid ophthalmopathy.

Other ocular findings in MG include ectropion of the lower eyelid due to orbicularis oculi weakness and the so-called peek sign, which occurs when the patient is asked to keep the eyes closed. The examiner can then see the patient's sclera "peek-

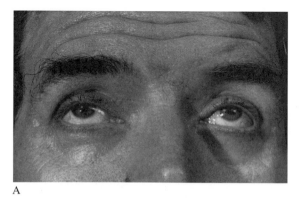
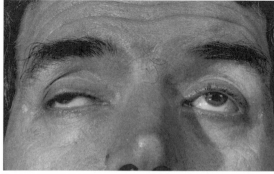

A   B

Figure 2.12 Patient with myasthenia gravis (**A**), who developed an outward deviation of the right eye from partial right internal rectus weakness and ptosis, on sustained upward gaze (**B**).

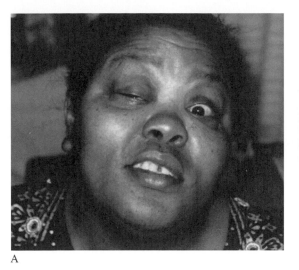
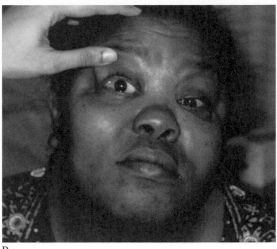

A   B

Figure 2.13 Patient with ptosis of the right eye **(A)** who developed ptosis of the left while the examiner held her right eyelid up to inhibit bilateral cortical control of the levator muscle (Hering's law) **(B)**.

ing" due to its inability to keep the eyelid closed. This is caused by weak orbicularis oculi muscles.[27]

Ptosis in MG can be reversed with the "ice test." In this test, a plastic bag or a glove filled with ice is placed over the eye for 30 seconds, which decreases the temperature and improves neuromuscular transmission.[28] Finally, the edrophonium test is used to observe the reversal of ptosis or muscle weakness from MG; this is the most important clinical diagnostic test in this disease. The test is discussed in detail in the section Edrophonium (Tensilon) Test.

Pupils

The pupils should also be examined carefully in neuromuscular disorders. As discussed before, a miotic pupil is seen in Horner's syndrome. Dilated pupils occur in botulism; diminished pupillary reflex can be seen in patients with autonomic dysfunction, and pharmacologic testing may be required to ascertain the exact nature and site of the pupillary paralysis.

Patients with LEMS can have small pupils, which may also be caused by anticholinesterase overmedication and organophosphate poisoning. Light-near dissociation, the "Argyll Robertson pupil," may occur not only in those with neurosyphilis but also in diabetic neuropathy and other neuropathies, such as lupus. Some patients with ganglioneuritis, CIDP, and GBS may manifest tonic pupils, as in the Adie's syndrome.[29,30]

Evaluation of Facial and Masticatory Muscles

During the evaluation of facial and masticatory muscles, the observer should determine whether there is symmetric or asymmetric weakness and whether it is peripheral or central, wherein the frontalis muscle is spared. It is worth remembering,

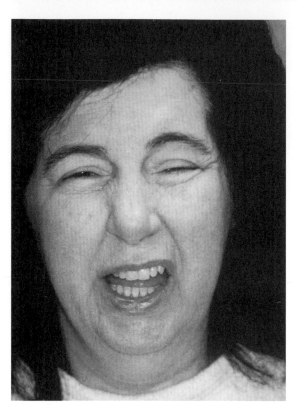

Figure 2.14 "Myasthenic snarl" in a patient with orbicularis oris weakness from myasthenia gravis. (Reprinted with permission from J Howard Jr. The myasthenic face and snarl. J Clin Neuromusc Dis 2000;1[4]:214.)

however, that damage of lower branches of the seventh nerve may produce paralysis of the lower facial muscle groups, mimicking a central paralysis.

When testing the orbicularis oculi, the patient should be observed for the presence of the Bell's palsy, in which both eyeballs roll upwards when attempting to tightly close the eyes. In psychogenic weakness, this phenomenon is absent. However, lack of eye elevation can also occur in MG. Patients with bilateral facial weakness, such as familial gelsolin amyloidosis and FSHMD,[31] may be unable to close the eyes tightly.

The orbicularis oris is evaluated by asking the patient to blow out his or her cheeks with the mouth closed and then to compress the cheeks gently. If air escapes, it is an indication of weakness. This muscle is also tested by asking the patient to repeat the sound "me, me, me" or by puckering the lips or whistling.

Facial muscle weakness can cause a downward deviation of the corners of the mouth with flattening of the nasolabial folds. A characteristic smile, referred to as the "myasthenic snarl" occurs in MG, giving the patient an angry look. The snarl is caused by horizontal contraction of the corners of the mouth with elevation of the weak central portion of the upper lip (Figure 2.14).[32] Dimples in the upper lip and a horizontal smile are other signs of facial weakness, which is characteristic of FSHMD (Figure 2.15).[23]

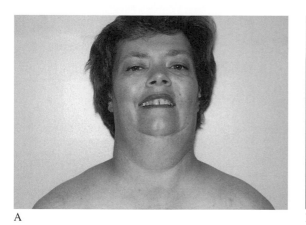

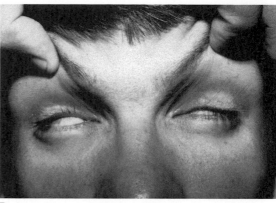

A   B

Figure 2.15 A. Horizontal smile in a patient with facioscapulohumeral dystrophy. **B.** Patient with fascioscapulohumeral dystrophy with a weak orbicularis oculi and
positive Bell's palsy (both eyeballs rolling upward).
C. Patient with fascioscapulohumeral dystrophy showing dimples of the upper lip from weakness of the orbicularis oris.

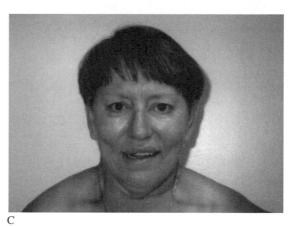

C

Facial muscle examination includes observation for fasciculations, which occur
in Kennedy's syndrome, Machado-Joseph disease, and advanced ALS. Facial myokymia can be seen in Schwartz-Jampel syndrome.

Patients with remote facial nerve lesion may also show evidence of aberrant
regeneration with contractions of the "wrong" muscles; for example, in the "jaw-
winking phenomenon," patients contract the orbicularis oris while blinking.

Temporalis muscle wasting and weakness occur in myopathies, such as MD
(Figure 2.16) and myotubular myopathy, whereas hypertrophy of the temporalis
and masseters can be seen in myotonia congenita and hypothyroidism. In some
patients, particularly those with MG, bilateral weakness of these muscles can
cause the "dropped-jaw" syndrome, in which the patient cannot maintain mouth
closure (Figure 2.17). To examine masticatory muscles, the patient is asked to
clench his or her teeth, and the temporalis and the masseters are palpated. The
patient is then asked to bite a tongue depressor while the examiner attempts to
pull it out of the mouth; this is done easily if these muscles are weak.

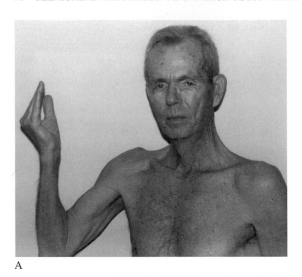
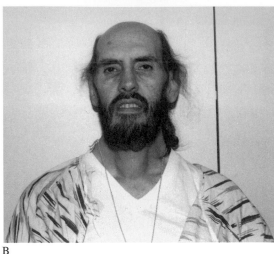

A   B

Figure 2.16 A. Patient with myotonic dystrophy showing "tapir lips," temporal wasting, and distal muscle wasting. **B.** Another myotonic dystrophy patient with balding, mild ptosis, temporal wasting, and a horizontal smile.

In some myopathies, such as those with rigid spine syndrome, contractures cause difficulty in opening the mouth. Unilateral weakness of pterygoid muscles causes a lateral deviation of the jaw to the weak side when opening the mouth.

The jaw jerk should also be elicited in patients with suspected motor neuron disease and corticospinal tract findings, because the presence of a brisk reflex argues against a cervical cord disease as a cause of the upper motor neuron signs.

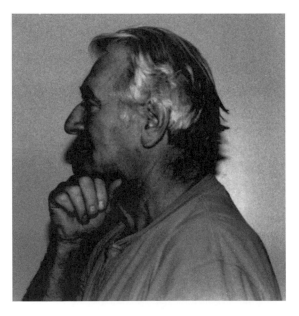

Figure 2.17 Patient with myasthenia gravis and a "dropped jaw." Note that the patient must use his fist to keep his mouth closed.

Palate and Tongue Muscles

Palatal weakness carries the risk of aspiration and hence is important to detect; for this, the examiner should observe the elevation of the palate when the patient says "ah." The ability of the patient to repeat the sound "gah, gah, gah" determines good palatal muscle movement. Deviation of the palate to the normal side is seen in unilateral lesions of the glossopharyngeal nerve. The "gag" reflex should also be performed, as this can be exaggerated in patients with ALS and decreased in bulbar palsy.

The tongue should be examined for atrophy and fasciculations for the diagnosis of motor neuron diseases (ALS, Kennedy's disease, and SMA). In MG and, sometimes, MD, the tongue may appear "forked" or may have triple furrows. Unilateral atrophy, causing the tongue to deviate to the paralyzed side when protruded, is seen in focal neuropathies that affect the hypoglossal nerve (Figure 2.18). Patients with tongue weakness have difficulty vocalizing the sound "la, la, la," and are unable to press the tongue against the cheeks. The examination should also include observation for atrophic fungiform papillae in pernicious anemia. Papillary atrophy is also a feature of Riley-Day syndrome. Tongue hypertrophy can occur in amyloidosis, hypothyroidism, DMD, sarcoidosis (see Figure 2.18), and Pompe's disease.

Axial and Limb Muscle Examination

The muscle examination must include a careful observation to determine whether there is focal or diffuse atrophy or hypertrophy. Proximal symmetric atrophy occurs in SMA (see Figure 2.5) and myopathies. Atrophy, however, sometimes can be asymmetric in these diseases (Figure 2.19). Distal atrophy and weakness are seen in polyneuropathies and some myopathies, as discussed in the section Distribution (Figure 2.20). In mononeuropathies and radiculopathies, weakness occurs in muscles innervated by the affected roots or nerves. The pattern of a selective or predominant involvement in some muscle groups is often helpful in the diagnosis—for example, a prominent atrophy of the quadriceps is seen in IBM and some muscular dystrophies, whereas trapezius muscle wasting with a "scapular hump" is characteristic of FSHMD (Figure 2.21).

Muscle hypertrophy may be seen in DMD and Becker's muscular dystrophy (BMD); myotonia congenita, particularly the autosomal recessive type; Schwartz-Jampel syndrome (Figure 2.22); some cases of amyloidosis; and parasitic infections, such as cysticercosis. Focal muscle hypertrophy may occur rarely in radiculopathies (Table 2.12).

Real versus Psychogenic Weakness. Frequently, the clinician has to determine whether the patient's weakness is real or psychogenic. An important clue is that patients with nonorganic disease usually perform functional tests better than when strength is tested by MMT.[2,3] For example, patients may be able to rise from a chair without difficulty, are not atrophic, and have normal reflexes, yet when the knee and hip extensors are tested, they appear very weak. A characteristic "give-away weakness" is also seen in nonorganic diseases. During testing, these patients initially resist the examiner and then the muscle collapses rapidly, sometimes in a staccato pattern. MG is sometimes difficult to differentiate from "functional" weakness, although the fact that the myasthenic weakness is present throughout the whole range of movement, without interruption, and increases only with repetitive contractions, may assist in the differentiation.

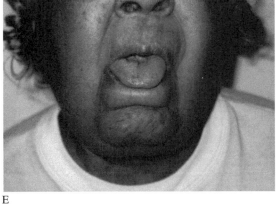

Figure 2.18 A. Patient with myasthenia gravis with a forked, triple furrowed tongue. **B.** Patient with amyotrophic lateral sclerosis showing tongue atrophy. **C.** Left tongue weakness with the tongue deviating to that side from left hypoglossal nerve paralysis. **D.** Patient with Duchenne's muscular dystrophy showing a large tongue. **E.** Partial hypertrophy on the left side of the tongue in a patient with sarcoidosis. (Note that the tongue is in the resting position and not protruded.)

Unilateral limb weakness is hard to fake if both arms are tested simultaneously. For example, a patient may have "weakness" when the examiner opposes the arm's adduction at the shoulder while the weak arm is extended. However, when both arms are tested simultaneously or when the patient is asked to extend the arms against resistance, the weakness is not apparent. Thus, the "weak" arm appears stronger than when the patient performs this task with each arm individually.

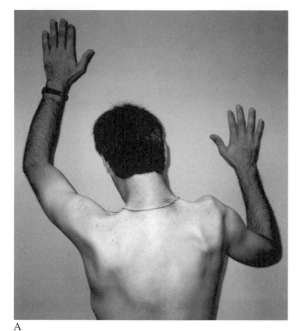

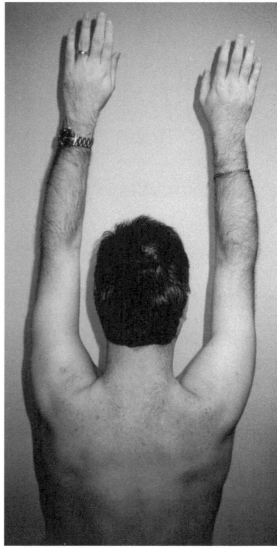

Figure 2.19 A. Patient with polymyositis with more severe wasting and weakness of the right shoulder girdle. **B.** Same patient raising both arms equally and normally after treatment.

The Hoover sign also helps to demonstrate "fake" unilateral leg weakness. In this test, the examiner places his or her hands under the patient's heels and asks the patient to lift the paralyzed limb off the bed. In real weakness, the patient presses down the opposite heel in an effort to raise the weak leg. Those with fake weakness make no effort, and, thus, no pressure is felt from the opposite heel.

Manual Muscle Testing. MMT is the technique used routinely in the evaluation of muscle strength. In this method, the examiner opposes the patient's forceful contraction, and the degree of resistance is graded accordingly.[3] Testing should also include evaluation of fatigue, particularly in proximal muscles if a disease of the neuromuscular junction is a consideration. All patients should, however, be tested for fatigue because this also occurs in other diseases (Figure 2.23). To test for fatigue, the examiner opposes the sustained contraction of the tested muscles,

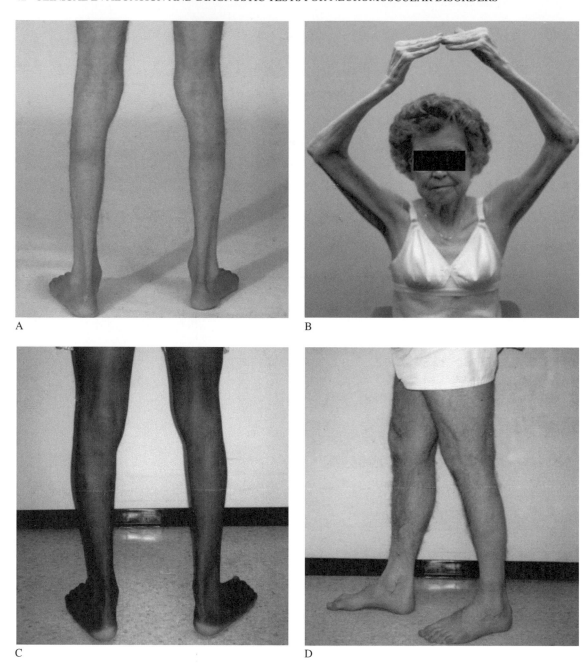

Figure 2.20 A. Distal leg wasting in a patient with peripheral neuropathy. **B.** Forearm and hand atrophy in a patient with inclusion body myositis. **C.** Calf atrophy in a patient with Miyoshi muscular dystrophy. **D.** Wasting of the left calf in a patient with postmyelopathy amyotrophy from a cornus medullaris lesion involving anterior horn cells of L5-S1 segments with chronic denervation on electromyography. (Reprinted with permission from P Narayanaswami, TE Bertorini. Progressive amyotrophy as a late complication of myelopathy. J Neurol Sci 2001;184:11–13.)

Figure 2.21 Patient with fascio-scapulohumeral dystrophy showing a scapular hump (prominent scapular bones seen due to wasting of the upper trapezius).

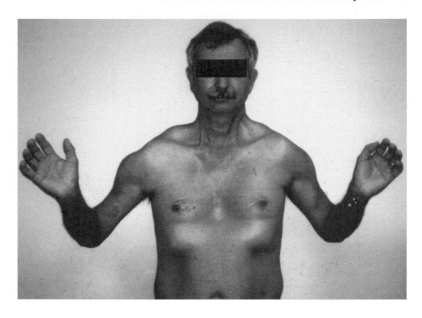

Figure 2.22 A. Muscle hypertrophy of thoracic muscles in a child with myotonia congenita. **B.** Muscle hypertrophy in a child with Schwartz-Jampel syndrome.

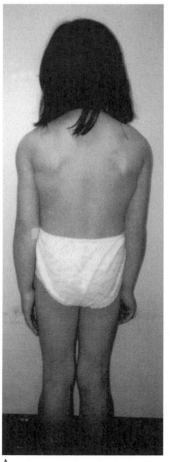

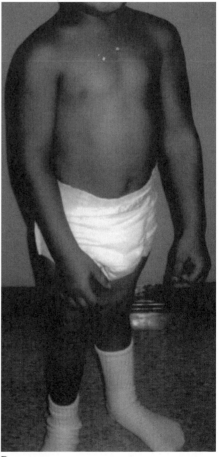

A

B

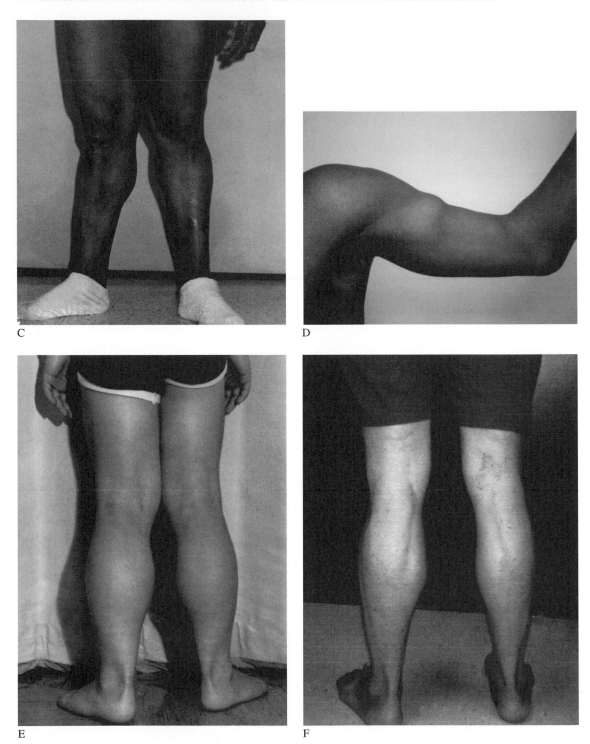

Figure 2.22 *Continued* **C.** Postpolio pseudohypertrophy of the legs. (Reprinted with permission from TE Bertorini, M Igarashi. Postpolio pseudohypertrophy. Muscle Nerve 1985;8:644–649.) **D.** Tendon rupture producing focal swelling of the biceps muscle. **E.** Bilateral calf hypertrophy in Duchenne's muscular dystrophy. **F.** Hypertrophy of the calf in a patient with S1 root damage from a tethered cord, with denervation with abundant complex high-frequency repetitive discharges. (Reprinted with permission from TE Bertorini, C Woodhouse, L Horner. Muscle hypertrophy secondary to the tethered cord syndrome. Muscle Nerve l994;17:331–335.)

Table 2.12 Neuromuscular Causes of Muscle Hypertrophy

Generalized hypertrophy
    Juvenile spinal muscular atrophy (usually early, mainly calves)
    Postpolio pseudohypertrophy
    Acromegaly
    Hypothyroid myopathy
    Schwartz-Jampel syndrome
    Isaac's syndrome
    Myotonia congenita
    Paramyotonia congenita
    Duchenne's muscular dystrophy (can be generalized but mainly in the calves)
    Becker's muscular dystrophy
    Limb-girdle muscular dystrophy (mainly in the calves)
    Flier syndrome
    Sarcoidosis (can be focal)
    Parasites (cysticercosis, schistosomiasis, trichinosis)
    Amyloidosis
Focal hypertrophy
    Sarcoidosis
    Radiculopathy or other causes of partial denervation (e.g., tethered cord)
    Tendon rupture

Source: Adapted from Evaluation of the Patient with Myopathy. In R Griggs, JR Mendell, RG Miller (eds), Evaluation and Treatment of Myopathies. Contemporary Neurology Series. Philadelphia: FA Davis, 1995;26.

such as the neck flexors or deltoids, hip flexor muscles, or those that the patient refers to as getting tired during the day; these muscles should then be examined after a period of exercise with repetitive contractions.

The grading system used most frequently in MMT is the Medical Research Council scale.[33] This grades muscle strength from 0 to 5. A grade of 0 indicates no

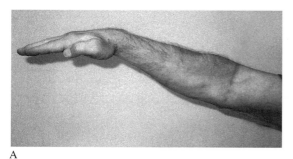

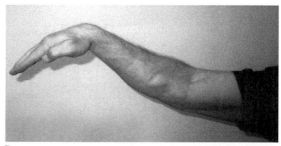

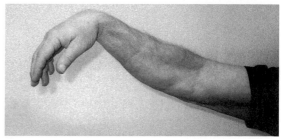

A

B

C

Figure 2.23 A. Patient with a multifocal motor neuropathy with wrist extended. **B.** Wrist extended for 10 seconds. **C.** Wrist drop after maintaining wrist extended for 15 seconds.

Table 2.13 Muscle Strength Gradings

FG	MRC	Modified/ MRC	Strength Assessment
N	5	10	Normal strength.
G+		9	Barely detectable weakness.
G	4	8	Holds test position against gravity and moderate resistance.
G–		7	Holds test position against gravity and mild resistance.
F+		6	Muscle moves joint fully against gravity—is capable of transient resistance but collapses abruptly.
F	3	5	Muscle moves joint fully against gravity but cannot hold against resistance.
F– and P+		4	Muscle moves joint against gravity but not the full possible extent of mechanical range.
P		3	Muscle moves joint when gravity eliminated through full extent of mechanical range.
P–	2	2	Muscle moves joint when gravity eliminated through partial extent of mechanical range.
Tr	1	1	A flicker of contraction felt in muscles; no joint motion.
O	0	0	No contraction felt in muscle.

F = fair; FG = functional grade; G = gravity; MRC = Medical Research Council; N = normal; O = no movement; P = poor; Tr = trace.

movement; grade 1 is a flicker of contraction; grade 2 is a movement that does not overcome gravity; grade 3 is a contraction that overcomes gravity but not resistance; grade 4 is a muscle that offers moderate resistance to the examiner; and grade 5 is a normal muscle. This is a simple method used clinically and in drug trials. A drawback of this system is that a muscle graded as level 4 indicates moderate weakness of varying degrees that cannot be differentiated. For this reason, some examiners[34] add a plus or a minus symbol to the score—for example, a 4– is a muscle that is overcome easily; a 4 is a weakness that is overcome without the examiner bracing himself; and a 4+ means the examiner must exert considerable effort.

Dr. W. K. Engel described a simple method to determine the level of grade 4 muscle weakness, subdividing this grade so that a subgrade 5 is a muscle that resists the examiner's five fingers, and a 4 resists only four fingers, and so on.[35] A system from 0 to 10 also allows the grading of intermediate levels of mild to moderate weakness.[36] This is shown in Table 2.13, which compares this grading system to the standard Medical Research Council grades and functional grading scores.[37]

These grading scales are nonlinear and therefore are not applicable for parametric statistical analysis, but in clinical trials, several muscle groups are graded. These values are added and divided by the number of muscles examined to arrive at an average score, providing data that behave as an interval and can be used for statistical analysis.[3,38] Many clinicians and investigators also use hand-held or fixed dynamometers to measure isometric contraction strength. (Chapter 15 discusses details of the use of MMT and dynamometry.)

Testing of Individual Muscle Groups. During routine evaluation, muscles are examined in groups according to their function. A more detailed, individual muscle testing should be performed in segmental diseases (i.e., radiculopathies, mononeuritis, or mononeuritis multiplex). The methods of individual muscle testing are not described here in detail, because many excellent textbooks with this information are available.[39,40] For proper localization, knowledge of the muscle innervation should be known; this information is listed in Table 2.14.[41–44]

NECK MUSCLES. Neck flexor strength is tested first by pulling the patient's arms to raise the trunk from the horizontal position to determine whether the patient has difficulty lifting his or her head while the examiner raises his trunk. The patient is then asked to raise his or her head from the supine position while the examiner pushes down on the patient's forehead.

The main neck flexor is the sternocleidomastoid, which is innervated by the spinal accessory nerve that arises from the cervical plexus, although other anterior neck muscles (e.g., the anterior longus colli, rectus capitis lateralis, and the anterior longus capitis) also contribute to this function. Weakness and atrophy of these muscles are seen in many myopathies, particularly in DMD patients who are usually unable to raise their head from a horizontal position (Figure 2.24). Other diseases that manifest with prominent neck flexor weakness include BMD, acid maltase deficiency, MD, PM, and DM. Neck flexor weakness is less prominent in IBM.

Neck extension is performed mainly by the splenius capitis and other paraspinal neck muscles, such as the longus capitis and rectus capitis posterior, which are examined as a group while the patient lies prone with his or her head on the edge of the table, and the examiner resists the patient's effort to raise the head by pressing the occipital area. As discussed previously in the section The History, neck extensor weakness may cause the "dropped head syndrome,"[45] which can be seen in a variety of conditions, such as ALS (Figure 2.25), PM, acid maltase deficiency, and MG, among others (Table 2.15).

RESPIRATORY MUSCLES. Respiratory muscles include mainly the diaphragm and intercostal muscles, and this function can be assessed at the bedside by having the patient blow at the examiner's hands placed 3–4 ft in front of him. Usually, the examiner can feel the blow at this distance. The patient is also asked to take a deep inspiration and count without taking a second breath. Usually, the ability to count to more than 30 indicates that the forced vital capacity (FVC) is at least 2 liters, and if the count is less than 20, the FVC is usually 1 liter or less. This is useful to monitor respiratory function at the bedside. During this evaluation it is also important to assess the patient's cough, which is a gross indication of respiratory muscle strength. More accurate measurement of respiratory function is performed by measuring the FVC with respirometers, as discussed later in the section Test of Pulmonary Function.

ANTERIOR ABDOMINAL MUSCLES. The anterior abdominal muscles are tested by asking the patient to sit up from the supine position. They can be weak in the early stages of disease in some myopathies, making it difficult to rise from the supine position, even when limb muscles are strong and their MMT scores are normal.

THORACIC AND LUMBAR PARASPINAL MUSCLES. Thoracic and lumbar paraspinal muscles are difficult to examine and grade clinically, but they are important, as their weakness contributes to the bent spine syndrome. They should be observed for atrophy and spasms in lumbosacral radiculopathy and the stiff-man syndrome.

SHOULDER MUSCLES. Among the shoulder muscles, the pectoralis muscles are tested by asking the patient to bring his or her hands together while the arms are raised to the horizontal. Weakness and atrophy of the pectoralis muscles occur in myopathies and in SMA, and these patients could have an oblique axillary skin fold from the periphery to the midline caused by pectoralis atrophy (Figure 2.26).

Table 2.14 Muscles of the Extremities and Their Innervation

Muscles, Innervation	Nerve	Cord	Trunk	Roots[a]	Activation
Upper extremity (shoulder and arm)					
Shoulder joint					
	Spinal accessory				
Trapezius		Not from brachial plexus	Not from brachial plexus	**C3, C4** (some branches)	Elevate shoulder
	Dorsal scapular				
Rhomboids		Directly from roots	Directly from roots	C4, **C5**	Retract scapula
Levator scapulae	**Dorsal scapular** + Twigs from C3, C4	Directly from roots	Directly from roots	C3, C4, **C5**	Elevate scapula
	Long thoracic				
Serratus anterior		Directly from roots	Directly from roots	C5, **C6, C7**[b]	Push forward against resistance
	Lateral pectoral				
Pectoralis major—clavicular		Lateral	Upper	**C5, C6,** (C7)[c]	Adduction of the shoulder
	Medial pectoral				
Sternal		Medial	Lower	**C7, C8,**[b] (T1)[c-e]	Extend and rotate the shoulder
	Lateral and medial pectoral				
Pectoralis minor		Lateral and medial	Upper, middle, and lower	C6, **C7,** C8	Depress scapula
	Suprascapular				
Supraspinatus and infraspinatus			Upper	(C4),[e] **C5,** C6	Abduct arm and external rotation of arm
	Thoracodorsal				
Latissimus dorsi		Posterior	Upper, middle, and lower	**C6,**[b] **C7,** C8	Internally rotate, adduct, and extend arm
	Subscapular				
Teres major		Posterior	Upper	C5, **C6,**[b] (C7)[e,f]	Abduct, internally rotate arm
	Axillary				
Teres minor		Posterior	Upper	(C4),[e] **C5,**[b] C6	Externally rotate arm
Deltoid		Posterior	Upper	**C5,** C6	Abduct, flex, and extend arm (posterior deltoid)
Arm					
	Musculocutaneous				
Biceps		Lateral	Upper	C5, **C6**[b]	Flex supinated forearm
Brachialis		Lateral	Upper	C5, **C6,** (C7)[e]	Flex supinated forearm
Coracobrachialis		Lateral	Upper and middle	(C5),[e] **C6,**[b] C7	Forward elevation of arm with elbow flexed
	Radial				
Triceps		Posterior	Middle and lower	C6, **C7, C8**[b]	Extend forearm

Upper extremity (forearm and hand)

Forearm

Radial

Muscle		Cord	Segment	Roots	Action
Brachioradialis		Posterior	Upper	C5, **C6**, (C7)^e	Flex forearm at semipronation
Extensor carpi radialis longus		Posterior	Upper and middle	C5, **C6**, (C7)^c-f	Extend and abduct hand at wrist
Anconeus		Posterior	Middle and lower	(C6)^c **C7**, **C8**, (T1)^e	Extend elbow
	Posterior interosseous				
Supinator		Posterior	Upper	(C5)^d-f **C6**,^b C7	Supinate forearm with elbow extended
Extensor carpi ulnaris		Posterior	Upper, middle, and lower	(C6)^c,d,f **C7**, **C8**^b	Extend and adduct hand at wrist
Extensor digitorum communis		Posterior	Middle and lower	(C6)^c,f **C7**, C8	Extension of metacarpophalangeal joints
Abductor pollicis longus		Posterior	Middle and lower	(C6)^c,f **C7**, **C8**^b	Abduct thumb at carpometacarpal joint
Extensor pollicis longus		Posterior	Middle and lower	**C7**, **C8**^b	Extend thumb at interphalangeal joint
Extensor pollicis brevis		Posterior	Middle and lower	(C6)^c,f **C7**, **C8**^b	Extend thumb at metacarpophalangeal joint
Extensor indicis proprius		Posterior	Middle and lower	**C7**, **C8**^b	Extend index finger with flexion of others
Median					
Pronator teres		Lateral	Upper and middle	C6, **C7**^b	Pronate forearm
Flexor carpi radialis		Lateral and medial	Upper, middle, and lower	C6, **C7**^b	Flex and abduct hand at wrist
Flexor digitorum superficialis		Lateral and medial	Middle and lower	**C7**, **C8**,^b T1	Flex fingers at proximal interphalangeal joint
Palmaris longus		Lateral and medial	Middle and lower	**C7**, **C8**, T1	Cup palm of hand
	Anterior interosseous				
Pronator quadratus		Lateral and medial	Middle and lower	**C7**, **C8**,^b T1	Pronate forearm
Flexor digitorum profundus I and II		Medial and lateral	Middle and lower	**C7**, **C8**, (T1)^c,e,f	Flex distal phalanx of index finger, third finger
Flexor pollicis longus		Lateral and medial	Middle and lower	**C7**, C8, (T1)^c,e,f	Flex distal phalanx of thumb

Table 2.14 *Continued*

Muscles, Innervation	Nerve	Cord	Trunk	Roots[a]	Activation
	Ulnar				
Flexor carpi ulnaris		Medial	Lower	C7, **C8**, T1	Flex and adduct hand at wrist
Flexor digitorum profundus III and IV		Medial	Lower	C7, **C8**, (T1)[c-f]	Flex distal interphalangeal joint
Hand					
	Median				
Abductor pollicis brevis		Medial	Lower	**C8,**[b] **T1**	Abduct thumb at right angle to palm
Flexor pollicis brevis (S)		Medial	Lower	**C8,**[b] **T1**	Flex thumb at metacarpophalangeal joint
Opponens pollicis		Medial	Lower	**C8,**[b] **T1**	Touch base of little finger with thumb
Lumbricals I and II		Medial	Lower	C8, **T1**	Extend finger at proximal interphalangeal joint
	Ulnar				
Abductor digiti minimi		Medial	Lower	**C8, T1**	Abduct little finger
Flexor digiti minimi		Medial	Lower	C8, **T1**	Flex little finger at metacarpophalangeal joint
Opponens digiti minimi		Medial	Lower	C8, **T1**	Oppose little finger to thumb
Adductor pollicis		Medial	Lower	C8, **T1**	Adduct thumb at right angle to palm
Flexor pollicis brevis (D)		Medial	Lower	**C8,**[b] **T1**	Flex thumb at metacarpophalangeal joint
Palmar interossei		Medial	Lower	C8, **T1**[b]	Adduct fingers
Dorsal interossei		Medial	Lower	C8, **T1**	Abduct fingers
Lumbricals III and IV		Medial	Lower	C8, **T1**[b]	Extend finger at proximal interphalangeal joint

Hip and thigh

Lower extremity (hip and thigh)

Muscle, Innervation	Nerve	Division	Plexus	Roots[a]	Activation
Femoral					
Iliopsoas	+N to psoas major, minor	Posterior	Lumbar	**L1, L2, L3**,[b] L4	Flexion of thigh
Quadriceps femoris		Posterior	Lumbar	L2, **L3, L4**	Extension of leg on the thigh
Pectineus		Posterior	Lumbar	**L2**,[b] L3, L4	Adduct thigh
Sartorius		Posterior	Lumbar	L2, **L3**, L4	Flexion, abduction of hip; flexion of knee
Obturator					
Adductor longus and brevis		Anterior	Lumbar	L2, **L3**, L4	Adduction of thigh
Adductor magnus	Also from sciatic	Anterior	Lumbar	L2, **L3, L4**[b]	Adduction of thigh
Gracilis		Anterior	Lumbar	**L2**,[b] L3, L4	Adduct thigh and flex knee
Superior gluteal					
Gluteus medius and minimus			Sacral	L4, **L5**, S1	Abduct thigh
Tensor fasciae latae			Sacral	L4, **L5**, S1	Flexion and internal rotation of thigh
Inferior gluteal					
Gluteus maximus			Sacral	**L5, S1, S2**[b]	Extend at the hip
Nerve to piriformis					
Piriformis			Sacral	(L5),[e] **S1**,[b] S2	Externally rotate thigh
Sciatic					
Adductor magnus	Also from obturator		Sacral	L2, L3, L4	Adduction of thigh
Obturator internus and gemellus superior	Obturator internus	Anterior	Sacral	L5, **S1**,[b] S2	Externally rotate thigh with extended leg

Table 2.14 *Continued*

Muscle, Innervation	Nerve	Division	Plexus	Roots[a]	Activation
Inferior gemellus	Quadratus femoris	Anterior	Sacral	L4, **L5**, **S1**, S2	Externally rotate thigh with extended leg
Quadratus femoris	Quadratus femoris	Anterior	Sacral	L4, **L5**, **S1**	Externally rotate thigh
Semitendinosus	(Tibial portion)	Anterior	Sacral	**L5**,[b] **S1**, S2	Flexion of knee
Semimembranosus	(Tibial portion)	Anterior	Sacral	(L4),[f] **L5**,[b] **S1**, S2	Flexion of knee
Biceps (long head)	(Tibial portion)	Anterior	Sacral	L5, **S1**, (S2)[e]	Flexion of knee
Biceps (short head)	(Common peroneal portion)	Posterior	Sacral	**L5**, **S1**, S2	Flexion of knee

Lower extremity (leg and foot)

Leg

Muscle, Innervation	Nerve	Division	Plexus	Roots[a]	Activation
	Tibial				
Gastrocnemius and soleus		Anterior	Sacral	**S1**,[b] **S2**[b]	Plantar flexion and inversion of foot
Tibialis posterior		Anterior	Sacral	L4, **L5**, (S1)[c,d,f]	Plantar flexion and inversion of foot
Flexor digitorum longus		Anterior	Sacral	L5, **S1**, **S2**, (S3)[e]	Flexion of toes
Flexor hallucis longus		Anterior	Sacral	L5, S1, **S2**,[b] (S3)[e]	Flex big toe
Popliteus		Anterior	Sacral	(L4),[c,e] **L5**, S1	Flex and internally rotate tibia
	Common peroneal				
Tibialis anterior	Deep peroneal	Posterior	Sacral	**L4**, L5, (S1)[c,f]	Dorsiflexion of foot
Extensor hallucis longus	Deep peroneal	Posterior	Sacral	(L4),[c,f] **L5**, S1	Dorsiflexion of distal phalanx of big toe
Extensor digitorum longus	Deep peroneal	Posterior	Sacral	(L4),[c,f] **L5**, S1	Dorsiflexion of toes
Peroneus tertius	Deep peroneal	Posterior	Sacral	**L5**, S1	Dorsiflexion and eversion of foot
Peroneus longus	Superficial peroneal	Posterior	Sacral	**L5**,[b] **S1**,[b] (S2)[d,e]	Eversion of foot
Peroneus brevis	Superficial peroneal	Posterior	Sacral	**L5**,[b] **S1**,[b] (S2)[d,e]	Eversion of foot

Foot

Muscle	Nerve	Division	Plexus	Roots	Action
Tibial					
Abductor hallucis	Medial plantar	Anterior	Sacral	(L5),[c,f] S1, S2, **S3**[b]	Plantar flexion abduction of the first toe
Flexor digitorum brevis	Medial plantar	Anterior	Sacral	(L5),[c,f] S1, S2, **S3**[b]	Flex middle phalanges of toes II–V
Flexor hallucis brevis	Medial plantar	Anterior	Sacral	(L5),[f] S1, S2, **S3**[b]	Flex metatarsophalangeal joint of big toe
Flexor digiti minimi	Lateral plantar	Anterior	Sacral	S1, S2, **S3**[b]	Flex metatarsophalangeal joint of little toe
Abductor digiti quinti	Lateral plantar	Anterior	Sacral	S1, S2, **S3**[b]	Abduct little toe
Adductor hallucis	Lateral plantar	Anterior	Sacral	(L5),[f] S1, S2, **S3**[b]	Adduct big toe
Interossei	Lateral plantar	Anterior	Sacral	S1, S2, **S3**[b]	Spread toes
Quadratus plantae	Lateral plantar	Anterior	Sacral	S1, S2, **S3**[b]	Flex toes
Common peroneal					
Extensor digitorum brevis	Deep peroneal	Posterior	Sacral	**L5, S1**, (S2)[e]	Dorsiflexion of proximal phalanges of toes

C = cervical; D = deep; L = lumbar; S = superficial; T = thoracic.

[a]Boldface letters in the Roots column indicate principal nerve roots as per Medical Research Council of the UK. Aids to the examination of the peripheral nervous system. London: Baillière Tindall, 1986.

[b]Indicates principal nerve roots as per PL Williams, R Warwick, M Dyson, LH Bannister. Gray's Anatomy. Edinburgh, UK: Churchill Livingstone, 1989. Superscript letters c–f indicate discrepancies and their references:

[c]As per J Goodgold. Anatomical Correlates of Clinical Electromyography. Baltimore: Williams & Wilkins, 1974.

[d]As per EF Delagi, J Iazzetti, A Perotto, A Marrison. Anatomic Guide for the Electromyographer. Springfield, IL: Charles C. Thomas, 1980.

[e]As per PL Williams, R Warwick, M Dyson, LH Bannister. Gray's Anatomy. Edinburgh, UK: Churchill Livingstone, 1989.

[f]As per AF Haerer. DeJong's: The Neurologic Examination. Philadelphia: Lippincott–Raven, 1992.

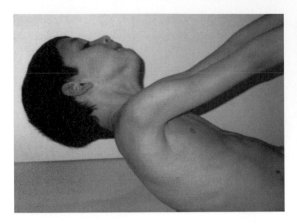

Figure 2.24 Patient with Duchenne's muscular dystrophy showing head lag when pulling up from the supine position due to prominent neck flexor weakness.

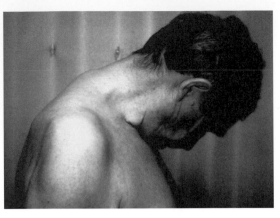

Figure 2.25 Head drop in a patient with amyotrophic lateral sclerosis due to neck extensor weakness.

Table 2.15 Conditions Associated with Cervical Paraspinal Muscle Weakness and Dropped Head Syndrome

Prominent, early paraspinal weakness in generalized processes
    Amyotrophic lateral sclerosis
    Myasthenia gravis
    Polymyositis/dermatomyositis
Isolated paraspinal muscle weakness
    Isolated neck extensor myopathy
    Bent spine syndrome
    Benign focal amyotrophy
Other diseases associated with paraspinal weakness or atrophy, or both
    Chronic inflammatory demyelinating polyneuropathy
    Lambert-Eaton myasthenic syndrome
    Inclusion body myositis
    Facioscapulohumeral dystrophy
    Nemaline myopathy
    Proximal myotonic myopathy
    Mitochondrial myopathy
    Acid maltase deficiency
    Carnitine deficiency
    Hypokalemic myopathy
    Hyperparathyroidism
Disorders that mimic dropped head syndrome
    Cervical dystonia (anterocollis)
    Fixed skeletal deformities of the spine

Source: From P Narayanaswami, T Bertorini. The dropped head syndrome. J Clin Neuromusc Dis 2000;2:106–112.

Figure 2.26 Pectoralis muscle atrophy and an oblique skin fold toward the midline on a patient with limb-girdle muscular dystrophy.

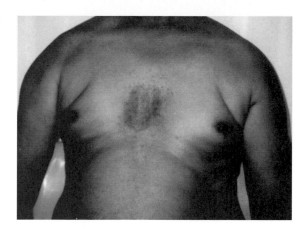

The upper trapezius is tested by opposing the patient's attempts to elevate the shoulders. This movement is affected in lesions of the cervical plexus or spinal accessory nerve, as in trauma or surgery of the lateral neck. Atrophy of the upper trapezius is noted when the patient is observed from the front and a prominent scapular bone is seen. In FSHMD, a characteristic hump is caused by a lack of fixation of the scapula when the patient raises his or her arms. During this maneuver, the bone becomes very prominent under a wasted trapezius muscle, giving the false appearance of a large trapezius (see Figure 2.21). To test the middle trapezius, patients are first evaluated from the back to observe for weakness that causes a lateral and upward displacement of the scapula with evidence of flaring and winging of its vertebral border. Elevation and abduction of the arms forward cause a more pronounced lateral deviation of the scapula (Figure 2.27). The patient is then asked to bring both

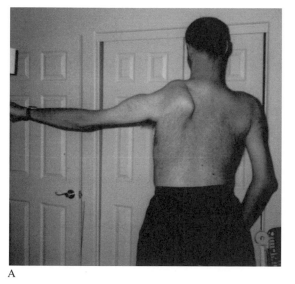

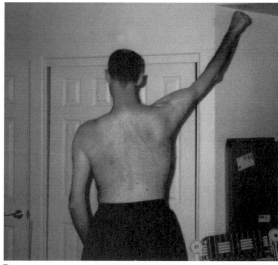

A   B

Figure 2.27 A. Patient with fascioscapulohumeral dystrophy with poor scapular fixation that causes inability to raise the left arm forward and winging of the scapula. **B.** Notice normal elevation of the right arm after surgical wiring of the scapula to the chest wall.

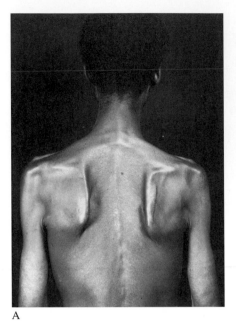
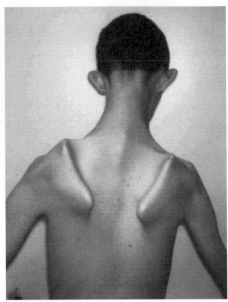

A   B

Figure 2.28 A. Atrophy of the scapular and trapezius muscles in a patient with polymyositis. **B.** Patient with congential myotonic dystrophy with prominent winging and inward rotation of the scapula.

scapulae together, and those with trapezius weakness have difficulty in bringing the scapula closer to the vertebral column.

Scapular fixation is brought about by not only the trapezius, but also the rhomboids and serratus muscles. Weakness of these muscles produces winging of the scapula, which is usually symmetric in most myopathies (Figure 2.28) and asymmetric in focal conditions, such as brachial neuritis, upper cervical radiculopathies, or plexopathies of the upper trunk. To differentiate true winging from the bony prominence seen in thin people, the examiner should ask the patient to raise his or her arms and press against the wall, which makes true winging more prominent. In lesions of the long thoracic nerve causing serratus weakness, the scapula is rotated medially and is closer to the vertebral column (Figure 2.29), with the angle of the winging becoming more prominent when the arms are stretched out and pushing forward. As described earlier, the scapula moves more laterally with this movement in trapezius weakness.

Lesions of the dorsal scapular nerve impair adduction of the shoulders from weakness of the rhomboids and the levator scapulae (which also raises this bone), whereas lesions of the suprascapular nerve cause weakness and atrophy of the supraspinatus or infraspinatus muscles, or both, which abduct and externally rotate the arm. This is seen in brachial neuritis, suprascapular nerve entrapment, and upper brachial plexus lesions.

The thoracodorsal nerve innervates the latissimus dorsi, which internally rotates, adducts, and extends the arms, whereas the subscapular nerve innervates the teres major, which also adducts the arms. All these muscles can be atrophic in myopathies (see Figure 2.28), SMA, and other motor neuron diseases.

Figure 2.29 Patient with brachial plexopathy and serratus anterior weakness causing winging of the scapula and medial deviation of the bone.

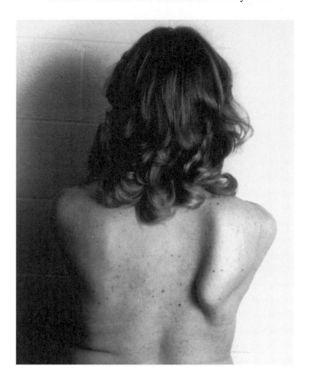

The deltoids are primarily responsible for shoulder abduction and elevation and are tested by opposing these movements. Weakness of these muscles is seen in myopathies and SMA. In some myopathies, such as FSHMD and BMD, the deltoids may be relatively spared whereas other shoulder girdle muscles are weak. Lesions of the axillary nerve, upper trunk and posterior cord of the brachial plexus, and C5 and C6 root disease cause unilateral deltoid weakness (Figure 2.30).

ARM FLEXION AND EXTENSION. The biceps and triceps muscles are tested by flexing and extending the arm, respectively. Flexion of the arm is also performed by the brachioradialis muscle; therefore, the examiner should be aware that patients with biceps weakness may compensate by using the brachioradialis to flex the arm. The action of the biceps should be tested with the forearm fully supinated while the brachioradialis flexes the semiprone forearm. Selective weakness of the biceps is seen in lesions of the musculocutaneous nerve (Figure 2.31) or the C5-6 roots, whereas the brachioradialis is affected in radial nerve lesions or in C5-6 radiculopathy. The biceps and brachioradialis are affected by lesions of the upper trunk and of the lateral or posterior cord of the brachial plexus, respectively. The triceps is affected in C6-8 radiculopathy, particularly C7, the middle trunk and posterior cord of the brachial plexors. Prominent, bilateral weakness of biceps and triceps is seen in some myopathies, especially in IBM, BMD, and Emery-Dreifuss muscular dystrophy.

FOREARM SUPINATION AND PRONATION. Pronation of the forearm is done by the pronator teres innervated by the median nerve and the pronator quadratus innervated by its anterior interosseus branch. Both can be weak in lesions of the main trunk of the median nerve, whereas the pronator quadratus is affected in lesions of its ante-

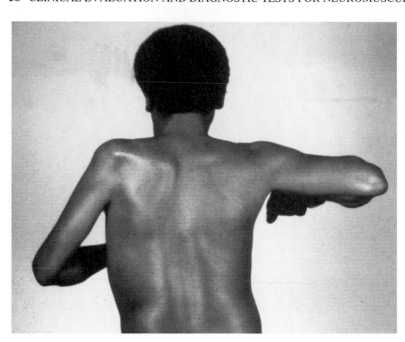

Figure 2.30 Patient with benign focal amyotrophy showing weakness and atrophy of the left deltoid and supra- and infraspinatus muscles. (Reprinted with permission from JC Metcalf Jr, JB Wood, TE Bertorini. Benign focal amyotrophy: metrizamide CT evidence of cord atrophy. Case Report. Muscle Nerve 1987;3:338–345.)

rior interosseous branch. Supination is performed by the supinator, a branch of the radial nerve, from the C6-7 roots.

WRIST FLEXION AND EXTENSION. Wrist flexion is brought about mainly by the median innervated muscles of the forearm (flexor carpi radialis and palmaris longus) and the flexor carpi ulnaris innervated by the ulnar nerve. Weakness of the median innervated muscles is also caused by lesions of C6 and C7 roots, whereas the ulnaris is affected by lesions of the C7-T1, mainly C8, nerve roots, the lower trunk, and medial cord of the brachial plexus. These muscles are usually weak in IBM, distal dystrophies

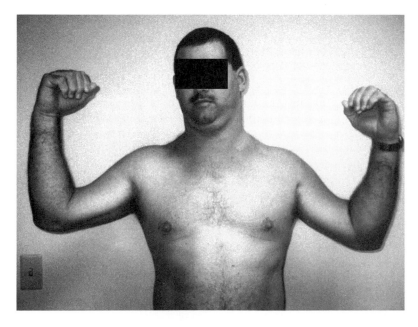

Figure 2.31 Patient with bilateral musculocutaneous atrophy apparently caused by compression of the musculocutaneous nerve during lower back surgery.

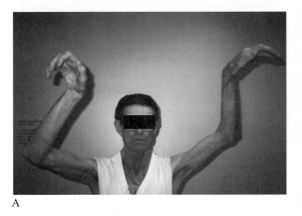
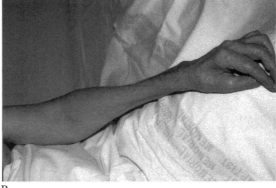

A   B

Figure 2.32 A. Prominent forearm wasting and wrist extensor weakness in a patient with Welander's muscular dystrophy.
B. Patient with inclusion body myositis showing wasting of the forearm muscles.

such as the Welander type, ALS, focal neuropathies of the median or ulnar nerves, and in polyneuropathies at more developed stages, as the hand muscles are affected first.

Wrist extension is performed by the extensor carpi radialis and ulnaris muscles, which are affected in the conditions that affect the C6-7 and C8 roots, or the radial nerve, which when compressed causes the characteristic wrist drop ("Saturday night palsy"). Lead poisoning is another cause of wrist drop. Bilateral weakness is seen in diseases that also affect the flexors (Figure 2.32), as described above.

FINGER FLEXION AND EXTENSION.   The flexor digitorum profundus, which is innervated by the C7, C8, and T1 roots; the median nerve through its anterior interosseous branch (second and third digit) (Figure 2.33); and the ulnar (forth and fifth digits) nerve flexes the distal phalanx, whereas the flexor digitorum superficialis innervated by the median nerve flexes the middle phalanxes and is tested by asking the patient to flex the middle or distal phalanges while holding the hand at the wrist or at the middle phalanx (see Figure 2.33). These muscles could be weak from lesions of their respective roots or nerves.

Finger extension of digits 2–5 at the metacarpophalangeal joints is performed by the extensor digitorum communis, extensor indices proprius, and extensor digiti minimi innervated by the radial nerve, which are thus weak in conditions that affect this nerve, particularly its posterior interosseus branch. Weakness of these muscles is also seen in lesions of the middle trunk and posterior cord of the brachial plexus, in C7 radiculopathies, and particularly in ALS, polyneuropathies, IBM, slow channel syndrome, and Welander's muscular dystrophy.

Extension of the proximal interphalangeal joints is performed by the extensor digitorum, the lumbricalis, and the palmar and dorsal interossei. The interossei and the third and fourth lumbricals are innervated by the ulnar nerve and C8-T1 roots, whereas the first and second lumbricals are innervated by the median nerve and C8 and T1 roots and the lower trunk and medial cord of the brachial plexus.

HAND MUSCLES.   The interossei muscles adduct (palmar interossei) and abduct (dorsal interossei) the fingers. Abduction is also done by the lumbricals. These mus-

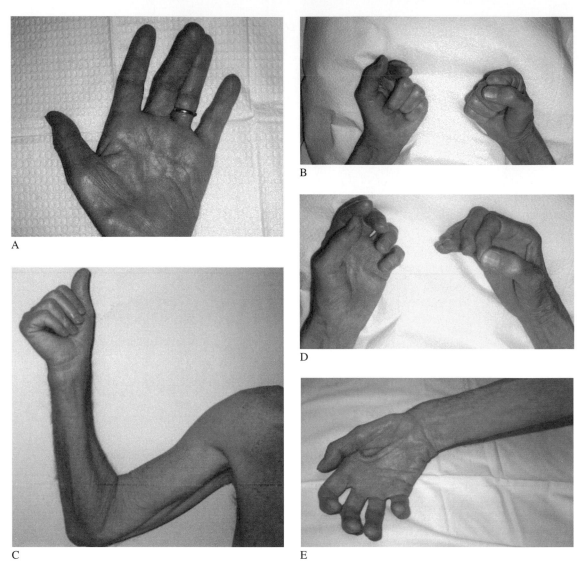

Figure 2.33 A. Median neuropathy causing thenar atrophy. **B.** Median neuropathy at the elbow causing weakness of flexion of first and second digits and partially of the third digit. **C.** Inability to flex distal phalanxes in a patient with myotonic dystrophy. **D.** Inability to produce the "O" or "OK" sign with the left hand in a patient with median neuropathy affecting predominantly the anterior interosseus innervated muscles. **E.** Clawhand and atrophy of the median and ulnar muscle.

cles could be weak in C8-T1 radiculopathies, diseases of the lower trunk and medial cord of the brachial plexus, diffuse neuropathies, median and ulnar mononeuropathies, and, frequently, ALS. The presence of a fasciculating limb with atrophic interosseous without numbness is highly suggestive of ALS. This presentation can also be seen in the rare adult form of debrancher enzyme deficiency (glycogenosis, type IV) in cervical spondylosis and syringomyelia.

A "clawhand" with prominent weakness of ulnar and median innervated muscle is seen in ALS and at later stages in polyneuropathies and distal dystrophies (see Figure 2.33). Ulnar neuropathy causes interossei wasting, and there is a partial flexion of the distal phalanx of the last two digits when the patient extends the wrist and

Figure 2.34 Patient with ulnar neuropathy attempting hand and finger extension. There is partial flexion of the last two digits.

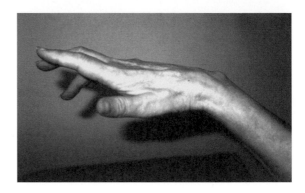

fingers.[40] This partial flexion of the last two digits is caused by weakness of the interossei and lumbricals, which, as discussed, are also extensors of the interphalangeal joints (Figure 2.34).

The median nerve innervates most of the thenar muscles of the thumb, including the abductor pollicis brevis, opponens and the superficial head of the flexor pollicis brevis, whereas the deep head of the flexor pollicis brevis and the adductor pollicis are innervated by the ulnar nerve, C8 and T1 roots, and lower trunk of the brachial plexus.[43] Flexion of the metacarpophalangeal joints of the thumb is performed by the flexor pollicis longus and brevis, whereas flexion of the distal phalanx is provided by the flexor pollicis longus, both median innervated. In proximal median and anterior interosseous neuropathy, weakness of the flexor pollicis longus causes the inability of the patient to flex the distal phalanx and to oppose it to the index finger (whose distal flexion can also be weak), making them unable to form the "O" or "OK" sign (see Figure 2.33). In median neuropathy, they are also unable to oppose the thumb to the fifth digit because of weakness of the opponens and flexor pollicis.

Abduction of the thumb is performed by the median innervated abductor pollicis brevis and also by the radial innervated abductor and extensor pollicis longus. Thumb adduction is performed by the first dorsal interosseous and the adductor pollicis, both of which are innervated by the ulnar nerve, C8, and T1. Weak adductors, from lesions to these nerves, produce the Froment's sign or "Signe de Journal" in which the patient cannot hold a paper between the thumb and index finger and has to flex the thumb with the median innervated flexor pollicis to compensate (Figure 2.35).[40] Extension of the thumb is performed by the extensor pollicis longus and brevis, both innervated by the radial nerve from C7-8 roots.

Figure 2.35 Froment's sign. Patient has to flex the distal phalanx to hold the paper from adductor weakness. Note also interosseus muscle atrophy of the first dorsal interosseus muscle (*left hand*).

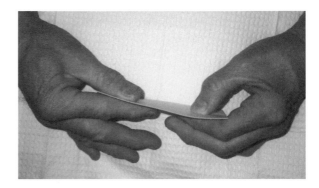

HIP MUSCLES.   The iliopsoas, which is the primary hip flexor, is innervated by the femoral nerve from the L1-3 roots. These muscles are tested by raising the leg from the horizontal position while supine, by flexing the leg while the knee is also flexed, or by raising the knee against resistance when the patient is sitting up straight. The tensor fascia lata, innervated by the superior gluteal nerve, also contributes to flexion and internal rotation of the thigh. The sartorius muscle, innervated by the femoral nerve, helps flex the hip, thigh and knee. Weakness of hip flexor muscles is common in myopathies and causes difficulty in ascending stairs.

The hip extensors, particularly the gluteus maximus, innervated by the L5-S1 roots and inferior gluteal nerve, are tested by extending the hip when the patient is prone or in the lateral decubitus position. The gluteus medius, innervated by the superior gluteal nerve from the L4-5 roots, abducts and externally rotates the thigh.

Weakness of the gluteus maximus and lumbar paraspinals causes difficulty in maintaining the erect position and in rising from the floor. This also contributes to the Gowers' maneuver in myopathies. Most hip muscles are weak early in myopathies.

THIGH FLEXION, EXTENSION, ADDUCTION.   The quadriceps, innervated by the femoral nerve and L2, L3, and L4 roots, is the main knee extensor. This muscle is best examined with the patient sitting and extending the knee with the examiner opposing this movement. The quadriceps is one of the most difficult muscles to grade clinically; even if the quadriceps is markedly weak functionally and unable to completely overcome gravity (a grade less than 3), the quadriceps is still hard to overcome by the examiner and is therefore usually graded 4 or higher.

The quadriceps muscles are selectively affected early in some myopathies such as IBM, SMA (see Figure 2.5), BMD, and the so-called quadriceps myopathy, which in most cases is a dystrophinopathy (Figure 2.36). Unilateral weakness is seen in compressive or traumatic femoral neuropathies, L2-3 radiculopathies, diabetic amyotrophy, and lumbar plexopathies.

The hamstring muscle group flexes the knee and is tested by resisting this movement while the patient is prone. These muscles are innervated mainly by L5-S1 roots and the sciatic nerve.

The adductor muscles of the thigh are innervated by the obturator nerve, although the adductor magnus is also partially innervated by the sciatic nerve. Their main action is the adduction of the thigh, whereas the gracilis muscle also assists in the flexion of the knee. Adductor weakness causes a tendency to swing the leg outward when walking. Evaluation of these muscles is very important to distinguish weak knee extension due to femoral neuropathy, in which they are spared, from an L2-3 radiculopathy or lumbar plexopathy, in which they are affected. They are especially weak early in adult and juvenile acid maltase deficiency.

DISTAL LEG AND FOOT MUSCLES.   Foot dorsiflexors, particularly the tibialis anterior, and the extensor hallucis longus muscles are innervated by L4 and, especially, L5 roots and the peroneal nerve. They are usually weak early in most neuropathies and in patients with focal peroneal nerve lesions causing foot drop and inability to walk on the heels. They are also selectively weak and wasted in the anterior compartment distal myopathy (Nonaka type). Weak dorsiflexors also occur in sciatic nerve and plexus lesions and upper motor neuron diseases; the foot evertors, peroneus longus and brevis, are weak in these disorders, and also in lesions of the peroneal nerve and of the L5-S1 roots and lumbosacral plexopathies.

The gastrocnemius-soleus group—innervated by the sciatic nerve with fibers from S1 and S2 roots—should be tested not only by MMT, but also by asking the patient to walk on the tiptoes, because they are hard to overcome when tested manually. These

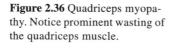

Figure 2.36 Quadriceps myopathy. Notice prominent wasting of the quadriceps muscle.

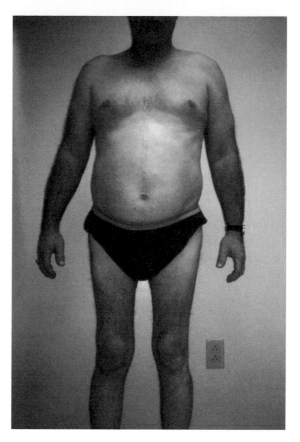

muscles are affected in most peripheral neuropathies, but usually later than the muscles of the anterior compartment, they are weak and atrophic early in the Miyoshi form of distal muscular dystrophy (see Figure 2.20). As discussed, prominent calf hypertrophy is seen in DMD (see Figure 2.22), BMD (see Figure 2.3), and some limb-girdle muscular dystrophies (LGMDs), as well as juvenile SMA. They can be weak unilaterally in lumbosacral radiculopathies and plexopathies.

The major foot invertor is the tibialis posterior, which is innervated by the tibial nerve and mainly by the L5 root.

Intrinsic foot muscles should be examined for atrophy and weakness. They are usually affected early in most neuropathies. In distal muscular dystrophy, the extensor digitorum brevis is spared, whereas the tibialis anterior or gastrocnemius may be atrophic (Figure 2.37), a pattern that is useful in differentiating these dystrophies from neuropathies.

Fasciculations. The clinician should carefully observe the patient while relaxed for the presence of fasciculations, which are small, localized muscle contractions or twitches produced by spontaneous depolarization of the whole or part of the motor unit. These are frequently accompanied by weakness in diseases of the lower motor neuron, occur in affected muscles in radiculopathies, and are prominent in some neuropathies, such as MMN. Fasciculations may be seen in the cramp fasciculation syn-

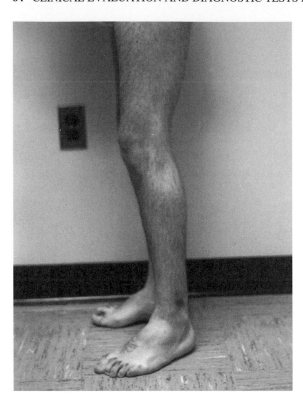

Figure 2.37 Patient with distal dystrophy showing wasting of the limb muscles, especially the lower leg with normal extensor digitorum brevis muscle.

drome, the distal legs in peripheral neuropathies, and adult debrancher enzyme deficiency. Myokymia, which are large rhythmic contractions of muscle, may be observed in some plexopathies and rarely in neuropathies. They occur diffusely in Isaacs' syndrome.

Reflexes. The examination of muscle stretch reflexes is a very important part of the neuromuscular evaluation. To help determine the location of the disease, the following grading system is routinely used: 0 (no reflex), 1 (trace or diminished reflexes), 2 (normal reflex), 3 (hyperactive but not necessarily abnormal), and 4 (increased reflexes with clonus). This system has limitations, and for this reason some authorities describe reflexes only as hyper- or hypoactive. Grading is important, however, to allow the examiner to determine whether there is asymmetry between sides, even when both are normal. Commonly tested reflexes include the following:

The biceps reflex is mediated by C5 and C6 roots, the upper trunk of the brachial plexus, and the musculocutaneous nerve. The triceps reflex tests C6-8 roots, particularly the C7 root and middle trunk of the plexus, and the radial nerve. The inverted triceps reflex described by Babinski is an important sign of C7 motor root involvement. In this reflex, tapping of the triceps tendon causes arm flexion rather than extension, because the tap simultaneously stimulates the C5 and C6 roots, causing a normal contraction of the biceps, which have intact innervation, but not the triceps, which motor roots affect. The brachioradialis reflex tests the C5 and C6 roots and the radial nerve. The pronator reflex, mediated by the median nerve and C7 and C8 roots, is obtained by tapping the posterior-inferior ulna with the arm flexed to produce pronation of the forearm. The finger flexor reflex, on the other hand, is tested by placing the palm over the patient's semiflexed fingers, tapping over it, and observing for flexion of fingers (mediated by the median and ulnar nerves and C7 and C8 roots). The Hoffman reflex is also important to test because its presence usually indicates hyperreflexia, although it is not necessarily pathologic unless asymmetric.

The quadriceps reflex tests the femoral nerve and L2, L3, and L4 roots, whereas the adductor reflex tests the obturator nerve and the same roots. The ankle jerk is mediated by the S1 and S2 roots and the tibial and sciatic nerves. Other reflexes such as deltoid, pectoralis, latissimus dorsi, or biceps femoris are also sometimes useful in the clinical diagnosis.

Toe extensor Babinski and Chaddock signs are important indicators of a pyramidal tract lesion. Other toe extensor signs, however, are usually not seen when a Babinski sign is not present.

The superficial and deep abdominal reflexes are also important in determining the presence of pyramidal tract lesions. Both can be lost in obese patients or after several pregnancies or surgery, but the absence of a superficial abdominal reflex with hyperactive deep abdominal reflexes usually suggests an upper motor neuron lesion.

In patients with good finger flexor strength, the presence of the Wartenberg reflex is an excellent indication of upper motor neuron disease affecting the upper extremity. This is elicited when the patient opposes flexion of the distal finger phalanges by the examiner. Normally, during this maneuver, there is a spontaneous flexion of the distal phalanx of the thumb, or partial adduction, whereas in the positive test there is flexion with opposition and adduction of the whole thumb across the hand (Figure 2.38).

Myotonia

Clinical *myotonia*, or delayed relaxation of a muscle after a voluntary contraction (e.g., closing the eyes or performing a grip), is seen in patients with some myopathies, particularly channelopathies. In testing for the presence of myotonia, the patient is asked to forcefully close the eyes and then rapidly open them, or to grip the examiner's fingers for approximately 10 seconds and then to relax. In myotonia, it takes several seconds for the patient to completely open the eyes or release the grip. Myotonia can also be elicited by percussion of the extensor carpi radialis or the thenar eminence, or by gently tapping the tongue while it rests on a blade (Figure 2.39). Normally, there is a quick extension of the wrist or contraction of thenar muscle or tongue, followed by prompt relaxation. In myotonia, relaxation is delayed, and the muscle remains contracted for a few seconds.

Myoedema, or a local persistent contraction of an area of a percussed muscle, is seen in patients with hypothyroidism.

Figure 2.38 Positive Wartenberg sign. Notice that the patient flexes the thumb while the examiner only flexes the distal phalanx.

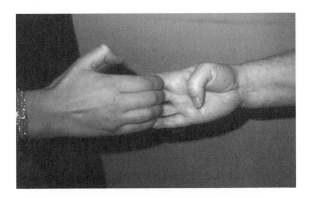

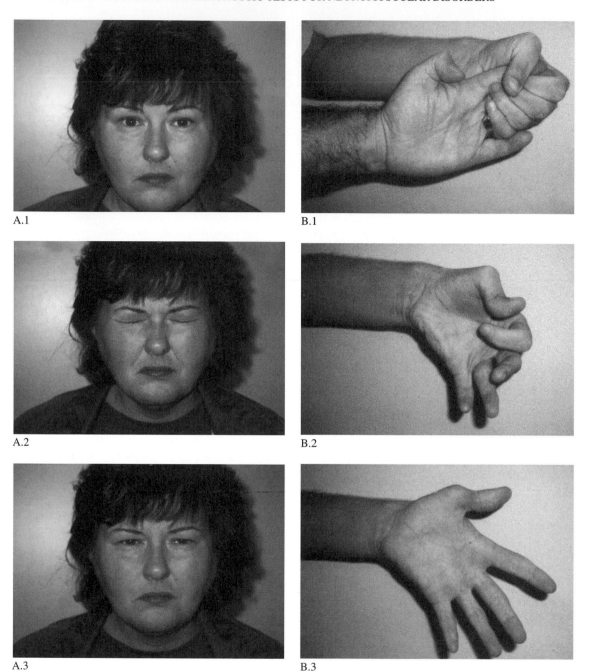

A.1

B.1

A.2

B.2

A.3

B.3

Figure 2.39 A. Myotonia of the eyelid and orbicularis oculi. Notice a patient showing difficulty opening her eyes after persistent closure for a few seconds. Eyes opened (**1**); eyes closed (**2**); delayed opening of the eye after closing a few seconds (**3**). **B.** Grip myotonia. Notice difficulty in opening of the handgrip. Gripping the examiner's hand (**1**); immediately after releasing it (**2**); after 10 seconds (**3**). **C.** Percussion myotonia of the tongue. Before percussion of the tongue (**1**). After percussion, the tongue remains contracted several seconds (**2**). **D.** Percussion of the thenar eminence. Notice that the thenar muscles remain contracted several seconds after percussion (**2**). Before percussion (**1**); after percussion (**2**). **E.** Percussion myotonia of the extensor carpi radialis showing a delayed relaxation of the wrist extension. Immediately after percussion (**1**); 5 seconds after percussion (**2**); 10 seconds after percussion (**3**).

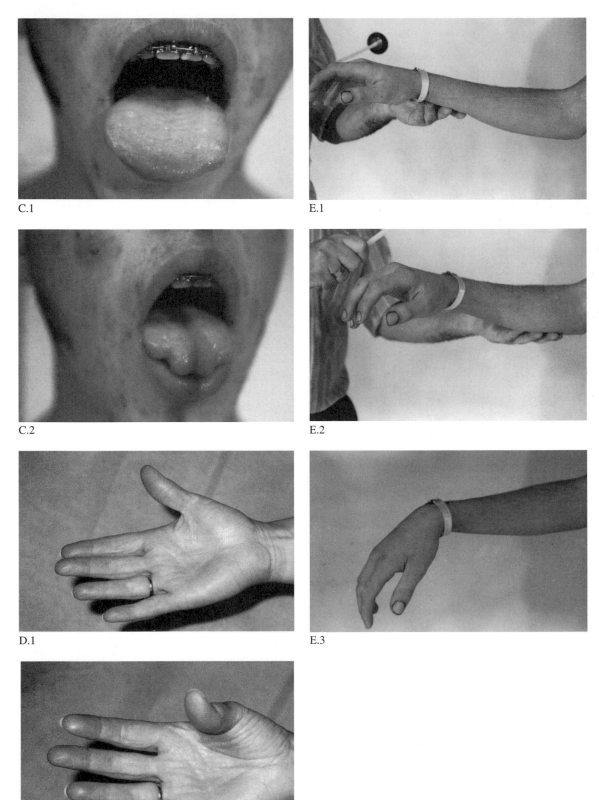

C.1

C.2

D.1

D.2

E.1

E.2

E.3

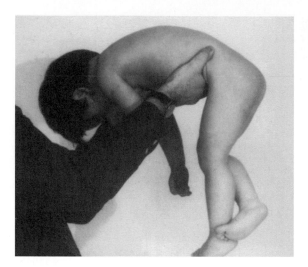

Figure 2.40 A floppy infant with infantile acid maltase deficiency. Note how limbs hang loosely and the chest is arched when the examiner holds the patient by the thorax.

Disorders of Muscle Tone (Hypotonia and Spasticity). *Hypotonia* is a common finding in myopathies and in SMA, and is characterized by a decrease in the resistance of a muscle to passive stretching. The hypotonic or floppy child has limp, hanging limbs when held by the trunk (Figure 2.40). These babies may also develop "abdominal breathing" and abduction of the hips when supine. Causes of floppy babies include particularly the infantile neuromuscular diseases (Table 2.16) and also diseases of the cen-

Table 2.16 Causes of Floppy Infants

Central nervous system disorders
    Cerebral palsy
    Mental retardation
Mixed (central and peripheral)
    Metachromatic leukodystrophy and other lipidosis
    Neuroaxonal atrophy
    Giant axonal neuropathy
    Fukuyama type congenital muscular dystrophy
Anterior horn cell diseases
    Infantile spinal muscular atrophy
Neuropathies
    Charcot-Marie-Tooth disease, particularly types 3 and 4
Diseases of the neuromuscular junction
    Congenital myasthenic syndromes
    Infantile botulism
    Neonatal transient autoimmune myasthenia gravis
Myopathies
    Infantile metabolic myopathies (e.g., acid maltase deficiencies or Pompe's disease, infantile phosphorylase deficiency)
    Congenital muscular dystrophy
    Other congenital myopathies (e.g., central core disease, myotubular myopathy, nemaline myopathy)
    Congenital myotonic dystrophy
    Myopathy from electrolyte and endocrine abnormalities

tral nervous system, or both, such as in MLD or some congenital myopathies. Muscle stretch reflexes are usually present or even exaggerated in central causes of floppy infant syndrome, whereas in neuromuscular disorders causing floppy infant syndrome, reflexes are diminished or absent. Those with diseases of the central nervous system also have other signs of cerebral dysfunction.

Spasticity, or the classical increase in passive resistance to stretching with a "clasp knife" characteristic, is seen in diseases that affect the upper motor neuron, such as ALS or primary lateral sclerosis. Spasticity is usually accompanied by hyperreflexia, and the Babinski sign.

Muscle Fibrosis and Contractures. *Muscle contractures* from fibrosis are common in chronic myopathies, particularly in the heel-cord and iliotibial band in DMD and BMD. They are also present in Bethlem myopathy and in some LGMDs and are prominent in Emery-Dreifuss muscular dystrophy (Figure 2.41A). Contractures occur in drug-induced muscle fibrosis, such as those caused by intramuscular injections of drugs like pentazocine, causing the "levitation sign,"[46] in which the patient's arm remains abducted and elevated while standing, instead of in the normal resting position (see Figure 2.41B).

Sensory Examination

Clinical sensory testing is most valuable in the evaluation of neuropathies, radiculopathies, and plexus lesions. To perform these tests, it is important that the clinician has a thorough knowledge of peripheral nerve anatomy to localize the site of the disease process. Knowledge of anatomy allows recognition of true deficits from malingering or psychogenic diseases. For instance, deficits in territories that do not follow a nerve or root distribution, a deficit that ends exactly at

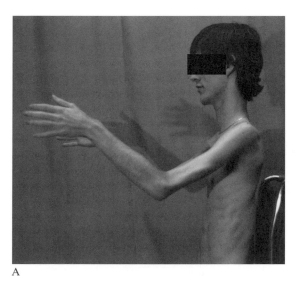
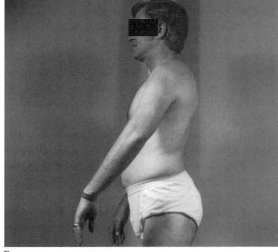

A   B

Figure 2.41 A. Muscle fibrosis in a patient with Emery-Dreifuss muscular dystrophy. **B.** Pentazocine myopathy causing fibrosis resulting in the levitation sign with the arm.

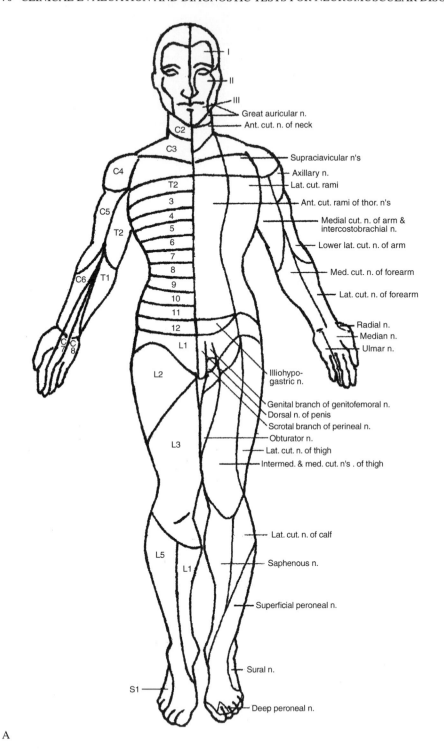

A

Figure 2.42 A. Dermatomal distribution in the body (frontal view). **B.** Back nerves and roots. (ant. = anterior; cut. = cutaneous; lat. = lateral; med. = median; n. = nerve; n's = nerves; post. = posterior; thor. = thoracic.) (Reprinted with permission from W Haymaker, B Woodhall. Peripheral Nerve Injuries. In Principles of Diagnosis. Philadelphia: Saunders, 1953.)

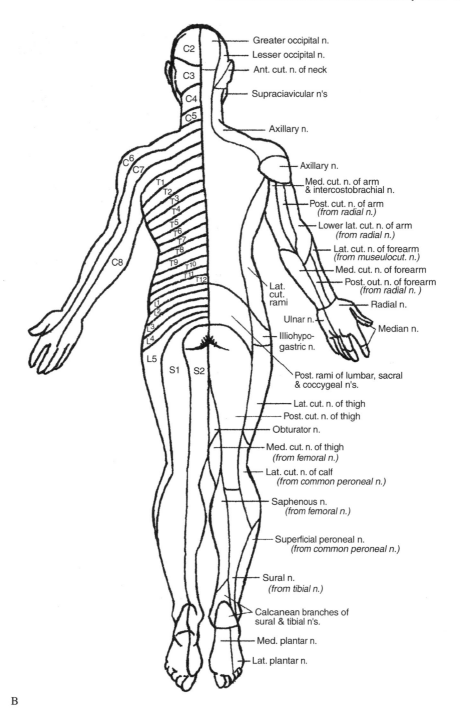

Greater occipital n.

Lesser occipital n.

Ant. cut. n. of neck

Supraciavicular n's

Axillary n.

Axillary n.

Med. cut. n. of arm
& intercostobrachial n.

Post. cut. n. of arm
(from radial n.)

Lower lat. cut. n. of arm
(from radial n.)

Lat. cut. n. of forearm
(from museulocut. n.)

Med. cut. n. of forearm

Post. out. n. of forearm
(from radial n.)

Radial n.

Median n.

Lat. cut. rami

Ulnar n.

Illiohypo-
gastric n.

Post. rami of lumbar, sacral
& coccygeal n's.

Lat. cut. n. of thigh

Post. cut. n. of thigh

Obturator n.

Med. cut. n. of thigh
(from femoral n.)

Lat. cut. n. of calf
(from common peroneal n.)

Saphenous n.
(from femoral n.)

Superficial peroneal n.
(from common peroneal n.)

Sural n.
(from tibial n.)

Calcanean branches of
sural & tibial n's.

Med. plantar n.

Lat. plantar n.

B

the midline (normally the midline has overlapping innervation from both sides), or a glove and stocking deficit affecting only one limb are suspected to be non-organic. Figure 2.42 illustrates the dermatomal distribution of roots and nerves, and Figures 2.43 and 2.44 demonstrate the root of origin of the nerves of the brachial and lumbosacral plexuses.

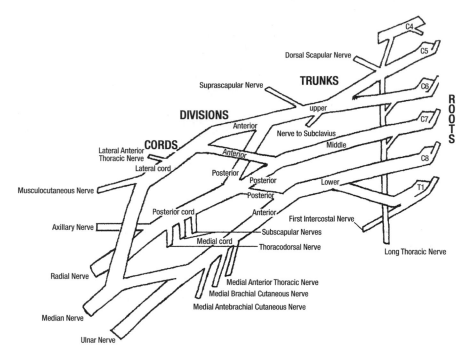

Figure 2.43 The brachial plexus.

It should be recognized that clinical sensory testing is imperfect; it is subjective and often not reproducible. It should be used only in screening and diagnosis, as fluctuations of the results can be caused, for example, by variations in the duration and intensity of the stimuli and by changes in temperature or thickness of the skin. Detailed quantitation requires sophisticated computerized devices, which are discussed in Chapter 4.

The sensory examination should determine whether the disorder is symmetric and distal, as in polyneuropathies, or whether it affects individual nerves or roots. For example, a distribution of sensory deficit in the last two digits could be secondary to a C8 radiculopathy or to an ulnar neuropathy, but in the latter the deficit usually splits the fourth digit and stops slightly above the wrist. Testing should include not only the limbs but also the anterior chest and abdomen, as a decreased sensation in these areas is seen in length-dependent polyneuropathies in a tear drop distribution.

Proprioception (Vibration and Position Sense)

This sensation originates through joint, periosteum, and cutaneous receptors. The most important are the pacinian corpuscles, but the Meissner's corpuscles also contribute, although the specificity of sensation of these receptors is not absolute. Proprioception is carried by large- and medium-sized myelinated axons whose neurons are located in the posterior root ganglia. These fibers travel through the posterior columns of the spinal cord to the nucleus gracilis and cuneatus of the medulla. The second order axons decussate in the medial lemniscus and end in the contralateral ventroposterolateral nucleus of the thalamus.

Position sense is tested by moving the patient's joints while his or her eyes are closed and asking for the direction of movement. Normally, the interphalangeal

Figure 2.44 The lumbosacral plexi. (Post. = posterior.)

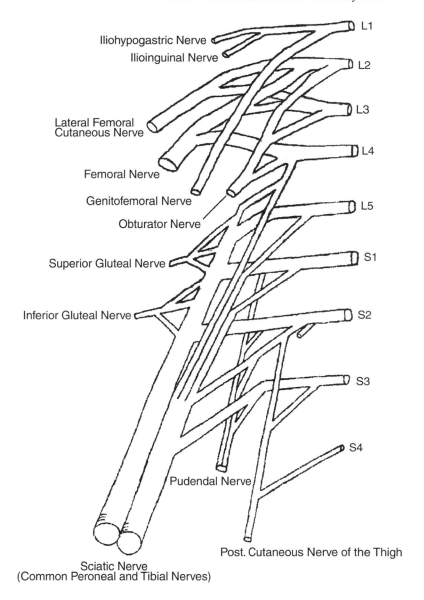

Iliohypogastric Nerve

Ilioinguinal Nerve

Lateral Femoral
Cutaneous Nerve

Femoral Nerve

Genitofemoral Nerve

Obturator Nerve

Superior Gluteal Nerve

Inferior Gluteal Nerve

Pudendal Nerve

Post. Cutaneous Nerve of the Thigh

Sciatic Nerve
(Common Peroneal and Tibial Nerves)

L1

L2

L3

L4

L5

S1

S2

S3

S4

joints require 5–10 degrees of movement for recognition. In the shoulder joint, less than 1 degree of passive movement can be recognized.

Vibration sensation, or pallesthesia, is tested with a 128-Hz tuning fork applied to the periosteum of toes, fingers, or malleoli, testing not only for the perception of the sensation but also for the length of time that it is perceived. The use of graduated tuning forks, like the Rydel-Seiffert model, allows for a better quantitation, but, even with their use, reproducibility of the results is low because the generation of the impulse for vibration varies with the intensity with which the tuning fork is hit by the examiner. To avoid this, we have designed a plastic device that fits on the end of a 128-Hz tuning fork. When it is removed, a vibration is created that is reproducible and less variable in intensity (Figure 2.45).[47] This device can be used routinely in clinical practice. More accurate and reproducible vibratory sense results are achieved with computerized equipment, but its use can be too cumbersome and expensive for routine evaluations.

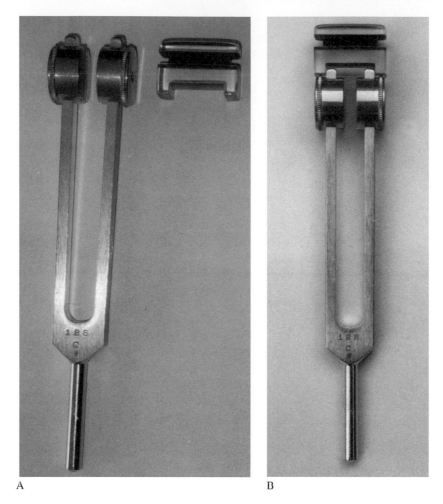

A   B

Figure 2.45 A small plastic device placed on the standard tuning fork that produces less variation in the intensity and duration of vibration. **A.** Before placement on the top of the tuning fork. **B.** After placement on the top of the tuning fork.

Normally, a person perceives the tuning fork vibrations for at least 20 seconds in the distal phalanx of the thumb and 10 seconds or more in the toe. Decreased vibration and position sense is seen in neuropathies affecting large myelinated fibers, either from demyelination or axonal loss. In these conditions, pain and temperature sensations are usually less affected, whereas in mixed neuropathies affecting both small and large fibers, all modalities are equally impaired.

Absent vibration sense in the legs but present in the iliac crest usually suggests a diagnosis of peripheral nerve disease. If vibration sensation is not detected over the iliac crest, a lesion in the spinal cord affecting the posterior columns should be considered. Testing vibration sense over the spinous processes of the vertebrae may then assist in detecting a sensory level for this modality.

Pain and Temperature

Pain and temperature are perceived by free nerve endings and carried through small myelinated (A-δ) and unmyelinated (C) fibers, whose neurons are located in the posterior root ganglion. They synapse in the spinal cord and decussate and travel in the contralateral spinothalamic tract to the ventroposterolateral nucleus of the thalamus and then to the somatosensory cortex. Pain sensation is tested with a sharp object, such as a pin. The use of a nondisposable pinwheel is discouraged because of the risk of infection. The test evaluates the territory of nerves or roots from limbs to detect a sensory level, and it should be done from the areas of diminished sensation toward the areas of normal sensation (i.e., from distal to proximal legs). The examiner evaluates whether the patient is able to differentiate a sharp versus a dull stimulus, using the point of a safety pin as the sharp object and its back as the dull object.

Temperature sensation is perceived by thermoreceptors, such as the Ruffini plumes (heat) and Krause end-bulbs (cold), and carried by the same type of fibers and pathways as pain sensation. Copper disks or hot and cold water in small test tubes are used to test temperature sense, but they are not used routinely. Having the patient perceive differences in the coldness of the tuning fork can be used for gross screening.

Light Touch Sensation

Touch sensation is carried through large and small myelinated axons by impulses generated by mechanical force applied to free nerve endings around hair follicles, the Merkel disks, and Meissner corpuscles. Their neurons are located in the dorsal root ganglion. The axons enter the spinal cord, ascend and descend several segments, and then decussate to travel in the ventral spinothalamic tract to the thalamus and then to the cortex. Fibers carrying discriminatory tactile sensitivity travel through the posterior columns to their nuclei in the medulla, after which they decussate in the medial lemniscus to the opposite thalamic nuclei and then to the somatosensory cortex.

Light touch is tested using a cotton swab. However, the use of the von Frey hairs or the Semmes-Weinstein monofilaments, which are nylon probes of varying diameters, provides an excellent screening method that allows quantitation. Numbers assigned to the different filaments represent the logarithm of 10 times the force in mg required to bend them. The 2.83 filaments are frequently used for screening sensory abnormalities, and kits of up to 20 filaments are used for detailed, quantitative testing. The use of only one or two is sufficient in routine clinical examination and has been proven useful in clinical trials of peripheral neuropathy.[48]

The two-point discrimination test evaluates the capacity to perceive touch in two different places simultaneously. This is a valuable test that can be useful in screening peripheral nerve disease, although it is discriminating and thus requires intact cortical function. For this test, a small graded caliper, such as the Weber compass, is frequently used. Discrimination of two points at 2–4 mm distance is normal on the fingertips, 4–6 mm on the dorsum of fingers, 7–10 mm on the distal thumb and wrist, 8–12 mm on the palm, and 20–30 mm on the dorsum of the hand.

Techniques to Reproduce Sensory Symptoms

Placement of the tuning fork in superficial areas of a nerve or a light tap over the nerve could cause pain in demyelinated axons in nerves damaged from stretching (Tinel's sign). The Phalen test or flexing the wrist for 30–60 seconds reproduces the pain and weakness in carpal tunnel syndrome. Root stretching with flexion or extension of the hip with an extended knee or leg, or moving the neck in the opposite direction is used to reproduce radicular pain.

Table 2.17 Causes of Elevation of Serum Creatine Kinase

Muscular dystrophy, including asymptomatic carriers of dystrophinopathy

Inflammatory myopathy (polymyositis, dermatomyositis, inclusion body myositis, sarcoid myopathy)

Trauma

Some toxins (e.g., alcohol)

Drugs (e.g., clofibrate)

Glycogen storage myopathy (e.g., acid maltase deficiency, myophosphorylase, phosphofructokinase, phosphorylase *b* kinase, phosphoglycerate kinase, B enolase deficiencies)

Lipid storage myopathy

Mitochondrial myopathy

Excessive exercise

Delirium, seizures

Trauma

Malignant hyperthermia

Idiopathic hyper-CKemia

McLeod syndrome

Hypothyroidism and hyperparathyroidism (mild elevation)

Some cases of spinal muscular atrophy and amyotrophic lateral sclerosis, particularly when cramps are prominent

Other causes of cramps and fasciculations (cramp fasciculation syndrome, postpolio syndrome)

LABORATORY STUDIES

Routine laboratory studies used in the evaluation of patients with neuromuscular disorders are discussed here. Other more specific tests, such as measurement of antibodies in autoimmune disorders and DNA testing in hereditary diseases, are covered in Chapters 3 and 20.

Muscle Enzymes

The most important blood test in the evaluation of patients with suspected myopathy is the measurement of serum creatine kinase (CK), which may be elevated from muscle necrosis (Table 2.17). The alanine aminotransferase (ALT), aspartate aminotransferase (AST), and lactate dehydrogenase (LDH) enzymes are also elevated in myopathies, although these may also reflect liver disease. To determine whether their abnormal elevation is from muscle damage, the gamma glutamyl transpeptidase (GGTP) levels should be measured, because this enzyme is elevated only in liver disease. Measurement of serum aldolase, which is produced primarily in muscle but also in the liver, is sometimes useful.

Although serum CK originates mainly in skeletal muscle, it is also produced in the myocardium and brain. To differentiate their origins, CK isoenzymes are helpful. In myopathies, the elevated isoenzymes are mainly from muscle (MM), but other isoenzymes can also rise, to a lesser degree, probably from regenerating immature muscle fibers.[49]

Very high CK levels are frequently seen in PM and DM, although not in all cases. Significant elevations are also seen in muscular dystrophy, particularly in dystrophinopathies, Miyoshi myopathy, some of the LGMDs, and in metabolic myopathies, especially after exercise when myoglobinemia or myoglobinuria can also develop.

CK elevation can also occur in other diseases, such as hypothyroidism; in patients without clearly recognized muscle disease, called "idiopathic hyper-CKemia,"[50] which may be a subclinical dystrophinopathy[23]; in the McLeod syndrome, after trauma; and occasionally in normal individuals, particularly after excessive exercise.[51] CK levels can also be elevated in female carriers of muscular dystrophy[23] and in those patients at risk of malignant hyperthermia,[52] and they may serve to detect but not to diagnose this conditions. Mild to moderate elevation can occur in motor neuron diseases,[53] especially in younger patients (see Table 2.17, which lists causes of CK elevation).

Serum CK determination is useful to evaluate response to treatment in inflammatory myopathies but should not be used as the only parameter of disease activity, because CK can decrease without clinical improvement.

Myoglobinemia and Myoglobinuria

Although elevation of serum myoglobin can be an indication of muscle breakdown in patients with myopathy and elevated CK, serum myoglobin levels above its renal threshold (2 mg/dl) manifest as myoglobinuria, which is expressed as darkly pigmented urine that is positive with the benzidine test. The methods of chromogen oxidation are routinely used for screening, but these are also positive in the presence of hemoglobinuria. Myoglobin is specifically measured with the ammonium sulfate test, electrophoresis, or immunoassay techniques.[54] Conditions that cause myoglobinuria are listed in Table 2.18.

Other Chemical Tests

Results of routine chemical tests may provide clues to the diagnosis of neuromuscular diseases. For example, elevated urea and creatinine may indicate renal failure in patients with myoglobinuria and may also diagnose chronic renal disease causing neuropathy as well as renal involvement in amyloidosis. Low creatinine, on the other hand, is caused by muscle wasting in myopathies. Abnormal liver function tests can suggest diffuse systemic disease or toxic effects of the immunosuppressants used to treat autoimmune diseases.

Electrolytes should be measured in evaluating patients with weakness (e.g., for hyper- or hypokalemia) and in determining the side effects of medications, such as hyponatremia from carbamazepine, corticosteroids, and diuretics.

A high venous CO_2 may indicate respiratory failure in patients with muscle weakness, but should be confirmed with estimation of arterial blood gases.

Random fasting serum glucose, 2-hour postprandial glucose, and sometimes glucose tolerance tests and measurement of glycosylated hemoglobin are necessary for the diagnosis of diabetes in the workup of neuropathies.

A determination of serum lactate is useful not only during the ischemic exercise test discussed in the section Forearm Exercise Test, but also in screening for possible mitochondrial myopathy, in which it may be elevated.

Phosphate, magnesium, and calcium should be measured in patients with weakness because the elevation of these elements can be the cause of the weakness,

Table 2.18 Causes of Myoglobinuria

Metabolic exhaustion

    Excessive exercise in healthy persons

    Seizures, delirium, tetanus, strychnine

    Heat stroke

    Cold exposure

    Metabolic myopathies, particularly during exercise: carnitine palmitoyl transferase deficiency, very-long-chain acyl-CoA deficiency, myoadenylate deaminase deficiency, mitochondrial diseases and glycogen storage diseases (phosphorylase, phosphofructokinase, phosphorylase kinase, phosphoglycerate mutase, phosphoglycerate kinase, lactate dehydrogenase, or deficiencies)

    Malignant hyperthermia

    Neuroleptic malignant syndrome, serotonin syndrome

    Diabetic acidosis

    Ischemia (coma, arterial occlusion)

    Trauma (crush syndrome)

    High voltage shock

Myopathies, nonmetabolic

    Dystrophinopathies

    Infectious myositis (influenza virus, human immunodeficiency virus, toxic shock, and bacterial infections: e.g., clostridium, legionnaires' disease)

    Autoimmune myositis (dermatomyositis, polymyositis)

Toxins, abused substances

    Alcohol

    Lysergic acid diethylamide

    Cocaine

    Plasmocid

    Methadone

    Heroin

    Phencyclidine

    Amphetamines

    Envenomations (e.g., wasps, spiders, snakes)

    Cicuta

    Haff disease

Medications

    Cholesterol-lowering drugs

    Hypokalemia-causing drugs (e.g., diuretics, amphotericin B), licorice

    Azidothymidine

    Salicylate overdose

    Azathioprine

    Theophylline

    Lithium

    Epsilon aminocaproic acid

Fluid, electrolyte imbalance

    Hypokalemia

    Hypernatremia

    Hyponatremia

    Hypophosphatemia

    Hyperosmolar states

    Water intoxication

CoA = coenzyme A.

Source: Modified from TE Bertorini. Myoglobinuria, malignant hyperthermia, neuroleptic malignant syndrome and serotonin syndrome. Neurol Clin 1997;15(3):649–671.

whereas hypocalcemia and hypomagnesemia are associated with tetany and thus are important in the evaluation of patients with muscle stiffness. Albumin levels should be determined simultaneously, with calcium levels, as this may be falsely low in hypoalbuminemia. Patients with hypercalcemia should have parathyroid hormone levels measured to detect hyperparathyroidism.

Elevated serum cholesterol and triglyceride levels may suggest hypothyroidism, a cause of muscle pains, high CK, and neuropathy, whereas low levels are associated with hyperthyroidism and abetalipoproteinemia. Hyperlipidemia is another reported cause of polyneuropathy,[55,56] and very-long-chain fatty acids in plasma are elevated in adrenomyeloneuropathy. Lipoprotein electrophoresis is useful for detection for the lack of α-lipoproteins in Tangier disease and for the diagnosis of abeta- or hypobetalipoproteinemia. Phytanic acid levels are elevated in serum in Refsum's disease and should be measured only when clinically suspected to diagnose this uncommon disease.

Arylsulfatase A is measured in blood to diagnose MLD, and urine studies are also used to detect metachromatic granules. Fabry's disease, on the other hand, is caused by a deficiency of α-galactosidase and requires an enzymatic assay in leucocytes.

Quantitative Immunoglobulins and Immunoelectrophoresis

Immunoglobulins are measured in the workup of neuropathy and before treatment with intravenous immunoglobulins, because hereditary immunoglobulin (Ig) A deficiency poses a risk of anaphylactic reaction to human blood products and is a contraindication to intravenous Ig use.

Routine serum protein electrophoresis is often used as initial screening for monoclonal gammopathy (Figure 2.46A); immunoelectrophoresis, however, is the most sensitive study for evaluation of these disorders, particularly when the immunofixation method is used (see Figure 2.46B).[57]

Complete Blood Cell Count, Erythrocyte Sedimentation Rate, and Folate Levels

A complete blood cell count is part of the workup of patients with peripheral neuropathy to determine the presence of anemia associated with chronic systemic disease or the basophilic stippling of red blood cells that occurs in lead and arsenic poisoning. Red blood cell analysis may show the presence of acanthocytes in McLeod syndrome or abetalipoproteinemia. The analysis should determine whether there is leukopenia (specifically whether the total number of granulocytes is low) in patients receiving immunotherapy; the total number of granulocytes should be monitored periodically.

Measurement of the erythrocyte sedimentation rate is important, as it can be markedly elevated in vasculitic neuropathies and PM; it is also most useful in the diagnosis of polymyalgia rheumatica.

Anemia with macrocytosis and hypersegmented neutrophils is suggestive of B_{12} or folate deficiency. B_{12} and folate levels, however, should be measured in those patients with peripheral neuropathy, even without anemia. If B_{12} or folate deficiency is suspected, methylmalonic acid and homocysteine should be measured, because both are elevated in pernicious anemia, whereas only homocysteine is elevated in folate deficiency.[58]

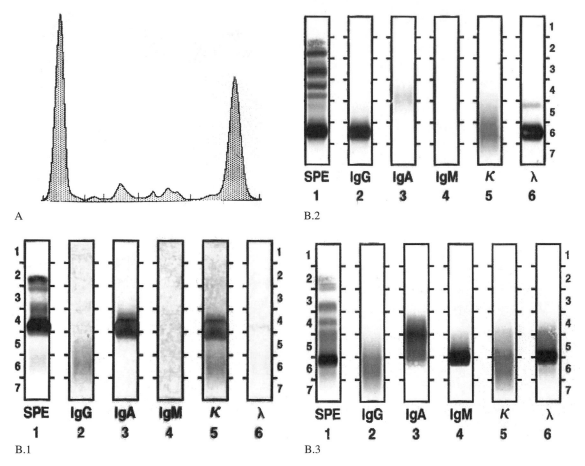

Figure 2.46 A. Protein electrophoresis in a patient with chronic inflammatory demyelinating polyradioneuropathy and monoclonal gammopathy. Notice prominent spikes of albumin and gammaglobulins. **B.** Immunoelectrophoretic patterns. **(1)** Immunoglobulin (Ig) A kappa monoclonal protein. IgA, 4,270 mg/dl (nl 70–312); IgG, 287 mg/dl (nl 640–1,350); IgM, 22 mg/dl (nl 56–352). **(2)** IgG lambda monoclonal protein with free λ light chains. IgA, 85 mg/dl; IgG, 4,800 mg/dl; IgM, 23 mg/dl. **(3)** IgM lambda monoclonal protein. IgA, 1,630 mg/dl; IgG, 942 mg/dl; IgM, 4,465 mg/dl. (SPE = serum protein electrophoresis.) (Courtesy of Dr. Richard McLendon.)

Schilling Test

The Schilling test is reserved for those patients who have borderline low serum B_{12} (cobalamine) levels, or if pernicious anemia is strongly suspected. The test is used to assess vitamin B_{12} absorption. In part one of the test, labeled B_{12} is administered intramuscularly, and the vitamin excretion is measured, as this is limited in patients with B_{12} deficiency due to increased utilization. Part two of the test consists of orally administering B_{12} with the addition of intrinsic factor. Decreased absorption of B_{12} in this part indicates malabsorption of cobalamine owing to gastrointestinal disease. In part three, the test is performed after treatment with antibiotics to eliminate gastrointestinal infection, which may impair absorption of this vitamin.[59]

Other Useful Laboratory Studies

Thyroid function tests are useful in patients with generalized weakness; in MG and periodic paralysis, which can be associated with thyroid disease; and in patients with muscle spasms or peripheral neuropathy and hyper-CKemia, as these can be caused by hypothyroidism.

Serum complement levels, particularly of C3 and C4, are usually low with systemic lupus erythematosus and should be measured in patients with elevation of fluorescent antinuclear antibody or extractable nuclear antigen titers (discussed in Chapter 3).

Serum cryoglobulin determination is important in patients who present with a mononeuritis multiplex or an undiagnosed predominantly sensory neuropathy, and especially in theose with known hepatitis infection. Cryoglobulins are proteins that precipitate in blood at low temperatures, as seen in macroglobulinemia, myeloma, leukemias, lupus, Sjögren's syndrome, and chronic hepatitis.[60]

Type I cryoglobulins are monoclonal immunoglobulins usually associated with liver disorders. Type II are a mixture of monoclonal IgM and polyclonal IgG associated with macroglobulinemia and chronic active hepatitis. Type III is a mixture of polyclonal IgM and polyclonal IgG.

Angiotensin-converting enzyme levels are measured in patients suspected for sarcoidosis, in which levels of this enzyme are elevated, or in those patients with undiagnosed neuropathy or myopathy, as these could be caused by sarcoidosis.

In young patients with a motor neuron disorder, serum hexosaminidase A assay is important, because hexoaminidase deficiency can have this presentation. Measurements of antibodies against GM-1 gangliosides should also be done if MMN is suspected as described in Chapter 3.

Elevated β_2-microglobulin is seen as a form of secondary amyloidosis, which, when associated with chronic renal disease, may present with carpal tunnel syndrome and thus could be useful to measure in those patients.[61]

Twenty-Four-Hour Urine Collection for Heavy Metals and Porphyrins

Measurement of the heavy metals, particularly lead and arsenic, can be valuable in the evaluation of peripheral neuropathy. Lead causes a predominantly motor neuropathy, whereas arsenic may produce a chronic or acute motor and sensory neuropathy that can sometimes be confused with GBS.

Arsenic poisoning is confirmed when urinary levels are elevated (25 µg per 24 hours),[62] but it should be taken under consideration that urinary arsenic levels can be mildly elevated in patients who have recently eaten seafood. If arsenic intoxication is strongly suspected and urine levels are normal, arsenic content should be measured in the nails or hair because it binds to keratin deposited in these tissues. Levels of 10 µg/g are considered diagnostic.[62] Occasionally, a chelating agent is used to release the arsenic from tissues, and arsenic is then measured in the urine to diagnose chronic poisoning.

Urinary porphyrin determination is used in the diagnosis of various types of porphyria,[63,64] which may manifest with a predominantly motor neuropathy that can be acute and confused with GBS.

Spinal Fluid Analysis

Spinal fluid analysis is useful in the evaluation of autoimmune demyelinating neuropathy. Marked elevation of albumin with albuminocytologic dissociation is seen in patients with GBS and CIDP. An elevation of protein with pleocytosis in a patient with a similar presentation is highly suggestive of a human immunodeficiency virus infection and should be diagnosed with serologic tests. Similar findings can be seen in sarcoidosis, acute poliomyelitis, and cytomegalovirus infections causing a lumbosacral plexopathy in patients with human immunodeficiency virus infection.

Lactate levels could be elevated in the spinal fluid of patients with mitochondrial encephalomyopathies and can help in their diagnosis. Cytology should be done when meningeal carcinomatosis causing weakness is considered and in patients with unexplained elevated spinal fluid lymphocyte counts to rule out lymphoma. Flow cytometry can be used in these patients to determine whether the lymphocytes are monoclonal (malignant), or polyclonal (inflammatory). Syphilis serology should always be performed, particularly when the number of cells is elevated. Similarly, angiotensin converting enzyme levels are used to diagnose sarcoidosis, and Lyme antibody titers are measured to diagnose Lyme disease.

CARDIAC EVALUATION, IMAGING

Electrocardiogram (ECG), echocardiogram, and Holter monitoring should be done when clinically indicated in patients with myopathies that involve cardiac muscle. These include muscular dystrophies, such as DMD, BMD, FSHMD, some types of LGMD, Emery-Dreifuss muscular dystrophy, MD, and acid maltase deficiency, particularly in the infantile form (Table 2.19). Abnormalities of ECG are also detected in some patients with PM. In muscular dystrophies, an ECG is performed annually or more frequently if clinically necessary.

Spinal radiograms are done periodically to measure the degree of scoliosis. With chronic muscle disease, particularly in DMD, SMA, and Friedreich's ataxia, the radiograms assist in determining the timing of scoliosis surgery.

Table 2.19 Neuromuscular Diseases That May Affect the Heart

Guillain-Barré syndrome

Amyloidosis—familial transthyretin amyloidosis (cardiomyopathy can also occur in other types of amyloidosis)

Dystrophinopathies (Duchenne's, Becker's)

Emery-Dreifuss muscular dystrophy

Myotonic dystrophy

Acid maltase deficiency (particularly infantile or Pompe's disease)

Myofibrillar or "desmin" myopathy

Limb-girdle muscular dystrophy

Facioscapulohumeral dystrophy

Periodic paralysis, particularly during attacks; periodic paralysis with cardiac arrhythmias (Andersen's disease)

Polymyositis and dermatomyositis

Mitochondrial myopathy

Autonomic neuropathies

Computerized axial tomography or magnetic resonance imaging of the chest is done in patients with MG, in patients with stiff-man and Isaacs' syndromes for the presence of thymoma. This is also done in patients with LEMS and idiopathic ganglioneuritis, and in older patients with PM and DM to rule out cancer of the lung. When negative, it should be followed by other proper tests to rule out a malignancy. Imaging of the spine and muscles is discussed in detail in Chpater 18.

Fluoroscopy or ultrasound studies are helpful in patients with respiratory failure to assess for diaphragmatic paralysis.

SPECIAL CLINICAL DIAGNOSTIC TESTS

Test of Pulmonary Function

Most clinics specializing in neuromuscular diseases use portable spirometers to measure FVC as a method to monitor respiratory muscle weakness. Measurements of FVC are also used during the performance of the edrophonium chloride (Tensilon) test in MG. More detailed and comprehensive testing is done in the pulmonary function laboratory in the hospital setting. However, simpler, portable spirometer equipment is a good compromise, as this determines other pulmonary function parameters; this can provide percentages of variations from normal, according to the patient's age and size.

The following is a description of some of the practical parameters used with this equipment.

Tidal volume is the volume of air moved during the inspiration and expiration of each regular breath; this is normally 0.35–0.50 liters. The air inspired when the patient takes a deep breath after a regular inspiration is called the *inspiratory reserve volume*, which is approximately 2.5–3.5 liters above the inspiratory tidal volume and represents the lungs' reserve for inhalation. Similarly, the volume obtained from a forced expiration after a normal expiration is called the *expiratory reserve volume*, which is normally between 1.0 and 1.5 liters.

The summation of the air that can be moved voluntarily with one breath from full inspiration to maximum expiration is the *FVC*. Normal FVC for males is 4–5 liters and for females is 3–4 liters.[65] These values, however, vary according to age, race, height, and sex, and much higher volumes are obtained in athletes and tall individuals. To determine the normal expected FVC for the patient's size, several formulas are available[65,66]:

For men, $[(0.052 \times \text{height in centimeters}) - (0.022 \times \text{age in years}) - 3.60] \pm 0.58$
For women, $[(0.0508 \times \text{height in centimeters}) - (0.032 \times \text{age in years}) - 3.02] \pm 0.52$

Other formulas for predicting FVC follow:

For men, $[(0.0583 \times \text{height in centimeters}) - (0.025 \times \text{age in years}) - 4.241]$
For women, $[(0.0453 \times \text{height in centimeters}) - (0.024 \times \text{age in years}) - 2.852]$
For male children, $[(0.078 \times \text{age in years}) + (0.05 \times \text{height in centimeters}) - 5.508]$
For female children, $[(0.092 \times \text{age in years}) + (0.033 \times \text{height in centimeters}) - 3.469]$

In addition to FVC, another useful method to assess pulmonary muscle function is the measurement of the *peak inspiratory pressure*, which normally should be −50 cc H_2O or more.

The *forced expiratory volume* (FEV) is measured when an inspiration is done rapidly and forcefully. The vital capacity obtained during this rapid expiration is slightly lower than that obtained if the measurement is done during slow expiration.

The *FEV at one second* (FEV_1) is the volume exhaled in 1 second, which normally should be approximately 80% or more than the FVC value. This percentage is decreased in patients with obstructive lung disease. In other words, if the vital capacity is low but the FEV_1 is 80% or more of the vital capacity, the patient likely has a restrictive lung disease, as that caused by muscle weakness. If the FVC is low and the FEV_1 is less than 80%, then the low FVC is caused by obstructive lung disease, or both obstructive and restrictive disease. In purely obstructive lung disease, the FEV_1 is much lower (usually below 70%).[66,67]

Predicted normal values for FEV_1 can be calculated as follows:

For men, [(0.0362 × height in centimeters) – (0.032 × age in years) – 1.26]
For women, [(0.035 × height in centimeters) – (0.025 × age in years) – 1.932]
For male children, [(0.045 × age in years) – (0.046 × height in centimeters) – 4.808]
For female children, [(0.085 × age in years) – (0.027 × height in centimeters) – 2.703]

Another important parameter to measure is the *forced expiratory flow rate*. The average flow rate measured at the middle of the forced expiration is 25–75%. This measurement may be closely related to the FEV_1 and is useful in supporting the diagnosis of primary obstructive lung disease.[67-69]

Maximum voluntary ventilation (MVV) is the volume of air exchanged during 15 seconds of rapid and deep breathing. This value is extrapolated and used to calculate what would be the volume if the patient continued breathing at this rate for 1 minute. This measurement is important to determine the patient's capacity to exercise when the demand for pulmonary ventilation increases. The test can be done with some portable respiratory testing equipment that may also provide normal values. If this is not available, the following formulas can be used to determine predicted normal values in liters per minute: for men, [(8.65 – 0.52 × age) × (body surface in m²)]; for women, [(71.3 – 0.474 × age) × (body surface in m²)].

The volume of air that remains in the lungs and cannot be exhaled after one exhales deeply is called residual lung volume (RLV), which is measured in the pulmonary function laboratory and is not determined directly with portable spirometers. The RLV is important because it allows an uninterrupted exchange of gas between the blood and the alveoli. Normal RLV averages between 1.0 and 1.2 liters for women and between 1.0 and 1.4 liters for men. The RLV value added to the FVC provides the total lung capacity. For these determinations, special gas dilution techniques are used, such as the helium or oxygen methods.

Edrophonium (Tensilon) Test

Edrophonium (Tensilon) is an acetylcholinesterase inhibitor that prolongs the half-life of acetylcholine at the neuromuscular junction and increases the probability of interacting with its receptor. This medication is used in the test, which is a very important clinical diagnostic tool in MG (Figure 2.47). The diagnosis of MG was initially described by McFarlane, Pelikan, and Unna,[70] and later by Westberger.[71]

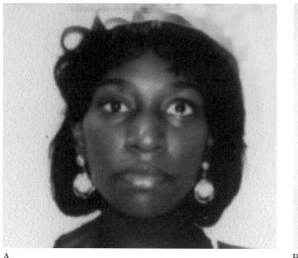

A

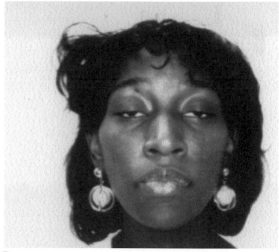

B

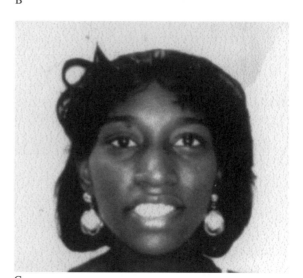

C

Figure 2.47 Positive intravenous edrophonium test in a patient with myasthenia gravis. Beginning of the test (**A**); after sustained upward gaze producing ptosis (**B**); improvement after 6 mg of intravenous edrophonium (**C**).

Osserman and Kaplan first reported its value in differentiating between myasthenic weakness and anticholinesterase overdose.[72]

Before testing, the patient should be carefully instructed of possible side effects, including arrhythmias, fasciculations, increased sweating, bradycardia, nausea and abdominal pain, increased lacrimation, and syncope. The test is usually performed by administering 2 mg of edrophonium intravenously, increasing the dose to 4–8 mg if no response is obtained. A 10-mg dose might be excessive and cause weakness in some myasthenic patients. It should be remembered that although the effect of Tensilon starts around 30 seconds and lasts 2–4 minutes, it may last as long as 20 minutes.[73]

In the pediatric population, 1 mg of edrophonium is used in children weighing less than 34 kg, and 2 mg for those more than 34 kg. Higher doses are used in larger children.

The patient should be blinded as to the drug to be used (saline placebo versus Tensilon). Some examiners perform a double-blind test, which is unnecessary if objective parameters are followed.

The test is performed after the clinician objectively determines a weak muscle to evaluate. The determination of improved strength with the drug should not be based solely on the patient's subjective feeling of improvement. For example, the examiner should observe for improvement in ptosis or extraocular movements. Other objective parameters include determination of neck flexor and shoulder muscle strength and measurement of FVC, especially in patients with generalized weakness.

It is recommended that two people participate in the performance of the test: one to check the patient's pulse and another to administer the drug and observe clinical effects. It is also advisable to have an Ambu bag available, particularly for patients with respiratory symptoms, and ECG monitoring should be used for older patients and for those with cardiovascular disease. The drug should not be given to patients with cardiac arrhythmia or asthma.

The Tensilon test can also be done using electrophysiologic and ophthalmologic evaluations, including measurement of neuromuscular jitter with single-fiber electromyography, the repetitive stimulation test, eye tonometry, and measurements of saccadic velocity and fatigue.

The following are the steps taken in the performance of the edrophonium test:

1. Explain the test to the patient.
2. Determine objective parameters to evaluate for improvement.
3. Have two 2-cc syringes available: one with normal saline and another with 1 mg of atropine (to use 0.5 mg per dose); have an Ambu bag available.
4. Obtain good venous access with a heparin lock.
5. Monitor pulse, record ECG when necessary.
6. Monitor vital capacity in patients with systemic weakness.
7. Examine for muscle weakness and fatigue.
8. Inject 1 cc of normal saline intravenously and observe for 1–2 minutes; this may be repeated once.
9. Inject 2 mg of edrophonium slowly and flush with normal saline.
10. Observe for improvement. If no improvement and no significant muscarinic effect is seen after 2 minutes, inject 4 mg of edrophonium and flush with saline.
11. If there is no improvement or increased weakness, wait 10 minutes and if no significant muscarinic effects are noted, inject 6–8 mg IV (if no weakness or muscarinic effects are noted, doses of 10 mg can be used after 30 minutes, if necessary).
12. Observe the patient for 5 minutes; when stable, remove the intravenous needle.
13. An objective improvement (positive test) is diagnostic of MG, although the test may produce positive results in other conditions, as listed in Table 2.20.
14. Atropine can be used if the patient develops significant side effects, particularly abdominal pain, syncope, and bradycardia.

Neostigmine (Prostigmin) Test

Intravenous neostigmine (Prostigmin) in doses of 0.5–1.0 mg can be used in patients needing longer observation periods because its effects last longer. This test is per-

Table 2.20 Possible Causes of a Positive Edrophonium (Tensilon) Test

Myasthenia gravis

Botulism

Lambert-Eaton myasthenic syndrome

Congenital myasthenic syndromes due to acetylcholine receptor deficiency; slow channel syndrome

Guillain-Barré syndrome

Amyotrophic lateral sclerosis

Some neuropathies

Brainstem glioma

formed only if the Tensilon test is negative; the effects of Prostigmin may begin in 15–30 minutes and last for 3–6 hours.

Forearm Exercise Test

The forearm exercise test is very valuable in the diagnosis of glycogen storage diseases and myoadenylate deaminase deficiency.[74–76] In normal individuals, there is up to threefold rise in serum lactate and ammonia after exercise, whereas lactate does not rise in some glycogen storage diseases, and ammonia does not rise in deaminase deficiency.

The use of ischemia during this test has been challenged, because patients with McArdle's disease might develop a compartment syndrome and myoglobinuria.[77] For this reason, others have recommended performing the forearm test without ischemia[78,79] or using a modified ischemic exercise,[80] which produces enough glycogenolysis and rise in lactate or ammonia in normal people to use for comparison in patients with suspected glycogen storage myopathies or deaminase deficiency in which this is abnormal. Munsat recommends standardization of the test by measuring strength with dynamometry.[81]

Normally during exercise, there is increased energy expenditure provided by glycogenolysis and, thus, increased production of lactate and pyruvate. There is also a rise in ammonia because of the adenylate kinase reaction that converts two molecules of adenosine 5'-diphosphate (ADP) to adenosine triphosphate (ATP) and adenosine monophosphate (AMP), which are converted by deaminase to ammonia and inosine monophosphate (IMP). As more ATP is depleted during exercise, more ammonia and IMP is produced, which is then converted to purine products, such as inosine and hypoxanthine.[65]

In some glycogen storage diseases, impaired glycogenolysis blocks the production of lactate and pyruvate with increased ATP degradation, causing a rise in ammonia and purines (Figure 2.48A).[82–85] This also occurs in CPT deficiency during fasting (see Figure 2.48).

In deaminase deficiency, there is lack of deamination of AMP to produce ammonia, so these patients have a normal rise in lactate but not of ammonia[74] or hypoxanthine[84] (Table 2.21). The examination should be performed as follows:

1. Inform the patient of the procedure and its possible complications (e.g., pain, swelling, ischemia, myoglobinuria).

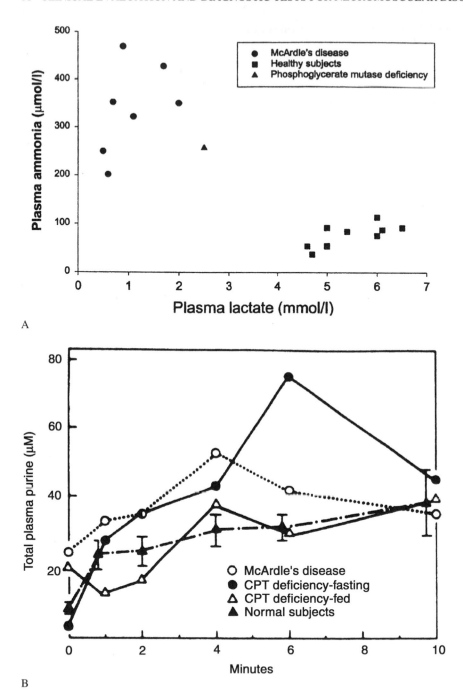

A

B

Figure 2.48 A. Peak plasma ammonia as a function of corresponding peak lactate responses to an ischemic forearm exercise test in seven patients with McArdle's disease, one patient with phosphoglycerate mutase deficiency, and nine healthy subjects. (Reprinted with permission from J Vissing, RG Haller. Metabolic Myopathies. In R Pourmand [ed], Neuromuscular Diseases: Expert Clinicians' Views. Butterworth–Heinemann, 2001.) **B.** Normal rise of purines during ischemic exercise in patients with carnitine palmitoyl transferase (CPT) and myophosphorylase deficiencies. (Reprinted with permission from TE Bertorini, V Shively, B Taylor, et al. ATP degradation products after ischemic exercise: hereditary lack of phosphorylase of carnitine palmityl transferase. Neurology 1985;35:1355–1357.)

Table 2.21 Findings in the Forearm Exercise Test in Various Myopathies

Normal rise in serum ammonia
    Normal controls and patients with glycogen storage disease
Decreased rise in serum ammonia
    Partial myoadenylate deaminase deficiency
Lack of rise in serum ammonia
    Myoadenylate deaminase deficiency
Normal rise in serum lactate
    Normal controls
    Myoadenylate deaminase deficiency
    Phosphorylase *b* kinase deficiency (if raised, this is usually blunted)
Decreased rise in serum lactate
    Some patients with myophosphorylase deficiency
    Phosphoglycerate mutase deficiency
Lack of rise in serum lactate
    Myophosphorylase deficiency
    Phosphofructokinase deficiency
    Phosphoglycerate kinase deficiency (if raised, this is blunted)
    Lactate dehydrogenase deficiency (this disease has a normal rise in pyruvate)

2. Obtain a good venous access in the antecubital vein with a 21-gauge needle or an Angiocath and place a heparin lock.
3. Obtain two baseline blood samples for lactate, pyruvate, and ammonia.
4. The exercise consists of repetitive grip contractions at a rate of 1 per second for 1 minute, or as tolerated, and should be stopped if the patient develops severe pain or muscle contractures.
5. Blood is drawn at cessation of exercise or when the cuff is deflated (if ischemia is used) and at 1, 2, 4, 6, and 10 minutes afterward for measurement of lactate, pyruvate, and ammonia levels. The heparin lock is filled with heparin between changes to prevent clotting. Blood and heparin left in the catheter are discarded at each drawing.

A normal rise in ammonia, hypoxanthine, pyruvate, and lactate should occur between 1 and 4 minutes and then return to baseline. A peak rise in lactate pyruvate occurs at 2 minutes with normals usually increasing to three times the baseline. Ammonia levels rise more slowly, peaking at 3–4 minutes. If ischemia is used, this is done by placing a blood pressure cuff inflated 40 mm Hg above systolic in the exercised arm; this should be done only in very select cases in which the nonischemic test was negative and the patient develops no pain during the test.

The measurement of venous oxygen content during the forearm exercise test was used by Wall et al.[86] in the diagnosis of mitochondrial myopathies. In mitochondrial myopathies, there was a significant rise in CO_2 that did not occur normally and thus correlated inversely with the arteriovenous O_2 difference.

Prolonged Fasting Test

This test is used to diagnose CPT deficiency. It is seldom necessary and is done mainly for research purposes because the diagnosis can be made with simpler, less risky methods such as biochemical analysis of muscle biopsy and DNA tests. Because CPT is involved in the β-oxidation of fatty acids, the normal rise in ketones seen with fasting is absent in patients with CPT deficiency; this occurs because the enzyme is also deficient in the liver, impairing ketone production.

The test is performed under close ECG monitoring and hourly monitoring of vital signs. Patients fast for 24–48 hours and are monitored for a rise in serum CK and ketones. Intravenous infusions of normal saline are used to keep patients hydrated, and blood and urine are checked every hour. The test is terminated if there is a rise in CK, if ketones appear in the urine or in serum, or if the patient develops weakness or muscle pains. Healthy persons do not develop muscle pains or elevated serum CK and ketosis develops within 24 hours (Figure 2.49).[13]

Provocative Oral Glucose Loading Tests for Patients Suspected of Hypokalemic Periodic Paralysis

Note: An experienced physician should do this and the following tests in the context of the clinical presentation and laboratory studies. The test should be explained in detail to the patient and informed consent should be obtained.

The provocative oral glucose loading test is useful in the diagnosis of hypokalemic periodic paralysis when other diagnostic tests, including DNA analysis, are negative.[87] Subjects should be monitored carefully for profound weakness and cardiac arrhythmia during the procedure.

After an overnight fast, with ECG monitoring and good venous access, an oral glucose load of 1.5 g/kg is given with a maximum of 100 g over 3 minutes. Blood

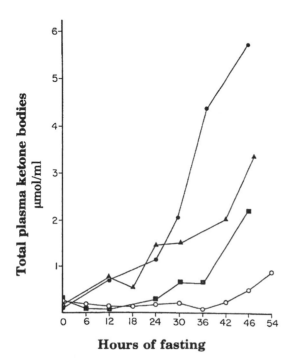

Figure 2.49 This figure illustrates lack of rise of ketones during prolonged fasting in a patient with carnitine palmitoyl transferase deficiency (*open circles*) compared with normals. (Reprinted with permission from TE Bertorini, Y Yeh, C Trevision, et al. Carnitine palmityl transferase deficiency: myoglobinuria and respiratory failure. Neurology 1980;30:263–271.)

should be obtained every 30 minutes from baseline up to 3 hours, then every 60 minutes for 5 hours for measurement of electrolytes, CO_2, and glucose.

The diagnosis of periodic paralysis is likely if the patient develops weakness and the serum potassium falls below 3.5 mEq/liter. The patient should then receive an oral potassium chloride supplement of 30–60 mEq in sugar-free solution every 30 minutes until the potassium level returns to normal and strength is regained. If the patient is nauseated or is severely weak, intravenous potassium chloride 35 mEq/liter with 5% mannitol can be used.

Intravenous Glucose and Insulin Test

After properly explaining the intravenous glucose and insulin test to the patient and using precautions similar to those of the oral glucose loading test, the patient receives insulin 20 mU/m^2 per minute and glucose infusion at a rate that maintains euglycemia over 2 hours.[88] The test should be performed with careful ECG monitoring, and serum, potassium, and glucose should be measured every 30 minutes due to mobilization of potassium to the intracellular space. Serum potassium normally falls over 30–60 minutes, after which it remains stable. Patients with hypokalemic paralysis may develop weakness, at which time the test should be discontinued and the patient treated intravenously with potassium chloride 35 mEq/liter with 5% mannitol, as in the oral test.

Hand Exercise Testing

In the hand exercise test,[89] the examiner records the amplitude and area of the compound muscle action potential (CMAP) of the hypothenar muscles using a supramaximal stimulus to the ulnar nerve every 30–60 seconds for 2–5 minutes to establish a baseline. Then the patient contracts the muscles isometrically for 15 seconds with a brief 3- to 4-second rest between contractions for a period of 2–5 minutes. The amplitude or area of the CMAP is recorded at the beginning and after each minute of exercise while the muscle is relaxed, and every 1–2 minutes after completion of the exercise for 30 minutes or until there is no longer a decrease in amplitude and the CMAP returns to normal.

The percentage of change in amplitude and area before and after exercise is calculated. A decrease of 40% of amplitude or area after 2–5 minutes of exercise is abnormal and is seen in periodic paralysis and in paramyotonia congenita.[89] Recently, Kuntzer et al. reported that this test can also be positive in other channelopathies.[90]

Regional Epinephrine Arterial Infusion Test

In the regional epinephrine arterial infusion test,[88] intraarterial infusion of epinephrine produces a regional decline in serum potassium, accompanied by weakness in affected individuals. Under careful ECG monitoring, epinephrine is injected at a rate of 2 μg per minute in the brachial artery for 5 minutes. Muscle strength is monitored clinically, and the hypothenar CMAP is recorded with supramaximal stimulation of the ulnar nerve at the wrist before, during, and 30 minutes after infusion. The test is considered positive if the amplitude or area of the CMAP declines by more than 30% within 30 minutes. Patients should be monitored carefully, and potassium chloride should be available to infuse or administer orally. This test should be done in specialized centers by experienced physicians.

Bicycle Ergometry Testing

In the bicycle ergometry test,[91] the patients first lie supine for 30 minutes, then an intravenous catheter is placed, and serum potassium levels are drawn at 10 and 5 minutes before exercise. Subjects pedal a bicycle ergometer (men, approximately 100 watts; women, approximately 80 watts) at a maintained pedal speed of 60 rpm up to 30 minutes. After the exercise, the patient rests supine for 10 minutes. Serum potassium is measured during exercise at 3, 6, 10, 20, and 30 minutes during the exercise and at 3 and 10 minutes after exercise. The test should be performed with ECG monitoring.

Normally, there is no weakness, and the serum potassium rises 0.8 ± 0.2 mEq/liter. Patients with hypokalemic periodic paralysis develop weakness after exercise, and the degree of rise of plasma potassium is lower. If the patient does not have an attack, a salt load preceding the exercise (2 g of aqueous sodium chloride in solution given orally every hour for 4 doses) may produce weakness.

Another useful test for the diagnosis of hypokalemic periodic paralysis is the measurement of in vitro muscle contraction strength, which is discussed in Chapter 15.

Potassium Loading Provocative Testing for Hyperkalemic Periodic Paralysis

The potassium loading provocative test[87] is useful in the evaluation of hyperkalemic periodic paralysis with otherwise negative diagnostic tests and DNA testing. After an overnight fast, 0.05 g of potassium chloride/kg in sugar-free solution is administered orally over 3 minutes, and the patient is observed for weakness.

Free-flowing arterialized blood is obtained every 15 minutes for the initial 2 hours to measure electrolytes and glucose, then every 30 minutes for the next 2 hours, if there is no weakness. If weakness develops, potassium levels should be measured every 10 or 15 minutes. If potassium elevation is mild, approximately 5.5 mEq/liter, 10 g of oral glucose should be given. If there is a rise in potassium above 6.5 mEq/liter, intravenous glucose should be administered, and if it is 7 mEq/liter or higher, then the patient should receive 10–20 units of insulin with glucose. Hyperkalemia usually resolves within 30–90 minutes.

During this test, the patient is monitored with ECG, and strength should be evaluated in proximal muscles. If the test is negative, the load can be repeated another day using a higher dose of potassium chloride (0.10–0.15 g/kg).

Exercise and Oral Potassium Test

Patients with suspected hyperkalemic paralysis who do not have weakness during the potassium load test, might require an exercise and oral potassium test.[88]

In this test, after an overnight fast, the patient exercises for 30 minutes on a stationary bicycle (at 100 watts for men and 80 watts for women) at a pedal rate of 60 rpm. After completion, the patient stays supine and receives oral potassium chloride, 0.10–0.15 g/kg, with very careful clinical ECG and electrolyte monitoring, as in the previous test.

In healthy individuals, there is a mild rise in potassium during exercise that returns to normal after 30–45 minutes. In patients with hyperkalemic periodic paralysis, there is a normal initial rise and fall in potassium after exercise, and potassium levels rise again within 30–90 minutes of exercise.

Forearm Cooling Exercise Test

During the forearm cooling exercise test,[92] muscle strength is quantitated using a grip dynamometer, and the development of electrical myotonia is assessed with needle electromyography to evaluate patients with hyperkalemic periodic paralysis and paramyotonia who can develop weakness or myotonia at low temperature.

The forearm and hand are placed in a trough in a supine position with the fingers flexed and attached to a force transducer. The forearm and hand are then secured so the patient isometrically contracts the flexor digitorum muscles. Electromyographic activity is recorded in the flexor digitorum profundus with intramuscular wire electrodes.

The patient exercises before the trough is filled with cold water (14–15°C) and again after the forearm is cooled for 30 minutes. The exercise consists of three 20-second isometric contractions interrupted by 10 seconds of rest, followed by 20 seconds of exercise and then 40 seconds of exercise.

In patients with paramyotonia congenita, there is a 20% fall in strength from baseline and myotonia, which may last for hours. Similar findings occur in patients with hyperkalemic periodic paralysis, but these patients recuperate promptly, usually in less than 60 minutes.

CONCLUSIONS

The explosion of new knowledge in muscle physiology, biochemistry, and genetics is making it increasingly difficult for the clinician to acquire an understanding of the multiple specialized areas that are needed to diagnose the various neuromuscular disorders. The clinical presentation, however, must first be recognized so the correct tests can be ordered to confirm a diagnosis for which the use of new methodologies may be necessary.

An ability to identify the symptoms and understand the clinical findings in the various diseases is of utmost importance. For example, the LGMDs are caused by many genetic abnormalities, yet they have similar phenotypes, and CMT disease has various forms of presentation and inheritance may require DNA studies for their diagnosis, yet one should first distinguish these diseases from other similar conditions for proper recognition and management.

Neuromuscular specialists are also frequently asked to diagnose segmental disorders, requiring knowledge of muscle innervation, proper clinical examination for selection of tests, and accurate interpretation of electrophysiologic and imaging techniques.

Standard MMT remains the most useful and simple method of evaluating the degree of impairment and disease progression in those with weakness. Thorough knowledge of the neuromuscular examination and of the basic and more specialized laboratory studies is valuable in arriving at the correct diagnosis.

Acknowledgments

For the excellent photographic work and assistance, I want to thank Richard Cherry and Joseph Martin from the Methodist Hospital of Memphis. I also would like to thank Zhigao Huang, Maritza Alfaro, and Felix Valdez, who, during their rotation in our laboratory, provided useful bibliographic help. Thanks also to Drs. Hani Rashed, Amado Freire, Paul Deaton, K. Senthilkumar, and Pushpa Narayanaswami for their participation and advice.

REFERENCES

1. Dubowitz V. Diagnosis and Classification of the Neuromuscular Disorders. In V Dubowitz (ed), Muscle Disorders in Childhood. Philadelphia: Saunders, 1996;1–33.
2. Griggs R, Mendell J, Miller R. Evaluation of the Patient with Myopathy. In R Griggs, J Mendell, R Miller (eds), Evaluation and Treatment of Myopathies. Contemporary Neurology Series. Philadelphia: FA Davis, 1995;17–78.
3. Brooke M. Clinical Evaluation of Patients with Neuromuscular Disease. In AHV Shapira, RC Griggs (eds), Muscle Diseases. Boston: Butterworth–Heinemann, 1999;1–30.
4. Griggs R, Mendell J, Miller R. Prevention and Management of Medical Complications of Myopathy. In R Griggs, J Mendell, R Miller, Evaluation and Treatment of Myopathies. Contemporary Neurology Series. Philadelphia: FA Davis, 1995;408–425.
5. Wolfe F, Smythe HA, Yunus MB, et al. The American College of Rheumatology 1990 criteria for the classification of fibromyalgia: report of the Multicenter Criteria Committee. Arthritis Rheum 1990;33(2):160–172.
6. Yunus M, Masi AT, Calabro JJ, et al. Primary fibromyalgia (fibrositis): clinical study of 50 patients with matched normal controls. Semin Arthritis Rheum 1981;11(1):151–171.
7. Brumback RA, Staton RD, Susag ME. Exercise-induced pain, stiffness and tubular aggregation in skeletal muscle. J Neurol Neurosurg Psychiatry 1981;44:250–254.
8. Masland RL. Cramp-fasciculation syndrome. Neurology 1992;42(2):466.
9. Levy LM, Dalakas MC, Floeter MK. The stiff-person syndrome: an autoimmune disorder affecting neurotransmission of gamma aminobutyric acid. Ann Intern Med 1999;131(7):522–530.
10. DiMauro S, Bresolin N. Phosphorylase Deficiency. In AG Engel, BQ Barker (eds), Myology, Basic and Clinical. New York: McGraw-Hill, 1986;1585–1601.
11. Fishbein WN, Armbrustmacher VW, Griffin JL. Myoadenylate deaminase deficiency. A new disease of muscle. Science 1978;200(4341):545–548.
12. Brody IA. Muscle contracture induced by exercise. A syndrome attributable to decreased relaxing factor. N Engl J Med 1969;281(4):187–192.
13. Bertorini T, Yeh YY, Trevison C, et al. Carnitine palmityl transferase deficiency: myoglobinuria and respiratory failure. Neurology 1980;30:263–271.
14. Salit IE. The chronic fatigue syndrome: a position paper. J Rheumatol 1996;23:540–544.
15. Fukuda K, Straus SE, Hickie I, et al. The chronic fatigue syndrome: a comprehensive approach to its definition and study. Ann Intern Med 1994;121:953–959.
16. Isaacs H. A syndrome of continuous muscle fiber activity. J Neurol Neurosurg Psychiatry 1961;24:319–325.
17. So YT, Zu L, Barraza C, et al. Rippling muscle disease: evidence for phenotypic and genetic heterogeneity. Muscle Nerve 2001;3:340–344.

18. Ochoa JL. Positive Sensory Symptoms in Neuropathy. Mechanisms and Aspects of Treatment. In AK Asbury, PK Thomas (eds), Peripheral Nerve Disorders. Oxford, UK: Butterworth–Heinemann, 1995;44–58.
19. Taylor DA, Carroll JE, Smith ME, et al. Facioscapulohumeral dystrophy associated with hearing loss and Coats syndrome. Ann Neurol 1982;12(4):395–398.
20. Purcell JJ, Rodrigues M, Chishti MI, et al. Lattice corneal dystrophy associated with familial systemic amyloidosis (Meretoga's syndrome). Ophthalmology 1983;90:1512–1517.
21. Ando E, Ando Y, Okamura R, et al. Ocular manifestation of familial amyloidotic polyneuropathy type I: long term follow up. Br J Ophthal 1997;81:295–298.
22. Brooke M. A Clinician's View of Neuromuscular Diseases. In M Brooke (ed), The Symptoms and Signs of Neuromuscular Disease. Baltimore: Williams & Wilkins, 1986;1–33.
23. Bertorini TE. Muscular Dystrophies. In R Pourmand (ed), Neuromuscular Diseases: Expert Clinicians' Views. Boston: Butterworth–Heinemann, 2001;227–294.
24. Barton JJ, Fouladvand M. Ocular aspects of myasthenia gravis. Semin Neurol 2000;20(1):7–20.
25. Gay AJ, Salmon ML, Windsor CE. Herring's law, the levators and their relationship in disease states. Arch Ophthalmol 1967;177:157–160.
26. Cogan D. Myasthenia gravis: a review of the disease and a description of lid twitch as a characteristic sign. Arch Ophthalmol 1965;74:217–221.
27. Osher RH, Griggs RL. Orbiculan's fatigue: the "peek" sign of myasthenia gravis. Arch Ophthalmol 1979;97:667–679.
28. Tas C, Arac M, Kumral N, Turcbay K. Ice test as a simple diagnostic aid for myasthenia gravis. Acta Neurol Scand 1994;89:227–229.
29. Anzai T, Uematsu D, Takahashi K, Katayama T. Guillain-Barré syndrome with bilateral tonic pupils. Intern Med 1994;33(4):248–251.
30. Waterschoot MP, Guerit JM, Lambert M, de Barsy T. Bilateral tonic pupils and polyneuropathy in Sjögren's syndrome: a common pathophysiological mechanism? Eur Neurol 1991;31(2):114–116.
31. Darras BT, Adelman LS, Mora JS, et al. Familial amyloidosis with cranial neuropathy and corneal lattice dystrophy. Neurology 1986;36:432–435.
32. Howard J Jr. The myasthenic face and snarl. J Clin Neuromuscul Dis 2000;1(4):214–215.
33. Medical Research Committee (MRC): AIDS in the Examination of the Peripheral Nervous System. Memorandum 45. London: Pedragon House, 1976.
34. Florence JM, Pandya S, King WM, et al. Clinical trials in Duchenne dystrophy. Standardization and reliability of evaluation procedures. Phys Ther 1984;64(1):41–45.
35. Engel WK. Finger force (FF): a simple rapid technique for one observer to reproducibly semiquantitate "grade A" muscle strength during drug testing. Muscle Nerve 1986;9(Suppl 5):270.
36. Bertorini TE. Clinical trials in Duchenne muscular dystrophy: the experience in Memphis, Tennessee. Ital J Neurol Sci 1984;(Suppl 1):153–158.
37. Lovett RW, Martin EG. Certain aspects of infantile paralysis with a description of a method of muscle testing. JAMA 1916;66:729–733.
38. Brooke MH, Griggs RC, Mendell JR, et al. Clinical trial in Duchenne dystrophy. The design of the protocol. Muscle Nerve 1981;4(3):186–197.
39. Reese BN, Lovelace-Chandler V, Soderberg GL. Muscle and Sensory Testing. Philadelphia: Saunders, 1999.
40. Haymaker W, Woodhall B. Peripheral Nerve Injuries. In Principles of Diagnosis. Philadelphia: Saunders, 1953.
41. Haerer AF, DeJong RN. DeJong's: The Neurologic Examination. Philadelphia: Lippincott–Raven, 1992.
42. Goodgold J. Anatomical correlates of clinical electromyography. Baltimore: Williams & Wilkins, 1974.
43. Delagi EF, Iazzetti J, Perotto A, Marrison A. Anatomic Guide for the Electromyographer. Springfield, IL: Thomas, 1980.
44. Williams PL, Warwick R, Dyson M, Bannister LH. Gray's Anatomy. Edinburgh, UK: Churchill Livingstone, 1989.
45. Narayanaswami P, Bertorini TE. The dropped head syndrome. J Clin Neuromusc Dis 2000;2(2):106–112.
46. Levin BE, Engel WK. Iatrogenic muscle fibrosis: arm levitation as an initial sign. JAMA 1975;234:621–624.
47. Bertorini TE, Boxman JR. A simple novel device to standardize vibratory sense testing at the bedside. Muscle Nerve 1998;1592(Abst).

48. Apfel SC, Schwartz S, Adornato BT, et al. (The rhNGF Clinical Investigator Group). Efficacy and safety of recombinant human nerve growth factor in patients with diabetic polyneuropathy. A randomized controlled trial. JAMA 2000;284(17):2215–2221.
49. Silverman LM, Mendell JR, Sahenk Z, Fontana MB. Significance of creatine phosphokinase isoenzymes in Duchenne dystrophy. Neurology 1976;26(6 pt 1):561–564.
50. Sunohara N, Takagi A, Nonaka I, et al. Idiopathic hyperCKemia. Neurology 1984;34:544–547.
51. Newham DJ, Jones DA, Edwards RH. Large delayed plasma creatine kinase changes after stepping exercise. Muscle Nerve 1983;6(5):380–385.
52. Bertorini TE. Myoglobinuria, Malignant Hyperthermia, Neuroleptic Malignant Syndrome, Serotonin Syndrome. In Neurology Clinics of North America. St. Louis: Saunders, 1997;649–671.
53. Welch KM, Goldberg DM. Serum creatine phosphokinase in motor neuron disease. Neurology 1972;22(7):697–701.
54. Jacobs DJ, DeMott W, Grady H, et al. Laboratory Test Handbook. Cleveland: Lexi Corp, 1990;669–672.
55. Fessel WJ. Fat disorders and peripheral neuropathy. Brain 1971;94(3):531–540.
56. Kaufman M. Triglycerides and neuropathy. Neurology 1995;45(11):2119–2120.
57. Karen DF. Immunofixation techniques, electrophoresis, and immunofixation techniques and interpretation. Boston: Butterworth, 1987;107–130.
58. Snow CF. Laboratory diagnosis of vitamin B_{12} and folate deficiency. A guide for the primary care physician. Arch Intern Med 1999;159:1289–1298.
59. Pruthi RK, Tefferi A. Pernicious anemia revisited. Mayo Clin Proc 1994;69(2):144–150.
60. Agnelio V. Mixed cryoglobulinemia and hepatitis C virus infection. Hosp Pract 1995;32:80–85.
61. Shirahama T, Skinner M, Cohen AS, et al. Histochemical and immunohistochemical characterization of amyloid associated with chronic hemodialysis as beta 2-microglobulin. Lab Invest 1985;53(6):705–709.
62. Widebank AJ. Metal Neuropathy. In PJ Dyck, PK Thomas (eds), Peripheral Neuropathy (3rd ed). Philadelphia: Saunders, 1993;1599–1570.
63. Albers J. Porphyria Neuropathy in the Diagnosis and Management of Peripheral Nerve Disorders. In JR Mendell, JT Kissel, PR Cornblath (eds), Contemporary Neurology Series. New York: Oxford University Press, 2001; 344–366.
64. Moore MR. Biochemistry of porphyria. Int J Biochem 1993;25(10):1353–1368.
65. Brooke MH. Clinical Measurements of Fatigue and Exercise in Neuromuscular Disease. In TL Munsat (ed), Quantification of Neurologic Deficit. Boston: Butterworth, 1989;101–118.
66. Clausen JL, Larins LP. Pulmonary Function Testing. Guidelines and Controversies. Orlando, FL: Grune & Stratton, 1983.
67. McArdle WP, Katch FI, Katch VL. Pulmonary Structure and Function. In Exercise Physiology. Philadelphia: Lea & Febiger, 1986;191–257.
68. Tests of Pulmonary Function. In JB West (ed), Respiratory Physiology—The Essentials. Baltimore: Williams & Wilkins, 1990;147–161.
69. Comroe JH Jr, Foster RE, Dubois AB, et al. The Lung Volumes (2nd ed). Chicago: Yearbook Medical Publishers, 1962;7–25.
70. MacFarlane DW, Pelikan EW, Unna KR. Evaluation of curarizing drugs in man. J Pharmacol Exp Ther 1950;100:382–392.
71. Westberger MR, Magee KR, Skideman FC. Effect of 3 hydroxyphesyl thylethyammonium chloride (Tensilon) in myasthenia gravis. Univ Michigan Med Bull 1951;17:311–316.
72. Osserman KE, Kaplan LI. Studies in myasthenia gravis. Arch Neurol Psychiatry 1953;70:385–396.
73. Rosenbaum RB, Bender AN, Engel WK. Prolonged response to edrophonium in Myasthenia Gravis. Trans Am Neurol Assoc 1975;100:233–235.
74. Valen PA, Nakayamn DA, Veum J, et al. Myoadenylate deaminase deficiency and forearm ischemic exercise test. Arthritis Rheum 1987;16(30):661–668.
75. Haller RC, Bertocci LA. Exercise Evaluation of Metabolic Myopathies. In AG Engel, C Franzini (eds), Myology. New York: McGraw-Hill, 1994;807–821.
76. Lewis SF, Haller RG. The pathophysiology of McArdle's disease: clues to regulation in exercise and fatigue. J Appl Physiol 1986(2);61:391–401.
77. Metabolic Myopathies. In RC Griggs, J Mendell, R Miller (eds), Evaluation and Treatment of Myopathies. Contemporary Neurology Series. Philadelphia: FA Davis, 1995;247–252.
78. Kazemi-Esfarjani P, Skomorowska E, Dysgaard-Jensen T, et al. No need for ischemia in the forearm exercise test for McArdle's disease. Neurology 2000;54(Suppl 3):A332(Abst).
79. Hogrel JY, Laforet P, Ben Yaon R, et al. A non-ischemic forearm exercise test for the screening of patients with exercise intolerance. Neurology 2001;56:1733–1736.

80. Bruno C, Bado M, Minetti C, Cordone G. Forearm semi-ischemic exercise test in pediatric patients. J Child Neurol 1998;13(6):288–290.
81. Munsat TL. A standardized forearm ischemic exercise test. Neurology 1970;20(12):1171–1178.
82. Bertorini TE, Shively V, Taylor B, et al. ATP degradation products after ischemic exercise: hereditary lack of phosphorylase of carnitine palmityl transferase. Neurology 1985;35:1355–1357.
83. Rumpf KW, Wagner H, Kaiser H, et al. Increased ammonia production during forearm ischemic work test in McArdle's disease. Klin Wochenschr 1981;59(23):1319–1320.
84. Brooke MH, Patterson VH, Kaiser KK. Hypoxanthine and McArdle's disease: a clue to metabolic stress in the working forearm. Muscle Nerve 1983;6:204–206.
85. Patterson VH, Kaiser KK, Brooke MH. Exercising muscle does not produce hypoxanthine in adenylate deaminase deficiency. Neurology 1983;33(6):784–786.
86. Wall A, Taivassalo T, Vissing J, Haller RG. Oxygen content of venous blood during aerobic forearm exercise: a diagnostic test in mitochondrial myopathy. Neurology 2000;54(Suppl 3):A331(Abst).
87. Moxley RT III. Channelopathies. Curr Treatment Options Neurol 2000;2:31–47.
88. Moxley RT. Hypo- and Hyperkalemic and Periodic Paralyses Diagnosis and Treatment. In Update in Myopathies, JT Kissell (Director). American Academy of Neurology Annual Meeting (Course #8ac#001), 1999.
89. McManis PG, Lambert EH, Daube JR. The exercise test in periodic paralysis. Muscle Nerve 1986;9(8):704–710.
90. Kuntzer T, Flocard F, Vial C, et al. Exercise test in muscle channelopathies and other muscle disorders. Muscle Nerve 2000;23(7):1089–1094.
91. Kantola IM, Tarsanen LT. Diagnosis of familial hypokalemic periodic paralysis: role of the potassium exercise test. Neurology 1992;42:2158–2161.
92. Ricker K, Lehmann-Horn F, Moxley RT III. Myotonia fluctuans. Arch Neurol 1990;47(3):268–272.

3

Autoantibody Testing

Pushpa Narayanaswami

The discovery by Patrick and Lindstrom[1,2] in 1973 that repeated immunization of rabbits using acetylcholine receptor protein obtained from electric eels caused muscular weakness was a milestone in the era of autoimmune neuromuscular diseases. The demonstration of humoral antibodies to the acetylcholine receptor; the correlation of weakness with antibodies attached to receptor sites; and the induction of weakness in normal animals by passive transfer of the antibodies defined myasthenia gravis (MG) as an autoantibody-mediated disorder.

Much water has passed under the bridge since this discovery. Potential antigens in the peripheral nervous system (PNS) continue to be defined, as do the association of disease processes with autoantibody responses to these antigens. In some instances, the presence of the autoantibody is linked to the pathogenesis of the disease. Examples of this include MG with antibodies to the postsynaptic acetylcholine receptor and Lambert-Eaton myasthenic syndrome (LEMS) with antibodies to the presynaptic P/Q voltage–gated calcium channel (VGCC). In other instances, the pathogenic role of the autoantibodies is not as clear. Instead, the autoantibody profile may serve to subtype the disease, providing insights into pathogenetic mechanisms and bearing prognostic implications. An example of this is the association of anti–GD-1a antibodies with acute motor axonal neuropathy, the axonal variant of Guillain-Barré syndrome (GBS).[3] Similarly, antibody to GM-1 ganglioside is associated with antecedent *Campylobacter jejuni* infection and axonal pathology in GBS.[4] A third group of autoantibodies is those associated with systemic autoimmune disorders, such as systemic lupus erythematosus and Sjögren's syndrome, to name a few, wherein nervous system involvement is a part of systemic involvement.

Target antigens in the nervous system may comprise structural intracellular proteins, ion channels, neurotransmitter receptors, intracellular enzymes, glycoproteins of peripheral myelin, gangliosides, and glycosphingolipids.[5,6] The following discussion is restricted to autoantibodies that are directed against antigenic determinants in the spinal cord and PNS and their clinical applications in the evaluation of neuromuscular diseases (Figure 3.1).

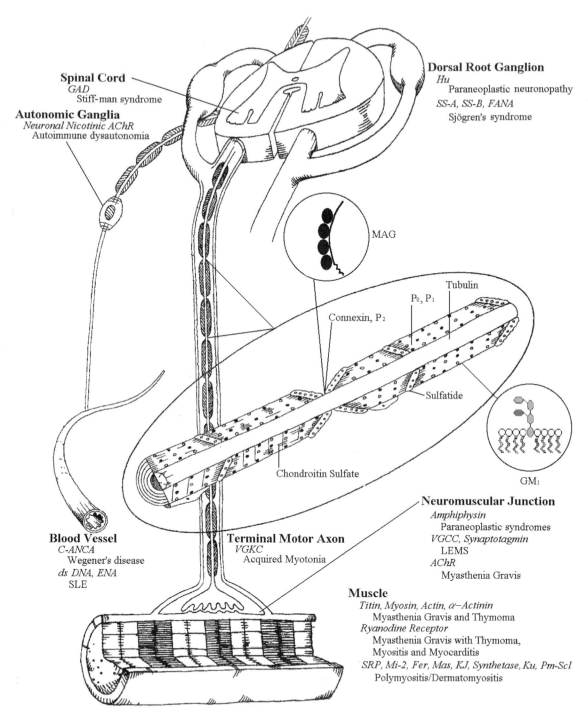

Figure 3.1 Antigenic determinants in the spinal cord and peripheral nervous system. (AChR = acetylcholine receptor; C-ANCA = antineutrophil cytoplasmic antibody; ds DNA = double-stranded deoxyribonucleic acid; ENA = extractable nuclear antibodies; FANA = fluorescent antinuclear antibody; GAD = glutamic acid decarboxylase; LEMS = Lambert-Eaton myasthenic syndrome; MAG = myelin-associated glycoprotein; SLE = systemic lupus erythematosus; SRP = signal recognition particle; SS-A = Sjögren's syndrome A antibody; SS-B = Sjögren's syndrome B antibody; VGCC = voltage–gated calcium channel; VGKC = voltage-gated potassium channel.)

Table 3.1 Autoantibodies in Disorders of the Spinal Cord and Neuromuscular Junction

Location	Antibody to	Clinical Syndrome
Spinal cord	Glutamic acid decarboxylase	SMS
NMJ (presynaptic)	Voltage-gated calcium channels, P/Q and N types	LEMS
NMJ (presynaptic)	Synaptotagmin	LEMS
NMJ (presynaptic)	Amphiphysin	Paraneoplastic syndromes (LEMS, SMS, sensory neuronopathy)
NMJ (postsynaptic)	Acetylcholine receptor (adult type)	MG, acquired slow channel syndrome
NMJ (postsynaptic)	Acetylcholine receptor (fetal type)	MG, arthrogryposis multiplex congenita
Muscle	Striational (titin)	MG with thymoma
Muscle	Ryanodine receptor	MG with thymoma, myositis/ myocarditis

LEMS = Lambert-Eaton myasthenic syndrome; MG = myasthenia gravis; NMJ = neuromuscular junction; SMS = stiff-man syndrome.

ANTIGENIC DETERMINANTS IN THE SPINAL CORD AND PERIPHERAL NERVOUS SYSTEM: ANATOMIC LOCALIZATION AND CLINICAL CORRELATIONS

Spinal Cord

Autoantibodies in disorders of the spinal cord and neuromuscular junction are listed in Table 3.1.

Stiff-Man Syndrome

Moersch and Woltman[7] first introduced the term *stiff-man syndrome* (SMS) in 1956 to describe 14 patients with progressive fluctuating muscular rigidity superimposed with episodic spasms. In 1988, Solimena and colleagues[8] reported the association of SMS with antibodies to glutamic acid decarboxylase (GAD), the rate-limiting enzyme for the synthesis of γ-aminobutyric acid. These antibodies are directed against the two isoforms of GAD, GAD-65 and GAD-67, in up to 65% of patients with SMS.[8–12] The demonstration by Dinkel and colleagues[13] that immunoglobulin (Ig) G anti-GAD antibodies in the serum and cerebrospinal fluid of patients with SMS inhibit GAD activity and affect the in vitro synthesis of γ-aminobutyric acid in crude extracts of rat cerebellum suggests that anti-GAD antibodies may play a pathogenetic role in the disease. It is proposed that loss of spinal inhibitory circuits enhances motor neuron hyperexcitability, resulting in the clinical syndrome.[14] Because GAD is also present in pancreatic cells, serum from anti-GAD–positive SMS patients also stains the β cells of the pancreas, and 30–70% of patients with SMS have diabetes mellitus.[15–17]

Table 3.2 Autoantibodies Associated with Peripheral Neuropathies and Neuromyotonia

Location	Autoantibody to	Clinical Association
Dorsal root ganglia	Hu	Paraneoplastic sensory neuronopathy
	SS-A/Ro, SS-B/La, fluorescent antinuclear antibody	Sensory neuronopathy associated with Sjögren's syndrome
Autonomic ganglia	Neuronal acetylcholine receptor	Autoimmune dysautonomia (idiopathic or paraneoplastic)
Peripheral nerve	Peripheral myelin protein 22	GBS, chronic inflammatory demyelinating polyneuropathy
	Myelin-associated glycoprotein	Demyelinating neuropathy associated with monoclonal gammopathy (mainly immunoglobulin M)
	GM-1, asialo GM-1	Multifocal motor neuropathy, ALS/MND, GBS with antecedent *Campylobacter jejuni* infection, AMAN
	GD-1a	AMAN, ALS/MND
	GD-1b	Sensory neuropathy, GBS, ALS/MND
	GQ-1b	Miller Fisher syndrome
	Gal*N*Ac–GD-1a	GBS, motor neuropathy
	GM-2	GBS with antecedent cytomegalovirus infection
Terminal motor axons	Voltage-gated potassium channel	Acquired neuromyotonia

ALS = amyotrophic lateral sclerosis; AMAN = acute motor axonal neuropathy; Gal*N*Ac–GD-1a = *N*-acetylgalactosaminyl–GD-1a; GBS = Guillain-Barré syndrome; MND = motor neuron disease; SS = Sjögren's syndrome.

SMS is characterized by progressive rigidity and stiffness of trunk and proximal limb muscles. There is exaggerated lumbar lordosis that persists in the supine position. Movement, fright, or sudden external stimuli, such as a loud noise, may precipitate episodic muscle spasms. Sphincter function is unimpaired. Dalakas[18] reports high serum anti-GAD antibody titers (greater than 32 μg/ml) in SMS. In this study, false-positive results were found in only 4 out of 47 patients (3 with MG and 1 with polymyositis) and were of low titer (100–1,000 ng/ml). The test is available commercially and is useful in the evaluation of patients presenting with axial rigidity and muscle spasms. The syndrome may be associated with various other autoimmune disorders, such as insulin-dependent diabetes mellitus,[8] thyroiditis,[19] pernicious anemia, and vitiligo.[20] Patients may have other autoantibodies, such as antiparietal cell, antinuclear, antithyroidal, anti–Jo-1, antiribonucleoprotein, and anti-intrinsic factor antibodies.[18]

Paraneoplastic SMS is discussed in the section Paraneoplastic Syndromes Involving the Peripheral Nervous System.

Dorsal Root Ganglia

Ganglioneuritis or sensory neuronopathy may be idiopathic or may occur as part of paraneoplastic syndromes or autoimmune diseases, such as Sjögren's syndrome

(Table 3.2). This is discussed in the section Paraneoplastic Syndromes Involving the Peripheral Nervous System.

Autonomic Ganglia

Antigenic Determinants

Although nicotinic acetylcholine receptors (AChRs) are best known as the targets of the autoimmune response at the neuromuscular junction in MG, they also mediate fast synaptic transmission in the autonomic ganglia of both sympathetic and parasympathetic systems (see Table 3.2).[21,22] Unlike the AChRs at muscle end plates, which have two α1, a-β1, δ, and γ/ε subunits (see the section Myasthenia Gravis: Antigenic Determinants), ganglionic AChRs express only α and β subunits (α3, 5, 7; β2 and 4).[23]

Clinical Correlation: Autonomic Neuropathy

Autonomic neuropathies may be inherited, degenerative, or autoimmune (idiopathic or paraneoplastic). Nonautoimmune acquired dysautonomia occurs in association with conditions such as diabetes and amyloidosis. Autoimmune dysautonomia is characterized by subacute onset with prominent symptoms of gastrointestinal dysmotility and pupillary dysfunction. Vernino and colleagues[24] found 5 out of 12 patients with subacute autonomic neuropathy to be seropositive for antibodies to ganglionic AChRs. Three of the five patients had underlying malignancies: small cell lung, bladder, and rectal cancers. In the same study, the authors found antibodies to neuronal AChR in several other disorders, including Isaacs' syndrome, LEMS, rapidly progressive dementia, and sensory neuronopathy. Fifty-eight percent of their patients had underlying cancers. The authors suggest that the presence of antibodies to neuronal AChR implies an autoimmune and potentially paraneoplastic etiology. These antibodies may also be responsible for the autonomic symptoms in LEMS. Pande and Leis[25] have reported antibodies to neuronal nicotinic AchR in a patient with seropositive MG, thymoma, and intestinal pseudo-obstruction. Gastrointestinal function normalized after treatment with plasma exchange and acetylcholinesterase inhibitors, suggesting a role for the antibodies in the pathogenesis of intestinal pseudo-obstruction in MG.

In a subsequent study of sera from patients with various forms of dysautonomia,[26] Verino and co-workers report ganglionic AChR binding antibodies in 41% of patients with idiopathic or paraneoplastic autonomic neuropathy and 9% of patients with other forms of dysautonomia, such as the postural tachycardia syndrome, idiopathic gastrointestinal dysmotility, and diabetic autonomic neuropathy. High titers correlated significantly with the severity of autonomic dysfunction, and titers decreased with clinical improvement. Because none of the patients with disorders such as pure autonomic failure or multisystem atrophy demonstrated these antibodies, it appears that they are specific for the autoimmune autonomic neuropathies. The authors suggest that a positive assay in the 9% of patients with other autonomic disorders, such as diabetic neuropathy, may imply an autoimmune basis for their symptoms. Thus, this assay may be useful in differentiating autoimmune autonomic neuropathy from other causes of dysautonomia and help to identify patients with autonomic neuropathy who require evaluation for underlying malignancies or those who may benefit from immunomodulatory therapies.

The assay may also prove useful in assessing response to treatment. At the present time, this assay is not available commercially.

Motor Neuron and Peripheral Nerve

Antigenic Determinants

Antibodies may be directed toward proteins or lipids of the myelin sheath. Neurofilaments have also been found to induce antibody formation (see Table 3.2).

Three major proteins—P0, P1, and P2—make up more than 70% of the total protein content of myelin.[27] P0 is thought to be involved in stabilizing the intraperiod line of compact myelin in the PNS.[5] P1 is identical to myelin basic protein in the central nervous system. P2 is found in the paranodal loops and Schmidt-Lanterman incisures.[28] Peripheral myelin protein 22 (PMP-22) is also present in compact myelin but accounts for less than 5% of the total protein.[5] Its role in normal myelin formation and maintenance is suggested by disorders such as Charcot-Marie-Tooth disease, Dejerine-Sottas disease (hereditary motor sensory neuropathy type 3), and hereditary neuropathy with susceptibility to pressure palsy, which result from abnormalities of the PMP-22 gene. Gabriel and co-workers[29] found antibodies to PMP-22 in 52% of patients with GBS, 35% of patients with chronic inflammatory demyelinating polyneuropathy (CIDP), and 3% of patients with other neuropathies. They suggest that an immune response against PMP-22 may play a role in the pathogenesis of inflammatory neuropathies.

Myelin-associated glycoprotein (MAG) is a well-known antigen for immunoglobulin M (IgM) antibodies associated with monoclonal gammopathies. It is localized in the periaxonal Schwann cell membranes and paranodal loops of myelin. It presumably acts as an adhesion molecule in Schwann cell–axon interactions.[30] Demyelinating neuropathy has been induced in experimental animals by transfer of human IgM anti-MAG antibodies, suggesting that these antibodies are indeed causally linked to neuropathy.[31,32]

Lipids constitute approximately 76% of the total nerve dry weight[28] and include gangliosides, cholesterol, galactocerebroside and the sulfated sphingolipids sulfatide, sulfated-3-glucuronyl paragloboside (SGPG), and sulfated glucuronyl lactosaminyl paragloboside (SGLPG). *Gangliosides* are acidic glycolipids composed of a lipid moiety, ceramide, linked to a complex oligosaccharide containing at least one sialic acid residue (*N*-acetylneuraminic acid in humans).[33–35] Their nomenclature is as follows: The first letter, *G*, stands for *ganglioside*. The second letter represents the number of sialic acid residues (M = 1, D = 2, T = 3, Q = 4). The numeral corresponds to the number of tetrasaccharide chains. The final lower case letter (*a* or *b*) denotes the isomeric position of the sialic acid residue (Figure 3.2). *Asialo GM-1* refers to GM-1 without a sialic acid residue. Gangliosides are situated in the membranes of neurons and supporting cells and are considered to have regulatory functions.[27] The complex gangliosides GM-1, GM-2, GD-1a, GD-1b, GT-1b, and GQ-1b have all been implicated as antigens in autoimmune peripheral neuropathy.

Differences in the regional distribution of gangliosides have been correlated with their clinical associations. For example, GM-1, which is located predominantly on motor nerves, is associated with multifocal motor neuropathy (MMN)[36] and the pure motor variant of GBS, acute motor axonal neuropathy.[3,27] This, however, may be an oversimpli-

Figure 3.2 Schematic representation of the structure of ganglioside GM-1. (Cer = ceramide; Gal = galactose; GalNAc = *N*-acetyl-galactose; Glc = glucose; NeuAc = *N*-acetyl-neuraminic acid.)

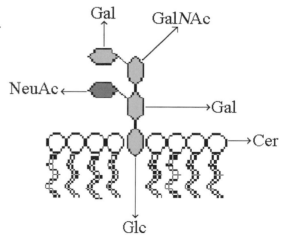

fication because there is evidence to suggest that GM-1 and related gangliosides may not be completely localized to motor fibers. It also appears that they are identified in the paranodal region of myelin as well as the axolemma.[37,38] Weber and colleagues[39] demonstrated that anti–GM-1 antibodies can reversibly block voltage-gated sodium channels, resulting in reversible conduction failure. It is therefore conceivable that these antibodies may cause a demyelinating or axonal neuropathy, although the clinical association of IgM anti–GM-1 antibodies is with the axonal form of GBS.[3, 27]

Sulfatide is a prominent component of central and peripheral myelin and is also present in the neuronal membrane of the dorsal root ganglia. The structure of sulfatide is similar to that of the gangliosides and consists of a lipid moiety, ceramide, linked to a hexose sugar. Instead of the sialic acid residue, a sulfate group attached to the sugar forms sulfatide.[40,41] Cell-to-cell adhesion and intercellular signaling are putative functions attributed to sulfatide. A genetic knockout mouse model of sulfatide deficiency has morphologically normal myelin, but the animals develop limb paralysis and tremor with aging.[40–42] The complex sphingolipids, SGPG and SGLPG, have also been implicated as antigens in peripheral neuropathies. SGPG is present in Schwann cell and neuronal membranes, including the myelin sheath and axolemma, and also in neural endothelial cells. It is believed to function in adhesion and cell-cell interactions.[43]

Antibodies may also be directed against intra-axonal antigens, although these are less accessible than the cell-surface antigens discussed above. IgM antibodies to β-tubulin have been reported in CIDP, GBS, and MMN.[44] They may, however, represent a secondary immune response to neural damage rather than a direct etiologic association. Antibodies that react with neurofilament proteins have also been described in amyotrophic lateral sclerosis (ALS), Alzheimer's disease, and Parkinson's disease.[45] In these disorders, the antibodies are polyclonal, primarily IgG, and directed at multiple epitopes on the target antigen. They resemble antibodies generated in a T-cell–dependent secondary immune response to a foreign antigen.

Chondroitin sulfates are sulfated glycosaminoglycans and are major components of connective tissues and basal laminae. Immunocytochemical studies demonstrate chondroitin sulfate in the Schwann cell basal lamina of the sciatic nerve as well as the extracellular matrix.[46,47] Antibodies to chondroitin sulfate S have been reported in peripheral neuropathy.

Clinical Correlations

Motor Neuron Disease. The localization of gangliosides to neuronal membranes makes it conceivable that autoantibodies directed against them may be present in patients with disorders of the motor neuron, such as ALS.[48,49] High titer (range 1:350–1:7,000) IgM anti–GM-1 antibodies occur in 5–10% of patients with ALS, whereas low titers (1:25–1:350) may be found in as many as 50% of patients.[50–52] Antibodies to other gangliosides, such as GD-1a and GD-1b, have also been described in these patients.[51,52] IgM antiganglioside antibodies have been reported in acute paralytic poliomyelitis as well as the postpolio syndrome.[53] Although ALS is not considered a disease involving the neuromuscular junction, electrophysiologic studies of muscle biopsies from ALS patients have revealed impairment of presynaptic transmission.[54] The application of IgG from patients with ALS to mouse muscle induced sensitivity to L-type calcium channels at motor end plates.[55] This suggests that ALS immunoglobulin may induce changes at nerve terminals that may be operative in eventual neuronal death. However, because none of these associations is sufficiently specific, the diagnosis of ALS remains based on the clinical features, electrophysiologic studies, and the exclusion of other disorders.[56,57]

Testing for antibodies to GM-1 ganglioside may be useful in patients with pure lower motor neuron syndromes in order to identify a subgroup of patients with MMN,[58,59] which may be amenable to immunomodulatory therapies. This is discussed further in the section Multifocal Motor Neuropathy. In this regard, the methodology used for the assay of these antibodies is an important concern. Kornberg and Pestronk, in an excellent review, discuss the interpretation of quantitative measurements of IgM anti–GM-1 antibodies.[60] Antibody titers above 1:6,000 are specific for distal motor neuropathy syndromes including MMN. Titers in the intermediate range (1:400–1:6,000) occur in motor neuropathies, other polyneuropathies, and ALS. Titers below 1:400 have little clinical significance. Testing for two other antigens, Histone H3 and NP-9, increases the specificity of the assay. Histone H3 is a nuclear deoxyribonucleic acid (DNA)–binding protein. NP-9 co-purifies with MAG during its isolation. High titers of IgM binding to GM-1 and NP-9 antigens and low binding to Histone H3 have over 90% specificity for MMN and distal asymmetric lower motor neuron syndromes without conduction block. This allows differentiation of these disorders from ALS. Other methodologic issues are discussed in the section Multifocal Motor Neuropathy.

In a recent report, Kaji and colleagues[61] describe three patients with a chronic motor axonal neuropathy, initially diagnosed as motor neuron disease, with elevated titers of antibodies to *N*-acetylgalactosaminyl–GD-1a (Gal*N*Ac–GD-1a). Two of these patients responded to intravenous immunoglobulin and cyclophosphamide.

Guillain-Barré Syndrome and Variants. Although the pathogenesis of GBS is not clearly understood, an autoimmune mechanism, possibly triggered by an infectious agent by way of molecular mimicry, has been proposed. To summarize briefly, the following autoantibodies have been identified in GBS:

1. Antibodies against several gangliosides, including GM-1, GD-1a, GD-1b, GT-1a, GT-1b, GM-2, GM-3, GD-2, GD-3, GQ-1b, Gal*N*Ac–GD-1a, and asialo GM-1[27]
2. Antibodies to glycolipids, such as sulfatide, galactocerebroside, sialosylparagloboside (SGP/LM1), and SGPG[28,62]

3. IgM antibodies to α- and β-tubulins[44]
4. Antibodies to the myelin proteins P0, P2, and PMP-22[27,29]

These antibodies have been correlated with several subtypes of GBS. The best-known association is that of antibodies to ganglioside GQ-1b with the Miller Fisher variant of GBS. Anti–GQ-1b antibodies are reported in 80–100% of patients with Miller Fisher syndrome (MFS), correlating with the abundant expression of GQ-1b in the paranodal regions of the extramedullary portions of the oculomotor nerves.[63,64] Although the pathogenesis of ataxia in MFS is debated (central versus peripheral), it has been related to selective staining of the cerebellar molecular layer by IgG from patients with high titer GQ-1b antibodies.[65] However, in a recent study, Carpo and others[66] detected GQ-1b antibodies in only 36% of patients with MFS, with the mechanisms underlying ophthalmoplegia and ataxia unclear in the majority of patients. An interesting, elegant study by Buchwald and co-workers[67] demonstrated that IgG anti–GQ-1b antibodies from patients with MFS induced both pre- and postsynaptic blockade at the neuromuscular junction in mouse hemidiaphragm and cultured mouse myotubes. The antibodies were not detectable after recovery, suggesting a pathogenetic role. The authors make an interesting observation as to the similarity in the pattern of cranial nerve involvement in MFS and botulism, a presynaptic disorder of neuromuscular transmission.

IgG GD-1a antibodies are associated with the pure motor form of GBS, acute motor axonal neuropathy.[3,68] Seropositivity for IgM or IgG anti–GM-1 ganglioside antibodies is closely associated with infection by *C. jejuni*.[69,70] The combination of *C. jejuni* infection and anti–GM-1 antibodies may correlate with greater axonal degeneration and degree of disability.[69] Carpo et al.[64] found that anti–GM-1 and GD-1a antibodies tended to be associated with worse disability at 6 months after GBS and, along with anti–GM-2 antibodies, with more frequent respiratory involvement. Patients with antibodies to GalNAc–GD-1a have a history of antecedent gastrointestinal infection, distal-dominant weakness, infrequent cranial nerve involvement, and pure motor involvement with axonal dysfunction.[71] The occurrence of anti–GM-2 antibodies in patients with antecedent cytomegalovirus infection is another association that may involve molecular mimicry[72,73] and has been reported with a form of GBS with severe sensory loss.[74] Predominantly sensory neuropathy is associated with antibodies to GD-1b, which is thought to be over-represented on sensory nerves.[30]

With the exception of the specific and relatively sensitive association between anti–GQ-1b antibodies and MFS,[63,64] it is at present not possible to predict the clinical course or outcome in GBS based on antibody testing. Two recent studies suggest that GBS patients with antibodies to GM-1 ganglioside may respond better to intravenous immunoglobulin as opposed to plasmapheresis.[75,76] However, more data are required to confirm this observation.

Chronic Inflammatory Demyelinating Polyneuropathy. Although the pathogenesis of CIDP, like GBS, is ascribed to immune mechanisms, the target antigens are yet to be defined. Elevated levels of antibodies to various gangliosides and sulfated glycolipids, such as SGPG, have been identified in patients with CIDP.[60,77] However, these associations are not consistent, as exemplified by the study by Melendez-Vasquez and co-workers,[78] in which there was no increase in the frequency of anti-glycolipid antibodies in 40 patients with CIDP as compared to patients with other peripheral neuropathies or normal controls. IgM antibodies to the cytoskeletal proteins α- and β-tubulins have also been described in some patients with CIDP.[44,79,80] However, none of these antibodies is specific or sensitive enough to be diagnostically or prognostically relevant at the present time.[44,81]

CIDP may be associated with monoclonal gammopathy of uncertain significance (MGUS), most often IgM-κ.[82] Patients with an underlying monoclonal gammopathy are generally older and have a more indolent and less severe illness with more sensory symptoms. Notermans and colleagues[83] have suggested diagnostic criteria for demyelinating neuropathy associated with monoclonal gammopathy. These patients are widely held to be less responsive to treatment than patients with CIDP without monoclonal gammopathy. Gorson and colleagues, however, found that the usual therapies for CIDP are just as effective in patients with CIDP associated with MGUS.[79,84]

CIDP has been described in association with melanoma and adenocarcinoma of the liver, colon, and pancreas.[85] Polyclonal IgM antibodies to GM-2, SGPG, and sulfatide have been reported in a patient with melanoma and CIDP, raising the possibility of molecular mimicry in this "paraneoplastic" form of CIDP.[86]

Multifocal Motor Neuropathy. The diagnosis of MMN is based on the clinical picture of progressive asymmetric, predominantly distal lower motor neuron weakness classically following the distribution of individual peripheral nerves, especially in the upper extremities, along with electrophysiologic evidence of multifocal motor demyelination with conduction blocks and normal sensory potentials. As discussed in the section Motor Neuron Disease, high titer IgM antibodies to GM-1 ganglioside—especially if associated with high titers of IgM binding to NP-9 antigen—and low binding to Histone H3 have over 90% specificity for MMN and distal asymmetric lower motor neuron syndromes without conduction block.[60] GM-1 antibody assay using covalent linkage of GM-1 to enzyme-linked immunosorbent assay plates (co–GM-1) is more sensitive than routine enzyme-linked immunosorbent assay techniques and, at high titers, is highly specific for immune-mediated motor neuropathies.[87] The antibodies are most often polyclonal IgM, but may be monoclonal in 20% of the cases.[36,88]

Although this assay is probably the most often used of the antibody assays in peripheral neuropathies, the implications of a positive assay should be interpreted in light of the clinical findings. The presence of conduction blocks establishes the diagnosis of MMN in the correct clinical context, regardless of a positive anti–GM-1 antibody assay.[89] In patients with lower motor neuron syndromes, the assay may be useful in identifying the small proportion of patients with motor neuropathy who do not have conduction block.[59] GM-1 antibody testing is often carried out in clinical practice in patients with pure lower motor neuron syndromes who do not fulfill the above criteria for MMN. Most commonly, these are patients with ALS who have yet to develop upper motor neuron signs. In these patients, a positive assay needs to be interpreted with caution, because low titer GM-1 antibodies are found in as many as 50% of patients with ALS.[50–52] It has been recommended that in the subgroup of these patients who do not develop upper motor neuron signs, high titer GM-1 antibodies should prompt immunomodulatory therapy, although studies to support this viewpoint are scarce. Pestronk and colleagues report improvement in four patients treated with plasma exchange followed by intravenous cyclophosphamide.[90] Serial determinations of anti–GM-1 antibody titers may be useful as a marker of therapeutic response to immunomodulation.[33] However, another study of 12 patients by Tsai and co-workers found no response to intravenous immunoglobulin despite a fall in GM-1 antibody titers.[91]

Sensory Neuropathies. Monoclonal or polyclonal antibodies that react with sulfatide have been reported in predominantly sensory neuropathies,[42,92] but these results are not consistent.[93,94] These antibodies have been associated with several subtypes of peripheral neuropathy, including predominantly sensory or sensorimotor axonal neuropathies and demyelinating neuropathy indistinguishable from CIDP. The sensory involvement may be either small fiber or mixed.[95]

Polyclonal antisulfatide antibodies are more often associated with painful axonal sensory neuropathies. There are isolated reports of immunomodulatory therapies in patients with neuropathy associated with antibodies to sulfatide.[96] Patients with prominent motor deficits accompanying the sensory changes and those with monoclonal antisulfatide antibodies may be more likely to respond to immunomodulation.[96,97] However, at this time, the implications of positive antisulfatide antibodies for etiology or treatment of sensory neuropathies is unclear. It has been recommended that testing for antisulfatide antibodies be restricted to a research setting at present.[98]

Paraproteinemia and Lymphoproliferative Disorders. Motor neuron disease, both lower motor neuron syndrome and typical ALS, has been associated with lymphoproliferative disorders and paraproteinemia.[99] The relationship of the monoclonal protein to the motor neuron disorder remains to be elucidated, although some of these patients have anti–GM-1 or GD-1b antibodies[48] and antibodies to SGPG.[100]

Several neuropathies are associated with the presence of excessive amounts of an abnormal immunoglobulin in the serum. The abnormal immunoglobulin may be present in a variety of disorders, such as MGUS, multiple myeloma, osteosclerotic myeloma, primary amyloidosis, cryoglobulinemia, non-Hodgkin's lymphoma, and the chronic leukemias. The abnormal blood proteins are usually monoclonal, hence the often-used collective term *monoclonal gammopathies* for these disorders. Some of the monoclonal proteins act as antibodies directed toward the myelin sheath or the axolemma of peripheral nerves and may, therefore, play a role in the pathogenesis of neuropathies associated with these disorders.

MONOCLONAL GAMMOPATHY OF UNCERTAIN SIGNIFICANCE. Almost two-thirds of patients with paraproteinemic neuropathies have an underlying MGUS.[101,102] These patients most frequently have an IgM-κ monoclonal gammopathy (60%) followed by IgG-κ (30%).[103] Men older than 50 years of age are most often affected. The neuropathy predominantly involves large sensory fibers. There may be associated pain and distal lower extremity weakness.[101–103] A pure motor disorder resembling motor neuron disease is described.[99,104]

Patients with IgM MGUS have more prominent tremor, sensory loss, and ataxia with electrophysiologic features of demyelination than those with IgG or IgA MGUS.[102,103] Approximately 50% of these patients with IgM MGUS have antibodies against MAG.[33,105] These patients comprise a relatively distinct subgroup, characterized by older age at onset, male predominance, and prominent sensory involvement with milder distal motor involvement. The disease is slowly progressive, with approximately half the patients eventually experiencing significant disability.[106] Electrophysiologically, there is evidence of predominantly distal demyelination.[78,95,102] Immunohistochemical staining of nerve biopsy specimens reveals deposition of anti-MAG IgM in the periaxonal regions.[107,108] Electron micrographs demonstrate wide spacing between the myelin lamellae owing at least in part to the intercalation of anti-MAG antibodies.[106–108] An inverse correlation between the distribution of MAG in peripheral nerve myelin and serum anti-MAG titers suggests that the deposition of the anti-MAG antibody may result in downregulation of MAG expression.[109] Nerve lesions, characterized by demyelination and remyelination and widening of myelin lamellae, have been produced experimentally in chicks by repeated intraperitoneal injection of human IgM anti-MAG.[32] Despite this evidence suggesting a direct association for anti-MAG and neuropathy, the relationship between the two is not clearly understood. Autopsy of a patient with anti-MAG antibodies and neuropathy revealed extensive anti-MAG deposits in cranial nerves without corresponding clinical findings. In the same study, sequential sural nerve biopsies did not reveal progressive demyelination despite the presence of anti-MAG deposits in both specimens.[108] Anti-MAG antibodies may cross-react with peripheral nerve sphingolipids, such as SGPG and SGLPG.[110]

Patients with IgG MGUS have a predominantly axonal neuropathy that may be sensory or sensorimotor.[111] In patients with sensory axonal neuropathy, antisulfatide antibodies have been identified.[42,112] A recent study[113] reported that patients with antisulfatide antibodies without paraproteinemia present more often with a pure sensory, painful axonal neuropathy, whereas patients with monoclonal gammopathy and antibodies to sulfatide more often have a demyelinating neuropathy with significant motor involvement. It is noteworthy that some anti-MAG antibodies cross-react with sulfatide.[114]

Antibodies to chondroitin sulfate S have been reported in patients with predominantly sensory axonal neuropathy associated with IgM monoclonal gammopathy.[113,115,116] Their role in the pathogenesis of these disorders is unknown.

PARAPROTEINEMIA ASSOCIATED WITH OTHER CONDITIONS. Multiple myeloma is associated with a symmetric, distal sensory, or sensorimotor axonal neuropathy. The paraprotein is usually IgM- or IgG-κ.[101] Osteosclerotic myeloma and the POEMS (*p*olyneuropathy, *o*rganomegaly, *e*ndocrinopathy, *M* protein, *s*kin changes) syndrome, in contrast, are associated with a symmetric, proximal, and distal sensorimotor areflexic demyelinating neuropathy that resembles CIDP. The monoclonal protein is usually IgG- or IgA-λ.[117] A symmetric, distal sensory, or sensorimotor demyelinating neuropathy may complicate Waldenström's macroglobulinemia and is usually associated with an IgM-κ monoclonal spike. Patients with primary (nonfamilial) systemic amyloidosis demonstrate an M protein, usually consisting of IgG-λ or light chains alone, with κ greater than λ.[102] The neuropathy is a predominantly small fiber axonal neuropathy with painful sensory and autonomic symptoms.[30] In a few patients with IgM monoclonal gammopathy and cryoglobulinemia, the M protein demonstrates anti-MAG activity.[107,118] Of the above conditions, osteosclerotic myeloma and amyloidosis are of particular interest to neurologists, because peripheral neuropathy may be a presenting feature of these conditions.[102]

In summary, the paraproteinemias may be associated with almost any kind of neuropathy, mild or progressive, sensory, motor or sensorimotor, involving small or large fibers. Serum immunofixation is the most sensitive clinical test for the detection of paraproteins.[119] Anti-MAG antibodies have been detected occasionally even in the absence of M protein, in slowly progressive sensorimotor demyelinating neuropathy.[120] Hence, anti-MAG assay may prove useful in establishing an autoimmune etiology in rare patients with peripheral neuropathy of unknown etiology. Although the presence of anti-MAG antibodies implies an immune-mediated pathogenesis, immunosuppressive therapy is often disappointing in patients with anti-MAG neuropathy.[107,121–123] Eurelings and colleagues, in a recent study of polyneuropathy associated with IgM monoclonal gammopathy, found that anti-MAG and anti-SGPG antibodies did not have prognostic value.[124] Assay of antisulfatide or anti–chondroitin sulfate C antibodies may provide insights into the pathogenesis of the neuropathies associated with these disorders but appears to carry no therapeutic or prognostic implications.

Gait Disorder Autoantibody Late-Age Onset Polyneuropathy. Pestronk and colleagues[125] have described a subset of patients with late-onset, disabling gait difficulty and predominantly distal sensorimotor neuropathy (GALOP syndrome). The electrophysiologic findings were variable and included both axonal and demyelinating neuropathies. These patients had high titers (>1:10,000) of antibodies that bound to central nervous system myelin antigens. Five of these patients improved with intravenous immunoglobulin, suggesting an immune pathogenesis. The assay is available commercially and may be useful in evaluating gait problems in the elderly.

Terminal Motor Axons

Acquired Neuromyotonia

Neuromyotonia is a heterogenous syndrome characterized by muscle fiber hyperactivity resulting in muscle stiffness at rest and continuous rippling fasciculations or myokymia.[126,127] Neuromyotonia may be hereditary or acquired. The two major syndromes of acquired neuromyotonia are Isaacs' syndrome and Morvan's syndrome. *Isaacs' syndrome* is characterized by persistent generalized muscle stiffness and weakness.[127,128] *Morvan's syndrome* is similar to Isaacs' syndrome, with the additional features of encephalopathy with insomnia, confusion, and hallucinations.[129,130] Acquired neuromyotonia has been described in isolation or in association with several autoimmune disorders, such as inflammatory demyelinating neuropathies,[131] thymoma with or without MG,[132] and as a paraneoplastic syndrome in association with bronchial carcinoma,[133] plasmacytoma with IgM paraproteinemia,[134] and Hodgkin's disease.[135] The diagnosis rests on the demonstration of spontaneous doublet, triplet, or multiplet high-frequency motor unit discharges on electromyography. These discharges increase with use, persist in sleep, and are abolished by curare.[136]

The voltage-gated potassium channel (VGKC) is one of the antigenic determinants in acquired neuromyotonia (see Table 3.2).[137] It consists of four transmembrane α subunits interacting with intracellular β subunits that are also tetrameric.[138] Six different VGKC α subunits have been described, each encoded by a different gene.[139] Hart and co-workers detected serum IgG antibodies in all of 12 patients with neuromyotonia.[140] The antibodies were heterogenous, varying in their immunoreactivity to the three VGKC α subunits studied. Their mechanism of action is unclear. There is no evidence at present that these antibodies directly block potassium channels.[137] Moreover, they are not detected in all patients with acquired neuromyotonia.

Neuromyotonia has been described in transgenic mice with a deletion or overexpression of the gene for PMP-22.[141,142] Thus, antigenic targets other than the VGKC may be involved in the pathogenesis of acquired neuromyotonia.

The detection of antibodies to the VGKC has added acquired neuromyotonia (Isaacs'[136] and Morvan's[129,130] syndromes) to the group of autoimmune channelopathies, along with LEMS and MG. Improvement in symptoms with plasmapheresis and immunosuppressive therapy suggests that the antibodies may be involved in the pathogenesis of the clinical syndrome.

Neuromuscular Junction

Autoantibodies in disorders of the neuromuscular junction are described in Table 3.1.

Lambert-Eaton Myasthenic Syndrome

Antigenic Determinants. The VGCCs in the neuromuscular junction are the antigenic determinants in LEMS. The VGCC consists of the voltage-sensing and pore-forming α-1 subunit, four transmembrane domains (the α2δ subunit, containing two proteins derived from the same gene and linked by a disulfide bond, and the γ subunit), and a cytoplasmic β subunit.[143] Several different α-1 subunits have been identified, each conferring unique electrophysiologic and pharmacologic properties on the channels.[143] The P-Q- and N-type VGCCs are all slowly inactivating and insensitive to dihydropyridines. They are expressed on nerve terminals and participate in neurotransmitter release.[144] P-Q-type VGCCs possess the α-1A subunit, whereas α-1B subunits are found in N channels.[143]

Approximately 95% of patients with LEMS have serum antibodies to P- and Q-type calcium channels. Antibodies against the N-type calcium channels are found in 50% of patients.[143] Engel and colleagues have demonstrated an autoantibody-mediated depletion of calcium channels at the motor nerve terminal in LEMS.[145] This results in a reduction of calcium-induced neurotransmitter release that is responsible for neuromuscular transmission. Passive transfer of the disease to mice is possible. Response to immunotherapy adds to the evidence that the antibodies are causally related to the disease.

Clinical Role of Autoantibody Testing in Lambert-Eaton Myasthenic Syndrome. Tests for antibodies to the VGCC are commercially available and are useful in the clinical setting when LEMS is suspected. In the paraneoplastic form of LEMS, antibodies to P/Q calcium channels are found in close to 100% of patients, whereas 74% of patients have antibodies to N-type calcium channels. In the primary autoimmune form of LEMS, these antibodies are found in 91% and approximately 40% of patients, respectively.[146] False-positive assays may be obtained in a small percentage (<3%) of patients with small cell lung cancer without LEMS, in less than 2% of healthy controls, in less than 5% of neurologic controls, and in approximately 10% of patients with cancers or hypergammaglobulinemia associated with autoimmune diseases (e.g., systemic lupus erythematosus, chronic liver diseases and infections) and owing to repeated freezing and thawing of serum.[147] Immunosuppressive therapy may result in false-negative results.[148] Approximately 13% of LEMS patients have coexisting AChR-binding antibodies.[148] However, these appear to be nonpathogenetic, as evidenced by the exclusively presynaptic lesion found microelectrophysiologically in several of these patients.[149,150] Coexisting LEMS and clinical MG, although rare, have been reported.[151]

Other autoantibodies, such as those against thyroglobulin, gastric parietal cells, and thyroid peroxidase (microsomal antibodies), are two to three times more common in patients with autoimmune LEMS and MG than in patients with other neurologic disorders.[148,152] A positive assay for these antibodies may be useful in supporting a diagnosis of LEMS in the absence of antibodies to VGCC.[147] Antinuclear, antimitochondrial, anti–smooth muscle antibodies, and rheumatoid factor are significantly more common in autoimmune LEMS than in paraneoplastic LEMS.[148] This may be useful in the evaluation of LEMS patients for the likelihood of underlying lung cancer.

Synaptotagmin is a synaptic vesicle protein acting as a cooperative calcium receptor during exocytosis.[153,154] Takamori and co-workers[155] found that sera from 12 of 47 patients with LEMS were positive for antibodies to synaptotagmin. Of the 12, four patients did not have antibodies to P/Q VGCC. An immune-mediated model of LEMS in rats by injection with synaptotagmin has been described.[156]

Assays of synaptotagmin antibodies are of doubtful clinical value. Neuronal AChR antibodies associated with paraneoplastic LEMS are discussed in the section Autonomic Ganglia. The foregoing assays are unavailable commercially at the present time.

Myasthenia Gravis

Antigenic Determinants. The nicotinic AChR forms the antigenic substrate for autoantibody-mediated damage at the neuromuscular junction in MG. The AChR is a heteropentamer; it has two identical α subunits, one β subunit, one δ subunit, and one γ subunit. The ϵ subunit replaces the γ subunit of the fetal AChR to form the adult AChR. These subunits extend through the cell membrane and are arranged around a channel.[157] The major antibody, the AchR-binding antibody, is directed toward the main immunogenic region, located on the distal portion of the extracellular part of the receptor.[158] The antibody appears to produce the neuromuscular transmission defect by several mechanisms. These include binding to the receptor with resultant functional changes, accelerated degradation, and complement-mediated lysis of the receptor.[159] Additional antibodies, such as AChR-modulating antibodies and AChR-blocking antibodies, may be detected in a smaller proportion of patients. The modulating antibodies, when applied to cell cultures, increase the degradation of AChR by cross-linking receptors; the blocking antibodies prevent the binding of α-bungarotoxin.[149]

The AChR-modulating antibodies are detected using cultured human muscle cells. In the presence of antibodies, there is accelerated endocytosis and degradation of the AChR. The reduction of AChR is detected by a decrease in I^{125}-labeled α-bungarotoxin binding.[147]

The AChR-blocking antibodies prevent the binding of bungarotoxin. The assay involves preincubating the antigen, usually skeletal muscle AChR or AChR from cultured muscle cells, with the serum to be tested and then incubating it with I^{125}-labeled α-bungarotoxin. A decreased level of bungarotoxin binding indicates the presence of blocking antibodies.[147,149]

Approximately 15–20% of patients with MG do not have detectable antibodies to AChR by immunoprecipitation of I^{125}-α-bungarotoxin-AchR complexes (seronegative MG [SNMG]). The clinical features in these patients are similar to, although less severe than, seropositive patients, and a larger proportion tends to be ocular.[160] Disease incidence in SNMG is equal in male and female patients across all ages, but males appear to be less severely affected. These patients are also less likely to have thymic abnormalities, and response to thymectomy may be less clear.[161]Vincent et al.[162] propose that in SNMG, there are antibodies of the IgM class that bind to an undefined muscle antigen and activate a second messenger pathway, resulting in

AChR phosphorylation and desensitization. Blaes and co-workers[163] have demonstrated antibodies in SNMG that bind to a muscle surface antigen other than the AChR, suggesting that SNMG may be a distinct subtype of MG.

Although genetic defects of the AChR, which alter channel properties, such as the slow channel syndrome, are well-described,[164] a rare immune-mediated disorder has been reported in which an antibody specific to the adult AChR alters channel properties, reducing total current and slowing closure. The name *acquired slow channel syndrome* has been proposed for this interesting disorder.[165] Routine assays of AChR antibodies use either partially denervated (ischemic) muscle from amputations, which contains mainly fetal AChR, or the human rhabdomyosarcoma cell-line TE671, which expresses only fetal AChR. In contrast to many MG patients whose sera bind fetal AChR as well as or better than adult AChR,[166,167] patients with the acquired slow channel syndrome possess autoantibodies that recognize specific epitopes of the ε subunit of the adult AChR.

Arthrogryposis multiplex congenita has been reported in infants of mothers with antibodies that bind specifically to the γ subunit of the fetal AChR.[168] The condition often coexists with lung hypoplasia and may be lethal. The mother may not have any symptoms or signs of MG, because the antibodies are directed against the fetal form of the AChR. Affected mothers, however, can give birth to normal babies if treated with thymectomy and immunosuppressants.[169]

Antibodies that react with the cross-striations of skeletal muscle (antistriational antibodies) are a reasonably sensitive predictor of thymoma in MG.[170,171] There is evidence to suggest that they react with titin, a giant skeletal muscle protein.[172,173] Gautel and co-workers[173] detected titin autoantibodies in 97% of patients with MG and thymoma. Antibodies to myosin, actin, α-actinin, and the sarcoplasmic reticulum have also been described in patients with MG and thymoma.[174,175] Recently, Mygland and colleagues[176] have distinguished between three groups of patients with thymoma-associated MG: (1) a group with myositis or myocarditis and antibodies to the ryanodine receptor (RyR); (2) a group with neuromyotonia without RyR antibodies; and (3) a group without myositis, neuromyotonia, or RyR antibodies.

Rare patients with MG also have rippling muscle disease as a part of the autoimmune response.[177] Autoantibodies from the sera of these patients are directed against high-molecular-weight muscle proteins. It is postulated that these antibodies may activate calcium channels, such as the dihydropyridine receptor or RyR, resulting in mechanosensitive activation of muscle contraction, causing the rippling muscle phenomenon.[178]

Clinical Role of Autoantibody Testing in Myasthenia Gravis. Antibody testing is in common clinical usage as a diagnostic tool in MG. The AChR-binding antibodies are characteristic of acquired MG in the context of the history and physical findings, electrophysiologic abnormalities, and response to edrophonium testing.[179] These antibodies are detected in 85–90% of patients with generalized MG and in 50–70% of patients with ocular MG, with a specificity of more than 99%.[180] AChR-binding antibody testing is the first choice assay for confirming the diagnosis of autoimmune MG.[149] The antibody titers do not correlate well with disease severity. However, in individual patients, a rough correlation exists between antibody titers and clinical severity, and titers usually fall in the course of long-term clinical improvement. Results may be negative in the first 6–12 months after disease onset or during immunosuppressive therapy.[147]

AChR-modulating antibodies are useful to confirm a diagnosis of MG when the AChR-binding antibody assay is negative, as in children or adults with MG of recent onset, ocular MG, or mild disease.[148,149] Lennon[148] suggests that this assay may be useful in MG patients aged 20 years or older in whom thymoma is a consideration, but imaging remains the investigation of choice in patients with suspected thymoma. The sensitivity of this assay is similar to the AChR-binding antibody assay.[149] False-positive results may occur owing to hemolysis, muscle relaxants, microbial growth, or exposure of the serum specimen to high ambient temperatures. A positive result in the AChR-modulating antibody assay in the absence of AChR-binding or blocking antibodies needs to be confirmed with a fresh serum specimen.[147]

AChR-blocking antibodies are found in 52% of patients with autoimmune MG and 30% of patients with ocular MG. They are present in only 1% of patients without detectable AChR-binding antibodies.[181] They are therefore not recommended as a screening test for MG. In addition, these antibodies bind near the receptor binding sites for α-bungarotoxin and cause apparent loss of AChR in the modulating antibody assay. Hence, testing for AChR-blocking antibodies is not indicated if the AChR-modulating antibody assay is normal.[147] Muscle relaxants can cause a false-positive result.[147]

A positive assay for antistriational antibodies supports a diagnosis of MG when tests for AChR antibodies are negative. Eighty percent of MG patients with thymoma have positive assays for antistriational antibodies.[181] Approximately 30% of adult patients with MG have antistriational antibodies. The frequency is higher in individuals who are older at disease onset, from 30% at ages 41–60 years to 55% at ages 61 years and older.[181] Testing for striational antibodies may also be useful in following thymoma patients after surgery, when a progressive rise in antibody titers may herald tumor recurrence.[182] false-positive results may be obtained in patients with autoimmune liver disease,[183] LEMS (6%),[152] and primary lung cancer (3%).[179]

Finally, in the clinical context, a positive result for antibodies against thyroglobulin, gastric parietal cells, or thyroid peroxidase (microsomal antibodies) may be useful in supporting a diagnosis of MG in patients who are negative for AChR antibodies but is not indicated in routine diagnostic evaluation. Antinuclear antibodies may be detected in MG patients with thymoma.[147]

Muscle

A listing of autoantibodies in muscle diseases is found in Table 3.3.

Inflammatory Myopathies

The inflammatory myopathies—polymyositis (PM), dermatomyositis (DM), and inclusion body myositis (IBM)—may occur in isolation or in conjunction with systemic autoimmune disease or malignancy.[184] Autoantibodies in inflammatory myopathies may be divided into two major groups: myositis-associated antibodies and myositis-specific antibodies.

Myositis-Associated Antibodies. A number of antibodies have been described in patients with myositis and other connective tissue disorders, such as anti-Ku and

Table 3.3 Autoantibodies in Muscle Diseases

Antibody	Clinical Syndrome
Myositis-associated antibodies	—
Anti-Ku	Myositis/scleroderma overlap syndrome
Anti–Pm-Scl	—
Anti–nuclear ribonucleoprotein	Mixed connective tissue disease
Myositis-specific antibodies	—
Antibodies to tRNA synthetases (anti–Jo-1, anti–PL-7, anti–PL-12, anti-OJ, anti-EJ, anti-KS)	"Antisynthetase syndrome": refractory PM/DM with interstitial lung disease, Raynaud's phenomenon, mechanic's hands, inflammatory arthropathy, fever
Antibodies to signal recognition particle	Refractory PM with congestive heart failure, poor response to corticosteroids, more common in blacks
Anti–Mi-2	DM, good response to corticosteroids
Anti-Mas	PM/DM, after alcoholic rhabdomyolysis
Anti-Fer	Nodular myositis
Anti-KJ	PM, pulmonary fibrosis
Antibody to chondroitin sulfate C moiety of decorin	Myopathy associated with Waldenström's macroglobulinemia

DM = dermatomyositis; PM = polymyositis; tRNA = transfer ribonucleic acid.

anti–Pm-Scl in myositis-scleroderma overlap syndromes,[185,186] and antibodies to nuclear ribonucleoprotein in mixed connective tissue disease.[187] Anti-Ku antibodies target Ku protein, a regulatory subunit of a DNA-dependent protein kinase.[188] The antigenic target for anti–Pm-Scl antibodies is a complex of 11–16 nuclear proteins whose function is unclear, although a role in periribosomal particle assembly is suggested. Antinuclear antibody testing gives a strong nucleolar staining pattern, consistent with the predominant nucleolar localization.[189,190] Other autoantibodies, such as antibodies to calpastatin, annexin XI, SS-A/Ro, and heat shock protein, have been described in patients with myositis. These are also found in other diseases, such as systemic lupus erythematosus, scleroderma, Sjögren's syndrome, and rheumatoid arthritis.[185,186,191] DM and PM have also been reported in association with the antiphospholipid antibody syndrome.[192] These antibodies are termed *myositis-associated antibodies.*

Myositis-Specific Antibodies. Myositis-specific antibodies are found only in patients with inflammatory myopathies (PM, DM) and target antigens involved in cellular protein synthesis. They may be divided into four major groups. The first group consists of autoantibodies to aminoacyl-transfer RNA synthetases. These synthetases catalyze the attachment of an amino acid to its transfer RNA (tRNA) in an adenosine triphosphate–dependent process during protein synthesis. Antibodies against several aminoacyl tRNA synthetases have been identified. These include anti–Jo-1 against histidyl tRNA synthetase, anti–PL-7 against threonyl tRNA synthetase, anti–PL-12 against alanyl tRNA synthetase, anti-OJ against isoleucyl tRNA synthetase, anti-EJ against glycyl tRNA synthetase, and anti-KS against asparaginyl tRNA synthetase.[193–198] Of these, the anti–Jo-1 autoantibodies are the most common.

The second group consists of antibodies directed against specific subunits of the signal recognition particle (SRP). The SRP is a small cytoplasmic RNA protein complex involved in regulating the translocation of newly synthesized proteins across the endoplasmic reticulum membrane.[199,200]

Antibodies against the Mi-2 antigen are almost exclusive to patients with dermatomyositis, including some patients with juvenile dermatomyositis.[201,202] The antigen is a 240-kDa protein that forms part of the molecular complex of several polypeptide chains.[203] The complementary DNA encoding this protein has been cloned and exhibits homology with helicase enzymes that are involved in regulating genomic replication, expression, and repair.[204]

Finally, there is a miscellaneous group of myositis-specific antibodies that is less well defined, such as anti-Fer, anti-Mas, and anti-KJ. Fer, Mas, and KJ are tRNA-related antigens. The exact role of these proteins is unclear. Anti-Fer is directed toward elongation factor 1-α. The target for anti-KJ is translation factor.[205]

Assays for these antibodies are probably not indicated in the initial evaluation of patients with inflammatory myopathies. These antibodies are found in 50% or fewer patients with DM and PM and are absent in IBM.[206] There is evidence that these antibodies may be involved in the pathogenesis of the disease.[207] In addition, several relatively homogenous clinical syndromes have been associated with some of these antibodies. The "antisynthetase syndrome" is comprised of PM or DM, interstitial lung disease, Raynaud's phenomenon, inflammatory arthropathy, fever, and "mechanic's hands" in association with anti–Jo-1 antibody. *Mechanic's hands* refers to hyperkeratosis and cracking of the skin over the palms and fingers. The clinical course is often characterized by refractory disease with relapses.[193,206]

Antibodies to the SRP are found in 5% of patients with PM. They are associated with severe, refractory myositis with both proximal and distal weakness and high serum creatine kinase levels. Blacks are disproportionately affected. Cardiac complications with congestive heart failure may occur, but features of the antisynthetase syndrome are absent. The response to corticosteroids is poor.[200] The 5-year survival in one study was only 25%.[194]

Although anti–Mi-2 antibodies are specific for DM, they are only seen in approximately 15–20% of patients.[200] This antibody is often associated with skin rash of two types: the "V" sign, involving the base of the neck and upper chest, and the "shawl" sign over the shoulder and upper back. These patients usually have a good therapeutic response to corticosteroids.[206]

Anti-Mas antibodies have been identified in patients with PM and DM after alcoholic rhabdomyolysis.[194,208,209] Anti-Fer antibody is associated with nodular myositis. The clinical association of anti-KJ antibody is PM with pulmonary fibrosis, similar to the antisynthetase syndrome.[208,209]

The anti–Pm-Scl antibody is associated with myositis that overlaps with systemic sclerosis and is found in 5–15% of patients with myositis.[186] The syndrome resembles the antisynthetase syndrome in its extramuscular manifestations. However, unlike the antisynthetase syndrome, the myositis associated with anti–Pm-Scl antibodies is often mild and corticosteroid responsive, with a good prognosis and high 5-year survival rate.[186,189,210]

Clinical Role of Autoantibody Testing in Inflammatory Myopathies. The diagnostic role of the myositis-specific antibodies in the clinical setting is limited at present. The low sensitivity (50%) makes it unlikely that they will replace conventional testing, such as muscle enzymes, electromyography, and biopsy, in patients with suspected PM or DM. However, they may be useful in certain clinical situations. It may be prudent to test patients with PM or DM for anti–Jo-1 antibodies before treatment with methotrexate, which is known to cause pulmonary fibrosis. In patients in whom the diagnosis of IBM versus PM is considered, the identification of a myositis-specific antibody rules out IBM. A positive test for these antibodies may be diagnostically useful in situations wherein the muscle biopsy is inconclusive. Targoff and colleagues have suggested adding testing for myositis-specific antibodies to the criteria for diagnosis of the inflammatory myopathies.[211] In addition, the myositis-specific antibodies help to delineate relatively homogenous patient populations with specific clinical features and prognostic implications, including response to corticosteroids, as previously discussed.

Other Myopathies

A noninflammatory myopathy with slowly progressive symmetric proximal weakness and high creatine kinase has been reported in association with Waldenström's macroglobulinemia. Monoclonal IgM from the patient's serum bound to the surface of muscle fibers.[212] The antigenic target was identified as muscle decorin, a proteoglycan found in the extracellular matrix of many tissues. Decorin is thought to have a role in extracellular matrix assembly and interaction.[213] The IgM antibody bound to the chondroitin sulfate C moiety of decorin. The test may be useful in identifying autoimmune myopathies, especially in the context of paraproteinemia. More information is necessary before the utility of this assay in the clinical setting can be determined.

PARANEOPLASTIC SYNDROMES INVOLVING THE PERIPHERAL NERVOUS SYSTEM

Antineuronal nuclear antibody type 1, also called anti-Hu antibody, was first reported by Croft and co-workers[214] in four patients with inflammatory sensory polyganglionopathy associated with small cell carcinoma of the lung and confirmed by a fluorescent antibody technique by Wilkinson and Zeromski.[215] These antibodies have since been reported in patients with paraneoplastic myelitis and autonomic dysfunction.[216] The antibodies react strongly with the nuclei and faintly with the cytoplasm of neurons in the brain, spinal cord, dorsal root ganglia. and myenteric plexus. They are targeted against a number of neuronal RNA-binding proteins, including HuD, HuC, and Hel-N1.[217–219] The great majority of small cell lung carcinomas express the Hu proteins, whether or not they are associated with a paraneoplastic syndrome. Intrathecal synthesis of anti-Hu antibody has been reported.[220] However, evidence of direct neuronal damage by the anti-Hu antibody has not yet been established.[221] The observation of infiltration by CD8+ lymphocytes in involved tissue suggests that cell-mediated immunity may be involved in neuronal damage.[222,223]

Subacute sensory neuronopathy may be paraneoplastic or nonparaneoplastic. The paraneoplastic form is associated with anti-Hu antibodies in the great majority of patients. The specificity and sensitivity of anti-Hu antibody testing for paraneoplastic sensory neuronopathy is high.[224,225] The test is available commercially and is invaluable in the evaluation of patients with subacute ataxic neuropathy. A positive assay mandates investigation for underlying cancer, most often small cell lung cancer. Sensory neuronopathy may also complicate Sjögren's syndrome, in which the only clue to the diagnosis may be markedly elevated antinuclear antibody titers.[226] SS-A/Ro and SS-B/La antibodies are found in 55% and 25–40% of patients with Sjögren's syndrome, respectively.

Motor neuron disease may rarely be associated with systemic cancer. Motor neuron involvement may be part of the paraneoplastic syndrome associated with anti-Hu antibodies. In patients in whom the motor neuron disorder is part of more extensive involvement with sensory abnormalities, ataxia, or autonomic dysfunction, testing for anti-Hu antibodies is appropriate.

Breast cancer is associated with an upper motor neuron syndrome resembling primary lateral sclerosis.[227] Ferracci and colleagues have reported a patient presenting with a lower motor neuron syndrome 4 months before developing breast cancer. This patient had autoantibodies directed against an undefined antigen concentrated at the axonal initial segments and nodes of Ranvier.[228]

Amphiphysin is a synaptic vesicle-associated protein that is related to endocytosis along with α-adaptin and dynamin, which are also expressed at presynaptic nerve terminals.[229] Antibody to amphiphysin has been reported in SMS associated with breast cancer.[230,231] Antoine and colleagues[232] have recently reported antiamphiphysin antibodies in sensory neuronopathy and encephalomyelitis, limbic encephalitis, LEMS, and paraneoplastic cerebellar degeneration. The cancers associated with the antibody were not specific and included breast cancer, small cell lung cancer, and ovarian carcinoma. Some patients also had other antibodies, such as antibodies to the VGCC in LEMS and anti-Hu antibody in limbic encephalitis. In contrast to anti-Hu antibodies that correlate strongly with the neurologic syndrome and the tumor association, antiamphiphysin antibodies do not appear to be specific for either one. In addition, the intracellular location of amphiphysin argues against a direct pathogenic role for the antiamphiphysin antibodies.

CONNECTIVE TISSUE DISORDERS, VASCULITIDES, AND OTHER SYSTEMIC DISEASES

Finally, PNS involvement as part of systemic involvement deserves brief mention. Autoimmune peripheral neuropathy may be a feature of diseases, such as necrotizing arteritis associated with systemic lupus erythematosus, Sjögren's syndrome, rheumatoid arthritis, systemic sclerosis, and the vasculitides, such as polyarteritis nodosa, microscopic polyangiitis, Wegener's granulomatosis, and allergic granulomatosis of Churg-Strauss.[233,234] In these conditions, the autoantibody association is that of the primary disease process. Antinuclear antibody and antibody to double-stranded DNA are useful in the diagnosis of systemic lupus erythematosus. Antineutrophil cytoplasmic antibody assay is positive in more than 90% of patients with Wegener's granulomatosis.[235] GM-1 ganglioside antibodies and cryoglobulins have been reported in systemic lupus erythematosus with peripheral neuropathy.[236,237] Peripheral neuropathy is a rare manifestation of systemic sclerosis.[238] The CREST syndrome (*c*alcinosis cutis, *R*aynaud's phenomenon, *e*sophageal dysmotility, *s*clerodactyly, *t*elangiectasia), a limited form of systemic sclerosis, may be associated with mononeuritis multiplex with vasculitic features.[239] These patients have anticentromere antibodies.[240]

Peripheral neuropathy and myopathy may complicate celiac disease. Neuromuscular symptoms may be the presenting feature of celiac disease without overt gastrointestinal symptoms. The diagnosis is made by the presence of antigliadin and antireticulin antibodies and small bowel biopsy.[241]

Although not autoantibody assays, there are other immunologic tests that are useful in the evaluation of patients with peripheral neuropathies. These include testing for hepatitis B and C antigenemia in patients with cryoglobulinemia, serologic testing for human immunodeficiency virus, human T-lymphotropic virus-1 (HTLV-1), cytomegalovirus, and Lyme disease in the appropriate clinical settings.

CONCLUSIONS

Advances in neuroimmunology result in the identification of an ever-increasing number of potential antigenic targets in the PNS. These advances enable insights into the pathogenesis of autoimmune disorders involving the nervous system as well as identify autoimmune disorders whose etiopathogenesis was previously unknown. The therapeutic implications are encouraging. However, in practice, the clinical syndrome should dictate relevant testing. Additionally, as with any laboratory test, it is important that the results be interpreted in light of the clinical and electrophysiologic data. Panels or profiles of autoantibodies for the evaluation of peripheral neuropathies are commercially available. However, the antibodies do not define clinical syndromes, and therapeutic decisions are not made solely on the basis of the results of autoantibody testing. There is also evidence to suggest that these commercially available "panels" are not cost-effective.[242] Hence, the routine use of these panels or profiles is discouraged. At the present time, the clinical applications of autoantibody testing in neuromuscular diseases may be summarized as follows:

- In patients with stiffness and muscle spasms, testing for anti-GAD antibodies assists in confirming the diagnosis of SMS, although a negative assay does not rule it out.
- Measurement of GM-1 ganglioside antibodies helps support a diagnosis of MMN in the correct clinical context. In patients with chronic lower motor neuron syndromes without detectable conduction blocks, high-titer IgM anti–GM-1 ganglioside antibodies in serum may identify patients with motor neuropathies that may be immune-mediated and responsive to immunomodulation. The specificity of low titer positivity of these antibodies is limited. Although the antibodies may be detected in acute motor neuropathies, such as GBS, their relevance in this setting is less clear.
- Serum anti–GQ-1b antibodies are highly sensitive and specific for Miller Fisher syndrome and suggest an immune-mediated pathogenesis responsive to immunomodulatory therapies. The assay is also useful in the evaluation of patients with acute ophthalmoparesis, in whom elevated titers suggest a variant of GBS.[243] However, decisions regarding therapy are usually made before the results of the assay are available.
- Anti-MAG antibodies suggest an immune-mediated neuropathy usually, but not invariably, associated with IgM paraproteinemia and mandate an evaluation for plasma cell dyscrasia. The response to immunosuppression is, however, not impressive.

- Patients with sensory neuronopathy should be evaluated for anti-Hu, SS-A, SS-B, and fluorescent antinuclear antibody. A positive anti-Hu assay should prompt investigation for an underlying malignancy.
- Testing for antibodies to the P/Q type VGCC is the single best way of confirming a diagnosis of LEMS. False-positive results are rare, and the clinical scenario is useful in differentiating them from LEMS.
- AChR-binding antibody assay is the most sensitive assay for MG, being positive in approximately 85% of patients with generalized MG and in 50–70% of ocular MG. In patients with a negative assay, the modulating antibody assay may increase the diagnostic yield. Striational antibodies may help make the diagnosis if the foregoing tests are negative. Striational antibodies may also serve to increase the suspicion of thymoma.
- The utility of myositis-specific antibodies for the diagnosis of PM and DM is limited. They may help to differentiate PM from IBM when the muscle biopsy is inconclusive and serve to identify relatively homogenous patient groups with respect to extramuscular manifestations, response to corticosteroids, and prognosis.

Acknowledgments

I dedicate this work to the memory of my father, Dr. V. Narayanaswami. I am indebted to my husband Rajan and my sister Padma for their help and encouragement, without which this chapter could not have been completed. I would like to thank Ronald F. Pfeiffer, M.D., Vice Chairman, Department of Neurology, University of Tennessee, Memphis, for his valuable suggestions.

REFERENCES

1. Patrick J, Lindstrom JP. Autoimmune response to acetylcholine receptor. Science 1973;180: 871–872.
2. Patrick J, Lindstrom JP, Culp B, McMillan J. Studies on purified eel acetylcholine receptor and acetylcholine receptor antibody. Proc Natl Acad Sci U S A 1973;70:3334–3338.
3. Ho TW, Willison HJ, Nachamkin I, et al. Anti-GD-1a antibody is associated with axonal but not demyelinating forms of Guillain-Barré syndrome. Ann Neurol 1999;45:168–173.
4. Hadden RD, Cornblath DR, Hughes RAC, et al. Electrophysiologic classification of Guillain-Barré syndrome: clinical associations and outcome. Plasma exchange/Sandoglobulin Guillain-Barré syndrome trial group. Ann Neurol 1998;44:780–788.
5. Quarles RH, Weiss MD. Autoantibodies associated with peripheral neuropathy. Muscle Nerve 1999;22(7):800–822.
6. Archelos JJ, Hartung HP. Pathogenetic role of autoantibodies in neurologic diseases. Trends Neurosci 2000;23:317–323.
7. Moersch FP, Woltman HW. Progressive fluctuating muscular rigidity and spasm ("stiff-man" syndrome): report of a case and some observations in 13 other cases. Mayo Clin Proc 1956;31: 421–427.
8. Solimena M, Folli F, Denis-Donini S, et al. Autoantibodies to glutamic acid decarboxylase in a patient with stiff-man syndrome, epilepsy and type I diabetes mellitus. N Engl J Med 1988;318: 1012–1020.
9. Solimena M, Folli F, Aparisi R, et al. Autoantibodies to GABA-ergic neurons and pancreatic beta cells in stiff-man syndrome. N Engl J Med 1990;322:1555–1560.
10. Solimena M, Butler MH, DeCamilli P. GAD, diabetes and stiff-man syndrome: some progress and more questions. J Endocrinol Invest 1994;17:509–520.
11. Vincent A, Grimaldi LM, Martino G, et al. Antibodies to 125I-glutamic acid decarboxylase in patients with stiff man syndrome. J Neurol Neurosurg Psychiatry 1997;62:395–397.

12. Ellis MT, Atkinson MA. The clinical significance of an autoimmune response against glutamic acid decarboxylase. Nat Med 1996;2:148–153.
13. Dinkel K, Meinck HM, Jury KM, et al. Inhibition of gamma-aminobutyric acid synthesis by glutamic acid decarboxylase autoantibodies in stiff-man syndrome. Ann Neurol 1998;44:194–201.
14. Floeter MK. Inhibitory pathways defined by electrophysiology. In LM Levy (moderator). The stiff-person syndrome: an autoimmune disorder affecting neurotransmission of γ-aminobutyric acid. Ann Intern Med 1999;131:523–524.
15. Daw K, Ujihara N, Atkinson M, Powers AC. Glutamic acid decarboxylase autoantibodies in stiff-man syndrome and insulin-dependent diabetes mellitus exhibit similarities and differences in epitope recognition. J Immunol 1996;156:818–825.
16. Solimena M, De Camilli P. Autoimmunity to glutamic acid decarboxylase (GAD) in stiff-man syndrome and insulin-dependent diabetes mellitus. Trends Neurosci 1991;14:452–457.
17. Brown P, Marsden CD. The stiff man and stiff man plus syndromes. J Neurol 1999;246:648–652.
18. Dalakas MC. Autoantibodies and immunopathogenesis of the stiff-person syndrome. In LM Levy (moderator). The stiff-person syndrome: an autoimmune disorder affecting neurotransmission of γ-aminobutyric acid. Ann Intern Med 1999;131:523–524.
19. Werk EE, Sholiton LJ, Marnell RT. The "stiff-man" syndrome and hyperthyroidism. Am J Med 1961;31:647–653.
20. Williams AC, Nutt JG, Hare T. Autoimmunity in stiff-man syndrome. Lancet 1988;2(8604):222.
21. Skok VI. Nicotinic acetylcholine receptors in the neurons of autonomic ganglia. J Auton Nerv Syst 1987;21:91–99.
22. Rust G, Burgunder JM, Lauterburg TE, Cachelin AB. Expression of neuronal nicotinic acetylcholine receptor subunit genes in the rat autonomic nervous system. Eur J Neurosci 1994;6:478–485.
23. Conroy W, Berg DK. Neurons can maintain multiple classes of nicotinic acetylcholine receptors distinguished by different subunit compositions. J Biol Chem 1995;270:4424–4431.
24. Vernino S, Adamski J, Kryzer TJ, et al. Neuronal nicotinic Ach receptor antibody in subacute autonomic neuropathy and cancer-related syndromes. Neurology 1998;50:1806–1813.
25. Pande R, Leis AA. Myasthenia gravis, thymoma, intestinal pseudo-obstruction, and neuronal nicotinic acetylcholine receptor antibody. Muscle Nerve 1999;22:1600–1602.
26. Vernino S, Low PA, Fealey RD, et al. Autoantibodies to ganglionic acetylcholine receptors in autoimmune autonomic neuropathies. N Engl J Med 2000;343:847–855.
27. Hartung HP, Willisen H, Jung S, et al. Autoimmune responses in peripheral nerve. Springer Sem Immunopathol 1995;18:97–123.
28. Hartung HP, Kieseier RC. Antibody responses in the Guillain-Barré syndrome. J Neurol Sci 1999;168:75–77.
29. Gabriel CM, Gregson NA, Hughes RAC. Anti-PMP22 antibodies in patients with inflammatory neuropathy. J Neuroimmunol 2000;104:139–146.
30. Ropper AH, Gorson KC. Neuropathies associated with paraproteinemia. N Engl J Med 1998;338(22):1601–1607.
31. Hays AP, Latov N, Takatsu M, Sherman WH. Experimental demyelination of nerve induced by serum of patients with neuropathy and an anti-MAG IgM protein. Neurology 1987;37:242–256.
32. Tatum AH. Experimental paraprotein neuropathy, demyelination by passive transfer of human IgM anti-myelin-associated-glycoprotein. Ann Neurol 1993;33:502–506.
33. Pestronk A. Motor neuropathies, motor neuron disorders and antiglycolipid antibodies. Muscle Nerve 1991;14:927–936.
34. Latov N. Antibodies to glycoconjugates in neuropathy and motor neuron disease. Prog Brain Res 1994;101:295–304.
35. Griffin JW. Antiglycolipid antibodies and peripheral neuropathies: links to pathogenesis. Prog Brain Res 1994;101:313–323.
36. Pestronk A, Cornblath DR, Ilyas AA, et al. A treatable multifocal neuropathy with antibodies to GM1 ganglioside. Ann Neurol 1988;63:28–34.
37. O'Hanlon GM, Paterson GJ, Veitch J, et al. Mapping immunoreactive epitopes in the human peripheral nervous system using human monoclonal anti-GM1 ganglioside antibodies. Acta Neuropathol 1998;95:605–618.
38. Sheikh KA, Deerinck TJ, Ellisman MH, Griffin JW. The distribution of ganglioside-like moieties in peripheral nerves. Brain 1999;122:449–460.
39. Weber F, Rudel R, Aulkemeyer P, Brinkmeier H. Anti-GM1 antibodies can block neuronal voltage-gated sodium channels. Muscle Nerve 2000;23:1414–1420.

40. Fredman P, Lekman A. Glycosphingolipids as potential diagnostic markers and/or antigens in neurological disorders. Neurochem Res 1997;22:1071–1083.

41. Fredman P. The role of antiglycolipid antibodies in neurological disorders. Ann N Y Acad Sci 1998;845:341–352.

42. Nemni R, Fazio R, Quatrini A, et al. Antibodies to sulfatide and to chondroitin sulfate C in patients with chronic sensory neuropathy. J Neuroimmunol 1993;43:79–85.

43. Jungalwala FB. Expression and biological functions of sulfoglucuronyl glycolipids (SGGLS) in the nervous system—a review. Neurochem Res 1994;19:945–957.

44. Manfredini E, Nobile-Orazio E, Allaria S, Scarlato G. Anti-alpha- and beta tubulin IgM antibodies in dysimmune neuropathies. J Neurol Sci 1995;133:79–84.

45. Braxton DB, Williams M, Kamali D, et al. Specificity of human anti-neurofilament autoantibodies. J Neuroimmunol 1989;21:193–203.

46. Aquino DA, Margolis RU, Margolis RK. Immunocytochemical localization of a chondroitin sulfate proteoglycan in nervous tissue. I. Adult brain, retina and peripheral nerve. J Cell Biol 1984;99: 1117–1129.

47. Aquino DA, Margolis RU, Margolis RK. Immunocytochemical localization of a chondroitin sulfate proteoglycan in nervous tissue. II. Role in the developing brain. J Cell Biol 1984;99:1130–1139.

48. Freddo L, Yu RK, Latov N, et al. Gangliosides GM1 and GD1b are antigens for IgM M-protein in a patient with motor neuron disease. Neurology 1986;36:454–458.

49. Niebroj-Dobosz I, Jamrozik Z, Janik P, et al. Anti-neural antibodies in serum and cerebrospinal fluid of amyotrophic lateral sclerosis (ALS) patients. Acta Neurol Scand 1999;100:238–243.

50. Pestronk A, Adams RN, Clawson L, et al. Serum antibodies to GM1 ganglioside in amyotrophic lateral sclerosis. Neurology 1988;38:1457–1461.

51. Pestronk A, Adams RN, Cornblath D, et al. Patterns of serum IgM antibodies to GM1 and GD1a gangliosides in amyotrophic lateral sclerosis. Ann Neurol 1989;25:98–102.

52. Shy ME, Evans VA, Lublin FD, et al. Antibodies to GM1 and GD1b in patients with motor neuron disease without plasma cell dyscrasia. Ann Neurol 1989;25:511–513.

53. Illa I, Leon-Monzon M, Agboatwalla M, et al. Antiganglioside antibodies in patients with acute polio and post-polio syndrome. Ann N Y Acad Sci 1995;753:374–377.

54. Masselli RA, Wollman RL, Leung C, et al. Neuromuscular transmission in amyotrophic lateral sclerosis. Muscle Nerve 1993;16:1193–1203.

55. Fratantoni SA, Weisz G, Pardal AM, et al. Amyotrophic lateral sclerosis IgG-treated neuromuscular junctions develop sensitivity to L-type calcium channel blocker. Muscle Nerve 2000;23:543–550.

56. Brooks BR. El Escorial World Federation of Neurology criteria for the diagnosis of amyotrophic lateral sclerosis. J Neurol Sci 1994;124(Suppl):96–107.

57. Revised criteria for the diagnosis of amyotrophic lateral sclerosis. World Federation of Neurology, 1998. Available at: http://www.wfnals.org/Articles/elescorial1998criteria.htm. Accessed February 2001.

58. Chaudhry V, Corse A, Cornblath DR, et al. Multifocal motor neuropathy: electrodiagnostic features. Muscle Nerve 1994:17:198–205.

59. Pakiam ASI, Parry GJ. Multifocal motor neuropathy without overt conduction block. Muscle Nerve 1998;21:243–245.

60. Kornberg AJ, Pestronk A. Chronic motor neuropathies: diagnosis, therapy and pathogenesis. Ann Neurol 1995:37(Suppl 1):S43–S50.

61. Kaji R, Kusunoki S, Mizutani K, et al. Chronic motor axonal neuropathy associated with antibodies monospecific for N-acetylgalactosaminyl GD1a. Muscle Nerve 2000;23:702–706.

62. Ilyas AA, Mithen FA, Dalakas MC, et al. Antibodies to acidic glycolipids in Guillain–Barré syndrome and chronic inflammatory demyelinating polyneuropathy. J Neurol Sci 1992;107: 111–121.

63. Chiba A, Kusonoki S, Shimizu T, Kanazawa I. Serum IgG antibody to ganglioside GQ1b is a possible marker of Miller-Fisher Syndrome. Ann Neurol 1992;31:667–669.

64. Chiba A, Kusonoki S, Obata H, et al. Serum anti-GQ1b antibody is associated with ophthalmoplegia in Miller-Fisher syndrome and Guillain-Barré syndrome: clinical and immunohistochemical studies. Neurology 1993;43:1911–1917.

65. Kornberg AJ, Pestronk A, Blume GM, et al. Selective staining of the cerebellar molecular layer by serum IgG in Miller-Fisher and related syndromes. Neurology 1996;47:1317–1320.

66. Carpo M, Pedotti R, Allaria S, et al. Clinical presentation and outcome of Guillain-Barré and related syndromes in relation to anti-ganglioside antibodies. J Neurol Sci 1999;168:78–84.

67. Buchwald R, Bufler J, Carpo M, et al. Combined pre- and post-synaptic action of IgG antibodies in Miller Fisher syndrome. Neurology 2001;56:67–74.

68. Yuki N, Yoshino H, Sato S, et al. Severe acute axonal form of Guillain-Barré syndrome associated with IgG anti-GD1a antibodies. Muscle Nerve 1992;15:89–903.

69. Rees JH, Gregson NA, Hughes RAC. Anti-ganglioside GM1 antibodies in Guillain-Barré syndrome and their relationship to *Campylobacter jejuni* infection. Ann Neurol 1995;38:809–816.

70. Sheikh KA, Nachamkin I, Ho TW, et al. *Campylobacter jejuni* lipopolysaccharides in Guillain-Barré syndrome: molecular mimicry and host susceptibility. Neurology 1998;51:371–378.

71. Kaida K, Kusunoki S, Kamakura K, et al. Guillain-Barré syndrome with antibody to a ganglioside, N-acetylgalactosaminyl GD1a. Brain 2000;123:116–124.

72. Irie S, Saito T, Nakamura K, et al. Association of anti-GM2 antibodies in Guillain-Barré syndrome with acute cytomegalovirus infection. J Neuroimmunol 1996;68:19–26.

73. Jacobs BC, van Doorn PA, Groeneveld JH, et al. Cytomegalovirus infections and anti-GM2 antibodies in Guillain-Barré syndrome. J Neurol Neurosurg Psychiatry 1997;62:641–643.

74. Visser LH, van der Meche FG, Meulstee J, et al. Cytomegalovirus infection and Guillain-Barré syndrome: the clinical, electrophysiologic and prognostic features. Dutch Guillain-Barré study group. Neurology 1996;47:668–673.

75. Jacobs PC, van Doorn PA, Schmitz PIM, et al. *Campylobacter jejuni* infections and anti-GM1 antibodies in Guillain-Barré syndrome. Ann Neurol 1996;40:181–187.

76. Kuwabara S, Mori M, Ogawara K, et al. Intravenous immunoglobulin therapy for Guillain-Barré syndrome with IgG anti-GM1 antibody. Muscle Nerve 2001;24:54–58.

77. Yuki N, Tagawa Y, Handa S. Autoantibodies to peripheral nerve glycosphingolipids SPG, SLPG and SGPG in Guillain-Barré syndrome and chronic inflammatory demyelinating polyneuropathy. J Neuroimmunol 1996;70:1–6.

78. Melendez-Vasquez C, Redford J, Choudhary PP, et al. Immunological investigation of chronic inflammatory demyelinating polyradiculoneuropathy. J Neuroimmunol 1997;73:124–134.

79. Connolly AM, Pestronk A, Trotter JL, et al. High-titer selective serum anti-beta-tubulin antibodies in chronic inflammatory demyelinating polyneuropathy. Neurology 1993;43:809–814.

80. Connolly AM, Pestronk A, Mehta S, et al. Serum IgM monoclonal autoantibody binding to the 301 to 314 amino acid epitope of beta-tubulin: clinical association with slowly progressive demyelinating polyneuropathy. Neurology 1997;48:243–248.

81. van Schaik IN, Vermeulen M, van Doorn PA, Brand A. Anti-beta-tubulin antibodies have no diagnostic value in patients with chronic inflammatory demyelinating polyneuropathy. J Neurol 1995;242:599–603.

82. Simmons Z, Albers JW, Bromberg MB, Feldman EL. Presentation and initial clinical course in patients with chronic inflammatory demyelinating polyradiculoneuropathy: comparison of patients without and with monoclonal gammopathy. Neurology 1993;43:2202–2209.

83. Notermans NC, Franssen H, Eurelings M, et al. Diagnostic criteria for demyelinating polyneuropathy associated with monoclonal gammopathy. Muscle Nerve 2000;23:73–79.

84. Gorson KC, Allam G, Ropper AH. Chronic inflammatory demyelinating polyneuropathy: clinical features and response to treatment in 67 consecutive patients with and without a monoclonal gammopathy. Neurology 1997;48:321–328.

85. Antoine JC, Mosnier JF, Lapras J, et al. Chronic inflammatory demyelinating polyneuropathy associated with carcinoma. J Neurol Neurosurg Psychiatry 1996;60:188–190.

86. Weiss MD, Luciano CA, Semino-Mora C, et al. Molecular mimicry in chronic inflammatory demyelinating polyneuropathy and melanoma. Neurology 1998;51:1738–1741.

87. Pestronk A, Choksi R. Multifocal motor neuropathy: serum IgM anti-GM1 ganglioside antibodies in most patients detected using covalent linkage of GM1 to ELISA plates. Neurology 1997;49:1289–1292.

88. Sadiq SA, Thomas FP, Kilidireas K, et al. The spectrum of neurologic disease associated with anti-GM1 antibodies. Neurology 1990;40:1067–1072.

89. Parry GJG. Antiganglioside antibodies do not necessarily play a role in multifocal motor neuropathy. Muscle Nerve 1994;17:97–99.

90. Pestronk A, Lopate G, Kronberg AJ, et al. Distal lower motor neuron syndrome with high-titer serum IgM anti-GM1 antibodies: improvement following immunotherapy with monthly plasma exchange and intravenous cyclophosphamide. Neurology 1994;44:2027–2031.

91. Tsai CP, Lin KP, Liao KK, et al. Immunosuppressive treatment in lower motor neuron syndrome with autoantibodies against GM1 ganglioside. Eur Neurol 1993;33:446–449.

92. Pestronk A, Li F, Griffin J, et al. Polyneuropathy syndromes associated with serum antibodies to sulfatide and myelin-associated glycoprotein. Neurology 1991;41:357–362.

93. Notermans NC, Wokke JHJ, Franssen H, et al. Chronic idiopathic polyneuropathy presenting in middle or old age: a clinical and electrophysiological study of 75 patients. J Neurol Neurosurg Psychiatry 1993;56:1066–1071.

94. Periquet M, Novak V, Collins MP, et al. Painful sensory neuropathy: prospective evaluation using skin biopsy. Neurology 1999;53:1641–1647.

95. Dabby R, Weimer LH, Hays AP, et al. Antisulfatide antibodies in neuropathy: clinical and electrophysiologic correlates. Neurology 2000;54:1448–1452.

96. Busis N, Pestronk A. Neuropathy with anti-sulfatide antibodies: response to treatment. Muscle Nerve 1994;17:1120.

97. Kincaid JC, Horak HA. Painful neuropathy and sulfatides: causation or coincidence. J Clin Neuromusc Dis 2000;1:159–163.

98. Griffin JW, Hsieh S-T, McArthur JC, Cornblath DR. Laboratory testing in peripheral nerve disease. Neurol Clin 1996;14:119–133.

99. Gordon PH, Rowland LP, Younger DS, et al. Lymphoproliferative disorders and motor neuron disease: an update. Neurology 1997;48:1671–1678.

100. Rowland LP, Sherman WL, Hays AP, et al. Autopsy-proven amyotrophic lateral sclerosis, Waldenstrom's macroglobulinemia and antibodies to sulfated glucuronic acid paragloboside. Neurology 1995;45:827–829.

101. Kissel JT, Mendell JR. Neuropathies associated with monoclonal gammopathies. Neuromuscul Disord 1996;6:3–18.

102. Gosselin S, Kyle RA, Dyck PJ. Neuropathy associated with monoclonal gammopathies of uncertain significance. Ann Neurol 1991;30:54–61.

103. Yeung KB, Thomas PK, King RH, et al. The clinical spectrum of peripheral neuropathies associated with benign monoclonal IgM, IgG and IgA paraproteinemia: comparative clinical, immunological and nerve biopsy findings. J Neurol 1991;238:383–391.

104. Younger DS, Rowland LP, Latov N, et al. Motor neuron disease and amyotrophic lateral sclerosis: relation of high CSF protein content to paraproteinemia and clinical syndromes. Neurology 1990;40:595–599.

105. Latov N, Hays P, Sherman WH. Peripheral neuropathy and anti-MAG antibody. Crit Rev Neurobiol 1988;3:301–332.

106. Mariette X, Chastang C, Clavelou P, et al. A randomised clinical trial comparing interferon-alpha and intravenous immunoglobulin in polyneuropathy associated with monoclonal IgM. The IgM-associated Polyneuropathy Study Group. J Neurol Neurosurg Psychiatry 1997;63:28–34.

107. Ellie E, Vital A, Steck A, et al. Neuropathy associated with "benign" anti-myelin-associated glycoprotein IgM gammopathy: clinical, immunological, neurophysiological, pathological findings and response to treatment in 33 cases. J Neurol 1996;243:34–43.

108. Mendell JR, Sahenk Z, Whitaker JN, et al. Polyneuropathy and IgM monoclonal gammopathy: studies on the pathogenic role of anti-myelin-associated glycoprotein antibody. Ann Neurol 1985;17:243–254.

109. Gabriel JM, Erne B, Miescher GC, et al. Selective loss of myelin-associated glycoprotein from myelin correlates with anti-MAG antibody titer in demyelinating paraproteinaemic polyneuropathy. Brain 1996;119:775–787.

110. van den Berg LH, Hays AP, Nobile-Orazio E, et al. Anti-MAG and anti-SGPG antibodies in neuropathy. Muscle Nerve 1996;19:637–643.

111. Notermans NC, Wokke JHJ, van den Berg LH, et al. Chronic idiopathic axonal polyneuropathy: comparison of patients with and without monoclonal gammopathy. Brain 1996;119:421–427.

112. Sherman WH, Latov N, Hays AP, et al. Monoclonal IgM kappa antibody precipitating with chondroitin sulfate C from patients with axonal polyneuropathy and epidermolysis. Neurology 1983;33:192–201.

113. Lopate G, Parks BJ, Goldstein JM, et al. Polyneuropathies associated with high titer antisulfatide antibodies: characteristics of patients with and without serum monoclonal proteins. J Neurol Neurosurg Psychiatry 1997;62:581–585.

114. Ilyas AA, Cook SD, Dalakas MC, Mithen FA. Anti-MAG IgM paraproteins from some patients with polyneuropathy associated with IgM paraproteinemia also react with sulfatide. J Neuroimmunol 1992;37:85–92.

115. Yee WC, Hahn AF, Hearn SA, Rupar AR. Neuropathy in IgM kappa paraproteinemia. Immunoreactivity to neural proteins and chondroitin sulfate. Acta Neuropathol 1989;78:57–64.

116. Briani C, Berger JS, Latov N. Antibodies to chondroitin sulfate S: a new detection assay and correlations with neurological diseases. J Neuroimmunol 1998;84:117–121.

117. Kelly JJ, Kyle RA, Miles JM, Dyck PJ. Osteosclerotic myeloma and peripheral neuropathy. Neurology 1983;33:202–210.

118. Thomas FP, Lovelace RE, Ding XS, et al. Vasculitic neuropathy in a patient with cryoglobulinemia and anti-MAG IgM monoclonal gammopathy. Muscle Nerve 1992;15:891–898.

119. Keren DF, Warren JS, Lowe JB. Strategy to diagnose monoclonal gammopathies in serum: high resolution electrophoresis, immunofixation and κ/λ quantification. Clin Chem 1988;34:2196–2201.

120. Nobile-Orazio E, Latov N, Hays AP, et al. Neuropathy and anti-MAG antibodies without detectable serum M-protein. Neurology 1984;34:218–221.

121. Notermans NC, Lokhorst HM, Franssen H, et al. Intermittent cyclophosphamide and prednisone treatment of polyneuropathy associated with monoclonal gammopathy of undetermined significance. Neurology 1996;47:1227–1233.

122. Ernerudh J, Brodtkorb E, Olsson T, et al. Peripheral neuropathy and monoclonal IgM with antibody activity against peripheral nerve myelin: effect of plasma exchange. J Neuroimmunol 1986:11:171–178.

123. Mariette X, Chastang C, Clavelou P, et al. A randomized clinical trial comparing interferon-alpha and intravenous immunoglobulin in polyneuropathy associated with monoclonal IgM. The IgM-associated polyneuropathy study group. J Neurol Neurosurg Psychiatry 1997:63:28–34.

124. Eurelings M, Moons KGM, Notermans NC, et al. Neuropathy and IgM M-proteins: prognostic value of antibodies to MAG, SGPG and sulfatide. Neurology 2001;56:228–233.

125. Pestronk A, Choksi R, Bieser K, et al. Treatable gait disorder and polyneuropathy associated with high titer serum IgM binding to antigens that co-purify with myelin associated glycoprotein. Muscle Nerve 1994;17:1293–1300.

126. Newsom-Davis J, Mills KR. Immunological associations of acquired neuromyotonia (Isaacs' syndrome). Brain 1993;116:453–469.

127. Isaacs H. A syndrome of continuous muscle-fiber activity. J Neurol Neurosurg Psychiatry 1961; 24:319–325.

128. Isaacs H. Continuous muscle-fiber activity in an Indian male with additional evidence of terminal motor fibre abnormality. J Neurol Neurosurg Psychiatry 1967;30:126–133.

129. Barber PA, Anderson NE, Vincent A. Morvan's syndrome associated with voltage-gated K+ channel antibodies. Neurology 2000;54:771–772.

130. Lee K, Maselli RA, Ellis WG, Agius MA. Morvan's fibrillary chorea: a paraneoplastic manifestation of thymoma. J Neurol Neurosurg Psychiatry 1998;65:857–862.

131. Vasilescu C, Alexianu M, Dan A. Muscle hypertrophy and a syndrome of continuous motor unit activity in prednisone-responsive Guillain-Barré polyneuropathy. J Neurol 1984;231:276–279.

132. Wakayama Y, Ohbu S, Machida H. Myasthenia gravis, muscle twitch, hyperhidrosis, and limb pain associated with thymoma: proposal of a possible new myasthenic syndrome. Tohoku J Exp Med 1991;164:285–291.

133. Waerness E. Neuromyotonia and bronchial carcinoma. Electromyogr Clin Neurophysiol 1974; 14:527–535.

134. Zifcu U, Drlicek M, Machacek E, et al. Syndrome of continuous muscle fiber activity and plasmacytoma with IgM paraproteinemia. Neurology 1994;44:560–561.

135. Caress JB, Abend WK, Preston DC, Logigian EL. A case of Hodgkin's lymphoma producing neuromyotonia. Neurology 1997;49:258–259.

136. Vincent A. Understanding neuromyotonia. Muscle Nerve 2000;23:655–657.

137. Hart IK. Acquired neuromyotonia: a new autoantibody mediated neuronal potassium channelopathy. Am J Med Sci 2000;319:209–916.

138. Wang H, Kunkel DD, Martin TM, et al. Heteromultimeric potassium channels in terminal and juxtaparanodal regions of neurons. Nature 1993;365:75–79.

139. Rettig J, Heinemann SH, Wunder F, et al. Inactivation properties of voltage-gated potassium channels altered by the presence of beta-subunit. Nature 1994;369:289–294.

140. Hart IK, Waters C, Vincent A, et al. Autoantibodies detected to expressed K+ channels are implicated in neuromyotonia. Ann Neurol 1997;41:238–246.

141. Toyka KV, Zielasek J, Ricker K, et al. Hereditary neuromyotonia: a mouse model associated with deficiency or increased gene dosage of the PMP22 gene. J Neurol Neurosurg Psychiatry 1997;63:812–813.

142. Zielasek J, Martini R, Suter U, Toyka KV. Neuromyotonia in mice with hereditary myelinopathies. Muscle Nerve 2000;23:696–701.

143. Greenberg DA. Neuromuscular disease and calcium channels. Muscle Nerve 1999;22:1341–1349.

144. Stanley EF. The calcium channel and the organization of the presynaptic transmitter release face. Trends Neurosci 1997;20:404–409.

145. Engel AG, Nagel A, Fukuoka T. Motor nerve terminal calcium channels in Lambert-Eaton myasthenic syndrome. Morphologic evidence for depletion and that the depletion is mediated by autoantibodies. Ann N Y Acad Sci 1998;560:278–290.

146. Lennon VA, Kryzer TJ, Griesmann GE, et al. Calcium-channel antibodies in Lambert–Eaton myasthenic syndrome and other paraneoplastic syndromes. N Engl J Med 1995;332:1467–1474.
147. Lennon VA. Serologic profile of myasthenia gravis and distinction from the Lambert-Eaton myasthenic syndrome. Neurology 1997;48(Suppl 5):S23–S27.
148. Lennon VA. Serological Diagnosis of Myasthenia Gravis and the Lambert-Eaton Myasthenic Syndrome. In R Lisak (ed), Handbook of Myasthenia Gravis. New York: Marcel Dekker, 1994;149–164.
149. Howard FJ, Lennon V, Finley J, et al. Clinical correlations of antibodies that bind, block or modulate human acetylcholine receptors in myasthenia gravis. Ann N Y Acad Sci 1987;505:526–538.
150. Sano M, Lambert EH, McCormick DJ, Lennon VA. Muscle acetylcholine receptors complexed with autologous IgG reflect seropositivity but not necessarily in vivo binding. Neurology 1992;42:218–222.
151. Newsom-Davis J, Leys K, Vincent A, et al. Immunological evidence for the co-existence of the Lambert-Eaton myasthenic syndrome and myasthenia gravis in two patients. J Neurol Neurosurg Psychiatry 1991;54:452–453.
152. Lennon VA, Lambert EH, Whittingham S, Fairbanks V. Autoimmunity in the Lambert-Eaton myasthenic syndrome. Muscle Nerve 1982;5:S21–S25.
153. Kelly RB. Synaptotagmin is just a calcium sensor. Curr Biol 1995;5:257–259.
154. Matteoli M, Takei K, Perin MS, et al. Exo-endo-cytotic recycling of synaptic vesicles in developing processes of cultured hippocampal neurons. J Cell Biol 1992;117:859–861.
155. Takamori M, Takahashi M, Yasukawa Y, et al. Antibodies to recombinant synaptotagmin and calcium channel subtypes in Lambert-Eaton myasthenic syndrome. J Neurol Sci 1995;133:95–101.
156. Takamori M, Hamada T, Komai K, et al. Synaptotagmin can cause an immune-mediated model of Lambert-Eaton myasthenic syndrome in rats. Ann Neurol 1994;35:74–80.
157. Synaptic and Junctional Transmission. In WF Ganong (ed), Review of Medical Physiology (18th ed). Norwalk, CT: Appleton & Lange, 1997;79–114.
158. Unwin N. Acetylcholine receptor channel imaged in the open state. Nature 1995;373:31–41.
159. Lindstrom JM. Acetylcholine receptors and myasthenia. Muscle Nerve 2000;23(4):453–477.
160. Sanders DB, Andrews I, Howard JF, Massey JM. Seronegative myasthenia gravis. Neurology 1997;48(Suppl 5):S40–S45.
161. Solliven BC, Lange DJ, Penn AS, et al. Seronegative myasthenia gravis. Neurology 1988;38:514–517.
162. Vincent A, Li Z, Hart A, et al. Seronegative myasthenia gravis: evidence for plasma factor(s) interfering with acetylcholine receptor function. Ann N Y Acad Sci 1993;681:529–538.
163. Blaes F, Beeson D, Plested P, et al. IgG from "seronegative" myasthenia gravis patients binds to a muscle cell line, TE671, but not to human acetylcholine receptor. Ann Neurol 2000;47:504–510.
164. Engel AG, Ohno K, Sine SM. Congenital myasthenic syndromes: recent advances. Arch Neurol 1999;56:163–167.
165. Wintzen AR, Plomp JJ, Molenaar PC, et al. Acquired slow channel syndrome: a form of myasthenia gravis with prolonged open time of the acetylcholine receptor channel. Ann Neurol 1998;44:657–664.
166. Somnier F. Anti-acetylcholine receptor (AChR) antibodies measurement in myasthenia gravis: the use of cell line TE671 as a source of AChR antigen. J Neuroimmunol 1994;51:63–68.
167. Vincent A, Newsom-Davis J. Acetylcholine receptor characteristics in myasthenia gravis. I. Patients with generalized myasthenia or disease restricted to ocular muscles. Clin Exp Immunol 1982;49:257–265.
168. Vincent A, Newland C, Brueton L, et al. Arthrogryposis multiplex congenital with maternal antibodies specific for a fetal antigen. Lancet 1995;346:24–25.
169. Jacobson L, Polizzi A, Morris-Kay GM, Vincent A. An animal model of antibody-mediated neurodevelopmental disease: arthrogryposis multiplex congenital caused by antibodies to fetal acetylcholine receptor. J Clin Invest 1999;103:1031–1038.
170. Lanska DJ. Diagnosis of thymoma in myasthenics using anti-striated muscle antibodies: predictive value and gain in diagnostic certainty. Neurology 1991;41:520–524.
171. Penn AS, Schotland DL, Lamme S. Antimuscle and antiacetylcholine receptor antibodies in myasthenia gravis. Muscle Nerve 1986;9:407–415.
172. Aarli JA, Gilhus NE, Hofstad N. CA-antibody: an immunologic marker of thymic neoplasia in myasthenia gravis? Acta Neurol Scand 1987;76:55–57.
173. Gautel M, Lakey A, Barlow DP, et al. Titin antibodies in myasthenia gravis: identification of a major immunogenic region of titin. Neurology 1993;43:1581–1585.

174. Williams CL, Lennon VA. Thymic B-lymphocyte clones from patients with myasthenia gravis secrete monoclonal striational autoantibodies reacting with myosin, alpha-actinin or actin. J Exp Med 1986;164:1043–1059.

175. Mygland A, Tysnes O-B, Aarli JA, et al. Myasthenia gravis patients with thymoma have antibodies against a high molecular weight protein in the sarcoplasmic reticulum. J Neuroimmunol 1992;37:1–7.

176. Mygland A, Vincent A, Newsom-Davis J, et al. Autoantibodies in thymoma-associated myasthenia gravis with myositis or neuromyotonia. Arch Neurol 2000;57:527–531.

177. Ansevin CF, Agamanolis DP. Rippling muscles and myasthenia gravis with rippling muscles. Arch Neurol 1996;53:197–199.

178. Walker GR, Watkins T, Ansevin CF. Identification of autoantibodies associated with rippling muscles and myasthenia gravis that recognize skeletal muscle proteins: possible relationship of antigens ads stretch-activated ion channels. Biochem Biophys Res Commun 1999;264:430–435.

179. Griesmann GE, Lennon VA. Detection of Autoantibodies in Myasthenia Gravis and Lambert-Eaton Myasthenic Syndrome. In NR Rose, E Conway DeMacario, JD Folds, et al. (eds), Manual of Clinical and Laboratory Immunology (5th ed). Washington, DC: ASM Press, 1997;983–988.

180. Somnier FE. Clinical implementation of anti-acetylcholine receptor antibodies. J Neurol Neurosurg Psychiatry 1993;56:496–504.

181. Lennon VA, Howard FM. Serological Diagnosis of Myasthenia Gravis. In RM Nakamura, MB O'Sullivan (eds), Clinical Laboratory Molecular Analysis: New Strategies in Autoimmunity, Cancer and Virology. New York: Grune & Stratton, 1985;29–44.

182. Cikes N, Momoi MY, Williams CL, et al. Striational autoantibodies: quantitative detection by enzyme immunoassay in myasthenia gravis, thymoma and recipients of D-penicillamine and allogenic bone marrow. Mayo Clin Proc 1988;63:474–481.

183. Hay JE, Lennon VA, Czaja AJ, et al. High frequency of acetylcholine receptor binding antibodies in autoimmune liver diseases. Clin Res 1989;37:538A(Abst).

184. Garlepp MJ, Mastaglia FL. Autoantibodies in inflammatory myopathies. Am J Med Sci 2000;319:227–233.

185. Von Muhlen CA, Tan EM. Autoantibodies in the diagnosis of systemic rheumatic diseases. Sem Arthritis Rheum 1995;24:323–358.

186. Marguerie C, Bunn CC, Copier J, et al. The clinical significance and immunogenetic features of patients with autoantibodies to nucleolar antigen PM-Scl. Medicine (Baltimore) 1992;71:327–336.

187. Sharp GC, Irvin WS, Tan EM, et al. Mixed connective tissue disease: an apparently distinct rheumatic disease syndrome associated with a specific antibody to an extractable nuclear antigen (ENA). Am J Med 1972;52:148–159.

188. Yamanishi Y, Maeda H, Katayama S, et al. Scleroderma-polymyositis overlap syndrome associated with anti-Ku antibody and rimmed vacuole formation. J Rheumatol 1996;23:1991–1994.

189. Oddis CV, Okano Y, Rudert WA, et al. Serum autoantibody to the nuclear antigen Pm-Scl. Arthritis Rheum 1992;35:1211–1217.

190. Reimer G, Scheer U, Peters JM, Tan EM. Immunolocalisation and partial characterization of a nucleolar autoantigen (Pm-Scl) associated with polymyositis/ scleroderma overlap syndrome. J Immunol 1986;137:3802–3808.

191. Rutjes SA, Vree Egberts WT, Jongen P, et al. Anti-Ro52 antibodies frequently co-occur with anti-Jo-1 antibodies in sera from patients with idiopathic inflammatory myopathy. Clin Exp Immunol 1997;109:32–40.

192. Sherer Y, Livneh A, Levy Y, et al. Dermatomyositis and polymyositis associated with the antiphospholipid syndrome—a novel overlap syndrome. Lupus 2000;9:42–46.

193. Miller FW. Myositis-specific autoantibodies. Touchstones for understanding the inflammatory myopathies. JAMA 1993;270:1846–1849.

194. Love LA, Leff RL, Fraser DD, et al. A new approach to the classification of idiopathic inflammatory myopathy: myositis-specific autoantibodies define useful homogeneous patient groups. Medicine 1991;70:360–374.

195. Hirakata M, Suwa A, Nagai S, et al. Anti-KS: identification of autoantibodies to asparaginyl-transferase RNA synthetase associated with interstitial lung disease. J Immunol 1999;162:2315–2320.

196. Targoff IN. Clinical manifestations in patients with antibody to PL-12 antigen (alamyl-tRNA synthetase). Am J Med 1990;88:241–251.

197. Targoff IN, Triem EP, Plotz PH, Miller FW. Antibodies to glycl-transferase RNA synthetase in patients with myositis and interstitial lung disease. Arthritis Rheum 1992;35:821–830.

198. Targoff IN, Arnett FC, Reichlin M. Antibodies to threonyl-transferase RNA-synthetase in myositis sera. Arthritis Rheum 1988;31:515–523.

199. Mimori T. Structures targeted by the immune system in myositis. Curr Opin Rheumatol 1996;8:521–527.
200. Targoff IN, Johnson AE, Miller FW. Antibody to signal recognition particle in polymyositis. Arthritis Rheum 1990;38:1361–1370.
201. Targoff IN. Humoral immunity in polymyositis/dermatomyositis. J Invest Dermatol 1993;100: 116S–123S.
202. Feldman BM, Reichlin M, Laxer RM, et al. Clinical significance of specific autoantibodies in juvenile dermatomyositis. J Rheumatol 1996;23:1794–1797.
203. Nilasena DS, Trieu EP, Targoff IN. Analysis of the Mi-2 autoantigen in dermatomyositis. Arthritis Rheum 1995;38:123–128.
204. Seelig HP, Moosbrugger I, Ehrfeld H, et al. The major dermatomyositis-specific Mi-2 autoantigen is a presumed helicase involved in transcriptional activation. Arthritis Rheum 1995;38:1389–1399.
205. Targoff IN, Arnett FC, Berman L, et al. A new antibody associated with the syndrome of polymyositis and interstitial lung disease. J Clin Invest 1989;84:162–172.
206. Lacomis D, Oddis CV. Myositis-specific and -associated autoantibodies: a review from the clinical perspective. J Clin Neuromusc Dis 2000;2:34–40.
207. Miller FW, Twitty SA, Biswas T, Plotz PH. Origin and regulation of a disease-specific autoantibody response. J Clin Invest 1990;85:468–475.
208. Mimori T. Autoantibodies in connective tissue diseases: clinical significance and analysis of target autoantigens. Intern Med 1999;38:523–532.
209. Targoff IN. Autoantibodies in polymyositis. Rheum Dis Clin North Am 1992;18:455–482.
210. Hausmanova-Petrusewicz F, Kowalska-Oledzka E, Miller FW, et al. Clinical, serological, and immunogenetic features in Polish patients with idiopathic inflammatory myopathies. Arthritis Rheum 1997;40:1257–1266.
211. Targoff IN, Miller FW, Medsger TA, Oddis CV. Classification criteria for the idiopathic inflammatory myopathies. Curr Opin Rheumatol 1997;9:527–535.
212. Al-Lozi MT, Pestronk A, Yee WC, Flaris N. Myopathy and paraproteinemia with serum IgM binding to a high-molecular-weight muscle fiber surface protein. Ann Neurol 1995;37:41–46.
213. Al-Lozi MT, Pestronk A, Choksi R. A skeletal muscle–specific form of decorin is a target antigen for a serum IgM M-protein in a patient with a proximal myopathy. Neurology 1997;49: 1650–1654.
214. Croft PB, Henson RA, Urich H, Wilkinson PC. Sensory neuropathy with bronchial carcinoma: a study of four cases showing serological abnormalities. Brain 1965;88:501–514.
215. Wilkinson PC, Zeromski J. Immunofluorescent detection of antibodies against neurons in sensory carcinomatous neuropathy. Brain 1965;88:529–583.
216. Rudnicki SA, Dalmau J. Paraneoplastic syndromes of the spinal cord, nerve and muscle. Muscle Nerve 2000;23:1800–1818.
217. Graus F, Cordon-Cardo C, Posner JB. Neuronal antinuclear antibody in sensor neuronopathy from lung cancer. Neurology 1985;35:538–543.
218. Graus F, Elkon KB, Cordon-Cardo C, Posner JB. Sensory neuronopathy and small cell lung cancer: antineuronal antibody that also reacts with tumor. Am J Med 1986;80:45–52.
219. Manley GT, Sillevis-Smitt P, Dalmau J, Posner JB. Hu Antigens: reactivity with Hu antibodies, tumor expression, and major immunogenic sites. Ann Neurol 1995;38:102–110.
220. Vega F, Graus F, Chen QM, et al. Intrathecal synthesis of the anti-Hu antibody in patients with paraneoplastic encephalomyelitis or sensory neuropathy: clinical-immunologic correlations. Neurology 1994;44:2145–2147.
221. Inuzuka T. Autoantibodies in paraneoplastic neurological syndrome. Am J Med Sci 2000;319(4): 217–226.
222. Graus F, Ribalta T, Campo E, et al. Immunohistochemical analysis of the immune reaction in the nervous system in paraneoplastic encephalomyelitis. Neurology 1990;40:219–222.
223. Yoshioka R, Ueda Y, Sakai K, et al. Immunohistochemical studies of paraneoplastic subacute sensory neuropathy—an analysis of antineuronal antibody and infiltrated lymphocytes. Rinsho Shinkeigaku 1992;32:397–404.
224. Chalk CH, Lennon VA, Stevens JC, Windebank AJ. Seronegativity for type 1 anti-neuronal nuclear antibodies (anti-Hu) in subacute sensory neuropathy patients without cancer. Neurology 1993;43:2209–2211.
225. Molinuevo JL, Graus F, Rene R, et al. Utility of anti-Hu antibodies in the diagnosis of paraneoplastic sensory neuropathy. Ann Neurol 1998;44:976–980.
226. Griffin JW, Cornblath DR, Alexander E, et al. Ataxic sensory neuropathy and dorsal root ganglionitis associated with Sjögren's syndrome. Ann Neurol 1990;27:304–315.

227. Forsyth PA, Dalmau J, Graus F, et al. Motor neuron syndromes in cancer patients. Ann Neurol 1997;41:722–730.
228. Ferracci F, Fassetta G, Butler MH, et al. A novel antineuronal antibody in a motor neuron syndrome associated with breast cancer. Neurology 1999;53:852–855.
229. David C, McPherson PS, Mundigl O, de Camilli P. A role of amphiphysin in synaptic vesicle endocytosis suggested by its binding to dynamin in nerve terminals. Proc Natl Acad Sci U S A 1996;93:331–335.
230. Folli F, Solimena M, Cofiell R, et al. Autoantibodies to a 128-kd synaptic protein in three women with the stiff-man syndrome and breast cancer. N Engl J Med 1993;328:546–551.
231. De Camilli P, Thomas A, Cofiell R, et al. The synaptic vesicle-associated protein amphiphysin is the 128-kD autoantigen of stiff-man syndrome with breast cancer. J Exp Med 1993;178:2219–2223.
232. Antoine JC, Absi L, Honnorat J, et al. Antiamphiphysin antibodies are associated with various paraneoplastic syndromes and tumors. Arch Neurol 1999;56:172–177.
233. Peyronnard JM, Charron L, Beaudet F, Couture F. Vasculitic neuropathy in rheumatoid arthritis and Sjögren's Syndrome. Neurology 1982;32:839–845.
234. Enevoldson TP, Wiles CM. Severe vasculitic neuropathy in systemic lupus erythematosus and response to cyclophosphamide. J Neurol Neurosurg Psychiatry 1991;54:468–469.
235. Moder KG. Use and interpretation of rheumatologic tests: a guide for clinicians. Mayo Clin Proc 1996:71:391–396.
236. Matsuki Y, Hidaka T, Matsumoto M, et al. Systemic lupus erythematosus demonstrating serum anti-GM1 antibody, with sudden onset of drop foot as the initial presentation. Intern Med 1999;38:729–732.
237. Sindern E, Stark E, Haas J, Steck AJ. Serum antibodies to GM1 and GM3 gangliosides in systemic lupus erythematosus with chronic inflammatory demyelinating neuropathy. Acta Neurol Scand 1991;83:399–402.
238. Lee P, Bruni J, Sukenik S. Neurological manifestations in systemic sclerosis (scleroderma). J Rheumatol 1984;11:480–483.
239. Dyck PJB, Hunder GG, Dyck PJ. A case-control and nerve biopsy study of CREST multiple mononeuropathy. Neurology 1997;49:1641–1645.
240. Rosenbaum R. Neuromuscular complications of connective tissue diseases. Muscle Nerve 2001;24:154–169.
241. Hadjivassiliou M, Chattopadhyay AK, Davies-Jones GA, et al. Neuromuscular diseases: a presenting feature of coeliac disease. J Neurol Neurosurg Psychiatry 1997:63:770–775.
242. Wolfe GI, El-Feky WH, Katz JS, et al. Antibody panels in idiopathic polyneuropathy and motor neuron disease. Muscle Nerve 1997;20:1275–1283.
243. Yuki N. Acute paresis of extraocular muscles associated with IgG anti-GQ1b antibody. Ann Neurol 1996;39:668–672.

4

Computerized Sensory Evaluation

Renato J. Verdugo and Alberto L. Dubrovsky

Peripheral nerve fibers carry sensory, motor, and autonomic impulses. Nerve fibers of somatic sensibility are classified according to diameter, conduction velocity, and related sensory modality. Cutaneous afferent fibers are divided into two groups: A (myelinated) and C (unmyelinated). Thick myelinated fibers with a diameter of approximately 10 μm and a conduction velocity of approximately 60 m per second are classified as A-β; these fibers mediate tactile and position senses. Thin myelinated fibers are classified as A-δ. They have a diameter of approximately 5 μm with a conduction velocity of approximately 15 m per second. They mediate cold sensation and sharp pain (A-δ nociceptors). The unmyelinated C fibers have a diameter of 1–2 μm with a conduction velocity of approximately 1 m per second. One group of C fibers mediates warm sensation, and another mediates burning pain sensation. A-δ and C fibers related to pain are known as *nociceptors*, because they respond only to intense stimulation in a range considered potentially harmful (Table 4.1).

Conventional nerve conduction studies and needle electromyography are reliable methods for studying peripheral nerve and muscle disorders. With these methods, it is possible to localize and characterize a peripheral nerve lesion as axonal or demyelinating, but they only evaluate function of motor and large-caliber afferent fibers, leaving unchecked the small afferent and autonomic fibers. Furthermore, due to the nature of nerve conduction, in which a volley of ectopically generated nerve impulses is induced by an external electrical stimulus, they are unsuitable for studying the pathophysiology of positive sensory symptoms, which are also the expression of dysfunction of large- and small-caliber afferent fibers.

Tactile paresthesias are common positive manifestations of large afferent fiber dysfunction, whereas burning and shooting spontaneous pains, mechanical and thermal hyperalgesias, and paradoxical temperature sensations are common positive symptoms of small-caliber afferent fiber dysfunction. These are frequently the patient's main complaints. This chapter summarizes the different laboratory methods of evaluation of sensory function that may complement conventional nerve conduction studies and needle electromyography.

Table 4.1 Simplified Classification of Cutaneous Afferent Fibers

Fiber Type	Diameter (μm)	Myelin	Conduction Velocity (m/sec)	Modality
A-β	6–20	Yes	40–80; avg. 60	Touch Proprioception Vibration
A-δ	1–5	Yes	5–30; avg. 15	Cold sensation Sharp pain
C	0.5–2.0	No	0.8–2.0; avg. 1	Warmth sensation Cold and heat pain

avg. = average.

MICRONEUROGRAPHY

Microneurography is a useful method to explore the functional mechanisms of positive sensory manifestations affecting both types of afferents, as well as autonomic fibers.[1] The technique consists of introducing a tungsten needle electrode of 200 μm, with a recording surface of a few microns, into a nerve fascicle, allowing it to record the discharges of a small group of fibers or only one fiber.

Important advances in the understanding of the physiology of sensation and autonomic function have been obtained with this technique. For example, microneurography allows the identification of sensations mediated at peripheral level by large- and small-caliber afferents in humans. More recently, it has also helped to identify abnormal mechanisms of pathologic sensation in the realm of peripheral nerve lesions, such as sensitization or ectopic discharge of nociceptors. Nevertheless, because the technique is time consuming, has a high percentage of false-negative results due to the small number of fibers possible to sample, and requires sophisticated equipment, microneurography cannot be recognized as a clinically useful method for the daily practice. At present, it is practiced only at a few centers in the world.

Different collision methods have been developed to evaluate the function of small-caliber afferent fibers. However, these techniques can only test for small myelinated fibers (A-δ); they cannot evaluate the substrate for positive sensory symptoms, are time consuming, and frequently meet with technical difficulties. For these reasons, they are rarely used in the routine clinical evaluation of A-δ fibers.

CLINICAL PSYCHOPHYSICAL EVALUATION OF SMALL-CALIBER AFFERENT PATHWAYS

Quantitative Somatosensory Thermal Tests

The quantitative somatosensory thermal tests (QSTs) are a useful group of techniques that evaluate the function of small afferent nerve fibers. These are psychophysical methods that determine the thresholds for different thermal sensations. They have become increasingly more popular, and guidelines for their use have been recommended to standardize their performance.[2] The value of these tests has been recognized by their application in clinical trials.[3–4]

Testing for the threshold of warm sensation evaluates the function of C-unmyelinated fibers, and testing for threshold of cold sensation allows for testing of small myelinated (A-δ) fibers. Testing for threshold for cold and heat pain evaluates function of unmyelinated C nociceptors.[5]

Different methods are applied to determine the various thermal thresholds. All are based on the sensation perceived by the patient as a response to a stimulating temperature applied to the skin. Some methods include the patient's reaction time, whereas others do not.[5]

The method of limits is one of the most commonly used techniques. Starting at a baseline temperature, usually approximately 30–32°C, a ramp of ascending or descending temperatures is applied on the skin of the subject, who acknowledges the sensation by pressing a switch. Several ramps of stimulating temperature are applied, and the threshold is considered as the average of the different responses. First, thresholds for cold and warm sensation are tested, and the patient must signal for the first thermal sensation felt. Then, thresholds for cold and heat pain are determined using ramps of stimulating temperatures at higher speeds to obtain a preferential stimulation of nociceptors. During this, the patient must signal for the first sensation of pain, independent of the thermal sensation. Heat pain sensation is usually tested at the end to prevent "after sensations" that may interfere with the next evaluation.

Normal values for these tests have been published[6] and are useful only for the precise area of the skin where they have been determined, and only when the same surface of stimulation, rate of change in temperature, and baseline temperature are used. A typical normal profile is displayed in Figure 4.1A. Each peak represents one ramp of stimulation; the increased threshold on successive ramps is most likely an expression of receptor fatigue, and its presence indicates good cooperation by the subject. On the other hand, erratic thresholds such as those in Figure 4.2C must call attention to the ability of the subject to adequately report the perceived sensations.

As a psychophysical method, the QST evaluates function not only of peripheral fibers, but also of the entire sensory pathway within the peripheral and central nervous system. This characteristic restricts the capacity of localizing an abnormal pattern, but it has the advantage of allowing for testing of central pathways, making this technique useful for evaluating sensory dysfunctions of peripheral and central origin. Another advantage of the psychophysical method is its ability to test both for diminution of function in the form of thermal hypoesthesia and evaluation of positive sensory manifestations in the form of thermal pain hyperalgesia.

A relatively common abnormal pattern seen in peripheral nerve disorders affecting small-caliber afferent fibers is warm hypoesthesia (see Figure 4.1B). In fact, the threshold for warm sensation increases in the feet with age.[6] Warm sensation is very dependent on spatial summation, and, therefore, a minor diminution of function of peripheral receptors is reflected as warm hypoesthesia. In simple terms, the diminution of receptors that mediate warm sensation results not only in a diminution of the area of thermal sensation, but also in a sensation of less warmth.

Spatial summation also exists for other thermal sensations, although to a much lesser degree. As the impairment of function of small afferents worsens, cold hypoesthesia and heat and cold pain hypoalgesia develop.

In disorders that affect predominantly small A-δ myelinated fibers, cold hypoesthesia develops before warm hypoesthesia. In this case, cold hypoesthesia is fre-

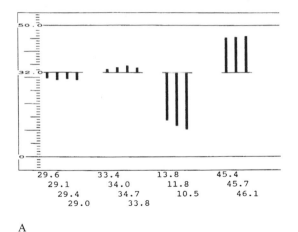

A

29.6	33.4	13.8	45.4
29.1	34.0	11.8	45.7
29.4	34.7	10.5	46.1
29.0	33.8		

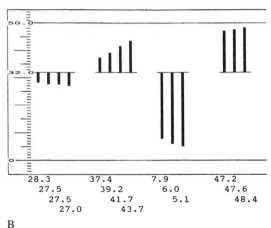

B

28.3	37.4	7.9	47.2
27.5	39.2	6.0	47.6
27.5	41.7	5.1	48.4
27.0	43.7		

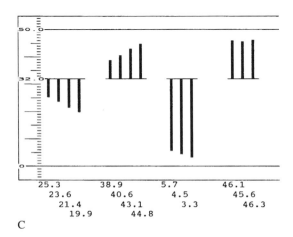

C

25.3	38.9	5.7	46.1
23.6	40.6	4.5	45.6
21.4	43.1	3.3	46.3
19.9	44.8		

Figure 4.1 A. Normal pattern. Each bar represents one ramp of stimulating temperature. The first four bars indicate thresholds for cold sensation. The second four bars correspond to threshold for warm sensation. The two last groups of three bars correspond to the thresholds for cold pain and heat pain, respectively. The temperatures (°C) signaled by the patient are indicated in the bottom of the figure. The average of the three or four stimuli is considered the threshold for each sensation. **B.** Pure warm hypoesthesia. There is increase in the threshold for warm sensation with relative preservation of cold threshold. **C.** Cold and warm hypoesthesia.

quently associated with cold pain hyperalgesia and paradoxical heat-burning sensation in response to low-temperature stimulation (see Figure 4.2B).[7]

A similar phenomenon occurs in normal subjects during selective blockade of myelinated fibers.[8] When cold hypoesthesia develops as a result of the blockade of A-δ fibers, cold hyperalgesia appears. The threshold for thermal sensation and the threshold for thermal pain in response to low temperature tend to be similar; the sensation reported is no longer "cold" but "hot burning" (see Figure 4.2B). This abnormal pattern of sensation indicates that normal cold pain sensation is probably the result of the combined discharge of cold-specific afferents and nociceptor fibers responding to low temperature. When the input from cold-specific fibers is no longer present, the nociceptive afference is released, and hot burning pain appears with mild lowering of the stimulating temperature (cold hyperalgesia), due to the discharge of nociceptors.

The QST may also demonstrate heat hyperalgesia as the expression of sensitization of peripheral C nociceptors.[9] In this case, there is heat pain with only mild elevation of the stimulating temperature. Frequently, heat hyperalgesia is combined with warm hypoesthesia due to the loss of unmyelinated, warm-specific fibers (see Figure 4.2A). When asked, the patients showing this pattern volunteer that they do not feel a gradual increase in the stimulating temperature, giving first the sensation

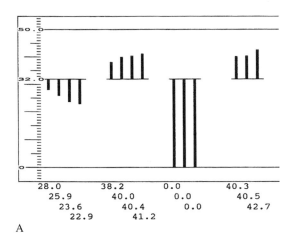

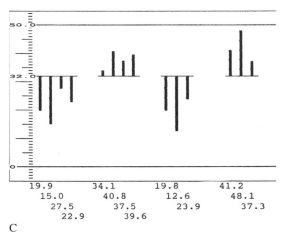

Figure 4.2 A. Warm hypoesthesia associated with heat hyperalgesia. Note that the thresholds for warm and heat pain sensations are similar. The patient frequently does not have warm sensation but sudden burning pain. The temperatures (°C) signaled by the patient are indicated in the bottom of the figure. **B.** Cold hypoesthesia with cold hyperalgesia. In this case, the patient frequently does not feel cold sensation but paradoxical hot burning sensation in response to low-temperature stimulation. **C.** Bizarre atypical pattern. The patient expresses erratic witnessing. Note that the threshold for thermal pain sometimes is lower than the threshold for temperature sensation.

of warmth and then burning pain. Instead, they feel a sudden development of burning sensation once the threshold of nociceptors is reached.

Patients with subcortical and thalamic vascular lesions displayed patterns of thermal hypoesthesia of variable severity.[10] In central pain after vascular lesions, a usually severe warm and cold hypoesthesia associated, in most cases, with thermal hypoalgesia has been described.[11] Obviously, in cases of supratentorial lesions, the thermal hypoesthesias may involve an entire hemibody, although the hemibody is affected with variable degrees of severity. In cases of lacunar infarction with sensory symptoms, the QST shows severe hypoesthesia for cold and warm sensation, as well as cold and heat hypoalgesia. Interestingly, in patients with "pure motor syndrome" after lacunar infarction, subclinical impairment of the spinothalamic pathway is revealed by the test.[12]

In cases of central pain after spinal cord injury, severe cold and warm hypoesthesia associated with relative preservation of the posterior column function has been found.[13] The QST is also useful in syringomyelia to demonstrate cold and warm hypoesthesia. The distribution of the abnormalities is not symmetric, correlating with the paramedian distribution of the syrinx. The thermal sensation deficits diminish after surgery.[14]

In cases of spastic paraparesis, a relatively selective impairment of cold sensation without development of cold hyperalgesia has been found. The lack of cold hyperalgesia distinguishes this pattern from the classical cold hypoesthesia of peripheral origin.[15] Sometimes these patients may also have paradoxical cold sensation in response to high-temperature stimulation, probably due to central mechanisms.

Finally, the test can also reveal abnormal patterns of characteristic nonorganic nature by showing bizarre and variable responses.[16,17] It can be concluded that the QST is a useful method for evaluating central and peripheral pathways mediating thermal and pain sensations. The interpretation of the results must agree with the clinical picture, and the localization of the level within the afferent channels where the abnormality resides should be the result of careful analysis of the distribution of the abnormal pattern found. Other methods to quantify sensation have been developed in an attempt to assess sensory abnormalities and to monitor, in an objective and reproducible manner, the changes during the course of any disease process involving sensory structures.

Other Methods of Sensory Evaluation

Current Perception Threshold

Current perception threshold (CPT) is a technique designed to measure the level of current perception, which is dependent on the integrity of different types of nerve fibers (myelinated and unmyelinated). The stimuli generated by the device are alternating currents with sinusoid waveforms at different frequencies, ranging from 5 to 2,000 Hz. Stimulus output intensities range from 0.01 to 9.99 mA. The physiologic basis for the test is the assumption that different frequency stimuli are capable of selectively depolarizing different diameter fibers. Transcutaneous electrical stimulation excites the nerve fibers directly, probably because they have low electrical resistance in comparison to the sensory end organs, such as Pacini corpuscles.

The possibility of depolarizing a nerve fiber depends on its refractory period, and this, in turn, depends on the number of ion channels in the nerve surface. Using different frequency stimuli, the CPT evaluations supposedly achieve sufficient neuroselectivity to stimulate each type of fiber.[17] The large-diameter fibers can respond to very rapid 2,000 Hz stimuli, whereas very small–diameter fibers only respond to 5 Hz.[18] The procedure is performed by trained technicians or by the physician. As in every psychophysical test, the patient must collaborate throughout the examination. The unit delivers electrical current stimuli, which are applied transcutaneously according to previously determined parameters. A pair of electrodes is attached to the skin with conductive gel in the selected place. Similar to the thermal testing, different algorithms can be used to examine sensory thresholds, selected according to the operator preferences or needs.

Basically, there are two different paradigms available for conducting the CPT evaluation: the double-blind, forced-choice method and the direct and more rapid method similar to the method of limits described for thermal sensation. The principles of the CPT methods are similar to those described for the thermal test. Typically, the test is performed in 2–6 sites and may take from 20 to 60 minutes. Normal values may be obtained from the manufacturers of the equipment or from studying sufficient numbers of normal subjects to obtain these values. Abnormally low CPT values indicate hyperesthetic conditions, whereas elevated CPT values are interpreted as hypoesthesia. As in any other neurophysiologic study, clinical correlation is necessary for appropriate interpretation of the data. The type and distribution of the sensory impairment is important.

CPT has been used in the study and identification of polyneuropathies,[19–21] radiculopathies,[22] and segmental nerve lesions.[23,24] The main criticism of this methodology is the lack of certainty that the different currents applied actually stimulate selectively the different types of afferents.

Biothesiometer

The biothesiometer is essentially an electrical tuning fork that can be used to more accurately evaluate vibratory sensation. Errors in measurement with the regular tuning fork are very common, and no quantitative assessment can be made. The peripheral fibers that are involved in this sensation modality are those subserving mechanosensation, which are A-β myelinated fibers. These fibers are responsible for the sensory potentials that are evoked in the nerve conduction studies. The vibration amplitude of the device can be predetermined or increased gradually until the sensation threshold is reached.

Although there are several models, one of the most important issues that applies to all models is that great care is needed regarding the pressure that the examiner applies to the vibrating tip; it must be constant to achieve reproducibility.[25]

As a simple method that can be managed by most physicians, the biothesiometer has been especially applied in the screening and evaluation of peripheral neuropathy in diabetics by endocrinologists.[26–29] Other devices can be purchased with the QST systems that measure vibratory thresholds, and the pressure with which the vibrating tip is applied to the test site is more standardized. With these devices, an increasing vibrating stimulus is applied until the patient perceives the sensation. In a second trial, a high-vibrating stimulus is applied and then decreased until the patient no longer perceives the vibration, establishing a threshold. Universal normal values are difficult to establish and should be obtained in each laboratory using its own equipment.

Semmes-Weinstein Monofilaments

The Semmes-Weinstein monofilament is a handheld instrument that consists of a series of nylon monofilaments of increasing diameters set in acrylic rods at 90-degree angles. The filaments are applied by the examiner to the region of the skin where sensation is to be evaluated. The filaments bend after a certain amount of pressure is exerted on each. A series of filaments are applied, and when sensation is perceived, the filament size is documented and can be quantitated. When used properly, the filaments have reproducible stimuli with acceptable standard deviations.[30]

Studies of sensation using these filaments have been done on the entire body of both control and diseased subjects to establish normal and abnormal values for each filament size.[31–33] The 2.83 filament serves as the index value for normality in men and women. The length of the filament, which should be constant, and its diameter are crucial in the accuracy of determination. The filaments, when appropriately managed, can provide a fairly sensitive measurement of sensory abnormality in the clinical setting.

CONCLUSIONS

QST are important psychophysiologic methods of assessing nerve fiber function, which is not usually studied with standard electrophysiologic methods. They have the advantage of providing reproducible quantitation that can be used for statistical analyses in clinical trials, but most have the disadvantage of being time consuming and, in particular, they are subjective and require the subject's cooperation. The application of these methods in clinical evaluation of patients with peripheral neuropathy, especially those affecting small nerve fibers, is becoming increasingly popular.

REFERENCES

1. Ochoa JL, Bell LA. Microneurography as a clinical research tool. In MJ Aminoff (ed), Electrodiagnosis in Clinical Neurology. Edinburgh, UK: 1999;291–301.
2. Dyck PJ. Quantitative sensory testing: a consensus report from the Peripheral Neuropathy Association. Neurology 1993;43(5):1050–1052.
3. Apfel SC, Kessler JA, Adornato BT, et al. Recombinant human nerve growth factor in the treatment of diabetic polyneuropathy. NGF Study Group. Neurology 1998;51(3):695–702.
4. Apfel SC, Schwartz S, Adornato BT, et al. Efficacy and safety of recombinant human nerve growth factor in patients with diabetic polyneuropathy. A randomized controlled trial. JAMA 2000; 284(17):2215–2221.
5. Yarnitsky D. Quantitative sensory testing. Muscle Nerve 1997;20:198–204.
6. Verdugo RJ, Ochoa JL. Quantitative somatosensory thermotest. A key method for functional evaluation of small calibre afferent channels. Brain 1992;115:893–913.
7. Ochoa JL, Yarnitsky D. The triple cold (CCC) syndrome: cold hyperalgesia, cold hypoesthesia and cold skin in peripheral nerve disease. Brain 1994;117:185–197.
8. Wahrén LK, Torebjörk HE, Jörum E. Central suppression of cold-induced C fibre pain by myelinated fibre input. Pain 1989;38:313–319.
9. Ochoa JL. The newly recognized painful ABC syndrome: thermographic aspects. Thermology 1986;2:65–107.
10. Boivie J. Sensory Abnormalities in Patients with Central Nervous System Lesions as Shown by Quantitative Somatosensory Tests. In J Boivie, P Hansson, U Lindblom (eds), Touch, Temperature, and Pain in Health and Disease: Mechanisms and Assessments. Progress in Pain Research and Management, Vol 3. Seattle: IASP Press, 1994;179–191.
11. Boivie J, Leijon G, Johansson I. Central post-stroke pain—a study of the mechanisms through analyses of the sensory abnormalities. Pain 1989;37:173–185.
12. Samuelsson M, Samuelsson L, Lindell D. Sensory symptoms and signs and results of quantitative sensory thermal testing in patients with lacunar infarct syndromes. Stroke 1994;25:2165–2170.
13. Beric A. Central pain: "new" syndromes and their evaluation. Muscle Nerve 1993;16:1017–1024.
14. Attal N, Brasseur L, Parker F, et al. Caractérisation des troubles sensitifs et des douleurs neuropathiques liés aux syringomyélies. Neurochirurgie 1999;45(Suppl 1):84–94.
15. Castillo JL, Cea JG, Verdugo RJ, Cartier L. Sensory dysfunction in HTLV-I associated myelopathy/tropical spastic paraparesis. A comprehensive neurophysiological study. Eur Neurol 1999; 42:17–22.
16. Verdugo RJ, Ochoa JL. Use and misuse of conventional electrodiagnosis, quantitative sensory testing, thermography, and nerve blocks in the evaluation of painful neuropathic syndromes. Muscle Nerve 1993;16:1056–1062.
17. Yarnitsky D, Sprecher E, Tamir A, et al. Variance of sensory threshold measurements: discrimination of feigners from trustworthy performers. J Neurol Sci 1994;125:186–189.
18. Dotson RM. Clinical neurophysiology laboratory tests to assess the nociceptive system in humans. J Clin Neurophysiol 1997;14:32–45.
19. Masson EA, Boulton AJ. The Neurometer: validation and comparison with conventional tests for diabetic neuropathy. Diabet Med 1991;8:S633–S666.

20. Katims JJ, Naviasky EN, Rendell MS, et al. Constant current sine wave transcutaneous nerve stimulation for the evaluation of peripheral neuropathy. Arch Phys Med Rehabil 1987;68:210–213.
21. Menkes D, Swenson M, Sander H. Current perception threshold: an adjunctive test for the detection of acquired demyelinating polyneuropathies. Electromyogr Clin Neurophysiol 2000; 40(4):195–204.
22. Katims JJ, Patil A, Rendell M, et al. Current perception threshold screening for carpal tunnel syndrome. Arch Env Health 1991;46:207–212.
23. Mironer YE, Somerville JJ. The current perception threshold evaluation in radiculopathy: efficacy in diagnosis assessment of treatment results. Pain Digest 1998;8:37–38.
24. Pelmear PL, Taylor W. Carpal tunnel syndrome and hand-arm vibration syndrome. Arch Neurol 1994;51:416–420.
25. Lowenthal LM, Hockaday TD. Vibration sensory thresholds depend on pressure of applied stimulus. Diabetes Care 1987;10(1):100–102.
26. Le Quesne PM, Fowler CJ. Quantitative evaluation of toxic neuropathies in man. In RJ Elligson, M Murray (eds), The London Symposium. EEG J Suppl 1987;39:347–354.
27. Bloom S, Till S, Sonksen P, Smith S. Use of a biothesiometer to measure individual vibration thresholds and their variation in 519 non-diabetic subjects. BMJ (Clinical Research Ed) 1984; 288(6433):1793–1795.
28. Ribera RL, Valls J, Gonzalez-Clemente JM, et al. Measurement of vibratory threshold in the diagnosis of diabetic neuropathy. Rev Clin Esp 1994;10:901–905.
29. Sosenko JM, Boulton AJ, Kubrusly DB, et al. The vibratory perception threshold in young diabetic patients: associations with glycemia and puberty. Diabetes Care 1985;8(6):605–607.
30. Bell Krotoski JA, Tomancik E. Repeatability of Semmes-Weinstein monofilaments. J Hand Surg (Am) 1987;12:155–161.
31. Weinstein S. Fifty years of somatosensory research: From the Semmes-Weinstein monofilaments to the Weinstein Enhanced Sensory Test. J Hand Ther 1993;6(1):11–28.
32. Weinstein S. Tactile sensitivity of the phalanges. Percept Mot Skills 1962;14:351–354.
33. Weinstein E, Seren E. Tactile sensitivity as a function of handness and laterality. J Comp Physiol Psychol 1961;54:665–669.

5

Nerve Conduction Velocity Tests: Their Clinical Applications*

Shin J. Oh

The measurement of nerve conduction is an expression of the physiologic or pathophysiologic state of nerve and is an essential tool for the study of neuropathy. This chapter discusses the basic and clinical aspects of the nerve conduction study (NCS) and the clinical applications of common and uncommon nerve conduction techniques in relation to the diagnostic workups for the neuromuscular diseases.

PHYSIOLOGIC BASIS OF NERVE CONDUCTION

The resting potential in the nerve is –70 mV. When the nerve is activated, brief positive changes (called the *action potential*) occur in the membrane potential. The action potential in a nerve cell always follows a constant sequence of depolarization and repolarization of the membrane, which occurs when the membrane is depolarized at or beyond the threshold level. The action potential in a nerve cell is therefore "all or none" in character and is said to obey the "all-or-none law" of excitation. Excitability is a typical property of nerves. The actual task of the nerve is the propagation of excitation (action potential). Once initiated, the action potential is self-propagating and spreads like a wave over the membrane until it has moved along the entire cell.

The mechanism of propagation of the action potential differs in unmyelinated and myelinated nerve fibers. There is "local circuit" conduction in unmyelinated fibers and "saltatory" conduction in myelinated fibers.[1] For an unmyelinated axon, during the peak of the action potential in a segment of nerve, the membrane potential reverses polarity, and the inside becomes positive in comparison with the outside. The reversal of polarity leads to a local current flow from positive to negative, as indicated by the arrows in Figure 5.1. The outward current flow through the resting membrane in front of the action potential—which is depicted

---

*Part of this chapter is an excerpt from SJ Oh. Clinical Electromyography: Case Studies. Baltimore: Williams & Wilkins, 1998, with permission.

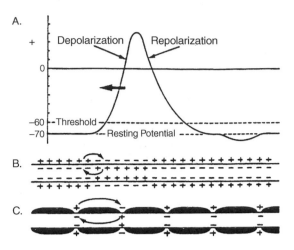

Figure 5.1 Phases of the action potential and its propagation. **A.** Terms for the various phases of the action potential. It also shows the action potential propagating from right to left. **B.** Mechanism of conduction in unmyelinated fiber: local circuit conduction. **C.** Mechanism of conduction in a myelinated fiber: saltatory conduction. (Reprinted with permission from SJ Oh. Clinical Electromyography: Nerve Conduction Studies [2nd ed]. Baltimore: Williams & Wilkins, 1993;7.)

as moving from right to left in Figure 5.1—depolarizes the membrane. The newly activated membrane, in turn, explodes into an action potential, generates local currents, depolarizes the next segment, and so on until the action potential has moved along the full length of the axon.

The conduction speed is determined by the diameter of the unmyelinated fibers. Larger fibers conduct more rapidly than small fibers because they have a lower resistance. Because of the continuous local circuit conduction, the nerve conduction velocity (NCV) of unmyelinated fibers is relatively slow. In human unmyelinated pain fibers, the NCV is 1 m per second. The giant axon of squid, which is 0.7 mm in diameter, has a speed of conduction of 25 m per second. In general, the NCV of unmyelinated fibers can be calculated by the following formula:

$$\frac{\text{NCV of unmyelinated}}{\text{fibers (m per second)}} = \sqrt{\frac{\text{diameter of unmyelinated}}{\text{fiber (axon)}(\mu m)}}$$

In myelinated fibers, the myelin sheath acts as an insulator and prevents transmembrane current flow in the internodes. The movement of the current occurs only at the nodes of Ranvier, spaced at intervals of approximately 2 mm in larger fibers. The impulse hops from one node to the next. This is called *saltatory conduction* in myelinated fibers. In vertebrates, all the fibers that conduct at velocities of propagation in excess of 3 m per second are myelinated. For myelinated fibers, the following formula is applied in the calculation of the NCV:

$$\frac{\text{NCV of myelinated}}{\text{fibers (m per second)}} = \frac{\text{conversion}}{\text{factor}} \times \frac{\text{outer diameter of}}{\text{myelinated fiber}(\mu m)}$$

The NCV that we measure in human subjects is predominantly contributed by the large-diameter fibers of the nerves. We do not have any good nerve conduction technique to measure the nerve conduction of smaller myelinated or unmyelinated fibers at this time. Thus, the NCV reflects the fastest conduction velocity of the nerve. The conversion factor varies according to the particular nerve and animal. It is 4.4 for the human sural nerve.[2] The conversion factor for humans is determined by comparing the NCV and the measurement of large-diameter fibers in the biopsied sural nerve.[2]

Slowing in NCV is caused by loss of large fibers or by segmental demyelination. When it is the axons that are predominantly affected by the disease process, the

NCVs are minimally affected. On the other hand, when it is the myelin that is predominantly involved, marked slowing in NCV is seen because of the loss of saltatory conduction. In fact, in axonal neuropathy, the NCVs are either normal or slowed by less than 40% of normal. In contrast, in demyelinating neuropathy the NCVs are slowed by more than 40% of normal.[1]

BASIC PRINCIPLES OF NERVE CONDUCTION

Basically, the nerve conduction can be studied in two ways: (1) by recording the compound muscle action potentials (CMAPs) from the muscle, and (2) by recording the compound nerve action potential (CNAP) from the tested nerve.[1] The *CMAP* refers to an action potential recorded in a muscle after stimulation of the nerve, whether motor, sensory, or mixed, and is obtained by a needle electrode or surface electrode. By recording the CMAP, motor nerve conduction, late responses (F waves and H reflexes), and reflex responses are studied. The *CNAP* refers to an action potential recorded in a nerve after stimulation of that nerve, either sensory or mixed, and is obtained by a needle electrode or surface electrode. In comparison with the CMAP, the CNAP is small in amplitude and short in duration. The sensory and mixed nerve conductions are thus studied by recording the CNAP.

Motor Nerve Conduction

The motor nerve conduction of a peripheral nerve is tested by stimulating the nerve with a single supramaximal stimulus at two proximal points along the course of the peripheral nerve and then recording the CMAP with a surface electrode from a muscle innervated by that nerve (Figure 5.2). For example, the median nerve may be

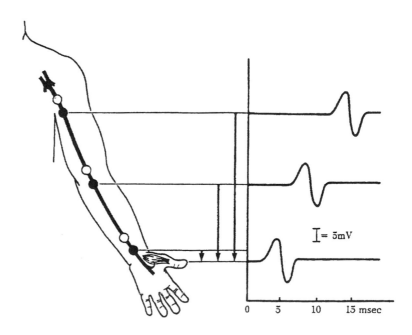

Figure 5.2 Motor nerve conduction study in the median nerve. The recording electrodes are placed in the belly of the abductor pollicis brevis muscle. The compound muscle action potentials (CMAPs) were obtained with stimulation at the wrist, elbow, and axilla. Latency (*arrows*) is measured at the onset of CMAP and amplitude, from peak-to-peak, or from the baseline to the negative peak. The motor nerve conduction velocity is calculated over the elbow-wrist and axilla-elbow segments. (Reprinted with permission from SJ Oh. Clinical Electromyography: Nerve Conduction Studies [2nd ed]. Baltimore: Williams & Wilkins, 1993;17.)

stimulated at the elbow and again at the wrist, with the recording electrode placed over the belly of the abductor pollicis brevis muscle. Latency, conduction time, and the CMAP amplitude, duration, and area are measured by most modern electromyography (EMG) machines.

Latency

Latency refers to elapsed time (milliseconds) from the stimulus onset to the beginning of the initial deflection of the CMAP. Thus, latency is a measure of the combined time for conduction of the nerve impulse from the point of stimulation to the axonal terminal, the neuromuscular transmission, and the depolarization of muscle fibers. When latency is obtained by stimulating at the most distal site possible along the nerve, it is termed *terminal* (distal) *latency.*

Amplitude

The negative-peak or peak-to-peak amplitude is measured. *Amplitude* is the rough estimation of the number of muscle fibers that are activated to nerve stimulation and, subsequently, of the number of nerve fibers that become excitable to nerve stimulation when neuromuscular transmission is normal. The amplitude of the negative deflection of the CMAP is said to reflect a measure of the number of active muscle fibers more accurately than the peak-to-peak amplitude. A more accurate measure would be a calculation of the area under the negative portion of the CMAP. Most modern EMG machines are capable of measuring the area of the CMAP. However, the normal value for the negative-peak amplitude or the negative-peak area is unavailable in most motor NCSs. Thus, the peak-to-peak amplitude is measured in practice.

The CMAP, which is obtained with a surface recording electrode or subcutaneous needle from the belly of the muscle, has a simple diphasic shape with an initial negative deflection. The surface electrode is the only reliable method for documenting conduction block and volume conduction. For these reasons, the surface recording electrode is essential in the motor nerve conduction. The motor NCS performed with an intramuscular needle electrode is usually not recommended because the response is recorded from a more limited area of the muscle, the shape of the CMAP is more complex, and the initial deflection of the potential is not always negative; however, it is sometimes necessary to use this test when the response obtained with the surface electrode is too small. The amplitude of the CMAP is an insensitive measure of mild impairment because of its wide variation among normal subjects. Thus, low CMAP amplitude represents a severe impairment of nerve conduction.

Duration

The duration of negative deflection (negative duration) or the duration of the entire CMAP (total duration) is measured. The duration of CMAP is compared with the duration of normal CMAPs or the duration of CMAPs at distal sites. It reflects the synchrony of discharges of the individual muscle fibers. When the muscle fibers are activated in near synchrony, the duration of the CMAP becomes short. If the conduction velocities vary widely among different nerve fibers, some muscle fibers are activated earlier than others, producing a longer-duration CMAP. Thus, the duration of the CMAP is related to the range of conduction velocities of the large-diameter

A

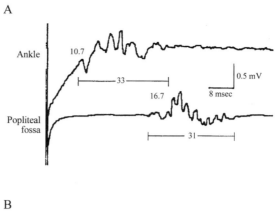

B

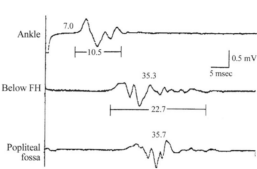

Figure 5.3 A. Dispersion phenomenon of the compound muscle action potential (CMAP) indicative of demyelination in the posterior tibial motor nerve conduction in a case of chronic sensory demyelinating neuropathy. Dispersion is obvious at the ankle as well as at the knee. Notice a long duration of CMAP (33 and 31 milliseconds) between two lines. Numbers above the CMAP refer to latency (milliseconds) at the ankle and nerve conduction velocity (m per second) at knee. **B.** Proximal dispersion phenomenon (temporal dispersion) indicative of focal demyelination between ankle and below-fibular head (FH) in the peroneal motor nerve conduction in a case of chronic inflammatory demyelinating polyneuropathy. Dispersion is obvious at below-fibular head compared with the distal CMAP duration (10.5 milliseconds). (Ankle = ankle stimulation; Popliteal fossa = popliteal fossa stimulation.)

motor nerve fibers. When the CMAP is split into numerous phases producing a long-duration abnormal temporal dispersion (dispersion phenomenon) (Figure 5.3), this represents a wide range of conduction velocities of the large-diameter motor nerve fibers and thus demyelination. Dispersion phenomenon is best determined by assessing total duration.

Area

The area represents the combination of the amplitude and duration of the CMAP and is thus the rough sum of the number of muscle fibers as well as a synchrony of the activated muscle fibers to nerve stimulation. It is consequently influenced by a change in the amplitude or duration of the CMAP. A decrease in the amplitude of the CMAP may simply result from the prolonged duration of the CMAP. This means that abnormal temporal dispersion alone produces a decrease in the CMAP amplitude, possibly mimicking a genuine "conduction block." In this case, there is no change in the area; thus, area measurement more accurately reflects the number of activated muscle fibers to nerve stimulation. This assumes that the phase cancellation of the components of the CMAP is not operative. In this context, phase cancellation refers to cancellation of positive and negative phases of individual motor unit action potentials that contribute to the formation of various components of the CMAP.[3]

Nerve Conduction Velocity

To obtain the conduction time from the proximal to the distal point of stimulation, the terminal latency is subtracted from the latency at the proximal point of stimulation. The distance between the proximal and distal points of stimulation is measured. NCV is determined by dividing this distance by the conduction time. The NCV represents the maximum conduction velocity of the fastest nerve fibers. Most motor nerve fibers must be slowed for the NCV to be diminished. Thus, the presence of a few intact motor fibers may yield an entirely normal NCV in patients with neuropathy. According to Gilliatt, it is necessary for approximately 75% of the large-diameter, fast-conduction fibers to be lost before there is any noticeable effect on the supramaximal NCV of the nerve.[4]

The motor nerve conduction procedure is limited to nerves that are accessible to stimulation. In the upper extremities, the most commonly tested nerves are the median, ulnar, and radial nerves; in the lower extremities, they are the sciatic, femoral, posterior tibial, and peroneal nerves.

Late Responses

There are two late responses that are commonly used in daily practice in the EMG laboratory: the H reflex and F wave.

H Reflex

The H reflex in the gastrocnemius soleus muscle is the electrophysiologic counterpart of the ankle reflex, thus measuring the latency over the monosynaptic reflex arc through the afferent Ia fibers and efferent α motor fibers of the S1 root. The *H reflex* is a late response with longer latency that has a threshold usually lower than that of direct CMAP (M wave) in motor NCSs. The H reflex is normally present at birth in the intrinsic hand and foot muscles but is present consistently only in the gastrocnemius soleus muscle after 12 months of age. In other muscles, the facilitation technique is needed to obtain the H reflex with some reliability. Other muscles that are sometimes tested are the flexor carpi radialis and ulnaris, extensor digitorum communis, vastus medialis, extensor digitorum longus, and anterior tibialis muscles.[1] The H reflex of the gastrocnemius soleus muscle is best obtained when the patient is placed in a prone position, with the feet suspended over the edge of the table or with a pillow placed under the ankles. It is easily obtained with the motor conduction setup by changing the sweep velocity to 10 milliseconds and the sensitivity to 500 μV. An active stimulating electrode should be placed closer to the spine (away from the recording electrodes). The H reflex is best elicited by a stimulus duration of 0.5–1.0 millisecond, which makes it more selective for the afferent Ia fibers. Stimulation should be random at the rate of once every 2 or more seconds to avoid any blocking. The H-reflex latency is measured from the start of stimulation to the onset of the initial deflection of the H reflex and is the most reliable index. The latency of the H reflex on the gastrocnemius soleus muscle is usually in the range of 25–34 milliseconds in normal individuals and is closely correlated with the patient's height. The H-reflex duration and amplitude are less clinically useful than the H-reflex latency.

The H-reflex latency in an individual must at least be compared with the normal value in relation to the body length. Normal histograms of H-reflex latency corrected to the height or lower leg length are readily available.[1,5] Because the H-reflex latency varies with height and, to a lesser extent, with age, a simple and practical way of judging abnormality is to compare the value with the H-reflex latency on the unaffected side. It ranges from 1.5 milliseconds in the gastrocnemius soleus muscle[6] to 3.6 milliseconds in the vastus medialis muscle.[7] This is only applicable when the H reflex is normal on the unaffected side. Thus, it is useful in the detection of a unilateral radiculopathy when it is prolonged or absent. This side-to-side comparison is critical in the H reflex because it is not always present in normal adults.

Differentiation between the H reflex and F wave is not always easy. The following guidelines are helpful in recognizing the H reflex (Figure 5.4). A late response is always the H reflex if it meets one of the following criteria[1]:

1. It is elicited by a subthreshold stimulus.
2. Its amplitude is higher than that of the M wave at a given stimulus.
3. Its amplitude is more than 50% higher than the maximum M-wave amplitude.

Conversely, a late response is always the F wave when it is elicited with a supramaximal stimulus. When the criteria are not met, the H reflex should be differentiated from the F wave by the classic change of amplitude of the H reflex in relation to the M wave with a change in stimulus intensity and by the shape and latency of the late responses. The H reflex is classically triphasic with an initial positive deflection and a large negative deflection in the gastrocnemius soleus muscle. The H-reflex latency is shorter than the F-wave latency. The latency classically varies with each F wave, while the latency of the H reflex is relatively constant. The H-reflex recording is helped by the trace contraction of plantar flexors and by the Jendrassik maneuver, in which the patient hooks his or her hands together with flexed fingers and attempts to pull his or her hands apart as forcefully as possible.

F Wave

Another late response is the F wave, which is evoked by supramaximal stimulation during the motor NCS. Originally considered to be a variant of the H reflex, the F wave is now considered to be a recurrent discharge of a few motor neurons activated by antidromic volleys in the motor fibers. The F wave is easily obtained by stimulating the distal portions of the median, ulnar, peroneal, and posterior tibial nerves using motor nerve conduction setups and changing the sweep velocity to 10 milliseconds and the sensitivity to 200 μV. It is difficult to obtain the F wave after proximal stimulation because the latter yields an F wave with a shorter latency, and the response is hidden in the CMAP (M wave). Again, an active stimulating electrode should be placed closer to the spine. Stimulate manually at the rate of once every 2 seconds (or more) to avoid the blocking response and obtain an F wave at least 10 times, preferably 20 times. Classically, the F-wave latency and shape varies with

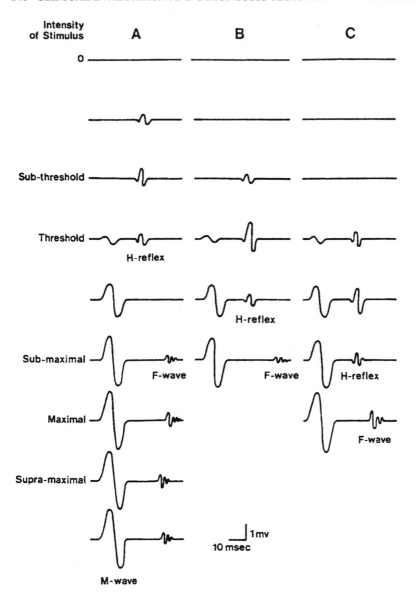

Figure 5.4 Differentiation between the H reflex and F wave. **A.** Any subthreshold late response is the H reflex. The highest amplitude is noted with the subthreshold stimulus. **B.** Any subthreshold late response that becomes higher than the M wave is the H reflex. **C.** Any late response that is higher than an M wave in amplitude at a given stimulus is the H reflex. Any supramaximal late response is the F wave.

each stimulation because the different motor neurons are activated. Rarely, one obtains the response between the M and F waves. This response is labeled as the axon-reflex because it is thought to be a recurrent discharge from another axon branch that is activated by antidromic volleys from the axons stimulated. The axon-reflex can easily be differentiated from the F wave on the basis of constant latency and shape. If the stimulating electrode is moved proximally, the axon-reflex latency is shortened. It is important to recognize the axon-reflex, otherwise the F-wave latency appear erroneously shortened, and its absence can be missed.

The F-wave latency is the most useful parameter and is measured from the start of the stimulus to the onset of initial deflection of the F wave with the shortest latency (minimal latency) among 10–20 F-wave latencies.[8,9] The latency of the F wave after distal stimulation is usually in the range of 23–33 milliseconds for median and ulnar nerves and 50–60 milliseconds for peroneal and posterior tibial nerves in normal individuals and is closely related with body height. Thus, it is essential to compare the F-wave latency obtained with the height-adjusted normal values.[1]

F-wave conduction velocity (FCV) is calculated by the following formula[10]:

$$\frac{\text{Distance (mm)} \times 2}{\text{F-wave latency} - \text{terminal latency} - 1 \text{ (millisecond)}}$$

Distance is measured from stimulus point to spinous process. The FCV is an extremely appealing method because, theoretically, it represents the NCV of the proximal segment of motor fibers. However, there is a potential flaw in the FCV value because of the introduction of two additional causes for error: distance measurement and "turnaround time." The error involved with distance measurement was discussed previously. The method for distance measurement introduced in the FCV is so imprecise that many technical errors can easily be introduced. Kimura assumed that 1 millisecond is needed for turnaround time in each motor neuron.[10] This assumption is based on animal data, indicating that this time is very close to 1.0 millisecond, and on the absolute refractory period (RP) of the fasted human motor fibers, which is also approximately 1.0 millisecond or slightly less.

F persistence is the number of definable F waves divided by the number of stimuli and can be obtained from 10 to 40 F waves.[8] Theoretically, F-wave persistence is of great importance in the detection of nerve conduction block in proximal segments of the peripheral nerves. This persistence in normal controls ranges from 60% to 100% in the ulnar, from 70% to 100% in the median, and from 15% to 100% in the peroneal and posterior tibial nerves in normal controls. Because of the wide range of responses in normal controls and the number of stimuli for the test, it has limited diagnostic value in daily practice.

F chronodispersion (CD) is the difference between minimum and maximum latency values in a series of F waves. To obtain a reasonably accurate value for CD, at least 60 waves must be recorded.[8] Theoretically, CD measures the range of conduction of the large motor fibers, and thus the sensitivity is high in patients with chronic demyelination.[11] Because of the large number of stimuli that must be administered to the patient, CD has limited value in everyday practice.

F tacheodispersion is the distribution of conduction velocities of statistically significant numbers of consecutively recorded F waves and is expressed as F-conduction velocity range and FCV mean. Panayiotopoulos and Chroni claimed that, by converting latency measurements to conduction velocities, F tacheodispersion allows comparison between subjects of different heights and facilitates statistical evaluation.[9] However, although the calculation and analysis of F tacheodispersion can be made by available EMG computer technology, the fact remains that this does not overcome the basic theoretical and technical flaws associated with FCV calculation as described previously.

Sensory Nerve Conduction

The sensory nerve conduction of a peripheral nerve may be tested orthodromically or antidromically (Figure 5.5). In the orthodromic method, the sensory nerve conduction is tested by stimulating the distal part of the nerve and recording the CNAP directly over the proximal part of the nerve. For example, conduction along the sensory fibers of the median or ulnar nerve can be tested by stimulating the digital

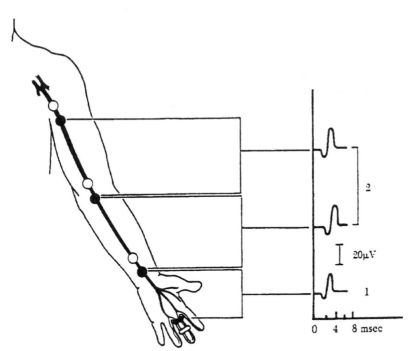

Figure 5.5 Sensory (1) and mixed (2) nerve conduction study in the median nerve. The compound nerve action potentials were obtained with the recording electrodes over the proximal part of the nerve and the stimulating electrodes over the distal part of the nerve. A reference stimulating electrode is placed distal to the active stimulating electrode. Latency is measured either to the onset or negative peak of the compound nerve action potential. The sensory nerve conduction velocity is calculated over the finger-wrist segment and the mixed nerve conduction velocity over the wrist-elbow and elbow-axilla segment. (Reprinted with permission from SJ Oh. Clinical Electromyography: Nerve Conduction Studies [2nd ed]. Baltimore: Williams & Wilkins, 1993;17.)

nerves at the fingers and recording the potential at the wrist. When the stimulating and recording electrodes are switched, this is called *antidromic stimulation*. The latency and conduction velocities are identical in the orthodromic and antidromic methods. Recorded with a surface electrode, the antidromic response is larger in amplitude than the orthodromic response. As a rule, the diagnostic yield of antidromic measurement is poorer than that of orthodromic measurement. A major disadvantage of the antidromic method is that the antidromic sensory CNAPs are obscured by the muscle potential from a neighboring contracting muscle.

Latency (Conduction Time)

The *latency* is a measure of the time required for conduction of the nerve impulse from the point of stimulation to the point of recording. Latency to the initial positive peak with the near-nerve needle and to the onset of the negative peak (this is preferred because of the frequent absence of an initial positive peak) with the surface electrode represents the time for the fastest sensory fibers. The negative peak latency includes the rise-time of the action potential and may therefore give an additional indication of temporal dispersion, thus representing the average conduction of the group Ia fibers. This author prefers the negative peak latency measurement in the surface electrode recording, because it gives more reliable and reproducible results than those obtained by measuring to the onset of the negative deflection.

Amplitude

The *amplitude* of the CNAP is the rough estimation of the number of large nerve fibers that are activated by nerve stimulation. With the surface electrode, the ampli-

Figure 5.6 Dispersion phenomenon of the sensory compound nerve action potential indicative of demyelination in near-nerve needle sensory nerve conduction of medial plantar nerve in a case of Guillain-Barré syndrome. Nerve conduction in the other nerves shows motor neuronopathy without any feature of demyelination. Notice the normal maximum and negative peak nerve conduction velocities (numbers at the positive and negative peaks) and the long duration (16 milliseconds) of the compound nerve action potential.

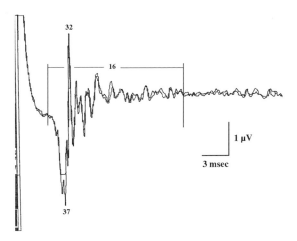

tude is heavily influenced by the distance of the recording electrode from the nerve. Thus, the amplitude is a less sensitive measure of mild impairment. With near-nerve electrodes, the amplitude is a more sensitive index of impairment. Low amplitude usually represents severe impairment of nerve conduction.

Duration

The *duration* is the range of NCVs of the various large-diameter sensory fibers. Thus, it is an index of temporal dispersion. Prolonged temporal dispersion is called *abnormal temporal dispersion* ("dispersion phenomenon"). Abnormal temporal dispersion is difficult or impossible to recognize with the surface electrode but is easily documented with the near-nerve needle and is typically observed in the presence of segmental demyelination (Figure 5.6).

Nerve Conduction Velocity

Unlike motor nerve conduction, the sensory nerve conduction time is equal to the latency in sensory nerve conduction. Thus, the NCV is determined by dividing the distance by the conduction time or latency. The NCV represents the maximum conduction velocity of the fastest sensory fibers when the latency is measured to the first positive peak. When the latency is measured to the negative peak with the surface electrode technique, it provides an estimate of conduction of the slower fibers. When the latency is measured to the smallest recognizable component with the near-nerve needle technique, the slowest NCV can be calculated. In some diseased nerves, the minimum NCV is slowed, whereas other parameters are normal. With the surface electrode and without the aid of a signal averager, a NCV slower than 20 m per second is seldom seen because beyond this point the CNAP is too small to register.

This procedure is used most often for studying the ulnar, median, sural, and radial nerves. Because a special technique is needed to obtain CNAP in the sciatic, posterior tibial, and peroneal nerves, this procedure is usually not used to study these nerves.

47.0 32.4

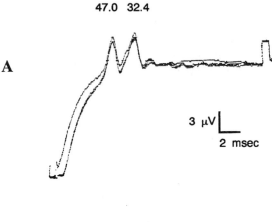

A

3 μV

2 msec

Figure 5.7 Mixed nerve conduction in the forearm segment in the ulnar nerve in a case of chronic inflammatory demyelinating polyneuropathy. **A.** Two peaks of mixed compound nerve action potential indicative of demyelination. Numbers at the top of two peaks represent nerve conduction velocities (m per second). Clearly, the nerve conduction velocity with the second negative peak is slow. **B.** Near-nerve needle mixed compound nerve action potential showing dispersion phenomenon. Numbers at the positive and negative peaks represent nerve conduction velocities (m per second).

42.6

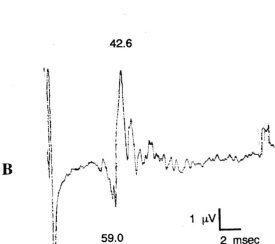

B

1 μV

59.0   2 msec

Mixed Nerve Conduction

The mixed nerve conduction of a peripheral nerve is tested by stimulating the distal part of the mixed nerve (sensory and motor fibers) and recording the CNAP directly over the proximal part of the nerve (see Figure 5.5). For example, conduction along the mixed fibers of the median and ulnar nerves can be tested by stimulating the mixed nerve at the wrist and recording the CNAP at the elbow. The methods of testing, measuring amplitude, and calculating velocity are identical to the orthodromic method of sensory nerve conduction; the only difference is that mixed (motor and sensory) nerve fibers are being stimulated. The clinical significance of mixed NCSs is also identical to that of the sensory NCSs (Figure 5.7).

FACTORS AFFECTING NERVE CONDUCTION TESTS

Among the various factors affecting nerve conduction tests, five are important: skin temperature, age, height, distance measurement, and filter settings.[1]

Temperature

Among the various physiologic factors, skin temperature is the most important factor affecting the nerve conduction test. Various studies have shown that the NCV increases linearly with the temperature within the physiologic range.[1] In motor nerve conduction, the rate of increase ranges from 1.1 to 2.4 m per second. In sensory nerve conduction, this rate ranges from 0.76 to 2.30 m per second. Among the various correction formulae, the most commonly used is the formula by DeJesus et al. that is based on the semilogarithmic relationship between NCV and temperature.[12] Their formula applies to motor as well as sensory fibers, offers a simple method of eliminating diagnostic error caused by temperature variation of the limbs, and requires only that the surface temperature be monitored. Thus, it is essential to measure skin temperature and adjust the NCV to the standard temperature if the skin temperature is below the desired level; otherwise, the surface of the area to be examined must be warmed to the standard temperature with a skin temperature–control unit or hot water immersion.

The distal motor latency is similarly influenced by changes in temperature: It increases by 0.2 millisecond per degree centigrade drop in temperature between 25° and 35°C. The amplitudes of the CMAP and CNAP increase linearly with decreasing temperature. However, there is no reliable correction formula for the amplitude change with temperature.

Age

Age is an important variable in the study of nerve conduction. The changes in nerve conduction are most important in the first 4 years of life and less marked in later years. The NCVs in motor, sensory, and mixed nerves are approximately 50% of the normal adult values in the full-term newborn, reaching approximately 75% of the adult value at 1 year of age, and nearing 100% at 4 years of age. The motor, sensory, and mixed NCVs increase in a logarithmic function. The increase in NCV during infancy and early childhood is most likely due to two factors: (1) the increase in the number of large fibers between birth and 8 years of age, when the number is the same as in adult nerves; and (2) the complete remyelination of nerve fibers by age 5 years. Thus, it is imperative to compare the NCV obtained in infants and babies with the normal values for that same age group.

In adults, the NCVs of motor, sensory, or mixed nerve conduction decrease with age beginning in the 20s. The amplitudes of the CMAP and CNAP are also affected by age, showing a gradual decline. However, this decline is so minimal up to 60 years of age that there is no need for correction. After age 60, however, the decrease is more prominent with age. Thus, minor corrections are needed if the normal adult data were pooled from individuals between 20 and 60 years of age, as is the case in our laboratory. When interpreting the results in patients older than age 60, a correction of 1 m per decade is allowed for the motor NCV and 2 m per decade for the sensory NCV measured with surface electrodes. For the amplitudes of CMAP and CNAP, the change in older individuals does not seem to be important in practice because of the wider range of CMAP and CNAP amplitudes in normal individuals.

Height

Height is not an important factor in the nerve conduction tests, but it is the most important factor in the study of F waves, H reflexes, and tendon reflexes. Because the nerve impulse has to loop through the efferent fibers of nerves, the spinal cord, and the long afferent pathway of nerves in these long latency tests, their linear relationship with body height is obvious and well documented. Thus, it should be customary to compare the obtained values with normal values for a given height. The body height does not affect NCV, but very tall individuals may have mildly slow nerve conduction.

Distance Measurement

Measurement of distance is the second most important factor affecting the nerve conduction tests. Because distance is affected by the position of the limbs (e.g., flexion or extension of the elbow in the ulnar nerve conduction) and contour of the anatomic part (e.g., thoracic outlet segment), it is essential to follow the recommended position of the limb being tested and use the recommended devices (caliper vs. flexible tape) for the distance measurement. Even when these obvious variables are accounted for, the possibility of examiner error is a serious problem in obtaining an accurate calculation of NCV. The shorter the distance, the more critical examiner error becomes. To minimize this influence, 10 cm is recommended as the shortest acceptable distance for the segmental NCV. Certainly, the short-segment NCS (inching technique) violates this rule, and this factor has to be considered in interpretation. One study showed that examiners may differ by up to 1 cm when measuring the distance between two points on a limb if instructed to lay the tape along the course of a nerve.[13] Distance error is primarily due to skin movement rather than to inaccurate reading of the tape measure. To reduce this error, it is best to measure the distance between the center of the stimulating cathode and the center of the active recording electrode using a flexible tape (unless stated otherwise) and to adhere to the recommended position of the limb being tested.

Machine Setups

A change in the machine setup is a possible source of error when measuring the latency and amplitude of the potentials. Although EMG machines are built to reproduce a response accurately with different sweep speeds and sensitivity settings, their measurement of these responses is subject to a certain amount of human error unless performed on a machine that automatically measures both amplitude and latency. Because of this, settings should be constant throughout each individual study whenever possible.

Filter

The filter selection of an amplifier is introduced to ensure distortion-free recording of actual potentials and to maintain the noise level as low as possible. Consequently, a high- or low-filter setting should be carefully chosen on the basis of the frequency characteristics of the CMAP or CNAP. In practice, the baseline shift, which is usually due to movement of the electrode or wire, can be minimized by increasing the low-filter setting from 2 to 20 Hz. When recording small nerve potentials (e.g., sensory or mixed CNAPs), the high-filter setting should be decreased to 2 kHz to reduce the high-frequency noise.

For the motor NCS, the recommended filter range is 12–10,000 Hz, and for the sensory and mixed NCSs, 20–2,000 Hz. These filter ranges have been selected to ensure exact reproduction of the responses. Thus, it is best to set the EMG machine to the standard filter settings for the motor nerve conduction as well as for the sensory and mixed nerve conduction, so that the examiner does not have to be concerned with them. This is because most normal values are obtained with the recommended standard filter settings.

It is obvious that a change in the filter range affects the amplitude and latency. If the change is excessive, the shape and duration of the potentials are also affected. In general, the narrower the frequency limit, the greater is the distortion noted in the potentials. In motor conduction, the lower-frequency limit affects the amplitude more than the high-frequency limit because of the longer duration of the potentials. On the other hand, with sensory and mixed nerve conduction, the high frequency is more important because of the shorter duration of the potentials. In principle, lowering the high filter limit eliminates the faster portions of the signal and, thus, artificially prolongs the signal's latency. Raising the lower filter limit has no effect on the latency. Either maneuver eliminates some of the signal and thus shortens the duration and the latency. In practice, according to our experience, reduction of the high-frequency limit is more critical in the NCS than is raising the lower-frequency limit.

With the near-nerve needle technique, the high-frequency limit might have to be set to 5 or 10 kHz to obtain nerve potentials with many short components. Under pathologic conditions, the CNAP may contain components with frequencies of 8–10 kHz. In such instances, excessive lowering of the upper frequency limit causes a reduction in amplitude of these short components. However, it is important to remember that the widening of the frequency range also introduces noise, which may be difficult to eliminate.

Change of Sensitivity

With the near-nerve needle technique in sensory nerve conduction, the initial positive peak used as the reference point for the latency is clearly identifiable. However, with surface recording in motor and sensory conduction, the point of reference for the latency is often curved, making it difficult to decide which point to measure. Recording with high sensitivity minimizes this difficulty but does not remove it. An error can occur when the sensitivity is changed during the performance of a NCS. Gassel[14] reported a tendency toward a slightly longer latency with low sensitivity than with higher sensitivity. Sensitivity changes can be expected to alter the examiner's judgment of where a reference point is. The sensitivity should be consistent for all stimulating sites of a nerve in the same test.

Change of Sweep Speed

Different sweep speeds can cause different latency measurements that can affect the distal latency and conduction velocity. There is a tendency for a slightly longer latency with higher sweep speeds. The sweep speed should be consistent for all stimulating sites of a nerve in the same test.

TECHNICAL REQUIREMENTS OF THE NERVE CONDUCTION

Supramaximal Stimulation

To obtain meaningful nerve conduction values, supramaximal stimulation is essential. A supramaximal stimulus can be achieved by increasing the intensity by 25–30% above maximal stimulation. The amplitude and latency of the potentials are affected by the intensity of the stimulus. With a gradual increase in stimulus intensity, the amplitude of potentials increases continuously up to the maximum (the maximal stimulation) and then does not increase with further stimulation up to the supramaximal. However, supramaximal stimulation beyond 30% above maximal stimulation is not recommended because the latency can be shortened artificially. This has been observed in motor as well as sensory nerve conduction with surface and needle recording electrodes. With a gradual increase of stimulus intensity, there is a continuous decrease in latency, which becomes still shorter after the CMAP has ceased to increase in amplitude.

Accurate Measurement of Distance

NCV is the most important parameter in the NCS. This can be influenced heavily by the distance measurement as discussed in the section Distance Measurement. To obtain the most reliable distance measurement, it is important to follow the instructions for the position of the limbs and the measuring equipment.

Temperature Control and Correction for Temperature Difference

As discussed in the section Temperature, temperature control is essential for the proper interpretation of NCV. Thus, it is important to control the skin temperature according to the specified temperature level of the particular method. In our laboratory, the skin temperature should be higher than 31°C. Without correction for temperature, NCVs obtained at lower temperatures can be interpreted as abnormal. Thus, if one can not control the skin temperature, one should correct the NCV to the standard temperature using the temperature conversion table (Table 5.1).

Surface Recording Electrodes and Tendon-Belly Placement of These Electrodes in the Motor Nerve Conduction

As discussed in the section Amplitude, the amplitude of the CMAP gives a rough estimation of the number of muscle fibers that respond to nerve stimulation. If the electrodes are arranged in the belly-tendon position with one electrode overlying the end-plate region and the other over the tendon, the CMAP

Table 5.1 Conversion Factors for the Temperature Difference in Nerve Conduction Velocity

Degree Difference	K*	Degree Difference	K*
0.5	1.021	5.5	1.259
1.0	1.043	6.0	1.286
1.5	1.065	6.5	1.313
2.0	1.087	7.0	1.341
2.5	1.117	7.5	1.369
3.0	1.134	8.0	1.398
3.5	1.157	8.5	1.428
4.0	1.183	9.0	1.458
4.5	1.207	10.0	1.520
5.0	1.233		

*Converted NCV = K × obtained nerve conduction velocity.
Source: Reprinted with permission from SJ Oh. Clinical Electromyography: Nerve Conduction Studies (2nd ed). Baltimore: Williams & Wilkins, 1993;44.

has a simple diphasic shape with an initial negative deflection. Thus, the surface electrode is the only reliable method for documenting the conduction block and the decremental response in the repetitive nerve stimulation test and for the objective measurement of the progressive degeneration of motor nerves. It is also useful for identifying the volume-conducted potential by the initial positive deflection. Therefore, we prefer the surface electrodes and placement of these electrodes according to the belly-tendon method for motor NCSs.

With this method, the initial deflection of the CMAP is upward (negative). If the initial deflection is not negative, the following possibilities exist (Figure 5.8)[1]:

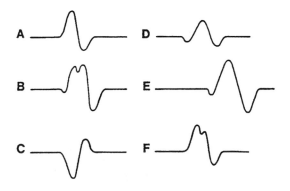

Figure 5.8 The various shapes of the compound muscle action potential. **A.** Normal compound muscle action potential is a diphasic wave with the initial negative deflection. **B.** Active recording electrode is away from the belly (motor point) and closer to the other neighboring muscle. **C.** The active and reference electrodes are reversed. **D.** Stimulation of the neighboring nerves by misplacement of the stimulating electrodes or by stimulus spread when the stimulus is too strong. **E.** Conduction of the nerve impulse through anomalous innervation. **F.** An active recording electrode is placed on the bellies of the two muscles innervated by the same nerve. (Reprinted with permission from SJ Oh. Clinical Electromyography: Nerve Conduction Studies [2nd ed]. Baltimore: Williams & Wilkins, 1993;41.)

- Incorrect placement of the active recording electrode on the desired muscle belly away from the motor point.
- Transposition of the active and reference recording electrodes.
- Stimulation of other neighboring nerves by misplacement of the stimulating electrodes. This technical error can easily occur in the axilla where the ulnar and median nerves are in close proximity. Thus, care must be taken to stimulate the ulnar or median nerves in isolation at the axilla.
- Stimulation of other nerves by stimulus spread when the stimulus has increased in duration and intensity. In severe carpal tunnel syndrome (CTS), this technical error commonly occurs with stimulation of the median nerve at the axilla and rarely occurs with stimulation at the wrist. Even with the correct placement of stimulation electrode at the median nerve, the ulnar nerve is stimulated due to the spread of increased stimulus intensity, which was required to get any response from the median nerve. This technical error can be avoided by careful inspection of the shape of CMAP and, additionally, in case of axilla stimulation, the unexpectedly faster nerve conduction in the axilla-elbow segment.
- Conduction of the nerve impulse through anomalous innervation. This is observed in patients with CTS and Martin-Gruber (median-ulnar nerve) anastomosis, the most common form of anomalous innervation (see the section Median-Ulnar Anastomosis of Motor Fibers).

The first three possibilities can be easily detected. For confirmation of the last two possibilities, careful study by an experienced physician is needed.

COMMON NERVE CONDUCTION TESTS

The median, ulnar, peroneal, posterior tibial (tibial), and sural nerves are tested most frequently in daily practice in the EMG laboratory to diagnose peripheral neuropathy and the common focal neuropathies. Most electromyographers should be proficient in the techniques and interpretation of the results of these tests (Table 5.2). In many laboratories, well-trained EMG technologists perform these procedures under technical supervision of electromyographers. In the workup of peripheral neuropathy, the tests should include: (1) motor, sensory, and mixed nerve conduction in one ulnar and one median nerve; (2) sensory nerve conduction in bilateral sural nerves; (3) motor nerve conduction in bilateral peroneal and posterior tibial nerves; and (4) F waves in median, ulnar, peroneal, and posterior tibial nerves. Because peripheral neuropathy is diffuse and predominantly involves the distal portions of the nerves, the abnormalities are also diffuse and more prominent in the distal segments. When the proximal segments of peripheral nerves are affected, only the F waves may show abnormalities. The most common focal neuropathies (CTS, ulnar neuropathy at the elbow, and peroneal neuropathy), and consequently the majority of neuropathies seen in daily practice, can be detected by one of the common nerve conduction tests.

ELECTROPHYSIOLOGIC RESPONSES IN DISEASED NERVES

Electrophysiologic responses in diseased nerves fall into three categories: (1) conduction slowing, (2) conduction block, and (3) reduced or absent excitability of the nerves. Nerve conduction slowing is the most important parameter in the NCS and is seen as prolonged latency or slow conduction time. This slowing may be

Table 5.2 Normal Nerve Conduction Data[a]

Anatomic Site	Terminal Latency (ms) and Nerve Conduction Velocity (m/s)[b]		Amplitude, Normal Limit	Demyelination Criteria[b]
	Mean ± Standard Deviation	Normal Limit		
Upper extremities				
Median nerve				
Sensory conduction[c]				
Palm-wrist	41.85 ± 3.90	34.05	10 µV	25.1
Finger-wrist	49.54 ± 4.14	41.26	10 µV	29.7
Mixed conduction[c]				
Wrist-elbow	55.99 ± 3.30	49.39	10 µV	33.6
Elbow-axilla	63.47 ± 4.76	53.95	10 µV	38.1
Motor conduction				
Terminal latency	2.78 ± 0.41	3.60	5 mV	4.2
Wrist-elbow	58.78 ± 4.41	49.96	—	35.3
Elbow-axilla	65.76 ± 4.90	55.96	—	39.5
F-wave latency	25.32 ± 2.19	29.70	—	38.0
Ulnar nerve				
Sensory conduction				
Finger-wrist	47.48 ± 4.11	39.26	8 µV	28.5
Mixed conduction				
Wrist-elbow	55.44 ± 3.99	47.46	10 µV	33.3
Elbow-axilla	57.14 ± 4.48	48.18	10 µV	34.3
Erb's point-axilla	64.09 ± 5.64	52.81	10 µV	38.5
Motor conduction				
Terminal latency	2.03 ± 0.24	2.51	5 mV	3.1
Wrist-elbow	61.15 ± 5.27	50.61	—	36.7
Across elbow	51.31 ± 4.25	42.81	—	30.8
Elbow-axilla	63.33 ± 5.47	52.69	—	38.0
Erb's point-axilla	68.36 ± 5.07	58.22	—	38.4
F-wave latency	25.68 ± 2.29	30.26	—	38.5
Radial nerve				
Sensory conduction (distal)	50.87 ± 3.28	44.31	10 µV	30.5
Lower extremities				
Peroneal nerve (motor)				
Terminal latency	3.72 ± 0.53	4.78	4 mV	5.6
Knee-ankle	49.51 ± 3.93	41.85	—	29.7
Knee-popliteal fossa	53.93 ± 7.11	39.11	—	32.4
F-wave latency	46.88 ± 4.25	55.38	—	70.3
Posterior tibial nerve (motor)				
Terminal latency	3.85 ± 0.63	5.11	5 mV	5.8
Knee-ankle	49.83 ± 4.60	40.63	—	29.9
F-wave latency	48.89 ± 4.19	57.27	—	73.3
H reflex on the calf muscle	28.02 ± 1.95	31.93	—	42.0
Sural nerve (sensory)				
Midcalf lateral malleolus	43.26 ± 4.29	34.68	6 µV	26.0

[a]Skin temperature, above 31°C; age range, 20–60; number of controls, 40.

[b]Terminal latency, F-wave latency, and H reflex are expressed in milliseconds. All other values represent nerve conduction velocity (m per second). Data were collected from the University of Alabama at Birmingham, May 1983.

[c]Orthodromic method.

Source: Reprinted with permission from SJ Oh. Clinical Electromyography: Case Studies. Baltimore: Williams & Wilkins, 1998;50.

attributed to three factors: (1) segmental demyelination, (2) loss of large-diameter fibers, and (3) metabolic abnormalities. With segmental demyelination, nerve conduction slowing occurs because of the loss of saltatory conduction in the demyelinated fibers. Slowing of the NCV parallels the degree of demyelination. Because the NCV is proportional to the outer fiber diameter of myelinated fibers, the loss of large-diameter fibers slows the nerve conduction, usually not more than 20% less than the normal mean. This is the pathologic basis of the minimal slowing seen in axonal neuropathy. Conduction block occurs with severe segmental demyelination. With mild segmental demyelination, slowing of conduction is a typical response. In more serious demyelination, many demyelinated fibers fail to conduct the nerve impulse, producing a conduction block. Conduction block is manifested by the reduction of amplitude of the CMAP, and CNAP and is best recognized as a dramatic reduction of amplitude across the site of the block.

Reduced or absent excitability of the nerve is observed when conduction block or axonal degeneration becomes severe. This is measured by the need for an increase in duration and intensity of the stimulus to generate the muscle or nerve action potential. If the conduction block or axonal degeneration is complete, the nerve eventually becomes inexcitable. This is observed best in wallerian degeneration, in which the nerve distal to the lesion becomes totally inexcitable 5 days after total separation.

ELECTROPHYSIOLOGIC CHARACTERISTICS IN AXONAL DEGENERATION AND SEGMENTAL DEMYELINATION

There are two major components in peripheral nerves—axon and myelin—and it is logical to classify a peripheral neuropathy according to the predominant pathologic involvement—axonal degeneration or segmental demyelination (Figure 5.9).[1] The pathophysiologic differences between axonal degeneration and demyelination are given in Table 5.3. Axonal degeneration or segmental demyelination can be recognized by the classic nerve conduction abnormalities (Table 5.4). In some diseased nerves, both processes may be present together.

Axonal Degeneration

The hallmark of nerve conduction abnormalities is the diminution of the amplitude of the CMAP in motor nerve conduction and of the CNAP in the sensory and mixed nerve conduction in the presence of normal or near-normal maximal NCVs and of normal shape and duration of the CMAP or CNAP.

In motor conduction, the following findings are typical of axonal degeneration:

- Unequivocal reduction of the amplitude of the CMAP in proportion to the severity of the axonal degeneration (Figure 5.10).
- Normal shape and duration of the CMAP.
- Minimal prolongation of the terminal latency by not more than 50% of the normal mean.

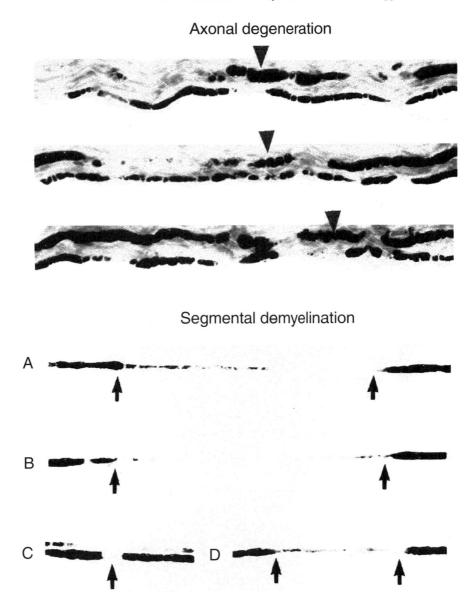

Figure 5.9 Teased nerve findings in axonal degeneration and segmental demyelination. Axonal degeneration: Arrowheads indicate many myelin ovoids indicative of active axonal degeneration in a case of vasculitic neuropathy (see Figure 19.64). Segmental demyelination: Arrows indicate segmental demyelination in **A** and **B** and paranodal widening in **C** and **D** (see Figures 19.68 and 19.69).

• Normal or near-normal NCV. NCV is normal or mildly slow but not more than 40% below the normal mean. This slowing is due to marked loss of large-diameter fibers because of axonal degeneration. The motor NCV in the median nerve is usually above 40 m per second, and in the peroneal nerve, above 35 m per second.

Table 5.3 Pathophysiology of Two Types of Peripheral Neuropathy

Type	Axonal Neuropathy	Demyelinating Neuropathy
Primary lesion	Axon	Myelin
Pathologic process	Axonal degeneration	Demyelination
Pathology by teasing preparation	Myelin ovoids	Segmental demyelination
Regeneration		
Mechanism	Axonal sprouting	Remyelination
Speed	Slow	Rapid
Nerve conduction		
Nerve conduction velocity	Mildly slow, above 30 m/sec	Markedly slow, below 30 m/sec
Compound muscle action potential	Low amplitude	Dispersion, conduction block
Needle electromyography		
Fibrillation and positive sharp waves	(+++)	(−) or (±)
Fasciculation	Absent	Present in chronic form
Neuropathies	Arsenic	Guillain-Barré syndrome
	Alcoholic	Chronic inflammatory
	Nutritional	demyelinating
	Vasculitic	polyneuropathy
	Giant axonal	Hypertrophic
	Thallium	Metachromatic
	Vitamin B_{12}	Tomaculous
	Gold	Leprosy
		Diphtheric

(+++) = prominent; (−) = absent; (±) = may be present.
Source: Reprinted with permission from SJ Oh. Clinical Electromyography: Case Studies. Baltimore: Williams & Wilkins, 1998;51.

In sensory conduction, the following findings are typical of axonal degeneration:

- Unequivocal reduction of the amplitude of the CNAP. With surface electrodes and without the use of signal averaging, the amplitude is so small that the CNAP is unrecordable. With the near-nerve needle electrode, the amplitude is significantly low in proportion to the severity of axonal degeneration.
- Normal shape and duration of the CNAP.
- Normal or near-normal NCV. Slowing of the NCV is less than 40% below the normal mean. The sensory NCV in the median nerve is usually above 35 m per second, and in the sural nerve, more than 30 m per second using the negative peak latency method.
- In cases of severe axonal degeneration, the nerve is inexcitable to obtain any CNAP, even with the near-nerve needle technique.

Table 5.4 Electrophysiologic Characteristics in Axonal Degeneration and Segmental Demyelination

Parameters	Axonal Degeneration	Segmental Demyelination
Motor nerve conduction (with surface electrodes)		
Amplitude	↓↓	N or ↓; conduction block
Duration	N	Dispersion phenomenon
Shape	N	N or multiphasic
Terminal latency	N or ↑ (<150%)	↑↑ (>150%)*
Conduction velocity	N or ↓ (>60%)	↓↓ (<60%)
Sensory nerve conduction		
With surface electrodes		
Amplitude	↓↓ or often absent response	N, ↓, or absent response
Duration	N	Rarely dispersion phenomenon
Shape	N	Rarely multiphasic
Conduction velocity	N or (>60%)	(<60%)
With near-nerve needle technique		
Amplitude	↓↓	N or ↓; conduction block
Duration	N	Prominent dispersion phenomenon
Shape	N	Multiphasic with many components
Conduction velocity	N or ↓ (>60%)	↓↓ (<60%)
F wave	↑ <150% or absent	↑ >150% or absent
H reflex	↑ <150% or absent	↑ >150% or absent

↑ = increased; ↑↑ = markedly increased; ↓ = decreased; ↓↓ = markedly decreased; N = normal.
*Percentage of normal means.
Source: Reprinted with permission from SJ Oh. Clinical Electromyography: Nerve Conduction Studies (2nd ed). Baltimore: Williams & Wilkins, 1993;483.

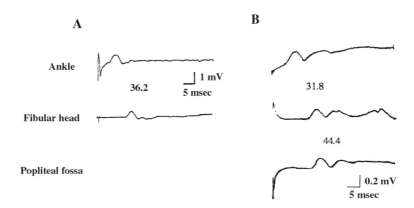

Figure 5.10 Low compound muscle action potential amplitude in peroneal motor nerve conduction in (**A**) (arsenic neuropathy) and in (**B**) (vasculitic neuropathy). Numbers between two compound muscle action potentials represent motor nerve conduction studies. (Ankle = stimulation at ankle; Fibular head = stimulation at below fibular head; Popliteal fossa = stimulation at popliteal fossa.)

Segmental Demyelination

The hallmarks of nerve conduction abnormalities in segmental demyelination are as follows:

- Conduction block. This is usually applied to motor nerve conduction.
- Abnormal temporal dispersion. This is usually applied to the CMAP in motor nerve conduction and to the CNAP in near-nerve sensory nerve conduction.
- Marked slowing in the NCV.

In motor conduction, the following findings are typical of segmental demyelination:

- Normal or reduced amplitude of the CMAP. Substantial slowing of the NCV in the presence of a normal amplitude is indicative of segmental demyelination. When the amplitude is reduced, this reduction is proportional to the degree of temporal dispersion of the CMAP and conduction block.
- Abnormal temporal dispersion or "dispersion phenomenon" (abnormal CMAP with multiple phases and prolonged duration). This is judged in comparison with the normal CMAP or with the CMAP at the distal site. We prefer the term *dispersion phenomenon* when comparing with the normal CMAP and "abnormal temporal dispersion" (see Figure 5.3) when comparing with the CMAP at the distal site. Abnormal temporal dispersion or dispersion phenomenon is typical of segmental demyelination.
- Marked prolongation of the terminal latency. The terminal latency is prolonged by more than 50% of the normal mean. Terminal latencies longer than 6 milliseconds in the median nerve and longer than 10 milliseconds in the peroneal nerve are indicative of segmental demyelination.
- Markedly slow NCV. Slowing of the NCV depends on the degree of segmental demyelination. NCV slowing by more than 40% less than the normal mean is indicative of segmental demyelination. Motor NCVs less than 35 m per second in the median nerve and less than 30 m per second in the peroneal nerve are indicative of segmental demyelination.
- Conduction block (Figure 5.11). The amplitude is somewhat lower with stimulation at more proximal sites in normal subjects. *Conduction block* is defined as being present when there is a greater than 50% reduction of CMAP amplitude and area with normal duration with proximal stimulation as compared with distal stimulation.

In sensory nerve conduction, the following findings are indicative of segmental demyelination:

- Normal or reduced amplitude of the sensory CNAP. Substantial slowing of the NCV in the presence of normal amplitude is indicative of segmental demyelination. When the amplitude is reduced, it is in proportion to the temporal dispersion and conduction block. With surface electrodes, the sensory CNAP is unobtainable in cases of severe segmental demyelination.
- Dispersion phenomenon or abnormal temporal dispersion (see Figure 5.6). Dispersion phenomenon is usually observed in the sensory nerve conduction, because sensory nerve conduction is tested in one segment in the routine study. On very rare occasions, this phenomenon can be documented with the surface electrode, but it is best documented with the near-nerve needle electrode after signal averaging.

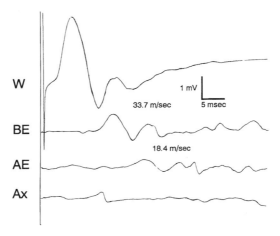

Figure 5.11 Conduction block in ulnar motor nerve conduction in a case with multifocal motor sensory demyelinating neuropathy. Partial conduction block in forearm and elbow segments, with total conduction block in the upper-arm segment and abnormal temporal dispersion in forearm and elbow segment. Numbers between the compound motor action potential responses represent nerve conduction velocity between the wrist (W) and below-elbow (BE) segment and across the elbow (AE). (Ax = axilla.) (Reprinted with permission from SJ Oh, GC Claussen, DS Kim. Motor and sensory demyelinating mononeuropathy multiplex [multifocal motor and sensory demyelinating neuropathy]: a separate entity or a variant of chronic inflammatory demyelinating polyneuropathy? J Peripher Nerv System 1997;2:363.)

When the sensory CNAP is markedly split and lengthened in duration with numerous smaller potential components after the main component, this is termed *dispersion phenomenon*, which is indicative of segmental demyelination.

• Marked slowing in NCV. Slowing of the sensory NCV depends on the severity of segmental demyelination. NCV slowing by more than 40% below the normal mean is indicative of segmental demyelination. Sensory NCV less than 30 m per second in the median nerve and less than 25 m per second in the sural nerve is indicative of segmental demyelination. It is rare to obtain an NCV less than 20 m per second with surface electrodes in severe segmental demyelination because the sensory CNAP is unobtainable due to the smaller amplitude.

• Conduction block. Because the sensory nerve conduction is tested in one segment in the routine NCS, conduction block cannot be documented by the routine sensory nerve conduction. This can only be demonstrated when the sensory fibers are orthodromically stimulated and the recording electrodes are placed in the short segment distal and proximal to the site of block, best seen with the near-nerve needle technique. In practice, because of these technical difficulties, it is almost impossible to demonstrate conduction block in sensory NCSs.

SPECIFIC PATTERNS OF NERVE CONDUCTION ABNORMALITIES

Although most peripheral neuropathies show mixed motor and sensory nerve conduction abnormalities in the NCS, there are certain patterns of abnormalities specific enough to be of value to clinicians in localizing the lesions to specific parts of the nerve axis and in suggesting the nature of a neuropathy (Table 5.5).[1]

Table 5.5 Characteristic Pattern in Nerve Conduction

Motor NCS	Sensory NCS	Pathology	Typical Diseases
Pure motor neuropathy			
Axonal neuropathy	Normal	Anterior horn cell	Motor neuron disease (amyotrophic lateral sclerosis)
		Polyradiculopathy	Axonal form of GBS
Demyelination	Normal	Pure motor neuropathy	Multifocal motor neuropathy
		Polyradiculoneuropathy	GBS (early stages)
Pure sensory neuronopathy			
Normal	Abnormal	Dorsal root ganglion	Friedreich's ataxia
			Sjögren's syndrome neuropathy
			Paraneoplastic subacute sensory neuropathy
Demyelinating mixed neuropathy			
Uniform demyelination	Abnormal	Hereditary neuropathy	Charcot-Marie-Tooth 1A
Nonuniform demyelination	Abnormal	Acquired demyelinating neuropathy	Chronic inflammatory demyelinating polyneuropathy, GBS
Axonal mixed neuropathy			
Axonal neuropathy	Abnormal	Axonal neuropathy	Alcoholic neuropathy, vasculitic neuropathy

GBS = Guillain-Barré syndrome; NCS = nerve conduction study.
Source: Reprinted with permission from SJ Oh. Clinical Electromyography: Nerve Conduction Studies (2nd ed). Baltimore: Williams & Wilkins, 1993;49.

With a pure motor neuropathy, the motor nerve conduction is abnormal, whereas the sensory nerve conduction is completely normal. This neuropathy can be classified into two categories: *axonal* and *demyelinating. Pure motor axonal neuropathy* is characterized by a low CMAP amplitude, mild motor NCV slowing, and normal sensory or mixed nerve conduction. This pattern is indicative of lesions in the anterior horn cells or ventral roots. The best examples of this pattern are seen in amyotrophic lateral sclerosis (ALS) and a few cases of the axonal form of Guillain-Barré syndrome (GBS). A *pure motor demyelinating neuropathy* is characterized by nerve conduction abnormalities typical of demyelination confined to the motor fibers. This pattern is indicative of demyelinating neuropathy involving the motor fibers alone and is typically seen in multifocal motor neuropathy and in some cases of GBS, especially in the early phases. With a *pure sensory neuronopathy*, the sensory nerve conduction is markedly abnormal, showing a pattern of axonal degeneration (extremely low or absent sensory CNAP with mild slowing of sensory NCV), whereas the motor nerve conduction is completely normal. This pattern is pathognomonic of a sensory neuronopathy involving the dorsal root sensory ganglia and is classically observed in Friedreich's ataxia, sensory neuropathy associated with Sjögren's syndrome, and paraneoplastic subacute sensory neuronopathy.

Uniform demyelinating neuropathy is a useful concept in differentiating between *hereditary motor sensory neuropathy* and *acquired chronic demyelinating neuropathy*. In uniform demyelinating neuropathy, the NCV is slowed "uniformly" to the same degree over all nerves and nerve segments. In addition, conduction block or abnormal temporal dispersion is absent because of the uniform demyelination of all fibers. This pattern is classically described in hereditary motor and sensory neuropathy type I (Charcot-Marie-Tooth disease [CMT] 1A) and familial neuropathies associated with metachromatic leukodystrophy, globoid leukodystrophy, and Cockayne's syndrome. In acquired demyelinating neuropathies, the nonuniform slowing of NCV over different nerves and nerve segments, conduction block, and abnormal temporal dispersion are typically observed.

DIAGNOSTIC VALUE OF MOTOR AND SENSORY NERVE CONDUCTION

Many studies have repeatedly shown that sensory conduction is a more sensitive indicator of a peripheral nerve lesion than motor conduction.[1] The advantages of testing sensory nerve conduction are based on the following factors: (1) sensory fibers are often affected earlier than motor nerves; (2) severe loss of nerve fibers can be discriminated more precisely in sensory than in motor fibers; and (3) a response from other than the fastest fibers can be recognized in sensory potentials. Increased temporal dispersion may be an early sign of impairment when conduction velocity along the fastest fibers and the amplitude of the potential are still within the range of normal.

The sensitivity of NCSs for identification of neuropathy is extremely high, being approximately 90% in most focal and diffuse neuropathies if the proper tests are selected for a given disorder and the tests are technically satisfactory.

Nerve conduction tests can identify axonal degeneration and segmental demyelination on the basis of nerve conduction characteristics. This distinction is important because it helps in understanding the basic pathologic process of disease without resorting to biopsy and in further identifying a definite etiology.

The NCS is helpful in identifying and localizing the site of individual nerve compression or entrapment. This information is crucial in the surgical management of many focal or entrapment neuropathies. A distinction can also be made by the NCS as to whether the neuropathy is multifocal (demyelinating or axonal) or diffuse. Multifocal demyelinating neuropathy is usually seen in multifocal motor neuropathy, and multifocal axonal neuropathy in vasculitic neuropathy. Diffuse neuropathy is typical of polyneuropathy.

The NCS can identify the specific pattern of nerve conduction abnormalities on the basis of nerve conduction characteristics. This enables the clinician to localize a lesion to a specific part of the nerve and helps in identifying a definite etiology.

In summary, the nerve conduction data can provide the clinician with invaluable information about the diseased nerve that cannot be obtained by any other means.

NERVE CONDUCTION ABNORMALITIES IN DISEASES

A discussion of nerve conduction abnormalities in each disease is beyond the scope of this chapter. Nerve conduction abnormalities in focal compression neuropathy and polyneuropathy in general are discussed here.[1]

Focal Compression Neuropathy

Focal neuropathies present a common diagnostic problem for the clinical electromyographer (Table 5.6). For the precise localization of a focal neuropathy, the NCS and needle EMG are essential. Among those with nontraumatic causes, the compression neuropathies, in which a nerve is compressed at an anatomically vulnerable site, are the most common. The basic pathologic process in focal compression neuropathies is focal segmental demyelination. In acute focal compression neuropathy, a mild focal demyelinating process is responsible for the conduction block that is the characteristic electrophysiologic finding and explains the complete paralysis of the involved muscle. Abnormal temporal dispersion and nerve conduction slowing may be present. The best examples of acute focal compression neuropathies are "Saturday night palsy" (radial nerve palsy), "crossed-leg palsy" (peroneal nerve palsy), and perioperative ulnar nerve palsy. In chronic focal compression neuropathy, focal demyelination by mechanical entrapment is responsible for the electrophysiologic evidence of chronic focal demyelination: marked focal slowing of the NCV. The presence of conduction block is less often demonstrable by nerve stimulation in chronic entrapment neuropathies than in acute compression neuropathy. Secondary wallerian degeneration is usually found in nerve segments distal to the site of compression.

To localize a focal demyelinating process, it is imperative to study the involved segment by means of the segmental NCS. In human entrapment neuropathy, it has been shown that the primary conduction abnormalities are confined to a short segment (often 5–10 cm) of the nerve. Most authorities regard 10 cm as the shortest acceptable distance for the segmental conduction study as discussed in the section Distance Measurement.

In focal neuropathies, focal slowing of NCV, conduction block, and temporal dispersion across the compression site are the characteristic nerve conduction abnormalities and are seen in more than 90% of cases of focal neuropathy.

Polyneuropathy (Diffuse Peripheral Neuropathy)

The NCS is an essential part of the workup in patients with a peripheral neuropathy. This study helps in the following: (1) confirming peripheral neuropathy, (2) determining the type of neuropathy (axonal neuropathy vs. demyelinating neuropathy) (Table 5.7), and (3) following the course of the disease. The NCS identifies neuropathy in 76–80% of patients with diabetic neuropathy and in 81–100% of patients with GBS. To obtain a greater diagnostic yield in the nerve conduction investigation of patients with peripheral neuropathy, it is important to follow two important guidelines. First, testing should be performed on several nerves. McLeod et al.[15] recommended several nerves in both upper and lower limbs. We recommend several nerves in one upper and both lower limbs. Secondly, the tests should include both

Table 5.6 Compression Site and Typical Clinical and Nerve Conduction Features of the Common Compression Neuropathies

Compression Syndrome	Entrapment Site	Typical Clinical Features	Classical EMG/NCS Findings
Median nerve			
Carpal tunnel syndrome	Carpal tunnel	Tinel's sign at the wrist; sensory impairment over the first 3.5 fingers; motor deficits on thenar muscles	Prolonged terminal latency; slow sensory NCV over finger- and palm-wrist segments
Anterior interosseous syndrome	At its origin from the median nerve	Pure motor weakness of the flexion of the middle phalanx of the first three fingers	Denervation in the flexor pollicis longus and pronator quadratus; abnormal anterior interosseous nerve conduction
Pronator syndrome	At the level of pronator teres	Entire median motor and sensory neuropathy with pronator teres spared; pronator muscle tenderness and Tinel's sign on it	Denervation in the median innervated muscles with pronator teres spared; slow motor and sensory-mixed NCS in the forearm and elbow
Ulnar nerve			
Tardy ulnar palsy and cubital tunnel syndrome	Elbow	"Claw hand"; motor deficit on hypothenar muscles; sensory impairment over the dorsal and palmar aspects of the last 1.5 fingers	Slow NCV across elbow; abnormal mixed and sensory NCS over finger-elbow
Guyon's canal	Wrist	Same as above except sensory impairment over palmar aspects of the last 1.5 fingers	Prolonged terminal latency; slow sensory NCV over finger-wrist segment
Thoracic outlet syndrome (brachial plexus)	Thoracic outlet	Sensory impairment over the ulnar side of the entire arm and hand; motor deficits in the hyper- and hypomuscles	Prolonged F wave; abnormal ulnar sensory NCS; low median compound muscle action potential; abnormal medial antebrachial NCS
Radial nerve			
Saturday night palsy	Spiral groove	Wrist drop	Denervation in the radial innervated muscles except triceps
Posterior interosseous syndrome	Arcade of Frohse	Finger drop	Denervation in the extensor digitorum communis and indices; extensor carpi and radials spared
Suprascapular nerve	Suprascapular foramen	Weakness in the supra- and infraspinatus muscles	Denervation in the supra- and infraspinatus muscles, prolonged latency when stimulating at Erb's point, and recording in the supra- or infraspinatus muscles; low-amplitude CMAP
Lateral femoral cutaneous nerve			
Meralgia paresthetica	Anterior iliac crest	Sensory impairment over the lateral thigh	Abnormal NCS in the lateral femoral nerve
Femoral nerve	Inguinal ligament	Weak knee extension and absent knee jerk	Abnormal femoral motor NCS
Peroneal nerve			
Crossed-leg palsy	Fibular head	Foot drop	Slow NCV across the fibular head
Posterior tibial nerve			
Tarsal tunnel syndrome	Tarsal tunnel	Sensory impairment over the palmar aspect of the foot; Tinel's sign at the ankle	Abnormal mixed NCV and sensory NCS in the medial and lateral plantar nerve
Morton's neuroma	III–IV interdigital nerve	Sensory impairment over the V-shaped area between III and IV toes	Dip phenomenon in the interdigital NCS

CMAP = compound muscle action potential; EMG = electromyography; NCS = nerve conduction study; NCV = nerve conduction velocity.

Table 5.7 Pathologic Classification of Peripheral Neuropathies

Axonal Degeneration	Segmental Demyelination
Hereditary neuropathies	
CMT 2; neuronal CMT (HMSN type II)	CMT 1A; hypertrophic CMT (HMSN type I)
Giant axonal sensory neuropathy	Refsum's disease (HMSN type IV)
Hereditary sensory autonomic neuropathy	Roussy-Lévy syndrome
Fabry's disease	Metachromatic leukodystrophy
Infantile neuroaxonal dystrophy	Krabbe's disease
Cerebral lipofuchsinosis	Hereditary neuropathy with liability to pressure
Mucopolysaccharidoses	palsy
Pelizaeus-Merzbacher disease	Cockayne's syndrome
	Adrenomyeloneuropathy
	Cerebroxanthomatosis
Autoimmune neuropathies	
Fisher's syndrome	Guillain-Barré syndrome
Chronic ataxic sensory neuropathy	CIDP
Neuropathy with serum autoantibody to sulfatide	Multifocal motor neuropathy
Neuropathy with anti-Hu antibody	Multifocal motor sensory demyelinating neuropathy
Sarcoid neuropathy	Chronic sensory demyelinating neuropathy
Vasculitic neuropathies	Anti–GM-1 ganglioside autoantibody neuropathy
	Myelin-associated glycoprotein–positive neuropathy
Paraneoplastic neuropathies	
Carcinoma	Lymphoma
Neuropathy with anti-Hu antibody	
Neuropathies with infectious diseases	
AIDS (late)	AIDS (early); Guillain-Barré syndrome or CIDP
Lyme disease	Diphtheric neuropathy
Neuropathy associated with tetanus	Leprosy
Hepatitis C	
Dysproteinemic neuropathies	
Multiple myeloma	MGUS neuropathy (IgM)
MGUS neuropathy (IgG or IgA)	Osteosclerotic myeloma
Cryoglobulinemia	Waldenström's macroglobulinemia
Amyloidosis	Angiofollicular lymph node hyperplasia
	POEMS syndrome
Metabolic neuropathies	
Uremia	Acromegaly
Diabetes mellitus	
Hypothyroidism	
Vitamin deficiency, including vitamin B_{12}	
Pyridoxin toxicity	
Acute porphyria	
Critical illness polyneuropathy	
Toxic neuropathies	
Lead (human)	Lead (animal)
Alcoholism	Tetrodotoxin, saxitoxin
Almost all drugs (except perhexiline, amiodarone)	Perhexiline, amiodarone
Almost all solvents, including hexane	
Arsenic	
Thallium	
Gold	
Cisplatinum	
Spanish toxic oil neuropathy	

AIDS = acquired immunodeficiency syndrome; CIDP = chronic inflammatory demyelinating polyneuropathy; CMT = Charcot-Marie-Tooth disease; HMSN = hereditary motor and sensory neuropathy; Ig = immunoglobulin; MGUS = monoclonal gammopathy of undetermined significance; POEMS = polyneuropathy, organomegaly, endocrinopathy, M protein, skin changes syndrome.

sensory and mixed NCSs in addition to motor nerve conduction. Abnormalities in sensory conduction are a more sensitive indicator of impairment than the motor response, as discussed above. A specific pattern of motor and sensory nerve conduction abnormalities is adequate to localize a lesion to specific parts of the nerve axis.

Nerve conduction abnormalities in peripheral neuropathy are usually diffuse. However, conduction abnormalities may not be observed in all nerves tested. When more than 50% of these nerves show evidence of abnormality, we interpret this as "indicative" of peripheral neuropathy. When fewer than 50% of nerves tested show abnormality, this is interpreted as "compatible" with peripheral neuropathy. The nerve conduction abnormalities in peripheral neuropathy depend on the nature of the pathologic process (axonal vs. segmental demyelination) and the site of the lesion, as discussed in the section Electrophysiologic Characteristics in Axonal Degeneration and Segmental Demyelination.

UNCOMMON NERVE CONDUCTION TESTS

Uncommon nerve conduction tests are those performed on uncommonly tested nerves. Considering the number of nerves in the human body and the possibilities of injury to these nerves, it is almost impossible to know the techniques and normal values for all uncommon nerve conductions. See the textbook for details of these techniques and normal data.[1]

The most common indication for performance of an uncommon NCS is confirmation of the diagnosis of a mononeuropathy. The most critical factors in this case are suspicion of neuropathy in a particular nerve and appropriate testing of that nerve. Accessory neuropathy as a cause of scapular winging is a good example of this, because it is commonly confused with paralysis of the serratus anterior muscle (long thoracic neuropathy), a more common cause for scapular winging. In accessory neuropathy, the trapezius muscle is always involved, producing shoulder drooping and winging of the upper scapula, which is accentuated by arm abduction at the shoulder level. In long thoracic neuropathy, the scapular winging is more prominent in the lower part of the scapula and is accentuated by forward elevation and pushing with outstretched arms. Almost all patients with accessory neuropathy in our EMG laboratory had previously been misdiagnosed as suffering from long thoracic neuropathy.

The second indication for an uncommon NCS is to aid in the diagnosis of a more proximal focal neuropathy. The best example of this is the medial antebrachial cutaneous nerve conduction in the diagnosis of neurogenic thoracic outlet syndrome (Figure 5.12). The medial antebrachial cutaneous nerve branches out from the medial cord proximal to the branching of the ulnar nerve and travels independently downward, exiting at the midportion of the upper arm and subserving sensation over the medial antebrachial area of the forearm. Thus, a nerve conduction abnormality of this nerve clearly localizes the lesion proximally at the lower trunk or medial cord of the brachial plexus, as this does not occur in ulnar neuropathy or in radiculopathy. In neurogenic thoracic outlet syndrome, the nerve conduction abnormality in this nerve is common.[16] Another example is the lateral antebrachial cutaneous nerve for the diagnosis of upper-trunk plexus neuropathy. Because this is the distal sensory branch of musculocutaneous nerve, the nerve

A

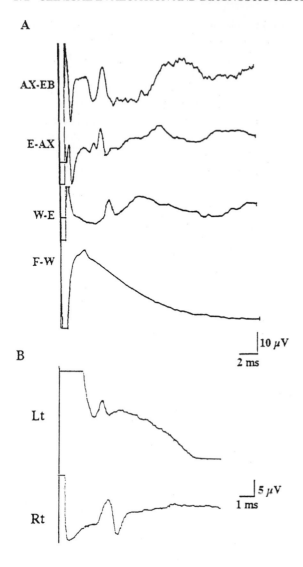

Figure 5.12 Sensory and mixed nerve conduction of ulnar nerve in a case of neurogenic thoracic outlet syndrome. **A.** Low compound nerve action potential amplitude in sensory nerve conduction in the finger-wrist (F-W) segment and in mixed nerve conduction in the wrist-elbow (W-E), elbow-axilla (E-AX), and axilla-Erb's (AX-EB) segments. **B.** Lower compound nerve action potential amplitude in the left (Lt) medial antebrachial cutaneous nerve compared with that on the right (Rt). (Reprinted with permission from SJ Oh. Principles of Clinical Electromyography: Case Studies. Baltimore: Williams & Wilkins, 1998;169.)

conduction abnormality in this nerve can help localize the lesion to the upper trunk in differential diagnosis from the C6 radiculopathy.

In performing the uncommon nerve conduction tests, the following tips are helpful in obtaining the motor or sensory responses successfully and interpreting the data meaningfully.[1]

1. Read through the method carefully from the standard textbook and follow the technical directions exactly.[1] Because the data from the patient must be compared with the published normal data of other laboratories, this rule becomes crucial. The skin temperature must also be controlled as suggested by the particular method. If the skin temperature is lower than the controlled temperature, it must be warmed by various techniques, or the measured NCV must be converted to the correct value for the controlled temperature using a correction formula.

2. Perform the NCS on the normal side, and use this as a technical control. Because the uncommon nerve conduction tests are rarely performed, it is difficult to master their techniques. Thus, it is a good idea to do the test on a normal nerve first and use this as a technical guide, comparing the data obtained with those from the abnormal side.

3. Position the recording and stimulating electrodes according to the anatomic guide in the text. If the CMAP or CNAP is not easily obtained, do not hesitate to move the electrodes, especially the stimulating electrode. One way to ensure the correct location of the stimulating electrode on the nerve being tested is to ask the patient whether there is paresthesia over the sensory nerve territory. Another way is to look for contraction of the muscles innervated by the tested motor nerve.

4. Use signal averaging liberally for the sensory nerve conduction. This is the surest way to obtain small abnormal sensory CNAPs.

PEDIATRIC NERVE CONDUCTION STUDIES

To achieve optimal results with the limited cooperation of a child, the following strategies are followed in our EMG laboratory.[1,17]

1. To reduce fear and elicit a child's cooperation, the presence of a parent in the examining room is usually helpful. We encourage the parent to participate by holding the child's hands or by having the child sit on the parent's lap for the study. However, this must be individualized because some parents cannot stand to watch their children having the electrodiagnostic test. Cooperation from the parent for the NCS can be improved by allowing the parent to experience a brief electrical stimulus on the palm before beginning the study with the child.

2. In general, the NCS can be performed without difficulty in a majority of pediatric patients. Thus, in the workup of suspected neuromuscular disorders in children, we recommend that the nerve conduction test be performed first. It often provides a definite diagnosis if the patient has peripheral neuropathy, and there is then no need for the more painful needle EMG study. Moreover, the nerve conduction test can be performed without much difficulty in infants and most older children. In small children who are not cooperative for the nerve conduction test, sedation is occasionally needed.

Because of their small body size, special technical considerations must be made for NCS in infants. For this procedure, we recommend the following guidelines:

1. A pediatric simulator should be used because the distance between the active and reference electrodes is shorter.

2. A ring electrode can be used as a reference-recording electrode for fingers or toes.

3. The posterior tibial nerve should be tested first because it shows the most reliable and technically satisfactory response.

4. Often, it is difficult to record the response from the extensor digitorum brevis (EDB) after stimulation of the peroneal nerve at the ankle in infants. This is due to the proximity of the stimulating electrode to the recording electrode. In this situation, the latency from the knee may be the only objective finding in the peroneal nerve.

5. In motor conduction studies of the median and ulnar nerves, the NCV can be calculated over the elbow-axilla segment if the response with wrist stimulation is unrecordable.

6. Sensory nerve conduction is easier to study in the median and ulnar nerves. If there is difficulty in obtaining the CNAP from the wrist after stimulation at the fingers, the recording electrodes should be placed on the elbow. Usually, no difficulty is encountered when obtaining the sensory CNAP at the elbow.

Once the nerve conduction data are obtained, these data must be compared with the normal values for the patient's age, as discussed above.

ANOMALOUS INNERVATION

Anomalous innervations may be a source of error in the nerve conduction if not recognized. Knowledge of a few common variations is crucial to the clinician in the performance of nerve conduction and electromyographic studies to prevent faulty interpretation of the electrophysiologic data.[1] In practice, the most important variations in the peripheral nerves are (1) median-ulnar anastomosis (Martin-Gruber anastomosis), and (2) an accessory deep peroneal nerve.

Median-Ulnar Anastomosis of Motor Fibers

Median-ulnar anastomosis is the most common form of anomalous innervation. Various NCSs have found an anastomosis in 15–39% of normal controls and in 8–26% of patients with CTS. This anastomosis involves axons leaving the main trunk of the median nerve or the anterior interosseous nerve, crossing through the forearm to join the main trunk of the ulnar nerve, and ultimately innervating the intrinsic hand muscles.

The Martin-Gruber anastomosis is best studied by recording the CMAP simultaneously in three muscles—the abductor digiti quinti, first dorsal interossei, and abductor pollicis brevis—with stimulation of the ulnar and median nerves at the wrist and elbow and by comparing the CMAP amplitudes.[1]

In practice, it is impossible to recognize the Martin-Gruber anastomosis in normal individuals with the setups for routine median and ulnar motor nerve conduction. In CTS, the Martin-Gruber anastomosis may produce additional electrophysiologic changes that make interpretation of the nerve conduction difficult unless the electromyographer is aware of this anomaly. Three different nerve conduction patterns are noted (Figure 5.13):

1. Median nerve stimulation at the elbow evokes a thenar CMAP with an initial positive deflection not seen on stimulation at the wrist.[18]

2. There is an erroneously normal proximal (elbow) motor latency in the median nerve with prolongation of the distal motor latency.

3. A thenar CMAP with two components is seen upon median nerve stimulation at the elbow.

Gutmann[18] reported a thenar CMAP with an initial positive deflection on median elbow stimulation as a pathognomonic electrophysiologic finding indicative of the Martin-Gruber anastomosis in the presence of CTS. Gutmann noted this change in

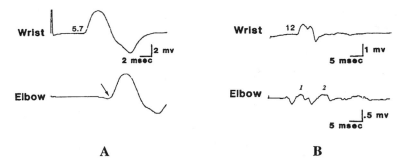

Figure 5.13 Two compound muscle action potential (CMAP) responses with wrist stimulation (Wrist) and elbow stimulation (Elbow) in median motor nerve conduction in two cases of carpal tunnel syndrome with Martin-Gruber anastomosis. **A.** The thenar CMAP on median elbow stimulation is preceded by a positive deflection (*arrow*) not seen on wrist stimulation. This was the cardinal clue indicative of Martin-Gruber anastomosis. **B.** The thenar CMAP with two components and the initial positive deflection on median elbow stimulation are prominent findings. The first component is the CMAP response through Martin-Gruber anastomosis (1) and the second component is the CMAP response through the median nerve (2). In this case, the latency from the elbow is shorter than the terminal latency. Numbers above the CMAP represent terminal latency.

20% of median nerves in 62 consecutive patients with bilateral CTS.[19] He gave the following reason for the thenar CMAP, preceded by an initial positive deflection, on elbow stimulation but not on wrist stimulation: Conduction in the median nerve axons going through the carpal tunnel and innervating thenar muscles is slower than in those median nerve axons crossing to the ulnar nerve and supplying the first dorsal interosseous, adductor pollicis, abductor digiti quinti, and flexor pollicis brevis.[19] The CMAP from the latter muscles, on median nerve stimulation at the elbow, is generated before that from the thenar muscles innervated by median axons going through the carpal tunnel. The earlier appearing CMAP is incorporated into the overall thenar CMAP, but, because it originates at some distance from the recording electrode, it produces an initial positive deflection. In fact, Gutmann suggested this initial positive deflection as an electrophysiologic diagnostic index for mild CTS.[20] He reported six cases of mild CTS in which motor and sensory nerve conductions were essentially normal, and a positive deflection preceding the thenar CMAP on elbow stimulation, but not on wrist stimulation, was the sole electrophysiologic abnormality.

Iyer and Fenichel[21] reported five cases of CTS in which near-normal latency was found on proximal stimulation of the median nerve, although the distal motor latency was prolonged. The presence of the Martin-Gruber anastomosis leads to partial or total sparing of the thenar muscles from the effects of compression of their nerve supply in a case of CTS. In cases of partial sparing, the distal latency of the median nerve is prolonged, but upon stimulation at the elbow, the latency is normal because the stimulus can travel along the noncompressed fibers constituting the anastomosis and can bypass the retinaculum via the ulnar nerve. This is the cause of the near-normal proximal latency resulting in the apparent short conduction time in the forearm segment of the median nerve and the spuriously high-calculated NCV. According to Gutmann,[19] this finding is less common in CTS in the presence of the anomaly. He observed this finding in only 1 of 63 consecutive patients studied and concluded that it is not a very useful finding.

Additionally, Lambert[22] described a thenar CMAP with two components on median nerve stimulation at the elbow, again related to the slower conduction in the median nerve at the wrist and the faster conduction in those axons that have crossed to the ulnar nerve. The ulnar nerve component is absent when the median nerve is stimulated at the wrist. According to our experience, this may be seen in severe CTS but also seems to be an uncommon finding.

Accessory Deep Peroneal Nerve

The accessory deep peroneal nerve is a common variant of the common peroneal nerve innervating the EDB. The EDB is usually innervated exclusively by the deep peroneal nerve, a main branch of the common peroneal nerve. However, in 19–22% of individuals, one or both of the EDBs are innervated partially by the accessory deep peroneal nerve, a branch of the superficial peroneal nerve.[23–25] The accessory deep peroneal nerve arises from the superficial peroneal nerve midway on the lateral aspect of the leg; it passes deep and posterior to the peroneus brevis tendon, behind the lateral malleolus, and subsequently innervates the lateral portion of the EDB. This anomaly seems to be inherited in an autosomal dominant mode. Awareness of this variation in innervation of the EDB is important for the correct clinical and electromyographic evaluation of peroneal nerve lesions.

This anatomic variation can be easily proved by stimulating the peroneal nerve at three locations: the deep peroneal nerve at the ankle, the common peroneal nerve at the fibular head (conventional method), and the accessory deep peroneal nerve posterior to the lateral malleolus (Figure 5.14).

This anatomic variation should be suspected when the CMAP amplitude in the EDB is considerably smaller when stimulating the deep peroneal nerve at the ankle as compared to stimulation of the common peroneal nerve at the knee. Normally, the CMAP amplitude of the EDB obtained by stimulating the deep peroneal nerve at the ankle should be 90–120% of that obtained by stimulating the common peroneal nerve at the knee.[19]

CLINICAL APPLICATION OF F WAVE

The F-wave test is known to be a sensitive test for polyneuropathy.[9,26] In general, the diagnostic sensitivity of F-wave latency is somewhat higher than that of motor NCS but equal to that of sensory NCS: abnormal late responses (F wave and H reflex) in 93–100% versus abnormal motor NCS in 73–83% and abnormal sensory NCS in 90–100% of patients.[11,27,28] This is the case in alcoholic neuropathy,[28] neuropathy with chronic renal failure,[27] and axonal neuropathy.[11] However, in demyelinating neuropathy, a different pattern emerges. In GBS and chronic inflammatory demyelinating polyradioneuropathy (CIDP), the F-wave latency is clearly more sensitive than the sensory NCS in view of the predominant motor involvement in these diseases[11,29]: Abnormal F-wave latency is observed in 70–98% of cases versus abnormal sensory NCS in 39–80%.

Figure 5.14 Accessory peroneal nerve in a patient with diabetes mellitus without neuropathy. **A.** Compound muscle action potential with peroneal stimulation at ankle. **B.** Compound muscle action potential with accessory peroneal nerve stimulation behind the lateral malleolus. **C.** Compound muscle action potential with peroneal nerve at the fibular head. (Reprinted with permission from SJ Oh. Clinical Electromyography: Nerve Conduction Studies [2nd ed]. Baltimore: Williams & Wilkins, 1993;329.)

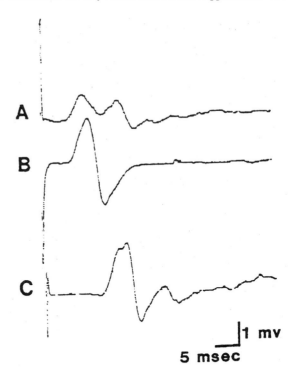

Among the various F-wave parameters, minimum latency is the most useful in polyneuropathy in general. Decreased persistence or absence of responses has a sensitivity comparable to minimum latency in GBS and CIDP, and chronodispersion has a sensitivity comparable with minimum latency only in CIDP.[11]

The F-wave test is most helpful in detection of neuropathy when it is abnormal in the presence of unremarkable routine NCS. This does occur but is rarer than once thought. The most quoted paper in this regard is that by Lachman et al., who reported abnormal late responses (H reflex and F wave) in 86% of cases in contrast to abnormal NCS in 72% of cases with various neuropathies.[30] This early study did not include the sural nerve conduction in the workup of peripheral neuropathy, which is a routine practice at this time.

The F-wave test is most useful diagnostically in polyneuropathies associated with prominent proximal involvement, which is not accessible by conventional methods. Under this circumstance, the F-wave latency can be abnormal even when the distal motor nerve conduction is unremarkable, as discussed previously in this section.[11,27,28,30] In this connection, the F-wave test is most useful in GBS. Kimura and Butzer used the F-wave conduction velocity as a measure of proximal conduction between the axilla and spinal cord in nine patients with mild GBS. In four of the nine patients, F-wave conduction velocity was slow, despite normal or borderline distal motor NCV.[31] King and Ashby, using a technique similar to Kimura's, also studied the F wave in motor fibers of the ulnar nerve in 11 patients with GBS.[32] They found that in two patients, the conduction velocity of the proximal segment was disproportionately reduced, whereas in one of these the NCV in the distal segment was within normal limits. Lachman et al. measured the F-wave latencies in the median nerve and the H-reflex latency to the soleus muscle in 11 patients with GBS.[30] In two patients, the F-wave latency was abnormal, although the distal motor NCV was normal. Walsh et al. found a prolonged F-wave latency in 8 of 17 GBS patients and in two of eight patients with normal motor NCS.[33] Thus, the F-wave study is of value in establishing the diagnosis in some GBS patients in whom the distal motor NCS is normal, especially early in the course of disease. On the other hand, in CIDP, the F-wave abnormality is as high as the motor nerve conduction abnormality.[11]

The F-wave test can be useful for the diagnosis of demyelinating neuropathy. Three criteria are used for the diagnosis of demyelinating neuropathy:

1. An F-wave latency longer than 150% of the normal mean or 120% of the upper normal limit.[1] This criterion was supported by later studies.[11,34,35]

2. The F chronodispersion. This is the F-wave counterpart of temporal dispersion and tends to be larger in demyelinating neuropathy than in axonal neuropathy.[11,36] Chronodispersion of more than 9 milliseconds was observed only in GBS and CIDP.[11] In CIDP, the F chronodispersion has a diagnostic sensitivity comparable to the F-wave latency.

3. Absence of F waves in nerves with normal CMAP amplitudes. Frazer et al. observed this situation only in 12 patients with GBS and CIDP and concluded that it provided evidence for proximal conduction block.[11]

Markedly prolonged F-wave latencies or absence of F wave in nerves with normal CMAP amplitude is highly specific for demyelination.[11] In contrast, the presence of F waves with normal or slightly delayed latencies favors an axonal rather than demyelinating process in chronic neuropathies when NCVs are slow and CMAP amplitudes are low.[9] On rare occasions, the diagnosis of demyelination can be made by the F-wave test alone. Olney and Aminoff observed 4 of 10 F-wave studies with prolonged latency in GBS to be longer than 120% of the normal upper limit, but the motor NCS also suggested demyelination in three of these.[29] Theoretically, the decreased F-wave persistence is indicative of partial conduction block in proximal segments of the peripheral nerves. However, this was not proven to be true. Fraser and Olney found that the decreased F-wave persistence occurred infrequently in demyelinating neuropathies as well as in axonal neuropathies and was always associated with prolonged minimum latency.[11]

The F-wave test is also helpful in diagnosis of chronic tetanus and stiff-man syndrome in which neuronal hyperexcitability is the physiologic hallmark due to failure of Renshaw-cell inhibition.[37] In normal individuals, the F-wave amplitude is less than 5% of the M-wave amplitude.[38] In chronic tetanus, huge F waves—as large as 75% of M-wave amplitudes—have been found.[37] In stiff-man syndrome, the F-wave amplitude was larger: 15% of the M-wave amplitude (Figure 5.15).[39] In myokymia-cramp syndrome, the repetitive discharge of F waves was helpful in recognizing repetitive discharge of CMAPs.[40]

The F wave is not useful in the diagnosis of more localized nerve lesions, such as radiculopathies or compression syndromes, in which conduction along the length of the nerve is otherwise normal. The F-wave latency is prolonged in ALS and is comparable to the degree of slowing of the motor NCV.[24]

CLINICAL APPLICATIONS OF THE H REFLEX

The H reflex is most useful in two rare conditions: Holmes-Adie syndrome and tabes dorsalis, in which the muscle stretch reflexes are abnormal in the presence

Figure 5.15 High amplitude of F wave (F/M ratio: 0.15 [normal <0.05]) in peroneal motor nerve (N) conduction in a case of stiff-man syndrome, indicating neuronal hyperexcitability. F/M is the ratio of the maximum amplitude of F wave to maximum M-amplitude.

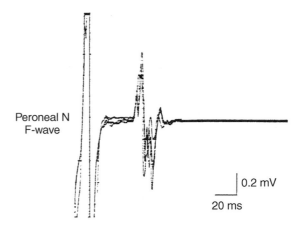

Peroneal N
F-wave

0.2 mV

20 ms

of normal NCS. In Holmes-Adie syndrome (tonic pupils and patchy areflexia), the H reflex was absent or virtually absent in patients with depressed reflexes, whereas the motor and sensory nerve conductions for the peroneal, posterior tibial, and sural nerves were normal,[41] indicating that the areflexia in Holmes-Adie syndrome is caused by loss of large spindle afferents or reduced effectiveness of their monosynaptic connections to motor neurons. This observation is partly compatible with the autopsy findings in Holmes-Adie syndrome, which reveal degeneration of dorsal root ganglion cells, fiber loss in the dorsal roots, and nerve fiber degeneration in the lumbosacral portions of the dorsal columns.[42,43] In tabes dorsalis, the H reflex and posterior tibial somatosensory evoked potentials were absent, whereas the motor and sensory nerve conductions were normal.[44] This observation correlates well with the known pathology of this disease in which the degeneration is confined to the dorsal roots, dorsal funiculi, and posterior columns of the lumbosacral and lower thoracic spinal cord, usually sparing the dorsal root ganglia.[45]

The H reflex is useful in cases of peripheral neuropathy in which only the H reflex is abnormal, whereas other nerve conduction parameters or the muscle stretch reflexes are normal. The H reflex is absent or prolonged in latency in the various polyneuropathies.[46–49] This is understandable in view of the frequent impairment of muscle stretch reflexes in peripheral neuropathy. The H reflex from the triceps surae was not obtainable in all patients with absent ankle reflexes.[28,30] On the other hand, normal muscle stretch reflexes do not guarantee normal H reflex. Kuruoglu and Oh found abnormal H reflexes in six patients with chronic demyelinating polyneuropathy who had intact muscle stretch reflexes,[50] fulfilling one of the diagnostic criteria of CIDP (areflexia or decreased reflexes).

There are a few studies comparing the conventional NCS and the H-reflex test in peripheral neuropathy. In 30 alcoholics, D'Amour et al. showed abnormalities in motor nerve conduction in 47% of cases, in late responses (F wave and H reflex) in 73% of cases, in sensory nerve conduction in median and ulnar nerves in 73% of cases, and in median, ulnar, and sural nerves in 90% of cases.[28] This study clearly indicates the greater diagnostic sensitivity of sensory nerve conduction in peripheral neuropathy compared with the late responses when sural nerve conduction is included. In 50 patients with various polyneuropathies, Lachman et al. found that the late responses (F wave in the median nerve and H reflex in the triceps surae) were abnormal in 18% of cases when the routine nerve conduction was normal.[30] Based on this, they claimed that the late responses are useful in early detection of peripheral neuropathy. However, their routine NCSs did not include sural nerve conduction, which is not acceptable to the present standard of electrophysiologic testing for peripheral neuropathy. More convincing evidence in this regard was presented by Schimsheimer et al., who observed the H reflex in the flexor carpi radialis to be abnormal in 13 (14%) of 93 polyneuropathy patients, whereas the median motor and sensory nerve conductions were normal in these 13 patients.[51] Thus, these studies indicate that there are a few cases of peripheral neuropathy in which only the late responses are abnormal although other nerve conduction parameters are normal. This is especially noted in early cases of GBS, which is known to involve predominantly the proximal nerve segments. Lachman et al. measured the F-wave latencies in the median nerve and the H-reflex latency to the soleus muscle in 11 patients with GBS.[30] In two patients (18%), the late responses were abnormal, although the distal motor NCV was normal. This is one instance in which the H-reflex test is helpful in the diagnosis of peripheral neuropathy. In chronic demyelinating neuropathy, there was no case in which the H reflex was abnormal when the posterior tibial motor NCS or sural NCS was normal.[50] Of 26 patients with chronic demyelinating neuropathy, the H reflex to the gastrocnemius soleus muscle was abnormal in 24 cases (92%): prolonged latency in nine patients and no potential in 15 cases. This is in contrast to abnormal posterior tibial motor NCS in 95% of cases, abnormal sural NCS in 88%, and abnormal T-reflexes in 96%. Electrophysiologic evidence of demyelination was better identified by the motor NCS than by the H reflex and T reflex: 58% of cases in the motor NCS, 8% in the H reflex, and 19% in the T reflex.

When the needle EMG test is normal or equivocal, the H reflex is useful in detecting radiculopathy in which the H reflex is the sole abnormality. This was observed in three of 100 patients with clinically diagnosed lumbosacral radiculopathy.[52] It has been well established that the H reflex in the gastrocnemius soleus (triceps surae) muscle is sensitive in the detection of S1 radiculopathy and helpful in differentiating it from L5 radiculopathy. The H reflex in the triceps surae is absent or prolonged in 50–100% of patients with S1 radiculopathy. On the other hand, in L5 radiculopathy the H reflex in the triceps surae is abnormal in 0–26% of cases. For the detection of L5 radiculopathy, the H reflex in the extensor digitorum longus muscle is the test of choice. This test was abnormal in 83% of patients with L5 radiculopathy, whereas it was abnormal in 33% with S1 radiculopathy. The H reflex in the vastus lateralis muscle successfully confirmed the diagnosis of L4 radiculopathy in all of 14 cases. The H reflex in the flexor carpi radialis is known to be helpful in detection of C6 or C7 radiculopathy, being abnormal in 68–90% of cases. Thus, these studies showed that the H reflex of the appropriate muscle can identify a radiculopathy involving the main root subserving that particular muscle. When using the H reflex test for radiculopathy, it is practical to perform side-to-side comparison as discussed in the section H Reflex, and the only practical H reflex that is reliable and simple is that in the gastrocnemius soleus muscle. A side-to-side latency difference greater than 1.5 milliseconds has been used to diagnose S1 radiculopathy.

The H-reflex test can be a valuable tool in differentiating between ALS and primary muscular atrophy or polyneuropathy. In ALS, it is possible to obtain the H reflex in muscles in which the H reflex is not normally obtainable without any facilitation technique, because the H reflex may be released from normal suppres-

Figure 5.16 Repetitive discharge in the H reflex in a case of myokymia-cramp syndrome. Repetitive discharge was not obvious in the compound motor action potential with normal sensitivity.

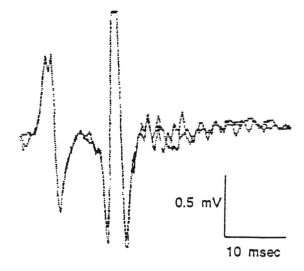

0.5 mV

10 msec

sion.[53] In fact, Norris found the H reflex present in almost all cases and in the hand and extensor digitorum muscles in 66–77% of 110 ALS patients.[54] In progressive muscular atrophy, he found the H reflex in the gastrocnemius in only seven patients and in other muscles in just 3 of 18 patients. These observations are in good contrast to patients with polyneuropathy, in whom the gastrocnemius-soleus H reflex was absent in almost all cases and in other muscles in all cases.

The H-reflex test can be useful for the objective measure of motor neuron hyperexcitability.[26] Although various techniques for this study have been introduced, the ratio of the maximum amplitude of H reflex to maximum M-amplitude ratio (H/M) is most practical because the technique is easier. Although there is considerable variability in H/M ratios, the H/M ratio for calf H reflexes is normally less than 0.7.[55] We found the motor neuron hyperexcitability test (H-reflex, T-reflex, and F-wave study) extremely helpful in diagnosing stiff-man syndrome[39] and an increase of H/M and F/M ratios in all three cases of this disorder.[17] The H-reflex test can also be helpful in diagnosing hyperexcitable peripheral nerve disorders, such as myokymia-cramp syndrome or Isaacs' syndrome, by demonstrating the repetitive discharge of H reflex (Figure 5.16).[40]

SPECIAL TECHNIQUES

Inching Technique

The ordinary NCS can localize the approximate site of compression in focal neuropathies. For this purpose, 10 cm is recommended as the shortest acceptable distance of the segmental NCV in the motor NCS.[1] This is because the error in the motor NCS is very high when conduction distances are 10 cm or less.[56] However, the more precise localization of focal slowing is possible by "inching" the stimulus in short increments along the course of the compressed segment of nerve. The "short-segment stimulation technique" (or the more commonly used

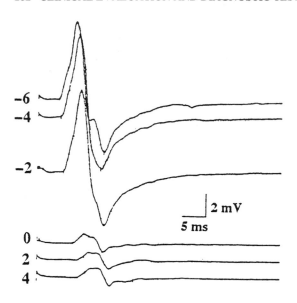

Figure 5.17 Compound muscle action potential responses at six different sites (inching technique) along the elbow sulcus in a case of ulnar neuropathy at elbow. Conduction block (89% decrease in the compound muscle action potential amplitude) and prolonged latency (2 milliseconds) between 2 cm (–2) distal and 0 cm to the medial epicondyle, confirming the diagnosis of epicondylar ulnar neuropathy.

term *inching technique*) of motor conduction has become a standard method of testing for this purpose.

This technique is used in three focal neuropathies: ulnar neuropathy at the elbow, peroneal neuropathy at the fibular head, and CTS. In practice, this technique is most useful in ulnar neuropathy at the elbow, because the precise localization of the compression dictates different therapeutic approaches. In the other two conditions, this technique is not of any practical value because it does not have any bearing on the choice of therapeutic management.

The inching technique of motor conduction has become a standard method of testing for ulnar neuropathy at the elbow. Campbell et al. used 1-cm segments,[57] and others have used 2-cm segments.[58,59] This technique can pinpoint a lesion to the exact site of compression and can distinguish cubital tunnel syndrome from tardy ulnar nerve palsy (epicondylar compression) (Figure 5.17). If the lesion is localized to more than 2 cm distal to the medial epicondyle, the diagnosis of cubital tunnel syndrome can be made.[57] On the other hand, if the lesion is localized to the medial epicondyle or proximal to it, epicondylar compression syndrome can be diagnosed. This distinction is important in determining therapeutic strategy: In cubital tunnel syndrome, decompression of the cubital tunnel is required, whereas for epicondylar compression syndrome, anterior transposition of the ulnar nerve is recommended.

Using this technique, Campbell et al.[57] were able to localize the lesion at the cubital tunnel in 6 of 19 cases and to the epicondylar sulcus in eight cases. In one case, the cubital tunnel and epicondylar sulcus were equally involved. In four cases, the test was nonlocalizing. By using this technique during surgery, they were able to pinpoint the lesion more accurately in six cases, including four patients with no localizing lesion. In 13 patients with ulnar compression neuropathy at the elbow, Kanakamedala et al.[59] localized the lesion by the 2 cm short-segment stimulation technique to the cubital tunnel in three cases, to the medial epicondyle in nine, and in both sites in one patient. These studies clearly show that there are two distinct compression syndromes involving the ulnar nerve at the elbow: (1) cubital tunnel syndrome, and (2) sulcal (epicondylar) compression syndrome. The studies also demonstrate that sulcal compression syndrome is more common. The near-nerve needle sensory nerve conduction technique may be needed in early ulnar nerve neuropathy, in which only sensory fibers are involved and the inching technique is not able to differentiate the lesion.[60] Odabasi[60] recorded the sensory or mixed nerve potential with the near-nerve needles at three sites: 6.0 cm and 1.5 cm below and 4.0 cm above the medial epicondyle, and he identified seven cases of epicondylar ulnar nerve palsy and one case of cubital tunnel syndrome. In three patients with epicondylar ulnar nerve palsy, the near-nerve needle technique accurately localized the lesion when other methods failed.

In peroneal neuropathy at the fibular head, Brown and Yates,[61] using an "inching" technique at an interval of 2 cm for motor conduction, were able to localize the major abnormalities at or adjacent to the fibular head. Using the short-segment stimulation technique, Kanakamedala and Hong found that a majority of the lesions were located just proximal to the fibular head.[62] Brown et al.[63] also performed the intraoperative motor nerve conduction in two patients with this disorder and found the most abnormal conduction to be proximal or distal to the entry of the common peroneal nerve into the peroneus longus muscle. These abnormalities were characterized by conduction block and delayed latency.

In CTS, Brown and Yates[63] studied the motor NCV during surgery in 23 median nerves. They obtained CMAPs from the thenar muscle after stimulation of the exposed median nerve 1–2 cm proximal to the origin of the flexor retinaculum and, in most instances, distal as far as the origin of the recurrent thenar motor branch. By measuring the amplitude of the CMAP, the latency, and the negative potential area, they were able to localize the most frequent sites of the abnormalities, as observed in 15 median nerves, to the first 1–2 cm distal to the beginning of the carpal tunnel. The maximum conduction abnormalities were located proximal to the flexor retinaculum, and in four median nerves, 2 cm distal. This is in sharp contrast to Kimura's study, which localized the most abnormal conduction to the 2–4 cm distal to the origin of the transverse carpal ligament in 52% of 91 affected nerves.[64] Kimura used the antidromic sensory NCV study after stimulation of the nonexposed nerve along the carpal tunnel in 1-cm increments. By using Kimura's technique, but in 2-cm increments, Brown et al.[63] found the worst conduction delays in patients with CTS toward the distal end of the flexor retinaculum, in agreement with Kimura's observation.[64] In a later study, Kimura performed an orthodromic sensory NCS by stimulating the digital nerve and recording the sensory nerve potential at multiple points, using a series of 10 electrodes mounted 1 cm apart on a specially constructed flexible strap.[65]

Near-Nerve Needle Technique in Sensory Nerve Conduction

Among the various uncommon nerve conduction techniques, the most sophisticated but neglected technique in this country is the near-nerve needle technique of sensory nerve conduction.[1] For the recording of sensory CNAP, early authors suggested the use of a pair of surface electrodes placed 2–3 cm apart along the nerve to be examined. This is still accepted as the standard method of testing worldwide because of its easier applicability. In 1966, Buchthal and Rosenfalck introduced the near-nerve needle technique of sensory nerve conduction in their classic monograph.[66] Since then, this technique has been widely accepted on the European continent. There is no question that the near-nerve needle technique provides an enormous wealth of valuable information that cannot be obtained with surface electrodes.

The sensory or mixed CNAPs are recorded with needle electrodes with clearly defined dimensions and characteristics and are specially made for the sensory CNAP near the nerve, not in the nerve. The reference electrode is placed subcutaneously at the same level as the active electrode at a transverse distance of 3–4 cm. Thus, this is a unipolar nerve conduction technique in contrast to the bipolar nerve conduction technique used with surface electrodes.

There are two critical technical details that must be followed to obtain the sensory CNAPs near the nerve[1]: (1) Special Teflon-coated steel needles (Medtronic 13L60–13L64 [Minneapolis, MN]) with uncoated tips should be used for the recording electrode (the active electrode has an uncoated tip of 2.0 mm in area and the reference electrode an uncoated tip of 3.5 mm); and (2) the needle should be placed near the nerve. In the mixed nerve, the active electrode is used to stimulate motor fibers, and its position is adjusted to the lowest threshold for the minimal motor response obtained. The lowest threshold is usually achieved with a stimulus intensity between 0.5 and 1.0 mA for a 0.2-millisecond stimulus and between 1 and 5 mA for a 0.05-millisecond stimulus. In the sensory nerve, the depth and direction of insertion are changed until the maximum amplitude of the sensory CNAP is obtained.

Major advantages of the near-nerve sensory nerve conduction techniques are listed below:

1. With surface electrodes, the sensory CNAP is unobtainable when the NCV is slower than 20 m per second. With the near-nerve needle technique, this small sensory CNAP can be obtained. Thus, an NCV slower than 20 m per second, a hallmark of demyelination, can be calculated.

2. The dispersion phenomenon can only be evaluated with the near-nerve needle technique. It can also identify multiple peaks, and thus the duration of CNAP can be clearly measured. With this technique, dispersion phenomenon, another hallmark of demyelination, can be identified. Axonal neuropathy can be clearly differentiated from demyelinating neuropathy, which is not possible to detect with surface recording electrodes.

In our laboratory, we use the near-nerve needle sensory nerve conduction technique in four clinical situations:

1. In the diagnostic workup of tarsal tunnel syndrome, medial and lateral plantar neuropathies, and interdigital neuropathy.[67–69] We found it difficult to record the sensory CNAP with surface recording electrodes in older patients and to use the near-nerve needle sensory nerve conduction technique to record these values reliably in the plantar nerves. With this technique, we are able to confirm the diagnoses of tarsal tunnel syndrome, medial and lateral plantar neuropathy, and interdigital neuropathy (Figure 5.18).

2. In distal sensory neuropathy, when the routine nerve conduction is normal. Usually, these patients were thought to have "small-fiber neuropathy" (SFN).[70] We tested the plantar nerves, the most distal nerves of the body, with the near-nerve needle technique; in this situation, we were able to diagnose large-fiber neuropathy in 65% of cases (Figure 5.19).

Figure 5.18 Sensory nerve conduction abnormalities in tarsal tunnel syndrome. The compound nerve action potentials are obtained with the near-nerve needle technique. Roman numerals indicate the stimulating digit; arabic numbers under each compound nerve action potential denote the maximum sensory nerve conduction velocity in m per second. No compound nerve action potential is obtained with V-digit stimulation. (Reprinted with permission from SJ Oh. Clinical Electromyography: Nerve Conduction Studies [2nd ed]. Baltimore: Williams & Wilkins, 1993;560.)

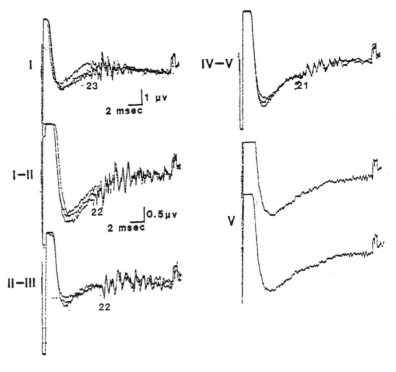

Figure 5.19 Compound nerve action potential responses with the near-nerve needle sensory nerve conduction of the digital and interdigital nerves of the plantar nerves. **A.** Axonal neuropathy. **B.** Demyelinating neuropathy. Both cases had distal sensory neuropathy with normal routine nerve conduction study. Roman numerals indicate the digit number. Arabic numbers under and above each compound nerve action potential denote maximum and negative peak nerve conduction velocity. Number between two arrows indicates compound nerve action potential duration. (Reprinted with permission from SJ Oh, AC Melo, DK Lee, et al. Large-fiber neuropathy in distal sensory neuropathy with normal routine nerve conduction. Neurology 2001;56: 1570–1572.)

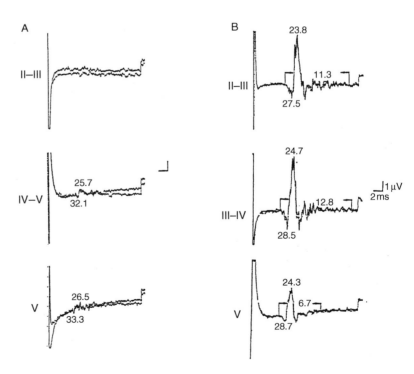

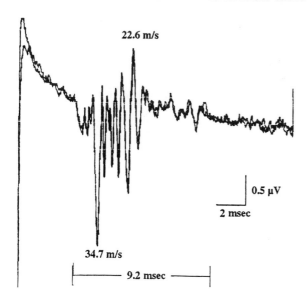

Figure 5.20 Dispersion phenomenon indicative of demyelinating neuropathy in the near-nerve needle sensory nerve conduction of the I–II interdigital nerve in a case of sensory Guillain-Barré syndrome with normal routine nerve conduction. Markedly slow (22.6 m per second) negative-peak nerve conduction velocity and long duration (9.2 m per second) of compound nerve action potential are indicative of demyelination.

3. When patients are suspected of having demyelinating neuropathy on clinical grounds, but the motor nerve conduction does not support this.[71] This is especially true in acute or chronic sensory demyelinating neuropathy (Figure 5.20).[34,72] For the detection of demyelination, the best and most common method is the motor nerve conduction because of the inherent limitation of the sensory nerve conduction with surface electrodes. In some cases of acute or chronic sensory demyelinating neuropathy, the motor nerve conduction is normal or nondemyelinating. In such cases, the only way to document the demyelinating nature of neuropathy is to use the near-nerve needle conduction technique, which can document the dispersion phenomenon (*vide infra*). With this technique, we were able to confirm the diagnosis of demyelinating neuropathy in a patient with sensory GBS, three patients with chronic sensory demyelinating neuropathy, and one patient with multifocal sensory demyelinating neuropathy.[73] The best example is a patient with multifocal motor neuropathy in whom the motor nerve conduction was unable to document any demyelination. In this case, the near-nerve plantar nerve study clearly documented the demyelination on the basis of the dispersion phenomenon, and immunotherapy was instituted with good response.

4. In focal neuropathies, when the motor nerve conduction is normal. This is especially useful for ulnar neuropathy at the elbow.[60] We have shown that this technique was able to differentiate cubital tunnel syndrome from tardy ulnar nerve palsy in a few patients with mild ulnar neuropathy (Figure 5.21).

Collision Technique

The *collision technique* in NCS refers to the procedure in which the response is obtained from the nerve by using two stimuli, usually at two different sites along the same nerve or in two different nerves, using "collision" of antidromic and orthodromic impulses. Two stimuli can be given simultaneously, or one stimulus can be delayed by a given interval from the other stimulus. Thus, this technique

Figure 5.21 Near-nerve sensory and mixed nerve conductions in a case with tardy ulnar sensory neuropathy. The most prominent change is noted with the sensory nerve conduction in BE(1.5)-AE segment: conduction block and slow nerve conduction velocity. Routine nerve conduction showed an absent mixed nerve compound nerve action potential at the elbow-axilla segment and normal motor nerve conduction study across the elbow. Inching technique was not able to localize the lesion. (AE = above elbow; BE = below elbow; VF = fifth finger; W = wrist.)

Near-nerve needle sensory nerve conduction

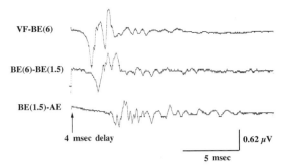

Near-nerve needle mixed nerve conduction

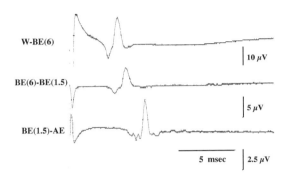

requires two stimulation units with delay capability. It is used solely in the motor nerve conduction.

The collision technique is based on two principles: (1) When a nerve fiber is stimulated, the nerve excitation travels orthodromically as well as antidromically; and (2) when the proximal and distal nerve action potentials meet between two points of stimulation, they cancel each other out. With this technique, the antidromic impulse set up in the nerve at a distal point cancels the orthodromic impulses of the proximal stimulation by collision; thus, the CMAP response from one nerve can be isolated from the unwanted or contaminated response from the other nerve, or the hidden response can be brought out by abolishing the CMAP response.

This collision technique has been used in four situations: (1) to record the F wave with stimulation at the proximal site of nerves, (2) to isolate the CMAP response of either the ulnar or median nerve from the other at the axilla in severe CTS or ulnar neuropathy at the elbow, (3) to isolate the median CMAP response from the ulnar response through Martin-Gruber anastomosis, and (4) to study the motor RP.

Kimura used the collision technique to record the F wave from axilla stimulation in the median and ulnar nerves.[10] In normal individuals, the F wave can be recorded in the median and ulnar nerves with wrist and elbow stimulation without difficulty. However, with axilla stimulation, the F wave is either non- or not clearly recognizable because of the extremely short difference between the M response and F wave. With the second stimulation at the wrist during the collision technique, the orthodromic impulse from the axilla is extinguished by collision with the antidromic impulse from the wrist, leaving the M response from the wrist and F wave from the axilla intact. Thus, the F-wave latency from the axilla is detected, and its latency is easily measured. By using this technique, Kimura was able to calculate the F-wave velocity in the central segment (axilla to spinal cord) in normal subjects and 10 CMT patients and found that it was approximately the same as the motor NCV in the proximal segment and slightly faster than the F-wave velocity in the distal segment in normal subjects. Similarly, he noted that it was comparable to that of motor NCV in the proximal and distal segments in CMT patients. Although this technique permits detection of the F wave elicited by proximal stimulation of the nerve, there has not been any clinical scenario reported in which this technique is indicated and useful.

The collision technique is also used for axillary stimulation of median and ulnar nerves in cases of CTS or tardy ulnar neuropathy.[74] In normal individuals, the stimulation of median and ulnar nerves in isolation at the axilla is not difficult with minimal adjustment of the stimulating electrode's position. However, in cases of severe CTS or ulnar neuropathy at the elbow, it is often difficult to stimulate the median or ulnar nerve in isolation at the axilla. This is because the two nerves lie in close proximity across the brachial artery at the axilla; higher stimulus intensity is required to elicit any response in the involved nerve in these focal neuropathies. Under this circumstance, stimulus spread to the normal nerve can elicit a CMAP response that is distorted by that from the recording muscle through volume conduction. For example, in severe CTS, with stimulation of the median nerve at the axilla, it is not unusual to record a higher-amplitude CMAP with a different shape from that obtained by elbow or wrist stimulation with a shorter latency and initial positive deflection (Figure 5.22). This response is mediated through the stimulation of the normal ulnar nerve at the axilla and recorded from the abductor pollicis brevis muscle by volume conduction. Unless this error is recognized, a faster NCV is obtained in the axilla-elbow segment. In this instance, the collision technique can be used to cancel the unwanted CMAP response from the ulnar nerve by stimulating the ulnar nerve at the wrist with the second stimulator. In this way, the orthodromic impulse from the axilla along the ulnar nerve is canceled by the antidromic impulse from the wrist and by muting the CMAP response through the ulnar nerve and recording the CMAP response through the median nerve in isolation. By this collision technique, the true NCV can be calculated over the axilla-elbow segment. In cases of ulnar nerve palsy at the elbow, a similar collision technique performed by stimulating the median nerve at the wrist can eliminate a potential source of error in the NCS by recording the CMAP response in isolation from the abductor digiti quinti muscle. In practice, this technical problem can be solved in a majority of cases by finding a more precise stimulation point for the involved nerve and adjusting the stimulus intensity. If this is not possible, the nerve conduction integrity can be studied by using the mixed nerve conduction technique over the elbow-axilla segment.

The collision technique has been used by Kimura to detect Martin-Gruber anastomosis by stimulating the median nerve simultaneously at the wrist and elbow.[74] In cases of Martin-Gruber anastomosis, elbow stimulation of the median nerve activates ulnar-innervated muscles in the thenar eminence through the communicating fibers. If these communicating fibers conduct faster than the median nerve, as in patients with CTS, the latency actually measured is erroneously short, and an unreasonably fast NCV from the elbow to the wrist is erroneously calculated. To

Carpal Tunnel Syndrome

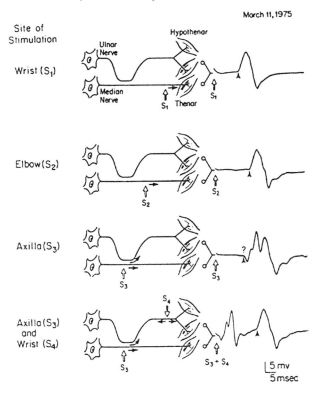

Figure 5.22 Collision technique in a patient with carpal tunnel syndrome. The median nerve was stimulated at the wrist (S$_1$), elbow (S$_2$), or axilla (S$_3$), and the compound muscle action potential (CMAP) was recorded by surface electrodes from the thenar eminence. Spread of axillary stimulation (S$_3$) to the ulnar nerve (*third tracing from top*) activated thenar muscles with shorter latency, obscuring the onset (*arrowhead*) of the CMAP under study. Another stimulus (S$_4$) applied to the ulnar nerve at the wrist (*bottom tracing*) blocked the proximal impulses by collision. The CMAP elicited by the wrist stimulation occurred much earlier without overlapping with the CMAP under study. The figures on the left show diagrammatically the orthodromic (*solid arrows*) and antidromic (*open arrows*) impulses of each stimulation. (Reprinted with permission from J Kimura. Collision technique. Physiologic block of nerve impulses in studies of motor nerve conduction velocity. Neurology 1976;26:681.)

isolate the CMAP response from the median nerve, a selective block can be achieved simply by delivering another stimulus at the wrist to the ulnar nerve. If more separation between these two responses is desirable, this can be accomplished by delivering the stimulus at the wrist a few milliseconds before the proximal stimulation. By this technique, Kimura reported Martin-Gruber anastomosis in 17% of unselected subjects.[75] For the study of Martin-Gruber anastomosis, a simpler technique, with the recording electrodes on three different intrinsic hand muscles and stimulation of the median and ulnar nerves separately at the wrist and elbow, is available and widely used.

The collision technique is also used and is essential for testing the RP of motor nerve conduction as discussed in the following section.

Refractory Period

A unique feature of nerve fiber is the period of inexcitability after the action potential. This period of inexcitability is termed the *RP*. The RP has two phases: the absolute RP followed by the relative RP. During the absolute RP, the fibers are totally inexcitable by the second stimulus, however intense, and during the relative RP, the fibers are excitable only by increasing stimulus intensity above the threshold level. The RP can be tested by paired stimulations in the sensory, mixed, and motor nerve fibers and can be used as a measure of nerve excitability.[1]

In the sensory or mixed nerve fibers, a technique for testing the RP in the median, ulnar, and sural nerves is available and rather straightforward.[1] This test is basically the sensory or mixed nerve conduction by paired stimulations with varying intervals between the paired stimulations using the conventional nerve conduction electrode placement. It is now easily performed with the automated programs on some commercial EMG machines. For the determination of absolute RP, the stimulus interval between the first and second stimulations is shortened consecutively by 0.1-millisecond decrements from 2.0 milliseconds to the critical interval at which the nerve ceases to conduct the second impulse (Figure 5.23). For the determination of relative RP, the stimulus interval is shortened consecutively by 0.25-millisecond decrements from 5.00 milliseconds. The *relative RP* is the stimulus interval at which the amplitude of the second response begins to decrease or the latency begins to be prolonged. Absolute RP in normal individuals ranges from 0.51 millisecond in the mixed ulnar nerve to 0.76 millisecond in the 40- to 60-year-old group in the sural nerve.[1] Normal relative RP ranges from 2.50 milliseconds by amplitude in the mixed ulnar nerve to 3.45 milliseconds in the ulnar sensory nerve.

In motor nerve conduction, testing the RP with the routine nerve conduction setups is impossible because the second CMAP is obscured by the long duration of the first CMAP. Antidromic collision must be used to separate the second CMAP from the first CMAP.[1] Two methods are available. Kimura's technique evaluates the RP at a proximal stimulation site with paired proximal stimuli and a single distal stimulus.[76] Ingram's technique evaluates the motor RP at a distal site; paired distal and paired proximal stimuli are applied simultaneously.[77] Ingram's test can be achieved easily with a commercially available automated program. Comparing the two techniques, Ruijten et al. concluded that Ingram's technique was better because it yielded a narrower RP distribution, displayed less interindividual variability, and was more reproducible and more sensitive in detecting abnormality in diabetic neuropathy.[78,79]

RP studies in the disease states are limited. All studies showed that the RP is more sensitive than conventional NCSs and that the relative RP is more sensitive than the absolute RP in detection of neuropathy. In 28 patients with diabetic neuropathy, Ruijten et al., using Ingram's technique, found an abnormal motor RP in 73% of cases and abnormal motor NCS in 46%.[78] In 22 patients with neuropathy, Lowitzsch et al. found that the relative RP in the mixed nerve conduction showed more prominent abnormality than the absolute RP or the NCV.[80] They were able to show abnormal RP (latency) in 12 patients with neuropathy who had normal NCVs, indicating that the relative RP study is more sensitive in detection of neuropathy than the NCV. Braune studied 30 diabetic patients without neuropathy and found a conventional sural nerve conduction abnormality in four patients and abnormal relative RP in the sural nerve in nine.[81] Schutt et al. studied 65 diabetic patients (30 of whom had neu-

Figure 5.23 Refractory period for the sensory median nerve. Paired stimuli of the median nerve, antidromic stimulation with recording at the third digit. Notice the first appearance of the second response (absolute refractory period) at the bottom (*long arrow*). The antidromic response becomes equal in amplitude to the first response at the top (*short arrow*). The time between the two stimuli that produced equal amplitude response is the relative refractory period. Calibration: 20 μV/cm; 2 milliseconds/cm. The stimulation was done at 0.5 millisecond (*bottom line*, 8), increasing up to 5-millisecond (*top line*, 1) interstimuli intervals. (Courtesy of Dr. Tulio E. Bertorini.)

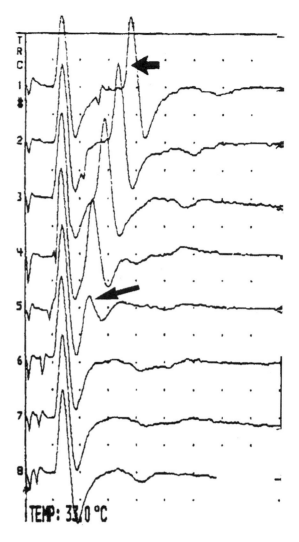

ropathy) and found, with a 3.0-millisecond interstimulus interval, a significant prolongation of the test response in paired stimulations in 21 of 30 patients with diabetic neuropathy and 16 of 35 with diabetes alone.[82] Slow sural NCV was found in 16 of 30 with diabetic neuropathy and in 4 of 35 patients with diabetes alone. Three studies reported abnormalities in the RP in patients with CTS. In 11 nerves of eight patients with CTS, Tachmann and Lehmann showed that the latency was more prolonged and the amplitude was more depressed in CTS than in normal subjects during the relative RP.[83] In 13 nerves of 10 patients with CTS, one study showed that the absolute RP was prolonged and that the relative RP at 50% reduction of amplitude was also prolonged.[84] Gilliatt and Meer studied the RP of transmission (measurement of the second CNAP with paired stimulations at fixed intervals) in 14 hands from 10 CTS patients using paired stimuli at intervals of 0.8 millisecond with stimulating electrodes just above the wrist and with recording electrodes at the fingers and elbow.[85] In CTS patients, the test response was abnormal (response absent or reduced in amplitude to less than 1 μV) in 79% of hands. In two cases, the sensory nerve conduction was normal.

T Reflex

The muscle stretch reflex test, the most important neurologic test, is a monosynaptic reflex elicited by a reflex hammer tap to the tendon and is used daily by neurologists as a measure of motor neuron excitability to differentiate between upper and lower motor neuron lesions. The reflex arc consists of Ia fibers as an afferent axon and alpha motor fibers as an efferent axon, and it is basically identical to the H-reflex arc. The muscle stretch reflex can be objectively documented by the T reflex, which can be elicited by an electronic hammer tap to the tendon.

Although the H reflex and T reflex have the same afferent and efferent pathways, there are, however, important distinctions between the two. The most obvious difference is the activation site of stimulation: For the H reflex, stimulation is directly on the Ia fibers, bypassing the muscle spindle organs, whereas for the T reflex, the stretch receptors (nuclear bags and chains) in the muscle spindle are activated after stretching the muscle fibers by tapping the tendon with a tendon hammer.

The recording electrodes are not placed according to the conventional belly-tendon method used for the NCS because such placement is associated with greater movement artifact caused by the tendon tap.[86] Certainly, the active recording electrode should be placed on the belly of the muscle. However, the reference electrode is placed either on the muscle tendon opposite the tapped tendon[86,87] or on a muscle 5–10 cm away from an active recording electrode.[88,89] As with any other reflex test, the superimposition of more than four or five recordings is essential for the accurate measurement of the shortest latency. Usually, a 5- to 10-millisecond sweep velocity and 500 to 1,000 μV sensitivity are the recommended EMG machine settings. The force with which the electronic hammer strikes the tendon does not produce any significant difference in latency as long as the onset of the initial negative deflection is clear. Reinforcement such as the Jendrassik maneuver increases the amplitude of the tendon response but does not change the latency. Alterations in the tension of the tendon provoke variations in the amplitude of the tendon response, but the reflex latency remains fairly stable.

Malcolm concluded that, as a quantitative measure of the reflex response, the visual observation was approximately as sensitive as the T reflex because a T-reflex response was not recorded when there was no visible reflex response.[90] Weintraub et al. studied the relationship between the ankle T reflex and the H reflex on the gastrocnemius soleus muscle in 400 limbs and found concordance in 86%.[91] When discordant, the ankle T reflex was almost always elicited, whereas the H reflex was not, indicating the technical superiority of the T reflex. We found the same results in our study of chronic demyelinating neuropathy.[89]

There have been only a few studies reporting normal data.[1] The ankle T reflex has been most studied. As expected from any late responses conducting through the long proximal nerve segments, the T-reflex latency is proportional to the height, arm length, or leg length.[1] Thus, it is important to compare the latency with the height. The latency difference between two sides is easier to compare. For the Achilles T reflex, it should not be more than 2 milliseconds according to Rico and Jonkman[88] and 3 milliseconds according to Kuruoglu and Oh.[89]

The T-reflex test has not been used very often in the clinical setting, probably because of the clinician's confidence in his or her own skill in identifying a segmental lesion in muscle stretch testing with the reflex hammer. The T-reflex test is useful in two clinical settings: (1) detection of cervical or lumbosacral radiculopathy, and (2) detection of peripheral neuropathy as a test for the proximal nerve conduction.

When the latency difference was compared between sides, the ankle T-reflex test was abnormal in 80–87% of patients with S1 radiculopathy.[88,90] Rico also showed that this test was more sensitive than the H-reflex test (65%) for the detection of S1 radiculopathy.[88] Stam found a unilateral absence of anterior tibialis reflex in 13 (72%) of 18 cases of L5 radiculopathy.[92] De Weerd and Jonkman found an abnormal side difference in 13 (60%) of 20 cases of L3 or L4 radiculopathy.[93] Koenig found a pathologic biceps and triceps T reflex in 11 (73%) of 15 patients with unilateral cervical C6 or C7 radiculopathy (prolongation of the latency for more than 2 milliseconds in 10 compared with the normal side and a significant amplitude reduction in one).[87] This was in contrast to the EMG abnormalities observed in 60% of cases. Thus, these studies showed that T-reflex testing is useful in the diagnosis of unilateral radiculopathy.

The usefulness of the T-reflex study in peripheral neuropathy is limited. Eisen et al. studied the T-reflex change in assessing peripheral nerve function after long-term therapy with diphenylhydantoin.[94] They found no significant difference in mean T-reflex latency between 45 seizure patients on diphenylhydantoin for more than 10 years and a control group. However, a prolonged T reflex was found in 65% of cases. This figure is comparable to the sensitivity figures for the H reflex, sural sensory, and peroneal motor nerve conduction tests. We have studied the T reflex test in 26 patients with chronic demyelinating polyneuropathy and found that the T-reflex latency was prolonged in 25 of 26 studied cases; the mean T-reflex latency was more than 150% beyond the normal mean, confirming demyelination as the basic pathologic process (Figure 5.24).[89] We found this test to be extremely useful in seven patients with CIDP, who had normal or brisk tendon reflexes, by documenting the prolonged T-reflex latency and satisfying one of the diagnostic criteria of absent or diminished reflex in CIDP.

Sympathetic Skin Response

Sympathetic skin response (SSR) is the potential generated by sweat in response to various stimuli.[95] Because the sweat gland is innervated by unmyelinated C fibers from the postganglionic sympathetic (cholinergic) neuron, SSR is considered to be a function of sympathetic nerve fibers. In such a sense, this is the only electrophysiologic autonomic test that can easily be performed with the regular EMG machine.

In theory, SSR can be obtained anywhere on the body surface where sweat glands are located. In fact, SSR is obtained from the forehead as well as from genitalia.[96,97]

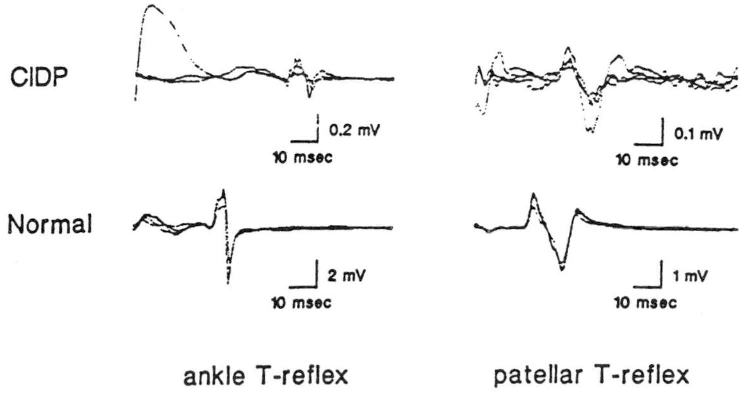

Figure 5.24 Ankle and patellar T-reflex responses in chronic inflammatory demyelinating polyneuropathy (CIDP), compared with normal control. Markedly prolonged latency of T-reflex response is obvious in CIDP. (Reprinted with permission from HR Kuruoglu, SJ Oh. Tendon-reflex testing in chronic demyelinating polyneuropathy. Muscle Nerve 1994;17:148.)

Most commonly, SSR is obtained from the hands and feet. An active recording electrode is placed on the palm of the hand and sole of the foot, and reference electrodes are positioned on the dorsum of the hand and foot.[1]

The most common stimulus used in most EMG laboratories is an electrical stimulation delivered to the median nerve at the wrist or the posterior tibial nerve at the ankle.[1] The stimulus duration is not different from that used for the motor nerve conduction and the stimulus intensity, between 10 and 30 mA. Auditory stimulation, deep breathing, and pudendal nerve stimulation have also been used. The stimulus must be delivered at irregular rates slower than one per minute to avoid any habituation of SSR because there is a tendency to habituation. Filter range should be set 0.1–2.0 Hz for the low filter and 4 kHz for the high filter. Sweep velocity should be set at 0.5 or 1.0 second.

SSR is in general biphasic or triphasic in shape and the amplitude of the response is variable, reaching a few millivolts. Amplitude of SSR is usually higher in the hands than in the feet. The latency of SSR, regardless of the stimulation site or stimulation parameters, is 1.3–1.5 seconds in the hand and 1.90–2.09 seconds in the foot.[98] The difference in the SSR latencies between the two limbs is insignificant. Shahani et al. tried to calculate the NCV by stimulating the proximal and distal parts of arms and legs: NCV value was calculated by dividing the distance between two spots by the latency difference.[98] According to this method, the NCV of sympathetic fibers ranged from 1.02[98] to 1.49 m per second[99,100] in the legs and 1.57 m per second in the arms.[98] These values are similar to those obtained from earlier direct determinations of NCV in skin sympathetic (sudomotor) nerves.[101,102] Physiologically speaking, however, these values are not the genuine NCV of unmyelinated fibers because the afferent pathways are different between the two stimulation sites and we are not testing the nerve connecting the two stimulating sites.

Because of habituation and great variability in the amplitude and morphology of the SSR, it is generally accepted that only an absent response should be considered abnormal, although others have used prolonged latency or lower amplitude as a criterion of abnormality.[103,104] No one advocates the use of NCV as a criterion for abnormality.

In neuropathy, Shahani et al.[98] and Van den Berg and Kelly[105] noted that SSR was absent in axonal neuropathies but present in demyelinating neuropathies. Shahani presented data showing that absence of SSRs correlated with preferential loss of the unmyelinated small fibers in a few biopsy-proven cases. Although the earlier study did not show any correlation between SSR absence and dysautonomia,[98] the later study showed that the SSR and P-R interval study (parasympathetic study) with deep breathing were helpful in assessing autonomic dysfunction.[106] In SFN, the SSR test was disappointing because low-amplitude SSRs were noted in only 10% of patients and absence of response was not observed in any patient.[104]

The most extensive studies were performed in diabetic neuropathy. Absent SSR was reported in 66–83% of cases.[107,108] Soliven et al. found a better correlation of absent SSR with severity of axonal damage than with demyelination and a more frequent absence of SSR in patients with dysautonomia.[107] Maselli et al. found high concordance between abnormal SSR and the quantitative sudomotor axon reflex test in patients with diabetic neuropathy.[109] However, Schondorf and Gendron noted a poor correlation among SSR, thermoregulatory sweat test, and pilocarpine-activated sweat gland silastic implant counts in patients with diabetic neuropathy.[110] Martin and Reid found an intact SSR in some patients with diabetic neuropathy with dysautonomia.[111] Levy et al. suggested that absent SSR is a finding in patients with advanced diabetic neuropathy because SSR was present in 96% of randomly selected diabetic patients.[103]

In familial amyloid polyneuropathy, SSR was absent in three of four fully developed neuropathy cases with abnormal NCS, and the SSR was low in four asymptomatic carriers with normal NCS.[112] Absent SSR was observed in 5 of 15 patients with CMT disease[113] and in the feet in 32 (53%) of 70 alcoholic patients; 28 of 32 had electrophysiologic evidence of neuropathy.[114]

SSRs have assisted in the study of male impotence. Ertekin et al. studied SSRs from the skin of genitalia of diabetic patients and concluded that the response may differentiate between organic and other causes of impotence.[97] Park et al. suggested that the absence of SSR in limbs after stimulation of the dorsal nerve of the penis could assist in the diagnosis of ejaculatory dysfunction.[115]

From this review, it is clear that the SSR is not helpful in SFN in which this test is most likely needed because the routine NCS was normal; however, it is helpful in another SFN, familial amyloid neuropathy. In other neuropathies, the SSR is not superior to the conventional NCS, and there is not a good correlation between absent SSR and dysautonomia.

Silent Period

A transient suppression of ongoing EMG activity during a sustained muscle contraction after sensory or mixed nerve stimulation is known as a "cutaneous silent period" (CSP).[116] To record the CSP, surface electrodes are placed over the contracting muscle, and a single shock is delivered to a cutaneous nerve. A sweep velocity of 20 milliseconds and a sensitivity of 500 μV are recommended for this test. The CSP latency onset and endpoint in small hand muscles typically occur at approximately 70 milliseconds and 120 milliseconds, respectively.[117] However, the CSP onset latency is reduced, and total duration increases with increased stimulus strength.[118] Most investigators agree that the CSP is generally accepted to be an inhibitory spinal reflex and the afferent impulses that generate the CSP are carried by the A-δ fibers.[117–119] In the mixed nerve silent period, which is induced by stimulation of a mixed nerve, there are two CSPs: the earlier one in the first 50–60 milliseconds and the later one in the last 50–70 milliseconds.[117] The evidence includes the observation that high-intensity stimulation, typically 10 times the perception threshold, is necessary to evoke the CSP.[119] In near-nerve needle recordings from the sural nerve, stimulation of this intensity produces nerve action potential components with a conduction velocity of 15–20 m per second.[118] Similar estimates of the afferent conduction velocity were calculated from CSPs produced by stimulating two points along a cutaneous nerve.[119–121] Finally, normal CSPs were reported in patients with sensory neuronopathies (no sensory nerve action potential but normal motor NCSs), indicating that large-diameter afferents are not essential for CSP recording.[117,121,122] Based on these observations, Leis stated that the CSP technique can be used to assess conduction in the smaller, slower conducting A-δ fibers, which are not tested by routine NCSs,[116] suggesting that this technique may be potentially useful for SFN. However, there has not been any consensus on what parameter of CSP should be used as the criteria of abnormality: Some have used an absent CSP[119,123,124]; others, a shortened[123] or prolonged CSP duration[124] or delayed onset of the CSP.[117] An absent silent period with normal conduction in large myelinated fibers has been reported as a characteristic finding in syringomyelia.[125]

Masseter inhibitory reflex

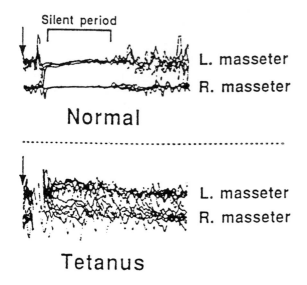

Figure 5.25 Masseter silent period produced by a tap on the chin while patient clenches teeth. The arrow represents a mechanical tap that initiates a sweep on the oscilloscope. Upper tracings depict a normal silent period; lower tracings demonstrate an absent silent period in a patient with tetanus. (L. = left; R. = right.) (Reprinted with permission from RG Auger. Diseases associated with excess motor unit activity. AAEE minimonograph #44. Muscle Nerve 1994; 17:1253.)

The study of the silent period is most useful in the assessment of tetanus.[126,127] In this connection, the silent period was also studied with the mechanical tap or T-reflex testing on the jaw (masseter inhibitory reflex).[126–128] In tetanus, a shortened or absent silent period in the jaw or in the mixed nerve silent period is an electrophysiologic hallmark, probably resulting from failure of Renshaw cell inhibition (Figure 5.25).[126–129] In nine cases of tetanus, the shortening or absence of the silent period after stretch reflex, electrical stimulation, or both was observed in all nine cases.[127] In contrast, the silent period is said to be normal in stiff-man syndrome.[130–132] However, in one case, the silent period was absent in the T-reflex test on the jaw.[39] These techniques are discussed in detail in Chapter 7.

Motor Unit Number Estimation

Motor unit number estimation (MUNE) was first introduced by McComas et al. in 1971.[133] With an improved understanding of the physiologic and technical problems of MUNE along with automated methods of MUNE measurement in recent years, the MUNE technique is now well accepted for the quantitative assessment of lower motor neuron survival and loss.

Supramaximal stimulation of a motor nerve activates all the functional motor axons within it. Thus, the CMAP represents the summated electrophysiologic activity of the simultaneously activated functional motor units within a given muscle. In theory, if a truly representative average single motor unit action potential (S-MUAP) is known, the approximate total number of motor units in a given muscle can be calculated by using the following formula:

$$MUNE = CMAP \text{ (amplitude or area) / average S-MUAP}$$

The available MUNE techniques are many but differ principally in the method used to derive the S-MUAP.[134] Each technique has its own merits and flaws. The size of S-MUAP can be measured by incremental,[133] multiple point stimulation,[135] statistical,[136] F-wave,[137] and spike-triggered averaging methods.[138] Some techniques are available on commercial EMG machines, making MUNE measurement easier in daily practice.[134] It is important to remember that none of these techniques can measure the size of a true S-MUAP and, thus, the MUNE by each technique represents the total number of "assumed S-MUAPs" by that particular technique. Therefore, it is not clear which of these techniques produces numbers that are the closest to the true values.[139]

MUNE is the only method that provides detailed quantitative assessment of lower motor neuron survival and loss[134]; therefore, it can be most reliably used in a neurogenic process such as ALS, where the reliability increases as the disease progresses.[140] In fact, this technique has been used as a means of objective assessment of motor unit loss in clinical trials of ALS and was found to be the most reliable method of measuring the loss of motor neurons.[141–143]

MUNE can be studied in any muscle in which the stimulation of innervating nerve and CMAP recording can be done reliably with surface electrodes. Thus, MUNE is most readily performed in distal muscles. Reproducibility is now comparable to that for CMAP.[144,145] Absolute MUNE values vary from technique to technique, from muscle to muscle, and from individual to individual. Thus, MUNE's greatest use is tracking motor unit loss over time via repeated longitudinal studies using the same technique in the same muscle group in a given individual. This subject is discussed in detail in Chapter 14.

*In Vitro Nerve Conduction Studies**

In vitro nerve conduction techniques allow for more detailed and precise studies of the various types of nerve fibers, and the results can be correlated with histologic findings. These techniques were initially performed on frog nerves by Erlanger and Gasser,[146,147] and they were later used in human nerve autopsy specimens after amputations[148] and in vivo during thoracic cordotomies.[149]

For in vitro NCSs, whole nerve segments, or single fascicles of approximately 4–5 cm are placed in a humidified, temperature-controlled chamber, and the nerve is stretched slightly with a small weight. The nerve segments are attached to small platinum or silver wire electrodes, stimulated at one end and recorded at the opposite end. Variations in the stimulus intensity, sweep speed, and recording time allow the study of the action potentials of the different nerve fibers.[150]

Characteristically, three peaks are easily identified. These are the large A-α potentials (approximately 60 m per second NCV) that correspond to large myelinated axons, the intermediate or small A-δ potentials (approximately 20 m per second NCV) that correspond to smaller myelinated fibers, and the late C poten-

---

*This portion of the chapter is co-authored with Dr. Tulio E. Bertorini.

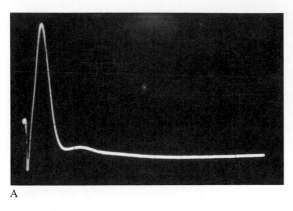 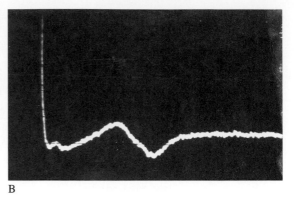

A   B

Figure 5.26 In vitro nerve conduction of a normal sural nerve recorded with a TECA-TE42 electromyography machine. **A.** A large response represents the A-α potential; a smaller response, the A-δ potential. Sweep velocity = 1 millisecond/cm; sensitivity = 1 mV/cm. **B.** C potential. Sweep velocity = 5 milliseconds/cm; sensitivity = 50 μV/cm. Nomenclature: EH Lambert, PJ Dyck. Compound Action Potentials of Sural Nerve In Vitro in Peripheral Neuropathy. In PJ Dyck, PK Thomas, EH Lambert (eds), Peripheral Neuropathy. Philadelphia: Saunders, 1975;427–441.

tials (1 m per second NCV) that correspond to unmyelinated axons, which require a higher stimulus intensity (Figure 5.26).[150,151] The CNAPs recorded with in vitro techniques depend on the fiber composition and the density of the fibers that produce each potential.[150,152] NCV and amplitude of the CNAPs are known to be proportional to fiber diameters.[152–154] However, within a given component of CNAP, the amplitude (or area of the component if its duration is not constant) is proportional to the density rather than to the total number of fibers that contribute to it.[150]

Dyck and collaborators performed detailed analyses of in vitro nerve conduction and correlated their findings with nerve histology.[150,155,156] These investigators identified the characteristics of the potentials in various neuropathies; for example, smaller or absent A-α potentials correspond to the absence of large myelinated fibers in Friedreich's ataxia. In addition, they found that an absent C potential and a markedly reduced A-δ potential correspond to the absence of unmyelinated fibers and to a preferential reduction of the small myelinated fibers in familial amyloidosis. Similarly, in hereditary sensory neuropathy type I, all potentials were reduced in amplitude and the reduction was more severe in A-δ and C potentials, corresponding to a marked reduction in unmyelinated or small myelinated fibers. In CIDP and CMT 1, a very small amplitude and dispersion of A-α potentials with very slow NCV were observed. In general, a reasonable correspondence between the fiber diameter histogram and the CNAP is found if degenerating and nonconducting fibers can be excluded. However, in demyelinating neuropathy, the fiber diameter histogram does not correlate well with the CNAP because the wide variation in diameter of successive internodes of a nerve fiber prevents reliable prediction of its conduction velocity.[150]

In vitro nerve conduction techniques are not widely used in clinical practice but could be valuable in experimental studies, particularly in the analysis of the effect of toxins on peripheral nerves, with determination of not only potential amplitudes and velocities, but also other parameters, such as RPs.

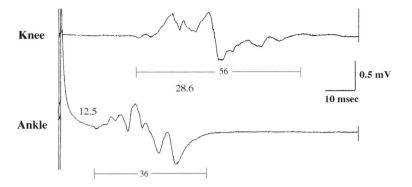

Figure 5.27 Low compound muscle action potential (CMAP) amplitude (1 mV) with ankle stimulation in the posterior tibial nerve in a case of multifocal motor sensory demyelinating neuropathy. Low CMAP is due to the dispersion phenomenon indicative of demyelination. Duration of CMAP was 36 milliseconds with ankle stimulation and 56 milliseconds with knee stimulation and multiphasic CMAP. Terminal latency was 12.5 milliseconds and nerve conduction velocity was 28.6 m per second.

COMMON PITFALLS IN THE NERVE CONDUCTION INTERPRETATION

1. Absent or low CMAP is not always due to axon loss. It is often incorrectly interpreted that an absent or low CMAP amplitude implies axon loss. This is because a low CMAP or CNAP amplitude is an electrophysiologic hallmark of axonal degeneration. Absent or low CMAP response can be due to a total or partial conduction block or to severe atrophy of the recording muscles. In peroneal nerve conduction, it is not unusual that the absent CMAP response is due to severe atrophy of the EDB muscle. Thus, the first step in cases of absent CMAP response is to palpate the extensor hallucis brevis muscle. Another rare cause of absent or low CMAP is conduction block due to demyelination in the distal segments (Figure 5.27). In cases of absent CMAP responses, one assumes that it is due to conduction block when other nerves show the electrophysiologic hallmarks of demyelination. When a low CMAP is recordable, the dispersion phenomenon is clearly an indication of demyelinating neuropathy.

2. F-wave prolongation is not always due to a proximal neuropathy. The F wave has been used as an electrophysiologic parameter of nerve conduction of the proximal segments of motor fibers. This is because the F-wave latency represents the conduction time over the afferent and efferent arcs of motor fibers from the stimulating site to the anterior horn cells. However, one has to remember that the F-wave pathway includes the terminal latency from the stimulating site to the recording muscle. Thus, when the terminal latency is markedly prolonged as in some cases of severe CTS, the F-wave latency is accordingly prolonged. In this case, the F-wave prolongation is not due to proximal neuropathy.

3. The presence of fibrillation and positive sharp waves in the needle EMG together with a slow NCV does not mean that the neuropathy is mixed (axonal and demyelinating). I have observed this conclusion repeatedly in EMG reports in my practice, especially in interpretations from inexperienced electromyographers. Such

an interpretation is based on the dictum that fibrillation and positive sharp waves physiologically represent axonal degeneration (wallerian degeneration) and that slow NCV indicates demyelination. Thus, to inexperienced electromyographers who do not know how to differentiate axonal neuropathy from demyelinating neuropathy, almost all neuropathy is mixed because fibrillations and positive sharp waves occur to some degree in almost all cases of neuropathy. In practice, such a conclusion does not serve a useful purpose because one cannot differentiate axonal neuropathy from demyelinating neuropathy.

4. Normal routine nerve conduction in sensory neuropathy is not indicative of SFN. *SFN* is defined by many physicians as when the routine NCS is normal in patients with distal sensory neuropathy that is often painful.[157–159] This is because pain, the symptomatic hallmark of SFN, is mediated by unmyelinated or small myelinated fibers, and the motor, mixed, and sensory nerve conduction reflects activity in the fastest-conducting, heavily myelinated fibers.[1] However, the routine NCS usually does not study the sensory nerve conduction of the sensory nerves below the ankles. Thus, it is possible that some patients with SFN may have a large-fiber neuropathy that remains undetected only because of the limitations of the routine NCS. In fact, our study using the near-nerve needle–nerve conduction of the plantar nerves found the large-diameter fiber neuropathy in 65% of cases.[70]

5. Nonuniform demyelinating neuropathy is not always an acquired demyelinating neuropathy. Uniform demyelinating neuropathy is the electrophysiologic hallmark of CMT 1A (hereditary motor and sensory neuropathy type 1) and other hereditary neuropathies. Thus, when conduction block or the dispersion phenomenon was observed in patients with hereditary neuropathy, it was once assumed that there was a superimposed acquired neuropathy (CIDP). In recent years, it has become clearer that nonuniform demyelinating neuropathy is the characteristic nerve conduction finding in Dejerine-Sottas disease, sex-linked CMT 1A, and hereditary neuropathy with liability to pressure palsy (Figure 5.28).

CONCLUSIONS

The following are important key points to consider in the performance interpretation of nerve conduction tests:

- Nerve conduction represents the physiologic status of fast-conducting, larger-diameter nerve fibers.
- Reduced amplitude of the CMAP in motor nerve conduction and of the CNAP in sensory and mixed nerve conductions in the presence of normal or near-normal maximal NCV is the hallmark of axonal degeneration.
- Demyelination is usually detected by the motor NCS.
- Conduction block and the dispersion phenomenon are two cardinal diagnostic hallmarks of demyelination.
- Absent sensory CNAP in the presence of normal motor nerve conduction is indicative of sensory neuronopathy (sensory ganglionopathy).
- Uniform slowing is strongly suggestive of hereditary neuropathy, especially in CMT 1A.
- Sensory nerve conduction is much more sensitive than motor nerve conduction in detection of neuropathy, either focal or diffuse.
- Focal segmental demyelination is the basic pathologic process in entrapment neuropathies. Thus, the diagnosis of an entrapment neuropathy can

Figure 5.28 Conduction block in the elbow-wrist segment and the axilla-elbow segment in median nerve conduction in a case of hereditary neuropathy with liability to pressure palsy. Temporal dispersion is also present in the compound muscle action potential with axilla stimulation. (Reprinted with permission from SJ Oh. Principles of Clinical Electromyography: Case Studies. Baltimore: Williams & Wilkins, 1998;318.)

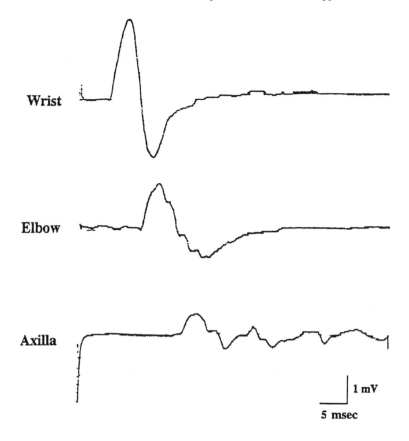

be confirmed by documentation of focal demyelination in the nerve conduction test.

- Nerve conduction abnormalities in peripheral neuropathy are usually diffuse. However, conduction abnormalities may not be observed in all nerves tested.
- Abnormal medial and lateral antebrachial cutaneous nerve conduction may localize the neuropathy to the brachial plexus.
- Martin-Gruber anastomosis may produce additional electrophysiologic changes that make interpretation of the nerve conduction difficult in CTS.
- The F-wave test is most useful in early GBS, when the F-wave abnormality may be the sole abnormality in the NCS.
- The markedly prolonged F-wave latency or absence of F waves in nerves with normal CMAP amplitude is indicative of proximal conduction block.
- The inching technique can distinguish cubital tunnel syndrome from tardy ulnar nerve palsy (epicondylar compression).
- In sensory nerve conduction, the diagnosis of demyelination can be made by the near-nerve needle sensory nerve conduction.
- Normal routine nerve conduction in sensory neuropathy is not always indicative of SFN. Large-fiber neuropathy can be documented by the near-nerve sensory nerve conduction of the plantar nerve.
- T-reflex testing can document prolonged T-reflex latency in demyelinating neuropathy, even when the reflexes are normal or brisk.
- Absence of silent period is the electrophysiologic hallmark of tetanus.

REFERENCES

1. Oh SJ. Clinical Electromyography: Nerve Conduction Studies. Baltimore: Williams & Wilkins, 1993.
2. Tackmann W, Spalka G, Oginszus HJ. Quantitative histometric studies and relations of number and diameter of myelinated fibres to electrophysiological parameters in normal sensory nerve of man. J Neurol 1976;212:71–84.
3. Rhee EK, England JD, Sumner AJ. A computer simulation of conduction block: effects produced by actual block versus interphase cancellation. Ann Neurol 1990;28:146–156.
4. Gilliatt RW. Nerve conduction in human and experimental neuropathies. Proc Royal Soc Med 1966;58:989–993.
5. Bradom RI, Johnson EW. Standardization of H reflex and diagnostic use in S1 radiculopathy. Arch Phys Med Rehabil 1974;55:161–166.
6. Jabre JF. Surface recording of the H-reflex of the flexor carpi radialis. Muscle Nerve 1981;4:435–438.
7. Verhagen WIM, Schrooten GJM, Schiphof PR, Van Ammers V. The H-reflex of the medial vastus muscle: a study in controls and patients with radiculopathy. Electromyogr Clin Neurophysiol 1988;28:421–425.
8. Fisher MA, Hoffen B, Hultimal C. Normative F-wave values and the number of recorded F-waves. Muscle Nerve 1994;17:1185–1189.
9. Panayiotopoulos CP, Chroni E. F-waves in clinical neurophysiology: a review, methodological issues and overall value in peripheral neuropathy. Electroencephalogr Clin Neurophysiol 1996;101:365–374.
10. Kimura J. F-wave velocity in the central segment of the median and ulnar nerves. A study in normal subjects and in patients with Charcot-Marie-Tooth disease. Neurology 1974;24:539–546.
11. Frazer JL, Olney RK. The relative diagnostic sensitivity of different F-wave parameters in various polyneuropathies. Muscle Nerve 1992;15:912–918.
12. DeJesus PV, Hausmanowa-Petrusewicz I, Barchi RL. The effect of cold on nerve conduction. Neurology 1973;23:1182–1189.
13. Gassel MM, Diamantopoulos E. Pattern of conduction times of the radial nerves: a clinical and electrophysiology study. Neurology 1964;14:222–231.
14. Gassel MM. Source of error in motor nerve conduction studies. Neurology 1964;14:825–835.
15. McLeod JS. Nerve Conduction Measurements for Clinical Use. In H Van Duijn, DNJ Donker, AC Van Hufflen (eds), Current Concepts in Clinical Neurophysiology. The Hague: NV Drukkenrij Trio, 1977;83–99.
16. Nishida T, Price S, Minieka M. Medial antebrachial cutaneous nerve conduction in true neurogenic thoracic outlet syndrome. Electromyogr Clin Neurophysiol 1993;33:285–288.
17. Oh SJ. Principles of Clinical Electromyography. Baltimore: Williams & Wilkins, 1998.
18. Gutmann L. Median-ulnar nerve communications and carpal tunnel syndrome. J Neurol Neurosurg Psychiatry 1977;36:899–990.
19. Gutmann L. Important Anomalous Innervations of the Extremities. AAEE Minimonograph #2. Muscle Nerve 1993;16;339–347.
20. Gutmann L, Gutierrez A, Riggs JE. The contribution of median-ulnar communications in diagnosis of mild carpal tunnel syndrome. Muscle Nerve 1986;9:319–321.
21. Iyer V, Fenichel GM. Normal median nerve proximal latency in carpal tunnel syndrome: a clue to coexisting Martin-Gruber anastomosis. J Neurol Neurosurg Psychiatry 1976;39:449–452.
22. Lambert EH. Diagnostic value of electrical stimulation of motor nerves. Electroencephalogr Clin Neurophysiol Suppl 1962;22:9–16.
23. Crutchfield CA, Gutmann L. Hereditary aspects of accessory peroneal nerve. J Neurol Neurosurg Psychiatry 1973;36:989–990.
24. Infante E, Kennedy WR. Anomalous branch of the deep nerve detected by electromyography. Arch Neurol 1970;22:162–165.
25. Lambert EH. The accessory deep peroneal nerve: a common variation in innervation of extensor digitorum brevis. Neurology 1969;19:1169–1176.
26. Fisher MA. H reflexes and F waves: physiology and clinical indications. AAEE minimonograph #13. Muscle Nerve 1992;15:1223–1233.
27. Ackil AA, Shahanni BT, Young RR, Rubin NE. Late response and sural conduction studies. Usefulness in patients with chronic renal failure. Arch Neurol 1981;38:482–485.
28. D'Amour ML, Shahani BT, Young RR, Bird KT. The importance of studying sural nerve conduction and late responses in the evaluation of alcoholic subjects. Neurology 1979;29:1600–1604.

29. Olney RK, Aminoff MJ. Electrodiagnostic features of the Guillain-Barré syndrome: the relative sensitivity of different techniques. Neurology 1990;40:471–475.
30. Lachman T, Shahani B, Young RR. Late responses as aids to diagnosis in peripheral neuropathy. J Neurol Neurosurg Psychiatry 1980;43:156–162.
31. Kimura J, Butzer JF. F-wave conduction velocity in the Guillain-Barré syndrome. Arch Neurol 1975;32:524–529.
32. King D, Ashby P. Conduction velocity in the proximal segments of a motor nerve in the Guillain-Barré syndrome. J Neurol Neurosurg Psychiatry 1976;39:538–544.
33. Walsh JC, Yiannikas C, McLeod JG. Abnormalities of proximal conduction in acute idiopathic polyneuritis: comparison of short latency evoked potentials and F-waves. J Neurol Neurosurg Psychiatry 1984;47:197–200.
34. Oh SJ, Joy JL, Kuruoglu R. "Chronic sensory demyelinating neuropathy": chronic inflammatory polyneuropathy presenting as a pure sensory neuropathy. J Neurol Neurosurg Psychiatry 1992;55:677–680.
35. Oh SJ, Claussen GC, Kim DS. Motor and sensory demyelinating mononeuropathy multiplex (multifocal motor and sensory demyelinating neuropathy): a separate entity or a variant of chronic inflammatory demyelinating polyneuropathy? J Peripher Nerv Syst 1997;2:362–369.
36. Shivde AJ, Fisher MA. F chronodispersion in polyneuropathy [abstract]. Muscle Nerve 1988;11:960.
37. Risk WS, Bosch EP, Kimura J, et al. Chronic tetanus: clinical report and histochemistry of muscle. Muscle Nerve 1981;4:363–366.
38. Eisen A, Odusote K. Amplitude of the F wave: a potential means of documenting spasticity. Neurology 1979;29:1306–1309.
39. Nicholas AP, Chatterjee A, Arnold MM, et al. Stiff-persons syndrome associated with thymoma and subsequent myasthenia gravis. Muscle Nerve 1997;20:493–498.
40. Smith KKE, Cluassen GC, Fesenmeier JT, Oh SJ. Myokymia-cramp syndrome: evidence of hyperexcitable peripheral nerve. Muscle Nerve 1994;17:1065–1067.
41. Miyasaki JM, Ashby P, Sharpe JA, Fletcher WA. On the cause of hyporeflexia in the Holmes-Adie syndrome. Neurology 1988;38:262–265.
42. Harriman DG, Garland H. The pathology of Adie's syndrome. Brain 1968;91:401–418.
43. Ulrich J. Morphological basis of Adie's syndrome. Eur Neurol 1980;19:390–395.
44. Donofrio P, Walker FO. Tabes dorsalis: electrodiagnostic features. J Neurol Neurosurg Psychiatry 1988;51:1097–1099.
45. Greenfield JG. Infectious Diseases of the Central Nervous System. In W Blackwood, WH McMenemey, A Meyer, et al. (eds), Greenfield's Neuropathology (2nd ed). Baltimore: Williams & Wilkins, 1963;164–181.
46. Mayer RF. Nerve conduction studies in man. Neurology 1963;13:1021–1030.
47. Blackstock E, Rushwirth G, Guth D. Electrophysiological studies in alcoholism. J Neurol Neurosurg Psychiatry 1972;35:326–334.
48. Mawsley C, Mayer RF. Nerve conduction in alcoholic polyneuropathy. Brain 1965;88:335–356.
49. Guiheneuc P, Bathien N. Two patterns of results in polyneuropathies investigated with the H reflex. J Neurol Sci 1976;30:83–94.
50. Kuruoglu HR, Oh SJ. Tendon-reflex testing in chronic demyelinating polyneuropathy. Muscle Nerve 1994;17(2):145–150.
51. Schimsheimer RJ, Ongerboer de Visser BW, Kemp B, Bour LJ. The flexor carpi radialis H-reflex in polyneuropathy: relations to conduction velocities of the median nerve and the soleus H-reflex latency. J Neurol Neurosurg Psychiatry 1987;50:447–452.
52. Kuruoglu R, Oh SJ, Thompson B. Clinical and electromyographic correlations of lumbosacral radiculopathy [letter]. Muscle Nerve 1994;17(2):250–251.
53. Teasdall RO, Park AM, Languth HW, Magladery JW. Electrophysiological studies of reflex activity in patients with lesions of the nervous system. II. Bull Johns Hopkins Hosp 1959;91:245–256.
54. Norris FH. Adult Spinal Motor Neuron Disease. In PJ Vinken, GW Bruyn (eds), Handbook of Clinical Neurology. Amsterdam: The Netherlands, 1975;22:1–56.
55. Delwaide PJ. Contribution of Human Reflex Studies to the Understanding of the Pyramidal Syndrome. In BT Shahani (ed), Electromyography in CNS Disorders: Central EMG. Boston: Butterworths, 1984;77–109.
56. Maynard FM, Stolov WC. Experimental error in determination of nerve conduction velocity. Arch Phys Med Rehab 1972;53:362–372.
57. Campbell WW, Sahni SK, Pridgeon RM, et al. Intraoperative electroneurography: management of ulnar neuropathy at the elbow. Muscle Nerve 1988;11:75–81.

58. Miller RG. The cubital tunnel syndrome: diagnosis and precise localization. Ann Neurol 1979;6:56–59.

59. Kanakamedala RV, Simons DG, Porter RW, Zucker RS. Ulnar nerve entrapment at the elbow localized by short segment stimulation. Arch Phys Med Rehabil 1988;69:959–963.

60. Odabasi Z, Oh SJ, Calussen GC, Kim DS. New near-nerve needle nerve conduction technique: differentiating epicondylar from cubital tunnel ulnar neuropathy. Muscle Nerve 1999;22:718–723.

61. Brown WF, Yates SK. Percutaneous localization of conduction abnormalities in human entrapment neuropathies. Can J Neurol Sci 1982;9:391–400.

62. Kanakamedala RV, Hong CZ. Peroneal nerve entrapment at the knee localized by short segment stimulation. Am J Phys Med Rehabil 1989;68:116–122.

63. Brown WF, Ferguson GG, Jones MW, Yates SK. The location of conduction abnormalities in human entrapment neuropathies. Can Neurol Sci 1976;3:111–122.

64. Kimura J. The carpal tunnel syndrome: localization of conduction abnormalities within the distal segment of the median nerve. Brain 1979;102:619–635.

65. Kimura J. Principles and pitfalls of nerve conduction studies. Ann Neurol 1984;16:415–429.

66. Buchthal F, Rosenfalck A. Evoked action potentials and conduction velocity in human sensory nerves. Brain Res 1966;3:1–120.

67. Oh SJ, Kim HS, Ahmad BK. The near-nerve sensory nerve conduction in tarsal tunnel syndrome. J Neurol Neurosurg Psychiatry 1985;48:999–1003.

68. Oh S, Lee K. Medial plantar neuropathy. Neurology 1987;1987:1408–1410.

69. Oh SJ, Kwon KH, Hah JS, et al. Lateral plantar neuropathy. Muscle Nerve 1999;22:1234–1238.

70. Oh SJ, Melo AC, Lee DK, et al. Large-fiber neuropathy in distal sensory neuropathy with normal routine nerve conduction. Neurology 2001;56:1570–1572.

71. Claussen GC, Odabasi Z, Oh SJ. Near-nerve sensory conduction study in chronic sensory demyelinating neuropathy. Muscle Nerve 1996;19:1219–1220.

72. Oh SJ, LaGanke C, Claussen GC. Sensory Guillain-Barré syndrome. Neurology 2001;56:82–86.

73. Oh SJ, Classen GC, Ryan H, Demirci M. Multifocal sensory demyelinating neuropathy: a heretofore unrecognized entity. 125th Annual Meeting of the American Neurological Association, October 15–17, 2000;79–80.

74. Kimura J. Collision technique. Physiologic block of nerve impulses in studies of motor nerve conduction. Neurology 1976;26:680–682.

75. Kimura J, Murphy MJ, Varda DJ. Electrophysiological study of anomalous innervation of intrinsic hand muscles. Arch Neurol 1976;33:842–844.

76. Kimura J. A method for estimating the refractory period of motor fibers in the human peripheral nerve. J Neurol Sci 1976;28:485–490.

77. Ingram DA, Davis GR, Swash M. The double collision technique: a new method for measurement of the motor nerve refractory period distribution in man. Electroencephalogr Clin Neurophysiol 1987;66:225–234.

78. Ruijten MW, De Haan GJ, Michels RP, et al. Motor nerve refractory period distribution assessed by two techniques in diabetic polyneuropathy. Electroencephalogr Clin Neurophysiol 1994;93(4):306–311.

79. Ruijten MWMM, Salle HJ, Kingma R. Comparison of two techniques to measure the motor nerve refractory period distribution. Electroencephalogr Clin Neurophysiol 1994;93:299–305.

80. Lowitzsch K, Hopf HC, Schlegel HJ. Conduction of Two or More Impulses in Relation to the Fiber Spectrum in the Mixed Human Peripheral Nerve. In JE Desmedt (ed), New Developments in Electromyography and Clinical Neurophysiology, Vol 3. Basel, Switzerland: Karger, 1973;3:272–278.

81. Braune HJ. Testing of the refractory period in sensory nerve fibres is the most sensitive method to assess beginning polyneuropathy in diabetics. Electromyogr Clin Neurophysiol 1999;39(6):355–359.

82. Schutt P, Muche H, Lehmann HJ. Refractory period impairment in sural nerves of diabetics. J Neurol 1983;229(2):113–119.

83. Tachmann W, Lehmann HJ. Relative refractory period of median nerve sensory fibers in the carpal tunnel syndrome. Eur Neurol 1974;12:309–316.

84. Holden L, Smith E, Palliyath S. Refractory studies of the median sensory nerve in carpal tunnel syndrome. Muscle Nerve 1987;10:652.

85. Gilliatt RW, Meer J. The refractory period of transmission in patients with carpal tunnel syndrome. Muscle Nerve 1990;13(5):445–450.

86. Dietrichson P, Sorbye R. Clinical method for electrical and mechanical recording of the mechanically and electrically elicited ankle reflex. Acta Neurol Scand 1971;47:1–21.

87. Koenig SK. T-wave response in cervical root lesions. Acta Neurol Scand 1991;84:273–276.

88. Rico RE, Jonkman EJ. Measurement of the Achilles tendon reflex for the diagnosis of lumbosacral root compression syndromes. J Neurol Neurosurg Psychiatry 1982;45:791–795.

89. Kuruoglu R, Oh SJ. Tendon-reflex testing in chronic demyelinating neuropathy. Muscle Nerve 1992;15:1178–1179.

90. Malcolm DS. A method of measuring reflex times applied in sciatica and other conditions due to nerve-root compression. J Neurol Neurosurg Psychiatry 1951;14:15–24.

91. Weintraub JR, Madalin K, Wong M, et al. Achilles tendon reflex and the H response: their correlation in 400 limbs. Muscle Nerve 1988;11:972.

92. Stam J. The tibialis anterior reflex in healthy subjects and in L5 radicular compression. J Neurol Neurosurg Psychiatry 1988;51:397–402.

93. De Weerd AW, Jonkman EJ. Measurement of knee tendon reflex latencies in lumbar radicular syndromes. Eur Neurol 1986;25:304–308.

94. Eisen AA, Woods JF, Sherwin AL. Peripheral nerve function in long-term therapy with diphenylhydantoin: a clinical and electrophysiologic correlation. Neurology 1974;24:411–417.

95. Gutrecht JA. Sympathetic skin response. J Clin Neurophysiol 1994;11:519–524.

96. Serra G, Guatrale R, Callengarini C, et al. Neurophysiological study of Horner's syndrome. Acta Neurol Scand 1991;84:411–415.

97. Ertekin C, Ertekin N, Mutulu S, et al. Skin potential (SP) recorded from the extremities and genital regions in normal and impotent subjects. Acta Neurol Scand 1987;76:258–267.

98. Shahani BT, Halperin JJ, Boulu P, Cohen J. Sympathetic skin response—a method of assessing unmyelinated axon dysfunction in peripheral neuropathies. J Neurol Neurosurg Psychiatry 1984;47:536–542.

99. Day TJ, Offerman D, Bajada S. Peripheral sympathetic conduction velocity calculated from surface potentials. Clin Exp Neurol 1986;22:41–46.

100. Elie B, Guiheneuc P. Sympathetic skin response: normal results in different experimental conditions. Electroencephalogr Clin Neurophysiol 1990;76:258–267.

101. Fagius J, Wallin BG. Sympathetic reflex latencies and conduction velocities in patients with polyneuropathy. J Neurol Sci 1980;47:433–448.

102. Fagius J, Wallin BG. Sympathetic reflex latencies and conduction velocities in normal man. J Neurol Sci 1980;47:449–461.

103. Levy DM, Reid G, Rowley DA, Abraham RR. Quantitative measures of sympathetic skin response in diabetes: relation to sudomotor and neurological function. J Neurol Neurosurg Psychiatry 1992;55:902–908.

104. Evans B, Lussyky D, Knezevic W. The peripheral autonomic surface potential in suspected small fiber peripheral neuropathy (abstract). Muscle Nerve 1988;11:982.

105. Van den Berg P, Kelly JJ. The evoked electrodermal response (EER) in peripheral neuropathies (abstract). Muscle Nerve 1986;9:656–657.

106. Shahani BT, Day TJ, Cros D, et al. RR interval variation and the sympathetic skin response in the assessment of autonomic function in peripheral neuropathy. Arch Neurol 1990;47:659–664.

107. Solivan B, Maselli R, Jaspan J, et al. Sympathetic skin response in diabetic neuropathy. Muscle Nerve 1987;10:711–716.

108. Niakan E, Harati Y. Sympathetic skin response in diabetic peripheral neuropathy. Muscle Nerve 1988;11:261–264.

109. Maselli RA, Jaspan JB, Soliven BC, et al. Comparison of sympathetic skin response with quantitative sudomotor axon reflex test in diabetic neuropathy. Muscle Nerve 1989;12:420–423.

110. Schondorf R, Gendron D. Evaluation of sudomotor function in patients with peripheral neuropathy (abstract). Neurology 1990;47:659–664.

111. Martin CN, Reid W. Sympathetic skin response (letter). J Neurol Neurosurg Psychiatry 1985;48:490.

112. Montagna P, Salvi F, Liguori R. Sympathetic skin response in familial amyloid polyneuropathy (letter). Muscle Nerve 1988;11:183–184.

113. Solders G, Anderson T, Persson A. Central conduction and autonomic nervous function in HMSN I. Muscle Nerve 1991;14:1074–1079.

114. Valls-Sole J, Monforte R, Estruch R. Abnormal sympathetic skin response in alcoholic subjects. J Neurol Sci 1991;102:233–237.

115. Park YC, Esa A, Sugiyama T, et al. Sympathetic skin response: a new test to diagnose ejaculatory dysfunction. J Urol 1988;139:539–541.

116. Leis AA. Cutaneous silent period. Muscle Nerve 1998;21:1243–1245.

117. Leis AA. Conduction abnormalities detected by silent period testing. Electroencephalogr Clin Neurophysiol 1994;93:444–449.

118. Shefner JM, Logigian EL. Relationship between stimulus strength and the cutaneous silent period. Muscle Nerve 1993;16:278–282.

119. Inghiller M, Berardelli A, Cruccu G, et al. Inhibition of hand muscle motor neurons by peripheral nerve stimulation in the relaxed human subject. Electroencephalogr Clin Neurophysiol 1995;97:63–68.

120. Leis AA, Ross MA, Emori T, ct al. Thc silent period produced by electrical stimulation of mixed peripheral nerves. Muscle Nerve 1991;14:1202–1208.

121. Uncini A, Kujirai T, Gluck B, Pullman S. Silent induced by cutaneous stimulation. Electroencephalogr Clin Neurophysiol 1991;81:344–352.

122. Leis AA, Kofler M, Ross MA. The silent period in pure sensory neuronopathy. Muscle Nerve 1992;15:1345–1348.

123. Syed NA, Sandbrink F, Luciano CA, et al. Cutaneous silent periods in patients with Fabry disease. Muscle Nerve 2000;23(8):1179–1186.

124. Aurora S, Ahmad B, Aurora T. Silent period abnormalities in carpal tunnel syndrome. Muscle Nerve 1998;21:1213–1215.

125. Kaneko K, Kawai S, Fuchigami Y, et al. Cutaneous silent period in syringomyelia. Muscle Nerve 1997;20(7):884–886.

126. Poncelet AN. Blink reflexes and the silent period in tetanus. Muscle Nerve 2000;23(9):1435–1438.

127. Steinegger T, Wiederkehr M, Ludin HP, Roth F. [Electromyography as a diagnostic aid in tetanus] [German]. Schweiz Med Wochenschr 1996;126(10):379–385.

128. Risk WS, Bosch EP, Kimura J, et al. Chronic tetanus: clinical report and histochemistry of muscle. Muscle Nerve 1981;4:363–366.

129. Struppler A, Struppler E, Adams RD. Local tetanus in man. Arch Neurol 1963;8:162–178.

130. Auger RG. Diseases associated with excess motor unit activity. AAEE minimonograph #44. Muscle Nerve 1994:17:1250–1263.

131. Mamoli B, Heiss WD, Maida E, Podreka I. Electrophysiological studies on the "stiff-man" syndrome. J Neurol 1977;217:111–121.

132. Ströhr M, Heckl R. Das stiff-man syndrome. Clinische, elektromyographische under pharmakologische efunde bei einem eigenen. Arch Psychiat Nervenkr 1977;223:17–180.

133. McComas AJ, Fawcett PRW, Campbell MJ, Sica REP. Electrophysiological estimation of the number of motor units within a human muscle. J Neurol Neurosurg Psychiatry 1971;34:121–131.

134. Gooch CL, Harati Y. Motor unit number estimation, ALS and clinical trials. Amyotrophic Lateral Sclerosis Other Motor Neuron Disord 2000;1:71–82.

135. Kadrie HA, Yates SK, Milner-Brown HS, Brown WF. Multiple point electrical stimulation of ulnar and median nerves. J Neurol Neurosurg Psychiatry 1976;39:973–985.

136. Daube JR. Estimating the number of motor units in a muscle. J Clin Neurophysiol 1995;12:585–594.

137. Stashuk DW, Doherty TJ, Kassam A, Brown WF. MUNE based on the automated analysis of F-responses. Muscle Nerve 1994;17:881–890.

138. Strong MJ, Brown WF, Judson AJ, Snow R. Motor unit estimates in the biceps-brachialis in amyotrophic lateral sclerosis. Muscle Nerve 1988;11:422–425.

139. Slawnych MP, Laszlo CA, Herschler C. A review of techniques employed to estimate the number of motor units in a muscle. Muscle Nerve 1990;13:1050–1064.

140. Felice KJ. Thenar motor unit number estimates using the multiple point stimulation technique: reproducibility studies in ALS and normal subjects. Muscle Nerve 1995;18:1412–1416.

141. Bromberg MB. Electrodiagnostic studies in clinical trials for motor neuron disease. J Clin Neurophysiol 1998;15:117–128.

142. Felice KJ. A longitudinal study comparing thenar motor unit number estimates to other quantitative tests in patients with amyotrophic lateral sclerosis. Muscle Nerve 1997;20:179–185.

143. Yuen EC, Olney RK. Longitudinal study of fiber density and motor unit number estimate in patients with ALS. Neurology 1997;49:573–578.

144. Lomen-Hoerth C, Olneyr R. A comparison of multipoint and statistical motor unit number estimation. Muscle Nerve 1999;22:1304.

145. Simmons Z, Epstein D, Kothari M, et al. Reproducibility of motor unit number estimation in individual subjects. Muscle Nerve 1999;22:1319.

146. Erlanger J. The interpretation of the action potentials in cutaneous and muscle nerves. Am J Physiol 1927;82:644.

147. Erlanger J, Gasser HS. Electrical Signs of Nervous Activity. Philadelphia: University of Pennsylvania Press, 1937.

148. Collins WF Jr, Nulsen FE, Randt CT. Relation of peripheral nerve fiber size and sensation in man. AMA Arch Neurol 1960;3:381.

149. Heinbecker P, Bishop GH, O'Leary J. Functional and histologic studies of somatic and autonomic nerves of man. Arch Neurol Psychiatry 1936;35:1233.

150. Lambert EH, Dyck PJ. Compound Action Potentials of Sural Nerve In Vitro in Peripheral Neuropathy. In PJ Dyck, PK Thomas, EH Lambert (eds), Peripheral Neuropathy. Philadelphia: Saunders, 1975;427–441.

151. Gasser HS. Effect of the method of leading on the recording of the nerve fiber spectrum. J Gen Physiol 1960;43:927.

152. Gasser HS, Erlanger J. The role played by the sizes of the constituent fibers of a nerve trunk in determining the form of its action potential wave. Am J Physiol 1927;80:522.

153. Gasser HS, Grundfest H. Axon diameters in relation to the spike dimensions and the conduction velocity in mammalian A fibers. Am J Physiol 1939;127:393.

154. Hursh JB. The conduction velocity and diameter of nerve fibers. Am J Physiol 1939;127:131.

155. Dyck PJ, Lambert EH. Compound nerve action potentials and morphometry. Electroencephalogr Clin Neurophysiol 1974;36:561.

156. Dyck PJ, Lambert EH, Nichols PC. Quantitative Measurement of Sensation Related to Compound Action Potential and Number and Sizes of Myelinated and Unmyelinated Fibers of Sural Nerve in Health. Friedreich's Ataxia, Hereditary Sensory Neuropathy and Tabes Dorsalis. In A Remond (ed), Handbook of Electroencephalography and Clinical Neurophysiology, Vol 9. Amsterdam, The Netherlands: Elsevier, 1971;83.

157. Stewart JD, Low PA, Fealey RD. Distal small fiber neuropathy: results of tests of sweating and autonomic cardiovascular reflexes. Muscle Nerve 1992;15(6):661–665.

158. Jamal GA, Hansen S, Weir AI, Ballantyne JP. The neurophysiologic investigation of small fiber neuropathies. Muscle Nerve 1987;10:537–545.

159. Smith SJM, Sli Z, Fowler CJ. Cutaneous thermal thresholds in patients with painful burning feet. J Neurol Neurosurg Psychiatry 1991;54:877–881.

6

Proximal Conduction Techniques: Somatosensory Evoked Potentials, Magnetic Stimulation, and Root Stimulation

Daniel L. Menkes

Other chapters have described some of the basic principles of electromyography (EMG) and nerve conduction studies (NCS) that are fundamental to the diagnosis of neuromuscular diseases. Although these techniques have vastly expanded the ability to accurately arrive at the correct diagnosis, they have their own unique limitations imposed on them by the anatomy and physiology of the peripheral nervous system. For example, routine NCS tend to emphasize the distal nerve segments. Motor NCS of the upper extremity are infrequently performed proximal to the mid-arm, and the lower extremity is infrequently conducted proximal to the knee. Sensory NCS are rarely performed more than 20 cm from the distal segment of the limb. Although late response studies, such as the F wave and H reflex, provide some information about proximal nerve function, they only assess a small portion of the nerve fibers examined by traditional NCS methodology.[1] Additional techniques must be used to adequately assess the proximal portions of the peripheral nervous system. These techniques include somatosensory evoked potentials, proximal motor conduction studies, and magnetic stimulation methodologies. Their use is better appreciated by reviewing the anatomic and physiologic organization of the nervous system.

ANATOMIC CONSIDERATIONS

Standard anatomy textbooks define the central nervous system as being composed of the brain and spinal cord, whereas the peripheral nervous system reflects those segments outside these regions. However, it should be recalled that the anterior horn cell and the origins of the motor nerve roots are actually physically located within the spinal cord. The sensory nerve cell body resides outside the spinal cord in the dorsal root ganglion (DRG). This sensory cell body receives sensory information from the periphery and projects it into the dorsal portion of the spinal cord. Standard anatomy textbooks illustrate these relationships that have important implications for clinical neurophysiology.

The anatomic arrangement of the sensory nervous system has important implications for NCS. Sensory deficits attributable to peripheral nervous system pathology may result from a lesion affecting the sensory fibers between their receptors and the dorsal root entry zone of the spinal cord where these axons first synapse. Lesions affecting sensory axons will result in wallerian degeneration distal to that site. In some instances, there may also be additional axon loss one or two nodes of Ranvier proximal to the pathologic site. Lesions that occur at or distal to the DRG should be reflected in the sensory nerve action potential (SNAP) once wallerian degeneration has occurred. However, lesions proximal to the DRG do not affect the distal segment and are not reflected in the SNAP. Other techniques must be used to examine the segment proximal to the DRG.

Lesions of the spinal cord that injure the anterior horn cells may result in wallerian degeneration down the entire length of the motor axon. Therefore, a reduction in the compound muscle action potential (CMAP) amplitude may result from a lesion anywhere along the pathway from the anterior horn cell to the target muscle. Because spontaneous activity on needle EMG confirms motor axon loss, primarily axonopathic processes affecting motor fibers can be readily detected. By contrast, demyelination without axonal loss has unique physiologic consideration, which is discussed later in this chapter.

It should be evident that proximal stimulation studies would be advantageous from an anatomic perspective for investigations of proximal nerve pathology. Although NCS can be performed transcutaneously from Erb's point (EP) distally, a thorough investigation of nerve segments proximal to EP requires invasive or indirect techniques. However, nerve physiology places additional limitations on the inherent difficulties of performing proximal conduction studies.

PHYSIOLOGIC CONSIDERATIONS

The differences between motor and sensory NCS must also be viewed from a physiologic perspective. It should be recalled that the amplitude of the CMAP from motor nerve stimulation tends to be three orders of magnitude greater than that of the SNAP observed from sensory fiber stimulation. It should also be recalled that there are several subpopulations of fiber types that contribute to these potentials. Over longer distances, the different conduction velocities of these subcomponent fiber types lead to a greater degree of temporal dispersion between the fastest and the slowest fibers contributing to the compound action potential. This phenomenon is responsible for the normal degree of temporal dispersion observed in routine NCS. Because proximal conduction studies are performed over greater distances, this magnifies the effects of the temporal dispersion phenomenon. In the case of the sensory NCS, the degree of temporal dispersion may result in an apparent loss of the SNAP in normal individuals when the stimulation is performed at EP.

Because only the largest, most heavily myelinated fibers are actually stimulated and recorded with these techniques, the less myelinated fibers and the unmyelinated fiber subtypes are not adequately evaluated by routine sensory NCS. The SNAP reflects the total number of large myelinated fibers that are excited by the electrical stimulus resulting in SNAP waveforms described in terms of their amplitude, duration, and area. The *amplitude* refers to the height of the wave and approximates the total number of excitable nerve fibers. The *duration* reflects the separation between the subpopulations of the most rapidly conducting and the least rapidly conducting fibers within the subpopulation excited by the electrical stimulus. The *area under the curve* (AUC) reflects the product of the amplitude and duration and provides a better approximation of the total number of excitable nerve fibers than the amplitude alone does. To reiterate, *temporal dispersion* is a natural phenomenon that occurs because of a greater degree of separation over distance. For example, one could visualize a group of cars that will start at the same time but travel at various speeds ranging from 40 to 60 miles per hour. After 10 seconds, there is minimal separation, but there will be a 20-mile separation after just 1 hour. The same number of cars is still present; they merely exhibit greater spacing between them. As in this analogy, the different fiber subtypes manifest greater degrees of separation over longer distances. In the upper extremity, fiber types have an average conduction velocity range of 40–60 m per second. After 1 millisecond, the most rapidly conducting myelinated fibers and the least rapidly conducting myelinated fibers are separated by 20 mm (2 cm). After 10 milliseconds, this distance increases to 200 mm (20 cm). Although the AUC is identical, the degree of temporal dispersion increases over greater distances. When the nerve action potential has a low amplitude and short duration distally, the waveform may not be easily recorded with proximal stimulation. This is especially true for sensory NCS that have a small AUC even with distal conduction studies. Nerve action potential recording requires separating the signal from a background awash with electrical noise. Irrespective of the techniques used, the signal must stand out from the background so that it may be accurately measured. Therefore, temporal dispersion over longer distances results in an action potential of lower amplitude and greater duration for the same AUC. Even with good recording techniques, low-amplitude SNAPs may be difficult to detect over the routine distances of 10–16 cm. The degree of temporal dispersion noted in routine sensory NCS is demonstrated in Figure 6.1. Because this degree of

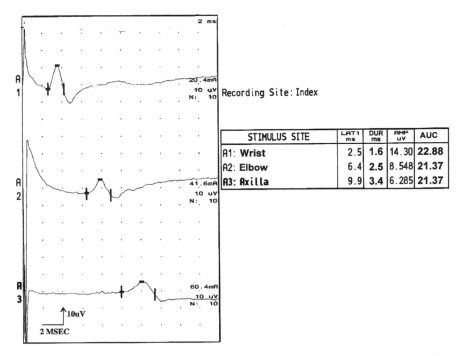

Recording Site: Index

STIMULUS SITE	LAT1 ms	DUR ms	AMP uV	AUC
A1: **Wrist**	2.5	1.6	14.30	**22.88**
A2: **Elbow**	6.4	2.5	8.548	**21.37**
A3: **Axilla**	9.9	3.4	6.285	**21.37**

Figure 6.1 Antidromic stimulation of the median nerve recording over the distal index finger. Note that the area under the curve remains relatively consistent. (AMP = amplitude; AUC = area under the curve; DUR = duration; LAT = onset latency.)

temporal dispersion is magnified over greater distances and with greater degrees of nerve pathology, one should be cautious about diagnosing conduction block in a sensory NCS. Although such instances have been reported, it is difficult to distinguish this finding from the natural degree of temporal dispersion. This phenomenon is of less concern for motor NCS, as their CMAPs are three orders of magnitude greater in amplitude and are less affected by this phenomenon. These physiologic effects must be considered in concert with signal processing and amplification techniques.

SIGNAL PROCESSING AND AMPLIFICATION

All electrical signals must be recorded from an environment that is awash in random electromagnetic activity or "noise." This unwanted activity or noise can be separated from the signal or the electrical activity of interest using amplification techniques, signal averaging techniques, Fourier transformation, and filters. Although standard textbooks of electrodiagnostic medicine treat these subjects in greater detail, several issues are worth revisiting. Although the mathematics underlying these concepts may be omitted, the concepts themselves should be understood.

Electromagnetism refers to the discipline involved with energy transformation and transfer. The first principle of thermodynamics states that the amount of energy in the universe remains the same; energy can be neither created nor destroyed. Although energy may be converted from one form to another, such as electrical energy to sound wave energy, the total amount of energy before and after the transformation is identical. The second principle of thermodynamics states that although energy may change forms, the transformation occurs imperfectly with some of the energy "lost" as heat or electromagnetic radiation. Basic principles of physics state that electromagnetic signals may be described by particle or wave theory. For the purposes of clinical neurophysiology, wave theory adequately explains most of the phenomena encountered in routine electrodiagnostic testing. Waves propagate as an electrical field that induces a magnetic field at a right angle to the original electrical field. This magnetic field then generates a second electrical field at right angle to itself, which results in another magnetic field being generated. Thus, magnetic fields are capable of inducing electrical fields and vice versa. This is the principle that underlies the magnetic stimulation techniques that are discussed later in the chapter. Any electromagnetic wave's behavior can be predicted on the basis of wave theory applied to combinations of fundamental sine and cosine waves.

All fundamental sine and cosine waves may be described in terms of their energy, which is related to their frequency and inversely proportional to their wavelength. The *wavelength* describes the distance traveled for the sine or cosine wave to complete one full cycle of 360 degrees. By contrast, the *frequency* describes how many cycles are completed in one second's time. The position of the wave within this repetitive 360-degree cycle is known as its *phase*. Two identical waves that are in the same portion of their cycle are said to be *in phase*, whereas those in different portions of their cycle are said to be *out of phase*. When these identical waves are 180 degrees apart, they are exact mirror images of one another and are *completely out of phase*. Two identical waves in phase are completely additive, whereas two identical waves 180 degrees out of phase completely cancel one another's effects. From a mathematic perspective, a flat ocean could represent either a net cancellation of two 400-ft tidal waves 180 degrees out of phase with one another or no wave activity at all; both will yield the same net result. Therefore, an absent waveform on the EMG oscilloscope screen could represent either complete cancellation of all waveforms or no activity at all. Lesser degrees of phase cancellation can result in various combinations of waveform dispersion and amplitude reduction. This may result in unusual-appearing waveforms. However, the underlying subcomponent waves that contribute to any signal can be identified through the use of Fourier analysis.

Fourier analysis is based on the mathematic concept that all waves, irrespective of their shape, can be decomposed into a summation of fundamental sine and cosine waves. Sine waves and cosine waves are, by definition, out of phase. Any waveform can be constructed by summating sines and cosines of different amplitudes and frequencies staggered into different phases. The decomposition of complicated waveforms into their subcomponent sine and cosine waves is known as *Fourier transformation,* whereas the opposite function of reintegrating the signal is known as *reverse Fourier transformation.* Most electrodiagnostic machines perform Fourier transformation to improve signal processing, as explained in the next paragraph. By contrast, the central nervous system performs reverse Fourier transformation to reintegrate incoming temporally dispersed signals. It is the central nervous system's ability to perform this function that underlies the use of somatosensory evoked potentials (SSEPs).

Electrodiagnostic medicine applies an electrical stimulus to an excitable tissue and records the result on an oscilloscope screen. The electrical activity generated from the excitable tissue is known as the *signal* to differentiate it from the unwanted background electromagnetic activity or noise. To differentiate the wanted signal from the unwanted noise, a variety of techniques must be used, including common mode rejection amplification, filtration, and, in some cases, signal averaging. These techniques are discussed briefly, as they are covered in greater detail in any standard textbook of electrodiagnostic medicine.

Common mode rejection is based on the principle that one electrode is placed adjacent to the signal generator (recording electrode) and the other is placed at a suitable distance from the signal generator (reference electrode). Both electrodes record the background noise, but proper placement of these electrodes should record the entire signal at the recording electrode and minimal to no signal at the reference electrode. The electrodiagnostic machine decomposes these inputs into a sum of sines and cosines by rapid Fourier transformation. Any wave that appears at both sites is rejected from further analysis, a process known as *common mode rejection.* Most modern machines have a common mode rejection ratio of 20,000 to 1 or greater. This excludes most of the background noise from further processing. The signal can then be refined by passing it through electrical filters.

Filters exclude electrical activity of a certain frequency. High frequency filters (HFF) eliminate higher frequencies or "pass" lower frequencies. Therefore, the terms *high frequency filter* and *low pass filter* may be used interchangeably. Conversely, a *low frequency filter* (LFF), or *high pass filter,* are similar terms and refer to a filter that eliminates frequencies less than the one selected. The *band pass* refers to the frequencies between the high pass and low pass filter settings. A *notch filter* eliminates one particular frequency and can be created by assigning the same value to the HFF and LFF. In reality, both the HFF and LFF eliminate approximately 70% of the frequency to which they are set, with greater degrees of noise elimination occurring at frequencies remote from their setting. Therefore, an HFF set to 2 kHz eliminates 70% of this frequency but close to 100% of a 10 kHz signal. It should be evident that proper filter settings are a prerequisite for proper proximal conduction studies.

Signals can also be amplified using averaging techniques. However, this technique works best when identical signals are averaged, as is the case with techniques that evaluate sensory fibers. It is more difficult to average motor unit action potentials, because there is always some variability in neuromuscular junction transmission time (the concept underlying single fiber EMG studies). In practice, sensory studies are the ones usually averaged. Averaging only improves the signal to noise ratio by a square root of the number of averages. Doubling this ratio requires four averages, tripling requires nine, and a tenfold increase requires 100 averages. Most SNAPs usually require nine or fewer averages to be recognizable. However, SSEP waveform recognition often requires 500–2,000 averages.

ELECTRODIAGNOSTIC CONSIDERATIONS

Although several techniques regarding antidromic sensory studies have been published, some caution is advised. The EMG machine amplifies any voltage difference detected between the recording and reference electrode. Figure 6.2 demonstrates what may occur when the median nerve is stimulated over the index finger, and the result is recorded over the medial portion of the wrist (the site where the ulnar SNAP is usually recorded). This result reflects a difference in electrical potential between the recording and reference electrodes. However, this difference in voltage was generated by a median nerve far-field potential and not from an ulnar nerve near-field potential. Thus, any electrical signal that is present at one electrode but not the other is amplified by the differential amplifier and displayed as a signal on the oscilloscope irrespective of the signal's generator (sensory or motor axons). Therefore, extreme care should be taken when stimulating a sensory nerve antidromically in the proximal portion of the limb,

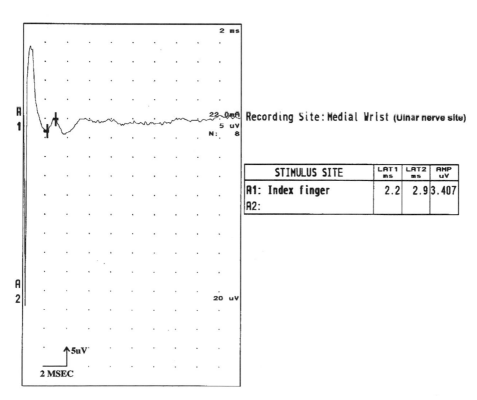

Figure 6.2 Stimulation of the index finger yields a recordable sensory nerve action potential from the site used to record an orthodromic ulnar sensory nerve action potential. (AMP = amplitude; LAT = onset latency.)

as inadvertent motor axon stimulation may occur simultaneously. The potential recorded over a distal digit may actually reflect distantly generated motor far-field potentials rather than a true SNAP. Such inadvertent stimulation results in a recordable potential that may not actually reflect sensory fiber function. Erroneous conclusions may result in such an instance. For reasons that are explained in the section Somatosensory Evoked Potentials, this situation may be avoided by using SSEPs.

The section Signal Processing and Amplification must also be considered when no waveform is observed on the oscilloscope screen. An absent waveform may represent complete phase cancellation of subcomponent waves or the absence of an electrical signal. These two entities cannot be differentiated with absolute certainty. Even if one were confident that the signal was truly absent, it would not be possible to distinguish myelin dysfunction from axon dysfunction.[2] Complete myelin dysfunction resulting in an inability to conduct a signal gives the same result as a stimulus applied to transected axons. Because CMAPs tend to be three orders of magnitude larger than SNAPs, complete phase cancellation in motor NCS is far less likely, as more subcomponent waves contribute to this response. Demyelination of motor fibers tends to result in some combination of reduced amplitudes and dispersed waveforms. However, demyelination of sensory nerves tends to result in apparently absent waveforms.

The disparate effects of myelin dysfunction on sensory and motor axons are not merely of arcane academic interest, because many treatable neuropathies manifest evidence of myelin sheath dysfunction. Immune-mediated demyelination tends to occur where there is a relative paucity of the blood-nerve barrier. This blood-nerve barrier is least robust at the nerve root level and the most distal segment of the axon.[3] This often results in demyelination occurring at opposite ends of the nerve with centripetal spread. Sensory NCS performed away from these segments may be normal early in the course of demyelination. This explains the "absent median, normal sural" phenomenon often seen in acquired demyelinating polyneuropathies.[4] Consider a case of demyelinating polyneuropathy when the demyelination has spread 6 cm from the opposite poles from the nerve root and the distal sensory axon. The distal segment of the sural nerve would be in the midfoot, whereas the median nerve pathology would be at the base of the second digit. In this paradigm, median nerve studies would traverse the site of demyelination, whereas sural nerve studies from the calf to the ankle would not. This would result in an absent median SNAP, whereas the sural SNAP would still be observed. However, this pattern could also be observed in a number of other conditions, including carpal tunnel syndrome with median nerve compression at the wrist. Therefore, sensory NCS cannot reliably distinguish between myelin dysfunction and axon loss when a SNAP is unrecordable. However, SSEPs may provide a means of distinguishing these entities owing to the process of central amplification and resynchronization explored in the next section.

SOMATOSENSORY EVOKED POTENTIALS

This technique uses many of the same principles involved in sensory NCS in that large-fiber sensory nerves are stimulated repeatedly to average similar signals. SSEPs and sensory NCS are similar in that they assess the same populations of the large myelinated fibers and do not provide information regarding lesser myelinated or unmyelinated fibers. The responses are recorded from electrodes placed along these pathways as the signal ascends through the peripheral nervous system,

Table 6.1 Upper Extremity Somatosensory Evoked Potentials

Evoked Potential	Alternate Name	Presumed Site of Origin	Maximum Latency (msec)
N9	Erb's point	Brachial plexus	12.0
PN/13	CVII	Cervical spine	16.3
N19	—	Thalamocortical relay	22.1
P22	—	Thalamocortical relay	25.9

Source: Summarized data from KH Chiappa (ed), Evoked Potentials in Clinical Medicine (3rd ed). New York: Raven Press, 1997.

traverses the spinal cord and brainstem, and terminates in the contralateral somatosensory cortex. These electrodes amplify voltage differences between the active and reference electrodes and are designated *far-field potentials*, because they are recorded at a distance from their source generator. All electrical signals dissipate as an inverse function of the distance from the source generator squared. A signal recorded at 2 cm from the source generator has 25% or one-fourth of the signal intensity measured at 1 cm. Therefore, these potentials are of significantly lower amplitude than the ones obtained from sensory NCS that record adjacent *near-field potentials*. To compensate for this lower amplitude, signal averaging techniques are used to magnify the signal to noise ratio. Because the signal to noise ratio improves as a function of the square root of the number of averages, between 500 and 2,000 averages are often required. At least two trials should be performed to demonstrate waveform reproducibility. The technical performance and interpretation of these studies is beyond the scope of this chapter but is covered extensively in Chiappa's textbook.[5] For purposes of this discussion, four important differences between SSEPs and sensory NCS need to be emphasized.

The first is that the far-field potential may be designated by its site of origin or in terms of its peak latency and usual polarity. Conventional neurophysiology terminology represents negativity as an upward deflection on an oscilloscope, whereas positivity is represented with a downward deflection. Therefore, one may describe the potential observed as a negative deflection with an average onset of 9 milliseconds from EP by its site of origin or by its waveform characteristics (e.g., N9 for negative deflection at an average of 9 milliseconds). These "average" SSEP values are based on normative data obtained from a sample population chosen to reflect the characteristics of the larger, regional population. Therefore, it is preferable to obtain site-specific normal values. If this is not feasible, then the technique should be performed in exactly the same manner as described for the set of reference standards that are being used. Upper extremity studies are usually performed on the median or ulnar nerves, whereas lower extremity studies are usually performed on the tibial or peroneal nerves. The most useful parameters are those derived from latency measurements, including absolute latency, interpeak latencies, and side-to-side latency comparisons. Amplitude data are more variable and tend to be less reliable. Normal values for these parameters depend on the population being evaluated. Tables 6.1 and 6.2 summarize the standard SSEP nomenclature, the presumed site of the waveform, and the upper limit of normal latency values for the tibial and median SSEPs.[5] An example of a normal median SSEP is depicted in Figure 6.3, and a normal tibial SSEP is depicted in Figure 6.4. The montages used to record these responses are listed in these figures.

A second significant difference between SSEPs and sensory NCS is that the amplitudes of these potentials are one order of magnitude smaller than the aver-

Table 6.2 Lower Extremity Somatosensory Evoked Potentials

Evoked Potential	Alternate Name	Presumed Site of Origin	Maximum Latency (msec)
Knee	PF	Tibial nerve	11.9*
Lumbar point	T12	Conus/Cauda	28.3*
N/P 37	—	Thalamocortical relay	47.8*
LP-N/P37	—	Interpeak latency	21.3*

*These values depend on lower extremity limb length and the patient's height. These data represent the extremes of normal.
Source: Summarized data from KH Chiappa (ed), Evoked Potentials in Clinical Medicine (3rd ed). New York: Raven Press, 1997.

age SNAP. Therefore, signal-averaging techniques are required to improve the signal to noise ratio. Because these waveforms are less distinct than most SNAPs, the peak latency is much more reliably identified than the onset latency. Sensory NCS may be calculated from either onset or peak latency. Onset latency represents the conduction velocity of the largest, most heavily myelinated subpopulation of the most heavily myelinated fibers. The peak latency, as used with evoked potentials, reflects the average velocity of this entire population. Therefore, greater degrees of demyelination must be present to result in a prolonged peak latency as opposed to an onset latency. Thus, a normal evoked potential peak latency does not exclude lesser degrees of demyelination within the large-fiber sensory pathways being examined.

Another significant difference between SSEPs and sensory NCS is that the central nervous system is capable of amplifying and resynchronizing the afferent sensory volleys. As explained previously, demyelination will result in temporal dispersion within the nervous tissue excited by the stimulus. Unlike the peripheral nervous system, the central nervous system can reintegrate these dispersed potentials into a recognizable cortical evoked potential. Although demyelinating pathology affecting the sensory fibers in a peripheral nerve may cause enough temporal dispersion to render it apparently absent on the EMG oscilloscope screen, a cortical SSEP may still be obtainable. Thus, SSEP studies should be considered when a SNAP is abnormal. A normal evoked potential obtained over EP should be interpreted as, "There is no electrophysiologic evidence of a conduction defect in the large-fiber sensory pathways between the wrist and Erb's point." However, it should be understood that "absence of evidence is not evidence of absence," as partial degrees of pathology may result in a normal study. A normal evoked potential only excludes significant degrees of large-fiber sensory pathway dysfunction. By contrast, an absent SNAP from antidromic EP stimulation has a variety of possible interpretations. These include sensory axon loss, demyelination between the stimulating and recording sites, or normal physiologic temporal dispersion. Even in the absence of any other evoked potential waveforms, the presence of a cortical potential obtained from SSEPs confirms that some of the sensory axons are in continuity between the site of stimulation and the somatosensory cortex. Therefore, SSEP studies may be used to demonstrate at least partial sensory axon continuity even when no SNAP is visible.

The final significant difference is that SSEPs evaluate the entire length of the large-fiber sensory pathways between the site of stimulation and the contralateral somatosensory cortex. Pathology affecting these pathways proximal to the DRG

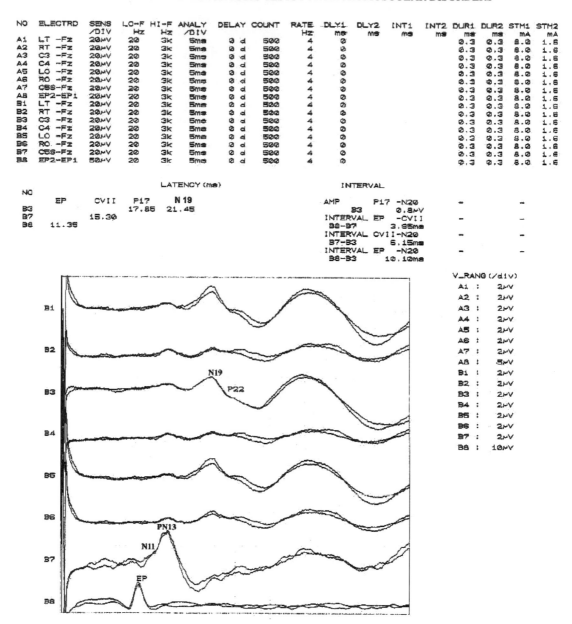

NO	ELECTRD	SENS /DIV	LO-F Hz	HI-F Hz	ANALY /DIV	DELAY	COUNT	RATE Hz	DLY1 ms	DLY2 ms	INT1 ms	INT2 ms	DUR1 ms	DUR2 ms	STM1 mA	STM2 mA
A1	LT -Fz	20μV	20	3k	5ms	0 d	500	4	0				0.3	0.3	8.0	1.6
A2	RT -Fz	20μV	20	3k	5ms	0 d	500	4	0				0.3	0.3	8.0	1.6
A3	C3 -Fz	20μV	20	3k	5ms	0 d	500	4	0				0.3	0.3	8.0	1.6
A4	C4 -Fz	20μV	20	3k	5ms	0 d	500	4	0				0.3	0.3	8.0	1.6
A5	LO -Fz	20μV	20	3k	5ms	0 d	500	4	0				0.3	0.3	8.0	1.6
A6	RO -Fz	20μV	20	3k	5ms	0 d	500	4	0				0.3	0.3	8.0	1.6
A7	C5S-Fz	20μV	20	3k	5ms	0 d	500	4	0				0.3	0.3	8.0	1.6
A8	EP2-EP1	20μV	20	3k	5ms	0 d	500	4	0				0.3	0.3	8.0	1.6
B1	LT -Fz	20μV	20	3k	5ms	0 d	500	4	0				0.3	0.3	8.0	1.6
B2	RT -Fz	20μV	20	3k	5ms	0 d	500	4	0				0.3	0.3	8.0	1.6
B3	C3 -Fz	20μV	20	3k	5ms	0 d	500	4	0				0.3	0.3	8.0	1.6
B4	C4 -Fz	20μV	20	3k	5ms	0 d	500	4	0				0.3	0.3	8.0	1.6
B5	LO -Fz	20μV	20	3k	5ms	0 d	500	4	0				0.3	0.3	8.0	1.6
B6	RO -Fz	20μV	20	3k	5ms	0 d	500	4	0				0.3	0.3	8.0	1.6
B7	C5S-Fz	20μV	20	3k	5ms	0 d	500	4	0				0.3	0.3	8.0	1.6
B8	EP2-EP1	50μV	20	3k	5ms	0 d	500	4	0				0.3	0.3	8.0	1.6

LATENCY (ms)

NO	EP	CVII	P17	N19
B3			17.85	21.45
B7		15.30		
B8	11.35			

INTERVAL

AMP	P17 -N20		
B3	0.8μV	–	–
INTERVAL EP -CVII			
B8-B7	3.95ms	–	–
INTERVAL CVII-N20			
B7-B3	6.15ms	–	–
INTERVAL EP -N20			
B8-B3	10.10ms	–	–

V_RANG (/div)

A1 :	2μV
A2 :	2μV
A3 :	2μV
A4 :	2μV
A5 :	2μV
A6 :	2μV
A7 :	2μV
A8 :	5μV
B1 :	2μV
B2 :	2μV
B3 :	2μV
B4 :	2μV
B5 :	2μV
B6 :	2μV
B7 :	2μV
B8 :	10μV

Figure 6.3 Normal median somatosensory evoked potential from wrist stimulation. (AMP = amplitude; DIV = division; DLY = delay; DUR = duration; EP = Erb's point; HI-F = high frequency; INT = interval; LO-F = low frequency; STM = stimulation.)

may be detected with SSEPs but will escape detection with sensory NCS. Therefore, SSEPs should be considered in those instances where pathology proximal to the DRG is suspected. SSEPs in concert with conventional EMG and NCS data may help differentiate between radiculopathies, dorsal root ganglionopathies, plexopathies, and mononeuropathies. In certain instances, SSEPs may provide indirect evidence to suggest an acquired demyelinating polyneuropathy. However, this statement can be made with confidence only in specific circumstances. Each of these indications is discussed in greater detail later in this chapter.

NO	ELECTRD	SENS /DIV	LO-F Hz	HI-F Hz	ANALY /DIV	DELAY	COUNT	RATE Hz	DLY1 ms	DLY2 ms	INT1 ms	INT2 ms	DUR1 ms	DUR2 ms	STM1 mA	STM2 mA
A1	LO -Fz	20µV	20	3k	10ms	0 d	531	3	0				0.3	0.3	15.0	1.0
A2	RO -Fz	20µV	20	3k	10ms	0 d	531	3	0				0.3	0.3	15.0	1.0
A3	C3 -Fz	20µV	20	3k	10ms	0 d	531	3	0				0.3	0.3	15.0	1.0
A4	C4 -Fz	20µV	20	3k	10ms	0 d	531	3	0				0.3	0.3	15.0	1.0
A5	Cz -Fz	20µV	20	3k	10ms	0 d	531	3	0				0.3	0.3	15.0	1.0
A6	Cz -C5S	20µV	20	3k	10ms	0. d	531	3	0				0.3	0.3	15.0	1.0
A7	X1 -X5	20µV	20	3k	10ms	0 d	531	3	0				0.3	0.3	15.0	1.0
A8	X3 -X7	20µV	20	3k	10ms	0 d	531	3	0				0.3	0.3	15.0	1.0
B1	LO -Fz	20µV	20	3k	10ms	0 d	705	3	0				0.3	0.3	15.0	1.0
B2	RO -Fz	20µV	20	3k	10ms	0 d	705	3	0				0.3	0.3	15.0	1.0
B3	C3 -Fz	20µV	20	3k	10ms	0 d	705	3	0				0.3	0.3	15.0	1.0
B4	C4 -Fz	20µV	20	3k	10ms	0 d	705	3	0				0.3	0.3	15.0	1.0
B5	Cz -Fz	20µV	20	3k	10ms	0 d	705	3	0				0.3	0.3	15.0	1.0
B6	Cz -C5S	20µV	20	3k	10ms	0 d	705	3	0				0.3	0.3	15.0	1.0
B7	X1 -X5	50µV	20	3k	10ms	0 d	705	3	0				0.3	0.3	15.0	1.0
B8	X3 -X7	20µV	20	3k	10ms	0 d	705	3	0				0.3	0.3	15.0	1.0

		LATENCY (ms)					INTERVAL	
NO	PF	T12	P31	N34	P35	N45	AMP	P35 -N45
B5					42.8	50.9	B5	2.1µV
B6			33.9	37.0			INTERVAL PF -T12	
B7		24.4					B8-B7	14.1ms
B8	10.3						INTERVAL T12 -P31	
							B7-B6	9.5ms
							INTERVAL T12 -P35	
							B7-B5	18.4ms
							INTERVAL PF -P35	
							B8-B5	32.5ms

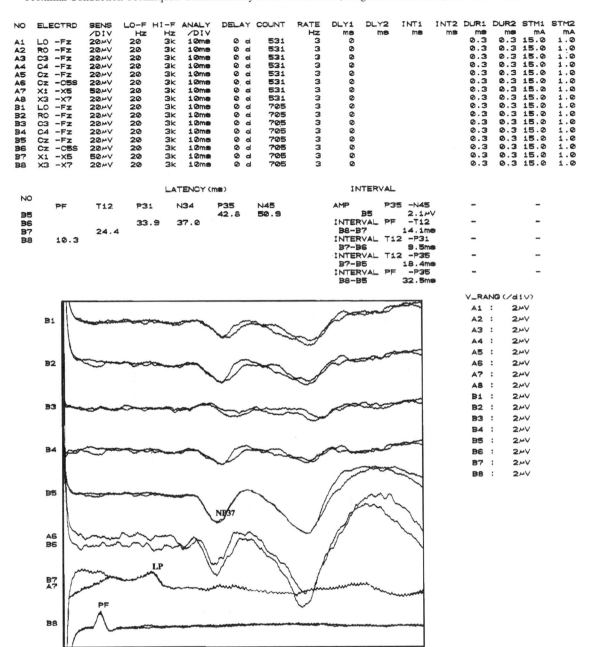

V_RANG (/div)	
A1 :	2µV
A2 :	2µV
A3 :	2µV
A4 :	2µV
A5 :	2µV
A6 :	2µV
A7 :	2µV
A8 :	2µV
B1 :	2µV
B2 :	2µV
B3 :	2µV
B4 :	2µV
B5 :	2µV
B6 :	2µV
B7 :	2µV
B8 :	2µV

Figure 6.4 Normal tibial somatosensory evoked potential from ankle stimulation. (AMP = amplitude; DIV = division; DLY = delay; DUR = duration; HI-F = high frequency; INT = interval; LO-F = low frequency; LP = lumbar point; PF = popliteal fossa; STM = stimulation.)

Somatosensory Evoked Potentials Interpretation

One common misconception is that SSEPs can only be used for the diagnosis of central demyelinating disease. It must be emphasized that this technique cannot differentiate central demyelination from central axon loss any more than an absent SNAP can distinguish between peripheral demyelination and peripheral axon loss. A properly obtained abnormal SSEP merely indicates the presence of pathology in the large-fiber sensory pathways, not the presence of demyelination. If an SSEP demonstrates a delay in peak latency but a normal amplitude, then myelin pathology is much more likely. If the peak latency is normal but the amplitude is reduced, then axon loss is more likely. However, such definitive statements should be made with caution. For example, consider a right median SSEP study in which the N9 latency is delayed. In this instance, the author would prefer to interpret this finding as "pathology affecting the large-fiber sensory pathways in the right median nerve between the wrist and Erb's point." This caveat exists because pathologic states other than acquired demyelination, including an inherited dysmyelinating neuropathy (e.g., Charcot-Marie-Tooth disease I), n-hexane exposure, and a nerve infarction, could potentially produce the same result.

Similar caution should be exercised when only a cortical evoked potential is observed. For example, consider a right median SSEP that demonstrates a delayed cortical potential with a normal amplitude. Although one might be tempted to label this as representing demyelination, that statement may not be correct for reasons stated previously. Moreover, even if one were certain that demyelination was causative, it could not be localized any more specifically than as occurring between the right wrist and contralateral cortex. In this instance, peripheral demyelination could not be differentiated from central demyelination.

Finally, consider an instance in which there is a dorsal root ganglionopathy, such as Friedreich's ataxia. The largest, most heavily myelinated fibers are gradually lost, leading to the proprioception deficits observed in this disorder. In such instances, the peripheral SNAPs may be absent, because the amplitude is so reduced that it cannot be distinguished from the background noise. If some sensory axons survive, they can be stimulated to produce an SSEP. Consider a case of Friedreich's ataxia in which 95% of the DRG cell bodies have been lost. This will result in an apparently absent SNAP in all sensory nerves tested. However, the central nervous system is capable of amplifying and resynchronizing impulses from the SSEP studies. The remaining fibers will conduct less robustly than in a normal person. Thus, a cortical potential with a prolonged latency will be observed. It would be incorrect to attribute this to a demyelinating lesion of the central nervous system. The correct interpretation would be that there is pathology affecting the large-fiber sensory pathways between the site of stimulation and the contralateral somatosensory cortex. Lesser degrees of axon loss coupled with central amplification and reverse Fourier transformation could yield a reproducible cervical spine potential. It would also be incorrect to interpret this delayed cervical potential as representing demyelination but reasonable to label it as representing pathology between the site of stimulation and the upper cervical spine. All of these caveats should be kept in mind throughout the subsequent paragraphs discussing SSEPs.

Somatosensory Evoked Potentials in Lesions Proximal to the Dorsal Root Ganglion

Because the SNAP can only assess sensory axon function between the DRG and the distal portion of its axon, SSEPs are the preferred neurodiagnostic method for assessing sensory pathology at, or proximal to, the DRG. As discussed, SSEPs are often viewed as "central nervous system" tests, but they can provide useful information regarding the peripheral nervous system. For example, SSEP studies are capable of differentiating incomplete sensory root lesions from complete lesions or sensory nerve root avulsions. Consider an instance of complete sensory nerve root avulsions at C6 and C7. Median and radial SNAPs will be normal despite the presence of complete anesthesia in these dermatomes. By contrast, a median SSEP would demonstrate a normal EP and no potentials rostral to this segment. If a cortical potential were present from either the median or radial SSEPs, then some sensory axons would remain in continuity, and the patient would have a better prognosis. However, it should be recalled that the median and radial nerve sensory pathways traverse two nerve roots. Although the presence of a cortical potential states that some of the sensory pathways are intact up to the cortex, no further statements regarding localization can be made with any degree of accuracy.

Somatosensory Evoked Potentials in Plexopathies

Brachial and lumbosacral plexopathies can usually be distinguished on the basis of EMG and NCS. Plexopathies involve multiple nerve territories distal to the dorsal root ganglia supplying the sensory axons to these nerves. In those cases in which sufficient sensory axons are lost, a plexopathy may be detected by noting a reduced SNAP in one of the limb nerves.[6] However, sufficient time must have elapsed for wallerian degeneration to occur. This axon loss has to enter segment where NCS are performed to detect axon loss. Otherwise, a normal SNAP may be obtained in the distal segment early in the course of the illness. Moreover, it may be difficult to obtain SNAPs in nerves with fewer sensory axons, such as the saphenous or the medial antebrachial cutaneous nerves.

Because SSEPs undergo central resynchronization and amplification, they can provide earlier identification of large-fiber sensory pathway pathology and differentiation of axon loss from demyelination.[7] An example of early detection would be a traumatic upper trunk and middle trunk brachial plexopathy in which all the sensory axons have been severed just proximal to EP. Sensory NCS performed in the radial or median nerves will be normal until wallerian degeneration has resulted in axon loss through the conducted segment. This may require 2–3 weeks. However, a median and radial nerve evoked potential ought to demonstrate a normal EP and no potentials rostral to this site, whereas an ulnar nerve SSEP would be completely normal. In the case of an incomplete brachial plexopathy, the presence of an evoked potential proximal to EP would indicate functional continuity of that nerve through the brachial plexus. Because surgical exploration is rarely performed so early in the course of a traumatic plexopathy, this particular use of SSEPs is of lesser clinical importance.

However, SSEPs have an advantage over sensory NCS when there is incomplete axon loss. Consider a lower trunk brachial plexopathy in which 95% of the sensory axons have been lost. The patient will describe sensory loss and paresthesias in the lower trunk distribution. Ulnar and medial antebrachial cutaneous SNAPs would be unobservable in this instance, as it would be difficult to amplify these few axons out of the background noise. The diagnosis of a lower trunk brachial plexopathy could be rendered on the basis of these "absent" SNAPs, but no statement could be made as to whether this represents subtotal or complete sensory axon loss. Ulnar SSEPs would be able to differentiate these two situations. The presence of a cortical potential, irrespective of the latency or amplitude, would provide irrefutable evidence that there was some degree of functional continuity in the ulnar nerve sensory fibers between the site of stimulation and the contralateral somatosensory cortex. This would portend a better prognosis than one in which there was no observable cortical potential.

Similar reasoning can be used in the case of a demyelinating brachial plexopathy. Consider the case of an upper trunk brachial plexopathy in which there was a significant degree of demyelination at EP but relatively little secondary axon loss. Sensory NCS could remain normal throughout the entire course of the illness so long as there was minimal secondary axon loss. By contrast, SSEPs from radial or median nerve stimulation might demonstrate a prolonged EP latency. One could be more confident regarding proximal demyelination as the cause if more than 3 weeks had elapsed. By this time, wallerian degeneration should have occurred and would have likely resulted in a reduced distal SNAP amplitude. If there were no alternative explanation for large-fiber sensory nerve pathology, one might consider the use of immunomodulating treatments.

Somatosensory Evoked Potentials in Polyneuropathies

One of the most challenging aspects of peripheral NCS is that of distinguishing compression-induced demyelination from demyelination due to other causes. This becomes even more challenging when the studies are conducted across a common site of compression, such as conducting the median nerve across the transverse carpal ligament. Median SSEPs are advantageous in this situation because they do not cross this segment. Consider a case of severe demyelination affecting the median nerve sensory fibers in the forearm in association with a carpal tunnel syndrome producing a second site of compression at the wrist. Stimulation of the median nerve either at the elbow or at the wrist would result in an absent SNAP recorded over the index finger. However, the concomitant carpal tunnel syndrome would not affect the median SSEPs. Stimulation of the wrist might demonstrate a delayed EP latency with milder degrees of demyelination. This would lead to the correct diagnosis.

More commonly, distally recorded SNAPs are absent because of demyelination spreading proximally from the distal end of the nerve segment. There is often associated demyelination in the sensory nerve roots as well. This results in the absence of all SSEP waveforms except for the cortical potential that results from central amplification and resynchronization. This is properly interpreted as pathology affecting the large fiber sensory pathways between the wrist and contralateral somatosensory cortex. However, peripheral demyelination can be deduced by stimulating the median nerve in the antecubital fossa. This second stimulation procedure results in a cortical SSEP of lesser latency because the stimulus is applied at a site that is more proximal. Because the distance between the elbow and the wrist is known, a conduction velocity can be calculated by subtracting the elbow latency from the wrist latency. A profoundly slow conduction velocity would be consistent with demyelination between the wrist and the elbow. This is the reverse of how a median nerve motor conduction velocity in the forearm is calculated.

Figures 6.5 and 6.6 illustrate how this method can be applied to tibial SSEPs. Figure 6.5 demonstrates that tibial nerve stimulation at the ankle yields no reproducible waveforms save for a cortical NP37 potential at 57.7 milliseconds. Figure 6.6 demonstrates an NP37 cortical potential with a latency of 33.8 milliseconds resulting from stimulation of the same tibial nerve at the knee, 475 mm proximal to the previous site. This latency is shorter because it is closer to the cortex and proximal to the site of myelin pathology. The conduction velocity is calculated by dividing the 475-mm segment by the latency difference of 57.7 milliseconds minus 33.8 milliseconds, or 23.9 milliseconds, that yields a conduction velocity of 20 meters per second, which is within the "demyelinating" range. This confirms peripheral demyelination because the only difference between these two stimulation sites is the tibial nerve between the knee and ankle, because all segments proximal to the knee are included in both studies.

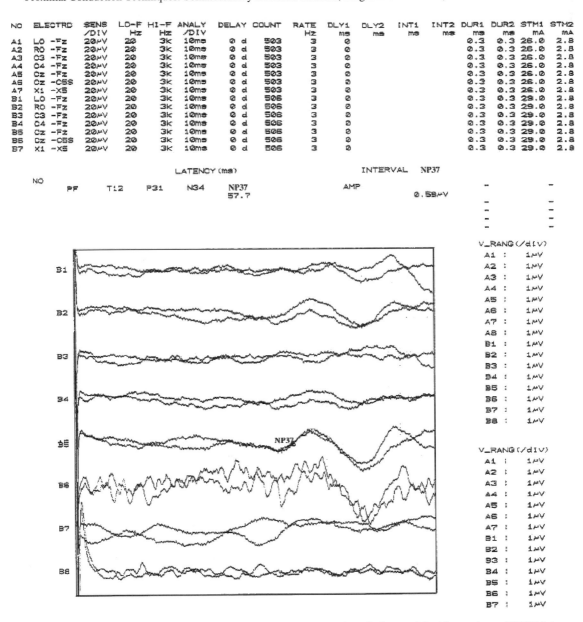

Figure 6.5 Stimulation of the tibial nerve at the ankle yields a dispersed cortical potential with a prolonged NP37 latency. (AMP = amplitude; DIV = division; DLY = delay; DUR = duration; EP = Erb's point; HI-F = high frequency; INT = interval; LO-F = low frequency; STM = stimulation.)

Somatosensory Evoked Potentials and Mononeuropathies

This indication for SSEPs probably has the least clinical applicability, although it can be used effectively in select instances. For example, consider two nearly identical cases of a radial neuropathy in the arm (Saturday night palsy). One patient has experienced complete axon loss, and the other has experienced incomplete axon loss. NCS could not readily differentiate these two patients until sufficient time had elapsed for wallerian degeneration to have occurred. However, evoked potentials

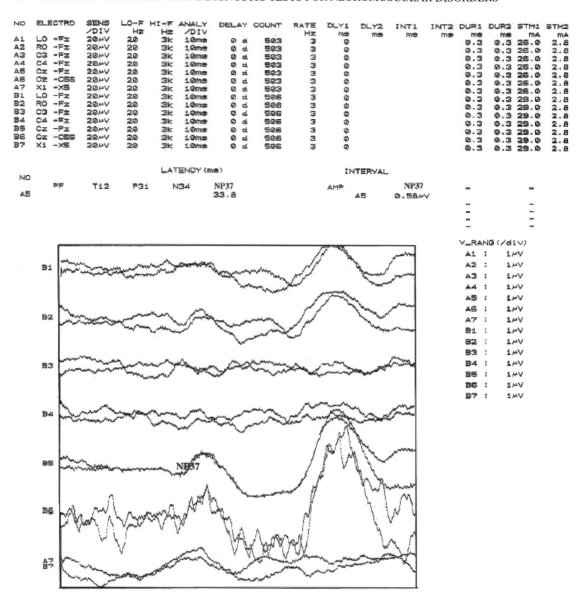

Figure 6.6 Restimulation of the same tibial nerve as in Figure 6.5 at the knee yields a more synchronized cortical potential with a shorter latency. (AMP = amplitude; DIV = division; DLY = delay; DUR = duration; HI-F = high frequency; INT = interval; LO-F = low frequency; LP = lumbar point; STM = stimulation.)

could readily differentiate these patients. Radial SSEPs would probably demonstrate a recordable cortical potential in the patient with incomplete loss of sensory axons, whereas the other would have an unrecordable cortical potential. However, it should be remembered that an absent cortical potential might be seen with complete sensory nerve conduction block that cannot be amplified and resynchronized by the central nervous system. The presence of a cortical evoked potential would portend a better prognosis, as some of the sensory axons are in continuity. However, this distinction rarely needs to be made, as surgical exploration is hardly ever performed before the period of wallerian degeneration has elapsed.[8]

Summary

SSEPs should be considered as complementary tests to the sensory NCS. Although they have numerous advantages over sensory NCS, they also have similar limitations in that they cannot assess thin or unmyelinated sensory fibers. Because they are able to assess the entire length of the large-fiber sensory pathways, they are useful in distinguishing axon loss from demyelination, irrespective of the pathologic site. They are also useful in determining whether there is functional continuity of these pathways between the site of stimulation and the somatosensory cortex. Unlike sensory NCS, SSEPs may be performed at any time after the pathologic insult. However, any delay in latency must be described as being between the last documented normal site and the first abnormal site. If only a delayed cortical potential is observed, then the delay is between the site of stimulation and the cortex. In these instances, the same nerve should be stimulated at a more proximal location to assess for peripheral nervous system pathology. If there is no evidence of a conduction delay between these two peripheral sites, then the pathology is rostral to the proximal stimulation site. However, this should not be interpreted as the absence of peripheral nervous system pathology. This statement may only be made if all the peripheral latencies are normal. In the upper extremities, this requires normal latencies of EP, cervical, and EP-cervical interpeak latencies. In the lower extremities, this requires normal latencies of the knee potential, lumbar point, and knee–lumbar point interpeak latency. Otherwise, the pathologic site cannot be precisely localized to be within the central nervous system. It should also be recalled that a normal evoked potential does not completely exclude pathology affecting the large-fiber sensory pathways. If a sufficient number of large-fiber sensory nerve fascicles are unaffected by the pathologic process, these fibers could generate an evoked potential of normal latency and amplitude. The absence of electrophysiologic evidence of large-fiber sensory nerve dysfunction does not mean that there is no pathology affecting that system.

PROXIMAL CONDUCTION STUDIES OF MOTOR NERVES

Analysis of the proximal portions of the motor nerves is less complicated than the sensory system because there is no intervening segment analogous to the DRG. Therefore, any motor nerve root pathology can be assessed more directly than can sensory nerve root abnormalities. Late response studies, such as the F wave and H reflex, may be used in this manner. However, these techniques only assess a small subpopulation of the largest, most heavily myelinated fibers. Because the H reflex evaluates the entire reflex arc, abnormalities may result from pathology, affecting the sensory afferent, interneurons, or motor efferent pathways. Because F waves only assess peripheral motor fibers, abnormalities can be attributed directly to motor fiber dysfunction. However, an absent F wave may result from either axon loss or demyelination. Because F waves only evaluate a small subpopulation of the large motor fibers, abnormalities may not be noted with lesser degrees of demyelination. Moreover, if only one fiber capable of generating an F wave generates a latency less than that required to diagnose demyelination, then the presence of proximal demyelination may be missed. Motor NCS assess the full population of the largest, most heavily myelinated fibers but only between the site of stimulation and the target muscle. In most instances, motor NCS tend to be performed along the distal half of the nerve. Root stimulation overcomes these limitations by assessing all of the large motor fibers from the axon hillock to the target muscle.[9] Stimulation may be performed with either an electrical or a magnetic stimulus that will excite the proximal motor fibers.

Clinically, these proximal conduction studies are used to evaluate the proximal portions of the motor nerves in suspected cases of demyelinating peripheral nerve pathology and in patients presenting with motor neuronopathies. Demyelinating neuropathies tend to affect the myelin sheath before the axons. Therefore, demyelination of the motor fibers leads to weakness out of proportion to the degree of atrophy. Greater degrees of proximal demyelination may lead to diminished or absent reflexes. Early or less fulminant cases of demyelination may present with normal motor NCS and F wave minimum latencies that do not meet published criteria for diagnosing demyelination. One study reported an increased sensitivity of detecting acquired demyelinating polyneuropathies using motor nerve root stimulation.[10] Conversely, this technique may be used to provide evidence against a diagnosis of proximal demyelination. Many clinicians can recall motor neuronopathy cases that had a superficial resemblance to amyotrophic lateral sclerosis that later proved to be a demyelinating motor neuropathy or neuronopathy. Root stimulation has been shown to differentiate motor neuron disease syndromes from demyelinating motor neuropathies.[11]

Motor Nerve Root Stimulation Techniques

Percutaneous electrical stimulation is performed by using a monopolar needle as the cathode, whereas the cathode is a ground electrode disc placed on the skin surface caudal to the needle. In this manner, the electrical field travels from the anode to the cathode, although they are separated by greater distances than usual. Cervical root stimulation is performed by inserting the monopolar needle at the C5-6 interspace, 1 cm lateral to the midline on the side to be stimulated, until it abuts the periosteum. The cathode is attached in the midline at T2. Lumbar root stimulation is similar, except the cathode is placed at L1, and the anode is placed at S1. Maximum output of the EMG machine is used or 100 mA with a duration of 1 millisecond. At least two stimulations must produce an identical waveform. Moreover, any drop in amplitude greater than 50% must be confirmed by repositioning the needle several times to demonstrate that the drop in amplitude is not due to technical factors.

Anatomic Considerations of Motor Nerve Root Stimulation

Cervical nerve root stimulation with recording at the intrinsic hand muscles was first conducted using a method of stimulation just rostral to the C8-T1 nerve roots by inserting a monopolar needle at C7. This technique does not provide different results from root stimulation performed between C5 and C6 but has an increased risk for inducing a pneumothorax.[12] For this reason, electrical nerve stimulation at C5-6 is preferred. Figure 6.7 demonstrates the typical waveforms observed when cervical root stimulation is performed while recording from the abductor pollicis brevis (APB), abductor digiti minimi (ADM), biceps brachii, and the triceps brachii. In certain instances discussed in the next paragraph, a collision technique is required when assessing for a proximal conduction block in the median nerve to the APB. For the lumbosacral region, stimulation at L1 is recommended to stimulate adjacent to the axon hillocks of the nerve roots. Stimulation below these levels activates the nerve roots of the cauda equina and does not examine the most proximal segments of these nerve roots. Because the target muscles usually examined are the tibialis anterior and the flexor hallucis brevis

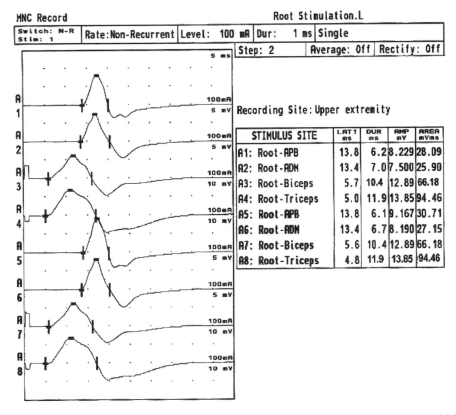

Figure 6.7 Cervical root stimulation at C5-6 recording left upper extremity target muscles. (ADM = abductor digiti minimi; AMP = amplitude; APB = abductor pollicis brevis; DUR = duration; LAT = onset latency; MNC = motor nerve conduction.)

(FHB), no collision technique is required, as the contribution of one muscle's CMAP to the other is negligible.

It should be recalled that the intrinsic hand muscles innervated by the median and ulnar nerves derive their innervation from the C8-T1 nerve roots. Therefore, stimulation of the C8-T1 nerve roots activates both the median and ulnar nerves at this level. A collision technique must be used to eliminate the contribution of the adjacent ulnar nerve–innervated muscles to the CMAP generated by the median nerve–innervated APB. This collision technique is only required when a proximal conduction block in the median nerve to the APB needs to be assessed. Figure 6.8 demonstrates a normal subject's APB CMAP waveform from stimulation at the wrist, whereas Figure 6.9 demonstrates the cervical root stimulation with collision technique and its results. The ulnar nerve is stimulated 6 milliseconds before stimulation at the cervical nerve roots. In this manner, the ascending ulnar nerve impulse collides with the descending root stimulation impulse eliminating the contribution of the ulnar nerve to the median nerve's APB CMAP.

Physiologic Considerations

To minimize the effect of axon loss on root stimulation studies, the distal amplitude should be greater than 1 mV. Moreover, the nerve must be tested above its

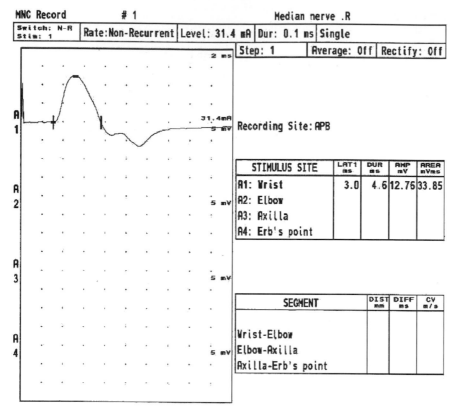

Figure 6.8 Stimulation of the right median nerve at the wrist. (AMP = amplitude; APB = abductor pollicis brevis; CV = conduction velocity; DIFF = difference; DIST = distance; DUR = duration; LAT = onset latency; MNC = motor nerve conduction; STIM = stimulation.)

common sites of entrapment. Conduction block criteria require that the significant decrease in amplitude and area cannot be the result of compression or entrapment. For example, the median nerve should be conducted above the wrist, and the ulnar nerve should be conducted above the elbow. Any drop in amplitude between the nerve roots, and this proximal site is far less likely to be due to an anomalous site of nerve compression. As with stimulation elsewhere in the peripheral nervous system, supramaximal stimulation is required at every site. Understimulation must be eliminated as a variable before a diagnosis of a proximal conduction block is rendered.

A proximal conduction block indicates pathology between the nerve root and the next site of stimulation along the nerve. Although this may confirm one's clinical suspicion of an acquired demyelinating polyneuropathy, several caveats are in order. The first is that this finding may be present with any process that interrupts nerve function along this pathway. For example, a traumatic motor nerve root avulsion could produce a similar finding known as *pseudoconduction block*. In this instance, motor nerve conduction studies performed immediately after the avulsion could demonstrate a normal CMAP from distal stimulation but no CMAP from nerve root stimulation. Nerve ischemia in the proximal segments of the nerve could also produce similar findings. Therefore, an isolated "conduction block" is a finding that should be interpreted with caution.

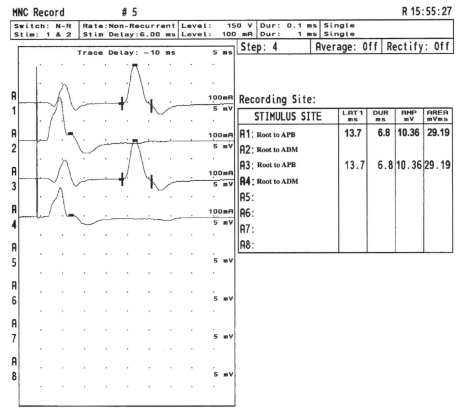

Figure 6.9 Stimulation at C5-6 6 milliseconds after stimulation of the ulnar nerve at the wrist. Note the trace delay of 10 milliseconds. Channels 1 and 3 demonstrate an abductor pollicis brevis (APB) compound muscle action potential, whereas channels 2 and 4 demonstrate the absence of an abductor digiti minimi (ADM) compound muscle action potential from the collision technique. (AMP = amplitude; DUR = duration; LAT = onset latency; STIM = stimulation.)

Magnetic Stimulation

The principles of magnetic stimulation are well beyond the scope of this chapter and are extensively discussed in reference textbooks on this subject.[13] The significant differences between magnetic and electrical stimulation may be summarized by recalling that magnetic fields are neither conserved nor resisted. Thus, there is no "impedance" or "resistance" to a magnetic field. This allows for noninvasive stimulation of excitable tissues. The magnetic field thus traverses all tissues and induces an electrical field at right angles to its direction of travel. This induces an electrical field within the excitable tissue, such as a nerve root or the motor cortex. Although magnetic stimulation techniques of the peripheral nervous system have been described, they are not clearly superior to conventional NCS.[14] They are even less reliable for EP stimulation and for motor nerve root stimulation.[15,16] Magnetic stimulation tends to result in understimulation of these nerve structures. As is discussed in subsequent sections, magnetic stimulation of the peripheral nervous system may be done as a screening examination. However, all abnormalities should be confirmed with conventional electrical stimulation techniques. Therefore, this technique is discussed only in relation to diagnosing central nervous system disorders.

Cortical Magnetic Stimulation

Before 1985, cortical stimulation had been performed with electrical stimulation applied to the brain itself during intraoperative corticography or through application of electrodes to the scalp. Because of the skull's impedance, transcranial electrical stimulation is painful and requires anesthesia or a tolerant subject. A significant breakthrough was achieved with the advent of transcranial magnetic stimulation (TMS).[17] The technique allows for the application of a magnetic pulse that is not attenuated or impeded by the skull. This tends to induce an electrical field within the brain in a direction opposite the magnetic field.[18] Some magnetic stimulators produce a unidirectional pulse (e.g., The Magstim Company Ltd., Whitland, UK; Jali Medical, Newton, MA), whereas others produce a decaying alternating direction sine wave pulse (e.g., Cadwell Laboratories, Kennewick, WA). Because the cortex responds better when a back to front stimulation is used, direction of stimulation is relevant for those producing a unidirectional pulse.

It should be noted that magnetic stimulation has the U.S. Food and Drug Administration's (FDA) approval only for peripheral stimulation. Stimulation of any site at or distal to the motor nerve roots has been approved. TMS has not been FDA approved for routine use at this time. The safety of TMS was recently reviewed in a publication by Wassermann et al.[19] This consensus statement concluded that single pulse or repetitive stimulation at frequencies less than 1 Hz should be considered nonsignificant risk, whereas repetitive stimulation at higher frequencies could pose significant risks, such as seizures. According to product bulletins on the magnetic stimulators manufactured by Cadwell Laboratories, the FDA no longer requires an investigational device exemption (IDE) on cortical stimulation with the low-frequency stimulator. However, the investigator must meet all requirements of the local institutional review board (IRB). If the IRB concurs that the project falls within the category defined as *nonsignificant risk*, then local approval of an IRB protocol is sufficient for its use. An IDE is still obligatory for repetitive TMS studies using rates exceeding 1 Hz. Although physicians may use medications and devices in a non–FDA-approved manner, the author cannot recommend this course of action. Until FDA approval occurs, TMS studies should probably be performed in medical centers in which there is significant experience with this technique under the auspices of their local IRB.

Physiologic Considerations

TMS differs from electrical stimulation in another important manner in that it activates cortico-cortical motor neurons (e.g., cortical neurons synapsing on pyramidal cells); unlike electrical stimulation techniques that directly activate pyramidal cells, magnetic stimulation only indirectly activates these cells.[20,21] Increasing the stimulus intensity increases the probability of activating sufficient numbers of pyramidal motor cells that result in a descending volley, which results in a CMAP over the target muscle. Although most muscles can be activated through this technique, it is easier to activate those with the greatest degree of cortical representation. For clinical purposes, most studies are conducted to intrinsic hand or foot muscles. The most useful parameters are those regarding thresholds, motor central conduction times, and inhibition studies. Each of these parameters requires a separate discussion.

Threshold Determination. *Motor threshold* is defined as the lowest percentage output of the magnetic stimulator that is capable of producing a response in the same target muscle in three out of six consecutive stimulations. For quantitative purposes, the CMAP is measured at a gain of 200 μV/division to verify that the CMAP latency is identical in these trials. Others merely use the presence or absence of a visible twitch in the target muscle. The author prefers the former, as it is more precise. Intrinsic hand muscles are best activated over the vertex, whereas the lower extremity muscles are optimally activated 4 cm anterior to the vertex. The upper extremity target muscles are the APB and ADM, whereas the lower extremity muscles are the tibialis anterior and the FHB. Normal values are 60% or less for the upper extremity and 85% for the lower extremity.[22] If there is no peripheral etiology for motor nerve inexcitability (e.g., conduction block, neuromuscular blockade), then this finding suggests upper motor neuron dysfunction. It should be emphasized that upper motor neuron pathology is not synonymous with motor neuron disease, as these findings could be noted with other diseases causing upper motor neuron dysfunction, such as multiple sclerosis or a stroke. As with any neurophysiologic test, it must be interpreted within the context of the patient's clinical presentation.

Central Motor Conduction Time. Central motor conduction time (CMCT) is especially useful for documenting evidence of corticospinal pathology. There are two methods by which the CMCT can be derived, known as the *direct* and *indirect methods.* In both situations, cortical magnetic stimulation techniques are identical. First, the threshold is determined to the target muscles. The output of the magnetic stimulator is then increased 25% above motor threshold. In the lower extremities, this may not always be possible to achieve, as some normal persons have a threshold less than or equal to 85%. In this particular instance, 100% of the magnetic stimulator output is used for supramaximal stimulation. The subject must be in a relaxed state, because anticipation of the magnetic pulse or contraction of the target muscle will shorten the CMCT.[16] At least two waveforms with the same latency and similar morphology must be generated to insure reproducibility. This latency represents the time required to travel from the cortex to the target muscle.

The peripheral conduction time may then be measured directly or indirectly. The direct method requires root stimulation techniques. Because magnetic stimulation techniques excite the nerve roots more distally than do electrical stimulation techniques, they should not be used for CMCT calculation. Although electrical nerve root stimulation is invasive, it allows for an accurate determination of CMCT. Figure 6.10 demonstrates a normal subject receiving TMS at 25% above motor threshold recording from the intrinsic hand muscles. Figure 6.11 demonstrates the peripheral conduction times obtained from cervical root stimulation. These two studies allow for a direct calculation of the CMCT to the APB (22.0 − 13.8 = 8.2 milliseconds) and to the ADM (21.2 − 13.4 = 7.8 milliseconds). These values are both within normal limits according to the normal CMCT values listed in Table 6.3. CMCT values that exceed these limits are consistent with corticospinal tract dysfunction.

The indirect method uses F waves to calculate a peripheral motor conduction time. Figure 6.12 demonstrates the result of TMS applied at 25% above motor threshold to the lower extremities recording from the FHB and tibialis anterior. The F-wave minimum latency is the time required to travel up to the axon hillock, the 1 millisecond required to depolarize the large fibers orthodromically, and the time required to travel back down the motor axons to the target muscle. If one subtracts this 1 millisecond time interval from the F-wave minimum latency and adds it to the distal motor latency, then this represents the amount of time for the impulse to travel the entire length of the motor nerve in both directions. This value is divided in half

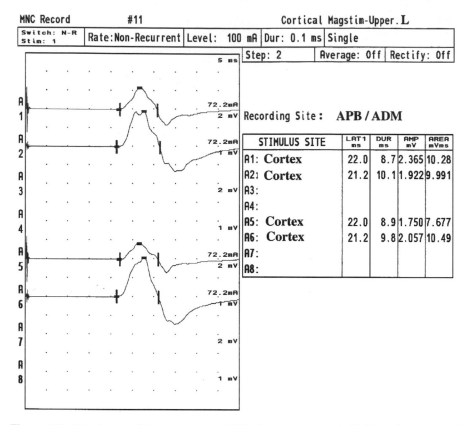

Figure 6.10 Stimulation of the motor cortex 25% above motor threshold. Note the compound muscle action potential amplitude variability. (ADM = abductor digiti minimi; AMP = amplitude; APB = abductor pollicis brevis; DUR = duration; LAT = onset latency; MNC = motor nerve conduction; STIM = stimulation.)

to obtain a peripheral conduction time. Figure 6.13 demonstrates a distal motor latency to the FHB of 5.0 milliseconds and an F-wave minimal latency of 50.7 milliseconds. One millisecond is subtracted from the F-wave minimal latency, yielding 49.7 milliseconds. This value is then added to the distal motor latency, yielding a time of 54.7 milliseconds to travel in both directions along the tibial nerve. Dividing this value in half yields a peripheral conduction time of 27.35 milliseconds. This value may then be subtracted from the total conduction time obtained from cortical stimulation to yield a CMCT to the FHB of 42.20 milliseconds minus 27.35 milliseconds, or 14.85 milliseconds, which is within normal limits. These data are from the same normal subject examined in Figures 6.10 and 6.11. Note that the CMCT to the lower extremity is approximately twice that to the upper extremity.

Irrespective of the method used, CMCT data can be used for the detection of corticospinal pathology. As with any other neurophysiologic test, a prolonged CMCT does not imply central demyelination. A slowed central conduction time may be seen with either demyelination or loss of faster conducting axons. As with SSEPs, a prolonged CMCT should be interpreted as pathology affecting the corticospinal tract between the cortex and the nerve roots that supply the target muscle. A prolonged CMCT to the intrinsic hand muscles should be interpreted as pathology between the

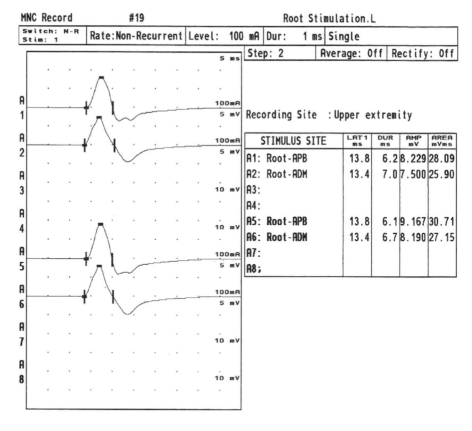

MNC Record	#19	Root Stimulation.L

Switch: N-R Stim: 1 | Rate:Non-Recurrent | Level: 100 mA | Dur: 1 ms | Single

Step: 2 | Average: Off | Rectify: Off

Recording Site : Upper extremity

STIMULUS SITE	LAT 1 ms	DUR ms	AMP mV	AREA mVms
A1: Root-APB	13.8	6.2	8.229	28.09
A2: Root-ADM	13.4	7.0	7.500	25.90
A3:				
A4:				
A5: Root-APB	13.8	6.1	9.167	30.71
A6: Root-ADM	13.4	6.7	8.190	27.15
A7:				
A8;				

Figure 6.11 Cervical root stimulation at C5-6 recording over abductor pollicis brevis and abductor digiti minimi. (ADM = abductor digiti minimi; AMP = amplitude; APB = abductor pollicis brevis; DUR = duration; LAT = onset latency; MNC = motor nerve conduction; STIM = stimulation.)

cortex and lower cervical spine, whereas prolongation to the lower extremities should be interpreted as pathology between the cortex and conus medullaris.

Persistent Inhibition. Persistent inhibition of the cortical silent period is another phenomenon that may be noted with corticospinal dysfunction.[23] The persistent inhibition technique evaluates a muscle that is under maximal contraction by the subject by using ongoing rectified EMG that is time-locked to the magnetic stimu-

Table 6.3 Central Motor Conduction Times

Target Muscle	Nerve Root Innervation	Central Motor Conduction Time Maximum (mean + 3 standard deviations) (msec)
Abductor pollicis brevis	C8-T1	10
Abductor digiti minimi	C8-T1	10
Tibialis anterior	L4-5	18
Flexor hallucis brevis	S1-2	20

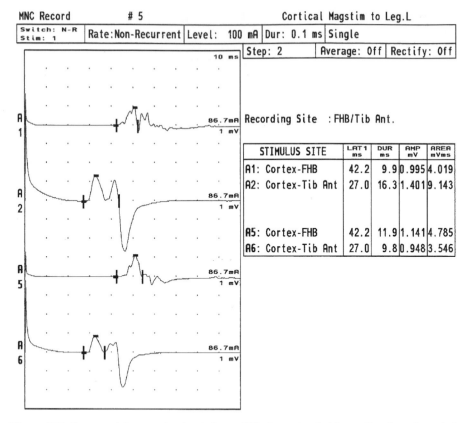

Figure 6.12 Transcranial magnetic stimulation at 25% above threshold recording from flexor hallucis brevis (FHB) and tibialis anterior (Tib Ant). (AMP = amplitude; DUR = duration; LAT = onset latency; MNC = motor nerve conduction.)

lus. Figure 6.14 demonstrates a normal subject maximally contracting the ADM with surface electrodes placed in the same location as for recording an ADM CMAP with TMS applied at 5% above motor threshold. These electrodes record averaged, rectified EMG obtained over at least six consecutive trials. This normal subject demonstrates that TMS produces a CMAP arising from the background rectified EMG activity after a latency of approximately 20 milliseconds. This is followed by an interval in which there is a relative paucity of rectified EMG activity known as the *cortical silent period*. When the cortical silent period ceases, there is resumption of rectified EMG activity. The amplitude of the CMAP and duration of the subsequent silent period are directly proportional to the intensity of the magnetic stimulus. As the intensity of the magnetic stimulus is reduced, the amplitude of the CMAP and the duration of the cortical silent period diminish. In normal persons, the CMAP disappears concurrently with the cortical silent period. Restated, a normal person should manifest a CMAP that is associated with a subsequent cortical silent period. Dissociation of the CMAP from the cortical silent period is thought to represent an imbalance of corticospinal inhibitory and excitatory circuitry. The presence of a CMAP without a subsequent CMAP has been interpreted as representing a relative increase in corticospinal excitability, whereas the converse would reflect a decrease in corticospinal pathway excitability (increased inhibition).

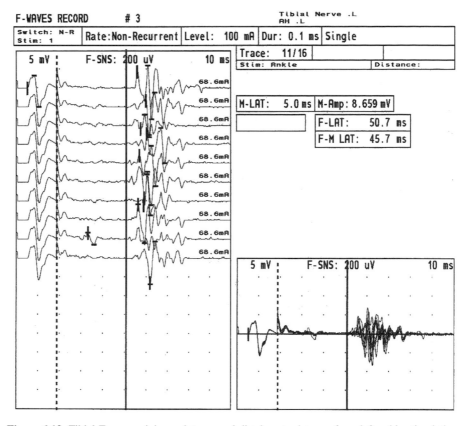

Figure 6.13 Tibial F-wave minimum latency and distal motor latency from left ankle stimulation. (AH = adductor hallucis; F-LAT = F-wave minimum latency; SNS = sensitivity; STIM = stimulation.)

Patients who manifest upper motor neuron dysfunction may demonstrate a dissociation of the CMAP from the cortical silent period. Some persons diagnosed with amyotrophic lateral sclerosis (ALS) demonstrate this "persistence of inhibition" that manifests with lower intensities of TMS wherein a cortical silent period is noted without an antecedent CMAP.[24,25] Although this finding is not infrequently noted in ALS, it may not be pathognomonic for this disorder. Additional studies of patients with diverse etiologies of corticospinal pathology need to be conducted before this finding can be designated as being sensitive and specific for ALS.

The converse has been demonstrated in patients with reduced cortical inhibition, such as stiff-man syndrome, a disorder thought to occur through an autoimmune-mediated dysfunction of gamma–aminobutyric acid–ergic (GABA-ergic) inhibitory neurons. Such persons tend to present with muscle stiffness produced by persistent, involuntary firing of motor units. One study of seven patients demonstrated shortened cortical silent periods in the leg muscles as well as decreased cortical inhibition and markedly increased facilitation with a paired pulse TMS paradigm.[26] At low TMS intensities, these patients may demonstrate a CMAP that occurs without a subsequent cortical silent period—a finding interpreted as a relative increase in the degree of cortical excitability. As noted previously, additional studies of corticospinal hyperexcitability states need to be conducted before stating that this finding is sensitive and specific for stiff-man syndrome. For those laboratories without TMS capability, vibration-

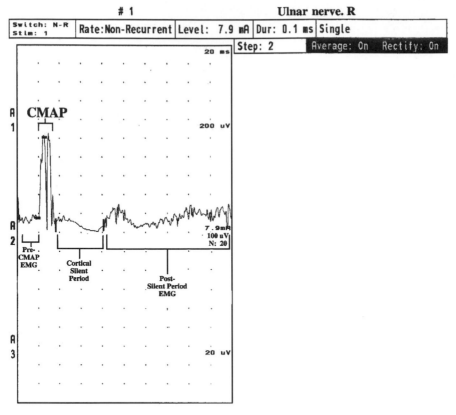

Figure 6.14 Averaged, rectified electromyography recorded from the abductor digiti minimi after transcranial magnetic stimulation was applied at 5% above motor threshold. (CMAP = compound muscle action potential; EMG = electromyography.)

induced H-reflex inhibition was noted in eight of nine patients with this disorder.[27] Either TMS or vibration-induced H-reflex inhibition studies may provide electrophysiologic evidence in support of this diagnosis, although neither should be considered to be absolutely specific for this disorder.

CONCLUSIONS

Proximal conduction studies should be more frequently performed in the neurophysiology laboratory because they may clarify the abnormalities noted on routine electrodiagnostic evaluations. Although some of these techniques, such as TMS, have yet to be approved by the FDA for general use, the other techniques are approved for use in the neurophysiology laboratory. These techniques can often provide useful information regarding less accessible portions of the nervous system. Somatosensory evoked potentials are able to assess the entire large-fiber sensory pathways from the site of stimulation to the contralateral cortex. Even when there are significant degrees of peripheral demyelination, the central nervous system is able to resynchronize these potentials and generate a cortical waveform. This phenomenon allows the practitioner to assess for peripheral as well as central nervous system demyelination. Root stimulation techniques permit a more complete assessment of the motor axon from the axon hillock to the target muscle. Although magnetic stimulation techniques are often sufficient, proximal conduction block should always be confirmed with electrical nerve root stimulation. Although these techniques are not often used in routine clinical practice, they are useful in certain selected indications.

Acknowledgments

The author would like to thank Dr. Tulio E. Bertorini for his assistance in preparing this manuscript. He would also like to acknowledge Ms. Stacie Mazerac-Walker, Medical Illustrator, for her assistance.

REFERENCES

1. Kimura J. Electrodiagnosis in Diseases of Nerve and Muscle (2nd ed). Philadelphia: F.A. Davis Co., 1989.
2. Cros D, Triggs WJ. There are no neurophysiologic features characteristic of "axonal" Guillain-Barré syndrome. Muscle Nerve 1994;17:675–677.
3. Kuwabara S, Ogawara K, Mizobuchi K, et al. Isolated absence of F waves and proximal axonal dysfunction in Guillain-Barré syndrome with antiganglioside antibodies. J Neurol Neurosurg Psychiatry 2000;68:191–195.
4. Bromberg MD, Albers JW. Patterns of sensory nerve conduction abnormalities in demyelinating and axonal peripheral nerve disorders. Muscle Nerve 1993;16:262–266.
5. Chiappa KH (ed), Evoked Potentials in Clinical Medicine (3rd ed). New York: Raven Press, 1997.
6. Wilbourn A. Brachial Plexus Disorders. In P Dyck, PK Thomas (eds), Peripheral Neuropathy (3rd ed). Philadelphia: WB Saunders, 1993.
7. Yiannikas C, Shahani B, Young R. The investigation of traumatic lesions of the brachial plexus by electromyography and short latency somatosensory evoked potentials. J Neurol Neurosurg Psychiatry 1983;46:1014–1022.
8. Kline DG, Hudson AR. Nerve Injuries: Operative Results for Major Nerve Injuries, Entrapments and Tumors. Philadelphia: WB Saunders 1995.
9. Berger AR, Busis NA, Logigian EL, et al. Cervical root stimulation in the diagnosis of radiculopathy. Neurology 1987;37:329–332.
10. Menkes DL, Hood DC, Ballesteros RA, Williams DA. Root stimulation improves the detection of acquired demyelinating polyneuropathies. Muscle Nerve 1998;21:298–308.
11. Raynor EM, Sheffner JM, Ross MH, et al. Root stimulation studies in the evaluation of patients with motor neuron disease. Neurology 1998;50:1907–1909.
12. Sander HW, Menkes DL, Triggs WR, Chokroverty S. Cervical root stimulation at C5/C6 excites C8/T1 roots and minimizes pneumothorax risk. Muscle Nerve 1999;22:766–768.
13. Chokroverty S (ed), Magnetic Stimulation in Clinical Neurophysiology. Boston: Butterworth, 1989;73–112.
14. Binkofsky F, Classen J, Benecke R. Stimulation of peripheral nerves using a novel magnetic coil. Muscle Nerve 1999;22:751–757.
15. Cros D, Gominak S, Shahani B, et al. Comparison of electric and magnetic coil stimulation in the supraclavicular region. Muscle Nerve 1992;15:587–590.
16. Cros D, Chiappa KH, Gominak S, et al. Cervical magnetic stimulation. Neurology 1990;49: 751–756.
17. Barker AT, Jalinous R, Freeston IL. Non-invasive magnetic stimulation of the human motor cortex. Lancet 1985;1:1106–1107.
18. Cohen LG, Roth BJ, Nilsson J, et al. Effects of coil design on delivery of focal magnetic stimulation. Technical considerations. Electroencephalogr Clin Neurophysiol 1990;75:350–357.
19. Wassermann EM. Risk and safety of repetitive transcranial magnetic stimulation: report and suggested guidelines from the International Workshop on the Safety of Repetitive Transcranial Magnetic Stimulation. Electroencephalogr Clin Neurophysiol 1998;108:1–16.
20. Amassian VE, Maccabee PJ, Cracco RQ, Cracco JB. Basic Mechanisms of Magnetic Coil Excitation of the Nervous System in Humans and Monkeys. Application in Focal Stimulation of Different Cortical Areas in Humans. In S Chokroverty (ed), Magnetic Stimulation in Clinical Neurophysiology. Boston: Butterworth, 1989:73–112.

21. Amassian VE, Quirk GJ, Stewart M. A comparison of corticospinal activation by magnetic coil and electrical stimulation of monkey motor cortex. Electroencephalogr Clin Neurophysiol 1990;77: 390–401.

22. Menkes DL, Ring SR, Chiappa KH, Cros D. Cortical Magnetic Stimulation to the Lower Extremities: Normal Controls and 14 Pathologic Cases (abstract). American Academy of Neurology; May 1994, Washington, DC.

23. Triggs WJ, Macdonnell RAL, Cros D, et al. Motor inhibition and excitation are independent effects of magnetic stimulation. Ann Neurol 1992;32:345–351.

24. Triggs WJ, Menkes DL, Onorato J, et al. Transcranial magnetic stimulation identifies upper motor neuron involvement in motor neuron disease. Neurology 1999;53:605–611.

25. Siciliano G, Manca ML, Sagliocco L. Cortical silent period in patients with amyotrophic lateral sclerosis. J Neurol Sci 1999;169:93–97.

26. Sandbrink F, Syed NA, Fujii MD, et al. Motor cortex excitability in stiff-person syndrome. Brain 2000;123:2231–2239.

27. Floeter MK, Valls-Sole J, Toro C, et al. Physiologic studies of spinal inhibitory circuits in patients with stiff-person syndrome. Neurology 1998;51:85–93.

7

Other Useful Electrodiagnostic Techniques: Blink Reflex, Masseter Reflex, and Silent Periods

Carlos A. Luciano

In addition to the traditional nerve conduction studies commonly used in the electrodiagnostic laboratory, there are a variety of complementary techniques that may be of value in the assessment of patients with neuromuscular diseases. These techniques allow the clinician to examine proximal and relatively inaccessible portions of the peripheral and central nervous system as well as nerve fiber populations different from those routinely assessed with conventional nerve conduction studies. They may also be of value in detecting abnormalities at the very early stages, when more diffuse changes are not apparent. This chapter reviews the use of some of these techniques in the investigation of patients with neuromuscular problems.

SPECIFIC TECHNIQUES

Blink Reflex

The electrophysiologic blink reflex (BR) is a reflex electromyographic response of the orbicularis oculi muscle that occurs after electrical stimulation of the trigeminal nerve branches in the periorbital region or after a mechanical tap over the glabella. It provides an assessment of trigeminal nerve afferent fibers and facial nerve fibers in their extracranial, intracranial, and central segments. It also provides information about the integrity of the brainstem connections between the trigeminal sensory and facial motor nuclei. The trigeminal nerve pathways constitute the afferent limb of the reflex, and the facial nerve constitutes its efferent limb. This dual sensory and motor testing capability makes the BR particularly valuable in the study of peripheral neuropathies or isolated cranial nerve abnormalities in the neuromuscular laboratory.

Anatomy and Physiology

The BR is usually elicited by electrical stimulation of the supraorbital nerve, a branch of the ophthalmic division of the trigeminal nerve, at the supraorbital notch.

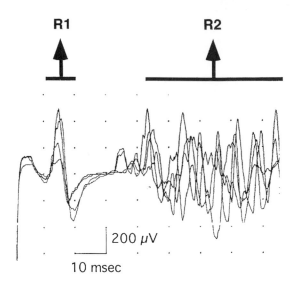

Figure 7.1 Blink reflex. Representative example showing an early (R1) component at 11 milliseconds and an intermediate response (R2) at approximately 32 milliseconds. Because it is more stable and reproducible, the R1 component is the one generally used for the study of peripheral pathways.

Although responses may be obtained after stimulating the infraorbital nerve and the mental nerve, they have not been used as frequently. The stimulus travels in a centripetal fashion through A-β myelinated afferent fibers of the trigeminal nerve before making connections in the brainstem nuclei. The waveform has two main components: an early response, occurring at approximately 10 milliseconds and designated as the R1 response, and an intermediate response, occurring at approximately 30 milliseconds and designated the R2 response (Figure 7.1). A much later response, occurring at approximately 80 milliseconds, the R3 response, is elicited with higher intensity and more painful stimuli[1] and is not normally used for routine electrodiagnostic assessment. The R1 response is relayed through an oligosynaptic pathway at the pons.[2,3] With electrical stimulation, this response usually appears only ipsilateral to the side of stimulation and is more reliably elicited with stimulation of the supraorbital than the infraorbital or mental nerves. With mechanical (tap to the glabella) or magnetic stimulation, the R1 response appears bilaterally, but with a mildly longer latency with mechanical stimulation. Because it is more stable and resistant to suprasegmental influences, the R1 response is used more commonly for the routine assessment of conduction of the peripheral pathways.

The R2 response is relayed through a more complex polysynaptic pathway via the spinal trigeminal nucleus and tract in the lateral medulla, with bilateral connections to the facial nuclei.[2,3] Unlike the R1 response, the R2 response appears in both sides after stimulating one side. This component has a more variable latency and is more prone to habituation, making it less reliable, though still useful, in the assessment of peripheral pathways. The R2 response is particularly valuable in differentiating an afferent from an efferent pathway abnormality.

Methodologic Aspects

Our preferred method of placement of the recording electrodes for the BR is shown in Figure 7.2. Briefly, the active recording electrodes are placed bilaterally in the lower portion of the orbicularis oculi, at the level of the rim of the orbit in the middle or lateral portions of the muscle. The reference electrode is placed over the temple (as shown in Figure 7.2) or on the side of the nose near the medial canthus.[4] If the

Figure 7.2 Electrode placement for blink reflex. Electrodes are placed bilaterally for simultaneous recordings with the active electrode on the outer third of the lower orbicularis oculi, and the reference electrode is placed on the temple (as shown) or on the side of the nose. The aim is to optimize activity from orbicularis oculi while minimizing contaminating muscle activity from other facial muscles.

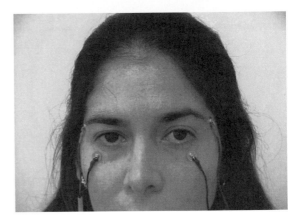

infraorbital nerve is stimulated, the active recording electrode is moved to the upper part of the orbicularis oculi.

To test the ophthalmic division of the trigeminal nerve, bipolar stimulation is applied near the supraorbital notch, on top of the supraorbital nerve. Stimuli of 0.1–0.2 millisecond are applied at intervals greater than 7 seconds to avoid habituation of the R2 component. The blink is best obtained while the subject is alert, supine, and resting, with the eyes opened and looking at a fixed spot directly in front of him or her. Latency values may be different with the eyes opened, as opposed to closed, implying that it is necessary to use to a specific eye-opening position when acquiring or comparing results to reference values.[5,6]

When the stimulus artifact is too large and obscures the R1 response, it is helpful to rotate the anode while keeping the cathode over the notch. In addition, it is sometimes impossible to obtain R1 responses in some healthy individuals. When this happens, R1 responses can be elicited using paired stimuli at 5-millisecond interstimulus intervals. These are not required to be both supramaximal: a first submaximal (conditioning) stimulus followed by a second supramaximal (test) stimulus suffices. When using paired stimuli, it is important to measure the latencies from the second stimulus artifact.

Although the supraorbital nerve is the one routinely stimulated, when symptoms are present in the second or third division of the trigeminal nerve, it is important to examine the maxillary and mandibular branches stimulating over the infraorbital or mental nerve. These generally elicit only an R2 response, and, in the case of mental nerve stimulation, it may be necessary to use stronger stimuli (0.2-millisecond duration) and longer intervals between stimuli (greater than 7 seconds) to elicit a reproducible response.[6]

It is advisable to also examine the facial nerve directly by stimulating at the stylomastoid foramen under the pinna or in the premastoid region and compare the latency of the direct response to the R1 response. Kimura[7] has suggested the use of the ratio between the R1 and the direct response latency (R/D ratio) as an additional conduction parameter and a way of distinguishing preferential distal versus proximal involvement of the facial nerve.

Normal parameters for the BR are summarized in Table 7.1. Latencies are usually measured to the initial deflection from the baseline and should be determined from a minimum of eight responses to ensure that an optimal response has been obtained. From each study, it is important to measure the following: (1) the minimal latencies for the R1 response and for the simultaneously acquired ipsilateral and contralateral

Table 7.1 Normal Values for Blink Reflex with Electrical Stimulation*

Parameter	Latency (msec, Mean ± SD)	Normal Limits (msec, Mean ± 3 SD)
Facial nerve motor latency	2.9 ± 0.4	4.1
R1 latency	10.5 ± 0.8	13.0
R2 latency (ipsi)	30.5 ± 3.4	40.0
R2 latency (contra)	30.5 ± 4.4	41.0
R1 latency difference between both sides	—	1.2
R2 latency, ipsi and contra difference, simultaneous recording	—	5.0
R2 latency difference, same side, ipsi and contra stimulation	—	7.0
R/D latency ratio	3.6 ± 0.5	2.6–4.6

Contra = contralateral; ipsi = ipsilateral; R1 = early response; R2 = intermediate response; R/D = ratio of R1 latency to direct facial nerve compound muscle action potential latency; SD = standard deviation.
*Values for 83 healthy subjects.
Source: Modified from J Kimura. The Blink Reflex. Electrodiagnosis in Diseases of Nerve and Muscle (3rd ed). New York: Oxford University Press, Inc., 2001;409–438.

R2 response from each side stimulated; (2) the latency difference between the R1 responses from each side; (3) the latency difference from the simultaneously recorded ipsilateral and contralateral R2 responses; and (4) the latency difference between the R2 responses recorded in the same side with ipsilateral and contralateral stimulation. Amplitudes are too variable and have not been proven to be of practical clinical value.

Clinical Applications in Neuromuscular Disease

The BR can be helpful in the investigation of signs and symptoms of facial sensory loss or pain or facial weakness. Among the various conditions that can affect the trigeminal or facial pathways, several are of particular importance for the neuromuscular specialist. Abnormalities of the BR have been observed in trigeminal neuropathies. These can be pure sensory or mixed sensory and motor and can occur as a result of trauma, dental procedures, infiltration or external pressure from tumor, exposure to neurotoxins (such as stilbamidine or trichloroethylene), secondary to various connective tissue diseases (scleroderma or mixed connective tissue disease, in particular), or from herpes zoster infection, among several possibilities.[8,9] Although peripheral lesions could be located anywhere in the peripheral trigeminal nerve, the trigeminal (gasserian) ganglion, or the intracranial fibers, the reflex abnormality, if present, would be the same: There could be a delayed or absent R1 response with or without delayed ipsilateral and contralateral R2 responses when stimulating the affected side.[9,10] If only the R1 response is absent, it is important to use paired stimuli, as previously mentioned, before assuming it is abnormal.

The yield of the BR could vary depending on the pattern of fiber damage (axonal versus demyelinating) and the extent of the lesion. In a series of patients with trigeminal neuropathies of mixed etiologies, Kimura[10] found an abnormal response in 10 of 17 (59%) patients; in another series of patients with symptomatic chronic trigeminal sensory neuropathy, an abnormal response was found in 8 of 17 (47%)

patients, with an afferent pattern of abnormality being the most common.[9] The BR has provided evidence that trigeminal sensory involvement is more common than suspected on a clinical basis in chronic inflammatory demyelinating polyneuropathy (CIDP) and diabetic polyneuropathy.[11,12] It can be particularly helpful in differentiating trigeminal neuralgia from other painful trigeminal neuropathies, because it is usually normal in trigeminal neuralgia.[13] In the evaluation of patients with motor neuronopathies, subclinical trigeminal sensory involvement with abnormal BRs has been observed in Kennedy's syndrome[14] (bulbospinal neuronopathy, spinal-bulbar sensory-motor neuronopathy, bulbospinal muscular atrophy), providing further evidence for coexistent involvement of sensory neurons and adding another differentiating feature from other motor neuronopathies.

One interesting observation is that the BR is usually normal in paraneoplastic sensory neuronopathy, in contrast to nonparaneoplastic sensory neuronopathy, where it is often abnormal.[15] Thus, an abnormal BR in a patient with a sensory neuronopathy would favor a nonparaneoplastic etiology. When sensory symptoms are restricted to the chin, the possibility of a mental, inferior alveolar, or mandibular division abnormality should be explored, because this may be a presenting feature of occult cancer. In this case, BRs with mental nerve stimulation as well as other complementary studies of the trigeminal system (discussed later in the chapter) should be performed for proper evaluation. Reference values and methodology for studying the BR with mental nerve stimulation have been previously published.[6]

Facial neuropathies can occur secondary to multiple and diverse etiologies, such as diabetes, sarcoidosis, infectious processes (e.g., Lyme disease, herpes zoster, and human immunodeficiency virus infection), or from direct invasion or external compression from a tumor. They can also be seen as a manifestation of a generalized peripheral nerve disorder, such as acquired or hereditary demyelinating polyneuropathies. In the latter types, the BR and the study of the direct facial nerve responses can be useful, particularly in patients in whom peripheral nerve conduction velocities are difficult to measure because of distal muscle atrophy. In isolation, the most common presentation is the idiopathic facial neuropathy or Bell's palsy. In the study of facial neuropathies, the BR offers the added advantage of testing the whole length of the nerve, including the intracranial and intraosseous segments, and providing additional information about the predominance of an axonal or demyelinating component. With unilateral facial neuropathies, the BR abnormality will show an abnormal "efferent pattern," in which the R1 and R2 responses are delayed or absent on the affected side but the simultaneously recorded contralateral R2 response is normal. In idiopathic facial neuropathy or Bell's palsy, the most common facial neuropathy, the BR can be a sensitive measure of diagnosis[16] and provide important information about prognosis[10,17–19] complementary to the side-to-side muscle action potential amplitude comparison of the direct facial responses and the clinical assessment. Two important issues must be considered when assessing prognosis in Bell's palsy: (1) that axonal degeneration can continue for several days after the onset of symptoms, and (2) that there is delay between irreversible acute axonal damage and the appearance of distal degeneration as determined by the direct facial response.

Typically in Bell's palsy, the R1 and R2 responses may be preserved within the first day or two after the onset of symptoms and then become progressively delayed or unobtainable in the following days, with a peak in the conduction delay at approximately 5 days (Figure 7.3). Because of this evolving process and the possibility of late degeneration, it is generally agreed that prognostic assessment cannot be made until after the end of the first week and that serial studies are more helpful.

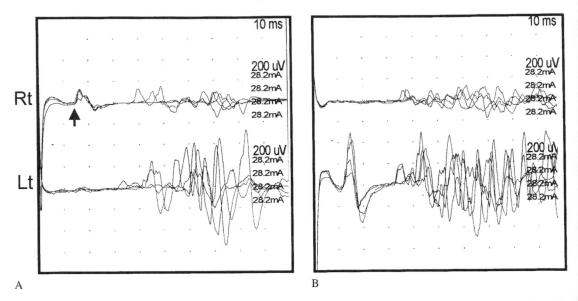

Figure 7.3 Blink reflex in Bell's palsy. Representative example of an abnormal blink reflex in a patient with a right Bell's palsy, 10 days after the onset of paralysis. On the right side (upper trace, **A** and **B**), the early response (R1) is delayed at 14 milliseconds (*arrow*), and the intermediate response (R2) shows a markedly reduced amplitude with stimulation on the right (**A**) or left (**B**) side. (Lt = left; Rt = right.)

The prognosis for recovery of function in Bell's palsy is considered favorable if the R1 component persists or reappears after the first week and unfavorable if the R1 and R2 remain absent after the first 3–4 weeks.[10,17,18] It is important to understand that the BR is complementary to the direct response and that both should be examined for prognostic purposes. These observations apply for Bell's palsy but do not necessarily apply to other facial neuropathies that may be mediated through other mechanisms.

The BR can also be of value in documenting and quantifying the presence of aberrant regeneration with synkinesis, after Bell's palsy. As shown in Figure 7.4, in these cases, the R1 and R2 responses can be recorded synchronously from other facial muscles where they are not normally present, after stimulation of the supraorbital nerve.[20–22] The BR can also be of value in the assessment of acquired or hereditary demyelinating polyneuropathies. It can be helpful in detecting evidence of demyelination affecting proximal nerve segments predominantly or when distal atrophy or marked reductions in compound muscle action potential amplitudes preclude proper assessment of distal limb segments. In a comprehensive series of patients with Guillain-Barré syndrome (GBS), almost one-half (46%) of all patients tested showed abnormalities of the BR in the form of a prolonged R1 response.[23] Abnormalities may also be seen in a significant proportion of patients without evidence of facial weakness, indicating subclinical involvement.[24] Comparisons of the R1 latency and the direct response latency have shown an increased ratio in GBS but not in other demyelinating polyneuropathies, such as CIDP and Charcot-Marie-Tooth disease I, providing further evidence of more prominent proximal involvement in GBS and a differentiating feature from other neuropathies with more prominent distal pathology.[10] The BR is particularly useful in GBS variants associated with facial weakness or facial sensory symptoms, such as polyneuritis cranialis[25] and the Miller Fisher syndrome. In this last variant, absent or prolonged R1 or R2 responses

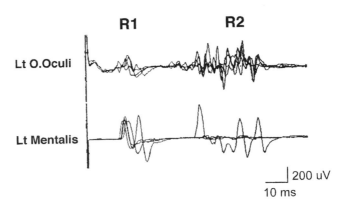

Figure 7.4 Synkinesis. Evidence of aberrant regeneration in a patient with a history of facial paralysis with residual weakness and synchronous twitches in the lower facial muscles on attempted blinking. There was evidence of a well-formed early response (R1) and a truncated intermediate response (R2) from the ipsilateral mentalis muscle when recording a blink reflex with stimulation of the supraorbital nerve. (Lt = left; O. Oculi = orbicularis oculi.)

have been observed in more than 50% of affected patients, usually when there is associated facial weakness.[26–28]

The BR has also been shown to be abnormal in hereditary neuropathies of the Charcot-Marie-Tooth type.[29,30] The abnormality may be in the afferent or efferent pathways in spite of the absence of symptoms and is more commonly observed with the demyelinating types. The BR may be helpful in these chronic neuropathies with marked distal atrophy, in which distinction between a demyelinating and an axonal process may be difficult. The BR has also been shown to be abnormal with prolonged R1 responses in the majority (>70%) of patients with familial amyloid neuropathy, Finnish type (gelsolin amyloidosis), in which facial weakness is one of the typical features.[31]

Masseter Reflex

The masseter reflex (jaw jerk, mandibular reflex) is the equivalent to the myotatic limb reflex for the masseter muscle. It is elicited by sudden stretching of the masseter muscle, a task usually accomplished with a tap on the chin with a reflex hammer. It provides an objective method of examining trigeminal motor and sensory pathways, particularly those from the mandibular division, and is complementary to the BR and the masseter inhibitory response.

Anatomy and Physiology

Although the jaw muscles are very similar to the limb muscles, they have specific adaptations to their particular functions, which are reflected in their neural organization.[32] One unique anatomic feature of this reflex is that the muscle spindle afferent neurons mediating the afferent limb of the reflex have their cell bodies located within the central nervous system—in the mesencephalic nucleus of the brainstem. In contrast, limb muscle spindle afferent and cutaneous afferent neurons have their cell bodies located in the spinal or gasserian ganglia—outside of the central nervous system. This discrepancy in location results in the possibility

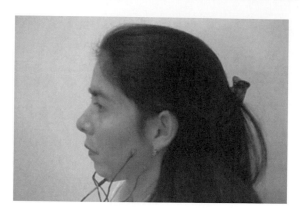

Figure 7.5 Electrode placement for the masseter reflex. The active electrode is placed over the lower third of the belly of the masseter muscle, and the reference electrode is placed 2 cm below the angle of the mandible. The aim is to optimize activity from the masseter muscle while minimizing contaminating muscle activity from facial muscles.

of differences in involvement between proprioceptive and cutaneous afferent neurons within the same nerve.

There is still debate about the path of the muscle spindle afferent fibers, with some investigators favoring the motor root,[33] whereas others favor the sensory root of the trigeminal nerve.[34] The spindle afferents provide collaterals to the ipsilateral trigeminal motor nucleus in the pons, which, along with the motor fibers, constitutes the efferent limb of the reflex. Unlike other brainstem reflexes, there are no connections across to the midline, resulting in uncrossed responses and allowing for the detection of side-to-side asymmetries.

Methodologic Aspects

Electrode placement for the masseter reflex is shown in Figure 7.5. The active electrode is best placed over the lower third of the belly of the masseter, and the reference electrode should be placed 2 cm below the angle of mandible.[4] The goal is to optimize the recording of the masseter response while minimizing activity from facial muscles. The standard method used in most laboratories uses one of several commercially available reflex hammers fitted with a microswitch that triggers the sweep of the electromyograph. The patient is seated upright, preferably in a chair with a headrest, and the patient's jaw is loose and slightly opened. Clenching the teeth may enhance the reflex. The response is strongly influenced by dental occlusion, position of the mandible, and central excitability, resulting in prominent variability of latency and amplitude between subjects and between successive trials in the same subject (Figure 7.6). Because of this, simultaneous, bilateral recordings from both masseters are used for diagnostic purposes. The latency is measured to the first deflection from the baseline and may range from 6 to 11 milliseconds. It is considered abnormal if there is a difference greater than 1 millisecond between the two simultaneously acquired responses or if the response is absent on one side.[4] Bilaterally absent responses can be seen, particularly in elderly individuals, and abnormalities may also be observed in craniomandibular disorders,[35] so these possibilities should be considered in the interpretation of abnormal results. In the presence of abnormal results, needle electromyography (EMG) of the masseter muscle may help to distinguish between an afferent (sensory) or efferent (motor) abnormality.

Figure 7.6 Masseter reflex. Representative example from a healthy volunteer showing the typical amplitude and latency variability. For diagnostic purposes, it is best to use latency differences from simultaneous bilateral recordings (normal = 1 millisecond). Upper trace shows right masseter reflex; lower trace shows left masseter reflex.

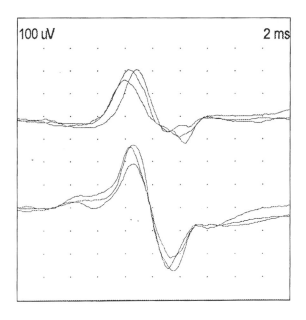

Clinical Applications in Neuromuscular Disease

Along with the BR and masseter inhibitory response, the masseter reflex has been a complementary and adjunct measure of trigeminal nerve involvement in patients with trigeminal neuropathies.[36,37] The masseter reflex has proven to be of value in discriminating between sensory neuronopathies and peripheral sensory or sensorimotor axonopathies when these involve the trigeminal territory. In a group of patients with Sjögren's syndrome and sensory neuronopathies, Valls-Solé et al.[38] found preservation of the masseter reflex in spite of abnormalities of the BR and the electrically elicited masseter inhibitory reflex (MIR), these last two reflexes being mediated through cutaneous sensory fibers. This provided evidence for damage at the neuronal level with selective involvement of cutaneous sensory neurons and sparing of masseter spindle afferent neurons located in the mesencephalic nucleus. In contrast, in patients with peripheral axonopathies involving the trigeminal nerve, they found abnormalities in all trigeminal reflexes, including the masseter reflex, providing a differentiating feature between trigeminal neuronal and axonal involvement. They concluded that an abnormal BR and cutaneous silent period, together with a normal masseter reflex and stretch-induced silent period, are characteristic signs of a lesion affecting gasserian ganglion neurons in pure sensory neuronopathy. This dissociation has been confirmed in patients with subacute idiopathic sensory neuronopathies and is presumed to be a result of the relatively protected environment of the centrally located neurons.[39] This distinct pattern is not unique to acquired or immune-mediated neuronopathies, nor to purely sensory neuronopathies, and it has also been observed in genetic conditions, such as Kennedy's syndrome[14] and Friedreich's ataxia.[40] The combination of a preserved masseter reflex with abnormalities of the blink and the masseter inhibitory reflex could serve as a differentiating feature between Kennedy's syndrome and other clinically similar motor-sensory axonopathies with nonspecific reductions in the limb sensory potentials.

Although the masseter reflex has also been used to detect subclinical involvement of the trigeminal nerve in polyneuropathies, such as CIDP and diabetic neuropathy, it has a lower sensitivity than the MIR or the BR.[11,12]

Silent Periods

The *silent period* is defined as a transient relative or absolute suppression in EMG activity during a volitional contraction or after a variety of stimuli, such as electrical stimulation of a mixed nerve[41] or cutaneous sensory nerve.[42] There are significant differences between the two types of nerve stimulation, and the resultant silent periods are currently divided into two distinct phenomena: the mixed nerve silent period and the cutaneous silent period. The *masseteric silent period* (MIR, exteroceptive suppression) is one variant of the silent period, which is used to study the trigeminal and brainstem pathways and is considered separately.

Anatomy and Physiology

The precise physiologic mechanisms and anatomic pathways involved in the generation of the silent period are still debated. It is important to understand that with mixed nerve stimulation, an ascending volley is generated with motor fibers stimulated antidromically and sensory fibers stimulated orthodromically. Current evidence suggests that the mixed nerve silent period is mainly dependent on afferent impulses in the ascending volley that are generated by the stimulation of the mixed nerve.[41] The mixed nerve silent period is a complex event that normally lasts from 100 to 200 milliseconds and is divided into three distinct periods, as shown in Figure 7.7A. The initial period of suppression is measured from the onset of suppression to the interruption by F waves, and when recorded from the hand muscles, the period of suppression ends approximately 30 milliseconds after the stimulus. This initial suppression is believed to result from collisions of the elicited antidromic and volitionally generated orthodromic motor impulses. The second period of suppression follows the F wave and, in hand muscles, lasts for approximately 30–75 milliseconds. The proposed mechanism for this period of suppression is believed to be the result of recurrent (Renshaw cell) inhibition from the antidromic motor volley.[43] The third period of suppression follows the long latency reflex, appears at 60–100 milliseconds, and is believed to result from the activation of high-threshold cutaneous afferent fibers similar to those activated in the cutaneous silent period with stimulation of a cutaneous nerve.[44] It is mediated through an oligo- or polysynaptic spinal reflex with an inhibitory interneuron.

The cutaneous silent period is produced by orthodromic activation of sensory fibers through stimulation of digital nerves or other cutaneous nerves, such as the sural or superficial radial. This can produce a silent period in muscles innervated by different nerves or spinal segments from those stimulated, and it lasts from 75 to 140 milliseconds when recorded from the hand muscles. It is elicited by supramaximal stimuli in the nociceptive range and is likely to be mediated by thinly myelinated, slow-conducting A-δ fibers.[42,45,46]

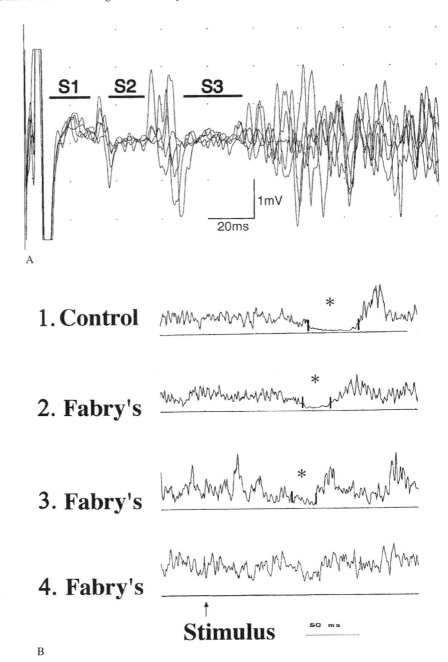

A

B

Figure 7.7 A. Mixed nerve silent period. Stimulation of the median nerve at the wrist results in three periods of suppression of electromyographic activity. The first period (S1) ends approximately 30 milliseconds after the stimulus with the appearance of the F waves. The second period (S2) follows the F waves and lasts from 30 to 75 milliseconds until the appearance of the long latency reflex. The third period (S3) follows the long latency reflex and is thought to be equivalent to the cutaneous silent period. **B.** Examples of waveforms showing the cutaneous silent period (CSP) over a period of 50 milliseconds in the lower extremity in control subject (1) and three patients with Fabry's disease (2–4). Each trace represents the rectified average of 10 CSPs. Markers indicate the beginning and end of the CSPs, also indicated by asterisks. The CSP was absent in patient 4 (4). (Reproduced with permission from N Ali Syed, F Sandbrink, CA Luciano, et al. Cutaneous silent periods in patients with Fabry's disease. Muscle Nerve 2000;23:1179–1186.)

Methodologic Aspects

To record the mixed nerve silent period, disk electrodes are placed over the contracting muscle while single shocks are delivered to the mixed nerve, innervating the muscle used for recording. In the upper limbs, it is common to record from the abductor pollicis brevis while stimulating the median nerve at the wrist or the elbow. The parameters that have been measured in studies of the silent period are (1) the onset and terminal latency, (2) the duration, and (3) the extent or magnitude of suppression of the EMG activity. Each of these is influenced by the stimulus strength and the level and type of contraction (isotonic vs. isometric), requiring the adherence to specific protocols for the acquisition of reproducible results that can be compared between groups. For isometric contractions, the extremity or the whole limb is held in position while the subject contracts to a predetermined level based on a percentage of his or her maximum force. This can best be accomplished using a force transducer or through the use of weights held against the muscle, although this process can be simplified by using maximum force.

For recording the mixed nerve silent period from the abductor pollicis brevis, the median nerve at the wrist is stimulated with square pulses of 0.1–0.2 millisecond with supramaximal stimulus intensities 20–25% above those required for the maximum M-response amplitude. For the cutaneous silent period, single shocks are delivered to cutaneous nerves, such as the median or ulnar sensory at the digit, at stimulus intensities of 10–12 times the perception threshold. To establish the onset and end of the silent period, it is better to average the rectified EMG signal and include a period of background EMG activity before the stimulus artifact (50–150 milliseconds). The initial period of baseline EMG activity is used to establish the mean amplitude of EMG activity. Because at times suppression is not complete, it is common practice to define the onset or offset of the silent period as the point at which the rectified EMG signal decreases or increases to a predetermined percent of the mean background EMG amplitude (i.e., 80% of the background EMG amplitude).

Clinical Applications in Neuromuscular Disease

The clinical use of the silent periods in the evaluation of neuromuscular diseases has focused mainly on the determination of continuity of proximal segments of motor and sensory fibers, the study of fiber populations not routinely examined with nerve conduction studies (e.g., the small myelinated A-δ fibers), and the detection of impaired inhibition in conditions with augmented muscle tone.

The cutaneous silent periods may be used to test the integrity of afferent pathways in conditions that involve radicular or proximal sensory pathways, such as radiculopathy or root avulsion.[46] This is more practical for the C6, C7, and C8 roots by stimulating the thumb, middle, or little finger, respectively. Disparate results in the cutaneous silent periods from patients with a similar clinical picture of profound sensory loss and absent sensory nerve action potentials have suggested differences in the type or pattern of afferent fiber involvement and the potential use of the silent period in discriminating between different types of sensory neuropathies.[47] We have shown that in patients with small-fiber neuropathies, the cutaneous silent period can be a useful adjunct measure in detecting small-fiber dysfunction, although it is not as sensitive as other psychophysical measures[48] (see Figure 7.7B). This has also been suggested in the evaluation of entrapment neuropathies.[49] It could also be a useful tool in the evaluation of conditions associated with spasticity or upper motor neuron signs, such as amyotrophic lateral sclerosis. Both incomplete inhibition of the middle period (S2) and a longer duration of the third period in the mixed nerve silent period have been observed in patients with amyotrophic lateral sclerosis,[50] suggesting its value as an objective measure of central nervous system dysfunction. In tetanus, the mixed nerve silent period can be shortened or absent and has been used to distinguish it from other conditions with excessive motor unit activity, such as the stiff-man syndrome, in which the silent period is normal.[51]

Masseter Inhibitory Reflex

Similar to what is observed in the limb muscles, when an electrical or mechanical stimulus is applied to the perioral region during forceful clenching of the jaw, a reflex inhibition is induced in the jaw-closing muscles. This inhibitory response is known as the *MIR*, or *masseteric silent period*. As shown in Figure 7.8, the inhibitory reflex is composed of two distinct periods of suppression, an early and a late period (silent periods 1 and 2 [SP1 and SP2], or exteroceptive suppression 1 and 2 [ES1 and ES2]). The reflex can provide important information about trigeminal afferent and efferent (motor) fibers as well as brainstem inhibitory interneurons, complementary to the blink and the masseter reflex (jaw-jerk).

Anatomy and Physiology

Afferent impulses elicited after electrical stimulation of the mental or infraorbital nerve travel orthodromically through the mandibular or maxillary roots of the trigeminal nerve. Current evidence suggests that each inhibitory period is mediated

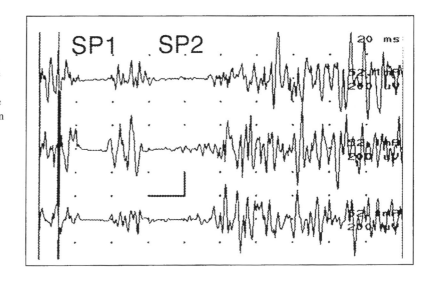

Figure 7.8 Masseter inhibitory reflex. Electrical stimulation of the mental nerve with maximal contraction of the masseter muscle results in early (SP1) and late (SP2) periods of electromyographic suppression. SP1 is more sensitive and is studied more often in the assessment of peripheral trigeminal pathways (sweep speed: 20 milliseconds/division; gain: 200 μV/division).

through two independent anatomic circuits. The SP1 response is mediated through an oligosynaptic pathway with an inhibitory interneuron at the level of the mid-pons, close to the trigeminal motor nucleus. The interneuron projects to both trigeminal motor nuclei. Afferent impulses for the SP2 response descend down the spinal trigeminal tract to the pontomedullary junction and connect through a polysynaptic path (located in the medullary lateral reticular formation) to an inhibitory interneuron that gives collaterals to both trigeminal motor nuclei.[3,52]

Methodologic Aspects

The reflex is recorded through surface electrodes applied to the masseter muscles bilaterally in the same manner as for the masseter reflex. It can be elicited by mechanical taps to the chin or electrical stimulation of the mental nerve, the gums, and the oral mucosa, among other areas. These two methods of stimulation assess two different afferent fibers, mainly proprioceptive muscle afferent fibers with the mechanical taps and cutaneous sensory fibers with electric stimulation. The placement of the electrodes also influences the size of the response, so it is important that electrode placement be done in a systematic and reproducible manner. The placement of electrodes for MIR is the same as that for the masseter reflex. The magnitude of EMG suppression is influenced by the level of contraction, so it is also advisable to use a uniform and reproducible contraction. In the absence of sophisticated force-measuring arrangements, maximal level of contraction can be used as the standard contraction. The patient clenches the teeth at maximum force, and stimuli of 0.1–0.2 millisecond of duration are applied to the mental or infraorbital nerve. The EMG suppression also varies with changing stimulus intensities, so it is important to quantify the intensities to compare results between patients and controls. Similar to what has been described for measuring the mixed nerve and cutaneous silent periods, the signal is full-wave rectified and averaged, and a predetermined decrease is used to mark the onset and duration of each of the suppression periods. The onset latency of the SP1 period is relatively stable and the parameter most commonly used for clinical purposes. An onset-latency difference between the two simultaneously acquired responses of more than 1.5 milliseconds would suggest an abnormality.[4] Because it is a test of inhibitory function, it may disclose abnormalities not apparent on the clinical examination. The other parameters used in studies of the cutaneous and mixed nerve silent periods can also be measured and studied with the MIR. Like the pattern of abnormalities described for the BR, it is possible to define afferent and efferent types of abnormalities from the MIR.[3] An afferent type of abnormality shows an abnormal ipsilateral and contralateral response on stimulation of one side and indicates a lesion in the trigeminal afferent fibers at any point before the crossing of impulses (peripheral or brainstem). A brainstem lesion is suggested by a mixed pattern with abnormal bilateral responses on stimulation of one side and an abnormal crossed response with contralateral stimulation. An efferent type of abnormality is an abnormal response confined to only one side, regardless of the side of stimulation. This pattern suggests an abnormality in the trigeminal motor root, although it has also been described in hemimasticatory spasm.[53]

Clinical Applications in Neuromuscular Disease

In the clinical laboratory, the MIR complements other techniques used in the assessment of the trigeminal pathways, such as the blink and the masseter reflex, by examining different segments and fiber populations. It may allow the distinction between axonal and demyelinating involvement or differentiate between a sensory ganglionopathy and a distal sensory neuropathy affecting trigeminal nerve fibers.

The MIR has been used extensively in the assessment of craniomandibular disorders.[54–56] It has been used to detect subclinical trigeminal nerve abnormalities in mild and severe diabetic polyneuropathy. In these cases, when studied in conjunction with other trigeminotrigeminal (masseter) and trigeminofacial (blink) reflexes, the MIR has been shown to be more sensitive than the other reflexes in detecting peripheral trigeminal nerve abnormalities.[11,12] Along with the masseter reflex, the MIR elicited by chin taps (proprioceptive stimuli) has been shown to be preserved in patients with a sensory neuronopathy associated with Sjögren's syndrome but not in peripheral neuropathies affecting trigeminal nerve fibers,[38] allowing the distinction between the two possibilities. The MIR can also be used to distinguish between axonal and demyelinating lesions or neuropathies. Using the chin-tap technique, Auger[57] demonstrated prolonged latencies in patients with CIDP but not in axonal neuropathies, suggesting its value in the differentiation between axonal and demyelinating polyneuropathies. More recently, Cruccu[11] showed similar findings in CIDP using electrically induced MIR and demonstrated similarly prolonged latencies in severe diabetic polyneuropathy. Cruccu's study also showed more frequent involvement of alveolomandibular nerve fibers compared to other trigeminal nerve divisions, suggesting an increased vulnerability of these fibers. The MIR can also be of value in the detection and study of trigeminal sensory neuropathies (Figure 7.9).[37,58] In tetanus, the MIR can be shortened or absent (see Figure 5.25), very much

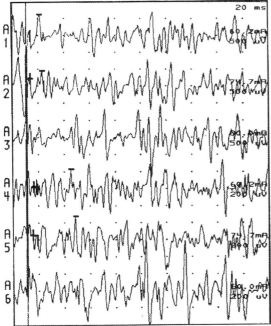
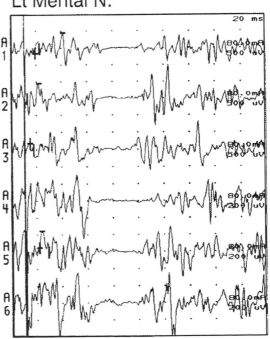
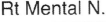

Figure 7.9 Bilateral trigeminal neuropathy and lymphoma. Example of an abnormal masseter inhibitory reflex in a patient with lymphoma and bilateral subacute facial sensory loss with no evidence of central nervous system involvement. The direct and crossed responses are abnormal with stimulation on either side: With stimulation of the right mental nerve, silent periods were absent on both masseter muscles, and with stimulation of the left mental nerve, silent period 1 (SP1) was absent, but a relatively preserved silent period 2 (SP2) could be observed on both sides. It has been suggested that SP1 is more susceptible than SP2 to extra-axial lesions, because it is mediated by a smaller number of afferents.[11] (A1–A3 = right masseter, 500 μV/division; A4–A6 = left masseter, 200 μV/division; Lt = left; N = nerve; Rt = right.)

like the mixed nerve silent period, and can be a distinguishing feature from other conditions characterized by excessive motor unit activity.[51,59,60]

CONCLUSIONS

In the patient with a suspected neuromuscular disease, the possibility of facial motor, motor-sensory, or pure sensory involvement can be studied through the use of various unconventional but well-established and sensitive neurophysiologic techniques. The elicited responses can serve as sensitive and quantifiable measurements of facial or trigeminal sensory and motor involvement and can provide valuable insight about the involved mechanisms or localization of the primary disease process. Furthermore, they may provide important information about selective or predominant involvement of specific axonal or neuronal populations in the peripheral or central nervous system. Measurement of the silent period of peripheral nerves also provides important information regarding the function of nerve fibers that are not studied during conventional electrodiagnostic tests. The techniques can be performed in the electrodiagnostic laboratory without the need of very sophisticated setups, and in view of the possibility of subclinical abnormalities, should not be limited to the presence of signs or symptoms. Together with the clinical examination and other laboratory data, the techniques could add valuable information leading to a more specific diagnosis.

REFERENCES

1. Rossi B, Risaliti R, Rossi A. The R3 component of the blink reflex in man: a reflex response induced by activation of high threshold cutaneous afferents. Electroencephalogr Clin Neurophysiol 1989;73:334–340.
2. Ongerboer de Visser B. Trigemino-Facial and Trigemino-Trigeminal Reflex Circuits. In J Valls-Solé, E Tolosa (eds), Brainstem Reflexes and Functions. Madrid: ENE Publicidad, S.A., 1998;67–78.
3. Cruccu G, Deuschl G. The clinical use of brainstem reflexes and hand-muscle reflexes. Clin Neurophysiol 2000;111:371–387.
4. Kimura J, Daube J, Burke D, et al. Human reflexes and late responses. Report of an IFCN committee. Electroencephalogr Clin Neurophysiol 1994;90:393–403.
5. Malin J-P. The human orbicularis oculi reflex. Electromyogr Clin Neurophysiol 1982;22:45–53.
6. Jääskeläinen S. Blink reflex with stimulation of the mental nerve. Methodology, reference values and some clinical vignettes. Acta Neuro Scand 1995;91:477–482.
7. Kimura J. The Blink Reflex. Electrodiagnosis in Diseases of Nerve and Muscle (3rd ed). New York: Oxford University Press, Inc., 2001;409–438.
8. Hughes R. Diseases of the Fifth Cranial Nerve. In P Dyck, P Thomas, J Griffin, et al. (eds), Peripheral Neuropathy, Vol 2. Philadelphia: W.B. Saunders, 1993;801–817.
9. Lecky B, Hughes R, Murray N. Trigeminal sensory neuropathy. Brain 1987;110:1463–1485.
10. Kimura J. The Blink Reflex as a Clinical Test. In M Aminoff (ed), Electrodiagnosis in Clinical Neurology (3rd ed). New York: Churchill Livingstone, 1992;369–402.
11. Cruccu G, Agostino R, Inghilleri M, et al. Mandibular nerve involvement in diabetic polyneuropathy and chronic inflammatory demyelinating polyneuropathy. Muscle Nerve 1998;21:1673–1679.
12. Urban P, Forst T, Lenfers M, et al. Incidence of subclinical trigeminal and facial nerve involvement in diabetes mellitus. Electromyogr Clin Neurophysiol 1999;39:267–272.
13. Cruccu G, Leandri M, Feliciani M, Manfredi M. Idiopathic and symptomatic trigeminal pain. J Neurol Neurosurg Psychiatry 1990;53:1034–1042.
14. Antonini G, Gragnani F, Romaniello A, et al. Sensory involvement in spinal-bulbar muscular atrophy (Kennedy's disease). Muscle Nerve 2000;23:252–258.
15. Auger R, Windebank A, Lucchinetti C, Chalk C. Role of the blink reflex in the evaluation of sensory neuronopathy. Neurology 1999;53:407–408.

16. Hill M, Midroni G, Goldstein W, et al. The spectrum of electrophysiological abnormalities in Bell's palsy. Can J Neurol Sci 2001;28:130–133.
17. Schenck E, Manz F. The Blink Reflex in Bell's Palsy. In J Desmedt (ed), New Developments in Electromyography and Clinical Neurophysiology, Vol 3. Basel, NY: S. Karger, 1973;678–681.
18. Ghonim M, Gavilan C. Blink reflex: prognostic value in acute peripheral facial palsy. ORL J Otorhinolaryngol Relat Spec 1990;52:75–79.
19. Celik M, Forta H. Electrophysiological investigations and prognosis in idiopathic facial palsy. Electromyogr Clin Neurophysiol 1997;37:311–315.
20. Celik M, Forta H, Vural C. The development of synkinesis after facial nerve paralysis. Eur Neurol 2000;43:147–151.
21. Kimura J, Rodnitzky R, Okawara S. Electrophysiologic analysis of aberrant regeneration after facial nerve paralysis. Neurology 1975;25:989–993.
22. Eekhof J, Aramideh M, Speelman J, et al. Blink reflexes and lateral spreading in patients with synkinesia after Bell's palsy and in hemifacial spasm. Eur Neurol 2000;43:141–146.
23. Ropper A, Wijdicks E, Shahani B. Electrodiagnostic abnormalities in 113 consecutive patients with Guillain-Barré syndrome. Arch Neurol 1990;47:881–887.
24. Neau J, Gil R, Boissonnot L, Lefevre J. The blink reflex and stimulus detection by the facial nerve in 50 cases of Guillain-Barré polyradiculitis. Acta Neurol Belg 1987;87:12–19.
25. Polo A, Manganotti P, Zanette G, Grandis D. Polyneuritis cranialis: clinical and electrophysiological findings. J Neurol Neurosurg Psychiatry 1992;55:398–400.
26. Calleja J, García A, de Pablos C, Polo J. Miller-Fisher syndrome: electrophysiological serial study of five patients. Rev Neurol 1998;27:60–64.
27. Fross R, Daube J. Neuropathy in the Miller Fisher syndrome: clinical and electrophysiologic findings. Neurology 1987;37:1493–1498.
28. Jamal G, Ballantyne J. The localization of the lesion in patients with acute ophthalmoplegia, ataxia and areflexia (Miller Fisher syndrome). A serial multimodal neurophysiological study. Brain 1988;111:95–114.
29. Kimura J. Conduction abnormalities of the facial and trigeminal nerves in polyneuropathy. Muscle Nerve 1982;5:S139–S144.
30. Malin J. Trigeminal and facial nerve involvement in Charcot-Marie-Tooth disease. An electrodiagnostic study. J Neurol 1981;226:101–109.
31. Kiuru S, Seppalainen A. Neuropathy in familial amyloidosis, Finnish type (FAF): electrophysiological studies. Muscle Nerve 1994;17:299–304.
32. Poliakov A, Miles T. Stretch reflexes in human masseter. J Physiol 1994;476(2):323–331.
33. Pennisi E, Cruccu G, Manfredi M, Palladini G. Histometric study of myelinated fibers in the human trigeminal nerve. J Neurol Sci 1991;105:22–28.
34. Ongerboer de Visser B. Afferent limb of the human jaw reflex: electrophysiologic and anatomic study. Neurology 1982;32:536–546.
35. Cruccu G, Frisardi G, van Steenberghe D. Side asymmetry of the jaw jerk in human craniomandibular dysfunction. Archs Oral Biol 1992;37:257–262.
36. Goor C, Ongerboer de Visser B. Jaw and blink reflexes in trigeminal nerve lesions: an electrodiagnostic study. Neurology 1976;26:95–97.
37. Auger R, McManis P. Trigeminal sensory neuropathy associated with decreased oral sensation and impairment of the masseter inhibitory reflex. Neurology 1990;40:759–763.
38. Valls-Solé J, Graus F, Font J, et al. Normal proprioceptive trigeminal afferents in patients with Sjögren's syndrome and sensory neuronopathy. Ann Neurol 1990;28:786–790.
39. Auger R. Role of the masseter reflex in the assessment of subacute sensory neuropathy. Muscle Nerve 1998;21:800–801.
40. Auger R. Preservation of the masseter reflex in Friedreich's ataxia. Neurology 1992;42:875–878.
41. Leis A, Ross M, Emori T, et al. The silent period produced by electrical stimulation of mixed peripheral nerves. Muscle Nerve 1991;14:1202–1208.
42. Uncini A, Kujirai T, Gluck B, Pullman S. Silent period induced by cutaneous stimulation. Electroencephalogr Clin Neurophysiol 1991;81:344–352.
43. Shahani B, Young R. Studies of the Normal Human Silent Period. In J Desmedt (ed), New Developments in Electromyography and Clinical Neurophysiology, Vol 3. Basel, NY: S. Karger, 1973.
44. Stetkarova I, Kofler M, Leis A. Cutaneous and mixed nerve silent periods in syringomyelia. Clin Neurophysiol 2001;112:78–85.
45. Shefner J, Logigian E. Relationship between stimulus strength and the cutaneous silent period. Muscle Nerve 1993;16:278–282.
46. Leis A. Cutaneous silent period. Muscle Nerve 1998;21:1243–1245.

47. Leis A. Conduction abnormalities detected by silent period testing. Electroencephalogr Clin Neurophysiol 1994;93:444–449.

48. Syed N, Sandbrink F, Luciano C, et al. Cutaneous silent periods in patients with Fabry disease. Muscle Nerve 2000;23:1179–1186.

49. Aurora S, Ahmad B, Aurora T. Silent period abnormalities in carpal tunnel syndrome. Muscle Nerve 1998;21:1213–1215.

50. Shefner J, Logigian E. The mixed silent period in normal subjects and patients with amyotrophic lateral sclerosis. Electromyogr Clin Neurophysiol 1998;38:505–510.

51. Poncelet A. Blink reflex and the silent period in tetanus. Muscle Nerve 2000;23:1435–1438.

52. Ongerboer de Visser B, Cruccu G, Manfredi M, Koelman J. Effects of brainstem lesions on the masseter inhibitory reflex: functional mechanisms of reflex pathways. Brain 1989;113:781–792.

53. Cruccu G, Pauletti G, Agostino R, et al. Masseter inhibitory reflex in movement disorders. Huntington's chorea, Parkinson's disease, dystonia and unilateral masticatory spasm. Electroencephalogr Clin Neurophysiol 1991;81:24–30.

54. Cruccu G, Frisardi G, Pauletti G, et al. Excitability of the central masticatory pathways in patients with painful temporomandibular disorders. Pain 1997;73:447–454.

55. Hussein S, McCall W. Masseteric silent periods electrically evoked in normal subjects and patients with temporomandibular joint dysfunction. Exp Neurol 1983;81:64–76.

56. Sharav Y, McGrath P, Dubner R. Masseter inhibitory periods and sensations by electrical tooth pulp stimulation in patients with oral-facial pain and mandibular dysfunction. Arch Oral Biol 1982;27:305–310.

57. Auger R. Latency of onset of the masseter inhibitory reflex in peripheral neuropathies. Muscle Nerve 1996;19:910–911.

58. Urban P, Keilmann A, Teichmann E, Hopf H. Sensory neuropathy of the trigeminal, glossopharyngeal, and vagal nerves in Sjögren's syndrome. J Neurol Sci 2001;186:59–63.

59. Fernandez J, Ferrandiz M, Larrea L, et al. Cephalic tetanus studied with single fibre EMG. J Neurol Neurosurg Psychiatry 1983;46:862–866.

60. Rick W, Bosch E, Kimura J, et al. Chronic tetanus: clinical report and histochemistry of muscle. Muscle Nerve 1981;4:363–366.

8

Autonomic Function Testing

Annabel K. Wang and Horacio Kaufmann

Involvement of the autonomic nervous system (ANS) is common in neuropathies due to systemic disorders such as diabetes and amyloidosis. In most neuropathies, however, autonomic fibers are not primarily affected. Recognition of autonomic dysfunction identifies a specific group of disorders and points to the correct diagnosis. Because autonomic dysfunction can be difficult to identify based on clinical history and examination alone, noninvasive autonomic testing is a useful diagnostic tool.

Noninvasive autonomic cardiovascular testing requires continuous systemic blood pressure and heart rate monitoring, as well as measurements of blood flow changes in particular vascular territories in response to various maneuvers. Noninvasive evaluation of the sympathetic sudomotor system uses a variety of methods that measure sweat. Cardiovascular and sudomotor tests assess small myelinated and unmyelinated fibers that cannot be assessed by conventional electromyographic studies.

Autonomic testing quantifies the extent of dysfunction and is useful for monitoring the course of the disease and assessing the effect of treatment. Autonomic testing identifies patients with increased morbidity and decreased life expectancy that may be susceptible to potentially dangerous complications during anesthesia and surgery.[1,2]

Inherited and acquired neuropathies may have symptoms of autonomic failure, both acute and chronic. Autonomic impairment may be diffuse or focal and with or without muscle weakness. Neuromuscular junction disorders, such as Lambert-Eaton myasthenic syndrome (LEMS) and botulism, may present with severe autonomic symptoms and signs.

In this chapter, we briefly review the anatomy of the peripheral ANS, noninvasive testing available to assess ANS function, and current knowledge of the most frequent neuromuscular disorders (i.e., neuropathies and neuromuscular junction disorders) with prominent autonomic dysfunction.

ANATOMY OF THE PERIPHERAL AUTONOMIC NERVOUS SYSTEM

The ANS is a complex network of neurons within the brain and spinal cord with peripheral afferent and efferent pathways and two major divisions: parasympathetic and sympathetic. Parasympathetic and sympathetic efferent systems consist of a two-neuron pathway with one synapse in peripheral autonomic ganglia. The soma of the preganglionic neuron is located centrally, whereas the ganglionic neuron is outside the central nervous system (CNS) and is referred to as *postganglionic*. Preganglionic axons, both parasympathetic and sympathetic, usually emerge from the CNS as small myelinated fibers, although preganglionic parasympathetic fibers can also be unmyelinated.[3] These small myelinated B fibers are approximately 3 μm in diameter and have conduction velocities ranging from 3 to 15 m per second. The main neurotransmitter for parasympathetic and sympathetic preganglionic to postganglionic synapses is acetylcholine. Postganglionic axons, both parasympathetic and sympathetic, are unmyelinated C fibers that are 0.3–1.3 μm in diameter with conduction velocities ranging from 0.7 to 2.3 m per second.[3] Cell bodies of parasympathetic preganglionic autonomic neurons are located within the brainstem and sacral (S2-4) regions (i.e., the craniosacral outflow). The main neurotransmitter in pre- and postganglionic parasympathetic neurons is acetylcholine. The cell bodies of sympathetic preganglionic neurons are located within the intermediolateral cell column of the thoracic and lumbar spinal cord (T1-L3) (i.e., the thoracolumbar outflow). The main neurotransmitter of postganglionic sympathetic neurons is noradrenaline (norepinephrine). Eccrine sweat glands are innervated by sympathetic neurons that use acetylcholine as a neurotransmitter.

Parasympathetic Nervous System

Axons of preganglionic parasympathetic autonomic neurons leave the CNS from the midbrain, pons, and medulla through the third, seventh, ninth, and tenth cranial nerves (Table 8.1). Preganglionic parasympathetic fibers are long and synapse in ganglia close to or within the innervated organs. The sacral division of the parasympathetic outflow exits from the second and fourth sacral roots (S2-4) and forms the pelvic splanchnic nerves, which innervate the lower colon, bladder, and genitals.

Sympathetic Nervous System

Monosynaptic connections to sympathetic preganglionic neurons in the intermediolateral cell column of the spinal cord originate in neurons of the paraventricular and lateral nuclei of the hypothalamus and the ventromedial and ventrolateral nuclei of the medulla. Myelinated sympathetic axons exit via the ventral roots of the tho-

Table 8.1 Parasympathetic Nervous System

Origin	Outflow	Function
Midbrain	CN III	Pupillary constriction, lens accommodation
Pons	CN VII	Lacrimation
Medulla	CN IX	Salivation, vasodilation
	CN X	Dorsal motor nucleus–respiratory and abdominal viscera; nucleus ambiguous–bradycardia, bronchial constriction, and secretion
Sacrum	S2-4 Plexus	Defecation, micturition, and erection

CN = cranial nerve.

Table 8.2 Sympathetic Nervous System

Origin	Outflow	Function
Sympathetic-paravertebral		
C1-4	SCG	Pupillary dilatation, vasoconstriction of head and neck, increase HR and SV, dilate coronary arteries
C5-6	MCG (may be absent)	Increase HR and SV, coronary arteries vasodilation, bronchial dilatation
C7-8	ICG	Increase HR and SV, coronary arteries vasodilation
T1-2	SG (may fuse with ICG)	Vasodilation, bronchial dilatation, sweat secretion, vasoconstriction and piloerection of upper extremity
Thoracic and lumbar cord	One pair per segment	Thoracic and abdominal end organs
Sympathetic-prevertebral		
Thoracic	Thorax	Cardiac and pulmonary plexuses
Lumbar	Abdomen	Celiac, renal, and superior or inferior mesenteric ganglia
	Pelvis	Superior and inferior hypogastric plexus
Sacrum	Four unpaired	Ganglion unpar

HR = heart rate; ICG = inferior cervical ganglion–fused C7-8; MCG = middle cervical ganglion–fused C5-6; SCG = superior cervical ganglion–fused C1-4; SG = stellate ganglion–fused T1-2; SV = stroke volume.

racic and lumbar regions of the spinal cord. The axons enter the white rami communicans to synapse with postganglionic neurons in the unpaired prevertebral ganglia or paired paravertebral chain ganglia that lie adjacent to the spinal cord. Postganglionic unmyelinated fibers join the spinal nerves through the gray rami communicans and synapse with sweat glands and smooth muscles in resistance arterioles and piloerector muscles. There are 24 pairs of paravertebral ganglia. The paired ganglia of the cervical region are fused into three ganglia (Table 8.2): superior, middle, and inferior cervical ganglion. The middle ganglion is often absent. The inferior cervical ganglion often fuses with the first and second thoracic ganglia to form the stellate ganglion. There is usually one pair of paravertebral ganglia for each thoracic and lumbar segment and four pairs of paravertebral ganglia in the sacral region. The unpaired prevertebral ganglia lie in plexuses anterior to the vertebral column in the thorax, abdomen, and pelvis (see Table 8.2).

AUTONOMIC FUNCTION

Clinical Evaluation

A wide range of symptoms may indicate abnormal function of the ANS. Characteristic autonomic symptoms are blurred vision due to defective pupillary accommodation; optic nerve or brain ischemia due to orthostatic hypotension; dry eyes or mouth due to impaired parasympathetic innervation to lacrimal or salivary glands; orthostatic lightheadedness with dull shoulder aching due to muscle ischemia as a result of hypotension; early satiety or alternating diarrhea and constipation due to gastrointestinal dysmotility; and urinary retention or sexual dysfunction due to sympathetic and parasympathetic den-

Table 8.3 Symptoms and Signs of Autonomic Dysfunction

Sympathetic	Parasympathetic
Orthostatic hypotension	Blurred vision
Blurred vision	Dilated pupils
Lightheadedness	Dry eyes
"Coat-hanger" pain	Dry mouth
Nonreactive pupils	Fixed heart rate
Sexual dysfunction	Resting tachycardia
Hypohidrosis	Abdominal pain
Anhidrosis	Early satiety
Heat intolerance	Nausea
Hyperhidrosis	Vomiting
	Constipation
	Ileus
	Diarrhea
	Urinary retention or frequency
	Incontinence
	Sexual dysfunction

ervation. Small fiber dysfunction, which can cause burning or lancinating pains of the hands or feet, may also cause hypohidrosis, anhidrosis, or compensatory hyperhidrosis (Table 8.3); patients with diabetic autonomic failure may also experience silent myocardial infarctions from the autonomic failure.[4] The onset, duration, and temporal profile of the autonomic symptoms should be ascertained. Information about current medications and concurrent illnesses, which may affect testing, should be obtained. Examination may reveal minimally reactive pupils, impaired blood pressure or heart rate control, distal anhidrosis, or decreased sensation to pain and temperature.

Laboratory Evaluation

Standard noninvasive laboratory assessment of autonomic function includes a battery of tests that evaluates cardiovascular and sudomotor reflexes.[5,6] Pupillary reflexes, evaluated using infrared and pharmacologic methods,[7] and gastrointestinal[8] and genitourinary[9] function evaluation are not discussed here. In general, for standard laboratory assessment of autonomic function, avoiding large meals, caffeine, and nicotine for at least 3 hours and alcohol for at least 12 hours before testing can facilitate the procedures and avoid potential confounding factors. Patients should be well hydrated, and those with diabetes should be euglycemic before testing. When possible, medications such as diuretics, fludrocortisone, anticholinergics, and sympatho- or parasympathomimetic agents should be discontinued for 48 hours before testing. Patients should be comfortable, and compressive clothing, such as Jobst stockings, should be removed and the bladder emptied before the onset of testing. Ideally, patients are allowed to relax in a quiet room for at least 10–20 minutes before testing.

Cardiovascular Autonomic Reflexes

The most commonly used tests of autonomic function are those that rely on cardiovascular changes: heart rate and blood pressure responses to deep breathing,

Table 8.4 Noninvasive Tests of Autonomic Function

Parasympathetic

Heart rate response to deep breathing

   (Standard deviation and MSSD of R-Ri)

   (E/I ratio* = longest R-Ri/shortest R-Ri)

Heart rate response to Valsalva maneuver

   (Valsalva ratio = longest R-Ri/shortest R-Ri)

Heart rate response to standing

   (30:15 ratio)

Sympathetic: vasomotor

Beat-to-beat BP responses to Valsalva maneuver

   $(BP_{phase\ IV} - BP_{phase\ before})$

Heart rate and BP responses to head-up tilt or active standing

Sympathetic: sudomotor

Quantitative sudomotor axon reflex test

Thermoregulatory sweat test

Sympathetic skin response

Silastic sweat imprint

BP = blood pressure; E/I ratio = expiratory/inspiratory ratio for the period of deep breathing; i = interval; MSSD = mean square of the successive differences.

*The E/I ratio is determined by dividing the longest R-R intervals (slowest heart rate) during expiration by the shortest R-R intervals (fastest heart rate) during inspiration.

Valsalva maneuver, and postural change. These tests are specific, sensitive, and safe and are widely used for diagnosis and monitoring of autonomic neuropathies (Table 8.4).

Testing these reflexes requires continuous electrocardiographic and blood pressure monitoring, now easily achieved with finger photoplethysmography (Finapres), which has accuracy comparable with intra-arterial pressure recordings. Beat-to-beat blood pressure and heart rate (R-R intervals) are analyzed in time and frequency domains.

Spectral analysis, using the fast Fourier transform algorithm, is widely used to quantify short-term oscillations in arterial pressure and heart rate. It is postulated that high-frequency bands (0.15–0.40 Hz) reflect mainly vagal influences on the sinus node, whereas low-frequency bands (0.02–0.15 Hz) reflect mainly sympathetic activity.

Paced Breathing. The increase in heart rate during inspiration and its decrease during expiration is known as *respiratory sinus arrhythmia*. This variability in heart rate is due to changes in vagal efferent nerve traffic and is accentuated during deep breathing. Both central and peripheral mechanisms are responsible for changing vagal efferent nerve traffic during the inspiratory and expiratory phases of breathing. Variability decreases with age and is affected by rate and depth of inspiration.[10] Heart rate response to deep breathing is the best noninvasive method to assess the integrity of cardiac vagal innervation[5] and is most often diminished in patients with autonomic neuropathies. The response to deep breathing can be measured as a change in heart rate or as a change in the R-R interval, which is the reciprocal of the instantaneous heart rate. R-R interval rather than heart rate should be used because it is most linearly related to cardiac

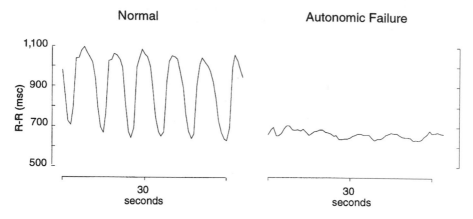

Figure 8.1 R-R intervals during paced breathing in a normal subject and in a patient with autonomic failure.

autonomic activity.[11,12] Patients are asked to breathe in a quiet and relaxed fashion for 5 minutes. They are then asked to breathe deeply for 1 minute at a rate of six breaths per minute (10 second cycle: 5 seconds of inspiration) (Figure 8.1). The standard deviation and the mean square of the successive differences of the R-R intervals are calculated for the period of quiet breathing.[13] The expiratory/inspiratory ratio is calculated for the period of deep breathing by dividing the longest R-R intervals (slowest heart rate) during expiration by the shortest R-R intervals (fastest heart rate) during inspiration ($R-R_{max}/R-R_{min}$). Values obtained from three cycles of six breaths a minute are averaged. The range of normal responses based on age from our laboratory is shown in Figure 8.2. Because these parameters decrease predictably in an age-related fashion, expiratory/inspiratory ratios are calculated and compared with plotted normal reference values for age.

Valsalva Maneuver. The Valsalva maneuver evaluates sympathetic and parasympathetic outflow. To perform the maneuver, the subject is asked to inhale deeply

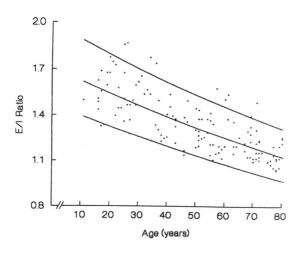

Figure 8.2 Expiratory/inspiratory (E/I) ratio during paced breathing in normal subjects according to age.

Figure 8.3 Muscle sympathetic nerve activity (MSNA), electrocardiogram (EKG), and blood pressure (BP) during the Valsalva maneuver in a healthy subject. The roman numerals at the top of the figure designate phases I–IV of the Valsalva maneuver.

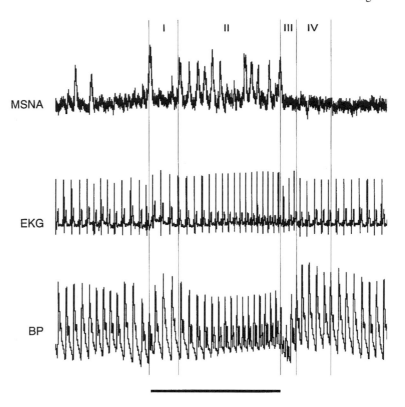

and then exhale forcibly into a leaky mouthpiece connected to a manometer and maintain a pressure of 40 millimeters of mercury (mm Hg) for 15–20 seconds. Blood pressure and heart rate are continuously recorded and four phases are identified (Figure 8.3)[14]:

Phase I: Mechanical compression of the aorta at the onset of expiration leads to the sudden rise of thoracic, abdominal, and blood pressure. Increased arterial pressure reduces heart rate for a few seconds due to a reflex increase in vagal efferent activity. This reduction in heart rate, however, does not always occur in normal individuals.

Phase II: Forcible exhaling against resistance increases intrathoracic pressure. Venous return is impeded, and blood pressure falls (early phase II). This fall in blood pressure triggers rapid tachycardia and vasoconstriction due to reflex parasympathetic withdrawal and increased sympathetic outflow, which leads to recovery in blood pressure (late phase II).

Phase III: After exhaling, the intrathoracic pressure returns to normal, which leads to a transient increase in pulmonary venous capacitance, which causes a fall in venous return. There is a further reduction in blood pressure while heart rate continues to increase.

Phase IV: Venous return increases, which leads to increased cardiac output. The vascular bed is still constricted due to increased sympathetic outflow during phases II and III leading to a systemic arterial pressure increase above baseline (i.e., "overshoot"), and there is reflex (i.e., "rebound") bradycardia due to reflex increase in vagal efferent activity.

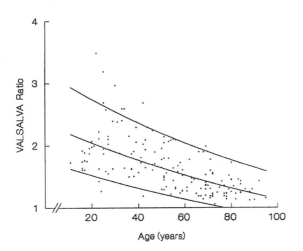

Figure 8.4 The Valsalva ratio in healthy subjects according to age.

Phases I and III are due to the mechanical factors, whereas Phases II and IV are due to changes in sympathetic and vagal outflow due to baroreflex activation. A deficiency in sympathetic outflow blunts the increase in blood pressure during phase IV[15]; therefore, there is no stimulus for increased vagal activity, which in turn will not produce bradycardia. In autonomic failure, subnormal sympathetic outflow leads to defective peripheral vasoconstriction. Blood pressure during phase II decreases markedly, and there is no blood pressure "overshoot" and no bradycardia during phase IV (see Figure 8.3). If vagal outflow is deficient, bradycardia does not occur. The *Valsalva ratio* is the ratio of the longest R-R interval during phase IV (bradycardia due to vagal activation) to the shortest R-R interval during phase II (tachycardia due to vagal withdrawal and sympathetic activation) (R-R_{max}/R-R_{min}). The Valsalva ratio is used as an index of cardiovagal function. The normal range in our laboratory is shown in Figure 8.4. Calculated Valsalva ratios are compared to normal ranges plotted by age. The Valsalva maneuver can be performed in the supine or sitting position. The cardiovascular and autonomic changes triggered by the maneuver are effort and position dependent and diminish with age.[10] Because forced expiration against resistance can increase the risk of retinal hemorrhage or lens dislocation, the Valsalva maneuver should be avoided in patients with proliferative retinopathy.[1]

Orthostatic Stress. Changes in blood pressure and heart rate induced by active standing or passive tilt provide valuable information. Orthostatic hypotension is the most characteristic symptom of sympathetic adrenergic dysfunction, particularly the splanchnic sympathetic outflow. Assuming an upright position by actively standing or using a tilt table (i.e., passive tilt) leads to a transient decrease in systolic, diastolic, and mean blood pressure due to the sudden venous pooling of blood in the legs, which lowers cardiac output and venous return. Baroreflex mechanisms lead to sympathetic activation and vagal withdrawal with vasoconstriction and tachycardia. Normally, a heart rate increase of 10–20 beats per minute and recovery of blood pressure occur within 1 minute of tilt. Using a tilt table is often advantageous in patients with weakness secondary to their neuromuscular disorders. Response to orthostatic stress is affected by food ingestion, time of day, state of hydration, ambient temperature, recent recumbency, postural

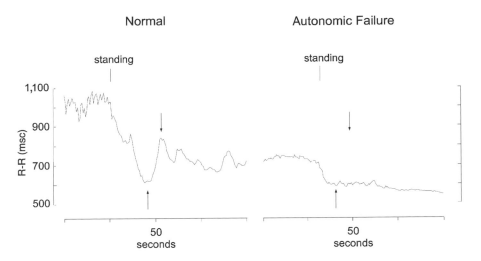

Figure 8.5 R-R intervals during active standing in a healthy subject and a patient with autonomic failure. Arrows show fifteenth and thirtieth heartbeat after standing.

deconditioning, hypertension, medications, gender, and age.[10] Blood pressure and heart rate are recorded after 1 and 5 minutes in the upright position. Greater changes are often seen when subjects are allowed to lie supine for 20 minutes before standing. *Orthostatic hypotension* is defined as a drop in systolic blood pressure of at least 20 mm Hg, a drop of diastolic blood pressure of at least 10 mm Hg, or both within 3 minutes of standing or using a tilt table at an angle of at least 60 degrees.[16] In some patients, a significant fall in blood pressure occurs only after a 10- to 20-minute period of standing.

Orthostatic hypotension may be symptomatic or asymptomatic, perhaps according to the efficacy of cerebral autoregulatory mechanisms. With active standing, the fastest heart rate or shortest R-R interval occurs around the fifteenth beat, whereas the maximal slowing of the heart rate or longest R-R interval occurs by the thirtieth beat.[17] The ratio between the longest to the shortest R-R should be greater than 1. If there is no change in heart rate, this ratio is less than or equal to 1. The 30 to 15 ratio (R-R interval at beat 30 divided by R-R interval at beat 15) is an index of cardiovagal function (Figure 8.5). The hallmark of diffuse autonomic failure, involving both sympathetic and parasympathetic systems, is a fall in blood pressure without compensatory tachycardia (Figure 8.6). A fall in blood pressure without heart rate changes indicates baroreflex abnormality. A prolonged tilt of 40 minutes is used to reproduce vasodepressor syncope. Infusion of pharmacologic agents, such as isoproterenol, is also used in some laboratories.

Pressor Stimuli. Normally, isometric exercise, cold stimulus, and mental stress all increase blood pressure through activation of sympathetic vasoconstrictor outflow, independent of the baroreflex. Before isometric exercise, the blood pressure is measured at rest. The subject is then asked to squeeze a handgrip dynamometer for as long as possible with the dominant hand (usually 1–2 minutes) at maximum effort to determine the maximum voluntary contraction. After 5 minutes of rest, handgrip is maintained at 30% of the maximum voluntary con-

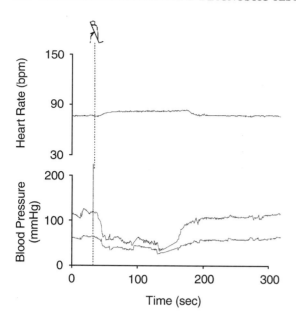

Figure 8.6 Blood pressure and heart rate response to passive head-up tilt (as depicted in the figure at the top of the graph) in a patient with autonomic failure. (bpm = beats per minute.)

traction or at least 3 minutes with continuous blood pressure and electrocardiograph monitoring. A normal response to isometric exercise is an increase in diastolic pressure of more than 15 mm Hg.[18] In the cold pressor test, cutaneous application of a cold stimulus is used to increase blood pressure and heart rate. Heart rate increases maximally during the first 30 seconds, whereas blood pressure rises steadily during 2 minutes. To perform the test, a hand is immersed in ice water (4°C) for 1 minute. Care is taken to avoid isometric contraction, breath-holding, or inadvertent Valsalva maneuvers, all of which can increase blood pressure. Of course, pain and temperature sensation must be intact for the reflex to occur. A normal response occurs within 1 minute with an increase in systolic blood pressure greater than 15 mm Hg and an increase in heart rate of 10 beats per minute. Testing is not sensitive, and it is frequently difficult to maintain the hand in ice water for a full minute. Mental stress, such as that induced by mental arithmetic,[19] unlike isometric exercise and the cold pressor test, does not use peripheral afferent pathways to increase sympathetic outflow and transiently increases blood pressure and heart rate. These changes, however, can be minor and are absent in many normal subjects. A normal response is an increase in blood pressure of 15 mm Hg and heart rate of 10 beats per minute above baseline values.

Venoarteriolar Reflex. Systemic vascular resistance increases with posture or limb dependency, due in part to local arteriolar constriction that occurs secondary to venous distension. This increase in vascular resistance is due to a local axon reflex (venoarterial reflex) of sympathetic C fibers that produce arteriolar vasoconstriction. The venoarteriolar reflex may be responsible for up to 40% of the total increase in limb vascular resistance elicited by standing. The venoarteriolar reflex is evaluated by measuring the change in blood flow in the dependent leg flexed at the knee with the subject recumbent. The reduction in flow is equivalent to the reflex vasoconstriction.[20,21]

Table 8.5 Sudomotor Innervation

Level	Innervation
T1-2	Ipsilateral face
T2-6	Upper limb
T5-12	Trunk
T10-L3	Lower limb

L = lumbar; T = thoracic.

Sudomotor Function

Sudomotor fibers can be activated locally by injection or by iontophoresis of a cholinergic agent in the skin or by a rise in body temperature that causes sweating over the entire body. Sudomotor function is assessed by the quantity or distribution of sweat output. The main neurotransmitter of sudomotor postganglionic fibers, unlike other postganglionic sympathetic nerves, is acetylcholine. Sudomotor function is affected by temperature, gender, and age. The total number of sweat glands is present at birth and regresses with age. Loss of sudomotor function correlates with the loss of unmyelinated nerve fibers. Because of multilevel skin innervation, sudomotor dermatomes are less precise than sensory dermatomes (Table 8.5). Sudomotor cholinergic unmyelinated fibers are frequently affected in small-fiber neuropathies.[22]

Quantitative Sudomotor Axon Reflex Test. The quantitative sudomotor axon reflex test (QSART) evaluates postganglionic sudomotor nerves using iontophoresis of acetylcholine, which stimulates an axon reflex in sudomotor nerves.[23] The iontophoresed acetylcholine activates a sudomotor sympathetic C fiber, which conducts an impulse antidromically to a branch point; then, the impulse travels orthodromically through a different sympathetic C fiber that releases acetylcholine and binds to muscarinic (M3) receptors in sweat glands (Figure 8.7).[24] The sweat released is cap-

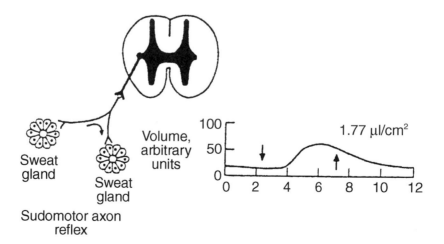

Figure 8.7 Quantitative sudomotor axon reflex. **Left:** Axon reflex (see text). **Right:** Representative axon-reflex sweat response. (Reprinted with permission from PA Low, TL Opfer-Gehrking, M Kihara. In vivo studies on receptor pharmacology of human eccrine sweat gland. Clin Auton Res 1992;2:29–34.)

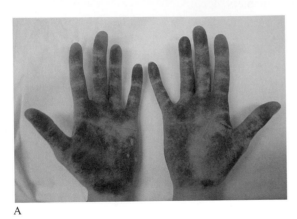
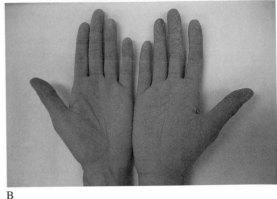

A   B

Figure 8.8 Thermoregulatory sweat test (see text). **A.** Hands of patient with palmar hyperhidrosis before treatment. **B.** Hands of the same patient after treatment.

tured using a multicompartmental cell, and its volume is calculated using a sudorometer. Capsules are placed at four sites: proximal foot, distal leg, proximal leg, and medial forearm. Reduced or absent sweat output indicates postganglionic sympathetic sudomotor failure. Polyneuropathies show loss of distal sweat volume or a distal to proximal gradient loss.[25] Exaggerated or persistent sweat activity has been shown to occur in the early stages of diabetic polyneuropathy, before the loss of sudomotor function.[26,27]

Thermoregulatory Sweat Test. Thermoregulation is primarily under sympathetic control involving sudomotor, vasomotor, and pilomotor nerves, with the sweat glands playing a major role. Sweat production induced by thermal stimuli is detected by covering the body surface with a chemical that changes color when moistened.[25] The thermoregulatory sweat test uses increases in blood and skin temperature to assess distribution of sweat production.[25] A mixture of alizarin red, sodium carbonate, and cornstarch is painted on the patient. The patient lies on a stretcher, which is then placed in a sweat cabinet. The temperature in the sweat cabinet is kept between 44 and 50°C with a relative humidity of 35–45%. Using overhead infrared lights, patients are monitored until their body temperatures rise to 38°C or increase by 1°C more than their baseline temperatures. A digital photograph is taken for semiquantitative analysis. A pixel counter is used to determine the amount or percentage of anhidrosis present. A correlation between the degree of autonomic neuropathy and percentage of anhidrosis has been demonstrated with thermoregulatory testing.[25] To demonstrate this method, digital photographs of the hands of a patient with hyperhidrosis before and after treatment with local intradermal injections of botulinum toxin are shown in Figure 8.8.[28] The areas in purple indicate excessive sweating, whereas the areas in yellow indicate an absence of sweating. Botulinum toxin blocks acetylcholine release from sympathetic postganglionic sudomotor nerves. After treatment, there is a marked reduction in sweating in the hands of the patient with palmar hyperhidrosis. Thermoregulatory testing is painless, noninvasive, and valuable in assessing areas of the body, such as the thoracic region, that are difficulty to test otherwise.

Silastic Imprint of Sweat Droplets. Iontophoresis of pilocarpine (2 mA for 5 minutes) over a centimeter squared (cm^2) area of skin over the dorsum of the foot is used to directly stimulate sweat droplet formation. Sweat droplets can be measured by spreading a silastic impression material over the skin, which creates a mold that retains the spherical contours of sweat droplets. The number, size, volume, and density of sweat droplets are measured using a dissection microscope, counting grid, and digitizer.[29] Histograms of sweat droplet size and sweat volume show age-dependent changes.[30] In patients with diabetes, a decrease in the number and volume of silastic sweat droplet imprints was found to correlate with clinical loss of pain sensation and abnormalities of cardiovascular reflexes.[30] Sweat droplets can still be detected when the QSART response is absent because pilocarpine stimulates the sweat glands directly. Mild or early QSART abnormalities, seen in early distal polyneuropathies, correspond to an over-representation of large droplets on silastic imprints.[27] Because the thermoregulatory sweat test evaluates pre- and postganglionic function, and the QSART and silastic imprint of sweat droplets specifically evaluate postganglionic function, the tests are complimentary and allow precise localization of the site of the lesion.

Tear Production. Dry eyes due to impaired innervation of lacrimal glands can be evaluated using Schirmer's test,[31] in which a strip of sterile filter paper is placed in the lower conjunctival sac to measure tear production (normal results are >5 mm of tear production in 5 minutes), or by placing Rose-Bengal dye[32] in the lower conjunctival sac, which stains to demonstrate areas of keratoconjunctivitis sicca.

Sympathetic Skin Response. The *sympathetic skin response* (SSR) is a transient change in the electrical potential of the skin owing to a change in electrical conductance as a result of sweat production. The SSR is based on the galvanic skin response, a test developed in 1888 to measure the change in skin resistance induced by pain and emotion.[33] The galvanic skin response was abandoned in most neurologic clinical neurophysiology laboratories because skin resistance was difficult to measure consistently.[33,34] The SSR is simple to elicit. Testing requires only standard electromyography equipment and can be evoked by different types of stimuli, including electrical stimulation, startle, deep inspiration, and cough. The responses are recorded using active electrodes in the palms and soles, referenced to electrodes over the dorsal surfaces of the hands and feet.[35] The SSR can be variable in size and form and has a tendency to habituate with repeated stimuli.[36] The SSR is affected by many factors, including temperature, age, stress, light, and medications. Criteria for abnormal SSR are controversial, but asymmetric or absent responses are considered abnormal. The SSR is correlated with changes in cardiovascular and sudomotor reflexes in patients with severe autonomic neuropathy.[37] It has been suggested that the afferent limb for the SSRs is in large-diameter myelinated fibers, which may be affected in severe polyneuropathies.[38] The SSR is discussed in detail in Chapter 5.

Other Tests of Autonomic Function

Infusion of pressor or depressor agents or a neck suction chamber that acts on carotid stretch receptors is used to evaluate baroreflex responses in specialized physiology laboratories. Limb plethysmography and laser Doppler flowmetry are used to evaluate sympathetic vasomotor function. Catecholamine measurements in plasma and urine are classic indicators of sympathetic adrenergic function. Newer tests, such as epidermal skin biopsy and autoantibody assays, may provide additional information about pathogenesis. Thermography is of uncertain value. Microneurography is too time consuming and invasive to be included in a standard battery of autonomic testing, but it is the only way to record directly from the autonomic nerve. In systemic disorders, such as diabetes and amyloidosis with cardiac and other end-organ damage, it is important to remember that noninvasive autonomic testing depends on end-organ responsiveness.

Microneurography. Noninvasive autonomic testing is indirect, evaluating the effector organs and not the autonomic nerves. Microneurography, however, has made it possible to record postganglionic sympathetic nerve activity directly. Although the technique has contributed significantly to our understanding of autonomic physiology, microneurography is invasive and time consuming and cannot be used in routine clinical assessments. Microneurography is discussed in detail in Chapter 4. Selective placement of tungsten microelectrodes with very small tip diameters in the appropriate nerve fascicles of easily accessible nerves, such as the peroneal or radial nerve, permits recording of multiunit sympathetic postganglionic electrophysiologic activity.[39] Both sympathetic nerves to blood vessels in striated muscle and the skin can be recorded.[40,41] Muscle sympathetic nerve recordings have a burst pattern, which is synchronous with the pulse. There is also increased burst frequency with expiratory breath-holds and phases II and III of the Valsalva maneuver (see Figure 8.3), but the activity does not respond to arousal or skin stroking. These features are used to discriminate between muscle and skin sympathetic nerve fibers. Results are expressed as bursts per minute or per 100 heartbeats. Because this technique is laborious and invasive and has tremendous interindividual variability, microneurography is a research tool that requires considerable expertise and cooperative patients. This technique is also valuable in the study of other small-caliber fibers (covered in Chapter 4).

Laser Doppler Flowmetry. Laser Doppler flowmetry is used to measure blood flow noninvasively without the changes in tissue compliance seen in limb plethysmography.[42] Blood flow is measured in fingers and toes because these areas only contain vasoconstrictor, and not vasodilator, fibers. Changes in blood flow of the fingers and toes are an index of arteriolar or local sympathetic activity. Inspiratory gasp, standing, cold pressor, and the Valsalva maneuver have all been to shown to cause an abrupt fall in blood flow.[21,42] Although distal blood flow can be affected by thermal and emotional stimuli, there appears to be good retest reliability if laser blood flow measurements are paired with arousal stimuli of peripheral sympathetic function such as an electrical stimulus, similar to the stimulus used in the SSR. These changes in blood flow, when paired with an arousal stimulus appear to be useful markers for early autonomic dysfunction in diabetes.[43]

Thermography. Thermography measures alterations in skin temperature using infrared and liquid crystal imaging. It is a painless and noninvasive test. In a controlled temperature environment, multiple photographs are taken of the affected and unaffected limb to determine temperature asymmetries using different colors for different temperatures. Thermography is less useful than electromyography or imaging studies in the diagnosis of entrapment neuropathies[44] and cervical[45] or lumbar radiculopathies.[46] It has been recommended that thermography be used only as an adjunct test in peripheral nerve injury, complex regional pain syndrome, focal autonomic neuropathies, and assessment of insensitive acral parts.[47]

Epidermal Skin Biopsy. Patients with small-fiber neuropathies often have distal anhidrosis due to degeneration of postganglionic unmyelinated sudomotor axons, which cannot be evaluated by conventional electrophysiologic studies.[48] Skin punch biopsies[49] or suction blisters[50] are inexpensive, minimally invasive techniques with low potential for scarring and infection.[51] Studies using skin biopsies have shown that C and possibly A-δ fiber densities are reduced in patients with small-fiber neuropathies, and this loss correlates with absent ankle jerks, absent sural sensory nerve action potentials,[52,53] and abnormalities on quantitative sensory testing.[54] Under confocal microscopy,[49] cutaneous nerves are best visualized using immunohistochemical staining for protein gene product 9.5.[55] This topic is also discussed and illustrated in Chapter 19.

Plasma and Urinary Catecholamines. Norepinephrine and its metabolites are accessible markers of sympathetic neural function, easily measured in the blood and urine. Circulating norepinephrine originates mostly in sympathetic nerves with only a small contribution (3–8%) from the adrenal medulla.[56] When sympathetic nerves are stimulated, approximately 10–20% of noradrenaline released into the synaptic cleft escapes neuronal reuptake and "spills over" into the bloodstream.[57] Plasma norepinephrine doubles with the upright posture in normal subjects, whereas in patients with autonomic failure, there is no change or a mild increase in noradrenaline in the upright posture.[58] In patients with autonomic neuropathies affecting postganglionic sympathetic fibers, like diabetes, noradrenaline at rest is usually low.[59] Plasma catecholamines are insensitive for detecting the presence of adrenergic failure but are essential in detecting dopamine β-hydroxylase (DBH) or related deficiencies.[60,61]

DISORDERS WITH AUTONOMIC INVOLVEMENT

Neuromuscular disorders with prominent autonomic involvement affect preganglionic autonomic neurons, postganglionic nerve bodies (located in sympathetic and parasympathetic ganglia), or postganglionic autonomic axons in peripheral nerves. Autonomic disorders can be classified according to the neurotransmitter of the affected postganglionic autonomic neuron: adrenergic (sympathetic), cholinergic (parasympathetic), or both, referred to as *pandysautonomia*. The main neurotransmitter in sympathetic postganglionic neurons is noradrenaline; acetylcholine is the main neurotransmitter in sympathetic sudomotor and all postganglionic parasympathetic neurons. Acetylcholine is also the main neurotransmitter in the neuromuscular junction. Thus, cholinergic disorders may present with autonomic dysfunction, muscle weakness, or both. The pandysautonomias are a combination of adrenergic and cholinergic dysfunction. The most common disorders with autonomic involvement are listed in Table 8.6.

Table 8.6 Disorders with Autonomic Nervous System Involvement

Adrenergic dysautonomias	Chronic small-fiber neuropathies
Pure adrenergic neuropathy	Diabetes
(Dopamine β-hydroxylase deficiency)	Amyloidosis
Cholinergic dysautonomias	Hereditary (HSAN-III, HSAN-IV, and
Acute cholinergic dysautonomia	Fabry's disease)
Chronic idiopathic anhidrosis	Infection (human immunodeficiency virus)
Adie's syndrome	Subacute or chronic sensory and autonomic
Chaga's disease	ganglionopathies
Botulism	Paraneoplastic
Lambert-Eaton myasthenic syndrome	Sjögren's syndrome
Pandysautonomias	
Ganglionic and postganglionic disorders	
Pure autonomic failure	
Acute and subacute neuropathies	
Acute pandysautonomia	
Guillain-Barré syndrome	
Paraneoplastic pandysautonomia	
Porphyria	
Toxins	
Drugs	

HSAN = hereditary sensory and autonomic neuropathy.

Adrenergic Dysautonomias

Pure adrenergic neuropathies are uncommon. The best examples are patients with the autosomal recessive disorder who have a deficiency of the enzyme that converts dopamine to noradrenaline. The human DBH gene has been localized to chromosome 9q34.[62] These patients have sympathetic adrenergic failure with preserved sympathetic cholinergic and parasympathetic function. Onset of this disorder is in childhood with postural hypotension, with or without ptosis and nasal stuffiness. Plasma levels of noradrenaline and adrenaline are undetectable, whereas dopamine levels are abnormally high.[63,64]

Cholinergic Dysautonomias

Acute or chronic cholinergic autonomic neuropathies occur as postinfectious or paraneoplastic syndromes. Symptoms of acute cholinergic neuropathies[65,66] are sudden loss of tear or saliva formation, anhidrosis, constipation, gastroparesis, paralytic ileus, abdominal pain, and urinary retention. When pupillary function is disrupted, vision is blurred. A rare disorder, chronic idiopathic anhidrosis,[67] is characterized by isolated loss of sudomotor function, due to pre- or postganglionic disruption of sympathetic cholinergic neurotransmission. Patients develop heat intolerance because of an inability to sweat when exercising or in response to increased ambient temperature.

Chaga's disease, a disorder endemic in South America, is caused by *Trypanosoma cruzi*, one of only two types of parasite that selectively invades and damages peripheral nerves.[68] The parasite enters the body orally or through broken skin or mucous membranes and invades cells of neuroectodermal (glial cells, nerve cells, and Schwann cells) or mesenchymal origin (adipose tissue and smooth and striated muscle). Circulating antibodies to β-adrenergic and muscarinic cholinergic receptors have been found and are thought to trigger an autoimmune reaction against β-adrenergic and muscarinic cells.[68] In the chronic stages of infection, these cells die and lead to characteristically enlarged hollow organs. Cardiomyopathy,[69] megaesophagus, and megacolon are characteristic of cell loss in parasympathetic cardiac ganglia and in ganglia within the Meissner's and Auerbach's plexuses. Cholinergic denervation is prominent with abnormalities of parasympathetic cardiac reflexes, pupillary responses,[70,71] and SSRs.[72] Vasomotor sympathetic function appears to be relatively spared.

Botulism and LEMS impair the release of acetylcholine in somatic and autonomic nerves, producing muscle weakness and cholinergic dysautonomia.[73] Botulism presents as an ascending, predominantly motor polyneuropathy with cranial nerve involvement, beginning 12–36 hours after ingesting food contaminated with the neurotoxins of the anaerobic bacteria *Clostridium botulinum*. The botulinum toxin impairs the presynaptic calcium-associated release of acetylcholine, leading to symptoms of cholinergic failure: dry eyes, dry mouth, blurred vision, dizziness, paralytic ileus, urinary retention, and anhidrosis.[74] Treatment is supportive with close monitoring as respiratory failure and cardiac arrhythmia can occur. Recovery is often protracted with autonomic dysfunction lasting as long as 6 months after onset.

Dry mouth, erectile dysfunction, proximal muscle weakness, and depressed tendon weakness are the most common symptoms of LEMS.[75–77] The syndrome is a paraneoplastic autoimmune disorder most commonly seen in association with small cell lung carcinoma. The risk of developing cancer is estimated to be 62% during the next 2 years after diagnosis; this risk decreases over time.[75] Autoantibodies to voltage-gated calcium channels, most commonly the P/Q type, have been found.[78] Autonomic dysfunction is worse in older patients with an underlying carcinoma[76] but improves with treatment of the underlying carcinoma.[77]

Pandysautonomias

Pandysautonomias involve sympathetic and parasympathetic neurons. *Pure autonomic failure*, a typical pandysautonomia, is a slowly progressive degenerative disorder of peripheral sympathetic and parasympathetic neurons.[79] Peripheral autonomic nerves in these patients contain α-synuclein–positive Lewy bodies, similar to those in Parkinson's disease patients.[80] Pandysautonomic neuropathies can be divided into *preganglionic demyelinating* and *postganglionic axonopathic*.[81] These neuropathies are acute or subacute with gradual but often incomplete recovery.[81,82] These acute and subacute neuropathies produce severe sympathetic and parasympathetic dysfunction: blurred vision, dry eyes and mouth, nausea, vomiting, abdominal pain, diarrhea, constipation, impotence, and loss of sweating. The acute pandysautonomias are uncommon and often affect healthy young individuals. Those with a protracted course and incomplete recovery are, more frequently, postganglionic axonal.[66,81] The preganglionic demyelinating pandysautonomia with involvement of the somatic nervous system may be on a spectrum ranging from pure pandysautonomia—with minimal somatic deficits—to classic Guillain-Barré syndrome (GBS)[83] and may have a better outcome than the postganglionic axonopathic pandysautonomia.[81] The cause of these pandysautonomias is unknown, but a postinfectious or other immune-mediated process is postulated. In the mid-1990s, reports showed complete recovery in a few patients with apparent postganglionic axonopathic pandysautonomia who were treated early with intravenous immunoglobulin therapy.[84] In some instances, paraneoplastic disorders may present as an acute pandysautonomic neuropathy,[73] and autoantibodies to ganglionic acetylcholine receptors have been identified.[85]

Signs of autonomic hyper- or hypoactivity are present in one- to two-thirds of patients with the acute inflammatory demyelinating polyradiculoneuropathy or GBS.[86] GBS classically presents as a symmetric ascending weakness, with or without cranial nerve involvement and areflexia; the degree of autonomic dysfunction does not necessarily correlate with the degree of somatic peripheral neuropathy.[87] In the majority of cases, there is mild autonomic hypoactivity with decreased pupillary function, resting tachycardia owing to decreased parasympathetic activity, and ileus. Urinary retention is less common. With autonomic hyperactivity, sweating is excessive, and there can be alternating hyper- or hypotension and alternating brady- or tachycardia. Measurements of R-R interval variability can be used to monitor autonomic dysfunction. Mortality is increased with significant dysautonomia.[88]

Neuropathies due to abnormal porphyrin metabolism are rare and only occur in the hepatic forms of porphyria (acute intermittent porphyria, hereditary coproporphyria, variegate porphyria, and delta-aminolevulinic acid dehydratase deficiency porphyria).[89] The clinical presentation is acute, and colicky abdominal pain, psychiatric disturbances, and acute polyneuropathy are present. The polyneuropathy can resemble GBS but can also be predominantly asymmetric or focal affecting proximal and distal muscles (e.g., wrist or foot drop). Sensory symptoms are mild. Facial weakness and dysphagia are common. Clinically, autonomic overactivity is frequent and may coexist with autonomic failure.[90] Symptoms include hypertension, pupillary dilatation, tachycardia, abdominal pain, constipation, diarrhea, urinary hesitancy and excessive sweating or anhidrosis.[73,89] Abnormalities seen in autonomic testing are usually reversible, although persistent abnormalities have been reported.[90] Heavy metal poisoning, such as thallium and arsenic, should also be considered in cases of acute abdominal pain and polyneuropathy. Blood and urine measurements of porphyrins and heavy metals can help distinguish these two entities.

Toxins and drugs cause a variety of autonomic neuropathies.[91] Cholinergic crises occur with organophosphate poisoning due to the anticholinesterase activity, which stimulates both sympathetic and parasympathetic activity. Sudomotor dysfunction occurs with chronic acrylamide,[92,93] arsenic,[93] or inorganic mercury poisoning. Orthostatic hypotension may occur with the use of perhexiline[94] and antineoplastic medications, such as cisplatin,[95] paclitaxel (Taxol),[96] and vincristine.[97] Victims of solvent intoxication have been shown to develop dizziness, vascular instability, palpitation, and erectile dysfunction, in addition to a sensory polyneuropathy.[98] Autonomic symptoms present fairly quickly with vincristine[91] but may be delayed in onset with thallium poisoning.[99]

Chronic small-fiber (postganglionic) neuropathies can be metabolic (diabetes or amyloidosis), inherited (hereditary and sensory autonomic neuropathy [HSAN]-III, HSAN-IV, and Fabry's disease) or infectious (e.g., human immunodeficiency virus [HIV]). Autonomic dysfunction in both amyloid and diabetes tends to involve all organ systems. Predominant autonomic failure (pronounced orthostatic hypotension and a fixed heart rate) may be the presenting feature. More frequently, patients show a mixed pattern of distal small-fiber autonomic and sensory neuropathy or predominantly small-fiber sensory neuropathy with only mild autonomic involvement. The autonomic symptoms may accompany, precede, or follow the somatic neuropathy.[73,100] Alternating diarrhea and constipation, explosive diarrhea, urinary retention, and anhidrosis or gustatory hyperhidrosis may be present. Erectile dysfunction is the most common autonomic symptom in diabetes,[18,101] and sudomotor changes may be the earliest sign in diabetic neuropathy.[26,102,103] Testing sudomotor function is particularly useful in the diagnosis of the diabetic thoracic polyneuropathy or diabetic lumbosacral radiculoplexus neuropathy—both of which are difficult to diagnosis with standard electrophysiologic testing.[25]

The ANS involvement in inherited disorders is best characterized in HSAN type III (Riley-Day syndrome), HSAN type IV, and Fabry's Disease. Riley-Day syndrome, also referred to as *familial dysautonomia* or *HSAN type III*, is a recessive disorder of Ashkenazi Jews due to a missense mutation in chromosome 9q31. Peripheral autonomic, motor, and sensory neurons are affected.[104] Infants present with poor feeding, unexplained fevers, abnormalities in lacrimation and salivation, excessive sweating, skin blotching, periodic vomiting, and difficulties in blood pressure and temperature control. Fungiform papillae of the tongue are absent. *HSAN-IV* is an autosomal recessive disorder seen in infancy. These children are described as having insensitivity to pain and can present with multiple mutilating injuries. They cannot distinguish between sharp and dull or hot and cold. Sweating is impaired; because of truncal anhidrosis, children can have high fevers with changes in ambient temperatures. There is no change in blood pressure to cold pressors. The neuropathy is due to a congenital loss of small and unmyelinated fibers.[105]

Fabry's disease is an X-linked disorder due to a deficiency of lysosomal α-galactoside A activity.[106] Young male patients often present with symptoms of small-fiber neuropathy with distal sharp, shooting, or burning pains in their hands and feet. Sweating is often impaired. Pupillary function is abnormal with abnormal tear and saliva production. Female carriers can also develop symptoms of small-fiber dysfunction later in life. Diagnosis can be made by genetic testing or by nerve or skin biopsies.[107,108]

Pandysautonomias are commonly associated with HIV and acquired immunodeficiency syndrome.[109] Peripheral neuropathies may be the most common complication of HIV-1 infection.[110] The autonomic dysfunction is frequent, often occurs in the presence of a distal sensory polyneuropathy, and worsens in the later stages of HIV infection.[111] Autonomic symptoms are present in up to 60% of patients. Bladder and sexual dysfunction are the most common symptoms. Testing reveals sympathetic and parasympathetic dysfunction.[112]

Chronic (or subacute) autonomic neuropathies or ganglionopathies are associated with paraneoplastic syndromes and Sjögren's syndrome. The chronic paraneoplastic autonomic neuropathies are similar to the acute and subacute pandysautonomias previously described.[73,113] Patients with anti-Hu antibody–related paraneoplastic syndrome presenting with progressive dysautonomia have been described, both with acute onset and subacute course of neurologic symptoms. Autonomic symptoms may improve with treatment of the underlying cancer. The neuropathies of Sjögren's syndrome are predominantly sensory polyneuropathies or ganglionopathies with superimposed mononeuropathies, autonomic and cranial neuropathies of variable severity. The pathophysiology is inflammatory or sometimes vasculitic in origin.[114,115] Autonomic dysfunction is mild, affecting sympathetic and parasympathetic fibers. Tonic pupils, sudomotor dysfunction, and isolated cases of cholinergic dysfunction and severe pandysautonomia have been reported.[116]

CONCLUSIONS

Autonomic dysfunction is symptomatic in various neuromuscular disorders. Early recognition leads to proper diagnosis and management. A battery of well-standardized cardiovascular and sudomotor tests is useful to evaluate ANS function and as secondary endpoints in clinical trials.[60,117] Noninvasive autonomic testing evaluates unmyelinated and small myelinated sympathetic and parasympathetic fibers that cannot be evaluated with other neurophysiologic tools. Autonomic dysfunction in patients with GBS and diabetes is associated with increased morbidity and mortality.[18,88] Noninvasive autonomic testing is particularly useful to evaluate the efficacy of novel therapies aimed at nerve regeneration in disorders like diabetes that typically affect distal small myelinated and unmyelinated nerve fibers.

REFERENCES

1. Ewing DJ, Clarke BF. Autonomic neuropathy: its diagnosis and prognosis. Clin Endocrinol Metab 1986;15:855–888.
2. Burgos LG, Ebert TJ, Asiddao C, et al. Increased intraoperative cardiovascular morbidity in diabetics with autonomic neuropathy. Anesthesiology 1989;70:591–597.
3. Brading A. The Autonomic Nervous System and Its Effectors. Oxford: Blackwell Science, 1999.
4. O'Sullivan JJ, Conroy RM, MacDonald K, et al. Silent ischaemia in diabetic men with autonomic neuropathy. Br Heart J 1991;66:313–315.
5. Assessment: clinical autonomic testing report of the Therapeutics and Technology Assessment Subcommittee of the American Academy of Neurology. Neurology 1996;46:873–880.
6. Ewing DJ, Martyn CN, Young RJ, Clarke BF. The value of cardiovascular autonomic function tests: 10 years experience in diabetes. Diabetes Care 1985;8:491–498.
7. Kawasaki A, Kardon RH. Disorders of the pupil. Ophthalmol Clin North Am 2001;14:149–168.
8. Camilleri M. Disorders of gastrointestinal motility in neurologic diseases. Mayo Clin Proc 1990; 65:825–846.
9. Fowler CJ. Neurological disorders of micturition and their treatment. Brain 1999;122:1213–1231.
10. Low PA. Effect of age and gender on sudomotor and cardiovagal function and blood pressure response to tilt in normal subjects. Muscle Nerve 1997;20:1561–1568.
11. Carlsten A, Folkow B, Hamberger C. Cardiovascular effect of direct vagal stimulation in man. Acta Physiol Scand 1957;41:68–76.
12. Koizumi K, Kollai M. Control of reciprocal and non-reciprocal action of vagal and sympathetic efferents: study of centrally induced reactions. J Auton Nerv Syst 1981;3:483–501.
13. Ewing DJ, Borsey DQ, Bellavere F, Clarke BF. Cardiac autonomic neuropathy in diabetes: comparison of measures of R-R interval variation. Diabetologia 1981;21:18–24.
14. Benarroch EE, Opfer-Gehrking TL, Low PA. Use of the photoplethysmographic technique to analyze the Valsalva maneuver in normal man. Muscle Nerve 1991;14:1165–1172.
15. Sandroni P, Benarroch EE, Low PA. Pharmacological dissection of components of the Valsalva maneuver in adrenergic failure. J Appl Physiol 1991;71:1563–1567.
16. The Consensus Committee of the American Autonomic Society and the American Academy of Neurology. Consensus statement on the definition of orthostatic hypotension, pure autonomic failure, and multiple system atrophy. Neurology 1996;46:1470.

17. Ewing DJ, Hume L, Campbell IW, et al. Autonomic mechanisms in the initial heart rate response to standing. J Appl Physiol 1980;49:809–814.

18. Ewing DJ, Campbell IW, Clarke BF. Assessment of cardiovascular effects in diabetic autonomic neuropathy and prognostic implications. Ann Intern Med 1980;92:308–311.

19. Locatelli A, Franzetti I, Lepore G, et al. Mental arithmetic stress as a test for evaluation of diabetic sympathetic autonomic neuropathy. Diabet Med 1989;6:490–495.

20. Moy S, Opfer Gehrking TL, Proper CJ, Low PA. The venoarteriolar reflex in diabetic and other neuropathies. Neurology 1989;39:1490–1492.

21. Schuller TB, Hermann K, Baron R. Quantitative assessment and correlation of sympathetic, parasympathetic, and afferent small fiber function in peripheral neuropathy. J Neurol 2000; 247:267–272.

22. Stewart JD, Low PA, Fealey RD. Distal small fiber neuropathy: results of tests of sweating and autonomic cardiovascular reflexes. Muscle Nerve 1992;15:661–665.

23. Low PA, Caskey PE, Tuck RR, et al. Quantitative sudomotor axon reflex test in normal and neuropathic subjects. Ann Neurol 1983;14:573–580.

24. Low PA, Opfer Gehrking TL, Kihara M. In vivo studies on receptor pharmacology of the human eccrine sweat gland. Clin Auton Res 1992;2:29–34.

25. Fealey RD, Low PA, Thomas JE. Thermoregulatory sweating abnormalities in diabetes mellitus. Mayo Clin Proc 1989;64:617–628.

26. Hoeldtke RD, Bryner KD, Horvath GG, et al. Redistribution of sudomotor responses is an early sign of sympathetic dysfunction in type 1 diabetes. Diabetes 2001;50:436–443.

27. Kihara M, Opfer-Gehrking TL, Low PA. Comparison of directly stimulated with axon-reflex-mediated sudomotor responses in human subjects and in patients with diabetes. Muscle Nerve 1993;16:655–660.

28. Saadia D, Voustianiouk A, Wang A, Kaufmann H. Treatment of primary palmar hyperhidrosis with botulinum toxin type A: a single-blind, two-dose, parallel group trial. Neurology 2001;56:A470–471.

29. Kennedy WR, Navarro X. Sympathetic sudomotor function in diabetic neuropathy. Arch Neurol 1989;46:1182–1186.

30. Kennedy WR, Sakuta M, Sutherland D, Goetz FC. The sweating deficiency in diabetes mellitus: methods of quantitation and clinical correlation. Neurology 1984;34:758–763.

31. Bjerrum KB. Test and symptoms in keratoconjunctivitis sicca and their correlation. Acta Ophthalmol Scand 1996;74:436–441.

32. Fox RI, Robinson CA, Curd JG, et al. Sjögren's syndrome. Proposed criteria for classification. Arthritis Rheum 1986;29:577–585.

33. Shaver BA, Brusilow SW, Cooke RE. Origin of the galvanic skin response. Proc Soc Exp Biol Med 1962;110:559–564.

34. Knezevic W, Bajada S. Peripheral autonomic surface potential. A quantitative technique for recording sympathetic conduction in man. J Neurol Sci 1985;67:239–251.

35. Shahani BT, Halperin JJ, Boulu P, Cohen J. Sympathetic skin response—a method of assessing unmyelinated axon dysfunction in peripheral neuropathies. J Neurol Neurosurg Psychiatry 1984;47:536–542.

36. Hoeldtke RD, Davis KM, Hshieh PB, et al. Autonomic surface potential analysis: assessment of reproducibility and sensitivity. Muscle Nerve 1992;15:926–931.

37. Shahani BT, Day TJ, Cros D, et al. RR interval variation and the sympathetic skin response in the assessment of autonomic function in peripheral neuropathy. Arch Neurol 1990;47:659–664.

38. Uncini A, Pullman SL, Lovelace RE, Gambi D. The sympathetic skin response: normal values, elucidation of afferent components and application limits. J Neurol Sci 1988;87:299–306.

39. Vallbo AB, Hagbarth KE. Activity from skin mechanoreceptors recorded percutaneously in awake human subjects. Exp Neurol 1968;21:270–289.

40. Macefield VG, Wallin BG. Respiratory and cardiac modulation of single sympathetic vasoconstrictor and sudomotor neurones to human skin. J Physiol 1999;516:303–314.

41. Macefield VG, Wallin BG. Firing properties of single vasoconstrictor neurones in human subjects with high levels of muscle sympathetic activity. J Physiol 1999;516:293–301.

42. Low PA, Neumann C, Dyck PJ, et al. Evaluation of skin vasomotor reflexes by using laser Doppler velocimetry. Mayo Clin Proc 1983;58:583–592.

43. Hilz MJ, Hecht MJ, Berghoff M, et al. Abnormal vasoreaction to arousal stimuli—an early sign of diabetic sympathetic neuropathy demonstrated by laser Doppler flowmetry. J Clin Neurophysiol 2000;17:419–425.

44. So YT, Olney RK, Aminoff MJ. Evaluation of thermography in the diagnosis of selected entrapment neuropathies. Neurology 1989;39:1–5.

45. So YT, Olney RK, Aminoff MJ. A comparison of thermography and electromyography in the diagnosis of cervical radiculopathy. Muscle Nerve 1990;13:1032–1036.
46. So YT, Aminoff MJ, Olney RK. The role of thermography in the evaluation of lumbosacral radiculopathy. Neurology 1989;39:1154–1158.
47. The American Academy of Neurology, Therapeutics and Technology Assessment Subcommittee. Assessment: thermography in neurologic practice. Neurology 1990;40:523–525.
48. McCarthy BG, Hsieh ST, Stocks A, et al. Cutaneous innervation in sensory neuropathies: evaluation by skin biopsy. Neurology 1995;45:1848–1855.
49. Kennedy WR, Wendelschafer-Crabb G, Carpenter C, Brelje T. A quantitative study of nerves in sweat glands in normal and diabetic subjects. Ann Neurol 1993;34:269–271.
50. Kennedy WR, Nolano M, Wendelschafer-Crabb G, et al. A skin blister method to study epidermal nerves in peripheral nerve disease. Muscle Nerve 1999;22:360–371.
51. McArthur JC, Stocks EA, Hauer P, et al. Epidermal nerve fiber density: normative reference range and diagnostic efficiency [see comments]. Arch Neurol 1998;55:1513–1520.
52. Holland NR, Stocks A, Hauer P, et al. Intraepidermal nerve fiber density in patients with painful sensory neuropathy. Neurology 1997;48:708–711.
53. Herrmann DN, Griffin JW, Hauer P, et al. Epidermal nerve fiber density and sural nerve morphometry in peripheral neuropathies [see comments]. Neurology 1999;53:1634–1640.
54. Spies JM, Sheikh KA, Gordon VM, et al. Comparison of quantitative sudomotor testing and epidermal nerve fiber density in patients with peripheral neuropathy. Neurology 1999;52:A388.
55. Kennedy WR, Wendelschafer-Crabb G, Brelje TC. Innervation and vasculature of human sweat glands: an immunohistochemistry-laser scanning confocal fluorescence microscopy study. J Neurosci 1994;14:6825–6833.
56. Axelrod J, Weinshilboum R. Catecholamines. N Engl J Med 1972;287:237–242.
57. Lake CR, Ziegler MG, Kopin IJ. Use of plasma norepinephrine for evaluation of sympathetic neuronal function in man. Life Sci 1976;18:1315–1325.
58. Ziegler MG, Lake CR, Kopin IJ. The sympathetic-nervous-system defect in primary orthostatic hypotension. N Engl J Med 1977;296:293–297.
59. Dejgaard A, Hilsted J, Christensen NJ. Noradrenaline and isoproterenol kinetics in diabetic patients with and without autonomic neuropathy. Diabetologia 1986;29:773–777.
60. Assessment: Clinical autonomic testing report of the Therapeutics and Technology Assessment Subcommittee of the American Academy of Neurology. Neurology 1996;46:873–880.
61. Lake CR, Ziegler MG, Coleman M, Kopin IJ. Lack of correlation of plasma norepinephrine and dopamine-beta-hydroxylase in hypertensive and normotensive subjects. Circ Res 1977;41:865–869.
62. Craig SP, Buckle VJ, Lamouroux A, et al. Localization of the human dopamine beta hydroxylase (DBH) gene to chromosome 9q34. Cytogenet Cell Genet 1988;48:48–50.
63. Robertson D, Goldberg MR, Onrot J, et al. Isolated failure of autonomic noradrenergic neurotransmission. Evidence for impaired beta-hydroxylation of dopamine. N Engl J Med 1986;314:1494–1497.
64. Mathias CJ, Bannister RB, Cortelli P, et al. Clinical, autonomic and therapeutic observations in two siblings with postural hypotension and sympathetic failure due to an inability to synthesize noradrenaline from dopamine because of a deficiency of dopamine beta hydroxylase. QJM 1990;75:617–633.
65. Hopkins IJ, Shield LK, Harris M. Subacute cholinergic dysautonomia in childhood. Clin Exp Neurol 1980;17:147–151.
66. Hart RG, Kanter MC. Acute autonomic neuropathy. Two cases and a clinical review. Arch Intern Med 1990;150:2373–2376.
67. Low PA, Fealey RD, Sheps SG, et al. Chronic idiopathic anhidrosis. Ann Neurol 1985;18:344–348.
68. Sterin-Borda L, Borda E. Role of neurotransmitter autoantibodies in the pathogenesis of chagasic peripheral dysautonomia. Ann N Y Acad Sci 2000;917:273–280.
69. Amorim DS, Mello de Oliveira JA, Manco JC, et al. Chagas' heart disease. First demonstrable correlation between neuronal degeneration and autonomic impairment. Acta Cardiol 1973;28:431–440.
70. Idiaquez J. Parasympathetic denervation of the iris in Chagas' disease. Clin Auton Res 1992;2:277–279.
71. Idiaquez J. Somatic and autonomic nerve studies in Chagas' disease. Muscle Nerve 1996;19:678–679.
72. Idiaquez J. ENMG and somatosensory evoked potential study in patients in the chronic phase of Chagas' disease (a reply). Muscle Nerve 1997;20:524.

73. McDougall AJ, McLeod JG. Autonomic neuropathy, II: specific peripheral neuropathies. J Neurol Sci 1996;138:1–13.

74. Chen JT, Chen CC, Lin KP, et al. Botulism: heart rate variation, sympathetic skin responses, and plasma norepinephrine. Can J Neurol Sci 1999;26:123–126.

75. O'Neill JH, Murray NM, Newsom-Davis J. The Lambert-Eaton myasthenic syndrome. A review of 50 cases. Brain 1988;111:577–596.

76. O'Suilleabhain P, Low PA, Lennon VA. Autonomic dysfunction in the Lambert-Eaton myasthenic syndrome: serologic and clinical correlates. Neurology 1998;50:88–93.

77. Khurana RK, Koski CL, Mayer RF. Autonomic dysfunction in Lambert-Eaton myasthenic syndrome. J Neurol Sci 1988;85:77–86.

78. Lennon VA, Kryzer TJ, Griesmann GE, et al. Calcium-channel antibodies in the Lambert-Eaton syndrome and other paraneoplastic syndromes. N Engl J Med 1995;332:1467–1474.

79. Hague K, Lento S, Morgello S, et al. The distribution of Lewy bodies in pure autonomic failure: autopsy findings and review of the literature. Acta Neuropathol 1997;94:192–196.

80. Kaufmann H, Hague K, Perl D. Accumulation of alpha-synuclein in autonomic nerves in pure autonomic failure. Neurology 2001;56:980–981.

81. Yokota T, Hayashi M, Hirashima F, et al. Dysautonomia with acute sensory motor neuropathy. A new classification of acute autonomic neuropathy. Arch Neurol 1994;51:1022–1031.

82. Suarez GA, Fealey RD, Camilleri M, Low PA. Idiopathic autonomic neuropathy: clinical, neurophysiologic, and follow-up studies on 27 patients. Neurology 1994;44:1675–1682.

83. Low PA, Dyck PJ, Lambert EH, et al. Acute panautonomic neuropathy. Ann Neurol 1983;13:412–417.

84. Smit AA, Vermeulen M, Koelman JH, Wieling W. Unusual recovery from acute panautonomic neuropathy after immunoglobulin therapy. Mayo Clin Proc 1997;72:333–335.

85. Vernino S, Low PA, Fealey RD, et al. Autoantibodies to ganglionic acetylcholine receptors in autoimmune autonomic neuropathies. N Engl J Med 2000;343:847–855.

86. Singh NK, Jaiswal AK, Misra S, Srivastava PK. Assessment of autonomic dysfunction in Guillain-Barré syndrome and its prognostic implications. Acta Neurol Scand 1987;75:101–105.

87. Tuck RR, McLeod JG. Autonomic dysfunction in Guillain-Barré syndrome. J Neurol Neurosurg Psychiatry 1981;44:983–990.

88. Winer JB, Hughes RA. Identification of patients at risk of arrhythmia in the Guillain-Barré syndrome. QJM 1988;68:735–739.

89. Meyer UA, Schuurmans MM, Lindberg RL. Acute porphyrias: pathogenesis of neurological manifestations. Semin Liver Dis 1998;18:43–52.

90. Laiwah AC, Macphee GJ, Boyle P, et al. Autonomic neuropathy in acute intermittent porphyria. J Neurol Neurosurg Psychiatry 1985;48:1025–1030.

91. Spencer PS. Biological Principles of Chemical Neurotoxicity. In PS Spencer, HH Schaumburg, AC Ludoph (eds), Experimental and Clinical Neurotoxicology. New York: Oxford University Press, 2000:3–54.

92. Auld RB, Bedwell SF. Peripheral neuropathy with sympathetic overactivity from industrial contact with acrylamide. CMAJ 1967;96:652–654.

93. Le Quesne PM, McLeod JG. Peripheral neuropathy following a single exposure to arsenic. Clinical course in four patients with electrophysiological and histological studies. J Neurol Sci 1977;32:437–451.

94. Fraser DM, Campbell IW, Miller HC. Peripheral and autonomic neuropathy after treatment with perhexiline maleate. BMJ 1977;2:675–676.

95. Rosenfeld CS, Broder LE. Cisplatin-induced autonomic neuropathy. Cancer Treat Rep 1984;68:659–660.

96. Jerian SM, Sarosy GA, Link CJ Jr, et al. Incapacitating autonomic neuropathy precipitated by Taxol. Gynecol Oncol 1993;51:277–280.

97. Hancock BW, Naysmith A. Vincristine-induced autonomic neuropathy. BMJ 1975;3:207.

98. Matikainen E, Juntunen J. Autonomic nervous system dysfunction in workers exposed to organic solvents. J Neurol Neurosurg Psychiatry 1985;48:1021–1024.

99. Nordentoft T, Andersen EB, Mogensen PH. Initial sensorimotor and delayed autonomic neuropathy in acute thallium poisoning. Neurotoxicology 1998;19:421–426.

100. Wang AK, Fealey RD, Gehrking TL, Low PA. Autonomic failure in amyloidosis. Neurology 1999;52:A388.

101. Dyck PJ, Kratz KM, Karnes JL, et al. The prevalence by staged severity of various types of diabetic neuropathy, retinopathy, and nephropathy in a population-based cohort: the Rochester Diabetic

Neuropathy Study (published erratum appears in Neurology 1993 Nov;43[11]:2345). Neurology 1993;43:817–824.

102. Fagius J. Microneurographic findings in diabetic polyneuropathy with special reference to sympathetic nerve activity. Diabetologia 1982;23:415–420.

103. Maselli RA, Jaspan JB, Soliven BC, et al. Comparison of sympathetic skin response with quantitative sudomotor axon reflex test in diabetic neuropathy. Muscle Nerve 1989;12:420–423.

104. Slaugenhaupt SA, Blumenfeld A, Gill SP, et al. Tissue-specific expression of a splicing mutation in the IKBKAP gene causes familial dysautonomia. Am J Hum Genet 2001;68:598–605.

105. Swanson AG. Congential insensitivity to pain with anhydrosis. Arch Neurol 1963;8:299–306.

106. Eng CM, Guffon N, Wilcox WR, et al. Safety and efficacy of recombinant human alpha-galactosidase A— replacement therapy in Fabry's disease. N Engl J Med 2001;345:9–16.

107. Scott LJ, Griffin JW, Luciano C, et al. Quantitative analysis of epidermal innervation in Fabry disease. Neurology 1999;52:1249–1254.

108. Ohnishi A, Dyck PJ. Loss of small peripheral sensory neurones in Fabry disease. Arch Neurol 1974;31:120–127.

109. Cohen JA, Laudenslager M. Autonomic nervous system involvement in patients with human immunodeficiency virus infection. Neurology 1989;39:1111–1112.

110. Wulff EA, Wang AK, Simpson DM. HIV-associated peripheral neuropathy: epidemiology, pathophysiology and treatment. Drugs 2000;59:1251–1260.

111. Ruttimann S, Hilti P, Spinas GA, Dubach UC. High frequency of human immunodeficiency virus-associated autonomic neuropathy and more severe involvement in advanced stages of human immunodeficiency virus disease. Arch Intern Med 1991;151:2441–2443.

112. Freeman R, Roberts MS, Friedman LS, Broadbridge C. Autonomic function and human immunodeficiency virus infection. Neurology 1990;40:575–580.

113. Sodhi N, Camilleri M, Camoriano JK, et al. Autonomic function and motility in intestinal pseudoobstruction caused by paraneoplastic syndrome. Dig Dis Sci 1989;34:1937–1942.

114. Mellgren SI, Conn DL, Stevens JC, Dyck PJ. Peripheral neuropathy in primary Sjögren's syndrome. Neurology 1989;39:390–394.

115. Grant IA, Hunder GG, Homburger HA, Dyck PJ. Peripheral neuropathy associated with sicca complex. Neurology 1997;48:855–862.

116. Wright RA, Grant IA, Low PA. Autonomic neuropathy associated with sicca complex. J Auton Nerv Syst 1999;75:70–76.

117. Olney RK. Clinical trials for polyneuropathy: the role of nerve conduction studies, quantitative sensory testing, and autonomic function testing. J Clin Neurophysiol 1998;15:129–137.

9

Repetitive Stimulation Tests

Emma Ciafaloni and Janice M. Massey

The repetitive nerve stimulation (RNS) test has its most useful application in the evaluation of defects affecting the neuromuscular junction (NMJ) because routine nerve conduction studies (NCSs) and electromyography (EMG) are frequently normal in these disorders. RNS is the most frequently used and widely available electrodiagnostic test for suspected cases of myasthenia gravis (MG) and Lambert-Eaton myasthenic syndrome (LEMS), and it should be considered in cases in which the compound muscle action potential (CMAP) amplitudes are diffusely low or fluctuating and when unstable motor units are detected by EMG in the absence of a neuropathic cause. RNS testing can be of value not only to confirm the diagnosis of NMJ diseases but also to localize the defect to the pre- or postsynaptic region and to assess the degree of disease severity and the response to treatment over time.

Although highly sensitive in detecting NMJ defects, RNS tests can sometimes be abnormal in other conditions such as motor neuron disease, multiple sclerosis, peripheral neuropathies, radiculopathy, and muscle disorders (myotonia). Therefore, RNS results need to be critically interpreted in conjunction with the overall clinical history and examination. Correct clinical interpretation of RNS studies also requires awareness of the possible technical pitfalls associated with the test as well as a precise understanding of the NMJ physiology under normal and abnormal circumstances.

THE NEUROMUSCULAR JUNCTION AND ITS PHYSIOLOGY

The NMJ (Figure 9.1) is a synaptic structure composed of the motor nerve terminal, the junctional cleft, and the muscle end plate with the folded postsynaptic membrane rich in acetylcholine (ACh) receptors (AChRs). There are many vesicles or quanta, each containing up to 10,000 ACh molecules, in the presynaptic axonal terminal. Approximately 1,000 quanta are available close to the cell membrane for immediate release, whereas 10,000 more quanta constitute the mobilization store and constantly move toward the membrane to replace released ACh. A third store of approximately 300,000 quanta lies in a reserve supply in which synthesis and packaging occur. There are two types of neurotransmitter releases in the NMJ: spontane-

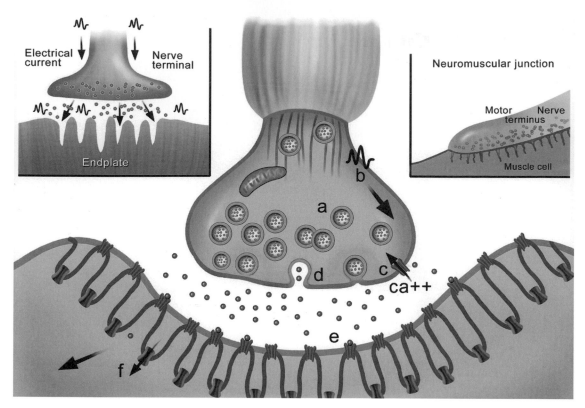

Figure 9.1 Diagram of the elements of neuromuscular transmission showing the following processes: vesicles with stored neurotransmitter (a); depolarization (b); depolarization causing opening of voltage-gated Ca^{++} channels (c); influx of calcium triggering fusion of vesicles with presynaptic membrane and releasing stored acetylcholine into the synaptic cleft (d); acetylcholine binding to receptor on postsynaptic membrane (e); and sodium channels opening and the muscle action potential initiating (f).

ous and evoked. The random spontaneous release of single quanta of ACh generates small, nonpropagating local depolarization of the postsynaptic membrane called *miniature end-plate potentials* (MEPPs). The amplitude of the MEPP is approximately 1 mV, far below the critical level needed for generation of a muscle action potential. MEPPs can be recorded by needle EMG electrodes and are recognized as the "seashell murmur" or "end-plate noise" when the needle is near the muscle end-plate zone. When an action potential propagates along the motor axon and arrives at the motor nerve terminus, the resulting depolarization opens the voltage-gated calcium channels, and calcium enters the presynaptic membrane. This initiates the calcium-dependent release of approximately 100–200 ACh quanta (immediately available pool) by exocytosis into the synaptic cleft. ACh diffuses across the 50-nm synaptic cleft and binds to AChRs, causing a Na$^+$ influx and a depolarizing end-plate potential (EPP) (see Figure 9.1). When the EPP reaches the 10–15 mV threshold, a muscle fiber action potential is initiated, causing a muscle contraction. Surface recording electrodes measure the temporal and spatial summation of all of the responding muscle fiber action potentials, the CMAP.

In normal situations, the amount of ACh quanta released by a nerve impulse is much greater than necessary to cause a depolarization of the end plate, accounting for a large "safety factor." With a train of RNS, the number of ACh quanta released decreases up to the fifth stimulus due to the use of the readily available ACh quanta (*depression*). Subsequently, the mobilization store of ACh quanta provides a constant release. With sustained voluntary muscle contraction or high-frequency nerve stimulation, the amount of AChRelease increases for several seconds to minutes due to the presynaptic intracellular accumulation of Ca^+ (*potentiation*). Potentiation is then followed by a period of *postactivation exhaustion* with decreased release of ACh due to overuse of the AChReserve supply. Because of the large safety factor in the normal NMJ, the EPP amplitude is always greater than the motor threshold; therefore, these events are not detected by electrophysiologic tests or clinical examination. Several components contribute to the safety factor: efficient synthesis and correct packaging and storage of ACh molecules, number of AChReceptors, intact synaptic cleft, concentration and transport of electrolytes, and integrity of membrane channels. A reduction of the safety factor and the subsequent failure of the EPP due to abnormality of any of the above components are the common denominators in all NMJ disorders.[1]

REPETITIVE NERVE STIMULATION TECHNIQUE AND PITFALLS

RNS is performed by stimulating a peripheral motor nerve with a train of supramaximal stimuli and recording the CMAP responses with an active surface electrode over the belly of the muscle. Correct placement of the recording electrode over the motor point is important to avoid technical artifacts. The electrode is correctly placed when a sharp negative deflection of the CMAP is recorded. The reference-recording electrode should be placed on a distal point where minimal electrical activity occurs. Supramaximal stimulation, 10–25% greater than the intensity needed to activate all the nerve fibers, must be used to avoid false-positive results due to "pseudodecrement." The stimulus duration should be no longer than necessary to obtain supramaximal stimulation, usually 0.1 millisecond for surface electrodes. This may vary with different stimulation sites. For deeper nerves, the intensity and duration of the stimulation pulses can be reduced by using needle electrodes: This produces less pain and is usually better tolerated. The CMAP amplitude reflects the number of muscle fibers activated by each nerve stimulus and is a marker of neuromuscular transmission efficiency. The size of the CMAP can be measured as peak-to-peak amplitude or as the area under the curve. Current EMG machines have the capability to automatically measure and store the amplitude, area, and duration of CMAPs and allow immediate interpretation or later analysis of the RNS results. The ability to display all the CMAPs of a train in a superimposed or rastered fashion is of great advantage in analyzing the results. Special attention should be given to the baseline of the single responses and to the overall shape of the train to recognize physiologically abnormal patterns from technical artifacts (Figure 9.2). Decrement in MG usually occurs gradually from the second through the fourth or fifth CMAP and frequently improves after the fifth or sixth potential, giving the classic envelope or saddle shape to the train. Sudden variations between responses that are irregular and not reproducible indicate technical artifact, usually from movement of the electrodes or the stimulator (see Figure 9.2). Changes in the relative positions of the recording electrode and the muscle during stimulation are usually more problematic at higher stimulation rates and in larger muscles. These

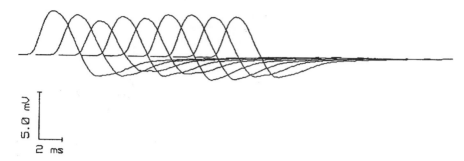

Figure 9.2 Movement artifact as noted by the variations in the baseline most obvious at the positive peaks of the waveforms. Repetitive nerve stimulation at 3 Hz stimulating the ulnar nerve and recording over the abductor digiti quinti: The 25% decrement between the first and third compound muscle action potentials is due to shifting of the recording electrode and not to true neuromuscular junction defect.

shifts can significantly alter the results of RNS and can be erroneously interpreted as abnormal decrements (see Figure 9.2). To minimize the risk of movement artifact, the examiner should effectively stabilize the electrodes and stimulator with tape and immobilize the limb by holding it or by using straps or clamps. The decrement should always be reproducible and gradual, and it usually improves or disappears after injection of edrophonium (Tensilon). Decrement and facilitation are defined by measuring the percent difference of the amplitude or area between the first and the fourth or fifth potential. Most electromyographers accept decrement greater than 10% and facilitation greater than 100% of the initial CMAP response as abnormal, although the criteria for abnormality vary some among different laboratories.

Effect of Medications

The use of cholinesterase inhibitors influences the results of RNS testing and, if safe for the patient, administration of anticholinesterase drugs should be discontinued 12 hours before testing to improve the sensitivity of the test.[2]

Temperature

Temperature is an important factor in neuromuscular transmission. It must be measured before starting RNS testing, then monitored frequently during the study. It is a well recognized, although not completely understood, clinical phenomenon that patients with NMJ diseases have worsening of fatigue and weakness in hot weather and that heat can exacerbate symptoms and even induce crisis in MG.[3] Local cooling increases the conduction velocities of the nerve impulse and duration and amplitude of the CMAP. This is the result of a prolonged opening time of the Ca^{++} channels and an increased release of ACh. Temperatures lower than 34°C also reduce acetylcholinesterase activity and increase AChR opening time, causing a net improvement in the NMJ safety factor.

Because cooling reduces the decremental response in MG and LEMS, distal muscles should be warmed before testing and maintained at 34°C or higher to obtain best diagnostic sensitivity (Figure 9.3). Falsely normal studies can occur if the hand

Figure 9.3 Temperature effect. **A.** Stimulation of median nerve at 3 Hz, recording from the abductor pollicis brevis: Decrement increases with higher temperature (**B**).

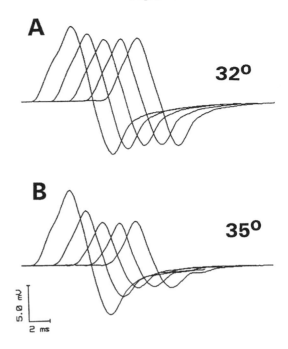

or foot muscles are cool, especially if the abnormality is mild. More proximal muscles are less prone to cooling and may not need to be warmed.

Muscle Selection

The diagnostic yield of RNS testing is greater if weak muscles are selected as recording sites and if several muscles are tested. The clinical history and examination are most useful in choosing the weaker muscles because the distribution and severity of weakness vary considerably among patients with MG. Often, proximal or facial muscles show greater abnormality than distal muscles. Proximal muscles are less subject to cooling than distal hand muscles, but stimulation of proximal sites for motor nerves is more painful and difficult, and stabilization of limbs is more challenging. A stimulating needle electrode inserted near the nerve may reduce discomfort and movement artifacts during stimulation trains and activation of proximal sites.

When possible, nerves involved by concomitant common disease processes like cervical radiculopathy or peripheral neuropathy should not be selected because decremental responses have been described in these conditions and may not represent a primary defect of NMJ transmission. Therefore, screening EMG and NCSs before RNS testing are usually indicated.

Proximal Muscles

Among the proximal muscles, the trapezius should always be tested in case of suspected MG disease because of its sensitivity in demonstrating a decremental response. Approximately 90% of patients with generalized MG show a decrement in the RNS of the spinal accessory nerve.[4] Testing is performed with the patient sitting on a low chair with the arm adducted, extended, and holding the bottom of the chair. The recording electrode is placed on the belly of the trapezius at the angle between the neck and the shoulder. The reference electrode is placed on the acromion. The spinal accessory nerve is stimulated at the posterior border of the sternocleidomastoid behind the ear where it is quite superficial. Activation of the trapezius is achieved by having the patient shrug the shoulder against resistance. The biceps is tested by stimulating the musculocutaneous nerve at the axilla between the coracobrachialis tendon and the axillary artery. Testing of the biceps is highly sensitive in demonstrating a decrement in moderately severe generalized MG. Stabilization of the arm can be accomplished by using an arm board. However, stimulation is usually uncomfortable and poorly tolerated by the patient, especially when using prolonged or high frequency trains. Stimulation of the Erb's point with recording from the deltoid shows abnormal decrement in a high percentage of patients with NMJ disease. It is technically challenging: Motion artifact is frequent; it is difficult to avoid stimulating nerves to other muscles; and the stimulation is painful.

Distal Muscles

Hand muscles are the most convenient to test but may demonstrate minimal or no decrement in up to 60% of moderately severe generalized MG. Recording is made from the thenar muscle stimulating the median nerve or from the hypothenar or first dorsal interosseous muscle stimulating the ulnar nerve at the wrist. Movement artifact can easily be avoided by immobilizing the hand with straps or clamps, but holding the patient's hand on the examining table is usually sufficient. Activation is produced by having the patient contract the tested muscle against resistance. Temperature needs to be carefully monitored throughout the test, as these distal muscles tend to cool easily. Testing in these muscles is less painful and better tolerated than in proximal muscles.

Facial Muscles

Facial muscles are most frequently affected in MG and can be tested by recording over the orbicularis oculi, orbicularis oris, or nasalis muscles with stimulation of the facial nerve anterior to the ear. Facial muscle testing may have a higher yield than limb muscle testing but is technically more difficult. Movement of recording and stimulating electrodes is significant, especially during activation, and patients usually tolerate the procedure poorly. Using a needle-stimulating electrode allows lower intensity and shorter duration of stimulation and can make the procedure more tolerable.

Masseteric nerve RNS has recently been described as a simple and well-tolerated procedure. It offers a new possibility in testing masticatory muscles, which are frequently affected in neuromuscular transmission disorders. Stimulation of the masseteric nerve is performed with a needle electrode inserted between the condyle and the coronoid process of the mandible, and the recording electrode is placed on the masseter muscle. This technique may be more sensitive in evaluating patients with predominant or limited weakness of bulbar muscles, and it is well tolerated.[5]

Proximal and Distal Lower Extremities

Lower extremities are less frequently used for RNS testing, and the sensitivity of femoral and peroneal nerve stimulation is unknown. Stabilization of the lower limb is problematic because of the strength of contracture. In addition, the stimulation of the femoral nerve in the inguinal region is painful. The peroneal nerve is stimulated at the fibular head, and recording is made from the tibialis anterior or

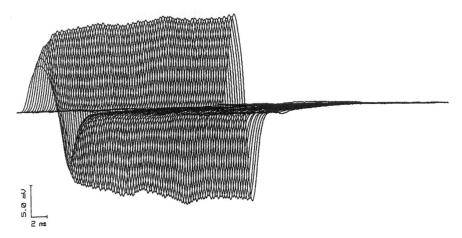

Figure 9.4 Pseudofacilitation. Median nerve stimulation at 20 Hz for 6 seconds recording from the abductor pollicis brevis. Note the increase in amplitude without change in area that occurs within the first 12 waveforms. Also notice mild movement artifact.

extensor digitorum brevis muscle. Activation is easier for the tibialis anterior, and clinical weakness of this muscle is frequently observed in MG.

Stimulation Rates and Activation Technique

Stimulation rates between 3 and 5 Hz are used in most RNS tests, as they are most likely to show a decremental response due to decreased quantal release of ACh after a train of stimuli.[6] Rates higher than 10 Hz are painful, can produce technical artifacts and pseudofacilitation, and should be avoided except when studying patients with suspected LEMS or botulism. An increase in CMAP amplitude without change in the negative peak area can be seen when using high-frequency nerve stimulation (usually higher than 10 Hz) or after voluntary muscle contraction in normal NMJ. This phenomenon is referred to as *pseudofacilitation* (Figure 9.4).[7] It is attributed to increased synchronization of the action potential propagation velocity in the muscle fibers and not to an increase in the number of activated muscle fibers as in true facilitation.

The most commonly used activation technique consists of having the patient maximally contract the muscle under study against resistance for 10–60 seconds. Alternatively, a train of tetanic stimuli can be delivered at 20–50 Hz for 1 second. Nerve activation produces an accumulation of Ca^{++} in the nerve terminal that facilitates AChRelease and increases the number of activated muscle fibers. In a presynaptic disorder such as LEMS, this induces a marked increase in CMAP amplitude, and this phenomenon is called *postactivation facilitation* (Figure 9.5). The greatest facilitation is seen within a few seconds after the end of activation. This is followed by a period in which a reduced amount of ACh is released by each nerve impulse. This phenomenon is maximal at 2–5 minutes after activation and is called *postactivation exhaustion*. Worsening of decremental response compared to the preactivation values or, in some patients, abnormal decrement not present before activation can be seen during the exhaustion stage. In individuals with normal NMJ, facilitation or exhaustion is not seen because of the large safety factor.

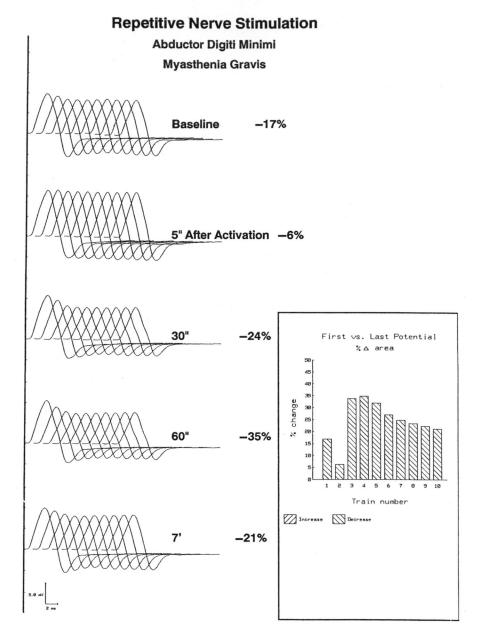

Figure 9.5 Activation cycle in myasthenia gravis. Stimulation of the ulnar nerve at 3 Hz recording over the abductor digiti minimi before and after 30 seconds of voluntary muscle contraction. There is 17% decrement of amplitude between the first and fourth compound muscle action potential; note the gradual decrease of amplitude and the typical envelope shape. Five seconds afterward, the decrement improved (facilitation) to 6% and worsened (exhaustion) to a maximum of 35% at 60 seconds with return to baseline by 7 minutes. (Δ = change.)

Enhancing Techniques

Using special activation techniques or provocative measures can enhance the diagnostic sensitivity of the RNS test. These techniques are indicated when no significant decrement is seen before and after activation in both proximal and distal muscles. If the clinical suspicion for NMJ defect remains high and a more sensitive test like single-fiber EMG (SFEMG) is not available, a prolonged stimulation protocol can be used. The median or ulnar nerve can be stimulated at 3 Hz for 4–5 minutes. The double-step RNS test can further improve the yield and is performed by applying prolonged stimulation in a hand muscle before and after ischemia of the limb.[8,9] A blood pressure cuff is placed around the upper arm and inflated to above systolic pressure during RNS of the ulnar or median nerve. This technique is painful and can be performed only in hand muscles.

Regional infusion of small doses of curare just before performing RNS test can further increase the chance of unmasking a NMJ transmission defect.[10] After a blood pressure cuff is placed around the upper arm and inflated to above systolic pressure, 0.2 mg of d-tubocurarine is injected in a distal vein of the same arm. The RNS test is then performed on a hand muscle. This technique must be used with caution. The electromyographer must be aware that patients with MG may experience exacerbation of generalized weakness after the blood pressure cuff is deflated.

Special techniques, as the ones described above, require experience and careful judgment for a correct interpretation.

USE OF REPETITIVE NERVE STIMULATION

Autoimmune Myasthenia Gravis

MG is an autoimmune disease clinically characterized by fluctuating weakness of ocular, bulbar, and limb muscles. Fatigability of ocular and limb muscles on examination and improvement after injection of edrophonium (Tensilon) are typical. Clinical diagnosis is confirmed by the presence of anti-AChR antibodies, but these are absent in approximately 20% of patients with the generalized form and in 50% of patients with the purely ocular form. Therefore, electrophysiologic tests are important in demonstrating a NMJ abnormality and in reaching a definite diagnosis.

In MG, the NMJ safety factor is compromised because of a decreased number of AChRs, rearrangement of the postsynaptic membrane, and direct blocking of AChRs by circulating antibodies. Sensory and motor NCSs are usually normal. The CMAP recorded from rested muscles is usually normal but can decrease if several supramaximal stimuli are delivered at short intervals in patients with severe disease.

RNS should be performed in clinically weak muscles if possible. Temperature in the tested limb should be maintained at 34°C or higher during the study as a decremental response can be masked by cooling (see Figure 9.3). Easily accessible distal muscles like the hypothenar or thenar muscles are usually tested first. Trains of nine supramaximal stimuli at 3 Hz are applied twice to the ulnar or median nerve at the wrist to demonstrate a reproducible response. The thenar or hypothenar muscles are then activated against resistance for 30 seconds, and trains of six to nine stimuli are applied at 5, 30, and 60 seconds after the end of activation to demonstrate facilitation and every minute thereafter for up to 5 minutes to demonstrate postactivation exhaustion. In normal controls, there is no change in the CMAP amplitude. A reproducible decrement of 10% or more in any train before activation or in the exhaustion phase of the activation cycle is indicative of a NMJ defect (see Figure 9.5). If no decrement is found in a hand muscle, a RNS study should be performed in a proximal muscle, usually the trapezius. The decrement seen on RNS test can be improved or reversed after injection of edrophonium (Tensilon). If no decrement is found in an RNS test of a proximal and distal muscle and the clinical suspicion of MG is high, one should consider SFEMG of the extensor digitorum communis, frontalis muscle, or both. SFEMG is a more sensitive test and is better in demonstrating a defect in patients with mild generalized or purely ocular forms of MG. Abnormal jitter is found in all patients with MG if a weak muscle is studied.[11] (SFEMG is discussed in detail in Chapter 13.)

Lambert-Eaton Myasthenic Syndrome

The clinical diagnosis of LEMS should be suspected in patients with progressive symmetric proximal weakness, hypoactive tendon reflexes, and dry mouth. Ocular and oropharyngeal symptoms are much less frequent than in MG. LEMS is associated with small cell carcinoma of the lung in approximately two-thirds of the cases. Clinically, the weakness and hyporeflexia may frequently, but not always, improve with exercise. The NMJ defect is presynaptic and consists of impaired release of ACh from the nerve terminal. Antibodies against the voltage-gated calcium channels in the presynaptic nerve terminal may be detected in the serum. Response to edrophonium is difficult to interpret and is less useful than in MG. Response to pyridostigmine (Mestinon) treatment alone is poor, but approximately 80% of patients have improvement of strength when taking pyridostigmine in combination with 3,4 diaminopyridine (DAP). Patients are very susceptible to exaggerated response to neuromuscular blocking agents and may have difficulties with extubation after surgery due to prolonged apnea.

Electrodiagnostic tests and RNS in particular are the most reliable diagnostic tools in confirming a clinical suspicion of LEMS, as the responses in this disease are highly characteristic. Low CMAP baseline amplitudes, decremental response to slow rates of RNS, and marked postactivation facilitation are typical. In the absence of myopathy or axonal neuropathy, one should consider this diagnosis if small CMAPs are found on routine NCSs or unstable motor unit potentials with variable morphology are seen on routine EMG.

Low CMAP amplitudes, often to less than 10% of normal, are found in at least one hand muscle in 97% of patients and represent a hallmark of the disease. F-wave amplitude may be higher than M-wave amplitude due to potentiation. The CMAP amplitude should be measured after supramaximal stimulation in a muscle rested and warmed to 34°C. The muscle is then maximally activated for 10 seconds and a supramaximal nerve stimulus delivered immediately after the end of muscle activation. An increment of 100% or more in CMAP amplitude is typical of LEMS (Figure 9.6).

After activation for 10 seconds or during repetitive stimulation at 20 Hz for 10 seconds, there is marked facilitation, greater than 100% in more than 70% of patients. Special attention must be taken not to exercise the muscle too long, as this depletes ACh release and masks facilitation. Rapid rates of stimulation may be used when studying LEMS patients to elicit facilitation but are less well tolerated than voluntary muscle contraction. Abnormal decrement to RNS at 2–5 Hz is seen in virtually all patients with LEMS.

Figure 9.6 Facilitation in Lambert-Eaton myasthenic syndrome. After 10 seconds of activation and 3 Hz stimulation, there is 260% facilitation of compound muscle action potential amplitude in the trapezius (**A**) and 130% in the abductor digiti quinti (**B**). Greater than 100% facilitation is typical of Lambert-Eaton myasthenic syndrome. The facilitation seen in myasthenia gravis is typically much less.

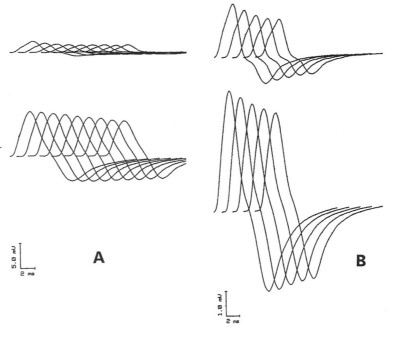

SFEMG studies demonstrate severely increased jitter and frequent blocking in most muscles tested.[12]

Congenital Myasthenic Syndromes

Congenital myasthenic syndromes are a rare heterogeneous group of genetically determined NMJ abnormalities with variable pre- and postsynaptic defects and without circulating AChR antibodies. Diagnosis frequently relies on sophisticated in vitro electrophysiologic studies and quantitative electron microscopy analysis performed in only a few specialized centers. The classification and genetic characterization of these disorders are still evolving and are discussed in detail in Chapter 10. We include here the ones in which the findings during repetitive stimulation tests are well characterized.

In familial infantile myasthenia, there is a defect in synaptic vesicle metabolism with abnormal resynthesis or packaging, or both, of ACh molecules. This disease is clinically characterized by fluctuating ptosis from birth, poor suck, cry, and difficulty feeding; recurrent episodes of apnea are typical during infection, vomiting, or excitement. The electrophysiologic findings are similar to the ones in muscles poisoned by hemicholinium (inhibitor of choline uptake). In weak muscles, a decremental response may be demonstrated with 3–5 Hz RNS. Prolonged stimulation at 3–5 Hz for 5 minutes followed by short trains of 3–5 Hz stimuli may be necessary to unmask a typical decrement. This decrement persists for 20–30 minutes and can be reversed by edrophonium (Tensilon).[13,14]

The slow-channel congenital myasthenic syndrome is inherited in an autosomal dominant fashion and is associated with a prolonged open time of the AChR ion channel. It is clinically characterized by variable onset in infancy, childhood, or adult life. Select involvement of cervical, scapular, and finger extensor mus-

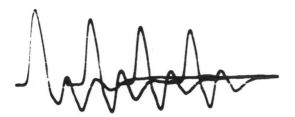

Figure 9.7 Afterdischarges in slow-channel congenital myasthenic syndrome. With 2-Hz stimulation of the ulnar nerve, there is a decrement of 20% between the first and fourth compound muscle action potential of the abductor digiti quinti muscle. There are afterdischarges as typically seen in slow-channel congenital myasthenic syndrome.

cles with mild to moderate weakness of eye muscles is typical. The affected muscles are atrophic and fatigue abnormally.[15,16] Motor nerve stimulation typically reveals repetitive discharges occurring 5–10 milliseconds after single nerve stimulation (Figure 9.7). Afterdischarges help to distinguish slow-channel congenital myasthenic syndrome from acquired MG but are not always seen in all muscles; therefore, motor nerve stimulation of several muscles is required.[17] The motor unit potentials fluctuate in morphology and amplitude during voluntary activation. RNS at 2–3 Hz demonstrates a decremental response in clinically weak muscles.

Congenital end-plate acetylcholinesterase deficiency is characterized by weakness and abnormal fatigability of facial, cervical, axial, and limb muscles present from birth or early childhood. Increased lordosis on standing due to severe axial muscle weakness is typical. The abnormality consists of a deficiency of ACh esterase at the NMJ. The RNS test shows a decremental response with 2-Hz stimulation. A repetitive CMAP response after a single nerve stimulus has been described in some patients and disappears at frequencies greater than 0.2 Hz or with mild activation.[15,18]

Botulism

Botulinum toxin is produced by the anaerobic bacterium *Clostridium botulinum*. Botulism may occur from ingestion of canned foods that have not been completely sterilized, or it may be wound related, predominantly occurring in drug abusers after subcutaneous injection of heroin.[19] Infantile botulism is caused by the growth of the bacterium in the gastrointestinal tract and the slow production of toxin over time.[20] The diagnosis is confirmed by wound or stool cultures or by serum assay for the toxin. Botulism causes a marked reduction in the number of ACh quanta released by autonomic and motor nerve terminals. Symptoms begin 12–36 hours after ingestion and consist of a descending paralysis with early ocular, bulbar, and pupillary weakness, followed by generalized weakness over a few days. Respiratory paralysis and autonomic symptoms are frequent. Clinical recovery in treated survivors is slow but usually complete. Some electrophysiologic abnormalities may persist despite clinical recovery.

The electrophysiologic findings vary with the severity and the time in the course of the disease and may be seen in only a few muscles at some time during the disease. This is in contrast to LEMS, in which an abnormality in RNS is usually demonstrated in most muscles. Reduced CMAP amplitude is not as severe as that seen in LEMS. At 2–3 Hz repetitive stimulation, a decremental response can be seen in severe cases; however, this finding is inconsistent and not a reliable sign. Tetanic and post-tetanic facilitation of at least 20% is highly sensitive and specific and, when seen in combination with low CMAP and absence of post-tetanic exhaustion, suggests the diagnosis of botulism. The persistence of facilitation for 2 minutes and up to 40 minutes is characteristic of botulism. When the above findings are seen, hypermagnesemia is also in the differential diagnosis.[21,22]

SFEMG shows markedly increased jitter and blocking and is abnormal in virtually all cases of botulism.[23]

CONCLUSIONS

Electrophysiologic studies are very useful and sensitive tools in the diagnostic evaluation of patients with suspected neuromuscular transmission defects. In patients with classic symptoms and examination, RNS tests are useful to (1) confirm the clinical diagnosis, (2) estimate the degree of severity, and (3) monitor the response to treatment. In patients in whom the diagnosis remains in doubt because of a less typical clinical presentation, equivocal edrophonium (Tensilon) test, and negative antibodies, RNS tests can be invaluable in establishing a diagnosis.

RNS testing, although less sensitive than SFEMG, is more widely available and often can be performed at the time of initial evaluation. A tensilon test may also be helpful in MG but is limited in patients with fatigue in whom there is no specific muscle weakness at the time of evaluation. Antibody titers are limited by the turnaround time. The sensitivity of RNS tests is increased by testing more than one muscle group, by discontinuing anticholinesterase medications, and by avoiding cooling of the tested muscles.

As always in electrophysiologic studies, correct interpretation of the results requires prompt recognition of technical artifacts and awareness of potential pitfalls. As in other aspects of the practice of neurology, the final diagnosis of NMJ disorders is the product of a critical and expert interpretation of clinical and electrophysiologic data.

REFERENCES

1. Engel AG. The Neuromuscular Junction. In AG Engel, C Franzini-Amstrong (eds), Myology (2nd ed). New York: McGraw-Hill, 1994;261–302.
2. Oh SJ, Eslami N, Nishihira T, et al. Electrophysiological and clinical correlation in myasthenia gravis. Ann Neurol 1982;12:348–354.
3. Borenstein S, Desmedt JE. Temperature and weather correlates of myasthenic fatigue. Lancet 1974;2:63–66.
4. Schumm F, Stohr M. Accessory nerve stimulation in the assessment of myasthenia gravis. Muscle Nerve 1984;7:147–151.
5. Pavesi G, Cattaneo L, Tinchelli S, et al. Masseteric nerve stimulation in the diagnosis of myasthenia gravis. Clin Neurophysiol 2001;112:1064–1069.
6. Desmedt JE. The Neuromuscular Disorder in Myasthenia Gravis. In JE Desmedt (ed), New Developments in Electromyography and Clinical Neurophysiology. Basel, Switzerland: Karger, 1973;241–304.
7. McComas AJ, Galea V, Einhorn RW. Pseudofacilitation: a misleading term. Muscle Nerve 1994; 17:599–607.

8. Desmedt JE, Borenstein S. Double-step nerve stimulation test for myasthenic block: sensitization of post-activation exhaustion by ischemia. Ann Neurol 1977;1:55–59.

9. Gilchrist JM, Sanders DB. Double-step repetitive stimulation in myasthenia gravis. Muscle Nerve 1987;10(3):233–237.

10. Horowitz SH, Sivak M. The regional curare test and electrophysiologic diagnosis of myasthenia gravis: further studies. Muscle Nerve 1978;1(5):432–434.

11. Sanders DB, Howard JF. AAEE minimonograph # 25: single-fiber electromyography in myasthenia gravis. Muscle Nerve 1986;9:809–819.

12. Tim R, Massey JM, Sanders DB. Lambert-Eaton myasthenic syndrome: electrodiagnostic findings and response to therapy. Neurology 2000;54(11):2176–2178.

13. Mora M, Lambert EH, Engel AG. Synaptic vesicle abnormality in familial infantile myasthenia. Neurology 1987;37:206–210.

14. Robertson WC, Chun RWM, Kornguth SE. Familial infantile myasthenia. Arch Neurol 1980;37(2): 117–119.

15. Engel AG, Lambert EH. Congenital myasthenic syndromes. Electroencephalograph Clin Neurophysiol 1987;39(Suppl):91–102.

16. Engel AG, Lambert EH, Mulder DM, et al. A newly recognized congenital myasthenic syndrome attributed to a prolonged open time of the acetylcholine induced ion channel. Ann Neurol 1982;11(6):553–569.

17. Bedlack RS, Bertorini TE, Sanders DB. Hidden afterdischarges in slow channel congenital myasthenic syndrome. J Clin Neuromuscul Dis 2000;1(4):186–188.

18. Vincent A, Cull-Candy SG, Newsom-Davis J, et al. Congenital myasthenia: end-plate acetylcholine receptors and electrophysiology in five cases. Muscle Nerve 1981;4(4):306–318.

19. Maselli RA, Ellis W, Mandler RN, et al. Cluster of wound botulism in California: clinical, electrophysiologic, and pathologic study. Muscle Nerve 1997;20(10):1284–1295.

20. Gutierrez AR, Bodensteiner J, Gutmann L. Electrodiagnosis of infantile botulism. J Child Neurol 1994;9(4):362–365.

21. Gutmann L, Pratt L. Pathophysiologic aspects of human botulism. Arch Neurol 1976;33(3): 175–179.

22. Cornblath DR, Sladky JT, Sumner JD. Clinical electrophysiology of infantile botulism. Muscle Nerve 1983;6(6):448–452.

23. Schiller HH, Stalberg E. Human botulism studied with single fiber electromyography. Arch Neurol 1978;35(6):346–349.

10

Role of In Vitro Intracellular Microelectrode Studies in the Diagnosis of Neuromuscular Disorders

Ricardo A. Maselli

Intracellular microelectrodes have been used for years to study disorders of the peripheral nervous system. Many conditions have been examined using microelectrode recordings, including motor neuron disorders,[1–3] neuropathies,[4,5] diseases of the neuromuscular junction (NMJ),[6,7] and myopathies.[5,8] At present, however, the main clinical application of this technique is in the study of diseases of the NMJ. Microelectrode recordings are also frequently used to investigate disorders of muscle membrane excitability, such as myotonias and periodic paralysis, but not as a diagnostic tool. In contrast, in one type of junctional disease, the congenital myasthenic syndromes (CMSs), in vitro microelectrode studies represent an indispensable instrument to diagnose these diseases.[9–11] In CMSs, the information generated by the in vitro microelectrode investigation, in conjunction with the ultrastructural analysis of the NMJ, provides fundamental guidance for subsequent diagnostic molecular genetic studies.

TECHNICAL CONSIDERATIONS

Selection of Muscle for Biopsy

Ideally, the muscle selected for biopsy should be short, flat, and easily dissociable into muscle bundles, and it should provide the least amount of discomfort and potential postoperative complications for the patient. Any muscle with these properties is potentially suitable for in vitro microelectrode studies. A short-length muscle is of paramount importance because to maintain an appropriate resting membrane potential and membrane excitability, the muscle fibers should be intact (uninterrupted from tendon to tendon). Furthermore, the short length of the muscle facilitates the localization of end plates.

The classic muscle used for microelectrode studies is the external intercostal muscle[12] (see Color Plate A9). The main advantage of this muscle is that it is short, and therefore it provides intact muscle fibers suitable for in vitro studies. An additional advantage of the intercostal muscle is that controls without neurologic diseases can be readily obtained from patients undergoing thoracic surgery. The intercostal muscle biopsy requires general anesthesia and can be potentially complicated with pneumothorax, but this complication is relatively rare.

The anconeus has been extensively used by our group[13] (see Color Plate A10). The main advantage of the anconeus is that it is short and can be easily separated into muscle bundles. Furthermore, the anconeus biopsy can be done under regional anesthesia as an outpatient procedure. We have performed biopsies of this muscle in severely debilitated patients and even in infants during the first weeks of life without any significant complications.

Several other muscles have been successfully used to perform in vitro microelectrode studies, including the peroneus brevis,[3] finger extensors,[14] abductor hallucis,[15] infraspinatus,[14] pyramidalis,[16] and vastus lateralis.[17] With long muscles, such as the deltoid and vastus lateralis, the studies are carried out using surgically sectioned fibers. The disadvantage of these recordings is that the continuous leakage of electrolytes through the open ends of the fibers often results in marked depolarization of the preparation, which, in turn, may compromise the excitability of nerve and muscle membranes.

Handling of the Biopsy Material

The success of the in vitro microelectrode studies depends, in large part, on the proper handling of the muscle biopsy material. The familiarity of the surgeon performing the biopsy with the anatomy of the muscle and with the need of collecting a minimally traumatized specimen is essential for the success of these studies. For best results, the individual performing the dissection of the muscle should collect the muscle specimen from the operating room. The specimen should be immediately washed out with oxygenated Tyrode's solution and pinned down under moderate tension to the bottom of a sylgarded chamber. This is done to remove any excess blood that may release intracellular potassium and depolarize the preparation. A gentle stretching of the muscle helps to avoid furrows and loops in the muscle fibers, which may also lead to damage of the muscle membrane and depolarization of the preparation. Although the metabolism of the muscle fibers is largely anaerobic, vigorous bubbling of the preparation with blood gas mixture is also essential to maintain the preparation in good condition.

The dissection of the preparation is always performed under the dissecting microscope. Several strategies of dissection can be followed to obtain a useful preparation. This usually depends on the types of recordings that are planned to be conducted. In general, the goal is to obtain a thin preparation that allows proper visualization of the end plates without damaging muscle fibers and distal intramuscular nerve branches.

During dissection, the muscle specimens are continuously washed to prevent accumulation of blood and electrolytes that may depolarize the preparation. In addition, this clears the NMJ from any minimal residual effect of drugs administered to the patient during induction and general anesthesia. Because surgery is done under general anesthesia, local anesthetics are not needed, and muscle relaxant drugs should be systematically avoided.

Types of In Vitro Microelectrode Studies

The in vitro intracellular microelectrode studies in human muscle biopsy material are best executed by placing the recording chamber on the stage of a straight-up microscope with a fixed stage, extra-long working distance lenses, and a hinged body to permit intermittent access to the preparation. A rectified image for correction of the image inversion introduced by the lenses and some form of contrast visualization (either Normansky or Hoffman interference contrast optics) are also highly desirable features of microscopes used for in vitro studies.

Voltage Studies

Microelectrode studies performed for diagnostic purposes in muscle biopsy material classically involve the recording of spontaneous and nerve-evoked synaptic potentials with a single intracellular electrode placed at the end plate (Figure 10.1A). The intracellular microelectrode registers changes of voltage across the muscle membrane. These changes are relatively sustained, as with the resting membrane potential, or transient, as with spontaneous miniature end-plate potentials (MEPPs).

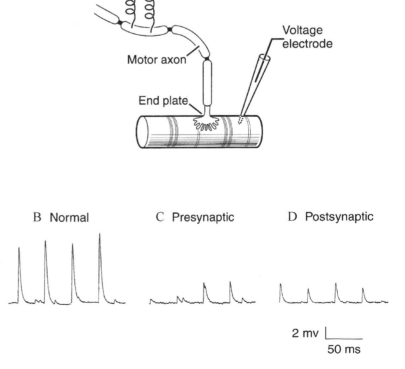

Figure 10.1 Diagram showing the principles of end-plate recordings. **A.** A microelectrode placed adjacent to the neuromuscular junction registers the resting membrane potential, spontaneous miniature end-plate potentials (MEPPs), and nerve-evoked end-plate potentials (EPPs). **B.** Example of a recording obtained from a control end plate. Four consecutive nerved-evoked EPPs are displayed. In between the EPPs, there are spontaneous MEPPs. Note that the amplitudes of the EPPs are much larger than the amplitudes of the MEPPs. **C.** Example of a recording obtained from a patient with a presynaptic disorder. As in (**B**), four consecutive nerve-evoked EPPs are displayed. The amplitudes of the first two EPPs are similar to the amplitudes of spontaneous MEPPs. This indicates that the quantal content of the first two EPPs was only one. **D.** Example of a recording obtained from a patient with a postsynaptic failure. Both EPPs and MEPPs are very small in amplitude, but the ratio between EPP and MEPP amplitudes is similar to that in the control muscle.

Spontaneous MEPPs result from the transient depolarization of the end plate secondary to the simultaneous opening of acetylcholine receptors' (AChR) ion channels. These ion channels are activated by thousands of molecules of acetylcholine (ACh) released into the synaptic cleft when a synaptic vesicle spontaneously fuses with the presynaptic membrane. The release of multiple synaptic vesicles into the synaptic cleft by the arrival of an action potential to the nerve terminal induces a much larger depolarization called the *end-plate potential* (EPP). Because the EPP results from multiple quanta of ACh, the magnitude of the EPP depends on the magnitude of a single quantum of ACh or MEPP and the number of quanta per EPP (see Figure 10.1B). The latter factor is called *EPP quantal content* and is represented by the letter *m*.

Calculation of the Quantal Content. There are many ways to calculate the EPP quantal content. However, the methods that can be implemented at the human NMJ are all indirect, and therefore, all can introduce potential bias. The simplest way to calculate the quantal content is by dividing the mean amplitude of EPPs by the mean amplitude of MEPPs recorded from the same end plate in the following way:

$$m = \frac{\text{EPP amp}}{\text{MEPP amp}}$$

This form of calculation of the EPP quantal content is easy and relatively accurate at low levels of quantal content.[18] However, at high levels of quantal content, it is complicated by nonlinear summation of quanta, which needs to be corrected by an additional set of equations.[19,20]

It is also possible to calculate low levels of quantal content by the method of the failures, which derives from predictions inherent in the Poisson distribution. In simple terms, the equation predicts that the magnitude of the quantal content is inversely related to the percentage of failures (nerve stimulations that fail to release any synaptic vesicle or quanta).

$$m = \ln\left(\frac{\text{number of impulses}}{\text{number of failures}}\right)$$

This method is also simple and does not require recording of MEPPs, but it cannot be implemented when there are no failures, as is usually the case in normal NMJs.

There is yet another traditional method to calculate the EPP quantal content. This method is based on the ratio between the EPP mean amplitude and the variability of the EPP amplitudes. This method is also simple and does not require values of MEPP amplitudes, although at high levels of quantal content, it produces a strong bias toward greater values of quantal content, which requires correction using additional equations.[21]

$$m = \frac{\text{mean EPP amplitude}}{\text{EPP amplitude SD}}$$

Because the quantal content *m* is a statistical term, it can also be represented as the product of the quanta available for immediate release (*n*) times the probability of release (*p*), a relation that is expressed as

$$m = np$$

At normal human NMJs and bathed with Tyrode's solution without curare or any other presynaptic or postsynaptic blocker, the mean quantal content (*m*) is approximately 20, and the probability of release (p) is approximately .5.[2] The quantal content m can also be represented as the product of the quantal store available for release (N) times the probability of mobilization and release from the quantal store (P).[2,22,23] As expected, the quantal store (N) is much larger than the pull of quanta available for immediate release (n). Conversely, the probability of mobilization and release (P) is smaller than the probability of release from the readily available pool (p).

It should be recognized that the quantal content at the human NMJ is significantly lower than that at NMJs of other species, notably the amphibian NMJ, where it is close to 100.[24] Perhaps this factor makes humans more susceptible to disorders of neuromuscular transmission. However, with normal postsynaptic function and normal resting membrane potential, only a few quanta are needed to trigger an action potential in the muscle membrane. This provides humans a comfortable safety factor in spite of the relatively low levels of quantal content.[25]

Voltage recordings of MEPPs and EPPs and the determination of the EPP quantal content are fundamental parts of the in vitro recordings because they permit one to ascertain whether there is failure of neuromuscular transmission. Moreover, they allow one to discriminate if the failure is presynaptic, postsynaptic, or both. In presynaptic conditions resulting from a decrease in the release of synaptic vesicles, the amplitudes of MEPPs are normal, but the amplitudes of EPPs are diminished (see Figure 10.1C). Furthermore, nerve stimulation often fails to release any quanta, and the EPP amplitudes are arranged according to the Poisson distribution. In contrast, in postsynaptic deficit, the amplitudes of EPPs and MEPPs are reduced, but the ratio between EPP and MEPP amplitudes is similar to that seen at the normal NMJs (see Figure 10.1D).

EPPs can also be obtained by pulse release of ACh, using an iontophoresis microelectrode placed near the end plate.[26,27] In theory, this is an excellent way to measure pure postsynaptic function, including populations of end-plate receptors, because it bypasses the presynaptic apparatus. In practice, the amplitudes of EPPs elicited by iontophoresis of ACh are heavily dependent on the accessibility of ACh to the end plate, the impedance of the iontophoresis electrode, and the distance between the electrode and the end plate. Because these factors are difficult to standardize, the amplitudes of the responses are extremely variable and unsuitable for clinical applications.

Microelectrode voltage studies performed outside the end-plate region are limited to the recording of action potentials. These studies provide little practical information and, therefore, are seldom used.

Voltage Clamp Studies

Important clinical information can be extracted from the decay phase of synaptic potentials, such as the opening time of the AChR ion channel and the functional status of the end-plate acetylcholinesterase (AChE). Nevertheless, the decay phase of voltage recorded synaptic potentials depends on many additional factors, including the resting membrane potential as well as the resistance and capacitance of the membrane lipid bilayer. These last two factors are also known as the *cable properties* of the membrane. A practical way to eliminate these unpredictable variables is by preventing the membrane from accumulating electrical charges.[28,29] This can be accomplished by injecting opposite charges to those recorded by the voltage electrode through a second electrode placed at the end plate (Figure 10.2A). The current-

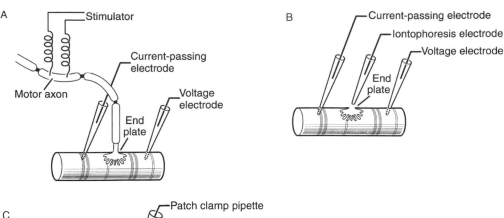

Figure 10.2 Schematic representation of the most important types of end-plate recordings. **A.** Two-microelectrode voltage clamp recording. **B.** Recording of end-plate noise during iontophoretic application of acetylcholine to voltage-clamped end plate. **C.** Tight-seal single-channel patch clamp recording using a firepolished pipette containing acetylcholine inside to activate the openings of acetylcholine receptor ion channels.

injecting electrode is connected to a negative feedback amplifier that reacts immediately in response to changes registered by the voltage-recording electrode. This permits the maintenance of the voltage at zero or at any other desired holding potential. At the end plate, neither MEPPs nor EPPs are recorded but, rather, the current that is needed to maintain the voltage constant during MEPPs or EPPs. These currents are called *miniature end-plate currents* (MEPCs) and *end-plate currents* (EPCs). In practice, owing to many technical factors including the limitations in the rate of transmission of current passing through the current electrode and the surface extension of the membrane or "space clamp," a perfect voltage clamp cannot be achieved. Nevertheless, this technique ameliorates significantly the bias introduced by the cable properties of the membrane.

Under voltage clamp conditions, it is also possible to derive basic properties of the AChR ion channel by using power spectral analysis of ACh-induced end-plate noise. Technically, power spectral analysis requires the placement of two microelectrodes to keep the end plate under voltage clamp and a third electrode for iontophoretic application of ACh (see Figure 10.2B). The end-plate noise observed during application of constant low concentrations of ACh arises from the random superposition of many elementary events corresponding to the opening and closing of discrete ion channels.[30,31] The frequency spectrum of the current fluctuations at fixed voltage obeys a relation of the Lorentz form. From the variance of the noise amplitude and the corner frequency of Lorentzian plots, it is possible to estimate the channel conductance and the channel open time.[32] Technically, in vitro studies of end-plate noise are challenging because they require the positioning of three microelectrodes in a small space. Furthermore, the much higher resolution provided by newer patch clamp techniques has rendered these types of studies obsolete.

Several voltage clamp studies have been performed in patients with disorders of muscle membrane excitability, including myotonic conditions and various types of periodic paralysis. Most of these studies have been conducted in patients with paramyotonia congenita,[33,34] adynamia episodica hereditaria,[35] and hypokalemic periodic paralysis[36] using external intercostal muscles. Voltage clamp recordings in muscle membrane disorders are far more informative than plain voltage recordings of action potentials, because they can dissect the different membrane currents. In addition, they can estimate the conductance of the currents across the membrane for different ions and provide voltage-current relationships. However, these studies are also demanding because they require the placement of at least three microelectrodes at 200- to 350-μm intervals to achieve an acceptable voltage clamp.[37] Patch clamp and molecular biology techniques, which allow the expression of ion channels and the recording of their activity in mammalian cell lines, have largely replaced microelectrode voltage clamp studies in disorders of muscle membrane excitability.

Patch Clamp Studies

The introduction of the patch clamp technique in the mid-1970s brought about a revolution in the field of cell physiology, because the patch clamp technique permitted the acquisition of electrophysiologic data from living cells in a way that was not possible before.[38,39] The patch clamp technique is based on the development of a high-resistance seal between a patch of cell membrane and the tip of a firepolished microelectrode or pipette, a maneuver that requires the application of negative pressure inside the pipette (see Figure 10.2C).

The high-resistance seal or gigaseal (from gigaohm resistance) obtained in patch clamp studies produces a dramatic increase of the signal to noise ratio that enables direct visualization of the opening and closing of single ion channels. This form of patch clamp recording is called *cell-attached configuration* or *on-cell configuration*. In another variant of patch clamp called *whole-cell recording,* the patch of the membrane is ruptured by the application of further negative pressure inside the pipette. This results in a continuity between the cell and the pipette that permits stable voltage clamp recordings even in small living cells.[40]

Early attempts to perform patch clamp recordings in human muscle biopsy material encountered insurmountable difficulties. A major obstacle to using a human biopsy muscle tissue is that a smooth, clean surface membrane is difficult to obtain, particularly at the end-plate region. Another vexing problem was the lack of attachment of muscle fibers to a rigid surface. This rigid attachment is important because it allows the application of mechanical pressure between the pipette and the membrane, which is required to initiate the seal. In spite of these initial technical difficulties, the neuromuscular group at the Mayo Clinic succeeded in the early 1990s in obtaining tight-seal patch clamp recordings from human muscle biopsy material.[41] These studies provided invaluable information about the kinetics of the AChR ion channels in several forms of CMS owing to mutations in genes encoding the AChR subunits.[42–45]

The technique of loose-patch voltage clamp has been successfully used for measurements of sodium currents and membrane capacitance in human intercostal muscles.[46,47]

Only a few studies using tight-seal patch clamp recordings have been performed in biopsy material of patients with disorders of membrane excitability.[48,49] Because of the large dimensions of human muscle fibers, whole-cell patch clamp recordings are not possible in biopsy material. For these types of recordings, aneural muscle cultures from human muscle biopsy material have been successfully used.[50]

Patch clamp studies can provide elegant data, particularly in the CMSs owing to mutations in genes encoding the AChR subunits. However, the rapid advances of molecular biology that allow for the expression of wild-type and mutant ion channel proteins in mammalian cell lines have reduced the pressure to conduct these technically challenging studies in fresh human muscle biopsy material.

CLINICAL APPLICATIONS

As discussed, the most important clinical application of in vitro microelectrode studies is in the study of primary disorders of neuromuscular transmission.

Disorders with Primary Failure of Neuromuscular Transmission

There are two major groups of primary disorders of neuromuscular transmission. The first is the CMS group, in which microelectrode studies play a fundamental diagnostic role. The other group is the acquired types of myasthenia, including autoimmune myasthenia gravis (MG) and the Lambert-Eaton myasthenic syndrome (LEMS). Although the classification of these diseases under primary disorders of neuromuscular transmission is appropriate, it should be noted that in some cases, these conditions are associated with other neurologic manifestations that may be even more important than the myasthenic symptoms.

Congenital Myasthenic Syndromes

CMSs represent a group of disorders that share as a common denominator an inborn defect of neuromuscular transmission. As in patients with MG, patients with CMS experience severe weakness and fatigability that could be severe. However, in contrast to adult acquired myasthenia, autoimmunity plays no role in the pathogenesis of CMS. The underlying causes of the CMSs are genetic defects that result in functional and structural abnormalities of the neuromuscular transmission system. Pioneering in vitro microelectrode studies conducted by Edward Lambert and Andrew Engel from the Mayo Clinic have played a pivotal role in the elucidation of the various pathogenic mechanisms underlying these disorders. Furthermore, the in vitro studies still represent indispensable diagnostic instruments to determine the type of CMS.

According to the site of primary deficit, CMSs are classified as presynaptic or postsynaptic. Table 10.1 delineates a classification of CMS of the most important CMSs known to date.

Congenital Myasthenia due to Abnormal Resynthesis of Acetylcholine. The most characteristic clinical features of congenital myasthenia due to abnormal resynthesis of acetylcholine, previously referred to as *familial infantile myasthenia,* are (1) recessive transmission, (2) onset soon after birth, (3) history of respiratory crisis (or even a fatal apnea) during infancy followed by spontaneous remissions, and (4) a unique form of precipitation of weakness and electromyographic abnormalities by exercise.[51–55] The electron microscopy of the NMJ is essentially normal in this condition.[56] Recently, at the Mayo Clinic, 10 different heteroallelic mutations in the

Table 10.1 Classification of Congenital Myasthenic Syndromes

Presynaptic conditions

Congenital myasthenia due to abnormal resynthesis of acetylcholine (also referred to as
 congenital myasthenic syndrome associated with episodic apnea)

Congenital myasthenia with paucity of synaptic vesicles

Congenital myasthenia with quantal release deficiency

Episodic ataxia with myasthenic weakness

Postsynaptic conditions

With kinetic abnormalities

    Slow channel congenital myasthenic syndrome

    Fast channel congenital myasthenic syndrome

Without primary kinetic abnormalities

    Receptor deficiency due to mutations in acetylcholine receptor genes

    Receptor deficiency due to mutations in rapsyn

Congenital end plate acetylcholinesterase deficiency

gene that encodes the choline acetyltransferase enzyme were identified in five patients with resynthesis abnormalities.[57] Expression studies in Cos cells have shown either no expression or low expression for four of the mutants. Enzymatic kinetic studies showed significantly impaired catalytic efficiencies of all bacterially expressed choline acetyltransferase mutants.

IN VITRO MICROELECTRODE STUDIES. Microelectrode studies performed by Lambert in the early 1970s were instrumental in the elucidation of the pathogenesis of this condition.[56] These studies revealed normal amplitudes of EPPs and MEPPs at rest (Table 10.2). However, the amplitudes of MEPPs and compound muscle action potentials (CMAPs) recorded in vitro from strips of intercostal muscles after sustained electrical nerve stimulation at 10 Hz were markedly reduced. Subsequent studies also showed that the EPP quantal content at rest and after sustained electrical stimulation was normal in this condition. The stimulation-induced reduction of MEPP amplitudes provided a strong lead in the elucidation of the pathogenesis of this condition, because it suggested an impaired mechanism of ACh resynthesis or packing of ACh molecules into synaptic vesicles. This original hypothesis, which was based on the in vitro microelectrode studies, was subsequently confirmed by the molecular genetic studies. In our experience, MEPP amplitudes are normal, but moderate reduction of EPP quantal content was present in the few patients who were studied (Figure 10.3).

Congenital Myasthenia with Paucity of Synaptic Vesicles. Only one patient has been reported with congenital myasthenia with paucity of synaptic vesicles.[58] The patient was a 21-year-old woman with bulbar and limb weakness since birth. Notably, she had variable ptosis, ophthalmoparesis, and facial weakness. Ultrastructurally, the NMJ revealed striking reduction of synaptic vesicles.

IN VITRO MICROELECTRODE STUDIES. The in vitro studies in the single patient reported with paucity of synaptic vesicles showed reduction of the EPP quantal content at the expense of a decrease of the quantal store available for immediate release. The probability of quantal release was normal. Amplitudes and frequencies of MEPPs were normal. We have encountered two patients with similar clinical in vitro physiology and electron microscopy of the NMJ (Figure 10.4). The cause of this syn-

Table 10.2 Most Common Electrophysiologic Findings in Neuromuscular Transmission Disorders

	Compound Muscle Action Potential	RNS at Slow Rate	RNS at Fast Rate	MEPP Amp	MEPP Frequency	EPP Quantal Content	MEPC
Lambert-Eaton myasthenic syndrome	↓ Amp	Decr	Incr	nl or ↓	nl or ↓	↓	nl
Botulism type A	↓ Amp	nl or decr	nl or incr	↓	↓	↓	nda
Botulism type B	↓ Amp	nl or decr	Incr	nl	nl	↓	nda
Abnormal acetylcholine resynthesis	nl	nl or decr[a]	nl, incr, or decr[a]	nl[b]	nl	nl or ↓	nl
Congenital myasthenia with quantal release deficiency	nl	nl or decr	nl, incr, or decr	nl	nl or ↑	↓	nl
Congenital myasthenia with paucity of synaptic vesicles	nl	Decr	Decr	nl	nl	↓	nl
Episodic ataxia type 2	nl	nl or decr	nl, incr, or decr	nl	nl or ↑	↓	nl
Myasthenia gravis	nl or ↓ amp	Decr	Decr	↓	nl	nl or ↓[c]	↓ Amp
Slow channel congenital myasthenic syndrome	Repet	nl or decr	nl or decr	↓	nl	nl or ↓	↓ Amp and prolonged
Fast channel congenital myasthenic syndrome	nl	Decr	Decr	↓ Or undet	nl	nl	↓ Amp and short
Severe acetylcholine-receptor deficiency	nl or ↓ amp	Decr	Decr	↓	nl	nl or ↓[c]	↓ Amp
Congenital end plate acetylcholinesterase deficiency	Repet or nl	Decr	Decr	nl or ↓	nl	↓	Prolonged

Amp = amplitude; decr = electromyographic decrement; EPP = end-plate potential; incr = increment; MEPC = miniature end plate current; MEPP = miniature end-plate potential; nda = no data available; nl = normal limits; repet = repetitive; RNS = repetitive nerve stimulation; undet = undetectable; ↑ = increase; ↓ = decrease.

[a]Decrement often present only after exercise.
[b]Reduced amplitude after sustained nerve stimulation at fast rates.
[c]Also reported to be increased at chronic stages of the disease.

drome is unknown; however, a reasonable assumption is that it may result from defects in genes involved in synaptic vesicle endocytosis and recycling, including the synaptotagmin gene.

Congenital Myasthenia with Quantal Release Deficiency. Quantal release deficiency has been recently described by our group.[59] Nevertheless, deficiency of quantal release as the sole manifestation of a CMS has also been encountered by other researchers.[60,61] Patients with this disorder had clinical histories of hypotonia and weakness since birth or infancy. Clinically, they differed from patients with abnormal acetylcho-

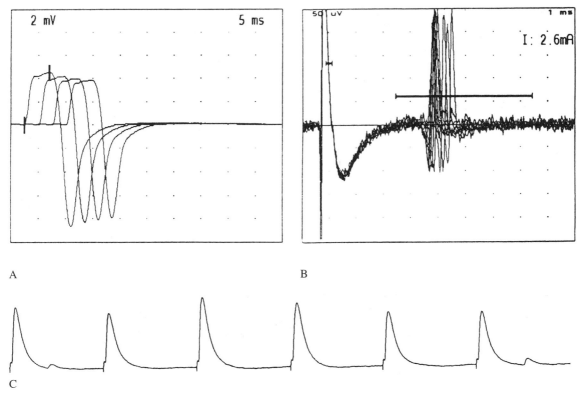

Figure 10.3 Electrophysiologic findings in a 16-month-old girl with a history of recurrent respiratory difficulties and bilateral eyelid ptosis. **A.** Repetitive nerve stimulation at 2 Hz of the left axillary nerve recording from the deltoid muscle showed 17% decrement of compound muscle action potential amplitudes. **B.** Stimulated single-fiber electromyography at 10 Hz in the left deltoid muscle showed increased jitter and impulse blocking in 18 muscle fibers. **C.** Except for mild reduction of the end-plate potential (EPP) quantal content, the microelectrode study showed no other abnormalities. In this example, six EPPs evoked by nerve stimulation at 1 Hz are displayed. The EPP amplitudes are mildly reduced, but the amplitudes of spontaneous MEPPs (shown next to the first and last EPP) are normal. The electron microscopy of the neuromuscular junction was normal, but mutational analysis of the *CHAT* gene revealed the presence of a missense mutation in exon 18 and a stop codon mutation in exon 15 that predicted truncations of the protein product.

line resynthesis in that they showed the following: (1) lack of evidence for an autosomal recessive transmission; (2) less conspicuous respiratory crisis or exercise-induced weakness; and (3) frequent additional neurologic findings including nystagmus, ataxia, and incoordination. The electron microscopy of the postsynaptic membranes is normal, but the axon terminal membrane often shows variable degrees of folding or invaginations. These folds occasionally form double-membrane–bound sacs containing synaptic vesicles. The number of synaptic vesicles is normal or even increased.

IN VITRO MICROELECTRODE STUDIES. The microelectrode studies show that the MEPPs are normal, but the mean EPP quantal content is markedly reduced. The latter becomes normal after exposing the end plates to high concentrations of calcium or diaminopyridine (Figure 10.5). MEPPs frequencies are normal or increased. Clearly, in congenital myasthenia with quantal release deficiency, failure of neuromuscular transmission results from impaired release of the neurotransmitter. At the level of the

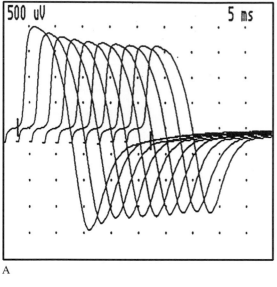

A

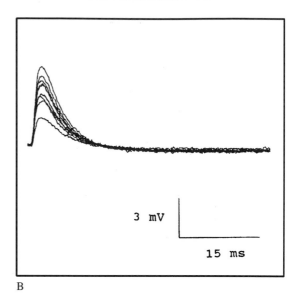

B

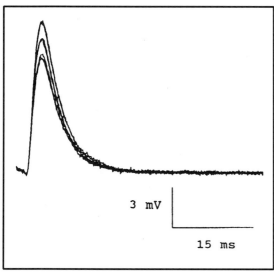

C

Figure 10.4 Electrophysiologic findings in a 10-year-old boy whose muscle biopsy showed almost complete depletion of synaptic vesicles. **A.** Repetitive stimulation at 20 Hz showing a clear decremental response. The decrement was less pronounced with stimulation at 2 Hz. **B.** Examples of small amplitude end-plate potentials recorded from the muscle biopsy of the same patient. **C.** Normal end-plate potentials recorded from a control.

in vitro microelectrode studies, patients with this condition show similarities to patients with episodic ataxia and LEMS.

Episodic Ataxia with Myasthenic Weakness. Episodic ataxia with myasthenic weakness is an autosomal dominant condition characterized by intermittent acetazolamide-responsive attacks of ataxia and interictal nystagmus.[62,63] The abnormal gene, *CACNA1A*, encodes the transmembrane subunit of the P/Q-type calcium channel, which is heavily expressed in the cerebellum and at the NMJ motor nerve terminal.[64,65] Some patients with episodic ataxia with myasthenic weakness also have weakness, fatigability, and markedly increased jitter on single-fiber elec-

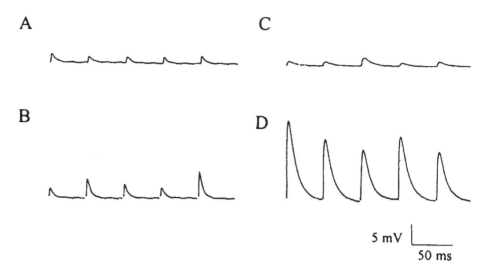

Figure 10.5 Examples of end-plate potentials (EPPs) and miniature EPPs (MEPPs) recorded from a patient with deficit of quantal release before and after exposing the muscle to high calcium solution. In physiologic calcium solution, the amplitudes of MEPPs are normal (**A**), but the amplitudes of EPPs recorded from the same end plate are severely reduced, which is consistent with low EPP quantal content (**B**). The amplitudes of MEPPs recorded from a different end plate after exposing the preparation to a high concentration of calcium (3.0 mM) are not different from those of MEPPs recorded in **A** (**C**); however, the amplitudes of EPPs at the same end plate are much larger than in (**B**), and the EPP quantal content is normal (**D**). (Reprinted with permission from Maselli R, Kong D, Bowe C, et al. Presynaptic congenital myasthenic syndrome due to quantal release deficiency. Neurology 2001;57:279–289.)

tromyography (SFEMG).[66] The electron microscopy of the NMJ is either normal or may show invaginated presynaptic membranes and an increased number of synaptic vesicles.

IN VITRO MICROELECTRODE STUDIES. The most striking abnormality of the electrophysiologic studies in patients with episodic ataxia with myasthenic weakness is the marked reduction of the EPP quantal content. MEPPs are normal or mildly reduced in amplitude, whereas the MEPP frequencies are normal or increased.[67] In contrast with controls and as in patients with deficiency of quantal release and LEMS, patients with episodic ataxia and neuromuscular transmission failure show no reduction of the EPP quantal content during fast rates of nerve stimulation (Figure 10.6). An additional finding is that the neurotransmitter release in these patients shows a novel sensitivity to N-type calcium channel blockade with ω-conotoxin not seen in controls.

Postsynaptic Conditions with Kinetic Abnormalities
SLOW CHANNEL CONGENITAL MYASTHENIC SYNDROME. Undoubtedly, the best characterized postsynaptic condition is the slow channel congenital myasthenic syndrome

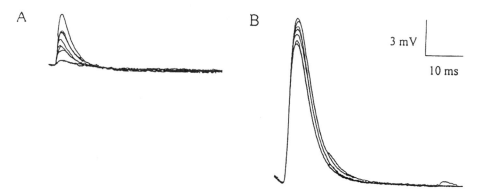

3 mV

10 ms

Figure 10.6 Examples of end-plate potentials recorded from a patient with episodic ataxia-2. **A.** Ten consecutive EPPs evoked by 1-Hz nerve stimulation are superimposed. The marked decrease and step-wise variation of EPP amplitudes are consistent with severe reduction of the EPP quantal content. **B.** Superimposed EPPs recorded from a control patient.

(SCCMS).[14] In this disease, structural abnormalities of the NMJ (often referred to as *end-plate myopathy*) are common, especially in the most severely affected patients. Failure of neuromuscular transmission results from reduction of EPP amplitudes and from staircase summation of prolonged EPP, which causes exercise-induced depolarization block.[68,69] Additional factors also contribute to failure of neuromuscular transmission, including an end-plate myopathy, which reduces the number of AChRs at the NMJ, and an accumulation of granular debris in the synaptic cleft, which interferes with the diffusion of ACh toward the AChR. At least 13 dominant mutations have been reported in different subunits and different domains of the AChR subunits in SCCMS.[70,71] All of these are missense mutations, and all result in pathologic gain of function; therefore, the condition is transmitted as a dominant trait. The classic electromyography findings are repetitive CMAP in response to a single nerve stimulation and decremental response to slow rates of nerve stimulation. However, the decremental response in some cases is totally absent.

In Vitro Microelectrode Studies. The most distinctive finding of the electrophysiologic studies is the marked prolongation of the decays of EPPs, MEPPs, and MEPCs (Figure 10.7). Noise analysis and single-channel recordings also confirm the presence of prolonged single-channel openings. MEPP and MEPC amplitudes are diminished. The EPP quantal content could be normal, but it is usually decreased as well. Repetitive nerve stimulation at fast rates with a DC-coupled amplifier readily demonstrates staircase phenomena resulting from the summation of prolonged EPP, which leads to stimulation-induced depolarization of the end plate.

Mutations that induce change of amino acids into the transmembrane M2 domain of the AChR subunits (nine mutations so far identified) produce the most dramatic slowing of the rate of channel closing. This results in the most severe prolongation of synaptic currents and end-plate myopathy.[72–74] Mutations in the M1 region of the subunits[75] also slow the channel closing time, but to a lesser extent than M2 mutations. On the other hand, mutations that introduce a change of an amino acid in the extracellular domain of the α subunit[76,77] produce less pronounced prolongation of synaptic currents and less damage of the end-plate region. These mutations tend to

Figure 10.7 Repetitive nerve stimulation and end-plate voltage clamp in a patient with slow channel congenital myasthenic syndrome (SCCMS). **A.** Marked decrement of compound muscle action potential (CMAP) amplitudes in response to repetitive stimulation of the right ulnar nerve at 2 Hz in a 9-year-old boy affected with SCCMS. Notice repetitive CMAP in response to a single nerve stimulus (*arrowhead*). **B.** Voltage clamp study. Averaged miniature end-plate currents (MEPCs) recorded from the patient (*arrow*) superimposed to an averaged MEPC recorded from a normal control (*arrowhead*). There is reduction of amplitude and marked prolongation of MEPC time constant in the patient.

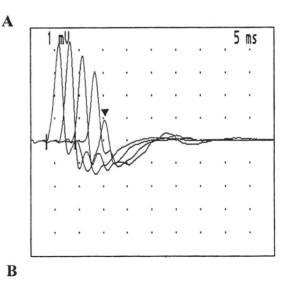

enhance the affinity of ACh for the receptor or decrease the rate of ACh dissociation from the binding site.

FAST CHANNEL CONGENITAL MYASTHENIC SYNDROME. In contrast with SCCMS in another type of CMS, the synaptic currents tend to be short. This condition results from a decreased affinity of AChR for ACh, and failure of neuromuscular transmission results from diminished EPP amplitudes. The end-plate ultrastructure in this condition is completely normal. Clinically, this patient can receive massive amounts of anticholinesterases without developing desensitization or depolarization block. At the molecular level, the common element in patients with this condition is replacement of the amino acid proline at position 121 in the ε subunit. Two heteroallelic AChR ε subunit gene mutations have been reported by Engel's group in two patients. One common εP121L mutation present in both patients combined with a signal peptide mutation (εG-8R) in one patient and a glycosylation consensus site mutation (εS143L) in the other patient.[78] We have encountered in our laboratory another patient with fast channel congenital myasthenic syndrome and similar clinical as well as molecular abnormalities.

In Vitro Microelectrode Studies. MEPPs and currents are small, often to the extent that miniature potentials and currents are unobtainable (Figure 10.8), although the quantal content of the EPP and the number of AChR per end plate are normal. The kinetic properties of AChR studied with analysis of ACh-induced current noise were fundamental in the elucidation of the pathogenesis of this syndrome.[79] These studies showed that mean single-channel conductance was nor-

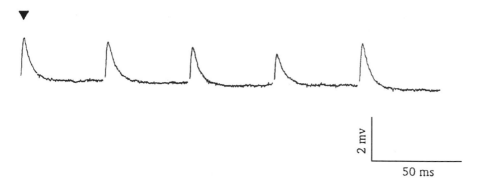

Figure 10.8 Voltage recordings in a patient with fast channel congenital myasthenic syndrome. Uniform reduction of amplitudes and shortening of decays of end-plate potentials (*arrowhead*) recorded from a 3-year-old girl carrying the εP121L mutation. Miniature end-plate potentials were unrecordable, and the electron microscopy of the neuromuscular junction was normal.

mal but that the noise power spectrum was abnormal, containing two components of different time course. These initial studies suggested an abnormal interaction between ACh and the AChR. Single channel patch clamp recordings have confirmed the presence of two different durations of channel openings with a major component being shorter than that in control patients. The most striking finding of the expression studies in human embryonic kidney cells is the completely normal expression of the εP121L mutant, which produces a dramatic reduction of ACh affinity for the receptor open channel. Because the other mutants showed severely reduced expression, εP121L defines the phenotype.

Other Forms of Fast Channel Congenital Myasthenic Syndrome. Patients with AChR subunit mutations other than εP121L have been presented as alternative forms of fast channel syndrome.[80,81] However, in contrast to εP121L, these cases showed a profound reduction in the number of radioactive alpha-bungarotoxin binding sites per end plate. This suggests that in these alternative cases, the primary mechanism of neuromuscular transmission failure is a deficiency in the number of AChRs per end plate. In addition, expression studies of a δ subunit mutant encountered in a patient with arthrogryposis multiplex have been predicted to result in a fast channel syndrome.[82] In vitro studies in a muscle biopsy of the patient carrying this interesting mutation are not available.

Postsynaptic Conditions without Primary Kinetic Abnormalities. Several forms of postsynaptic CMAPs have been described. The common denominator of all these conditions is a severe reduction of MEPP amplitudes with a variable degree of simplification of postsynaptic foldings and reduction of AChR count per end plate. A great deal of genetic heterogeneity underlies these disorders.[83–85] In most cases, the mutations are heterozygous, except in large consanguineous families or when the mutation is in the promoter region[86] of the ε subunit in which homozygous mutations are more common. In the majority of the instances, mutational analysis reveals the presence of a stop codon or a frame-shifting premature chain termination (nonsense mutations) combined with missense mutations (compound heterozygous).[87] The majority of these mutations are located in

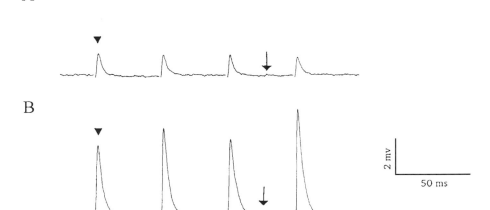

Figure 10.9 Voltage recordings in a 3-year-old boy with severe deficiency of acetylcholine receptors and markedly simplified postsynaptic folding pattern. **A.** End plate with severe reduction of amplitudes of end-plate potentials (EPPs) (*arrowheads*) and miniature EPPs (MEPPs) (*arrows*). **B.** End plate with less pronounced reduction of amplitudes of EPPs and MEPPs suggesting variable expression of acetylcholine receptors with normal physiologic characteristics. The molecular genetic and the expression studies in HEK cells revealed a compound heterozygous defect in the acetylcholine receptor–subunit gene with a null allele and variable (as well as deficient) expression of an allele, which resulted in physiologically normal acetylcholine-receptor ion channels.

the ε subunit, especially at the long cytoplasmatic loop between the M3 and M4 regions. A possible explanation is that the ε subunit, which is the subunit expressed in innervated muscles from adult individuals, can be rescued by the γ subunit, which is the subunit expressed during the fetal stage or in denervated muscle. This substitution provides patients a means for survival that cannot occur if the null mutation is in subunits that cannot be replaced by other subunits. This mechanism has been confirmed by means of immunohistochemistry. Nevertheless, other alternative explanations for the survival of these patients have been proposed.[88]

IN VITRO MICROELECTRODE STUDIES. The most characteristic sign of postsynaptic conditions without primary kinetic abnormalities is the marked reduction of amplitudes of MEPPs and MEPCs (Figure 10.9). The EPP quantal content is usually normal, but it has been reported to be increased in some cases, perhaps owing to increased presynaptic area at mature sprouted end plates or as a compensatory mechanism.[84] In addition, the increased EPP quantal content may result, in part, from the method of calculation of the quantal content. As described earlier, some methods of calculation of the quantal content, such as the one using the variance of the EPP amplitudes, may result in a bias toward high levels of quantal content.

In spite of the small amplitude of MEPCs, it is often possible to resolve two components of MEPC decays, which suggests the presence of more than one population of channels. Noise analysis and single-channel patch clamp recordings often show that the conductance of a slowly closing channel is diminished and consistent with that of a fetal type of AChR channel formed by the γ subunit in replacement of the ε subunit. In other cases, single-channel recordings in cells carrying the mutants suggest that one of the components of the MEPC decays reflects the kinetics of one of the mutant alleles.

It should be realized that the minimal kinetic changes resulting from either mutant or rescuer channels are overshadowed by the severe deficiency of AChR present at the end plate of these patients.

END-PLATE ACETYLCHOLINE-RECEPTOR DEFICIENCY DUE TO MUTATIONS IN RAPSYN. In a small number of patients with CMS with clear reduction of AChR count per end plate and a variable degree of simplification of postsynaptic folds, no mutations can be detected in the AChR subunit genes. Recently, Ohno et al.[89] demonstrated that in some of these patients, the AChR deficiency is secondary to mutations in the gene that encodes rapsyn. The findings of the microelectrode studies are essentially the same as in patients with AChR deficiency due to mutations in the AChR subunit genes.

Congenital End-Plate Acetylcholinesterase Deficiency. *Congenital end-plate AChE deficiency* (CEAD) is a recessive condition characterized by severe reduction of end-pate AChE, small nerve terminals (often encased by the Schwann cell), focal degeneration of the end-plate folds, diminished action potential–evoked release of a neurotransmitter, and prolonged decay of synaptic potentials and currents.[90] Clinically, these patients are hypotonic, show a profound scoliosis, and often have sluggishly reactive pupils. The electromyography shows (as in the SCCMS) repetitive CMAPs in response to a single nerve stimulation, although this is less pronounced than in the SCCMS, and sometimes it can be completely absent. Repetitive nerve stimulation usually shows decremental response. In this condition, the normal asymmetric type of AChE is absent from muscle. Failure of neuromuscular transmission occurs as a result of depolarization block and diminished release of a neurotransmitter. Mutational analysis of the gene encoding the AChE catalytic (AChET) subunit revealed normal sequence and mRNA splicing. At least 16 mutations (either homozygous or compound heterozygous) have been encountered in the gene encoding the collagen tail subunit (ColQ) of the AChE.[91–94] The human ColQ gene is composed of 17 exons and is mapped to chromosome 3 (3p25). There is marked heterogeneity in the pathogenic mutations of ColQ. The majority are stop-codon or frame-shifting premature chain termination mutations resulting in a truncated protein. Missense mutations as well as splice donor mutations resulting in exon skipping have also been encountered. Studies performed in Cos cells showed that these mutations result in severe reduction of AChE expression, indicating that they are indeed pathogenic. According with the site, these mutations can (1) cancel the attachment of ColQ to AChET when they are located in the proline-rich attachment domain, (2) prevent triple helix formation of ColQ (truncated protein), (3) prevent triple helix formation at the C-terminal (i.e., frame-shift with change of amino acid sequence), or (4) abolish insertion of the ColQ to the basal membrane (missense and truncation mutations in the C-terminal region).

IN VITRO MICROELECTRODE STUDIES. The findings of the microelectrode studies are quite heterogeneous, but there are distinctive elements that permit an easy recognition of this syndrome. MEPP amplitudes could be normal but are usually depressed as a result of focal degeneration of synaptic folds and loss of AChR. The frequency of MEPPs is diminished owing to the reduced size of the nerve ter-

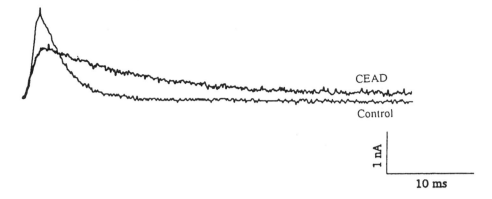

Figure 10.10 Prolongation of synaptic current in congenital end-plate acetylcholinesterase deficiency (CEAD). Example of an averaged miniature end-plate current (MEPC) recorded from a 10-year-old boy with CEAD. Note the reduction of the amplitude and the prolongation of the time constant of the MEPC from a CEAD in comparison with a MEPC from a control.

minal and decreased number of synaptic vesicles readily available for release. The duration and half-decay time of MEPPs and time constants of MEPCs are prolonged, and prostigmin has no additional effect (Figure 10.10). As in the SCCMS, repetitive nerve stimulation at fast rates demonstrates a staircase phenomenon resulting from the summation of prolonged EPP. This suggests that stimulation-induced depolarization of the end plate plays a role, at least in part, in the pathogenesis of this condition. Analysis of ACh-induced current noise shows that the kinetics of the AChR ion channel are essentially normal. The quantum content of the EPP is decreased owing to a reduced store of quanta immediately available for release, but the probability of release is normal.

Acquired Disorders of Neuromuscular Transmission

Although acquired disorders of neuromuscular transmission are more common than CMS, in vitro microelectrode studies are seldom required to make the diagnosis of these conditions. For their diagnosis, other electrophysiologic methods are routinely used, as discussed in previous chapters. Nevertheless, at times, the in vitro studies are needed to differentiate some acquired forms of neuromuscular transmission failure from CMS.

Only the most important acquired disorders of neuromuscular transmission have been studied with microelectrode recordings. In almost all instances, the microelectrode recordings played a fundamental role in the elucidation of the pathogenesis of these disorders.

Botulism. *Botulism* is an acquired presynaptic disorder of neuromuscular transmission resulting from the action of a toxin produced by the anaerobic, spore-forming organism *Clostridium botulinum*. Types A and B are the most important serotypes of the seven types so far identified. These toxins cleave key proteins that enable the fusion of synaptic vesicles to the nerve terminal. Type A cleaves the presynaptic membrane protein SNAP-25, whereas type B cleaves the synaptic vesicle VAMP or synaptobrevin.[95,96] The rest of the toxin types cleave the same proteins at different cleavage sites. Neuromuscular transmission fails as a result of a reduced synaptic vesicle release. In food-borne botulism, the toxin is ingested with contaminated food. In wound botulism, the toxin is produced locally at tissues contaminated with *C. botulinum*. In infant botulism, the disease results from the ingestion of spores that germinate and colonize the immature intestinal tract of infants. The most characteristic electrodiagnostic findings in botulism are reduction of CMAP amplitudes and incremental response to repetitive nerve stimulation at high rates, particularly with botulism type B.

IN VITRO MICROELECTRODE STUDIES. Several cases of wound and food-borne botulism type A have been investigated with in vitro microelectrode recordings.[97,98] The most consistent findings are the decline of the EPP quantal content and the reduction of MEPP amplitudes and frequencies (Figure 10.11). These findings are similar to those found in human denervation,[2] suggesting that botulism type A fundamentally induces ultraterminal pharmacologic denervation. In contrast, in type B intoxication, there is less decrease of MEPP amplitudes and frequencies but equal or even more reduction of EPP quantal content than in type A.[15] In addition, in type B, there is marked desynchronization of EPP onsets or *EPP jitter* (Figure 10.12). These findings suggest that toxin type B interferes with the release of synaptic vesicles primed by the impulse-evoked peak entry of Ca^{2+} into the nerve terminal. On the other hand, toxin type A appears to interfere with the release of both synaptic vesicles primed by the impulse-evoked peak entry of Ca^{2+} and those that spontaneously fuse with the presynaptic membrane.

Lambert-Eaton Myasthenic Syndrome. *LEMS* is a presynaptic disorder of neuromuscular transmission that is characterized by a reduced quantal release from peripheral motor and autonomic nerve terminals as a result of an autoimmune attack of presynaptic voltage-gated calcium channels. The serum immunoglobulin G fraction from LEMS patients reacts mainly against epitopes located in the transmembrane and regulatory subunits of the P/Q-type calcium channel.[99,100] This also reacts with other types of calcium channels and even with proteins associated with calcium channels, such as synaptotagmin.[101] In half of the patients with this syndrome, there is an associated small cell carcinoma of the lung. The most characteristic electromyographic findings are the generalized reduction of CMAP amplitudes and the often dramatic increment of CMAP amplitudes in response to high-frequency nerve stimulation (30–50 Hz). Decremental response to slow rates of nerve stimulation is quite constant and present in both proximal and distal muscles.[102]

IN VITRO MICROELECTRODE STUDIES. The findings with LEMS are similar to those encountered in congenital myasthenia with quantal release deficiency and episodic ataxia type 2. The amplitudes and frequencies of MEPPs are normal or moderately reduced, but the EPP quantal content, which depends on the rapid entry of calcium into the nerve terminal during the arrival of an action potential, is severely reduced. The mean EPP quantal content in LEMS patients is approximately five times smaller than the quantal content determined in adult control patients.[2,98] In LEMS muscles, there is great variability of EPP amplitudes, which are distributed according to the Poisson distribution (Figure 10.13). Statistical calculations performed on binomial-distributed EPPs demonstrated that the reduction of the EPP quantal content (*m*) in LEMS is due to a reduction of both the quanta

Figure 10.11 Electrophysiologic findings in a case of botulism type A intoxication. **A.** Repetitive nerve stimulation at 30 Hz in a 44-year-old patient intoxicated with type A botulinum toxin showing moderate incremental response. **B.** End-plate potentials (EPPs) recorded from the muscle biopsy of the same patient demonstrating marked reduction and variability of EPP amplitudes (**inset**). The EPP amplitudes follow a gaussian curve with a mean of approximately 1 mV. The bar on the left represents stimuli that failed to elicit EPPs. The probability of release is low but not as low as in Lambert-Eaton syndrome, in which EPP amplitudes at the majority of the end plates are arranged following Poisson distribution.

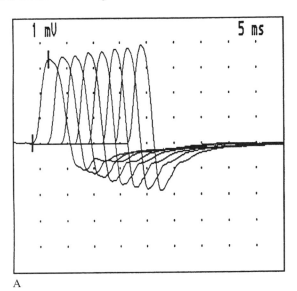

A

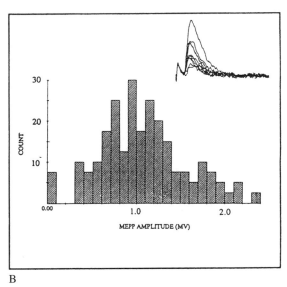

B

available for immediate release (n) and the probability of release (p). Because n closely reflects the number of synaptic vesicles positioned at the active zones, the reduction of n in LEMS correlates well with the demonstrated depletion and disorganization of active zones by freeze fracture microscopy at the nerve terminal of patients with this disease.[103] On the other hand, because p depends on the sudden elevation of calcium concentration at the nerve terminal during an action potential, the reduction of p in LEMS indicates an impairment of calcium entry into the nerve terminal. As in patients with congenital myasthenia with quantal release deficiency and episodic ataxia type 2, fast rates of nerve stimulation fail to depress

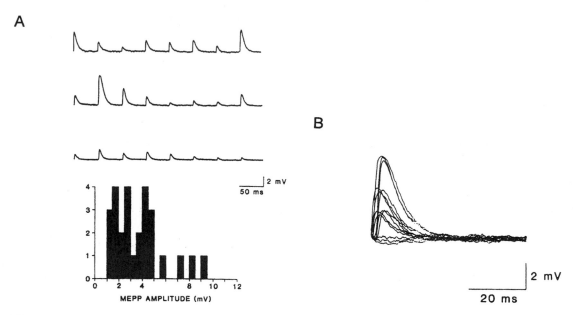

Figure 10.12 Voltage recording in botulism type B intoxication. **A.** Examples of spontaneous miniature end-plate potentials (MEPPs) (*top*) and the corresponding amplitude frequency distribution (*bottom*). MEPPs were recorded from a single end plate in the muscle biopsy of an 8-week-old girl intoxicated with botulinum toxin type B. Notice the large amplitude of some of the MEPPs, which are often referred to as *giant MEPPs*. Neither the frequency nor the amplitudes of the MEPPs were significantly reduced. **B.** Stepwise variation of small amplitudes of end-plate potentials (EPPs) recorded from the same patient. Notice also the prominent variation of EPP onsets or *EPP jitter*. (Reprinted with permission from Maselli RA, Burnett ME, Tonsgard JH. In vitro microelectrode study of neuromuscular transmission in a case of botulism. Muscle Nerve 1992;15[3]:273–276.)

the EPP quantal content. The increments of EPP amplitudes during tetanic nerve stimulation are usually modest, suggesting that additional factors may play a role in the generation of prominent electromyographic increments of CMAP amplitudes during high rates of nerve stimulation in LEMS.

Myasthenia Gravis. The pathogenesis of MG involves an autoimmune attack directed against the AChR, which leads to a reduction of the number of receptors at the motor end plate.[104–106] As a result of the reduced number of postsynaptic receptors, the amplitudes of synaptic potentials (i.e., MEPPs and EPPs) decrease, producing failure of neuromuscular transmission. Immune complexes, including immunoglobulin G and complement components, can be demonstrated at the NMJ of MG patients.[107–109] In addition, circulating antibodies directed against the AChR are present in 85–90% of patients with MG. As in the animal model of MG (referred to as *experimental autoimmune myasthenia gravis*), inflammatory cell reaction at the NMJ is often detected at early stages of the human disease.[110,111] Later on, the most constant ultrastructural finding is a simplification of postsynaptic fold pattern.[112] In the 10–15% of patients with generalized MG and absent circulating antibodies against the AChR, the physiologic and ultrastructural findings (i.e., reduction of synaptic potential amplitudes and simplification of the postsynaptic membranes) are similar to those seen in seropositive MG patients. However, in a small percentage of patients with seronega-

Figure 10.13 Electrophysiologic findings in Lambert-Eaton myasthenic syndrome. **A.** Repetitive nerve stimulation at 50 Hz showing prominent incremental response in a patient with Lambert-Eaton myasthenic syndrome. **B.** EPPs recorded from the muscle biopsy of the same patient showing reduction and stepwise variation of end-plate potential (EPP) amplitudes (**inset**). The EPP amplitudes are arranged following Poisson distribution. Stimulations resulted in failures (*left bar*), EPPs of about 1 mV amplitude (first gaussian), EPPs of 2 mV amplitude (second gaussian), or EPPs of 3 mV amplitude (third gaussian).

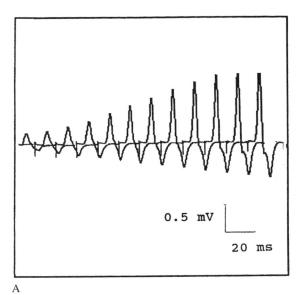

A

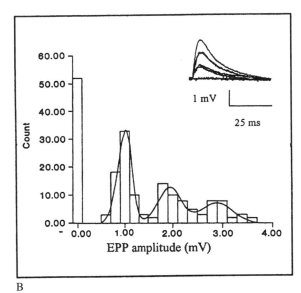

B

tive MG, the characteristic ultrastructural abnormalities of MG are surprisingly absent. It has been postulated that the serum antibodies of these patients may be directed against different antigens from those of seropositive MG.[113]

IN VITRO MICROELECTRODE STUDIES.   MG was the first disorder of neuromuscular transmission studied with in vitro microelectrode recordings. The cardinal finding of the in vitro studies in MG is a marked reduction of amplitudes of MEPPs and EPPs without significant change of the normal ratio between the amplitudes of EPPs and MEPPs (Figure 10.14). Initially, these findings were interpreted as a presynaptic

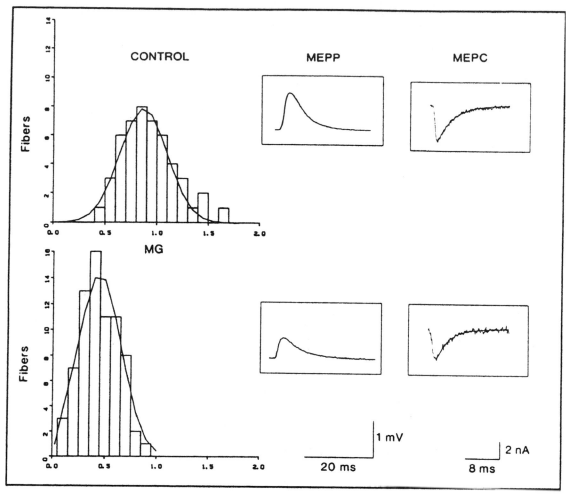

Figure 10.14 Distribution of miniature end-plate potential (MEPP) amplitudes from patients with myasthenia gravis (MG). Normal gaussian distribution of MEPP amplitudes in controls and MG patients with marked shift of amplitudes toward the low end in the MG patients. The insets show examples of averaged MEPPs and miniature end-plate currents (MEPCs) from controls (*top*) and MG patients. Notice that there is no difference in the duration of MEPCs from controls and MG patients. (Reprinted with permission from Maselli RA, Richman DP, Wollmann RL. Inflammation at the neuromuscular junction in myasthenia gravis. Neurology 1991;41[9]:1497–1504.)

failure owing to insufficient packing of ACh molecules into individual quanta.[114,115] However, subsequent studies, which included the measurement of receptor sensitivity to iontophoretic application of ACh, correctly suggested a postsynaptic cause.[116] Using analysis of ACh-induced end-plate noise, it was later demonstrated that in spite of the severe reduction of amplitudes of MEPPs and MEPCs, the AChR ion channel, conductance, and channel open time are normal in MG.[117] These results clearly indicated that in MG the amplitudes of MEPPs and MEPC are reduced as a result of a reduction in the number of AChR ion channels but that the unitary current flowing through a single AChR channel is normal.

Because the ratio between the amplitudes of EPP and MEPPs is normal, the EPP quantal content is not significantly changed in MG. Nevertheless, some studies have reported an increase in quantal content,[118] whereas others have presented evidence of a moderate decrease.[111] This variability of EPP quantal content in MG probably reflects changes of the quantal content occurring in reinnervating sprouts. At small immature reinnervating sprouts, the quantal content is reduced, but it may be actually increased at well-developed sprouts owing to an expansion of the presynaptic surface and the resultant increase in the number of active zones. This explanation may apply to other disorders of neuromuscular transmission, including CMS.

Other Autoimmune Disorders of Neuromuscular Transmission: Combined Acquired Presynaptic and Postsynaptic Disorders and the "Acquired Slow Channel Syndrome"

Some forms of invasive thymomas produce not only antibodies against the AChR but also autoantibodies to a variety of neuromuscular antigens, including titin, skeletal muscle, calcium channels, presynaptic voltage-gated calcium channels, and voltage-gated potassium channels.[119] The clinical syndromes resulting from the expression of these multiple autoantibodies are variable and frequently quite complex.[120] In addition to the myasthenic symptoms, patients with these syndromes often have evidence of myositis, myocarditis, polyneuropathy, dysautonomia, and electromyographically proven neuromyotonia. When these symptoms are combined with signs of central nervous system dysfunction (e.g., insomnia, delirium, and hallucinations) there is overlapping with a rare condition referred to as *Morvan's syndrome* (Maladie de Morvan), which comprises neuromyotonia, hyperhydrosis, and sleep abnormalities.[121–122] These syndromes respond well to plasmapheresis and a surgical removal of the tumor.

In Vitro Microelectrode Studies

In a single reported case of Morvan's syndrome and myasthenia secondary to an invasive thymoma, there were signs of combined postsynaptic and presynaptic failure.[121] The amplitude of MEPPs and the EPP quantal content were both severely reduced (Figure 10.15). The in vivo studies showed that the neuromyotonia was resistant to nerve block, suggesting an origin at the motor nerve terminal. This patient showed serum antibodies to AChR, titin, N-type calcium channels, and voltage-gated potassium channels.

Acquired Slow Channel Syndrome

A recent paper postulated the attractive possibility that some forms of autoimmune MG may show some of the characteristic signs of SCCMS.[123] In this paper, a single patient was studied with microelectrode recordings, and the study showed prolonga-

A

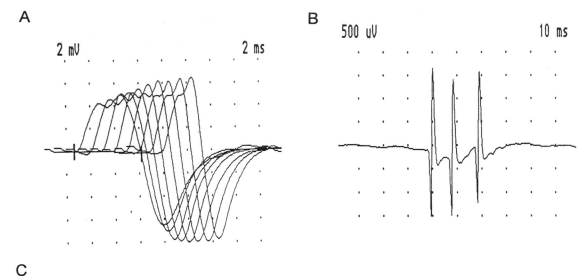

B

C

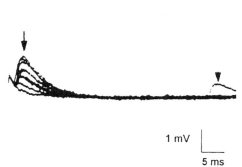

Figure 10.15 Electrophysiologic findings in a patient with a malignant thymoma and autoantibodies against multiple presynaptic and postsynaptic epitopes. **A.** Incremental response of 42% to repetitive stimulation of the right ulnar nerve at 30 Hz. **B.** Spontaneous burst of repetitive motor unit potentials with an intraburst frequency of 100 Hz consistent with neuromyotonia. **C.** Stepwise variation and reduction of end-plate potential amplitudes (*arrow*) consistent with presynaptic failure. The arrowhead points to a miniature end-plate potential that is also mildly reduced in amplitude.

tion of half-decays of EPPs and MEPPs. However, no voltage clamp or patch clamp recordings were performed; therefore, it is not possible to draw any definite conclusions. Future voltage clamp and patch clamp studies are needed to validate the existence of this potentially interesting condition.

Disorders with Secondary Failure of Neuromuscular Transmission

Numerous disorders of the peripheral nervous system show evidence of failure of neuromuscular transmission as indicated by the presence of decremental response to repetitive nerve stimulation or increased jitter on SFEMG. Only motor neuron diseases, such as amyotrophic lateral sclerosis (ALS) and the postpolio syndrome (PPS), have been studied in some detail with in vitro microelectrode recordings. These studies were conducted not only to define the nature of the neuromuscular failure but also as an effort to elucidate the underlying pathogenesis of these disorders.

Amyotrophic Lateral Sclerosis

Several studies have documented failure of neuromuscular transmission in ALS. These studies showed electromyographic features of presynaptic and postsynaptic failure.[124,125] SFEMG studies also suggested that failure of neuromuscular transmission (i.e., increased jitter) is most prominent in rapidly progressing cases displaying modest amounts of reinnervation (i.e., modest increase of fiber density).[126]

In Vitro Microelectrode Studies. Only two in vitro studies of neuromuscular transmission have been conducted in ALS.[1,2] The first study, which was limited to the recording of spontaneous MEPPs, demonstrated a generalized reduction of MEPP amplitudes. A subsequent, more complete study, which included recordings of MEPPs, nerve-evoked EPPs, and MEPCs under voltage clamp conditions, demonstrated not only a reduction of MEPP amplitudes but also a severe reduction of EPP quantal content. The MEPP frequencies were highly variable in ALS patients, but the average MEPP frequency was not different from that in control patients. An interesting and surprising finding in this study was that in spite of the reduction of the EPP, quantal content, and the quanta available for immediate release (n), the probability of quantal release (p) was normal or even increased, suggesting an excitability component at the nerve terminals of ALS patients (Figure 10.16). Subsequent in vivo studies using analysis of peristimulus histograms demonstrated findings suggestive of similar increased excitability at the central motor pathway synapse during early stages of ALS.[127,128] The molecular abnormalities responsible for these physiologic abnormalities in ALS remain unknown.

Postpolio Syndrome

For years, several clinical and electrodiagnostic features of PPS have captivated the attention of clinicians and investigators alike. The onset of progressive weakness and persistence of electromyographic signs of denervation several decades after a successful recovery from an attack of polio, as well as the relationship, if any, between PPS and ALS, have generated a significant amount of interest among neuromuscular researchers. Single-fiber and macro electromyography have shown marked changes in the architecture of the motor neuron consistent with prominent reinnervation and, often, maximal increase of the number of muscle fibers driven by single motor neurons.[129,130] Failure of neuromuscular transmission in PPS can be easily demonstrated by the presence of marked increments of SFEMG jitter. However, repetitive nerve stimulation usually fails to demonstrate failure of neuromuscular transmission even in significantly affected muscles.

The most generally accepted theory on the pathogenesis of PPS postulates a continuous remodeling process taking place at motor units that have maximized their sprouting capabilities. This results in a delicate balance between denervation and reinnervation, which later in life (perhaps as a result of premature aging) tilts toward retraction of reinnervating sprouts and attrition of the motor unit size and denervation.[131]

In Vitro Microelectrode Studies. A single in vitro study performed in 10 PPS patients encountered no homogeneous findings.[132] The MEPP frequencies were generally normal, but as in other conditions with underlying denervation, MEPP amplitudes ranged from normal to severely reduced. The EPP quantal content was also quite variable, being normal in two patients, decreased in five patients, and actually increased in three patients (Figure 10.17). These findings, rather

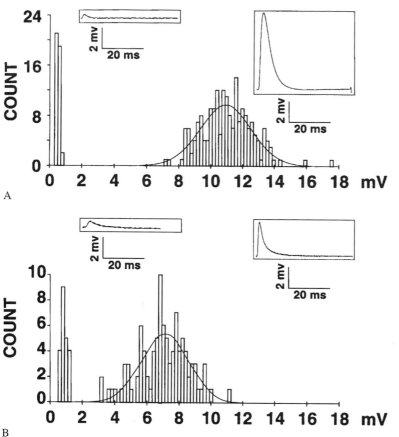

Figure 10.16 Neurotransmitter release at the neuromuscular junction in amyotrophic lateral sclerosis (ALS). Amplitude distributions of end-plate potentials (EPPs) and miniature EPPs (MEPPs) recorded from a control (**A**) and from a patient with ALS (**B**). The corresponding averaged MEPPs and EPPs are displayed in the insets. There is marked shift of the EPP amplitude distribution toward the low-amplitude end without similar shift of the MEPP amplitudes. This is consistent with low quantal content. However, in spite of the low quantal content, the amplitudes of the EPPs are distributed normally with a narrower dispersion in comparison with the control. This indicates high probability of neurotransmitter release at the neuromuscular junction of the ALS patient. (Reprinted with permission from Maselli RA, Wollman RL, Leung C, et al. Neuromuscular transmission in amyotrophic lateral sclerosis. Muscle Nerve 1993;6[11]:1193–1203.)

than uncovering a common pathophysiologic mechanism for PPS, appear to reflect the efficiency of neuromuscular transmission at reinnervating sprouts during different stages of maturation. Thus, the in vitro studies correlated well with the electromyographic findings of persistent denervation and failure of neuromuscular transmission demonstrated only at individual NMJs by SFEMG. The findings are also consistent with the current theory of the attrition of the motor unit in PPS described previously.

Disorders of Muscle Membrane Excitability

In contrast to primary disorders of neuromuscular transmission, intracellular microelectrode studies play relatively minor roles in the diagnosis of disorders of muscle membrane excitability. Most of these conditions are dominantly inherited and usually result in well-defined clinical features.[133,134] These facts have enabled a proper identification of affected individuals and the implementation of neurogenetic studies using conventional linkage analysis. Currently, the diagnosis of these disorders heavily depends on mutational analysis performed in positional candidate genes. The patho-

Figure 10.17 Quantal release in postpolio syndrome. Examples of end-plate potentials (EPPs) (*arrows*) and miniature EPPs (MEPPs) (*asterisks*) recorded from three different patients with postpolio syndrome. **A.** Relatively normal amplitudes of EPPs and MEPPs and normal quantal content. **B.** Increased EPP amplitudes with reduced MEPP amplitudes resulting in very high quantal content. **C.** Reduced amplitudes of EPPs and MEPPs consistent with postsynaptic failure. (Reprinted with permission from Maselli RA, Wollmann R, Roos R. Function and ultrastructure of the neuromuscular junction in post-polio syndrome. Ann N Y Acad Sci 1995;753:129–137.)

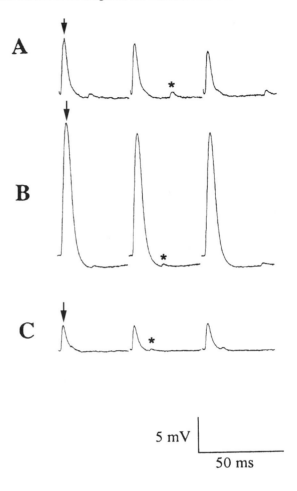

genic nature of identified mutations is tested using whole-cell patch clamp techniques conducted in mammalian cell lines expressing wild-type and mutant DNA.

CONCLUSIONS

In vitro microelectrode techniques represent invaluable tools for the study of neuromuscular diseases, especially primary disorders of neuromuscular transmission. They provide a way to evaluate a number of clinically important physiologic parameters that are not possible to assess with routine electromyographic studies. These include the EPP quantal content (which allows one to differentiate presynaptic from postsynaptic failure), the mechanism of synthesis and repacking of ACh into synaptic vesicles, the AChR channel open time, and the status of the end-plate AChE. Thus, the in vitro studies are especially indicated when facing a disorder of neuromuscular transmission of unclear etiology, a relatively common situation in CMS.

The high sophistication of some of the in vitro techniques, such as single-channel patch clamp recordings, provides the unique opportunity to carry the electrodiagnostic analysis all the way to the molecular level.

REFERENCES

1. Highstone HH, Colton RP, Norris FH. Amyotrophic Lateral Sclerosis: Changes in Motor Nerve Terminal Function. In WG Bradley, MD Gardner, JN Walton (eds), Recent Advances in Myology. Amsterdam: Excerpta Medica, 1975;542–545.
2. Maselli RA, Wollman RL, Leung C, et al. Neuromuscular transmission in amyotrophic lateral sclerosis. Muscle Nerve 1993;6(11):1193–1203.
3. Maselli RA, Wollmann R, Roos R. Function and ultrastructure of the neuromuscular junction in post-polio syndrome. Ann N Y Acad Sci 1995;753:129–137.
4. Lambert EH, Dyck PJ. Compound action potentials of human sural nerve biopsies. Electroencephalogr Clin Neurophysiol 1968;25(4):399–400.
5. Haynes J. Miniature end-plate potentials in neuromuscular disease: an electrophysiological investigation of motor-point muscle biopsies. J Neurol Neurosurg Psychiatry 1971;34:521–526.
6. Elmqvist D, Hofmann WW, Kugelberg J, Quastel DMJ. An electrophysiological investigation of neuromuscular transmission in myasthenia gravis. J Physiol (Lond) 1964;174:417–434.
7. Elmqvist D, Lambert EH. Detailed analysis of neuromuscular transmission in a patient with the myasthenic syndrome sometimes associated with bronchogenic carcinoma. Mayo Clin Proc 1968;43(10):689–713.
8. Gruener R, Stern LZ, Markovitz D, Gerdes C. Electrophysiologic properties of intercostal muscle fibers in human neuromuscular diseases. Muscle Nerve 1979;2(3):165–172.
9. Vincent A, Cull-Candy SG, Newsom-Davis J, et al. Congenital myasthenia: end-plate acetylcholine receptors and electrophysiology in five cases. Muscle Nerve 1981;4(4):306–318.
10. Engel AE. 73rd ENMC International Workshop: congenital myasthenic syndromes. 22–23 October, 1999, Naarden, The Netherlands. Neuromuscul Disord 2001;11(3):315–321.
11. Ohno K, Engel AG. Congenital myasthenic syndromes: gene mutations. Neuromuscul Disord 2000; 10(7):534–536.
12. Stern LZ, Gruener R, Anderson RM. External intercostal muscle biopsy. Arch Neurol 1975;32(11): 779–780.
13. Maselli RA, Mass DP, Distad BJ, Richman DP. Anconeus muscle: a human muscle preparation suitable for in-vitro microelectrode studies. Muscle Nerve 1991;14(12):1189–1192.
14. Engel A, Lambert E, Mulder D, et al. A newly recognized congenital myasthenic syndrome attributed to a prolonged open time of the acetylcholine-induced ion channel. Ann Neurol 1982;11:553–569.
15. Maselli RA, Burnett ME, Tonsgard JH. In vitro microelectrode study of neuromuscular transmission in a case of botulism. Muscle Nerve 1992;15(3):273–276.
16. Coffield JA, Bakry N, Zhang RD, et al. In vitro characterization of botulinum toxin types A, C and D action on human tissues: combined electrophysiologic, pharmacologic and molecular biologic approaches. J Pharmacol Exp Ther 1997;280(3):1489–1498.
17. Slater CR, Lyons PR, Walls TJ, et al. Structure and function of neuromuscular junctions in the vastus lateralis of man. A motor point biopsy study of two groups of patients. Brain 1992;115(Pt 2):451–478.
18. del Castillo J, Katz B. Quantal components of the end-plate potential. J Physiol 1954;124:560–573.
19. Martin AR. A further study of the statistical composition of the end plate potential. J Physiol 1955;130:114–122.
20. Stevens C. A comment on Martin's Relation. Biophys J 1976;16:891–895.
21. McLachlan EM, Martin AR. Non-linear summation of end-plate potentials in the frog and mouse. J Physiol 1981;311:307–324.
22. Elmqvist D, Quastel DM. A quantitative study of end-plate potentials in isolated human muscle. J Physiol 1965;178(3):505–529.
23. McLachlan E. The Statistics of Transmitter Release at Chemical Synapses. In R Porter (ed), International Review of Physiology Neurophysiology III, Vol 17. Baltimore: University Park Press, 1978;83–115.
24. Herrera A. Polyneuronal innervation and quantal transmitter release in formamide-treated frog sartorius muscles. J Physiol 1984;355:267–280.
25. Wood SJ, Slater CR. Safety factor at the neuromuscular junction. Prog Neurobiol 2001; 64(4):393–429.
26. Kuffler SW, Yoshikami D. The number of transmitter molecules in a quantum: an estimate from iontophoretic application of acetylcholine at the neuromuscular synapse. J Physiol 1975;251(2):465–482.

27. Van Helden DF, Gage PW, Hamill OP. Conductance of end-plate channels is voltage dependent. Neurosci Lett 1979;11(2):227–232.
28. Takeuchi A, Takeuchi N. Active phase of frog's end-plate potential. J Neurophysiol 1959;22: 395–411.
29. Gage PW, Armstrong CM. Miniature end-plate currents in voltage-clamped muscle fibre. Nature 1968;218(139):363–365.
30. Katz B, Miledi R. Membrane noise produced by acetylcholine. Nature 1970;226:962–963.
31. Katz B, Miledi R. The characteristics for "end-plate noise" produced by different depolarizing drugs. J Physiol 1973;230:707–717.
32. Anderson CR, Stevens CF. Voltage clamp analysis of acetylcholine produced end-plate current fluctuations at frog neuromuscular junction. J Physiol 1973;235(3):655–691.
33. Lehmann-Horn F, Rüdel R, Dengler R, et al. Membrane defects in paramyotonia congenita with and without myotonia in a warm environment. Muscle Nerve 1981;4(5):396–406.
34. Lehmann-Horn F, Rüdel R, Ricker K. Membrane defects in paramyotonia congenita (Eulenburg). Muscle Nerve 1987;10(7):633–641.
35. Lehmann-Horn F, Küther G, Ricker K, et al. Adynamia episodica hereditaria with myotonia: a non-inactivating sodium current and the effect of extracellular pH. Muscle Nerve 1987;10(4):363–374.
36. Hofmann WW, Smith RA. Hypokalemic periodic paralysis studies in vitro. Brain 1970;93(3): 445–474.
37. Adrian RH, Chandler WK, Hodgkin AL. Voltage clamp experiments in striated muscle fibres. J Physiol 1970;208(3):607–644.
38. Neher E, Sakmann B. Single-channel currents recorded from membrane of denervated frog muscle fibres. Nature 1976;260(5554):799–802.
39. Neher E, Sakmann B, Steinbach JH. The extracellular patch clamp: a method for resolving currents through individual open channels in biological membranes. Pflugers Archiv 1978;375(2):219–228.
40. Hamill OP, Marty A, Neher E, et al. Improved patch-clamp techniques for high-resolution current recording from cells and cell-free membrane patches. Pflugers Archiv 1981;391(2):85–100.
41. Milone M, Hutchinson DO, Engel AG. Patch-clamp analysis of the properties of acetylcholine receptor channels at the normal human endplate. Muscle Nerve 1994;17(12):1364–1369.
42. Engel AG, Ohno K, Milone M, et al. New mutations in acetylcholine receptor subunit genes reveal heterogeneity in the slow-channel congenital myasthenic syndrome. Hum Mol Genet 1996;5(9): 1217–1227.
43. Engel AG, Ohno K, Milone M, Sine SM. Congenital myasthenic syndromes. New insights from molecular genetic and patch-clamp studies. Ann N Y Acad Sci 1998;841:140–156.
44. Milone M, Ohno K, Fukudome T, et al. Congenital myasthenic syndrome caused by novel loss-of-function mutations in the human AChR epsilon subunit gene. Ann N Y Acad Sci 1998;841:184–188.
45. Engel AG, Ohno K, Sine SM. Congenital myasthenic syndromes: recent advances. Arch Neurol 1999;56(2):163–167.
46. Ruff RL, Whittlesey D. Na$^+$ currents near and away from endplates on human fast and slow twitch muscle fibers. Muscle Nerve 1993;16(9):922–929.
47. Ruff RL. Sodium channel slow inactivation and the distribution of sodium channels on skeletal muscle fibres enable the performance properties of different skeletal muscle fibre types. Acta Physiol Scand 1996;156(3):159–168.
48. Burton F, Dörstelmann U, Hutter OF. Single-channel activity in sarcolemmal vesicles from human and other mammalian muscles. Muscle Nerve 1988;11(10):1029–1038.
49. Lerche H, Mitrovic N, Dubowitz V, Lehmann-Horn F. Paramyotonia congenita: the R1448P Na$^+$ channel mutation in adult human skeletal muscle. Ann Neurol 1996;39(5):599–608.
50. Wieland SJ, Gong QH, Fletcher JE, Rosenberg H. Altered sodium current response to intracellular fatty acids in halothane-hypersensitive skeletal muscle. Am J Physiol 1996;271(1 Pt 1):C347–C353.
51. Greer M, Schotland M. Myasthenia gravis in the newborn. Pediatrics 1960;26:101–108.
52. Conomy JP, Levinsohn M, Fanaroff A. Familial infantile myasthenia gravis: a cause of sudden death in young children. J Pediatr 1975;87:428–430.
53. Fenichel GM. Clinical syndromes of myasthenia in infancy and childhood. Arch Neurol 1978;35: 97–103.
54. Robertson W, Chun R, Kornguth S. Familial infantile myasthenia. Arch Neurol 1980;37:117–119.
55. Engel A. Congenital myasthenic syndromes. Myasthenia gravis and myasthenic syndromes. Neurol Clin 1994;12(2):401–437.
56. Mora M, Lambert E, Engel A. Synaptic vesicle abnormality in familial infantile myasthenia. Neurology 1987;37:206–214.

57. Ohno K, Tsujino A, Brengman J, et al. Choline acetyltransferase mutations cause myasthenic syndrome associated with episodic apnea in humans. Proc Natl Acad Sci U S A 2001;98(4):2017–2022.

58. Walls TJ, Engel AG, Nagel AS, et al. Congenital myasthenic syndrome associated with paucity of synaptic vesicles and reduced quantal release. Ann N Y Acad Sci 1993;681:461–468.

59. Maselli R, Kong D, Bowe C, et al. Presynaptic congenital myasthenic syndrome due to quantal release deficiency. Neurology 2001;57:279–289.

60. Vincent A, Newsom-Davis J, Wray D, et al. Clinical and experimental observations in patients with congenital myasthenic syndromes. Ann N Y Acad Sci 1993;681:451–460.

61. Engel AG, Ohno K, Sine SM. Congenital Myasthenic Syndromes. In AG Engel (ed), Myasthenia Gravis and Myasthenic Disorders. New York: Oxford University Press, 1999;251–297.

62. Tournier-Lasserve E. CACNA1A mutations: hemiplegic migraine, episodic ataxia type 2, and the others [editorial; comment]. Neurology 1999;53(1):3–4.

63. Guida S, Trettel F, Pagnutti S, et al. Complete loss of P/Q calcium channel activity caused by a CACNA1A missense mutation carried by patients with episodic ataxia type 2. Am J Hum Genet 2001;68(3):759–764.

64. Stea A, Tomlinson WJ, Soong TW, et al. Localization and functional properties of a rat brain alpha 1A calcium channel reflect similarities to neuronal Q- and P-type channels. Proc Natl Acad Sci U S A 1994;91(22):10576–10580.

65. Protti DA, Reisin R, Mackinley TA, Uchitel OD. Calcium channel blockers and transmitter release at the normal human neuromuscular junction. Neurology 1996;46(5):1391–1396.

66. Jen J, Wan J, Graves M, et al. Loss-of-function EA2 mutations are associated with impaired neuromuscular transmission. Neurology 2001;57(10):1843–1848.

67. Maselli RA, Jen J, Graves M, et al. Patients with CACNA1A mutations and associated myasthenic weakness have presynaptic failure of neuromuscular transmission [abstract]. Neurology 2001; 56(8)(Suppl 3):A60.

68. Maselli RA, Soliven BC. Analysis of the organophosphate-induced electromyographic response to repetitive nerve stimulation: paradoxical response to edrophonium and D-tubocurarine [see comments]. Muscle Nerve 1991;14(12):1182–1188.

69. Maselli RA, Leung C. Analysis of anticholinesterase-induced neuromuscular transmission failure. Muscle Nerve 1993;16(5):548–553.

70. Engel AG, Ohno K, Milone M, Sine SM. Congenital myasthenic syndromes. New insights from molecular genetic and patch-clamp studies. Ann N Y Acad Sci 1998;841:140–156.

71. Engel AG, Ohno K, Sine SM. Congenital myasthenic syndromes: recent advances. Arch Neurol 1999;56(2):163–167.

72. Ohno K, Hutchinson DO, Milone M, et al. Congenital myasthenic syndrome caused by prolonged acetylcholine receptor channel openings due to a mutation in the M2 domain of the epsilon subunit. Proc Natl Acad Sci U S A 1995;92(3):758–762.

73. Gomez CM, Maselli R, Gammack J, et al. A beta-subunit mutation in the acetylcholine receptor channel gate causes severe slow-channel syndrome. Ann Neurol 1996;39(6):712–723.

74. Milone M, Wang HL, Ohno K, et al. Slow–channel myasthenic syndrome caused by enhanced activation, desensitization, and agonist binding affinity attributable to mutation in the M2 domain of the acetylcholine receptor alpha subunit. J Neurosci 1997;17(15):5651–5665.

75. Engel AG, Ohno K, Milone M, et al. New mutations in acetylcholine receptor subunit genes reveal heterogeneity in the slow-channel congenital myasthenic syndrome. Hum Mol Genet 1996;5(9): 1217–1227.

76. Sine SM, Ohno K, Bouzat C, et al. Mutation of the acetylcholine receptor alpha subunit causes a slow-channel myasthenic syndrome by enhancing agonist binding affinity. Neuron 1995; 15(1):229–239.

77. Croxen R, Newland C, Beeson D, et al. Mutations in different functional domains of the human muscle acetylcholine receptor alpha subunit in patients with the slow-channel congenital myasthenic syndrome. Hum Mol Genet 1997;6(5):767–774.

78. Ohno K, Wang HL, Milone M, et al. Congenital myasthenic syndrome caused by decreased agonist binding affinity due to a mutation in the acetylcholine receptor epsilon subunit. Neuron 1996; 17(1):157–170.

79. Uchitel O, Engel AG, Walls TJ, et al. Congenital myasthenic syndromes: II. Syndrome attributed to abnormal interaction of acetylcholine with its receptor. Muscle Nerve 1993;16(12):1293–1301.

80. Milone M, Wang HL, Ohno K, et al. Mode switching kinetics produced by a naturally occurring mutation in the cytoplasmic loop of the human acetylcholine receptor epsilon subunit. Neuron 1998;20(3):575–588.

81. Wang HL, Milone M, Ohno K, et al. Acetylcholine receptor M3 domain: stereochemical and volume contributions to channel gating. Nat Neurosci 1999;2(3):226–233.
82. Brownlow S, Webster R, Croxen R, et al. Acetylcholine receptor delta subunit mutations underlie a fast-channel myasthenic syndrome and arthrogryposis multiplex congenita. J Clin Invest 2001;108(1):125–130.
83. Engel AG, Ohno K, Bouzat C, et al. End-plate acetylcholine receptor deficiency due to nonsense mutations in the epsilon subunit. Ann Neurol 1996;40(5):810–817.
84. Ohno K, Quiram PA, Milone M, et al. Congenital myasthenic syndromes due to heteroallelic nonsense/missense mutations in the acetylcholine receptor epsilon subunit gene: identification and functional characterization of six new mutations. Hum Mol Genet 1997;6(5):753–766.
85. Quiram PA, Ohno K, Milone M, et al. Mutation causing congenital myasthenia reveals acetylcholine receptor beta/delta subunit interaction essential for assembly. J Clin Invest 1999; 104(10):1403–1410.
86. Nichols P, Croxen R, Vincent A, et al. Mutation of the acetylcholine receptor epsilon-subunit promoter in congenital myasthenic syndrome. Ann Neurol 1999;45(4):439–443.
87. Croxen R, Young C, Slater C, et al. End-plate gamma- and epsilon-subunit mRNA levels in AChR deficiency syndrome due to epsilon-subunit null mutations. Brain 2001;124(Pt 7):1362–1372.
88. Croxen R, Newland C, Betty M, et al. Novel functional epsilon-subunit polypeptide generated by a single nucleotide deletion in acetylcholine receptor deficiency congenital myasthenic syndrome. Ann Neurol 1999;46(4):639–647.
89. Ohno K, Engel AG, Shen XM, et al. Rapsyn mutations in humans cause endplate acetylcholine-receptor deficiency and myasthenic syndrome. Am J Hum Genet 2002;70(4):875–885.
90. Engel AG, Lambert EH, Gomez MR. A new myasthenic syndrome with end-plate acetylcholinesterase deficiency, small nerve terminals, and reduced acetylcholine release. Ann Neurol 1977;1(4): 315–330.
91. Ohno K, Brengman J, Tsujino A, Engel AG. Human endplate acetylcholinesterase deficiency caused by mutations in the collagen-like tail subunit (ColQ) of the asymmetric enzyme. Proc Natl Acad Sci U S A 1998;95(16):9654–9659.
92. Donger C, Krejci E, Serradell AP, et al. Mutation in the human acetylcholinesterase-associated collagen gene, COLQ, is responsible for congenital myasthenic syndrome with end-plate acetylcholinesterase deficiency (type Ic). Am J Hum Genet 1998;63(4):967–975.
93. Ohno K, Brengman JM, Felice KJ, et al. Congenital end-plate acetylcholinesterase deficiency caused by a nonsense mutation and an A→G splice-donor-site mutation at position +3 of the collagenlike-tail-subunit gene (COLQ): how does G at position +3 result in aberrant splicing? Am J Hum Genet 1999;65(3):635–644.
94. Ohno K, Engel AG, Brengman JM, et al. The spectrum of mutations causing end-plate acetylcholinesterase deficiency. Ann Neurol 2000;47(2):162–170.
95. Schiavo G, Benefenati F, Poulain B, et al. Tetanus and botulinum-B neurotoxins block neurotransmitter release by a proteolytic cleavage of synaptobrevin. Nature 1992;359:832–835.
96. Blasi J, Chapman ER, Link T, et al. Botulinum neurotoxin A selectively cleaves the synaptic protein SNAP-25. Nature 1993;365:160–163.
97. Lambert EH, Engel AG, Cherington M. End-plate potentials in human botulism [abstract]. Excerpta Med (Amsterdam) 1974;334:65.
98. Maselli RA, Ellis W, Mandler RN, et al. Cluster of wound botulism in California: clinical, electrophysiologic, and pathologic study. Muscle Nerve 1997;20(10):1284–1294.
99. Motomura M, Lang B, Johnston I, et al. Incidence of serum anti-P/O-type and anti-N-type calcium channel autoantibodies in the Lambert-Eaton myasthenic syndrome. J Neurol Sci 1997; 147(1):35–42.
100. Takamori M, Iwasa K, Komai K. Antibodies to synthetic peptides of the alpha1A subunit of the voltage-gated calcium channel in Lambert-Eaton myasthenic syndrome. Neurology 1997;48(5): 1261–1265.
101. Takamori M, Komai K, Iwasa K. Antibodies to calcium channel and synaptotagmin in Lambert-Eaton myasthenic syndrome. Am J Med Sci 2000;319(4):204–208.
102. Tim RW, Massey JM, Sanders DB. Lambert-Eaton myasthenic syndrome (LEMS). Clinical and electrodiagnostic features and response to therapy in 59 patients. Ann N Y Acad Sci 1998;841: 823–826.
103. Fukunaga H, Engel AG, Osame M, et al. Paucity and disorganization of presynaptic membrane active zones in the Lambert-Eaton myasthenic syndrome. Muscle Nerve 1982;5:686–697.

104. Appel SH, Anwyl R, McAdams MW, et al. Accelerated degradation and acetylcholine receptor from cultured rat myotubes with myasthenia gravis sera and globulins. Proc Natl Acad Sci U S A 1977;74:2130–2134.
105. Drachman DB, Adams RN, Stanley EF, et al. Mechanisms of acetylcholine receptor loss in myasthenia gravis. J Neurol Neurosurg Psychiatry 1980;43:601–610.
106. Drachman DB, Adams RN, Josifek EF, et al. Antibody-mediated mechanisms of ACh receptor loss in myasthenia gravis. Clinical relevance. Ann N Y Acad Sci 1981;377:175–188.
107. Engel AG, Lambert EH, Howard FM. Immune complexes (IgG and C3) at the motor end-plate in myasthenia gravis. Ultrastructure and light microscopic localization and electrophysiological correlations. Mayo Clin Proc 1977;52:267–280.
108. Engel AG, Sahashi K, Fumagalli G. Part II. Effect of anti-acetylcholine receptor anti-bodies on acetylcholine receptor structure and function: the immunopathology of acquired myasthenia gravis. Ann N Y Acad Sci 1987;377:158–174.
109. Engel AG, Sahashi K, Lambert EH, et al. The ultrastructural localization of the acetylcholine receptor, immunoglobulin G and the third and ninth complement components at the motor end-plate and the implications for the pathogenesis of myasthenia gravis. Excerpta Medica International Congress Series 1979;455:111–122.
110. Pascuzzi RM, Campa JF. Lymphorrhage localized to the muscle end-plate in myasthenia gravis. Arch Pathol Lab Med 1988;112:934–937.
111. Maselli RA, Richman DP, Wollmann RL. Inflammation at the neuromuscular junction in myasthenia gravis. Neurology 1991;41(9):1497–1504.
112. Engel AG, Santa T. Histometric analysis of the ultrastructure of the neuromuscular junction in myasthenia gravis and in the myasthenic syndrome. Ann N Y Acad Sci 1971;183:46–63.
113. Hoch W, McConville J, Helms S, et al. Auto-antibodies to the receptor tyrosine kinase MuSK in patients with myasthenia gravis without acetylcholine receptor antibodies. Nat Med 2001;7(3):365–368.
114. Dahlback O, Elmqvist D, Johns TR, et al. An electrophysiologic study of the neuro-muscular junction in myasthenia gravis. J Physiol (Lond) 1961;156:336–343.
115. Elmqvist D, Hofmann WM, Kugelberg J, et al. An electrophysiological investigation of neuromuscular transmission in myasthenia gravis. J Physiol (Lond) 1964;174:417–434.
116. Albuquerque EX, Rash JE, Mayer RJ, et al. An electrophysiological and morphological study of the neuromuscular junction in patients with myasthenia gravis. Exp Neurol 1976;51:536–563.
117. Cull-Candy SG, Miledi R, Trautmann A. End-plate currents and acetylcholine noise at normal and myasthenic human end-plates. J Physiol 1979;287:247–265.
118. Cull-Candy SG, Miledi R, Trautmann A, Uchitel OD. On the release of transmitter at normal, myasthenia gravis and myasthenic syndrome affected human end-plates. J Physiol 1980;299:621–638.
119. Vincent A, Jacobson L, Plested P, et al. Antibodies affecting ion channel function in acquired neuromyotonia, in seropositive and seronegative myasthenia gravis, and in antibody-mediated arthrogryposis multiplex congenita. Ann N Y Acad Sci 1998;841:482–496.
120. Mygland A, Vincent A, Newsom-Davis J, et al. Autoantibodies in thymoma-associated myasthenia gravis with myositis or neuromyotonia. Arch Neurol 2000;57(4):527–531.
121. Maselli RA, Agius M, Lee EK, et al. Morvan's fibrillary chorea. Electrodiagnostic and in vitro microelectrode findings. Ann N Y Acad Sci 1998;841:497–500.
122. Lee EK, Maselli RA, Ellis WG, Agius MA. Morvan's fibrillary chorea: a paraneoplastic manifestation of thymoma. J Neurol Neurosurg Psychiatry 1998;65(6):857–862.
123. Wintzen AR, Plomp JJ, Molenaar PC, et al. Acquired slow-channel syndrome: a form of myasthenia gravis with prolonged open time of the acetylcholine receptor channel. Ann Neurol 1998;44(4):657–664.
124. Norris FH. Adult Spinal Neuron Disease Progressive Muscular Atrophy (Aran's Disease) in Relation to Amyotrophic Lateral Sclerosis. In PJ Vinken, GW Bruyn (eds), Handbook of Clinical Neurology: Systems Disorders and Atrophies, Vol 22. New York: Elsevier, 1975;1–56.
125. Denys EH, Norris FH. Amyotrophic lateral sclerosis. Impairment of neuromuscular transmission. Arch Neurol 1979;36:202–205.
126. Stålberg E, Schwartz MS, Trontlej JV. Single fiber electromyography in various process affecting the anterior horn cell. J Neurol Sci 1975;24:403–415.
127. Mills KR. Motor neuron disease. Studies of the corticospinal excitation of single motor neurons by magnetic brain stimulation. Brain 1995;118(Pt 4):971–982.
128. Kohara N, Kaji R, Kojima Y, et al. Abnormal excitability of the corticospinal pathway in patients with amyotrophic lateral sclerosis: a single motor unit study using transcranial magnetic stimulation. Electroencephalogr Clin Neurophysiol 1996;101(1):32–41.

129. Maselli RA, Cashman NR, Wollman RL, et al. Neuromuscular transmission as a function of motor unit size in patients with prior poliomyelitis. Muscle Nerve 1992;15(6):648–655.

130. Grimby G, Stålberg E, Sandberg A, Stibrant Sunnerhagen K. An 8-year longitudinal study of muscle strength, muscle fiber size, and dynamic electromyogram in individuals with late polio. Muscle Nerve 1998;21(11):1428–1437.

131. Dalakas MC. Pathogenetic mechanisms of post-polio syndrome: morphological, electrophysiological, virological, and immunological correlations. Ann N Y Acad Sci 1995;25(753):167–185.

132. Maselli RA, Wollmann R, Roos R. Function and ultrastructure of the neuromuscular junction in post-polio syndrome. Ann N Y Acad Sci 1995;753:129–137.

133. Jurkat-Rott K, Lerche H, Mitrovic N, Lehmann-Horn F. Teaching course: ion channelopathies in neurology. J Neurol 1999;246(9):758–763.

134. Lehmann-Horn F, Jurkat-Rott K. Voltage-gated ion channels and hereditary disease. Physiol Rev 1999;79(4):1317–1372.

11
Routine Needle Electromyography

Jun Kimura

Electromyography tests the integrity of the upper and lower motor neurons, neuro-muscular junction, and muscle, with seven possible sites of involvement that may cause muscle weakness (Figure 11.1). Electromyography consists of multiple sampling at rest and during different degrees of voluntary contraction in each muscle of interest. The patient's symptoms and signs guide the optimal selection of specific muscle groups.[1,2] Thus, the studies must be conducted as an extension of the physical examination rather than as a laboratory procedure.[3,4] No routine approach with a predetermined list of muscles suffices, because the findings in the initially tested muscles dictate the course of subsequent exploration.

In an unstable denervated muscle, individual fibers fire independently in the absence of neural control. The detection of these spontaneous single-fiber potentials constitutes one of the most important findings in electromyography. Diseases of the nerve or muscle also cause structural or functional disturbances of the motor unit, the smallest functional element of volitional contraction. These in turn lead to alterations in the waveform and discharge patterns of their electrical signals or motor unit potentials. Other biological and nonbiological factors, however, have important influences on the recorded signals. For example, the size of an action potential detected in the external field varies considerably depending on the spatial relationship between the source and the tip of the needle electrode. Thus, when recorded by an electrode with a small leadoff surface, the amplitude falls off sharply to less than 10% at a distance of 1 mm from the generator.

A patient treated with anticoagulants should undergo appropriate laboratory tests as a screen for bleeding tendency. With heparin infusion, a criterion for needle study calls for partial thromboplastin time less than 1.5 of control value. With warfarin (Coumadin) therapy, the international rating should not exceed 2.0. The same precautions must apply to those with other coagulopathy, such as hemophilia.[5] For thrombocytopenia, local pressure can usually accomplish hemostasis if the platelet count remains above 20,000 platelets/mm.[6] Testing a superficial muscle first for bleeding tendency helps to determine the feasibility of further study. External compression often cannot counter bleeding adequately in deeper muscles.

Certain muscle diseases, such as muscular dystrophy and polymyositis, increase serum creatine kinase; this also occurs in other conditions, such as cardiac ischemia, hypothyroidism, and sustained athletic participation. The combination of elec-

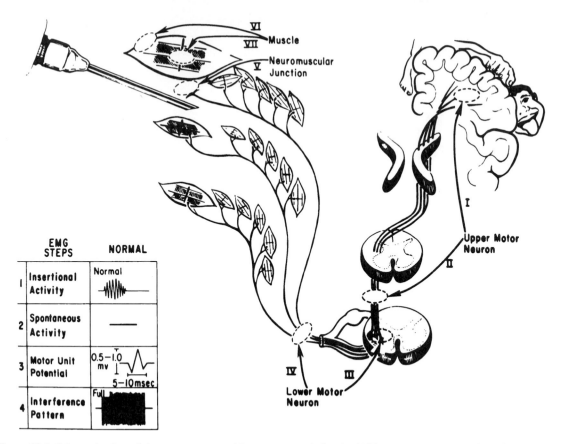

Figure 11.1 Schematic view of the motor system with seven anatomic levels: (I, II) upper motor neuron from the cortex to the spinal cord; (III, IV) lower motor neuron with the anterior horn cell and nerve axon; (V) neuromuscular junction; and (VI, VII) muscle membrane and contractile elements. The insert illustrates diagrammatically four steps of electromyographic (EMG) examination and normal findings. (Adapted from FH Netter. The Ciba Collection of Medical Illustrations, Vol 1. Summit, NJ: Ciba Pharmaceutical Company, Medical Eduction Division, 1983.)

tromyography, diurnal variation, and prolonged exercise[7,8] may also alter the level considerably even in normal muscles. Needle examination by itself, however, should not elevate the enzyme to a misleading level.

Electromyography examines neuromuscular integrity in four steps:

1. Insertional activity caused by needle movement with the muscle at rest
2. Spontaneous activity recorded with the needle stationary in a relaxed muscle
3. Motor unit potentials activated individually by mild voluntary contraction
4. Recruitment pattern during progressively stronger contraction leading to interference pattern at the maximum level

The needle electrode registers muscle action potentials only from a restricted area of the muscle, necessitating frequent needle repositioning in small steps to allow multiple sampling for adequate survey. Exploration in four directions from a single puncture site minimizes the patient discomfort. Studies of larger muscles require additional insertions in proximal, central, and distal portions. The four steps of electromyography help to categorize motor dysfunction into upper and lower motor neuron disorders and myogenic lesions. The illustrations in Figure 11.2 emphasize typical findings in each entity at the risk of oversimplification.

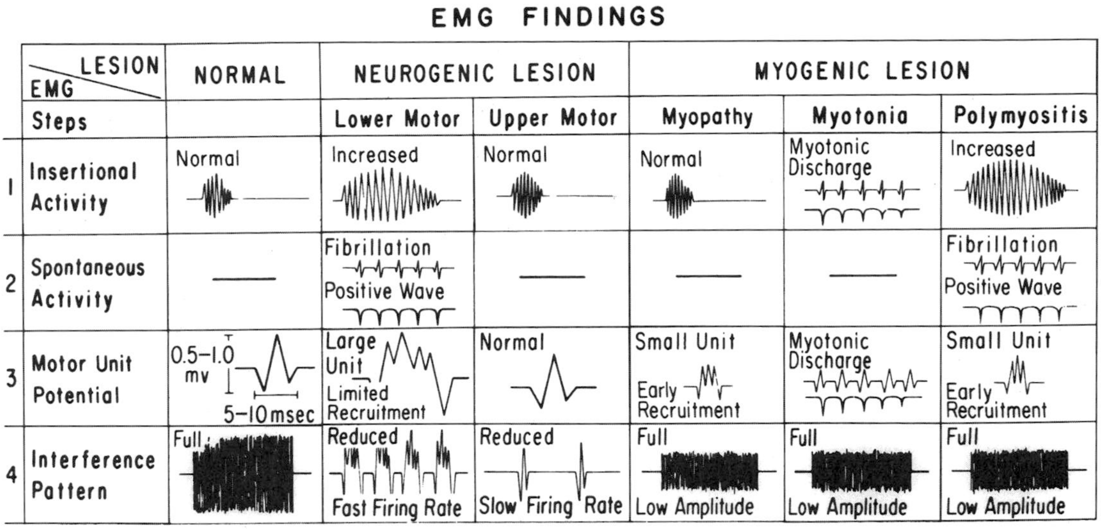

EMG FINDINGS

LESION EMG	NORMAL	NEUROGENIC LESION		MYOGENIC LESION		
Steps		**Lower Motor**	**Upper Motor**	**Myopathy**	**Myotonia**	**Polymyositis**
1 Insertional Activity	Normal	Increased	Normal	Normal	Myotonic Discharge	Increased
2 Spontaneous Activity	—	Fibrillation / Positive Wave	—	—	—	Fibrillation / Positive Wave
3 Motor Unit Potential	0.5-1.0 mv / 5-10 msec	Large Unit / Limited Recruitment	Normal	Small Unit / Early Recruitment	Myotonic Discharge	Small Unit / Early Recruitment
4 Interference Pattern	Full	Reduced / Fast Firing Rate	Reduced / Slow Firing Rate	Full / Low Amplitude	Full / Low Amplitude	Full / Low Amplitude

Figure 11.2 Typical findings in lower and upper motor neuron disorders and myogenic lesions. Myotonia shares many features common to myopathy in general, in addition to myotonic discharges triggered by insertion of the needle or voluntary effort to contract the muscle. Polymyositis shows combined features of myopathy and neuropathy, including (1) prolonged insertional activity; (2) abundant spontaneous discharges; (3) small-amplitude, short-duration, and polyphasic motor unit potentials; and (4) early recruitment leading to low-amplitude, full-interference pattern. (EMG = electromyography.) (Reprinted with permission from J Kimura. Electrodiagnosis in Diseases of Nerve and Muscle: Principles and Practice [3rd ed]. New York: Oxford University Press, 2001.)

INSERTIONAL ACTIVITY

Insertion of a needle electrode into the muscle for each repositioning normally gives rise to a brief burst of electrical discharges. The insertional activity slightly exceeds the movement of the needle, on the average, lasting a few hundred milliseconds. The magnitude and speed of the needle movement, among other things, dictate the level of response. As an important measure of muscle excitability, semiquantitative analysis typically shows reduced activity in fibroses, and exaggerated response in denervated muscle or inflammatory processes. Functionally inexcitable muscle fibers also show reduced insertional activity, for example, during attacks of familial periodic paralysis. An abnormally prolonged insertional activity outlasts the cessation of needle movement in irritable muscle with instability of the muscle membrane, as might be seen in denervation, myotonic disorders, or myositis.[9] During the early stages of denervation, 10 days to 2 weeks after nerve injury, a briefly sustained run of positive waves may follow insertional activity. These early abnormalities of denervation seen before the appearance of spontaneous activity resemble a normal insertional activity that may also take the form of positive sharp potentials. Denervated muscles, however, show reproducible trains of activity lasting several seconds to minutes after cessation of the needle movement (Table 11.1).

END-PLATE ACTIVITIES

In normal resting muscles, needles held stationary detect no electrical activity except at the end-plate region. A dull pain, which the patient reports in association with end-plate activities, dissipates with slight withdrawal of the needle. End-plate activities consist of

Table 11.1 Origin of Spontaneous and Evoked Discharges

Muscle fiber	
Insertional positive waves	Briefly sustained single muscle fiber discharges triggered by needle movement
Myotonic discharge	Repetitive single muscle fiber discharges triggered by needle movement
Fibrillation potential	Spontaneous single muscle fiber discharges, negative type
Positive sharp waves	Spontaneous single muscle fiber discharges, positive type
Complex repetitive discharge	A group of emphatically activated spontaneous single muscle fiber discharges
End-plate noise	Miniature end-plate potentials recorded extracellularly at motor point
End-plate spikes	Single muscle fiber discharges triggered by needle movement at motor point
Lower motor neuron	
Fasciculation potential	Spontaneous motor unit discharges involving a single unit, totally or fractionally
Myokymic discharge	Clusters of repetitive firing of the same motor unit, usually from demyelination
Neuromyotonic discharge	Continuous high-frequency discharges involving many motor units
Cramp discharges	Briefly sustained high-frequency discharges involving many motor units
Hemifacial spasm	Intermittent unilateral contraction of facial muscles, either idiopathic or post–Bell's palsy
Hemimasticatory spasm	Intermittent unilateral contraction of masseter muscle
Upper motor neuron	
Stiff-man syndrome	Sustained contraction of motor units in many agonistic and antagonistic muscles
Involuntary movement	Tremor, chorea, hemiballismus, athetosis, dystonia, myoclonus, epilepsia partialis continua

two components, which may occur conjointly or independently: low-amplitude, undulating *end-plate noise* and high-amplitude, *intermittent spikes* (Figure 11.3). The end-plate noise comprises frequently recurring, irregular negative potentials, 10–50 μV in amplitude and 1–2 milliseconds in duration, representing extracellularly recorded miniature end-plate potentials (MEPP). Over the loudspeaker, the end-plate noise produces a characteristic sound much like a live seashell held to the ear. The end-plate spikes consist of repetitive discharges of single muscle fibers,[10,11,12] 100–200 μV in amplitude and 3–4 milliseconds in duration. They fire irregularly at 5–50 Hz, typically showing an initial negativity because the spikes originate at the tip of the recording electrode. Fibrillation potentials have the same waveform with an initial negativity when recorded at the end-plate region, but they fire more regularly at a slower rate.

MYOTONIC DISCHARGE

A sustained contraction of the muscle follows voluntary or stimulus-induced muscle fiber discharge in myotonia congenita, myotonia dystrophica, paramyotonia congenita,[13] and hyperkalemic periodic paralysis.[14,15] Clinical myotonia usually accompanies *myotonic discharges* triggered by insertion of the needle electrode but outlasting the external source of excitation (Table 11.2). The reverse does not neces-

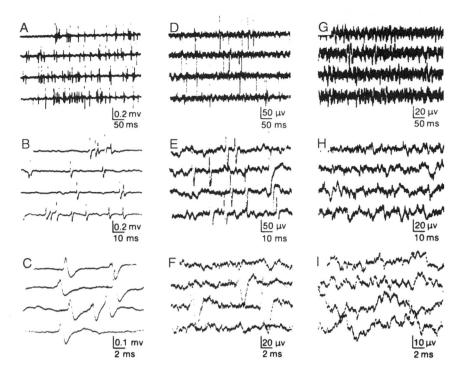

Figure 11.3 End-plate activities recorded from the tibialis anterior in a healthy subject. Two types of potentials shown represent the initially negative, high-amplitude end-plate spikes (**A–C**) and low-amplitude end-plate noise (**G–I**). The spikes and end-plate noise usually, though not necessarily, appear together (**D–F**). (Reprinted with permission from J Kimura. Electrodiagnosis in Diseases of Nerve and Muscle: Principles and Practice [3rd ed]. New York: Oxford University Press, 2001.)

sarily hold because electromyography may uncover myotonic discharges in the absence of clinical myotonia in a variety of disorders. These include polymyositis, type II glycogen storage disease with acid maltase deficiency,[16] some forms of myopathy (e.g., cytoplasmic body myopathy resembling myotonic dystrophy),[17] and other conditions with chronic denervation.

Depending on the spatial relationship between the recording surface of the needle electrode and the discharging muscle fibers, myotonic discharge takes one of two types of sustained activity: (1) a run of sharp positive waves, each followed by a low-amplitude negative component of much longer duration, or (2) a run of negative spikes with a small initial positivity (Figure 11.4). The positive waveforms, like those of denervation, probably represent recurring single-fiber potentials recorded from an injured area of the muscle membrane, whereas negative spikes resemble fibrillation potentials. Of the two patterns, the positive sharp waves usually follow needle insertion, whereas the negative spikes tend to occur at the beginning of slight volitional contraction. Both forms of discharge typically wax and wane in amplitude over the range of 10 µV to 1 mV, often, although not always, varying inversely to the rate of firing. Their frequency may increase or decrease within the range of 50–100 Hz, giving rise to a characteristic noise over the loudspeaker, reminiscent of an accelerating or decelerating motorcycle or chain saw.

Table 11.2 Disorders with Myotonic Discharges

With clinical myotonia	Without clinical myotonia
Myotonia dystrophica	Myositis
Myotonia congenita	Acid maltase deficiency
Paramyotonia congenita	Cytoplasmic body myopathy
Hyperkalemic periodic paralysis	Hyperthyroidism
Proximal myotonic myopathy	Hypothyroidism
	Familial granulovacuolar lobular myopathy
	Malignant hyperpyrexia
	Multicentric reticulohistiocytosis
	Myopathies induced by
	Glycyrrhizin
	Hypocholesterolemic agent
	Colchicine

SPONTANEOUS ACTIVITY

Basic types of spontaneous activity comprise *fibrillation potentials, positive sharp waves, complex repetitive discharges, fasciculation potentials*, and *myokymic discharges* (Table 11.3). Isolated visible muscle twitches over a localized area may accompany fasciculation potentials and complex repetitive discharges, but neither fibrillation potentials nor positive sharp waves.

Both fibrillation potentials and positive sharp waves result from single fiber activation.[3,18–21] In contrast, complex repetitive discharges represent rapid firing of cluster of muscle fibers in sequence, driven ephaptically at a point of lateral contact between neighboring units.[22–24] A spontaneously activated single muscle fiber serves as a pace-

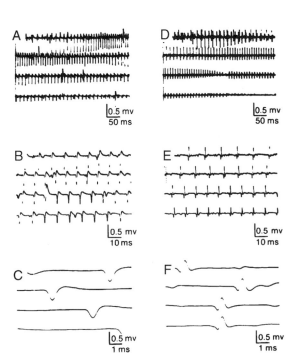

Figure 11.4 Myotonic discharges from the right anterior tibialis in a 39-year-old man with myotonic dystrophy. The tracings show two types of discharges: trains of positive sharp waves (**A–C**) and negative spikes with initial positivity (**D–F**). The discharges in (**A**) and (**D**) reveal waxing and waning quality. (Reprinted with permission from J Kimura. Electrodiagnosis in Diseases of Nerve and Muscle: Principles and Practice [3rd ed]. New York: Oxford University Press, 2001.)

Table 11.3 Common Types of Spontaneous Discharges

Fibrillation potentials and positive sharp waves	Fasciculation potentials
Neuropathic condition	Motor neuron disease
Muscular dystrophy	Radiculopathy
Myositis	Entrapment neuropathy
Complex repetitive discharges	Muscular pain-fasciculation syndrome
Motor neuron disease	Healthy subjects
Radiculopathy	**Myokymic discharges**
Chronic polyneuropathy	Guillain-Barré syndrome
Polymyositis	Radiation plexopathy
Muscular dystrophy	Spinal stenosis
Myxedema	Nerve root compression
Schwarz-Jampel syndrome	Bell's palsy
	Multiple sclerosis
	Syringobulbia

maker, regulating the frequency and pattern of discharge by two different, usually independent, mechanisms: rate of rhythmic depolarization of the denervated muscle fiber and circus movements of currents among muscle fibers.[25]

Fasciculation potentials are isolated spontaneous discharges of a motor unit, whereas *myokymic discharges* represent repetitive firing of a motor unit, as the name, *grouped fasciculation potentials*, indicates. Fasciculation potentials give rise to local muscle twitches, or *fasciculations*, whereas myokymic discharges seen in cramp syndromes cause sustained segmental contraction, called *myokymia*. In contrast, more generalized muscle spasms characterize the syndrome of neuromyotonia, representing peripheral nerve hyperexcitability. Patients with the stiff-man syndrome also experience similar involuntary muscle contraction, although responsible discharges originate in the central nervous system.

A numeric grading scale serves to semiquantify each of these spontaneous activities:

+1 Rare spontaneous potentials recordable in one or two sites only after some search. This category includes abnormally sustaining insertional positive sharp waves elicited after moving the needle electrode.
+2 Occasional spontaneous potentials registered in more than two different sites.
+3 Frequent spontaneous potentials that are recordable regardless of the position of the needle electrode.
+4 Abundant spontaneous potentials nearly filling the screen of the oscilloscope.

Fibrillation Potentials

Fibrillation potentials range from 1 to 5 milliseconds in duration and from 20 to 500 μV in amplitude when recorded with a concentric needle electrode.[11] They usually have diphasic or triphasic waveforms with initial positivity (Figure 11.5). Close scrutiny of a train of fibrillation potentials reveals no change in shape between the first and the last discharges. Voluntarily activated single-fiber potentials and fibrillation potentials have the same shape and amplitude distribution when studied with single-fiber electromyography.[26] These findings indicate that fibrillation potentials originate from single muscle fibers, a view consistent with the observation that they represent the smallest unit recorded by the needle electrode.[27,28]

Over the loudspeaker, fibrillation potentials produce a crisp clicking noise reminiscent of the sound caused by wrinkling tissue paper. Fibrillation potentials, typically triggered by spontaneous oscillations in the membrane potential, usually fire in a regular pattern at a rate of 1–30 Hz with an average frequency of 13 Hz,[11,29] although occasional units may discharge irregularly in the range of 0.1–25.0 Hz.[30,31] The appearance of an irregular firing pattern seen in profound denervation represents discharges from more than one fiber.

Positive Sharp Waves

Positive sharp waves, which also result from single-fiber activation, have a sawtooth appearance with the initial positivity and a subsequent slow negativity. They are much lower in amplitude and longer in duration compared to fibrillation potentials (see Figure 11.5). They often follow insertion of the needle, which damages the membrane. Sustained standing depolarization at this point then precludes the generation of a negative spike. Thus, propagating action potential only approaches the site of injury, giving rise to a sharp positive discharge, followed by low-amplitude negative deflection. When positive sharp waves fire spontaneously, the absence of a negative spike implies recording near the damaged part of the muscle fiber. As discussed earlier, positive sharp waves may form part of myotonic discharges, triggered by insertion of the needle or mild vol-

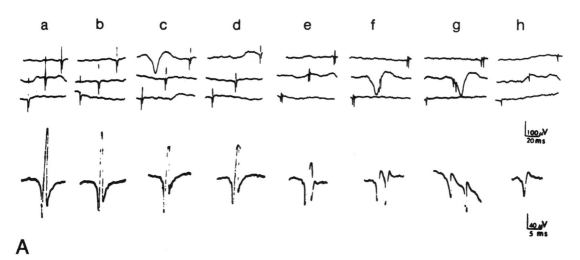

Figure 11.5 A. Spontaneous single-fiber discharges recorded from the denervated tibialis anterior in a 67-year-old man with acute onset of a footdrop. Note the gradual alteration of the waveform from triphasic spike with major negativity to paired positive potentials and finally to single positive sharp wave over the time course of 8 seconds (a–h) without movement of the needle. This fortuitous recording provides direct evidence that the same single-fiber discharge can be recorded either as fibrillation potentials or positive sharp waves. Long duration positive deflections (c, f, g) represent a pulse artifact. (Reprinted with permission from J Kimura. Electromyography and Nerve Stimulation Techniques: Clinical Applications. Tokyo: Igaku-Shoin, 1990.) **B.** Spontaneous single-fiber activity of the anterior tibialis in a 68-year-old woman with amyotrophic lateral sclerosis. The tracings show two types of discharges: positive sharp waves (a–c) and fibrillation potentials (d–f). **C.** Spontaneous single fiber activity of the paraspinal muscle in a 40-year-old man with radiculopathy, consisting of positive sharp waves (a–c) and fibrillation potentials (d–f). **D.** Spontaneous single-fiber activity of the deltoid (a–c) and tibialis anterior (d–f) in a 9-year-old boy with a 6-week history of dermatomyositis with two types of discharges: positive sharp waves (a–c) and fibrillation potentials (d–f). **E.** Spontaneous single-fiber activity of the tibialis anterior in a 7-year-old boy with Duchenne's muscular dystrophy, showing positive sharp waves (a–c) and fibrillation potentials (d–f). (Reprinted with permission from J Kimura. Electrodiagnosis in Diseases of Nerve and Muscle: Principles and Practice [3rd ed]. New York: Oxford University Press, 2001.)

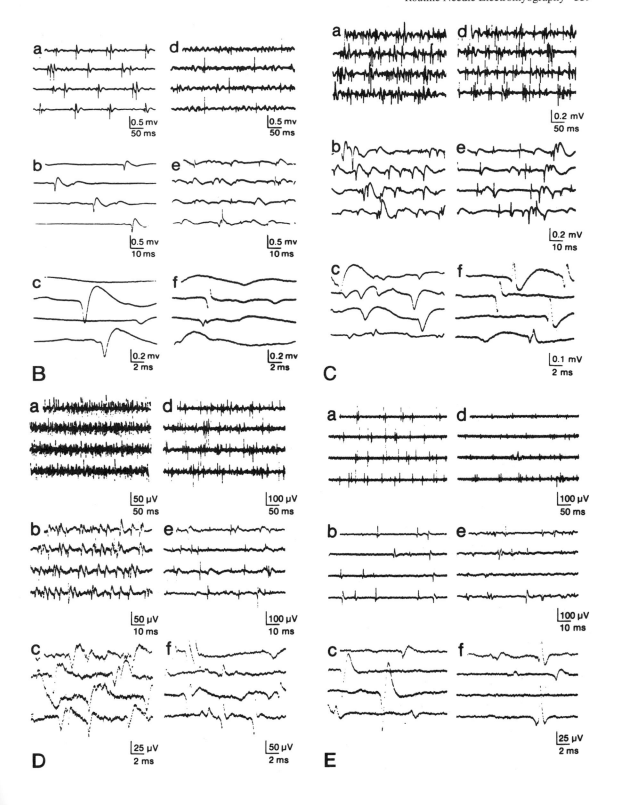

untary contraction. Despite close resemblance in waveform, myotonic discharges, which characteristically wax and wane, do not appear spontaneously.

Spontaneous Single-Fiber Discharges as a Clinical Measure

Spontaneous single-fiber activity, if reproducible in at least two muscles, provides the most useful sign of abnormality in clinical electromyography. Its presence usually implies lower motor neuron disorders, such as diseases of anterior horn cells, radiculopathies, plexopathies, and axonal polyneuropathies. Its absence, however, does not exclude denervation during the early weeks of nerve injury because of the latent period of 2–3 weeks. The distribution of spontaneous potentials in disorders of the lower motor neuron can aid in localizing lesions of the spinal cord, root, plexus, or peripheral nerve. Spontaneous discharges are also found in certain myopathic processes, such as muscular dystrophy, dermatomyositis, or polymyositis. Fibrillation potentials in patients with progressive muscular dystrophy[11] probably result from denervation secondary to muscle necrosis.[32] Similarly, polymyositis may cause focal degeneration, separating a part of the muscle fiber from the end-plate region.[33] Alternatively, spontaneous activity may suggest increased membrane irritability[34] or inflammation of intramuscular nerve fibers.[35]

Less consistently, diseases of neuromuscular junction also give rise to fibrillation potentials, as do many other disorders.[36,37] These include facioscapulohumeral dystrophy, limb-girdle muscular dystrophy, oculopharyngeal dystrophy,[38] myotubular (centronuclear) myopathy,[39] and trichinosis.[40]

Complex Repetitive Discharges

A group of muscle fibers fires in near synchrony to form *complex repetitive discharges*, which range from 50 μV to 1 mV in amplitude and up to 50–100 milliseconds in duration (Figure 11.6). The entire sequence repeats itself at slow or fast rates, usually in the range of 5–100 Hz. These discharges typically begin suddenly, maintain a constant rate of firing for a short period, and cease as abruptly as they started. The polyphasic and complex waveform remains uniform from one group of discharges to another, with a periodic shift to a new pattern mimicking the sound of a machine gun over the loudspeaker. The unique repetitive pattern once prompted the use of now discarded terms, *bizarre high frequency discharges* and *pseudomyotonia*. The firing pattern showing an identical waveform from one burst to the next makes the complex repetitive discharges distinct from myokymia, neuromyotonia, and cramp syndromes despite their superficial resemblance (see Table 11.3).

This discharge may occur in some myopathies (e.g., muscular dystrophy or polymyositis) and a wide variety of chronic denervating conditions (e.g., motor neuron disease, radiculopathy, chronic polyneuropathy, myxedema, and the Schwarz-Jampel syndrome sometimes associated with neurogenic muscle hypertrophy).[41] In a large series,[22,23] an overall analysis showed its highest prevalence in Duchenne's muscular dystrophy, spinal muscular atrophy, and Charcot-Marie-Tooth disease. Women with urinary retention may have profuse activity of this type in the striated muscle of the urethral sphincter.[42] Incidental findings of the complex repetitive discharges in apparently healthy subjects probably imply the presence of foci of a clinically silent irritative process, which tends to involve deeper muscles in general and the iliopsoas in particular.

Figure 11.6 Complex repetitive discharges of the left quadriceps in a 58-year-old man with a herniated lumbar disk. The tracings show two types of discharges: trains of single- or double-peaked negative spikes (**A–C**) and complex positive sharp waves (**D–F**). In **F**, each sweep, triggered by a recurring motor unit potential, shows remarkable reproducibility of the waveform within a given train. (Reprinted with permission from J Kimura. Electrodiagnosis in Diseases of Nerve and Muscle: Principles and Practice [3rd ed]. New York: Oxford University Press, 2001.)

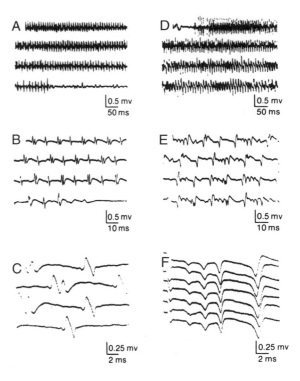

Fasciculation Potentials and Myokymic Discharges

A fasciculation potential results from spontaneous discharges of a group of muscle fibers representing either a whole or possibly part of a motor unit. This type of discharge usually induces a visible muscle twitch, although electromyography may reveal a fasciculation potential in the depth of the muscle without clinically detectable movement. Unlike normal voluntary motor unit potentials, which maintain constant shape as long as the needle remains stationary, fasciculation potentials may undergo slight changes in amplitude and waveform from time to time. Attempts to volitionally control the discharge pattern by mildly contracting agonistic or antagonistic muscles fail to alter the firing rate. Although the neural discharge may originate in the spinal cord or anywhere along the length of the peripheral nerve,[43] the existing evidence favors a distal site of origin at or near the motor terminals.[44] Fasciculation potentials, although typically associated with diseases of anterior horn cells, also occur in other neuropathic conditions, such as radiculopathy, entrapment neuropathy, and the muscular pain-fasciculation syndrome.[45]

Patients with cervical spondylotic myelopathy may have fasciculation potentials in the lower limbs, presumably secondary to loss of inhibition, vascular insufficiency, cord traction, or denervation. Although these hypotheses lack anatomic or physiologic evidence, spontaneous discharges do abate after cervical decompression.[46,47] Fasciculation potentials are also seen in some metabolic derangements, such as tetany, thyrotoxicosis, and overdoses of anticholinesterase medication.[47] Simultaneous occurrences of fasciculation potentials from multiple units tend to show frequent association with amyotrophic lateral sclerosis and progressive spinal muscular atrophy but are also seen in other degenerative diseases of the anterior horn cells, such as poliomyelitis and syringomyelia. Synchronous fasciculations seen in muscles supplied by different nerves or in homologous muscles on opposite sides possibly suggest an intraspinal mechanism[48] or a reflex in origin via spindle afferent, activated by the arterial pulse.[49]

Single or grouped spontaneous discharges occur commonly in otherwise normal muscle,[50] sometimes, but not always, causing cramps. These benign fasciculations do not imply an ominous prognosis as a prelude to progressive motor neuron disease. To avoid the serious implications, a number of investigators have sought to differentiate benign types of fasciculations from those associated with motor neuron disease on the basis of waveform characteristics, such as amplitude, duration, and number of phases.[51,52] No single method, however, reliably distinguishes the two categories, although the frequency of discharge may possibly help: irregular firing at an average interval of 3.5 seconds in motor neuron disease compared to 0.8 seconds in asymptomatic individuals.[52,53] Fasciculations in amyotrophic lateral sclerosis characteristically arise proximally early in the disease and distally in the later stages.[53] In conclusion, healthy subjects may have fasciculation potentials, which, therefore, by themselves cannot provide absolute proof of abnormality. When in doubt, electromyographic detection of concomitant fibrillation potentials or positive sharp waves clarify the nature of fasciculation potentials, which now imply disease of the lower motor neuron with the origin at any level from the anterior horn cells to axon terminals.

In contrast to isolated discharges of one motor unit, more complex bursts of repetitive discharges cause vermicular movements of the skin called *myokymia*.[54] Repetitive firing of the same motor units usually occurs in bursts at regular intervals of 0.1–10.0 seconds, with 2–10 spikes discharging at 30–40 Hz in each burst (Figure 11.7). Myokymic discharges commonly, although not specifically, involve facial muscles in patients with brainstem glioma or multiple sclerosis (see Table 11.3). Myokymic discharges also favor certain chronic demyelinative neuropathic processes, such as Guillain-Barré syndrome[54] and radiation plexopathies.[56–58] Hyperventilation induces hypocalcemia, which in turn amplifies axonal excitability and myokymic bursts generated ectopically in a demyelinated segment of motor fibers.[59]

Continuous Muscle Fiber Activity

Continuous muscle fiber activity, or prolonged spontaneous motor unit activity, may occur in a heterogeneous group of central or peripheral disorders.[60] Of these, stiff-man syndrome represents a rare but well-recognized entity characterized by sustained involuntary discharges of central origin. Electromyography shows normal motor unit potentials producing a sustained interference pattern in the agonists and antagonists simultaneously. These discharges abate with peripheral nerve or neuromuscular block, after spinal or generalized anesthesia, or during sleep. The administration of diazepam, but not phenytoin or carbamazepine, also abolishes or attenuates the activity.

Neuromyotonia, or continuous muscle fiber activity of peripheral origin,[61] characterizes various, probably related, disease entities such as Isaacs' syndrome, quantal squander, generalized myokymia, pseudomyotonia, and normocalcemic tetany.[62,63] These syndromes vary in their clinical and electrophysiologic presentations despite the shared feature of sustained involuntary motor activity. The generator site responsible for neuromyotonia varies from proximal segments of the nerve to the intramuscular nerve terminals.[64–66] Excess motor unit activity remains during sleep and after general or spinal anesthesia, confirming its peripheral origin. Neuromuscular blocking agents totally abolish the abnormal activity, whereas procaine injection of the peripheral nerve counters only the discharges originating in the more proximal segment.

Patients show undulating movements of the overlying skin and a delay of relaxation after muscle contraction. Motor units characteristically discharge at high fre-

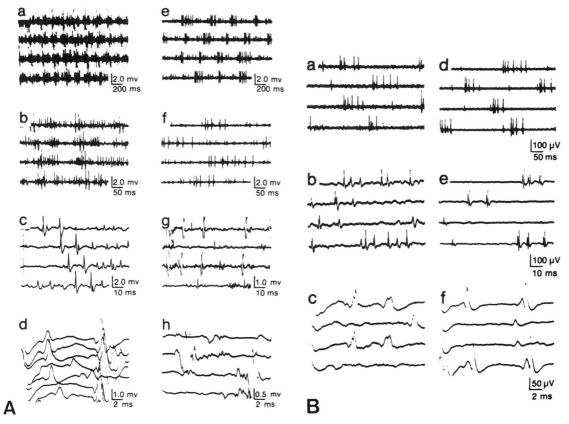

Figure 11.7 A. Myokymic discharges in a 21-year-old woman with multiple sclerosis. The patient had visible undulating movement of the facial muscles on the right side of her face associated with characteristic bursts of spontaneous activity recorded from the orbicularis oris (a–d) as well as orbicularis oculi (e–h). In d, each sweep, triggered by a recurring spontaneous potential, shows a repetitive but not exactly time-locked pattern of the waveform. **B**. Myokymic discharges in a 57-year-old man with a 2-week history of Guillain-Barré syndrome and a nearly complete peripheral facial palsy. Despite the absence of visible undulating movement, rhythmically recurring spontaneous discharges appeared in the upper (a–c) and lower (d–f) portions of the left orbicularis oris. In c and f, each sweep triggered by a recurring spontaneous potential shows the repetitive pattern. (Reprinted with permission from J Kimura. Electrodiagnosis in Diseases of Nerve and Muscle: Principles and Practice [3rd ed]. New York: Oxford University Press, 2001.)

quencies (often reaching 300 Hz) and produce a typical "pinging" sound over the loudspeaker. The firing motor unit potentials decline in amplitude slowly or rapidly as an increasing number of single muscle fibers fails to follow the high rate of repetitive pattern. The high frequency discharge accentuates with ischemia or electrical nerve stimulation but usually not with voluntary contraction. Phenytoin or carbamazepine effectively reduces involuntary movements in most patients.

Cramps

Cramps may develop either as normal phenomena or as a sign of abnormality in patients with neuromuscular disorders. After severe cramps, the pain may persist for days. The impulses responsible for these sustained involuntary muscle contractions—in part or in their entirety—originate in the peripheral nerve. Although the exact underlying mechanism remains unknown, cramps may result from mechanical excitation of motor nerve terminals during muscle shortening.[44,67–69] Spinal or general anesthesia has no effects on cramp discharges, but peripheral nerve block often abolishes the activity. Needle recording shows repetitive discharges of normal motor unit potentials at a high rate in the range of 200–300 Hz, beginning with single potentials or doublets and gradually spreading to involve other areas of a muscle. Several different sites may be activated simultaneously or sequentially. The discharges may wax and wane for several minutes, then abate spontaneously.

MOTOR UNIT ACTION POTENTIAL

The *motor unit* consists of a group of muscle fibers innervated by a single anterior horn cell. The factors that determine its anatomic and physiologic properties include the innervation ratio, fiber density, propagation velocity, and integrity of neuromuscular transmission. These characteristics vary not only from one muscle group to another but also with age for a given muscle. Motor unit potentials result as the sum of all single muscle fiber spikes that occur nearly synchronously within the recording radius of the electrode. According to principal components analysis, three elements determine 90% of the variance of the data set: changes in the size of the motor units, variations in the arrival time at the recording electrode, and loss of muscle fibers within the motor unit territory.[70] In addition to the inherent properties of the motor unit itself, many other physiologic factors influence the shape of motor unit potentials. These include the resistance and capacitance of the intervening tissue and intramuscular temperature.[71,72] Finally, the spatial relationships between the needle and individual muscle fibers play a crucial role in determining the waveform.[73] Thus, slight repositioning of the electrode alters the spacial orientation and introduces a new motor unit potential profile for the same motor unit.

A wide range of neuromuscular disorders affects the measures that define a motor unit potential (i.e., amplitude, rise time, duration, phases, stability, and territory) (Figure 11.8). Characteristic combinations of such abnormalities help to distinguish primary muscle diseases from disorders of the neuromuscular junction and lower motor neurons (Table 11.4). In myopathies, a random loss of individual fibers decreases the spike duration and amplitude of motor unit potentials.[74] In contrast, surviving fibers with sprouting after a loss of axons give rise to a larger potential than normal in neuropathies or anterior horn cell diseases. Thus, taken together with abnormalities of insertional and spontaneous activities and recruitment pattern, changes in the size of the motor unit potential play essential roles in the classification of weakness in diseases of the nerve and muscle.[75,76] In addition, serial assessment helps to monitor the disease process based on the established correlation between physiologic and histologic alteration of the motor unit.[77]

Amplitude and Area

With activation of one axon, all the individual muscle fibers belonging to the motor unit discharge in near synchrony. Of these, only a limited number located near the tip of the recording electrode contributes to the amplitude of a motor unit potential. Thus, the recorded amplitude varies greatly with the position of the needle electrode relative to the discharging unit. With the use of an ordinary concentric needle, mus-

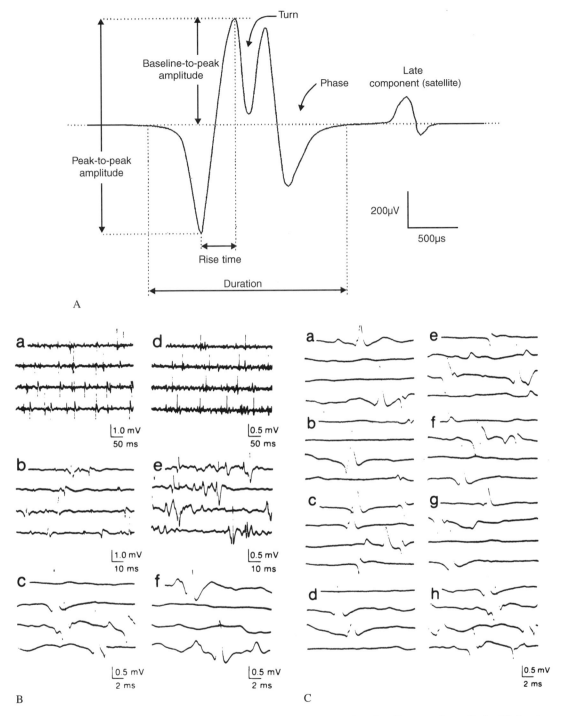

Figure 11.8 A. Profile of motor unit potential determined by (1) peak-to-peak or baseline-to-peak amplitude; (2) rise time, or the time interval from the onset of a change to its peak; (3) turn, or point of change in direction; (4) phase, portion of a waveform between departure from and return to the baseline; and (5) late component, or satellite potential, separated from the main motor unit potential. (Courtesy of David Walker, M.S.E.E.) **B.** Normal motor unit potentials from minimally contracted biceps in a 40-year-old healthy man (a–c) and maximally contracted tibialis anterior in a 31-year-old woman with hysterical weakness (d–f). In both patients, low firing frequency indicates weak voluntary effort. **C.** Normal variations of motor unit potentials from the same motor unit in the biceps of a healthy subject. Tracings a–h represent eight slightly different sites of recording, with the patient maintaining isolated discharges of a single motor unit. (Reprinted with permission from J Kimura. Electrodiagnosis in Diseases of Nerve and Muscle: Principles and Practice [3rd ed]. New York: Oxford University Press, 2001.)

Table 11.4 Types of Motor Unit Potentials

Brief duration, small amplitude, early recruitment	Long duration, large amplitude, late recruitment
Muscular dystrophy	Motor neuron disease
Congenital myopathy	Radiculopathies
Metabolic myopathy	Plexopathies
Endocrine myopathy	Polyneuropathies
Myositis	Entrapment syndromes
Myasthenia gravis	
Myasthenic syndromes	

cle fiber potentials fall off in amplitude to less than 50% at a distance of 200–300 μm from the source and to less than 1% a few millimeters away from the source.[78,79] Selecting a motor unit potential with a short rise time of 500 microseconds or less guarantees its proximity to the recording surface (see Figure 11.8A).

The number of single muscle fibers within the recording radius from the tip of the needle determines the size of the negative spike. Specifically, fewer than 5–10 muscle fibers lying within a 500-μm radius of the electrode tip contribute to the high voltage spike of the motor unit potential.[80,81] The muscle fibers lying closer together near the recording surface give rise to a higher amplitude. Computer simulation indicates that the proximity of the closest muscle fiber to the recording electrode determines the amplitude.[82–84] These findings indicate that, in general, the measure of amplitude aids in determining the muscle fiber density, not the motor unit territory.

The same motor unit can give rise to many different profiles depending on the position of the recording electrode. The amplitude of a motor unit potential normally varies from several hundred microvolts to a few millivolts. The use of a monopolar needle substantially increases the average amplitude of motor unit potentials compared to those recorded with a concentric needle.[85] The ratio between area and amplitude measures the "thickness" of the potential, which varies much less with changes in electrode position.[86] The combination of amplitude and the area-amplitude ratio improves discrimination considerably, detecting approximately 70% of neurogenic changes compared to only 15–30% by duration criteria alone.[87]

Rise Time

The *rise time*, defined as a time lag from the initial positive peak to the subsequent negative peak, is used to estimate the proximity of the discharging motor unit to the recording tip of the electrode. A distant unit has a greater rise time, reflecting the resistance and capacitance of the intervening tissue, which acts as a high-frequency filter. Such a discharge produces a dull sound over the loudspeaker, indicating the need to reposition the electrode closer to the source. In general, a rise time less than 500 microseconds ensures recording from within the motor unit territory,[88] although some argue for less restrictive criteria.[89] A sharp, crisp sound over the loudspeaker provides an important clue for the proximity of the discharging unit to the electrode. The measurement of the rise time confirms the suitability of the recorded potential for quantitative assessment of the amplitude.

Duration

The duration of a motor unit potential is measured from the initial takeoff to the return to the baseline (see Table 11.1). It reflects the length, conduction velocity, and degree of synchrony of many individual muscle fibers with variable membrane excitability.[90] Unlike the spike amplitude, which represents only a small number of muscle fibers near the electrode, the duration of a motor unit potential reflects the activity from a greater number of muscle fibers. In a concentric needle, the uptake area of the recording surface extends approximately 2.5 mm from the core.[80,83] Therefore, distant units not contributing to the amplitude of the negative spike add to the motor unit duration, increasing the time of the initial and terminal positivity. Although the motor unit duration serves as a measure of a larger part of the muscle fiber population, it still does not cover the entire motor unit territory, which measures 1–2 cm.

A slight shift or rotation of the needle influences the duration much less than the amplitude.[91] The duration normally varies from 5 to 15 milliseconds, depending on the age of the subject (Table 11.5). The use of a wide-open amplifier bandpass combined with enhanced signal-to-noise ratio results in a much longer duration, approaching 30 milliseconds recorded either with a single-fiber or macroelectrode. Under this circumstance, the total time of single action potential from end-plate zone to musculotendinous junction may dictate overall duration of motor unit action potential.[92]

Phases

A *phase* is defined as that portion of a waveform between the departure from and return to the baseline. The number of baseline crossings plus one equals the number of phases, determined by counting negative and positive peaks to and from the baseline. Most normal motor unit potentials have four or fewer phases. Desynchronized discharges of individual muscle fibers lead to polyphasic potentials with more than four phases, reflecting either fiber size variability or random loss of fibers (Figure 11.9). These potentials comprise between 5% and 15% of the total population in a healthy muscle when recorded with a concentric needle electrode. The use of a monopolar needle tends to increase polyphasic activities, although no studies have established the exact incidence. Some action potentials show several "turns" or directional changes without crossing the baseline.[93] In one study,[94] these irregular potentials appeared more commonly in acute process. These serrated action potentials or, less appropriately, complex or pseudopolyphasic potentials also indicate desynchronization among discharging muscle fibers.

Abnormalities of Motor Unit Potentials

The following discussion deals with the contrasting features of the motor unit potential seen in myopathies and lower motor neuron disorders. Each type of change occurs as a common feature in a number of disease categories. Thus, such abnormalities per se often fail to establish a specific diagnosis.

Most motor unit potentials are diphasic or triphasic in normal muscles. The number of polyphasic units having four or more phases increases in myopathy,

Table 11.5 Mean Action Potential Duration (ms) in Various Muscles at Different Ages (Concentric Electrodes)*

Age (yrs)	Arm Muscles						Leg Muscles				Facial Muscles	
	Deltoideus	Biceps Brachii	Triceps Brachii	Extensor Digitorum Communis	Opponens Pollicis; Interosseus	Abductor Digiti Quinti	Biceps Femoris; Quadriceps	Gastrocnemius	Tibialis Anterior	Peroneus Longus	Extensor Digitorum Brevis	Orbicularis Oris Superior; Triangularis; Frontalis
0	8.8	7.1	8.1	6.6	7.9	9.2	8.0	7.1	8.9	6.5	7.0	4.2
3	9.0	7.3	8.3	6.8	8.1	9.5	8.2	7.3	9.2	6.7	7.2	4.3
5	9.2	7.5	8.5	6.9	8.3	9.7	8.4	7.5	9.4	6.8	7.4	4.4
8	9.4	7.7	8.6	7.1	8.5	9.9	8.6	7.7	9.6	6.9	7.6	4.5
10	9.6	7.8	8.7	7.2	8.6	10.0	8.7	7.8	9.7	7.0	7.7	4.6
13	9.9	8.0	9.0	7.4	8.9	10.3	9.0	8.0	10.0	7.2	7.9	4.7
15	10.1	8.2	9.2	7.5	9.1	10.5	9.2	8.2	10.2	7.4	8.1	4.8
18	10.4	8.5	9.6	7.8	9.4	10.9	9.5	8.5	10.5	7.6	8.4	5.0
20	10.7	8.7	9.9	8.1	9.7	11.2	9.8	8.7	10.8	7.8	8.6	5.1
25	11.4	9.2	10.4	8.5	10.2	11.9	10.3	9.2	11.5	8.3	9.1	5.4
30	12.2	9.9	11.2	9.2	11.0	12.8	11.1	9.9	12.3	8.9	9.8	5.8
35	13.0	10.6	12.0	9.8	11.7	13.6	11.8	10.6	13.2	9.5	10.5	6.2
40	13.4	10.9	12.4	10.1	12.1	14.1	12.2	10.9	13.6	9.8	10.8	6.4
45	13.8	11.2	12.7	10.3	12.5	14.5	12.5	11.2	13.9	10.1	11.1	6.6
50	14.3	11.6	13.2	10.7	12.9	15.0	13.0	11.6	14.4	10.5	11.5	6.8
55	14.8	12.0	13.6	11.1	13.3	15.5	13.4	12.0	14.9	10.8	11.9	7.0
60	15.1	12.3	13.9	11.3	13.6	15.8	13.7	12.3	15.2	11.0	12.2	7.1
65	15.3	12.5	14.1	11.5	13.9	16.1	14.0	12.5	15.5	11.2	12.4	7.3
70	15.5	12.6	14.3	11.6	14.0	16.3	14.1	12.6	15.7	11.4	12.5	7.4
75	15.7	12.8	14.4	11.8	14.2	16.5	14.3	12.8	15.9	11.5	12.7	7.5

*The values given are mean values from different subjects without evidence of neuromuscular disease. The standard deviation of each value is 15% (20 potentials for each muscle). Therefore, deviations up to 20% are considered within the normal range when comparing measurements in a given muscle with the values of the table.
Source: Reprinted with permission from F Buchthal. An Introduction to Electromyography. Copenhagen: Scandinavian University Books, 1957.

Figure 11.9 Polyphasic motor unit potentials from the anterior tibialis in a 52-year-old man with amyotrophic lateral sclerosis recorded at different sweep speeds (**A–C**). Temporal variability of repetitive discharges in waveform suggests intermittent blocking of some axon terminals. (Reprinted with permission from J Kimura. Electrodiagnosis in Diseases of Nerve and Muscle: Principles and Practice [3rd ed]. New York: Oxford University Press, 2001.)

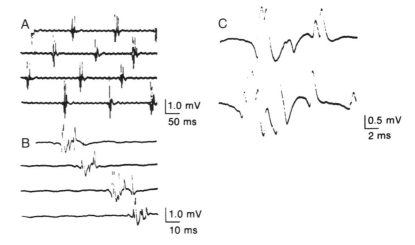

neuropathy, or motor neuron disease (see Figure 11.9), indicating abnormal temporal dispersion of muscle fiber potentials within a motor unit. Such desynchronization probably implies unequal alteration of conduction time along the individual terminal branch of the nerve or muscle fibers. In addition to polyphasic activities, some motor units may have extrapotentials clearly separated from the main *unit potential*, or a *satellite potential*.[95–97] Satellite potentials also occur in neuropathy or myopathy, both having five times higher incidence compared to normal muscles.[98] During neurapraxia or an acute stage of axonotmesis, motor unit potentials, if recorded at all, show normal waveforms, indicating the integrity of the surviving axons.

Motor units normally discharge semirhythmically, with successive potentials showing nearly identical configuration. Fatigue causes irregularity and reduction in the firing rate without altering its waveform. Defective neuromuscular transmission causes fluctuation in amplitude of a repetitively firing motor unit from intermittent blocking of individual muscle fibers within the unit. Increased jitter of the constituent single-fiber potentials also leads to waveform variability of the motor unit potential.[99] Motor unit evaluation plays an important role in documenting deficiency of neuromuscular transmission, especially in muscles not accessible by conventional nerve stimulation techniques. Such an instability of motor unit potential, termed *jiggle*,[100] however, may imply a large group of disorders. These include myasthenia gravis, myasthenic syndrome, botulism, motor neuron disease, poliomyelitis, and syringomyelia as well as early stages of reinnervation. In myotonia congenita, a characteristic decline in amplitude of the successive motor unit discharges reflects changes that affect single-fiber muscle action potentials, which typically recover during continued contraction.

Lower Motor Neuron versus Myopathic Disorders

Disorders of the lower motor neuron include motor neuron disease, poliomyelitis, and syringomyelia as well as diseases of the peripheral nerve (e.g., chronic neuropathy and reinnervation after nerve injury).[87] In these disorders, anatomic reorganization of denervated muscle fibers during reinnervation leads to the increased size of motor unit potential (Figure 11.10). Sprouting axon terminals usually remain within their own motor unit territory, failing to reach the denervated muscle fibers outside this boundary. Thus, the consequences of reinnervation relate primarily to an increased number of muscle fibers within the territory of the surviving axon after incorporation of denervated fibers. More specifically, increased amplitude indicates a greater muscle fiber density, whereas an increased duration probably results from abnormal variability in length and conduction time of regenerating axon terminals, as predicted by computer simulation.[101] Two or more motor units may discharge simultaneously with abnormal synchronization at the cord level or with ephaptic activation at the root level[102] or near the terminal axons.[103] A monopolar or concentric needle, inherently restricted by a small recording radius, fails to identify the enlarged territory of motor unit potentials. A macro study serves better for delineating the size of simultaneously discharging units.

In general, primary myopathic disorders have reduction in amplitude and duration of the motor unit potential (Figure 11.11). These disorders include muscular dystrophy, congenital myopathies, periodic paralysis, myositis, and disorders of neuromuscular transmission such as myasthenia gravis and myasthenic syndromes. In all these entities, muscle degeneration, inflammation, metabolic change, or failure of neuromuscular activation causes a random loss of functional muscle fibers from each motor unit. A reduction in amplitude and duration of motor unit potentials results from a lower fiber density reflecting a decrease in the number of muscle fibers. In extreme cases, voluntary contraction activates only a single muscle fiber, and a motor unit potential becomes indistinguishable from a fibrillation potential. The short spikes, 1–2 milliseconds in duration, produce a high-frequency sound reminiscent of spontaneously discharging fibrillation potentials over the loudspeaker. Unlike some inherited disorders of muscle, metabolic or toxic myopathies may cause reversible changes.[73] Mild metabolic and endocrine myopathies characteristically show little or no alteration in duration or amplitude of the motor unit potential.

Myopathies and lower motor neuron disorders generally show contrasting changes in the waveform of motor unit potentials,[104,105] albeit with equivocal distinction in some cases.[106] Sick axon terminals in distal neuropathy may result in random loss of muscle fibers within a motor unit. Similarly, during early reinnervation, immature motor units consist of only a few muscle fibers. Motor unit potentials may then show a low amplitude and short duration. In both instances, changes classically regarded as consistent with a myopathy result from a neuropathic process.[107] Conversely, motor unit potentials may have a long duration in myopathies with regenerating muscle fibers, erroneously suggesting a neuropathic process.[32,108,109] These potentials may appear quite distinct from the main unit, thus giving rise to the terms *satellite* or *late component*. Complex potentials with normal or increased duration may appear in myopathy, reflecting increased variability of fiber diameter.[70] Additionally, an increased fiber density during regeneration leads to a change in amplitude in a range much greater than ordinarily expected for myopathy. Hence, abnormalities of motor unit potentials may not necessarily correlate with the oversimplified clinical dichotomy between myopathy and neuropathy.[110,111] Nonetheless, electromyography and histochemical findings from muscle biopsies have an overall concordance of 90% or greater.[76,104,105,112]

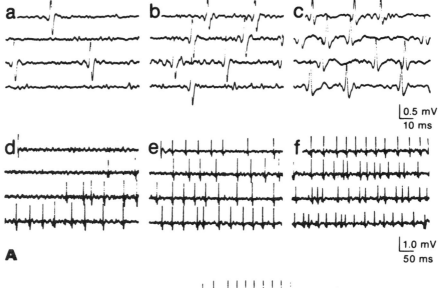

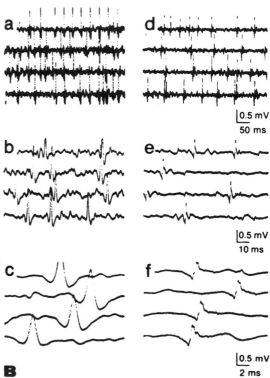

Figure 11.10 A. Motor unit potentials from the extensor digitorum communis in a 20-year-old man with partial radial nerve palsy. Minimal (a, d), moderate (b, e), and maximal voluntary contraction (c, f) recruited only a single motor unit, which discharged at progressively higher rates. **B.** Motor unit potentials from the extensor carpi ulnaris (a–c) and extensor carpi radialis longus (d–f) in the same subject. Maximal voluntary contraction recruited only a single motor unit firing at a high discharge rate. (Reprinted with permission from J Kimura. Electrodiagnosis in Diseases of Nerve and Muscle: Principles and Practice [3rd ed]. New York: Oxford University Press, 2001.)

Discharge Pattern of Motor Units

Recruitment

With a mild voluntary contraction, a healthy subject can initially discharge only one or two motor units at a rate of five to seven impulses per second (see Figure 11.8) before recruiting additional units in a fixed order.[113] The units activated early consist primarily of small, type I muscle fibers according to the size principle.[114–117]

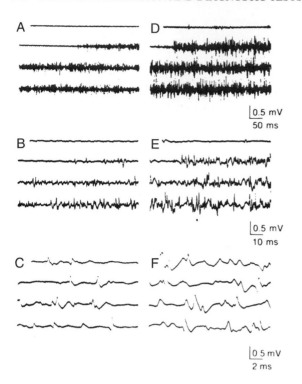

Figure 11.11 Low-amplitude, short-duration motor unit potentials from the biceps (**A–C**) and tibialis anterior (**D–F**) in a 7-year-old boy with Duchenne's muscular dystrophy. Minimal voluntary contraction recruited an excessive number of motor units in both muscles. (Reprinted with permission from J Kimura. Electrodiagnosis in Diseases of Nerve and Muscle: Principles and Practice [3rd ed]. New York: Oxford University Press, 2001.)

Despite constant contraction, these motor units typically discharge semirhythmically, with slowly increasing and then decreasing interspike intervals. At such minimal levels of muscle contraction, changes in firing rate grade the muscle force (rate coding). Greater muscle force is achieved by two separate but related changes in the pattern of motor unit discharge: (1) recruitment of previously inactive units, and (2) more rapid firing of already active units. Which of the two plays a greater role is not known, but both mechanisms operate simultaneously. A normal recruitment pattern implies an appropriate number of discharging motor units for the muscle force generated by the effort. In a reduced or increased recruitment, a fewer or greater number of units discharge than expected. A loss of motor units results in late and reduced recruitment with increased rates of firing to compensate for a smaller number of available units (see Figure 11.10). In contrast, a random loss of muscle fibers from each motor unit gives rise to early or increased recruitment at minimal and moderate levels of effort (see Figure 11.11). For accurate assessment, the examiner must know the approximate number of active motor units expected for a given force being exerted. In basal ganglia disorders such as parkinsonism, motor units may fire irregularly in groups at or near the rates of tremor.[118] Upper motor neuron lesions, such as spinal cord injury, may alter motor unit forces and recruitment patterns.[119]

The *recruitment frequency* is defined as the firing frequency of the initially activated unit at the time an additional unit is recruited. In healthy subjects, this measure of the pattern of motor unit discharge averages 5–10 Hz, depending on the types of motor units under study.[120–122] Patients with neuromuscular disorders often deviate from the normal range,[123] although reported values show a considerable overlap with healthy subjects. The ratio of the average firing rate to the number of active units also serves as a practical measure of recruitment.[3] In healthy subjects, this ratio should not exceed 5 with, for example, three units firing less than 15 Hz each. A ratio greater than 10, with two units firing over 20

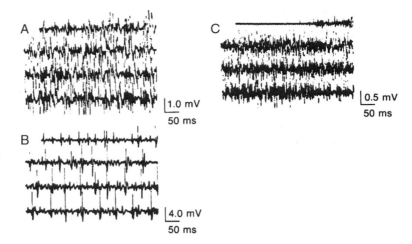

Figure 11.12 Interference patterns seen in the triceps of a 44-year-old healthy man (**A**), tibialis anterior of a 52-year-old man with amyotrophic lateral sclerosis (**B**), and quadriceps of a 20-year-old man with limb-girdle muscular dystrophy (**C**). Discrete single motor unit discharge in (**B**) stands in good contrast to abundant motor unit potentials with reduced amplitude in (**C**). (Reprinted with permission from J Kimura. Electrodiagnosis in Diseases of Nerve and Muscle: Principles and Practice [3rd ed]. New York: Oxford University Press, 2001.)

Hz, indicates a loss of motor units. With greater contraction (Figure 11.12), simultaneous activation of many different units precludes recognition of individual motor unit potentials, hence the name *interference pattern*, which can be described by the spike density and the average amplitude of the summated response. Its analysis provides a simple quantitative means of evaluating the number of firing units and the muscle force exerted with maximal effort. This measure, however, reflects the complex interaction among descending input from the cortex, the number of motor neurons capable of discharging, the firing frequency of each motor unit, the waveform of individual potentials, and the probability of phase cancellation.

Measurements of Turns and Amplitude

Individual motor unit potentials evaluated during weak voluntary effort mainly comprise low-threshold type I muscle fibers. Quantitative assessment of the interference pattern during strong muscle contraction relates to a wider range of motor units.[124] An automated technique is designed to count the number of "turns" or directional changes of a waveform that exceeds a minimum excursion without necessarily crossing the baseline.[125] This method selects potential changes greater than 100 μV, measuring the amplitude from a point of change in direction to the next, during a fixed-time epoch, with the subject maintaining constant levels of muscle contraction.[126,127] Reported measures include turns' frequencies,[128] the maximal ratio of turns to mean amplitude or peak ratio, and the number of time intervals between turns.[129] Turns and spectral analyses of interference patterns, although efficient, only indirectly relate to the physiologic properties of the motor units.[130] With increasing voluntary contraction from low to moderate levels, the number of turns accelerates faster than does the mean amplitude change between turns, but the pattern reverses at higher force levels.[131] Consequently, shape of the "normal cloud," which shows the relationship between the turns and amplitude, critically depends on the level of effort at which recordings are made. For example, an increment from 10% to 30% maximal voluntary contraction significantly increased the mean firing rate, number of turns, amplitude, and rise rate.[131] Clinical studies, therefore, must control contractile force precisely as a major determinant of waveform and firing properties (this is discussed in detail in Chapter 15).

In one study,[132] mean amplitudes, durations, and numbers of turns all increased linearly with age in both low-threshold and high-threshold motor units, suggesting an ongoing process of denervation and reinnervation. An increased ratio of turns to mean amplitude in myopathy, especially at 10–20% of maximum force, stands in contrast to a decreased ratio in neurogenic disorders, mainly at a force of 20–30%.[133] Similarly, the ratio of root mean square voltage to turns increases in chronic neuropathies.[134] Quantitative measurements of recruitment patterns also help to differentiate primary muscle disease from neurogenic lesions in infants and young children.[135,136] Evaluation of individual potentials allows precise description of normal and abnormal motor units and their temporal stability. Analysis of recruitment reveals an overall muscle performance by demonstrating the number and discharge pattern of all the motor units (this is discussed in detail in Chapter 12).

Lower and Upper Motor Neuron Disorders

The recruitment pattern depends primarily on the number of functional motor units and the average force contributed by each unit. In disorders of the motor neuron, root, or peripheral nerve, a reduced number of excitable motor units leads to limited recruitment despite increased effort to contract the muscle. Surviving motor neurons must fire at an inappropriately rapid rate to compensate for the loss in number. A single motor unit potential may discharge at frequencies as high as 50 Hz, producing a discreet "picket fence" appearance at maximal effort (see Figures 11.10 and 11.12). In contrast, the excited motor units discharge more slowly in a late recruitment caused by failure of descending impulses in disorders of the upper motor neuron. Studies of the temporal discharge pattern of single motor units may also elucidate characteristic firing behavior in patients with upper motor neuron lesions.[137,138] In one study of 15 stroke patients with paretic tibialis anterior, low-threshold motor units fired within the lower end of the normal range, whereas high-threshold motor units, if recruited at all, discharged below their normal range.[139] Patients with hemiparesis showed two characteristic patterns: compression in the range of motor neuron recruitment forces and failure to discharge motor units at a higher rate during increased voluntary effort to contract the paretic muscles.[140] Thus, a lower motor neuron weakness with a rapid rate of discharge stands in good contrast to an upper motor neuron or hysterical paralysis with a slow rate of discharge, although both show a reduced interference pattern. In addition, hysterical weakness or poor cooperation often produces irregular, tremulous firing of motor units not seen in a genuine paresis unless the patient also experiences an essential or other type of tremor.

Myopathy

In myopathy, each motor unit potential, low in amplitude and short in duration, contributes less force. Therefore, many units must discharge early to functionally compensate in quantity for the smaller force per unit. In general, the less efficient is the discharge from each motor unit, the greater is the number of units required to maintain the same force. With slight voluntary effort, many axons fire almost instantaneously in typical myopathies (see Figure 11.11). A full interference pattern develops at less than maximal contraction, but it is of low amplitudes, reflecting a decreased fiber density of individual motor units (see Figure 11.12). For the same reason, the motor units also show early recruitment in diseases of neuromuscular transmission, reaching a full interference prematurely. In advanced myogenic disorders, however, loss of whole motor units rather than individual muscle fibers may show a limited recruitment, leading to an incomplete interference pattern. This finding mimics a neuropathic change, characterized by a reduced number of motor units.

Involuntary Movement

Electromyography helps to characterize involuntary motor symptoms. In tremors, bursts of motor unit potentials repeat at a fairly constant rate. Many motor units, firing in a group during each burst, show no fixed temporal or spatial relationships varying in amplitude, duration, and waveform. Despite the changing appearance and rhythmic pattern, a subclinical tremor burst may mimic a polyphasic motor unit potential. Electromyographic recordings can delineate different types of tremor on the basis of their rate, rhythm, and distribution.[141] In hemifacial spasm or after aberrant regeneration, synkinesis gives rise to unintended activation of motor units in the muscles not under voluntary contraction. Simultaneous recording from multiple muscles can confirm the presence of time-locked discharge of aberrant motor unit potentials. This technique, therefore, helps to distinguish between pathologic synkinesis and associated movement or cocontraction of different muscles seen during normal voluntary activity without a precise time relationship.

PRINCIPLES OF LOCALIZATION

Proximal lesions at the level of the root or plexus affect either the motor or sensory fibers, or both. The features of motor involvement include weakness and atrophy of the muscle, hyporeflexia, fatigue, cramps, and fasciculations. Electrophysiologic studies help to delineate the distribution of the affected muscles, localize the level, and elucidate the extent and chronicity of the lesion.[142] A combination of clinical, laboratory, and electrodiagnostic features determines the level of a radicular involvment.[143] Some studies report a high correlation among electromyographic evidence of denervation, myelographic abnormalities, and surgical findings.[144] In one series,[145] however, electromyography and magnetic resonance imaging agreed in only 60% of patients, and one of the studies showed abnormality in the remaining 40%, suggesting that they provide complementary diagnostic information. Some advocate application of a computer-aided expert system to brachial plexus injuries.[146]

Broad and frequently anomalous segmental innervations challenge the clinician in attributing any pattern of clinical or electromyographic findings to a specific spinal level.[147] Nonetheless, electromyographic studies provide an objective means to corroborate clinical diagnosis of a radicular lesion. The deep cervical muscles receive innervation from the posterior as opposed to anterior rami of the spinal nerves. Evidence of denervation here, therefore, indicates an intraforaminal lesion affecting the root or spinal nerve before the division into the two rami. Studies of paraspinal muscles thus help to document the involvement of the posterior rami, confirming a radicular as opposed to a plexus lesion. Other muscles innervated proximally to the brachial plexus include the rhomboids supplied by the dorsal scapular nerve and the serratus anterior subserved by the long thoracic nerves.

Spontaneous activity in these muscles also serves to distinguish between root and plexus lesions.

In the affected muscle, needle examination initially reveals poor recruitment of motor unit potentials, indicating structural or functional loss of axons. Subsequent appearance of fibrillation potentials and positive sharp waves in 2–3 weeks suggest axonal degeneration. Low-amplitude, polyphasic motor unit potentials have temporal instability during active regeneration of motor axons. In contrast, high-amplitude, long-duration motor unit potentials with stable configuration appear after completion of reinnervation. The length-dependent delay of nerve degeneration[31] predicts the appearance of denervation potentials first in the paraspinal muscle. In one study,[148] however, multivariate estimates showed no correlation between paraspinal muscle spontaneous activity and symptom duration. In practice, therefore, this time relationship may not necessarily hold.[149] Clinical findings should dictate which muscles to examine (Table 11.6) for the optimal identification of the involved root.[150] Structural abnormalities do not necessarily coincide with functional deficits uncovered by electrophysiologic studies.[151]

In the upper limbs, motor deficits are more reliable localizing signs than are sensory impairments. The reverse seems to hold in the lower limbs because anatomic peculiarity makes clinical and electrophysiologic localization of radicular lesions more difficult. In conus lesions, electromyographic studies usually reveal symmetric abnormalities involving multiple roots. A cauda equina lesion resembles a conus medullaris lesion showing bilateral involvement of the level ordinarily unaffected by a herniated lumbar disk. Electromyographic studies show fibrillation potentials and large motor unit potentials in the distribution of several lumbosacral roots, including paraspinal muscles[152] and urethral sphincter.[153] These findings mimic those of an intrinsic conus involvement except for an asymmetric distribution of the abnormalities with spread above the sacral myotomes.

Disk protrusion involves the L4-5 and L5-Sl interspaces, in most cases, and the L3-4 space much less frequently. The protruding disk tends to compress the lumbosacral roots slightly above the level of their respective foramina before their lateral deviation toward the exit. Needle studies help to confirm the diagnosis and identify the damaged root (Table 11.7). As in the cervical region, denervation of the paraspinal muscles implies a lesion located proximal to the origin of the posterior ramus. The absence of denervation here, however, does not necessarily exclude the possibility of root compression. The multifidus muscles are innervated by a single root, in contrast to the polysegmental innervation of the rest of the paraspinal muscle mass.[154] Nonetheless, paraspinal abnormalities usually fail to provide the exact location of the involved segment on this basis alone.[155] Determination of the precise level of lesion, therefore, depends on careful exploration of the affected muscles in the lower limbs. In addition to the diagnostic use, series of studies can guide the management by substantiating clinical progression or improvement.[156]

When radiologic and clinical findings conflict, electrodiagnosis plays a particularly important role in justifying surgical exploration.[157] For example, extraforaminal compression of the L5 root by lumbosacral ligaments may cause denervation despite a normal myelogram and other imaging studies.[158] Conversely, asymptomatic subjects may have abnormal magnetic resonance scans of the lumbar spine, making it imperative to seek a physiologic and clinical correlation.[159] To supplement the electrophysiologic evaluations of functional deficits, T2-weighted and short time to inversion recovery magnetic resonance

Table 11.6 Innervation Patterns of the Cranial, Shoulder Girdle, and Upper Limb Muscles

Nerves	Muscles	C2	C3	C4	C5	C6	C7	C8	T1
Anterior primary rami									
Cervical plexus									
Spinal accessory nerve	Sternocleidomastoid	■	■						
	Trapezius, upper, middle, lower		■	■					
Phrenic nerve	Diaphragm		■	■					
Brachial plexus									
Dorsal scapular nerve	Rhomboid				■				
Suprascapular nerve	Supraspinatus				■	▨			
	Infraspinatus				■	▨			
Axillary nerve	Teres minor				■	■			
	Deltoid, anterior, middle, posterior				■	■			
Subscapular nerve	Teres major				■	■			
Musculocutaneous nerve	Brachialis				■	▨			
	Biceps brachii				■	■			
	Coracobrachialis					▨	■		
Long thoracic nerve	Serratus anterior				■	■	■		
Lateral pectoral nerve	Pectoralis major (clavicular part)				■	■			
Medial pectoral nerve	Pectoralis minor						▨	■	■
Radial nerve	Brachioradialis				▨	■			
	Extensor carpi radialis				▨	■			
	Triceps, long, lateral, middle heads					▨	■	▨	
	Anconeus						■	▨	
Posterior interosseous nerve	Supinator				■	■			
	Extensor carpi ulnaris						■	▨	
	Extensor digitorum						■	▨	
	Extensor pollicis brevis						■	▨	
	Extensor indicis						■	▨	
Median nerve	Pronator teres					▨	■		
	Flexor carpi radialis					▨	■		
	Abductor pollicis brevis							▨	■
Anterior interosseous nerve	Flexor digitorum profundus (I and II)						▨	■	
	Pronator quadratus						▨	■	
	Flexor pollicis longus						▨	■	
Ulnar nerve	Flexor digitorum profundus (III and IV)						▨	■	
	Flexor carpi ulnaris						▨	■	
	Adductor pollicis							▨	■
	Abductor digiti minimi							▨	■
	Interossei, volar (I–III), dorsal (I–IV)							▨	■
Posterior primary rami	Cervical erector spinae				■	■	■	■	■

■ = primary innervation; ▨ = secondary innervation.

Table 11.7 Innervation Patterns of the Hip Girdle and Lower Limb Muscles

Nerves	Muscles	L2	L3	L4	L5	S1	S2
Anterior primary rami							
Lumbosacral plexus							
Femoral nerve	Iliopsoas	■	■				
	Sartorius	■	■	■			
	Rectus femoris		■	■			
	Vastus lateralis, medialis		■	■			
Obturator nerve	Gracilis	■	■	▨			
	Adductor longus, brevis, magnus	■	■	■			
Superior gluteal nerve	Gluteus medius			■	■	■	
	Gluteus minimus			▨	■	▨	
	Tensor facie latae			▨	■	■	
Inferior gluteal nerve	Gluteus maximus				▨	■	■
Sciatic nerve							
Tibial division	Semitendinosus, semimembranosus				■	■	■
	Biceps femoris, long head				▨	■	▨
Peroneal division	Biceps femoris, short head				▨	■	■
Common peroneal nerve							
Deep peroneal nerve	Tibialis anterior			■	■		
	Extensor digitorum longus				■	■	
	Extensor digitorum brevis				■	■	
	Extensor hallucis longus				▨	■	
Superficial peroneal nerve	Peroneus longus				■	■	
	Peroneus brevis				■	■	
Tibial nerve	Tibialis posterior			■	■		
	Flexor digitorum longus				■	■	▨
	Flexor hallucis longus				■	■	■
	Gastrocnemius, medial head					■	▨
	Gastrocnemius, lateral head					▨	■
	Soleus				▨	■	■
Medial plantar nerve	Abductor hallucis					■	■
Lateral plantar nerve	Abductor digiti minimi					■	■
	Interossei					■	■
Posterior primary rami	Lumbosacral erector spinae	■	■	■	■	■	■

■ = primary innervation; ▨ = secondary innervation.

imaging sequences can be used to detect denervated skeletal muscle, which shows increased signal intensity. In one study,[160] this abnormality corresponded closely with spontaneous activities on electromyographic examination.

CONCLUSIONS

Electromyographic studies analyze the propagating muscle action potentials extracellularly. Except for the end-plate activities and brief injury potentials coincident with the insertion of the needle, a relaxed muscle is electrically silent. Several types of spontaneous discharges seen at rest, therefore, signal diseases of the nerve or muscle, although they do not necessarily carry the same clinical implications. Both fibrillation potentials and positive sharp waves result from excitation of individual muscle fibers, whereas complex repetitive discharges comprise high-frequency spikes derived from multiple muscle fibers, which discharge sequentially maintaining a fixed order.

A *motor unit* is the smallest functional element of volitional contraction. In conventional electromyography, isolated discharges of single motor axons give rise to motor unit potentials. Diseases of the nerve or muscle cause structural or functional disturbances of the motor unit, which in turn lead to alterations in the waveform and discharge patterns of their electrical signals. Because certain characteristics of such abnormalities suggest a particular pathologic process, the study of motor unit potentials provides information useful in elucidating the nature of the disease.

Electromyography serves as a clinical tool only if the examiner interprets the findings in light of the patient's history, physical examination, and other diagnostic studies. In fact, the study constitutes an extension of physical examination rather than an independent laboratory test. As such, studies are most useful if conducted by a physician thoroughly familiar with the clinical findings, which provide an overall orientation for subsequent physiologic evaluation.

REFERENCES

1. Geiringer SR. Anatomic Localization for Needle Electromyography. Philadelphia: Hanley & Belfus, 1994.
2. Perotto A, Delagi EF, Iazzetti J, Morrison D. Anatomical Guide for the Electromyographer, the Limbs and Trunk (3rd ed). Springfield, IL: Charles C. Thomas, 1994.
3. Daube JR. AAEE minimonograph #11: needle examination in clinical electromyography. Muscle Nerve 1991;14:685–700.
4. Stålberg E, Falck B. The role of electromyography in neurology. Electroencephologr Clin Neurophysiol 1997;103:579–598.
5. Scranton PE, Hasiba U, Gorenc TJ. Intramuscular hemorrhage in hemophiliacs with inhibitors. JAMA 1979;241:2028–2030.
6. Bouisset S. EMG and Muscle Force in Normal Motor Activities. In JE Desmedt (ed), New Developments in Electromyography and Clinical Neurophysiology, Vol 1. Basel, NY: S. Karger, 1973;547–583.
7. Brooke MH, Carroll JE, Davis JE, Hagberg JM. The prolonged exercise test. Neurology 1979;29:636–643.
8. Pedinoff S, Sandhu RS. Electromyographic effect on serum creatine phosphokinase in normal individuals. Arch Phys Med Rehabil 1978;59:27–29.
9. Kugelberg E, Petersen I. "Insertion activity" in electromyography: with notes on denervated muscle response to constant current. J Neurol Neurosurg Psychiatry 1949;12:268–273.
10. Brown WF, Varkey GP. The origin of spontaneous electrical activity at the endplate zone. Ann Neurol 1981;10:557–560.
11. Buchthal F, Rosenfalck P. Spontaneous electrical activity of human muscle. Electroencephalogr Clin Neurophysiol 1966;20:321–336.
12. Heckmann R, Ludin HP. Differentiation of spontaneous activity from normal and denervated skeletal muscle. J Neurol Neurosurg Psychiatry 1982;45:331–336.
13. Weiss MD, Mayer RF. Temperature-sensitive repetitive discharges in paramyotonia congenita. Muscle Nerve 1997;20:195–197.
14. Buchthal F, Engbaek L, Gamstorp I. Paresis and hyperexcitability in adynamia episodica hereditaria. Neurology 1958;8:347–351.
15. Morrison JB. The electromyographic changes in hyperkalemic familial periodic paralysis. Ann Phys Med 1960;5:153–155.
16. Hudgson P, Gardner-Medwin D, Worsfold M, et al. Adult myopathy from glycogen storage disease due to acid maltase deficiency. Brain 1968;91:435–462.

17. Nakano S, Engel AG, Waclawik AJ, et al. Myofibrillar myopathy with abnormal foci of desmin positivity. I. Light and electron microscopy analysis of 10 cases. J Neuropath Exp Neurol 1996;55:549–562.

18. Dumitru D. Single muscle fiber discharges (insertional activity, end-plate potentials, positive sharp waves, and fibrillation potentials): a unifying proposal. Muscle Nerve 1996;19:221–226.

19. Dumitru D, King JC, Rogers W, Stegeman DF. Positive sharp wave and fibrillation potential modeling. Muscle Nerve 1999;22:242–251.

20. Kraft GH. Fibrillation potentials and positive sharp waves: are they the same? Electroencephalogr Clin Neurophysiol 1991;81:163–166.

21. Kraft GH. Are fibrillation potentials and positive sharp waves the same? No. Muscle Nerve 1996;19:216–220.

22. Emeryk B, Hausmanowa-Petrusewicz I, Nowak T. Spontaneous volleys of bizarre high frequency potentials (b.h.f.p.) in neuro-muscular diseases. Part I. Occurrence of spontaneous volleys of b.h.f.p. in neuro-muscular diseases. Electromyogr Clin Neurophysiol 1974;14:303–312.

23. Emeryk B, Hausmanowa-Petrusewicz I, Nowak T. Spontaneous volleys of bizarre high frequency potentials (b.h.f.p.) in neuro-muscular diseases. Part II. An analysis of the morphology of spontaneous volleys of b.h.f.p. in neuromuscular diseases. Electromyogr Clin Neurophysiol 1974;14: 339–354.

24. Stålberg E, Trontelj JV. Single Fiber Electromyography. Surrey, UK: The Mirvalle Press Limited, Old Woking, 1979.

25. Jablecki C, Knoll D. Fibrillation potentials and complex repetitive discharges [abstract]. Electroencephalogr Clin Neurophysiol 1980;50:242.

26. Stålberg E, Ekstedt J. Single Fiber EMG and Microphysiology of the Motor Unit in Normal and Diseased Human Muscle. In JE Desmedt (ed), New Developments in Electromyography and Clinical Neurophysiology, Vol 1. Basel, NY: S. Karger, 1973;113–129.

27. Denny-Brown D, Pennybacker JB. Fibrillation and fasciculation in voluntary muscle. Brain 1938;61:311–332.

28. Jasper H, Ballem G. Unipolar electromyograms of normal and denervated human muscle. J Neurophysiol 1949;12:231–244.

29. Thesleff S. Fibrillation in Denervated Mammalian Skeletal Muscle. In WJ Culp, J Ochoa (eds), Abnormal Nerves and Muscle as Impulse Generators. Oxford, UK: Oxford University Press, 1982;678–694.

30. Buchthal F. Fibrillations: Clinical Electrophysiology. In WJ Culp, J Ochoa (eds), Abnormal Nerves and Muscles as Impulse Generators. Oxford, UK: Oxford University Press, 1982;632–662.

31. Miller RG. AAEE minimonograph #28. Injury to peripheral motor nerves. Muscle Nerve 1987;10:698–710.

32. Desmedt JE, Borenstein S. Regeneration in Duchenne muscular dystrophy. Electromyographic evidence. Arch Neurol 1976;33:642–650.

33. Simpson JA. Handbook of Electromyography and Clinical Neurophysiology, Vol 16. Neuromuscular Diseases. Amsterdam: Elsevier, 1973.

34. Bohan A, Peter JB. Polymyositis and dermatomyositis. N Engl J Med 1975;292:344–347.

35. Richardson AT. Clinical and electromyographic aspects of polymyositis. Proc R Soc Med 1956;49:111–114.

36. Fusfeld RD. Electromyographic abnormalities in a case of botulism. Bull Los Angeles Neurol Soc 1970;35:164–168.

37. Petersen I, Broman AM. Elektromyografiska fynd frèn ett fall av botulism. Nordisk Med 1961;65:259–261.

38. Heifernan L, Rewcastle NB, Humphrey JG. The spectrum of rod myopathies. Arch Neurol 1968;18:529–542.

39. Spiro AJ, Shy GM, Gonatas NK. Myotubular myopathy: persistence of fetal muscle in an adolescent boy. Arch Neurol 1966;14:1–14.

40. Waylonis GW, Johnson EW. Electromyographic findings in induced trichinosis. Arch Phys Med Rehabil 1965;615–625.

41. Rowin J, Meriggioli MN. Complex repetitive discharges: cause or effect of neurogenic muscle hypertrophy? Muscle Nerve 1999;22:1603–1606.

42. Fowler CJ, Kirby RS, Harrison MJG. Decelerating burst and complex repetitive discharges in the striated muscle of the urethral sphincter, associated with urinary retention in women. J Neurol Neurosurg Psychiatry 1985;48:1004–1009.

43. Wettstein A. The origin of fasciculations in motoneuron disease. Ann Neurol 1979;5:295–300.

44. Layzer RB. The origin of muscle fasciculations and cramps. Muscle Nerve 1994;17:1243–1249.

45. Hudson AJ, Brown WF, Gilbert JJ. The muscular pain-fasciculation syndrome. Neurology 1978;28:1105–1109.

46. Kadson DL. Cervical spondylotic myelopathy with reversible fasciculations in the lower extremities. Arch Neurol 1977;34:774–776.
47. King RB, Stoops WL. Cervical myelopathy with fasciculations in the lower extremities. J Neurosurg 1963;20:948–952.
48. Norris FH Jr. Synchronous fasciculation in motor neuron disease. Arch Neurol 1965;13:495–500.
49. Roth G, Egloff-Baer S. ECG-related fasciculation potential. Electroencephalogr Clin Neurophysiol 1997;105:132–134.
50. Mitsikostas DD, Karandreas N, Coutsopetras P. Fasciculation potentials in healthy people. Muscle Nerve 1998;21:533–535.
51. Richardson AT. Muscle fasciculation. Arch Phys Med Rehabil 1954;35:281–286.
52. Trojaborg W, Buchthal F. Malignant and benign fasciculations. Acta Neurol Scand 1965;41(Suppl 13):251–254.
53. de Carvalho M, Swash M. Fasciculation potentials: a study of amyotrophic lateral sclerosis and other neurogenic disorders. Muscle Nerve 1998;1:336–344.
54. Conrad B, Jacobi HM, Prochazka VJ. Unusual properties of repetitive fasciculations. Electroencephalogr Clin Neurophysiol 1973;35:173–179.
55. Mateer JE, Gutmann L, McComas CF. Myokymia in Guillain-Barré syndrome. Neurology 1983;33:374–376.
56. Aho K, Sainio K. Late irradiation-induced lesions of the lumbosacral plexus. Neurology 1983;33: 953–955.
57. Albers JW, Allen AA, Bastron JA, Daube JR. Limb myokymia. Muscle Nerve 1981;4:494–504.
58. Daube JR, Kelly JJ Jr, Martin RA. Facial myokymia with polyradiculoneuropathy. Neurology 1979;29:662–669.
59. Brick JF, Gutmann L, McComas CF. Calcium effect on generation and amplification of myokymic discharges. Neurology 1982;32:618–622.
60. Eisen A. The physiologic basis and clinical applications of needle EMG in neuromuscular abnormalities. Principles and pitfalls in the practice of EMG and NCS. American Academy of Neurology 49th Annual Meeting; April 12–19, 1997; Boston.
61. Garcia-Meriono A, Cabello A, Mora JS, Liano H. Continuous muscle fiber activity, peripheral neuropathy and thymoma. Ann Neurol 1991;29:215–218.
62. Isaacs H. Continuous muscle fiber activity. J Neurol Neurosurg Psychiatry 1961;24:319–325.
63. Newsom-Davis J. Immunological associations of acquired neuromyotonia (Isaacs' syndrome). Report of five cases and literature review. Brain 1993;116:453–469.
64. Magistris MR, Roth G. Motor axon reflex and indirect double discharge: ephaptic transmission? A reappraisal. Electroencephalogr Clin Neurophysiol 1992;85:124–130.
65. Roth G. Repetitive discharge due to self-ephaptic excitation of a motor unit. Electroencephalogr Clin Neurol 1994;93:1–6.
66. Torbergsen T, Stålberg E, Brautaset NJ. Generator sites for spontaneous activity in neuromyotonia. An EMG study. Electroencephalogr Clin Neurophysiol 1996;101:69–78.
67. Layzer RB. Muscle Pain, Cramps, and Fatigue. In AG Engel, C Franzini-Armstrong (eds), Myology (2nd ed). New York: McGraw-Hill, 1994;3462–3497.
68. Layzer RB, Rowland LP. Cramps. N Engl J Med 1971;285:30–31.
69. Obi T, Mizoguchi K, Matsuoka H, et al. Muscle cramp as the result of impaired GABA function—an electrophysiological and pharmacological observation. Muscle Nerve 1993;16:1228–1231.
70. Nandedkar SD, Sanders DB. Principal component analysis of the features of concentric needle EMG motor unit action potentials. Muscle Nerve 1989;12:288–293.
71. Bertram MF, Nishida T, Minieka MM, et al. Effects of temperature on motor unit action potentials during isometric contraction. Muscle Nerve 1995;18:1443–1446.
72. Denys E. The influence of temperature in clinical neurophysiology. Muscle Nerve 1991;14:795–811.
73. Buchthal F. The General Concept of the Motor Unit. In RD Adams, LM Eaton, GM Shy (eds), Neuromuscular Disorders. Baltimore: Williams & Wilkins, 1960.
74. Buchthal F, Rosenfalck P. Electrophysiological Aspects of Myopathy with Particular Reference to Progressive Muscular Dystrophy. In GH Bourne, MN Golarz (ed), Muscular Dystrophy in Man and Animals. New York: Hafner Publishing Company, 1963.
75. Emeryk-Szajewska B, Kopec J, Karwanska A. The reorganization of motor units in motor neuron disease. Muscle Nerve 1997;20:306–315.
76. Hausmanowa-Petrusewicz I, Jedrzejowska H. Correlation between electromyographic findings and muscle biopsy in cases of neuromuscular disease [abstract]. J Neurol Sci 1971;13:85–106.
77. Stålberg E. Invited review: electrodiagnostic assessment and monitoring of motor unit changes in disease. Muscle Nerve 1991;14:293–303.

78. Ekstedt J, Stalberg E. How the size of the needle electrode leading-off surface influences the shape of the single muscle fibre action potential in electromyography. Comput Programs Biomed 1973;3:204–212.

79. Griep PAM, Gielen FLH, Boom HBK, et al. Calculation and registration of the same motor unit action potential. Electroencephalogr Clin Neurophysiol 1982;53:388–404.

80. Stålberg E, Nandedkar SD, Sanders DB, Falck B. Quantitative motor unit potential analysis. J Clin Neurophysiol 1996;13:401–422.

81. Thiele B, Bohle A. Number of spike-components contributing to the motor unit potential. EEG EMG Z Elektroenzephalogr Elektromyogr Verwandte Geb 1978;9:125–130.

82. Dumitru D, King JC, Nandedkar SD. Motor unit action potentials recorded with concentric electrodes: physiologic implications. Electroencephologr Clin Neurophysiol 1997;105:333–339.

83. Nandedkar SD, Sanders DB, Stålberg EV, Andreassen S. Simulation of concentric needle EMG motor unit action potential. Muscle Nerve 1988;11:151–159.

84. Stashuk DW. Detecting single fiber contributions to motor unit action potentials. Muscle Nerve 1999;22:218–229.

85. King JC, Dumitru D, Stegeman D. Monopolar needle electrode spatial recording characteristics. Muscle Nerve 1996;19:1310–1319.

86. Nandedkar SD, Barkhaus PE, Sanders DB, Stålberg EV. Analysis of amplitude and area of concentric needle EMG motor unit action potentials. Electroencephalogr Clin Neurophysiol 1988;69:561–567.

87. Sonoo M, Stålberg E. The ability of MUP parameters to discriminate between normal and neurogenic MUPs in concentric EMG: analysis of the MUP "thickness" and the proposal of "size index." Electroencephalogr Clin Neurophysiol 1993;89:291–303.

88. International Federation of Societies for Electroencephalography and Clinical Neurophysiology. Recommendations for the Practice of Clinical Neurophysiology. Amsterdam: Elsevier, 1983;143.

89. Barkhaus PE, Nandedkar SD. On the selection of concentric needle electromyogram motor unit action potentials: is the rise time criterion too restrictive? Muscle Nerve 1996;19:1554–1560.

90. Dumitru D, King JC. Motor unit action potential duration and muscle length. Muscle Nerve 1999;22:1188–1195.

91. Nandedkar SD, Dumitru D, King JC. Concentric needle electrode duration measurement and uptake area. Muscle Nerve 1997;20:1225–1228.

92. Dumitru D, King JC, Nandedkar SD. Comparison of single-fiber and macro electrode recordings: relationship to motor unit action potential duration. Muscle Nerve 1997;20:1381–1388.

93. Nandedkar SD, Sanders DB, Stålberg EV. On the shape of the normal turns-amplitude cloud. Muscle Nerve 1991;14:8–13.

94. Zalewska E, Rowinska-Marcinska K, Hausmanowa-Petrusewicz I. Shape irregularity of motor unit potentials in some neuromuscular disorders. Muscle Nerve 1998;21:1181–1187.

95. Daube JR. Electrodiagnosis of Muscle Disorders. In AG Engel, C Franzini-Armstrong (eds), Myology (2nd ed). New York: McGraw-Hill, 1994;764–794.

96. Finsterer J, Mamoli B. Satellite potentials: definition normal values and validity in the detection of mild myogenic lesions. EEG EMG Z Elektroenzephalogr Elektromyogr Verwandte Geb 1992;23:20–28.

97. Trojaborg W. Quantitative electromyography in polymyositis: a reappraisal. Muscle Nerve 1990;13:964–971.

98. Finsterer J, Mamoli B. Satellite potentials as a measure of neuromuscular disorders. Muscle Nerve 1997;20:585–592.

99. Payan L. The blanket principle: a technical note. Muscle Nerve 1978;1:432–436.

100. Stålberg E, Sonoo M. Assessment of variability in the shape of the motor unit action potential, the "jiggle," at consecutive discharges. Muscle Nerve 1994;17:1135–1144.

101. Lester JM, Soule NW, Bradley WG, Brenner JF. An augmented computer model of motor unit reorganization in neurogenic diseases. Muscle Nerve 1993;16:43–56.

102. Cholachis SC, Pease WS, Johnson EW. Polyphasic motor unit action potentials in early radiculopathy: their presence and ephaptic transmission as an hypothesis. Electromyogr Clin Neurophysiol 1992;32:27–33.

103. Roth G, Magistris MD. Ephapse between two motor units in chronically denervated muscle. Electromyogr Clin Neurophysiol 1985;25:331–339.

104. Buchthal F. Diagnostic Significance of the Myopathic EMG. In LP Rowland (ed), Pathogenesis of Human Muscular Dystrophies. Durango, CO: Proceedings of the Fifth International Scientific Conference of the Muscular Dystrophy Association, June 1976. Amsterdam: Excerpta Medica, 1977.

105. Buchthal F. Electrophysiological signs of myopathy as related with muscle biopsy. Acta Neurol (Napoli) 1977b;32:1–29.

106. Engel WK. Brief, small, abundant motor-unit action potentials: a further critique of electromyographic interpretation. Neurology 1975;25:173–176.
107. Nakashima K, Tabuchi Y, Takahashi K. The diagnostic significance of large action potentials in myopathy. J Neurol Sci 1983;61:161–170.
108. Lang AH, Partanen VSJ. "Satellite potentials" and the duration of motor unit potentials in normal, neuropathic and myopathic muscles. J Neurol Sci 1976;27:513–524.
109. Pickett JB. Late components of motor unit potentials in a patient with myoglobinuria. Ann Neurol 1978;3:461–464.
110. Engel WK, Warmolts JR. The Motor Unit. Diseases Affecting It In Toto or In Partia. In JE Desmedt (ed), New Developments in Electromyography and Clinical Neurophysiology, Vol 1. Basel, NY: S. Karger, 1973;141–177.
111. Warmolts JR, Mendell JR. Open-biopsy electromyography: direct correlation of a pattern of excessively recruited, pathologically small motor unit potentials with histologic evidence of neuropathy. Arch Neurol 1979;36:406–409.
112. Black JT, Bhatt GP, DeJesus PV, et al. Diagnostic accuracy of clinical data, quantitative electromyography and histochemistry in neuromuscular disease: a study of 105 cases. J Neurol Sci 1974;21:59–70.
113. Henneman E. Relation between size of neurons and their susceptibility to discharge. Science 1957;126:1245–1247.
114. De Luca CJ, Erim Z. Common drive of motor units in regulation of muscle force. Trends Neurosci 1994;7:299–305.
115. Erim Z, De Luca CJ, Mineo K. Rank-ordered regulation of motor units. Muscle Nerve 1996; 19:563–573.
116. Henneman E, Mendell LM. Functional Organization of Motoneuron Pool and Its Inputs. In JM Brookhart, VB Mountcastle (eds), Handbook of Physiology, Vol 2. Bethesda, MD: American Physiological Society, 1981;423–507.
117. Scutter SD, Turker KS. Recruitment stability in masseter motor units during isometric voluntary contractions. Muscle Nerve 1998;21:1290–1298.
118. Dengler R, Wolf W, Schubert M, Struppler A. Discharge pattern of single motor units in basal ganglia disorders. Neurology 1986;36:1061–1066.
119. Thomas CK, Broton JG, Calancie B. Motor unit forces and recruitment patterns after cervical spinal cord injury. Muscle Nerve 1997;20:212–220.
120. Gunreben G, Schulte-Mattler W. Evaluation of motor unit firing rates by standard concentric needle electromyography. Electromyogr Clin Neurophysiol 1992;32:103–111.
121. Petajan JH. Antigravity posture for analysis of motor unit recruitment: the "45 degree test." Muscle Nerve 1990;13:355–359.
122. Petajan JH. AAEM minimonograph #3: motor unit recruitment. Muscle Nerve 1991;14:489–502.
123. Fuglsang-Frederiksen A, Smith T, Hogenhaven H. Motor unit firing intervals and other parameters of electrical activity in normal and pathological muscle. J Neurol Sci 1987;78:51–62.
124. Shochina M, Vatine JJ, Mahler Y, et al. Diagnostic value of computer analysis of multipeaked EMG spikes. Electromyogr Clin Neurophysiol 1992;32:113–117.
125. Willison RG. Analysis of electrical activity in healthy and dystrophic muscle in man. J Neurol Neurosurg Psychiatry 1964;27:386–394.
126. Hayward M. Automatic analysis of the electromyogram in healthy subjects of different ages. J Neurol Sci 1977;33:397–413.
127. Hayward M, Willison, RG. The Recognition of Myogenic and Neurogenic Lesions by Quantitative EMG. In JE Desmedt (ed), New Developments in Electromyography and Clinical Neurophysiology, Vol 2. Basel, NY: S. Karger, 1973;448–453.
128. Junge D. Turns and averaging as static and dynamic measures of masseter EMG activity. Electromyogr Clin Neurophysiol 1993;33(1):11–18.
129. Liguori R, Dahl K, Fuglsang-Frederiksen A. Turns-amplitude analysis of the electromyographic recruitment pattern disregarding force measurement. I. Method and reference values in healthy subjects. Muscle Nerve 1992;15:1314–1318.
130. Dorfman LJ, McGill KC. AAEE minimonograph #29: automatic quantitative electromyography. Muscle Nerve 1988;11:804–818.
131. Dorfman LJ, Howard JE, McGill KC. Influence of contractile force on properties of motor unit action potentials: ADEMG analysis. J Neurol Sci 1988;86:125–136.
132. Howard JE, McGill KC, Dorfman LJ. Age effects on properties of motor unit action potentials: ADEMG analysis. Ann Neurol 1988;24:207–213.
133. Fuglsang-Frederiksen A, Monaco M, Dahl K. Turns analysis (peak ratio) in EMG using the mean amplitude as a substitute of force measurement. Electroencephalogr Clin Neurophysiol 1985;60:225–227.

134. Fisher MA. Root mean square voltage/turns in chronic neuropathies is related to increase in fiber density. Muscle Nerve 1997;20:241–243.

135. Smyth DPL. Quantitative electromyography in babies and young children with primary muscle disease and neurogenic lesions. J Neurol Sci 1982;56:199–207.

136. Smyth DPL, Willison RG. Quantitative electromyography in babies and young children with no evidence of neuromuscular disease. J Neurol Sci 1982;56:209–217.

137. Fang J, Shahani BT, Bruyninckx FL. Study of single motor unit discharge patterns using 1/F process model. Muscle Nerve 1997;20:293–298.

138. Yan K, Fang J, Shahani B. Motor unit discharge behaviors in stroke patients. Muscle Nerve 1998;21:1502–1506.

139. Frontera WR, Grimby L, Larsson L. Firing rate of the lower motoneuron and contractile properties of its muscle fibers after upper motoneuron lesion in man. Muscle Nerve 1997;20:938–947.

140. Gemperline JJ, Allen S, Walk D, Rymer WZ. Characteristics of motor unit discharge in subjects with hemiparesis. Muscle Nerve 1995;18:1101–1114.

141. Shahani BT, Young RR. The Blink, H, and Tendon Vibration Reflexes. In J Goodgold, A Eberstein (eds), Electrodiagnosis of Neuromuscular Diseases (2nd ed). Baltimore: Williams & Wilkins, 1977;245–263.

142. Wilbourn AJ, Aminoff MJ. AAEM minimonograph #32: the electrodiagnostic examination in patients with radiculopathies. Muscle Nerve 1998;21:1612–1631.

143. McGonagle IK, Levine SR, Donofrio PD, Albers JW. Spectrum of patients with EMG features of polyradiculopathy without neuropathy. Muscle Nerve 1990;13:63–69.

144. Levin KH, Maggiano HJ, Wilbourn AJ. Cervical radiculopathies: comparison of surgical and EMG localization of single root lesions. Neurology 1996;46:1022–1025.

145. Nardin RA, Patel MR, Gudas TF, et al. Electromyography and magnetic resonance imaging in the evaluation of radiculopathy. Muscle Nerve 1999;22:151–155.

146. Fisher WS III. Computer-aided intelligence: application of an expert system to brachial plexus injuries. Neurosurgery 1990;27:837–843.

147. Phillips LH II, Park TS. Electrophysiologic mapping of the segmental anatomy of the muscles of the lower extremity. Muscle Nerve 1991;14:1213–1218.

148. Pezzin LE, Dillingham TR, Lauder TD, et al. Cervical radiculopathies: relationship between symptom duration and spontaneous EMG activity. Muscle Nerve 1999;22:1412–1418.

149. Dillingham TR, Pezzin LE, Lauder TD. Cervical paraspinal muscle abnormalities and symptom duration: a multivariate analysis (short report). Muscle Nerve 1998;21:640–642.

150. Lauder TD, Dillingham TR. The cervical radiculopathy screen: optimizing the number of muscles studies (short report). Muscle Nerve 1996;19:662–665.

151. Trojaborg W. Clinical, electrophysiological, and myelographic studies of 9 patients with cervical spinal root avulsions: discrepancies between EMG and X-ray findings. Muscle Nerve 1994;17:913–922.

152. Bartleson JD, Cohen MD, Harrington TM, et al. Cauda equina syndrome secondary to long-standing ankylosing spondylitis. Ann Neurol 1983;14:662–669.

153. Fowler CJ, Kirby RS, Harrison MJG, et al. Individual motor unit analysis in the diagnosis of disorders of urethral sphincter innervation. J Neurol Neurosurg Psychiatry 1984;47:637–641.

154. Campbell WW, Vasconcelos O, Laine FJ. Focal atrophy of the multifidus muscle in lumbosacral radiculopathy. Muscle Nerve 1998;21:1350–1353.

155. Haig AJ, Talley C, Grobler LJ, LeBreck DB. Paraspinal mapping: quantified needle electromyography in lumbar radiculopathy. Muscle Nerve 1993;16:477–484.

156. Johnson EW, Fletcher FR. Lumbosacral radiculopathy: review of 100 consecutive cases. Arch Phys Med Rehabil 1981;61:321–323.

157. Tullberg T, Svanborg E, Isacsson J, Grane P. A preoperative and postoperative study of the accuracy and value of electrodiagnosis in patients with lumbosacral disc herniation. Spine 1993;18:837–842.

158. Olsewski JM, Simmons EH, Kallen FC, Mendel FC. Evidence from cadavers suggestive of entrapment of fifth lumbar spinal nerves by lumbosacral ligaments. Spine 1991;16:336–347.

159. Boden SD, Davis DO, Dina TS, et al. Abnormal magnetic-resonance scans of the lumbar spine in asymptomatic subjects. Am J Bone Joint Surg 1990;72(3):403–408.

160. Carter GT, Fritz RC. Electromyographic and lower extremity short time to inversion recovery magnetic resonance imaging findings in lumbar radiculopathy (short report). Muscle Nerve 1997;20:1191–1193.

12

Quantitative Analysis: Objective and Interactive Assessment in Electromyography

Sanjeev D. Nandedkar and Paul E. Barkhaus

The neuromuscular system functions in a smooth and efficient manner because of the closed-loop feedback organization of its components (Figure 12.1). The command for voluntary muscle contraction is initiated in the upper motor neuron. It arrives at the lower motor neuron, located in the anterior horn of the spinal cord, in the form of an "excitatory" input. This is indicated as "+" in Figure 12.1. When excitatory inputs to the motor neuron exceed a threshold level, the motor neuron discharges. The neuron generates an action potential (AP) that propagates along the axon (i.e., motor nerve fiber) to the terminal axon branches, arriving at the neuromuscular junction (also called *end plate* or *synapse*).

This excitatory input is transmitted to the muscle fiber (MF) by release of acetylcholine (ACh). When ACh binds to the receptors on the postsynaptic muscle membrane, it depolarizes the membrane locally to produce an end-plate potential. When the end-plate potential exceeds a threshold, the MF membrane is excited and, in turn, generates its own AP. The MF AP propagates from the end plate to the tendons and excites the mechanical apparatus within the MF. Thus, the excitation of a motor neuron results in MF contraction to generate force and also its electrical activity. Each motor neuron activates a collection of MFs that is termed a *motor unit* (MU).

Interspersed among the MFs are specialized spindle MFs that monitor the mechanical output. This is relayed back to the motor neurons to complete a feedback loop. Feedback is also received from sensory neurons and their peripheral afferents that monitor the sensory inputs to the body (e.g., touch, displacement, pain). Each afferent providing feedback may further excite the neuron (positive feedback) or inhibit it (negative feedback). This balance of excitatory and inhibitory inputs controls motor neuron behavior. In a stable system, overall feedback is negative.

Disease processes that affect one or more components of the previously mentioned feedback system ultimately affect the normal neuromuscular function. One may assess function by measuring the physical outputs from the neuromuscular sys-

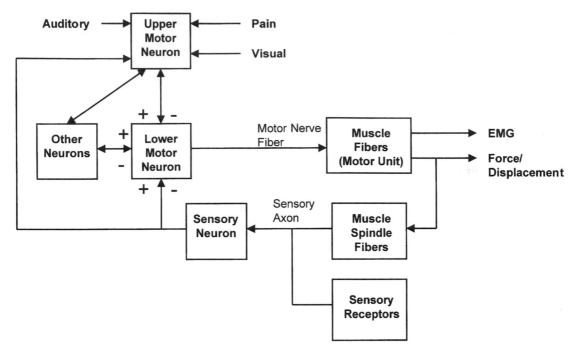

Figure 12.1 The organization of the neuromuscular control is shown as a block diagram. From an engineering viewpoint, the closed-loop feedback system makes the system stable and easy to manipulate. The excitatory and inhibitory inputs are indicated by + and –, respectively. (EMG = electromyogram.)

tem. Force is measured routinely by manual muscle testing or quantitative muscle testing using strain gauges or similar devices. Displacement is assessed via the range of motion. These measurements reflect the overall function of a single muscle or muscle group. Both measure the output of the system. The electrical activity generated with the muscle contraction within this system—namely, the portions involving depolarization of the MFs—is the electromyogram. The electromyogram is very easy to record and offers the ability to study detailed aspects of the neuromuscular system. It also allows us to study the individual components of the feedback system described in Figure 12.1. Therefore, it is an important tool in the diagnosis of neuromuscular diseases.

The routine needle electromyography (EMG) examination is performed with a concentric needle (CN) or a monopolar needle (MN) electrode. The details of their construction are shown in Figure 12.2. The CN contains a 150-μm diameter wire inserted into a hollow metal cylinder called the *cannula*. The tip of the assembly is ground to expose an elliptical recording surface called the *core*. The core is the active recording surface and the cannula serves as the reference. An MN electrode is made from an insulated metal wire. The tip of the wire is ground to expose a cone-shaped recording tip that serves as the active recording surface. A remote surface electrode is used for reference.

The signals are assessed from a free-running display of signals on an oscilloscope-type screen. The operator relies heavily on the subjective assessment of the signal waveforms and their sound. The details of assessment are described in Chapter 11. This approach is quite adequate when the abnormalities are obvious.

Figure 12.2 Microphotograph of the monopolar needle (MN) and concentric needle (CN) tips shows the details of needle construction. (Courtesy of Oxford Instruments.)

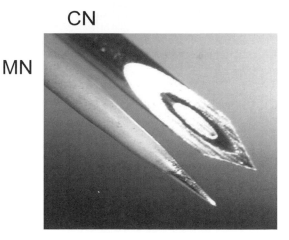

When findings are equivocal, or when conflicting abnormalities (e.g., neuromyopathy) are seen, it can be difficult to assess the underlying pathophysiology. Subjective assessment also makes it difficult to assess dynamic changes in the MUs as the disease progresses. It is in these situations that quantitative analysis (QA) is extremely useful.

Although many consider QA quite distinct from routine EMG, we believe that there is only a thin line that separates them. All rules that guide the routine EMG examination have been derived from quantitative studies, some performed more than half a century ago. QA is the predecessor of routine EMG and hence is essential for interpretation of EMG findings. This is especially true when the EMG findings do not fit the mold of neuropathic or myopathic findings. Such categorization is discouraged by specialists in clinical neurophysiology and also by histopathologists.[1–3] QA can also be useful when there is less concordance between muscle biopsy and routine EMG studies. For example, in a study by Bertorini et al.,[4] the biopsy showed significant MF predominance that could support reinnervation that was not seen by EMG. The predominance was found histochemically to be from a normal distribution of fiber subtypes. The quantitative analysis of fiber density[5] measurements showed normal values.

The knowledge of QA gives us a better appreciation of the relationship between MU pathophysiology and EMG measurements. It can be used to extract more information about the disease processes (e.g., active vs. inactive, acute vs. chronic). It may also allow us to make some comments on prognosis. The methods of QA can be incorporated within the routine EMG examination to better document the MU abnormalities. We call this approach the *objective-interactive EMG.*[6,7]

This chapter is divided into four main sections: (1) The principles and methods of QA are reviewed. The techniques are restricted to those of motor unit action potential (MUAP) and interference pattern (IP) analysis of CN or MN EMG signals. (2) The QA findings in patients with neuromuscular diseases are summarized. (3) The relationship between the EMG measurements and the MU is illustrated from computer simulation studies. Finally, (4) the concepts are applied to explain the typical and atypical findings for patients with neuromuscular diseases. Due to the close relationship between QA and routine EMG in our interpretations, some concepts are also replicated in Chapter 11.

WHAT IS QUANTITATIVE ANALYSIS?

The principles of QA are quite simple and involve three basic steps. First, the EMG signal is recorded using a standard protocol. This implies standardized settings of the instrument (e.g., recording devices). Second, the signal is quantified by a variety of measurements. These may be made manually or by using computer-aided, automated systems. Measurement criteria must be well defined. Recordings are performed from different sites in the tested muscle to obtain a statistically valid sample for analysis. In EMG, a sample of 20 recordings is usually considered adequate. Third, measurements of the various features (e.g., amplitude, area, duration) are compared against appropriate reference values to identify abnormality.

QA does not imply computerized EMG. Indeed, many analysis techniques can be used without automated analysis methods. Similarly, some EMG measurements are yet to be automated and require the operator to make all measurements. QA is only as good as the quality of signals that are processed. Automated methods work on the GIGO principle (*garbage in, garbage out*). There is no substitute for good quality EMG recordings.

Reference Values

Perhaps the most critical part of QA is the comparison of EMG measurements in the patient against the reference values. We deliberately use the term *reference* instead of *normal* to describe the criteria for assessment. Subjects used in the development of reference values are considered normal based on their own description. It is not unusual, however, to find subclinical abnormalities in some normal or healthy subjects. The decision to include or exclude them is often subjective. Secondly, the reference range is often defined as ±2 standard deviations from the mean. Assuming a Gaussian distribution of values (which may not be true), this range contains 95% of the tested healthy subjects. Thus, there is always a slight chance that a normal subject may have an abnormal measurement. No matter what type of analysis technique is used, the electrodiagnostic consultant should not use published reference values without ascertaining their validity for his or her own laboratory.

Reference values depend not only on the technique of analysis but also on the needle type (CN vs. MN), age, gender, and muscle. Most reference values described in this chapter are based on the CN.

Strategies for Assessment

Two strategies have been developed to assess measurements. The first method uses mean and standard deviations of a set of measurements. The second method analyzes each measurement individually. This is illustrated using MUAP amplitude as an example (Figure 12.3). In the first, traditional method of approach, the mean value of amplitude from 20 different MUAPs is computed. This is compared against reference values derived from normal subjects. Along with the mean values, one can also compute the standard deviation (SD) of the measurements. This reflects the scatter of data points. Together, the mean and SD can be used to assess the significance of change in amplitude between serial investigations.

Figure 12.3 Strategies for assessing quantitative measurements. The amplitude distribution from 20 motor unit potentials (MUPs) is shown, and the dotted line indicates the mean value. The triangles define the upper and lower limits of the mean value. The arrows represent the upper and lower limits for "outlier" MUPs. The study in (**A**) is normal. In (**B**), the amplitude is increased. In (**C**), the study is abnormal despite normal mean values.

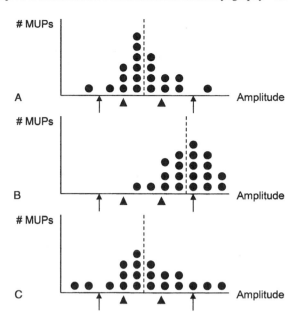

This strategy is quite different from the routine EMG examination in which one quickly recognizes potentials that are rarely seen in normal muscles (e.g., very-high-amplitude ["giant"] MUAPs). If such MUAPs are seen rarely in a tested muscle, these are ignored as a chance phenomenon. But when these MUAPs are seen on a few occasions, it convinces the electrodiagnostic consultant of abnormality. To quantitate this, Stålberg and co-workers[8] defined the upper and lower limits of amplitude for individual MUAPs. When the amplitude is outside the reference range, it is an *outlier*. A normal muscle can have no more than 10% outlier recordings. Thus, a study with 20 recordings can have two abnormal MUAPs. When three or more MUAPs with abnormality are found, the test is considered abnormal. This could occur within the first five or six recordings within a muscle. At this point, the procedure has reached diagnostic significance in the tested muscle. Hence, further evaluation in that muscle may be stopped and the next muscle studied.

The outlier-based method of analysis was first introduced in single-fiber EMG analysis.[5] Recently, it has been applied to routine needle EMG recordings. This strategy reduces the time of an EMG examination because it is not be necessary to record 20 different MUAP signals. A small MUAP sample may be adequate to define abnormalities. However, from a statistical standpoint, the small sample will also give it a high SD value. In serial investigations, it is important have low SD values to assess changes in the tested muscle. Therefore, regardless of the analysis technique (i.e., mean values or outliers), one must analyze more than 20 MUAPs to assess changes in serial QA studies.[9]

A study is considered abnormal when the mean value is outside the reference range, when more than 10% recordings are outliers, or both (see Figure 12.3B,C). Conversely, a normal study has mean values within the reference range *and* less than 10% of recordings are outliers (see Figure 12.3A). In general, an abnormal study based on mean values is also abnormal by outlier criterion, and vice versa (see Figure 12.3B). In using the outlier approach, one looks for similar patterns of abnormality in the muscles tested. If the outliers occur owing to very high and very low values in the same muscle, it is possible that the mean value will remain normal (see

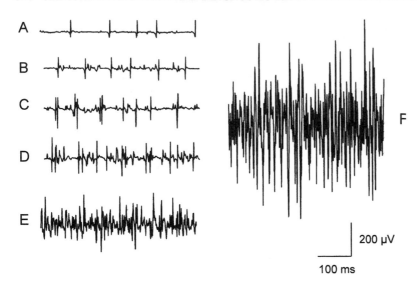

Figure 12.4 The concentric needle electromyography recording illustrates the change in electromyographic signal when the force of contraction is increased. In (**A**), discharges of a single motor unit potential are seen. Its firing rate is increased in (**B**), and recruitment of motor units is seen in (**C**) and (**D**). The signal in (**E**) and (**F**) contains discharges of several motor units to produce the interference pattern.

Figure 12.3C). This combination is often described as *mixed findings*, implying presence of myopathy and neuropathy in the tested muscle. As described later, this description may be misleading, requiring further analysis.

Generation of the Electromyography Signal

An MU consists of all MFs innervated by one motor neuron. When the neuron discharges, all MFs respond by producing an AP, which leads to the twitch of the MU. The electrical activity of the MFs registered by the CN or MN electrode is the MUAP. At minimal contraction, a single MU discharges in a relatively rhythmic pattern. The MUAP shape reflects the *MU structure* (Figure 12.4A).

When the force of contraction is increased, the firing rate of the discharging MU increases, and new MUs are recruited (see Figure 12.4B,C). This is recognized by additional MUAP waveforms in the EMG signal. The firing rates of MU in relationship to the number of recruited MUs reflects the *MU coordination*.

As the force of contraction is increased further to reach maximum effort, the individual MUAPs can no longer be seen (see Figure 12.4D,E). The IP is assessed from the number of spikes and their amplitudes (see Figure 12.4F). This signal reflects the *number of MUs* in the tested muscles and also their MUAP waveforms.

Methods of Electromyography Quantitation

The methods of QA aim to assess the *structure* and *number* of MUs, and also their activation pattern (i.e., *coordination*). These methods are briefly discussed here, and measurements to the generators of the MUAP and IP are described later.

Manual Motor Unit Action Potential Analysis

Buchthal and colleagues pioneered MUAP analysis in the 1950s.[10,11] CN EMG signals were analyzed manually from printed recordings. They characterized the MUAP wave-

Figure 12.5 Motor unit action potential waveform characterization. **A.** Simple. **B.** Polyphasic. **C.** Serrated. **D.** Unstable. **E.** Linked potential. The arrows indicate the beginning and end of the motor unit action potential. In **(E)** the horizontal line with the arrowheads indicates the motor unit action potential spike duration.

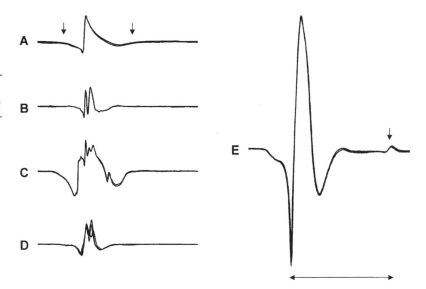

form by three defined features still in use today: amplitude, duration, and phases (Figure 12.5). MUAP amplitude is measured from maximum negative to maximum positive deflection. The beginning of MUAP occurs when the signal deviates from the baseline. When the signal returns to the baseline and remains there, it represents the end of the MUAP. These are indicated by the arrows in Figure 12.5A. The beginning and end points are assessed at a standard display setting (usually 100 μV–500 μV/division). The time interval between these points is the MUAP duration. A phase represents a deviation from, and return to, the baseline. It can be assessed quite easily: Determine the number of baseline crossings and add 1 to the value. A MUAP is defined as polyphasic when it has more than four phases (see Figure 12.5B). A simple MUAP has four or fewer phases (see Figure 12.5A). The mean value of the MUAP amplitude (all MUAPs sampled), mean value MUAP duration (using only simple [nonpolyphasic] MUAPs),[12] and percentage of polyphasic MUAPs are used for assessment.

The reference values of MUAP features for some of the muscles are described in Tables 12.1 and 12.2. MUAP duration values that deviated by more than 20% from the mean values in Table 12.1 were considered abnormal. Most normal muscles had less than 12% polyphasic MUAPs. Buchthal and co-workers have described a very extensive set of reference values.[13,14] The set is quite impressive and described extensively in the literature. Nevertheless, these reference values have some limitations that must be recognized. Although the duration values are presented for more than 20 different age groups, the overall number of subjects participating in the study was quite small for many muscles. Most likely, a linear regression–type analysis was used to predict the reference values. This may explain the similar rate of MUAP duration increase in many muscles. Furthermore, MUAP duration values are often identical for different muscles in all age groups.

Manual MUAP analysis works best when the recording contains discharges of a single MUAP at low activation (Figure 12.6A). This requires greater patient cooperation. Weak cooperative patients with myopathy may not be able to maintain sufficient slight and steady contraction. When several MUAPs discharge, it becomes too time consuming to identify the individual discharges (see Figure

Table 12.1 Mean Motor Unit Action Potential Duration in Different Muscles

Age (yrs)	Vocalis	Frontalis	Abductor Pollicis Brevis	Abductor Digiti Minimi	First Dorsal Interosseus	Biceps	Triceps	Soleus	Gastrocnemius	Extensor Digitorum Brevis	Tibialis Anterior	Vastus Lateralis
0	2.1	4.1	6.2	6.2	7.7	7.7	9.0	7.7	7.2	7.2	9.5	9.7
3	2.3	4.4	6.8	6.8	8.2	8.2	9.6	8.2	7.7	7.7	10.1	10.3
5	2.5	4.5	7.3	7.3	8.5	8.5	9.9	8.5	8.0	8.0	10.5	10.7
8	2.8	4.7	7.9	7.9	8.9	8.9	10.3	8.9	8.4	8.4	11.0	11.2
10	3.0	4.8	8.3	8.3	9.1	9.1	10.6	9.1	8.6	8.6	11.2	11.5
13	3.2	5.0	8.7	8.7	9.4	9.4	11.0	9.4	8.8	8.8	11.6	11.8
15	3.3	5.1	9.0	9.0	9.5	9.6	11.2	9.6	8.9	8.9	11.7	12.1
18	3.4	5.2	9.2	9.2	9.3	9.8	11.4	9.8	9.2	9.2	12.1	12.3
20	3.4	5.3	9.2	9.2	10.0	10.0	11.6	10.0	9.4	9.4	12.3	12.6
25	3.4	2.8	9.2	9.2	10.3	10.3	11.9	10.3	9.7	9.7	12.7	13.0
30	3.4	2.8	9.3	9.3	10.6	10.6	12.0	10.6	10.0	10.0	13.1	13.4
35	3.4	2.8	9.3	9.3	10.9	10.9	12.1	10.9	10.2	10.2	13.4	13.7
40	3.4	2.8	9.3	9.3	11.1	11.1	12.2	11.1	10.4	10.4	13.6	14.0
45	3.5	2.9	9.4	9.4	11.2	11.2	12.3	11.2	10.5	10.5	13.8	14.1
50	3.5	2.9	9.4	9.4	11.4	11.4	12.4	11.4	10.7	10.7	14.0	14.4
55	3.5	5.6	9.4	9.4	11.6	11.6	12.5	11.6	10.9	10.9	14.3	14.6
60	3.5	5.7	9.5	9.5	11.9	11.9	12.6	11.9	11.2	11.2	14.7	15.0
65	3.5	5.7	9.5	9.5	12.2	12.2	12.7	12.2	11.5	11.5	15.0	15.4
70	3.5	5.8	9.5	9.5	12.4	12.4	12.8	12.4	11.7	11.7	15.3	15.3
75	3.5	5.8	9.5	9.5	12.6	12.6	12.8	12.6	11.8	11.8	15.5	15.5
80	3.5	5.9	9.5	9.5	12.8	12.8	12.8	12.8	12.0	12.0	15.7	15.7
Number of subjects	32	49	13	36	36	238	23	24	15	11	30	12

Source: Adapted from F Buchthal. Electromyography in the Evaluation of Muscle Diseases. In A Fuglsang-Frederiksen (ed), Methods in Clinical Neurophysiology, Vol 2. Skovlunde, Denmark: DANTEC Elektronik, 1991.

Table 12.2 Concentric Needle Motor Unit Action Potential Amplitude (µV) in Adult Subjects

Muscle	Subjects	Mean	Standard Deviation	Range
Deltoid	8	212	147	150–304
Triceps	9	340	—	—
Biceps	57	180	—	120–390
Extensor digitorum communis	34	210	115	—
Abductor digiti minimi	23	350	—	—
Abductor pollicis brevis	11	260	—	—
Vastus medialis	10	230	—	150–360
Vastus lateralis	9	260	—	210–370
Rectus femoris	9	170	—	130–215
Gastrocnemius	10	160	95	—
Tibialis anterior	19	220	—	—
Extensor digitorum brevis	11	460	—	—

Source: Adapted from F Buchthal. Electromyography in the Evaluation of Muscle Diseases. In A Fugl-sang-Frederiksen (ed), Methods in Clinical Neurophysiology, Vol 2. Skovlunde, Denmark: DANTEC Elektronik, 1991.

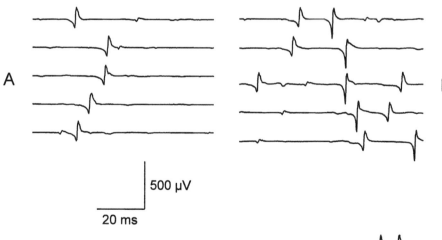

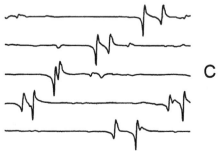

Figure 12.6 Manual motor unit action potential (MUAP) analysis. In (**A**), discharges of the first recruited MUAP are recognized quite easily. In (**B**), the second motor unit is recruited. The MUAPs of the two motor units are not superimposed. Later in the same recording (**C**), superimposition of two MUAPs produces waveforms that appear polyphasic and of long duration. However, they do not repeat.

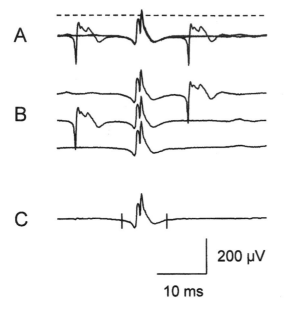

Figure 12.7 Amplitude trigger and delay line are used to time-lock discharges of one motor unit action potential on screen. In (**A**), five consecutive discharges are superimposed. The dashed horizontal bar indicates the amplitude level. In (**B**), three discharges of the triggered potential are shown in raster mode. The averaged motor unit action potential is shown in (**C**). The vertical tick marks represent the beginning and end of the motor unit action potential as defined by the computer.

12.6B). One must recognize the MUAP waveform repeating at least three times before considering it a MUAP.[15]

Chance superimposition of two or more MUAPs may result in spuriously enlarged or polyphasic waveforms with long duration (as may be seen in pathology). The trick in readily identifying the superimposed MUAPs is that they do not subsequently recur in the recording as would a bona fide MUAP; hence, they are excluded from analysis (see Figure 12.6C). This method of analysis can be performed on any basic EMG instrument so long as it has the capacity to make a printout. The disadvantage is that only three basic MUAP features may be measured and that it may require 30 or more minutes to capture 20 different MUAPs. Additional time is required to derive mean values for MUAP amplitude and duration and to calculate the percent of polyphasic waveforms.

Muscle Unit Action Potential Analysis by Amplitude Trigger, Delay Line, and Averager

Amplitude trigger, delay line, and averager are software features (hardware devices on older systems) that allow one to select a single MUAP for analysis.[16] Like manual analysis, recordings are performed at minimal voluntary effort. The user selects an amplitude "trigger" level at some point above (or below) the baseline such that only one MUAP waveform crosses it (Figure 12.7A). When this happens, the sweep is triggered. To allow complete visualization of the waveform, the trigger point is moved from the left edge of the screen, or "delayed," placing it three to four divisions to the right. This allows the whole MUAP to be displayed on the screen. With this instrumentation, the discharges of the triggering MUAP appear "time-locked" on the display (i.e., they recur at the same point on the screen on subsequent discharges). Other EMG activity appears randomly on successive sweeps (see Figure 12.7B). In a sense, this is similar to the noise and interference seen on the sensory nerve conduction studies. Averaging such time-locked discharges reduces background activity and noise. Averaging is stopped after a predefined number of sweeps, or when the baseline appears noise-free by visual inspection (see Figure 12.7C). If the baseline appears noise-free, yet the MUAP waveform over consecutively recorded discharges shows loss of amplitude or loss of complexity, then variability or instability of the MUAP should be suspected and the MUAP re-evaluated at special settings (discussed in the section Blanket Principle [or Poor Persons' Single-Fiber Electromyography]).

In routine EMG studies, the trigger can be used to assess MUAPs. It is not necessary to average them. Superimposing a few discharges can check the quality of the recording. A good quality recording shows a high level of congruence of the MUAPs as they superimpose on each other. This method was used to show most of the MUAPs in subsequent figures in this chapter. The disadvantage is that one loses the MUAP's perspective with respect to other MUAP activity.

Stewart and co-workers used this approach for MUAP analysis in the biceps brachii muscle.[17] The averaged MUAP was quantified using an automated, computer-based algorithm. The beginning and endpoint of the MUAP were manually adjusted when they differed significantly from visual assessment. In addition to the three basic MUAP features (amplitude, duration, and phases) described earlier, they also measured the area under the rectified MUAP waveform. The MUAP area to amplitude ratio was used to quantify MUAP thickness (particularly in the main spike) that is often subjectively assessed on routine EMG examination.[18] Turns in MUAP were also counted. A turn occurred at the peak of a MUAP. To exclude peaks generated by noise, the signal amplitude changed by at least 50 μV between successive turns. A MUAP was *serrated* when it contained more than five turns (see Figure 12.5C). A MUAP was called *complex* when it was polyphasic or serrated.

The mean values for MUAP amplitude, area, and area to amplitude ratio turns were used for analysis (Figure 12.8). The mean MUAP duration was computed from only the simple MUAPs (phases <5 and turns <6). It showed a slight increase with age. The upper and lower reference limits were approximately 30% above and below the mean value, respectively. This represents a wider range compared to 20% variation used by Buchthal and co-workers. These investigators found up to 20% complex MUAPs in normal biceps brachii muscle. The change in MUAP duration with age was less pronounced compared to the change seen in Table 12.1.

This technique can easily be performed on most modern EMG systems. Unlike the manual method, the signal may contain discharges of more than one MUAP. However, by inherent design of the instrumentation, one extracts only the highest amplitude MUAP from the signal. When different MUAPs of similar amplitudes are discharging concurrently in the signal, it is difficult to trigger on a single MUAP. One must manipulate the needle electrode position to maximize the amplitude of one MUAP to ensure its selection by the amplitude trigger. By maximizing amplitude, the rise time of the MUAP is reduced. Collectively, these factors bias amplitude measurements to higher values in this technique. During acquisition, the electrodiagnostic consultant must continually adjust (i.e., interact) needle position, trigger level, and other controls on the instrument. This requires practice. Generally, only one MUAP per site can be acquired; although with practice, one may adjust the patient's level of activation or manipulate the needle electrode to acquire a second, different MUAP. One can acquire and analyze 20 MUAPs in approximately 20–30 minutes.

Some modern instruments offer two amplitude levels to define the trigger point. The signal must exceed the lower amplitude level but not the higher one. This allows the user to trigger on smaller amplitude MUAPs. Although quite useful to study

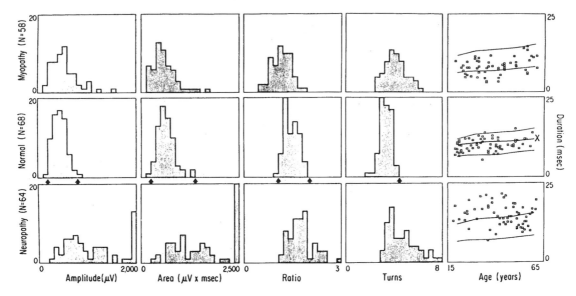

Figure 12.8 Motor unit action potential analysis in normal subjects (*middle row*) and in patients with myopathy (*top row*) and neuropathy (*bottom row*). The mean values of motor unit action potential measurements are indicated. The arrows in the middle row indicate the upper and lower limits of normal. The mean motor unit action potential duration values are plotted against the subjects' ages. The top and bottom horizontal lines represent the upper and lower normal limits, respectively. The line indicated by *x* in the middle plot shows the mean value. (Reprinted with permission from C Stewart, SD Nandedkar, JM Massey, et al. Evaluation of an automatic method of measuring features of motor unit action potentials. Muscle Nerve 1989;12:141–148.)

smaller MUAPs, the technique requires even more user manipulations. As seen in the next sections, the modern automated methods do this triggering automatically.

Multi-Motor Unit Analysis

With access to fast digital computers, signal-processing algorithms can be used to extract and analyze MUAPs in a truly automated fashion. Signals are recorded at a minimal, constant force of activation and may contain discharges of one to four different MUAPs (as may be visualized on routine or subjective EMG). The computer identifies portions that contain EMG spikes. These are called *templates*. The templates are compared with each other, and similar templates are grouped. When a group contains several templates (>10), it is considered to represent discharges from a single MUAP. The templates in the group are averaged to extract and quantify the MUAP. This technique is termed *multi-motor unit analysis* (MMA) to emphasize that it measures multiple discharges of the same, and different, MUs.[19,20] The MMA algorithms focus on extracting sufficient discharges of MUAP to extract its waveform with adequate signal quality. There is little effort to resolve superimpositions. Some discharges of a MUAP may not be identified.

MMA at one site in the vastus lateralis muscle of a patient with myopathy is shown in Figure 12.9. Each "cell" on the left contains discharges of the MUAP displayed in a "trigger-and-delay" fashion (i.e., superimposed). The averaged MUAP is overlaid in black. The vertical tick marks on the MUAP represent its beginning and end, thus denoting duration. Measurements are shown in each cell and also in the

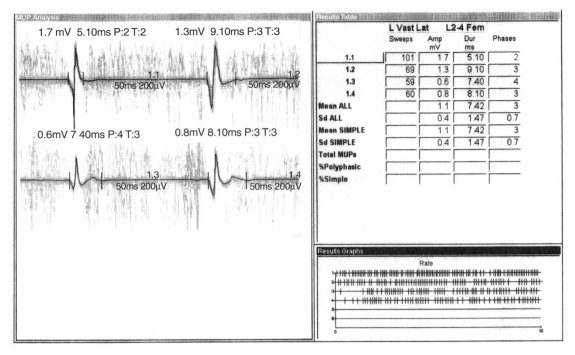

Figure 12.9 The multi-motor unit analysis technique was used to analyze electromyography recordings from the vastus lateralis muscle (L Vast Lat) of a patient with myopathy. (See text for details.) (Amp = amplitude; Dur = duration; Fem = femoral; MUP = motor unit potential; Sd = standard deviation.)

results table to the right. Mean values of measurements are shown at the end of the table. The MUAP firing pattern is indicated in the bottom right corner. The horizontal line represents a 10-second epoch. Each vertical tick mark along this line indicates a single discharge of this MUAP. Gaps in the firing pattern reflect the portions of the signal where the MUAP discharge could not be extracted or resolved due to superimposition with other discharging MUAPs. Gaps may also occur if the MUAP stops firing.

MMA requires special software that is not available on all EMG systems. If very few MUAP discharges are averaged, the baseline may be noisy. This may result in erroneous placement of markers used for duration. Measurements that appear inappropriate must be corrected manually. It is possible that the discharges of a single MUAP may be represented in two or more cells. This typically occurs when the MUAP waveform changes during the recording (e.g., electrode movement, MUAP instability) or when the MUAP is complex. In such instances, the operator must edit such MUAPs manually. Nevertheless, the method of analysis is very rapid. A 10-second epoch may be analyzed in less than 2 seconds. The software allows the operator to save all analyses for subsequent review and editing. Hence, 30 MUAPs may be quickly acquired for future editing. In anticipation of a few unacceptable signals, a residual number of at least 20 should be easily available. This reduces recording time and patient discomfort. With practice and experience, it is possible to acquire and analyze more than 20 MUAPs in 5–10 minutes!

Table 12.3 Reference Values for Mean Motor Unit Action Potential Features Based on Multi-Motor Unit Analysis*

Muscle	Amplitude (µV)			Duration (msec)			Thickness (Area/Amplitude)		
	Mean ± SD	Max	Min	Mean ± SD	Max	Min	Mean ± SD	Max	Min
Deltoid	550 ± 110	1,831	162	10.4 ± 1.3	18.4	4.2	1.56 ± 0.22	2.94	0.65
Biceps	436 ± 115	1,414	178	9.9 ± 1.4	16.4	4.2	1.46 ± 0.2	2.09	0.56
First dorsal interosseus	752 ± 247	2,301	188	9.4 ± 1.3	18.0	4.0	1.38 ± 0.22	2.61	0.49
Vastus lateralis	687 ± 239	1,954	172	11.7 ± 1.9	21.6	4.6	1.72 ± 0.23	3.11	0.6
Anterior tibialis	666 + 254	1,572	194	11.4 + 1.2	18.4	4.6	1.67 + 0.23	2.81	0.58

Max = maximum; Min = minimum; SD = standard deviation.

*Max and min refer to the upper and lower limits for individual motor unit action potential measurements used in "outlier" assessment.

Source: Adapted from C Bischoff, E Stålberg, B Falck, K Eeg-Olofsson. Reference values of motor unit action potentials obtained with multi-MUAP analysis. Muscle Nerve 1994;17:842–851.

Stålberg et al.[20] and, independently, Nandedkar et al.[19] developed the MMA technique. Their findings in normal subjects are shown in Tables 12.3 and 12.4.[21,22] The duration values in those studies showed less dependence on age between the second and sixth decade.[22,23] Stålberg and co-workers added two more features to the analysis. The spike duration is usually measured between the first and last peak of the MUAP (see Figure 12.5E). In simple MUAPs, spike duration is less than total MUAP duration. In pathology, the MUAP waveform may be divided into two or more sections that are separated by baseline. In these recordings, the MUAP onset and endpoint are determined for the section that gives the longer duration. The other

Table 12.4 Mean and Standard Deviation of the Mean Values of Motor Unit Action Potential (MUAP) Features in Normal Subjects

Muscle	Number of MUAPs	Amplitude (µV)	Area (µV × msec)	Area/ Amplitude	Duration (msec)	Firing Rate (Hz)	Turns	Polyphasic (%)
Biceps	593	370 ± 151	622 ± 307	1.8 ± 0.2	10.4 ± 1.1	10.7 ± 1.2	2.1 ± 0.2	4.7 ± 3.7
Medial cervical	387	534 ± 91	689 ± 194	1.3 ± 0.2	8.8 ± 1.2	7.9 ± 0.9	2.6 ± 0.3	7.4 ± 4.8
Medial thoracic	363	588 ± 147	812 ± 141	1.5 ± 0.3	9.7 ± 1.5	8.2 ± 1.1	2.7 ± 0.2	7.4 ± 6.2
Medial lumbar (multifidus)	369	563 ± 114	851 ± 317	1.5 ± 0.3	9.3 ± 1.4	7.4 ± 1.0	2.6 ± 0.3	6.3 ± 6.9
Lateral lumbar (longissimus)	396	462 ± 41	795 ± 76	1.8 ± 0.1	10.8 ± 1.0	7.5 ± 0.8	2.5 ± 0.2	4.6 ± 5.3

Source: Adapted from PE Barkhaus, MI Periquet, SD Nandedkar. Quantitative motor unit action potential analysis in paraspinal muscles. Muscle Nerve 1997;20:272–275.

Figure 12.10 In (A), the motor unit action potential (MUAP) is recorded from a distant motor unit. In (B), the MUAP rise time is 300 microseconds. In (C), the MUAP has a rise time of 900 microseconds owing to serration in the rising edge. The amplitude calibration is 100 μV for these three MUAPs. In (D), the amplitude calibration is 2 mV. Although the pathologic MUAP has a rise time that was 1.5 milliseconds, we accept this MUAP for analysis due to the high rate of voltage change.

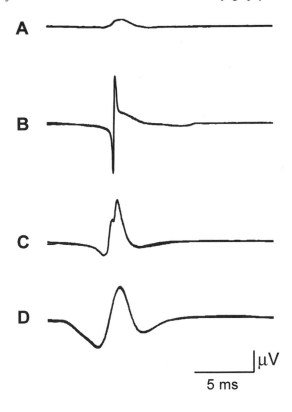

component(s) of the MUAP isolated by baseline are called *linked potentials* or *satellites*. When such potentials are recorded, one would expect the spike duration to be longer than the MUAP duration. The area to amplitude ratio depends on the MUAP amplitude. Sonoo and Stålberg[24] adjusted this dependence mathematically to yield the so-called size index.

In MMA, the needle position is adjusted to record signals that sound "sharp" and "crisp" on the audio monitor. No attempt is made to maximize the amplitude of any specific potential. Therefore, the reference limits of amplitude are smaller compared to those seen in Figure 12.8. In MMA, the EMG spikes are detected when the rate of change of voltage is high. This is similar to, but not synonymous with, rise time. The high rate of voltage change occurs when the MUAP has a short rise time (Figure 12.10B), high amplitude (see Figure 12.10D), or both. Traditionally, only a rise time of less than 500 microseconds has been used for MUAP acceptance (see Figure 12.10B). It implies that the recording electrode is close to the MFs within the MU. If the electrode is distant from the MU, the MUAP has low amplitude, long rise time, and a bi- or monophasic waveform (see Figure 12.10A). The 500-microsecond criterion may not be fulfilled when the MUAP has a complex waveform or serrations along the rising edge (see Figure 12.10C). In patients with large reinnervated MUs, the rise time may be inherently high due to summation of hundreds of APs (see Figure 12.10D). In such recordings, we do relax the criterion and accept MUAPs with rise time greater than 500 microseconds.[25] Furthermore, we do not accept MUAPs of amplitude less than 50 μV for CN recordings because they may be recorded by the cannula of the needle.

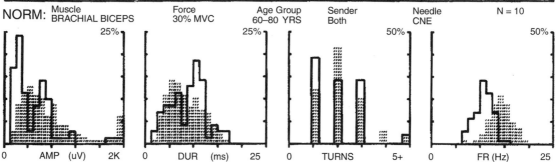

Cumulative Properties for 70 MUAPs from 10 Insertions.						
	Mean Values				Standard Deviation	
Amp (uV)	506	818 ±	305	387	564 ±	271
DUR (ms)	8.8	8.7 ±	1.1	3.5	3.7 ±	0.4
TURNS	2.0	2.3 ±	0.3	1.0	1.1 ±	0.2
FR (Hz)	10.7	14.5±	1.4	1.8	2.9 ±	0.4

NORM: Muscle BRACHIAL BICEPS — Force 30% MVC — Age Group 60–80 YRS — Sender Both — Needle CNE — N = 10

Figure 12.11 Automatic decomposition electromyography analysis in a patient with progressive lateral sclerosis shows normal motor unit action potential (MUAP) waveform measurements but a reduced firing rate. The shaded area represents the findings in healthy subjects. (AMP = amplitude; CNE = concentric needle electrode; DUR = duration; FR = frequency; MVC = maximal voluntary contraction; NORM = normal.) (Reprinted with permission from L Dorfman, J Howard, K McGill. Clinical Studies Using Automatic Decomposition Electromyography (ADEMG) in Needle and Surface EMG. In JE Desmedt [ed], Computer Aided Electromyography and Expert Systems. Clinical Neurophysiology Updates. Amsterdam: Elsevier, 1989;189–204.)

Automated Decomposition of Electromyography

As the name implies, the automated decomposition of EMG method aims to completely decompose an EMG signal into its constituent MUAP discharges.[26] The strategy is quite similar to MMA, except the algorithm makes a more aggressive effort to resolve superimposition. It can extract MUAPs from EMG signals recorded at moderate effort. Mean values of amplitude, duration, and turns are used for MUAP analysis. In addition, MUAP firing rate is also measured. The rate is calculated as the mean number of MUAP discharges per second. The findings are displayed as histograms. The distribution seen in reference subjects is indicated in the background of the plot (Figure 12.11).

This technique requires special software that is not available on all instruments. The time for analyzing one epoch used to be almost 1 minute. However, this has been considerably shortened owing to faster computers. One must always validate individual MUAP waveforms and their measurements. This is critical for small-amplitude MUAPs that cannot be recognized by visual assessment. The mean values of MUAP amplitude, duration, and rate are used for analysis. Some reference values for these features are summarized in Table 12.5.[27] The MN electrode gives slightly higher amplitude and greater incidence of complex MUAPs compared to the CN recordings. The duration values are similar for both needle types,[27,28] although some investigators have reported higher duration values for the MN electrode.[29]

In all MUAP analysis techniques, one must consider the effect of technical factors on the MUAP waveform. Some of these factors are illustrated using the MUAP recording in Figure 12.12. The individual MUAP discharges are shown in superimposed fashion in Figure 12.12E and indicate a component that is missing in some discharges. If a MUAP is unstable, the averaged waveform has lower amplitude and complexity compared to

Table 12.5 Motor Unit Action Potential Measurements at Different Force Levels

Muscle	Feature	Concentric Needle			Monopolar Needle		
		Threshold	10%	30%	Threshold	10%	30%
Biceps	Amplitude (µV)	422 ± 122	463 ± 139	638 ± 190	689 ± 192	798 ± 166	1,172 ± 331
	Duration (ms)	10.9 ± 1.0	9.4 ± 1.3	7.9 ± 0.8	10.6 ± 1.4	9.5 ± 1.4	7.4 ± 0.8
	Turns	1.7 ± 0.3	1.8 ± 0.4	2.2 ± 0.3	2.1 ± 0.3	2.4 ± 0.3	2.6 ± 0.3
	Rate (Hz)	10.6 ± 0.9	12.3 ± 1.2	16.0 ± 1.2	10.7 ± 0.9	12.1 ± 1.4	16.3 ± 1.4
Anterior tibialis	Amplitude (µV)	573 ± 111	586 ± 178	693 ± 211	1,040 ± 344	1,116 ± 340	1,228 ± 337
	Duration (ms)	12.6 ± 1.3	10.8 ± 1.1	9.2 ± 0.7	12.8 ± 1.9	11.2 ± 1.7	9.6 ± 1.6
	Turns	2.3 ± 0.3	2.5 ± 0.4	2.7 ± 0.6	3.3 ± 0.5	3.6 ± 0.2	3.8 ± 0.1
	Rate (Hz)	8.4 ± 0.8	9.9 ± 0.9	12.2 ± 1.3	8.5 ± 0.6	9.7 ± 0.7	11.9 ± 0.1

Source: Adapted from JE Howard, KC McGill, LJ Dorfman. Properties of motor unit action potentials recorded with concentric and monopolar needle electrodes: ADEMG analysis. Muscle Nerve 1988;11:1051–1055.

individual MUAP discharges (see Figure 12.12A). Reducing the high-frequency setting of the band pass filter (e.g., from 10 kHz to 2 kHz) reduces the MUAP amplitude and increases its rise time (see Figure 12.12B). Increasing the low-frequency setting (e.g., from 20 Hz to 100 Hz) reduces the duration also (see Figure 12.12C). Therefore, one must use standardized filter settings in MUAP recordings. The MUAP duration assessed at low gain (500 µV/division) (see Figure 12.12D) instead of at 200 µV/division (see Figure 12.12A) has low numeric values. The computers are not biased by display gain and, hence, automated methods are more reproducible. However, if the duration markings must be corrected, one should use a standardized display gain.

Blanket Principle (or Poor Person's Single-Fiber Electromyography)

The single-fiber EMG electrode[5] is very sensitive in assessing the efficacy of neuromuscular transmission and distribution of MFs within the MU. The technique is

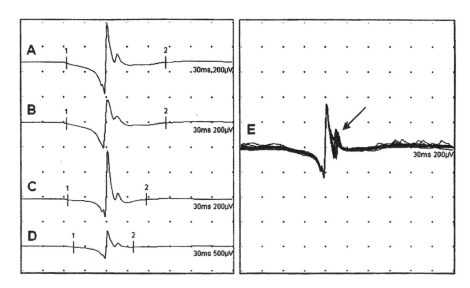

Figure 12.12 A–E. Technical factors affecting the motor unit action potential are shown. The markers 1 and 2 represent the beginning and end of motor unit action potential by visual assessment. The arrow in (**E**) indicates a component that is blocked in some discharges. See text for details.

called *selective* because the electrode can record from just one or two MFs of the MU. The high selectivity is realized by using a very small recording surface and by increasing the low-frequency setting of the band pass filter to 500 Hz (compared to 10–20 Hz in routine EMG). In contrast, a macro EMG electrode[30] is nonselective and records from the entire MU. The CN and MN electrodes have intermediate selectivity, and they record from a moderate portion of the MU.[31] When these techniques are used together, they provide complementary information about the MU.[32] Although quite fascinating, this is not always practical. It would be useful if the selectivity of the electrode could be modulated. This is analogous to converting a standard camera lens (CN or MN needle) to a zoom lens (single-fiber EMG) or a wide-angle lens (macro EMG) without actually changing lenses.

One can increase the selectivity of the CN and MN electrode by increasing the low-frequency setting of the band pass filter to 500 Hz (or even 2 kHz) as in single-fiber EMG. This change attenuates the APs of distant MFs and thus enhances the APs of the closest of MFs of the MU. Payan[33] described this simple trick using a metaphor of a statue. When covered with a blanket, one cannot appreciate the intricacies and shape of the underlying structure. When the blanket is removed (i.e., increasing low-frequency setting), the finer details of its shape can be easily appreciated.

At the increased selective setting, the MUAP is recorded using an amplitude-triggered delay line, and succeeding sweeps are superimposed. To improve visual assessment, the sweep speed is increased to 0.5–2.0 milliseconds per division. By this simple change in instrumentation and without changing electrodes, the variability and stability of the MUAP waveform is assessed with greater confidence. If the waveform remains relatively constant, it is called a *stable MUAP* (Figure 12.13A,B; see Figure 12.5A). If unstable (see Figures 12.5D and 12.13C,D), the MUAP waveform changes significantly in amplitude of the main spike (variability) or by changes in the intervals between individual spikes (interpotential interval) that approximate the jitter in single-fiber EMG.

Unstable MUAPs are rarely seen in normal subjects. A highly unstable MUAP may be difficult to trigger. The variability or instability may also be recognized by its sound on the audio monitor. Confirmation is readily made by freezing several triggered or delayed (superimposed or rastered), free-running sweeps to observe the MUAP waveform on successive discharges.

Stålberg and Sonoo[34] introduced a new parameter called *jiggle* to measure MUAP variability. MUAP discharges were recorded using an amplitude trigger delay line. A 2.5-millisecond portion about the MUAP peak was used for analysis. The median value of amplitude change in successive sweeps at each point on the MUAP was measured.

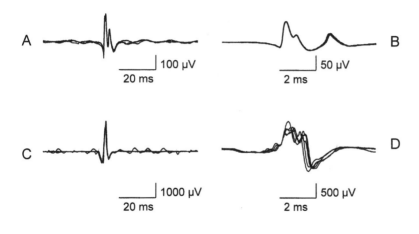

Figure 12.13 Discharges of two motor unit action potentials are shown in superimposed fashion when the low-frequency setting of the band pass filter is 20 Hz (**A,C**) and 500 Hz (**B,D**). The motor unit action potential in (**A**) and (**B**) is stable. The instability of MUAP in (**C**) is better seen in (**D**).

The area under this plot was normalized to the MUAP area. The result is called *consecutive amplitude difference*. A stable MUAP has a very small consecutive amplitude distance value.

Although this instrumentation adjustment approximates single-fiber EMG technique, the CN or MN can never substitute for a single-fiber EMG electrode in some instances, such as in making fiber density measurements. Although spikes may represent APs of single MFs, they cannot be assumed to represent them because of the inherent physical characteristics of the recording electrodes. Nevertheless, observation of the "spikiness" of the signal at these settings may suggest early or mild remodeling of an MU.

Onset and Recruitment Frequency

The MU firing rate can be measured in many different ways. A simple technique is to freeze a 500-millisecond epoch on the screen and count the MU discharges. Multiplying this by 2 gives the firing rate (Figure 12.14A). The time interval between successive discharges is called the *interdischarge interval* (IDI). The reciprocal of IDI is the *firing rate*. If the IDI is measured in milliseconds, the firing rate is obtained by the following formula:

$$\text{Firing rate (Hz)} = \frac{1,000}{\text{IDI (milliseconds)}}$$

When EMG signals are displayed in rastered sweeps, the rate can be assessed qualitatively. In Figure 12.14B–D, the total sweep duration is 100 milliseconds. The traces are drawn from top to bottom. If the firing rate is 10 Hz, the IDI is 100 milliseconds—the duration of one sweep. Therefore, the MUAP discharges appear roughly at the same location on the sweep (see Figure 12.14C). If the MUAP appears to shift right, the firing rate is less than 10 Hz. Occasionally, it may not be seen on a single sweep at all (see Figure 12.14B). If the firing rate is greater than 10

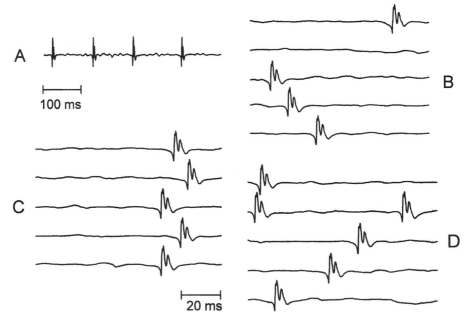

Figure 12.14 A–D. Assessment of firing rate. See text for details.

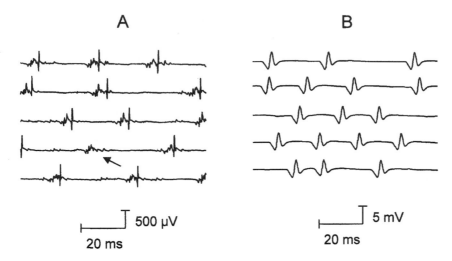

A   B

500 µV   5 mV

20 ms   20 ms

Figure 12.15 Reduced recruitment. Single fast-firing motor units are recorded in severely weak muscle of a patient with myopathy (**A**) and a patient with neuropathy (**B**). The potential in (**A**) is complex and unstable. The missing large-amplitude spike of the motor unit action potential is indicated by the arrow. Very-low-amplitude motor unit action potentials from other motor units can be seen if the display gain is increased. In (**B**), the motor unit action potential has a very high amplitude and is considered "giant." It appears small due to the display setting of 5 mV/division.

Hz, the MUAP appears to shift left on successive sweeps. On some sweeps, the MUAP may recur twice (see Figure 12.14D). If a MUAP recurs two or more times on *each* sweep, the firing rate is greater than 20 Hz (Figure 12.15).

The onset frequency is the MU's firing rate when it is first activated. This is usually measured when MU discharges are sustained through graded activation and not from their occasional and sporadic firings (Figure 12.16A). As force is increased, an MU increases its firing rate. Its firing rate just before recruitment of a new MU is called the *recruitment frequency* (see Figure 12.16B). This is computed from the IDI of the first MU just before the second MUAP is seen. The onset and recruitment interval measurements in different normal muscles are summarized in Table 12.6.[35]

Firing rate assessment can be performed on most electromyographs as shown in Figure 12.16. The difficult part of this analysis is the patient's ability to recruit individual MUs in a very controlled manner. This requires a high level of patient cooperation compared to basic MUAP measurement. In myopathic disorders, the fine recruitment of MUs may not be possible even when the patient makes every effort to perform the necessary activation (Figure 12.17). There is no automated program for detecting the recruitment; therefore, it must be performed manually. This can be time consuming.

Recruitment Ratio

The recruitment ratio method is useful when the patient cannot activate a single MU to assess its firing rate or the recruitment frequency. Rather, the EMG is recorded so that it contains discharges of three or more different MUs. The number of discharging MUs is divided into the firing rate of the fastest MU to obtain the recruitment ratio.[36] In Figure 12.17A, three MUs are recognized, and the fastest one is discharging at approximately 10 Hz. This gives a recruitment ratio of 3.3. In normal muscles, the ratio is less than 5 and corresponds to three MUs firing at less than 15 Hz. Two MUs discharging at more than 15 Hz indicate reduced recruitment as seen in neuropathy.

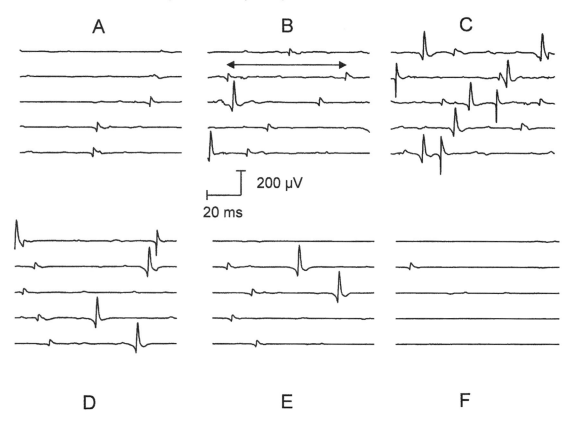

Figure 12.16 Electromyographic recordings in the biceps muscle of a subject demonstrates orderly recruitment and release of motor units (MUs) when the force of contraction was gradually increased and then decreased. **A.** The first MU is activated, and the onset frequency is approximately 10 Hz. **B.** The second MU is recruited and recruitment frequency is measured (approximately 12 Hz). The recruitment interval is shown on the second trace (*line with arrowheads*). **C.** The third MU is recruited. **D.** The third MU stops discharging as the patient relaxes. **E.** The second recruited MU is released. **F.** The first recruited MU stops discharging as the muscle is completely relaxed.

This method is conceptually simple but requires detection of individual MUAPs and their firing rates. When several MUs are discharging (e.g., myopathy), this can be tedious to perform manually (see Figure 12.17B). The MMA methods of MUAP assessment can simplify the calculations by automatically identifying MUAPs and their discharge frequencies. In Figure 12.9, the four MUAPs are firing at less than 9 Hz. This corresponds to a recruitment ratio of 2.25.

To demonstrate normal recruitment, the EMG signal must contain discharges of at least three MUs. For example, if one measured the ratio just when the second MU is recruited at 12 Hz, the numeric value of ratio would be 6 and considered abnormal. Two MUs discharging at more than 15 Hz is considered evidence of reduced recruitment.

Antigravity Test

MU recruitment and firing rate depend on the force of contraction. In the antigravity test, the *force* is simply defined as that which is required to overcome gravity.[37] For example, the biceps brachii muscle is tested with the forearm flexed and maintained at a 45-degree angle from the surface of the examination table. The EMG signal is analyzed manually to identify MUs and to measure their firing rates. To simplify the

Table 12.6 Recruitment and Onset Interval*

Muscle	Onset Interval	Recruitment Interval	Number of Motor Units
Frontalis	102 ± 29	46 ± 15	72
Orbicularis oris	70 ± 19	34 ± 10	58
All facial muscles	86 ± 29	40 ± 16	130
Deltoid	116 ± 23	84 ± 16	53
Biceps	124 ± 21	86 ± 14	56
Triceps	132 ± 36	84 ± 17	49
Brachioradialis	116 ± 22	78 ± 18	36
Pronator teres	132 ± 38	88 ± 19	35
First dorsal interosseus	142 ± 39	98 ± 21	51
Multifidus	152 ± 33	102 ± 20	39
Vastus lateralis	126 ± 30	88 ± 18	80
Gluteus maximus	128 ± 30	88 ± 16	48
Tibialis anterior	124 ± 26	90 ± 13	85
Biceps femoris	132 ± 29	92 ± 16	64
Medial gastrocnemius	156 ± 29	110 ± 23	54
Extensor digitorum brevis	138 ± 29	98 ± 13	43
Normal muscles	132 ± 32	90 ± 19	693
Neuropathy	48 + 17	36 + 12	
Myopathy	65 + 11	45 + 8	
Amyotrophic lateral sclerosis	64 + 30	42 + 22	

*The data from normal subjects are indicated at the top. The results from different subject groups are indicated in the bottom four rows.

Source: Adapted from JH Petajan, BA Phillips. Frequency control of motor unit action potentials. Electroencephalogr Clin Neurophysiol 1969;27:66–72.

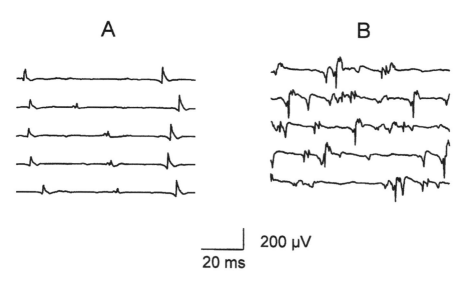

Figure 12.17 Recruitment ratio (see text). In (**A**), the recording from a normal biceps muscle contains discharges of three motor unit action potentials firing at approximately 10 Hz, giving a recruitment ratio of 3.3. The low-amplitude motor unit action potential could be missed on visual assessment. In (**B**), the recording from a patient with myopathy shows discharges of many motor unit action potentials, even at minimal effort. It is difficult to measure the recruitment ratio.

Table 12.7 Results of the Antigravity Test of Recruitment

Subject Group	Number of Motor Units	Number of Spikes/Sec
Control	4.2 ± 1.6	40 ± 20
Neuropathy	3.2 ± 1.7	29 ± 20
Dystrophy	8.3 ± 2.4	122 ± 42
Polymyositis	6.8 ± 2.6	76 ± 29

Source: Adapted from J Petajan. Antigravity posture for analysis of motor unit recruitment: the 45 degree test. Muscle Nerve 1990;13:355–359.

procedure, the number of spikes with amplitudes more than 100 μV was measured. The findings in normal subjects and patients are described in Table 12.7.

The analysis was initially performed manually and was time consuming. With access to techniques such as MMA, it should be easier to identify MUAPs and to make the above measurements. The technique of turns and amplitude (TA) (described later in the section Turns and Amplitude) can count the number of spikes with more than a 100-μV amplitude.

Firing Rate Variability

The firing rate of an MU is never constant. It fluctuates slightly even when the patient appears to maintain a steady contraction. The variability can be quantified by the standard deviation of instantaneous firing rate or by the IDI values.[38] This represents a long-term change in firing rate. The short-term changes can be studied by correlating successive IDIs. In healthy subjects, a negative correlation is found that corresponds to a long IDI after a short IDI and vice versa.[39] This is easily recognized when one records extra discharges of MUAPs. The methods for quantifying IDI variability are not commercially available.

Interference Pattern at Maximal Effort

Buchthal and Kamieniecka[11] described a very simple semiquantitative method to assess the IP signals recorded at maximal effort. They described the signal by its fullness, which reflects the density of spikes in the signal. A full pattern contains many MUAP spikes that obscure the baseline (Figure 12.18A,B). In a reduced pattern, the number of spikes is reduced, and the signal baseline may be seen (see Figure 12.18C, bottom trace). In a discrete pattern, individual MUAP discharges can be recognized. The amplitude was quantified from the "envelope" of the spikes. The envelope was defined by connecting the positive peaks and negative peaks and measuring the amplitude difference between them. Solitary spikes were excluded from this measurement (see Figure 12.18B). Criteria for abnormality are as follows:

- A full pattern in a weak or wasted muscle, or both, with reduced amplitude (<2 mV for adults) is consistent with myopathy (see Figure 12.18A).
- A discrete pattern with increased amplitude indicates neuropathy (see Figure 12.18C).

These criteria can be applied quite easily within the routine needle EMG examination. Amplitude measurement remains somewhat subjective. The fullness should be assessed at standardized sweep duration settings. Using a very slow sweep (e.g., 50 milliseconds/ division) compresses the signal and may create a spurious appearance of fullness.

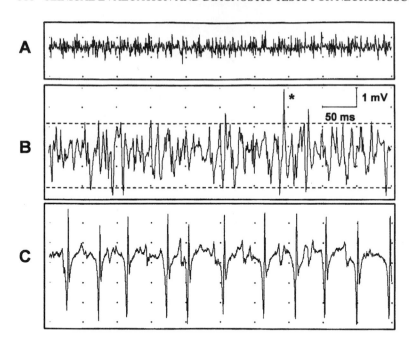

Figure 12.18 The interference pattern signal at maximal effort in biceps muscle of a patient with myopathy (**A**), a healthy subject (**B**), and a patient with neuropathy (**C**). In (**B**), the solitary spike is indicated by the asterisk, and the dashed horizontal lines define the envelope.

Power Spectrum Analysis

The change in EMG signal waveform can also be heard on an audio monitor. This led Walton to quantify the EMG signal using an audio spectrometer.[40] The concept in this analysis is quite simple. Any signal (Figure 12.19A) can be represented as the sum of harmonically related sinusoids. This calculation is performed using the so-called Fourier Transform.[41] In Figure 12.19B, the fundamental frequency is 10 Hz. The higher frequencies are integer multiples of the fundamental (i.e., harmonics). The power spectrum is

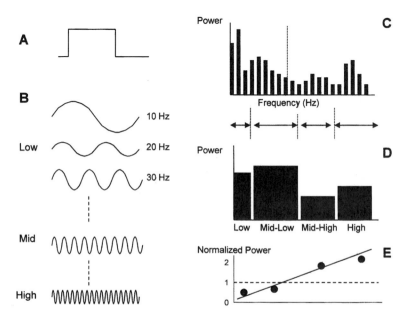

Figure 12.19 Power spectrum analysis. **A.** A rectangular pulse is used as a signal. **B.** The pulse is represented as a sum of sinusoids. **C.** The power spectrum is constructed and looks like the display of a graphic equalizer on a high-fidelity audio amplifier. The dotted line indicates median frequency. **D.** The lines with arrowheads define four bands. The power in each band is used for broad band analysis. **E.** Normalized power (*solid circles*) shows a positive slope indicating a shift to high frequency.

Figure 12.20 Interference pattern analysis in a healthy subject. The signal at top was recorded at maximal effort. The baseline is completely obscured with electromyography spikes; hence, it is considered to be full. The power spectrum of this epoch is shown to the middle right. The quantitative analysis using turns and amplitude (*middle left*) and expert's quantitative interference pattern analysis (EQUIP) (*bottom*) show more than 90% of data points within the normal cloud. (Amp = amplitude.) (Reprinted with permission from DB Sanders, EV Stålberg, SD Nandedkar. Analysis of electromyographic interference pattern. J Clin Neurophysiol 1996;13:385–400.)

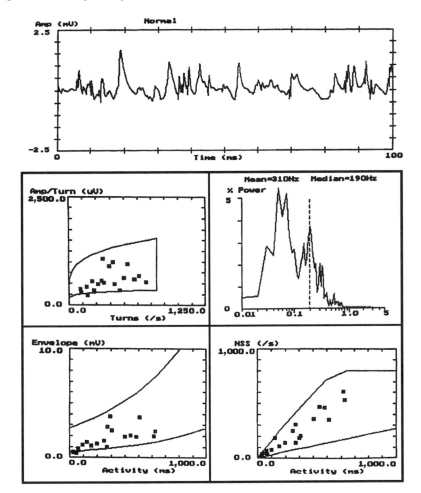

obtained by plotting the power in the sinusoids against their frequency (see Figure 12.19C). When the signal changes, the shape of the spectrum also changes.

The power spectrum is characterized by a variety of features.[42–44] The sum of powers in all frequencies is the total power. High signal amplitude gives more power. The median frequency divides the spectrum in half. Therefore, 50% of the total power is found in sinusoids below the median frequency, and the other half occurs above it. The mean frequency is computed as

$$\text{Frequency} = \frac{\text{power} \times \text{frequency}}{\text{total power}}$$

The spectrum shifts to high frequency in patients with myopathy (Figures 12.20 and 12.21). This gives higher values of mean and median frequencies and corresponds to the high-pitch sound of the signal. An opposite pattern is seen in patients with neuropathy (see Figure 12.20; Figure 12.22). There is a paucity of reference values for this analysis technique. However, it is useful to study muscle fatigue.[45,46]

Broad Band Filter Analysis

The power spectrum analysis breaks down the signal in hundreds of sinusoids. Therefore, it is difficult to compare the spectra other than by using measurements

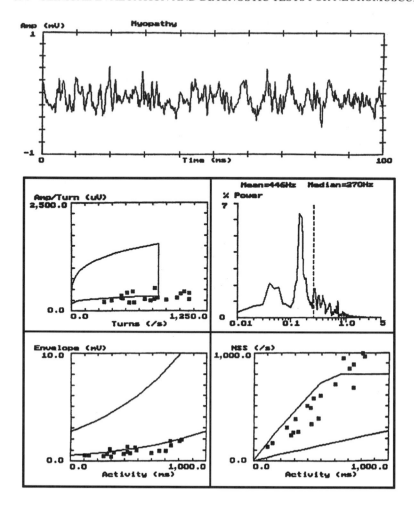

Figure 12.21 Interference pattern analysis in a patient with myopathy. The signal at top was recorded at maximal effort. The baseline is completely obscured with electromyography spikes; hence, it is considered to be full. The power spectrum of this epoch is shown to the middle right. The quantitative analysis using turns and amplitude (*middle left*) and expert's quantitative interference pattern analysis (*bottom*) show more than 10% of data points outside the normal cloud. (Amp = amplitude; NSS = number of short segments.) (Reprinted with permission from DB Sanders, EV Stålberg, SD Nandedkar. Analysis of electromyographic interference pattern. J Clin Neurophysiol 1996;13:385–400.)

such as total power, median frequency, and so forth. For a simpler description of the spectrum, Sandstedt and Henriksson[47] measured the power in four nonoverlapping frequency bands (see Figure 12.19D). The measured power values were divided by the mean values from subjects. If the tested muscle is normal, the normalized value should be 1 (see Figure 12.19E, dotted line). A shift towards high frequency gives values greater than 1 at high frequency and values less than 1 at low frequency. The line connecting these data points has a positive slope value. The greater the shift to high frequency, the higher the slope value is. An opposite pattern should result in patients with neuropathy. The slope value can be used to follow the disease progression. This technique is not commercially available. In computerized form, this technique should be quite easy to perform.

Turns and Amplitude

A signal rich in high frequencies should have many peaks. This simple concept probably led Willison[48] to define a *turn* in the EMG signal as follows (Figure 12.23A):

- A turn occurs at the peak of the signal.
- If a turn occurs on a positive going peak, its previous and next turns occur on negative going peaks and vice versa.

Figure 12.22 Interference pattern analysis in a patient with neuropathy. The signal at top was recorded at maximal effort. The number of spikes is reduced; however, the baseline is obscured. The power spectrum of this epoch is shown to the middle right. The quantitative analysis using turns and amplitude (*middle left*) and expert's quantitative interference pattern analysis (*bottom*) show more than 10% of data points outside the normal cloud. (Amp = amplitude; NSS = number of short segments.) (Reprinted with permission from DB Sanders, EV Stålberg, SD Nandedkar. Analysis of electromyographic interference pattern. J Clin Neurophysiol 1996;13:385–400.)

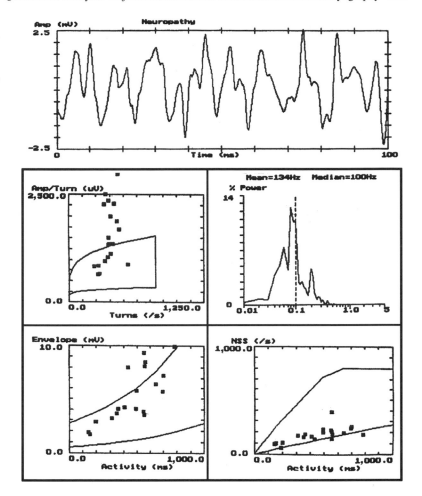

- To exclude peaks generated by noise, successive turns are separated by at least 100 µV amplitude change.

Willison and co-workers designed an analog device that could count the number of turns (NT) per second in the IP. Later, the mean amplitude (MA) change between successive turns was added to the IP parameter.

As force of contraction is increased, new MUs are recruited, and the firing rate of all MUs increases. The NT increases until the force reaches nearly 50% of maximum. With further increase in force, NT increases much less or may even decrease. MA increases at all force levels (see Figure 12.23B). Therefore, force of contraction must be standardized to analyze these parameters.[49]

Willison and co-workers used a fixed load for resistance—2 kg—for the biceps brachii.[48,50–52] Fuglsang-Frederiksen and co-workers argued that a fixed load represents a different relative force for different subjects (e.g., 50% for a weak muscle vs. 10% for a normal or strong muscle). Therefore, they standardized the force level to 30% of the subject's maximum force. In addition to the NT and MA, they analyzed the ratio of these parameters and incidence of short intervals between successive turns.[53,54]

Force measurements add another level of complexity to the EMG test procedure. Not only does the electrodiagnostic consultant require the appropriate instrumentation, but an increased level of cooperation from the patient is also essential. This is

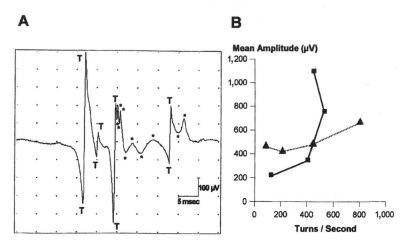

Figure 12.23 A. Turns (T) are identified from an electromyography signal epoch. The small-amplitude peaks that did not qualify as turns are indicated by asterisks. **B.** The change in number and turns and mean amplitude with increased force of contraction is shown. Data points from two different sites (*triangles* and *squares*) are connected by lines.

certainly difficult, and sometimes impossible, in children. Therefore, Smyth[55] and later Smyth and Willison[56] ignored the force of contraction in their recordings. The mean value of the NT/MA ratio was used for assessment. Gilchrist et al.[57] also used this approach for testing biceps brachii muscle in adult subjects.

Many investigators later monitored the NT/MA ratio as the force of contraction was increased.[58,59] In healthy subjects, the ratio increased and reached maximal value at moderate force. The maximum value of this parameter at the tested site was used for analysis. All of the above investigations used the mean values of the IP measurements from the different tested sites in the muscle.

Stålberg and co-workers[60] presented a different way of analyzing the NT and MA data (see Figures 12.20–12.22; Figure 12.24). In this method, now known as *turns*

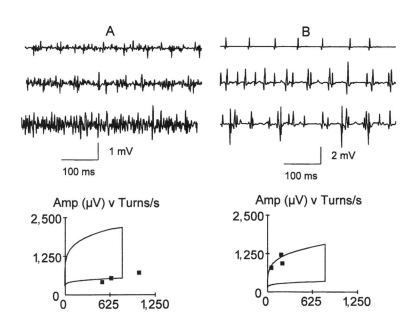

Figure 12.24 Interference pattern analysis in tibialis anterior muscle of a patient with myopathy (**A**) and biceps muscle of a patient with neuropathy (**B**). The signals recorded at minimal, moderate, and maximal effort are shown in order at the top of the figures. Note the different amplitude (Amp) calibrations. The number of turns and mean amplitude values for those signals are shown graphically at the bottom along with the normal clouds. Note the difference in recruitment between these two patients.

Figure 12.25 Normal clouds for concentric needle electromyography recordings are shown. The larger clouds are used for patients older than 60 years. (EDC = extensor digitorum communis.) (Reproduced with permission from E Stålberg, J Chu, V Bril, et al. Automatic analysis of the EMG interference pattern. Electroencephalogr Clin Neurophysiol 1983;56:672–681.)

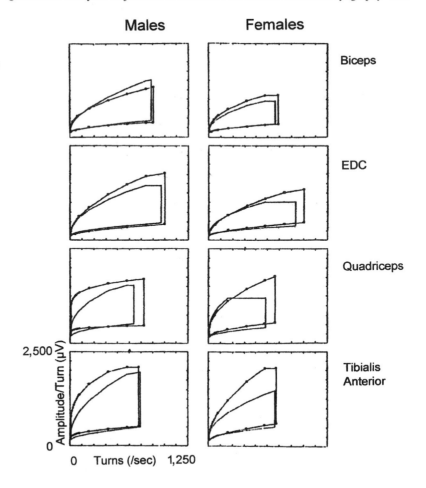

and amplitude (TA), they recorded the IP at different force levels ranging from minimum to maximum at each of the tested sites (see Figure 12.20). The MA and NT were measured from each signal and presented as a plot of MA versus NT. An area on this plot was defined that contained more than 95% of data points in every normal subject. This is called a *normal cloud*. In a typical study, IP is recorded from 6 to 10 sites to obtain 20 data points. A normal study has more than 90% of data points inside the cloud (see Figure 12.20). For a sample of 20 epochs, two points outside the cloud are acceptable for a normal muscle. But when three or more data points are outside the cloud, the muscle is considered abnormal (see Figures 12.21 and 12.22).

The clouds depend not only on the tested muscle (Figure 12.25) but also on the type of needle electrode used (CN vs. MN), gender, and age (older than or younger than 60 years). Clouds may also vary on the technique of muscle activation. Stålberg and co-workers used manual resistance in their study. Nandedkar et al.[61] had the subjects pull against a strain gauge to generate force. A much larger cloud was found by the latter, and the difference was seen mainly at maximal effort.

This technique is quite easy to perform but requires special software that is not available on every instrument. A study can be finished within minutes. Normal clouds are defined for just a few muscles but are not readily available.

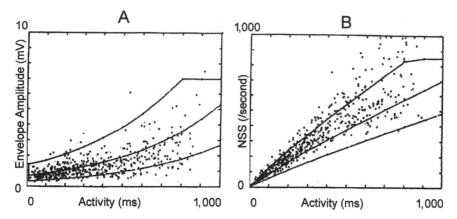

Figure 12.26 Expert quantitative interference pattern analysis in female patients with polymyositis. The measurements from several subjects are pooled and plotted. In (**A**), some data points are on the upper side of the normal cloud. This is usually seen in patients with neuropathy. Reduced amplitude values are seen when activity values are more than 400 milliseconds (i.e., at moderate and high effort) (**B**). The number of short segments (NSS) is increased at all force levels. (Reprinted with permission from PE Barkhaus, SD Nandedkar, D Sanders. Quantitative EMG in inflammatory myopathy. Muscle Nerve 1990;13:247–253.)

Expert's Quantitative Interference Pattern Analysis

The previous techniques of IP quantitation are very different from subjective IP assessment. Therefore, Nandedkar and co-workers[62] defined three new parameters of the IP. *Activity* measures the portion of a 1-second IP epoch containing the spike component of the MUAP. This reflects the fullness of the IP. When the activity values are greater than 500 milliseconds, the IP appears full by visual inspection. At very high activity values, the IP appears dense.

The signal amplitude was quantified from the envelope amplitude.[62,63] The number of short segments (NSS) measured the low-amplitude, short-duration spikes in the signal. They are not appreciated on visual inspection but can readily be heard by their high-pitched sound on the audio monitor. The signals are recorded and analyzed as described in the TA method (see Figures 12.20–12.22; Figure 12.26).[64] EQUIP (*ex*pert's *qu*antitative *i*nterference *p*attern analysis) requires special software that is not available on all electromyographs, and there is a paucity of reference values for this method.

QUANTITATIVE ANALYSIS IN NEUROMUSCULAR DISEASES

Structure of Motor Units

Over the last five decades, a variety of techniques have been used to quantify individual MUAPs. Regardless of the approach, all studies have given similar patterns of abnormality.[11,17,65–67] In our experience, the increased incidence of polyphasic MUAPs is the earliest abnormality on MUAP analysis.[17,68,69] This is seen in patients with neuropathy and myopathy. Hence, it is considered a non-specific finding.

The MUAP duration is increased in patients with neuropathy and reduced for patients with myopathy. This makes duration abnormalities a specific finding. In patients with myopathy, the reduced duration values are better reflected in simple MUAPs.[12,68] The polyphasic MUAPs may have long duration, sometimes in excess of 20–30 milliseconds, as in muscular dystrophy. Therefore, we exclude polyphasic MUAPs in our calculations of mean duration. Long duration polyphasic MUAPs in myopathy may reflect a chronic disease process; however, there is no consensus in literature.[69–71] Although duration changes are specific, they are not a sensitive feature in MUAP analysis. Mean MUAP duration is often normal in muscles that are mildly affected.[17] As a corollary, muscles with abnormal duration are moderately affected. Such muscles are more suitable for muscle biopsy than end-stage muscles. In this fashion, QA can aid histologic studies.

The MUAP amplitude is increased in patients with neuropathy. However, a mild amplitude increase (less than twice the normal upper limit) may also be seen in some patients with myopathy (see Figure 12.8). Therefore, mild increase in amplitude is a nonspecific finding on MUAP analysis. In patients with myopathy, the MUAPs with increased amplitude often have a thin appearance—that is, reduced area to amplitude ratio. In contrast, this ratio is normal or increased for patients with neuropathy. Therefore, reduced area to amplitude ratio is specific to myopathy.[18] It is particularly useful when the MUAP amplitude is mildly increased.

Unstable MUAPs are characteristic of patients with neuromuscular junction disorders. However, they are often seen in patients with neuropathy in which there is ongoing reinnervation. Unstable MUAPs may also be recorded in some patients with myopathy (e.g., inflammatory myopathy) but are uncommon (see Figure 12.15A).

Coordination of Motor Units

In patients with neuropathy, the recruitment frequency and recruitment ratio are increased (see Table 12.6). This is easier to demonstrate in muscles with extensive MU loss (see Figure 12.24B). The number of spikes and number of active MUs are also reduced in the antigravity test (see Table 12.7). At steady contraction, the MU firing rate is increased compared to normal. This is described as *reduced recruitment* and refers to the number of MUs and not their firing rates. In patients with upper motor neuron disease, the MU firing rate is reduced. Furthermore, the firing pattern is not rhythmic—that is, the IDI values vary considerably from one discharge to another. This is often described as *irregular firing*. The sequential IDIs may not have the negative correlation as seen in normal subjects.[72]

Patients with myopathy activate more MUs than expected for the force of contraction (see Figure 12.24A). This is described as *increased recruitment* and makes is quite difficult to quantify the recruitment ratio or recruitment frequency. Under steady contraction, automated decomposition of EMG reveals a slightly higher MU firing rate.[65] In moderately or severely weak muscle, one may observe few fast firing MUs, as commonly seen in patients with neuropathy (see Figure 12.15). This should not be misinterpreted as evidence of a neurogenic involvement.[69]

Number of Motor Units

When IP is recorded in a normal muscle at maximal effort, it appears full. In patients with neuropathy (see Figures 12.22 and 12.24B), the IP at maximal effort shows a reduced or discrete pattern with increased amplitude. In the TA method, the data points fall on the upper side of the normal cloud. In EQUIP, the activity values may remain less than 500 milliseconds, indicating a reduced pattern. The data points fall on the upper side of the envelope-activity cloud indicating higher signal amplitude. The data points lie on the lower side of the NSS activity cloud indicating the dull sound of the EMG signal and a shift of power spectrum to low frequency.

A reduced pattern may also result if the subject fails to give maximal effort due to pain. Therefore, one must be careful when assessing a pattern that is not full. If the muscle is normal, we expect to see normal MUAPs and recruitment at minimal force. In patients with neuropathy, the recruitment frequency is increased and the MUAP waveform may also be abnormal. A patient with upper motor neuron disease produces a reduced pattern, but the firing pattern of MUs is irregular.

In patients with myopathy (see Figures 12.21 and 12.24), the IP is full and has reduced amplitude. On TA, the data points fall on the lower side of the normal cloud. The NT to MA ratio is increased. In EQUIP, the activity values are usually more than 500 milliseconds, corresponding to a full pattern. In the envelope-activity plot, many data points are below the normal cloud. This is seen mainly at high force levels. Some data points also fall on the upper side of the cloud (see Figure 12.26). This gives the mixed appearance to recordings in some patients with myopathy. In the NSS-activity plot, the data points fall on the upper side of the cloud. This indicates a high-pitched sound of the EMG signal and a shift of its power spectrum to high frequency.

CONCEPTS OF ELECTROMYOGRAPHY MEASUREMENTS IN UNDERSTANDING THE MOTOR UNIT ARCHITECTURE

Structure of Motor Units

An MU consists of all MFs innervated by one motor neuron (Figure 12.27). The MU size reflects the number and diameter of MFs in the MU. The size of the MU, and in turn its MUAP, varies considerably among different muscles. Small muscles used in fine movements (e.g., hand, laryngeal, extraocular) contain fewer MFs in their MUs compared to larger, proximal limbs used for forceful activity. The latter may contain several hundred MFs in an MU.[73] Due to differences in the MU size, one must use appropriate reference values in QA.

The MFs in an MU are distributed randomly within a roughly circular territory.[5,74,75] In normal MUs, there is no tendency for MFs to form subgroups or clusters. The MFs of an MU may often be separated from each other by 300 μm or more. Owing to this distribution of MFs, a cross section of muscle examined under low power containing up to 100 MFs may be represented by 20–30 different MUs. Larger MUs have larger territories. This gives the same density of MFs for both large and small MUs (see Figure 12.27A,B).

The diameter of an MF may vary from 30 to 80 μm with a mean value of 50–60 μm.[76] The AP propagation velocity increases proportionately with the MF diameter. In the biceps brachii muscle, the AP propagates at approximately 2–6 m per

Figure 12.27 The motor unit (MU) architecture is illustrated schematically. The large circle represents the MU territory. Solid circles represent individual muscle fibers. The normal MU in (**A**) is altered to simulate myopathy (**C**) and neuropathy (**D**). The architecture of a large normal MU is shown in (**B**).

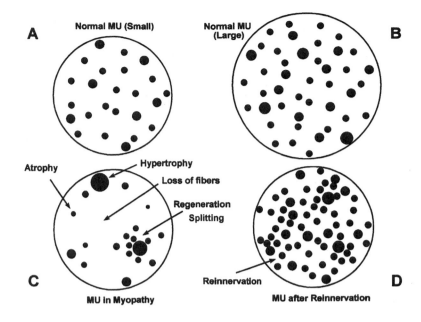

second with a mean value of 3.7 m per second.[77] The end plates of the MFs are usually located in an equatorial zone near the center of the MFs. This end-plate zone varies considerably among different muscles due to the organization of MFs within it.[78] In the biceps brachii muscle, used frequently in QA, the end plates are located within a 5- to 10-mm zone at the muscle's center where MFs may reach 10 cm in length (Figure 12.28).

When the motor neuron discharges, all MFs in the MU respond by producing an AP. These are shown schematically in Figure 12.28C. There are three important characteristics of these potentials that are essential to interpret the MUAP waveform. First, the APs are recorded from extracellular space. They usually have a

Figure 12.28 A motor unit (MU) is shown schematically in a longitudinal (**A**) and cross-sectional view (**B**). The individual action potentials recorded by the needle are shown in (**C**), and their sum is the motor unit action potential (**D**).

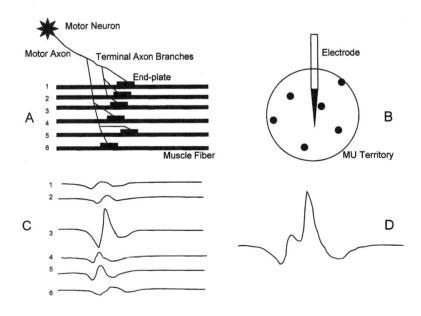

triphasic waveform that is quite different from the roughly monophasic intracellular AP. The initial positive (i.e., down-going) deflection denotes the arrival of AP from the end plate to the recording site where the electrode is located. The positive-to-negative deflection occurs as the AP passes in front of the needle electrode. As the AP moves away from the electrode, the AP produces a small positive deflection before returning to baseline.

Second, the shape of the AP varies considerably among the MFs of a given MU. As the AP passes the electrode, some MFs (e.g., fiber no. 3 in Figure 12.28) are quite close to the recording surface (i.e., <500 μm). Thus, their APs are recorded as having higher peak-amplitude with short rise time. As the radial distance to the MFs increases (i.e., 1–2 mm), the APs from these MFs are recorded from a commensurately greater distance. This is reflected in higher rise time and lower amplitude of the APs from these more distant MFs. This disparity is not present for the initial and terminal slow-positive deflections. If the electrode is 1–2 cm away from the end-plate zone, all of the end plates will be roughly equidistant from the electrode. Therefore, the initial positive deflection, although low in amplitude, is similar for all MFs. For the same reason, the terminal positive phase is likewise similar for all MFs.

Finally, the positive-to-negative spikes of the APs are not synchronous (see Figure 12.28C). This is because the APs of the single MFs pass the needle electrode's recording surface at different times. This variation in time is termed *temporal dispersion*. It is the result of many anatomic characteristics of the MU. The AP traveling down the motor neuron's axon must go through terminal axon branches of different lengths. AP propagation velocity may vary among these branches. As a result, the AP arrives at the presynaptic terminal at different times. The time for synaptic transmission varies slightly among different end plates. It also varies from one discharge to another within the same end plate. This forms the basis for single-fiber EMG jitter analysis.[5] Once the end-plate potential is generated in the MF, its distance to the electrode site varies owing to the end-plate zone size and distance to the electrode. Finally, the AP propagation velocity depends on MF diameter.

To summarize, the MUAP is the sum of all of the APs of all MFs in the MU recorded by the electrode (see Figure 12.28D). It is obvious that it is affected by the MU's architecture. This includes not only the actual size of the MFs, but also their distribution within the MU territory, MF length, end-plate zone size, etc. Neuromuscular disease processes affect the MUAP and IP measurements in a slightly different fashion depending on how they affect the structural integrity of the MU.

Based on simulations of CN electrode EMG,[79] the peak-peak amplitude of the MUAP depends mainly on those MFs within 0.5 mm of the needle electrode tip (Figure 12.29A). Only fibers in front of the core affect the MUAP amplitude. This represents a very small portion of the MU territory. Therefore, MUAP amplitude is strongly influenced by the size and distance of the MFs closest to the recording surface. Slight changes in needle electrode position significantly affect the MUAP amplitude.[18,79] This is a very common observation in the routine needle electrode examination.

The spike component of the MUAP depends on the temporal dispersion of APs of MFs within 1 mm and in front of the core of the CN (see Figure 12.29A). This usually represents 5–10 MFs of the MU.[80] The number of phases and turns and the spike duration characterize the spike component. The greater the tempo-

Figure 12.29 The uptake area of concentric (**A**) and monopolar needles (**B**) is superimposed on a motor unit cross section. Note the semicircular territory for the amplitude and spike component for the concentric needle electrode. The fibers within the enclosed area principally define the corresponding motor unit action potential feature.

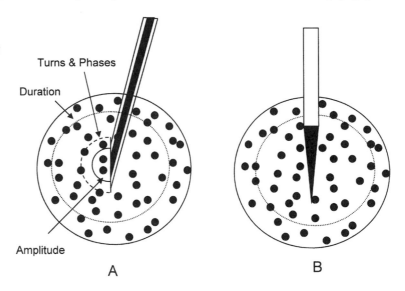

ral dispersion, the higher the numeric values of these features are. Simulations indicate that loss of MFs does not change a simple MUAP waveform to polyphasic shape.[81] This is contrary to the previous explanation of polyphasic MUAPs in myopathy. In fact, when most MFs are lost, there may be just one MF near the needle tip. This produces a simple triphasic MUAP.

MUAP duration is measured from the beginning of initial positive to the end of the terminal slow components of the waveform. As described earlier, all individual MFs have similar waveforms for the initial and terminal positive portions of their AP (see Figure 12.28C). Summating these small, but approximately equal, contributions from each of the MFs within the MU generates the initial and terminal components of the MUAP. Simulation studies indicate that MUAP duration depends on the number and size of MFs that are within 2.5 mm of the CN core. MFs that are behind the cannula (i.e., on the opposite side of the core) also contribute to the duration.[82] This circular area represents a large percentage of the MU territory, even in larger muscles. Hence, MUAP duration can be used to assess change in the number of MFs. Furthermore, those few MFs closest to the electrode's recording surface do not affect MUAP duration. Slight changes of the needle electrode's position within the MU territory do not significantly affect the duration values.[18,79] This makes it a very robust feature of the MUAP. This is also appreciated quite easily in the routine needle EMG examination.

The MN electrode has a circular uptake area (see Figure 12.29B). Therefore, it records the spike component from more MFs near the tip than does the CN electrode. This gives MN EMG higher MUAP amplitude and a greater incidence of polyphasic MUAP. For duration measurements, the CN and MN have similar uptake area. Some differences in duration can occur owing to cancellation by the signal recorded by the cannula.

The MUAP waveform is also affected by the position of the needle electrode within the MU.[83] If the needle is in the end-plate area (Figure 12.30A, position 3), the approaching volley of APs is not recorded. Hence, the MUAP does not have an initial positive deflection (see Figure 12.30B, MUAP 3); rather, it has a negative

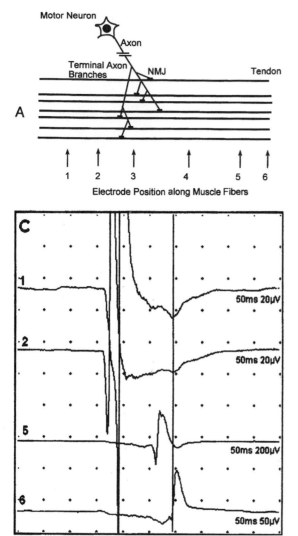

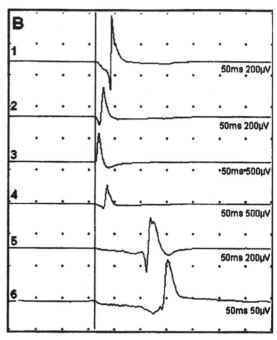

Figure 12.30 Motor unit action potentials were recorded at different positions along the longitudinal axis of the motor unit. Based on their waveforms shown in (**B**), the electrode positions in the motor unit are shown schematically in (**A**). Some motor unit action potentials in (**B**) are shown in (**C**) at a higher display gain. The vertical cursors are used to compare the onset and positive dips in the terminal phase of the motor unit action potentials. (NMJ = neuromuscular junction.)

takeoff. As the electrode is moved off the end-plate zone (see Figure 12.30A, positions 2 and 4), a small initial deflection is seen (see Figure 12.30B, MUAPs 2 and 4). The duration of this phase is longer (see Figure 12.30B, MUAPs 1, 5, and 6) when the electrode is moved further away from the end-plate zone (see Figure 12.30A, positions 1, 5, and 6).

In the terminal phase of MUAP, one may observe a low-amplitude positive going dip. This dip occurs at the same location in the MUAP, regardless of the needle position in the MU. This corresponds to the arrival of the AP at the tendon. The waveform after this dip represents the extinction of the AP. This dip is better seen on the MN EMG recordings and when the display gain is increased (see Figure 12.30C). At high gain, one can also notice that the onset of the MUAP also occurs at the same time at all recording positions of the needle electrode! In other words, the MUAP duration is constant at all recording positions. Indeed, this is the case if one uses a very high display gain to assess the MUAP duration. Furthermore, the duration value represents the time of AP propagation, duration of the AP, and time for its extinction. This measurement approaches approximately 30 milliseconds in the biceps muscle, and it is called the *physiologic duration*.[84] This measurement depends on the muscle length and AP propagation velocity. Hence, it is the same in normal muscle and also in the muscles of most patients with diseases!

In practice, the duration is assessed using a display gain of 100–500 µV per division. In this setting, a 10–20 µV amplitude threshold is applied to detect the onset, rather than the absolute beginning, of the signal from baseline.[19,85] This strategy quantifies the amplitude of initial and terminal slow components and gives duration measurements that are clinically useful.

Coordination of Motor Units

A normal muscle contains MUs of different sizes. Under normal conditions and at minimal force, the neuromuscular system initially activates the smaller, type I MUs. As force is increased, the MU firing rate is increased and new MUs are recruited (see Figure 12.16A–C). The latter recruited MUs also have a larger size. The activation of MUs based on their size is called *the size principle*.[86–88] When the patient relaxes, the MUs are released in the reversed order of recruitment—that is, the last recruited MU stops discharging first. The first activated MU is the last to stop firing just before the muscle is completely relaxed (see Figure 12.16D–F).

This dynamic process is elegantly demonstrated by a technique called *precision decomposition*.[89] A special electrode with four recording surfaces is used to simultaneously record three channels of EMG activity from the recording site. The signals are decomposed into their constituent MUAP discharges. Additional channels make it easier to identify individual MUAPs with greater confidence. It also allows one to resolve the superimposition of individual MUAPs. The method is partially automated and may require a few minutes to a few hours to analyze a 10-second epoch.

In a typical experiment, the subject gradually increases the force of contraction and then relaxes the tested muscle. A plot of individual MU firing rate and force is constructed as shown in Figure 12.31.[90] The orderly recruitment and release of MUs is seen quite easily. This pattern can also be observed using standard recording needle electrodes. This would, however, require hours of analysis that cannot be justified in the routine clinical EMG setting. By the time the force exceeds minimal effort, several MUs are discharging, and it becomes impossible to identify individual MUAPs and their firing rates. In the standard clinical EMG recording, one can assess MU firing rate only at its lower discharge rates (5–15 Hz). Precision decomposition demonstrates that these MUs may fire at much higher rates (25–40 Hz) at higher force levels in normal muscle. Most electrodiagnostic consultants do not generally appreciate this high end of the spectrum of normal MU discharge rates.

Although each MU fires at a different rate, all MUs show a concurrent change (increase or decrease) in the firing rate. This is called the *central drive* and represents the coordination in activation of the motor neurons. When a new MU is recruited, it suddenly increases the total force output. This is immediately and partially compensated by a slight decrease in the firing rate of earlier recruited MUs. This reflects the feedback loop of the neuromuscular control illustrated in Figure 12.1.

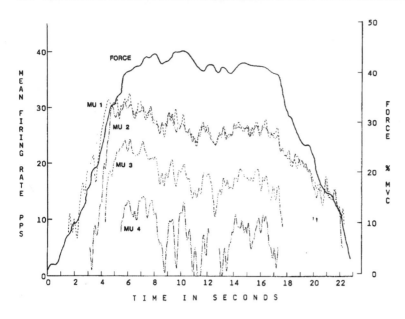

Figure 12.31 Precision decomposition. The healthy subject increased the force of contraction and then relaxed the tested muscle over the 22-second recording epoch. The variation in force and firing pattern of four motor units (MUs) is shown. Note the high motor unit firing rate, which is usually not appreciated in routine electromyography studies. (MVC = maximum voluntary contraction; PPS = pulses per second.) (Reprinted with permission from D Stashuk, CJ Deluca. Update on the Decomposition and Analysis of EMG Signals. In JE Desmedt [ed], Computer Aided Electromyography and Expert Systems. Clinical Neurophysiology Updates. Basel, Switzerland: Karger, 1989;39–53.)

The concept of recruitment is demonstrated using a simple hydraulic analogy. The tank in Figure 12.32 represents the neuromuscular system. The water level represents the level of excitation (see Figure 12.1), and each tap represents an MU. When the level reaches the first tap, we see water flowing out. The flow rate is low. This corresponds to the recruitment of the first MU and its low discharge frequency (see Figures 12.16A and 12.32A-1). When the water level is increased, the flow rate

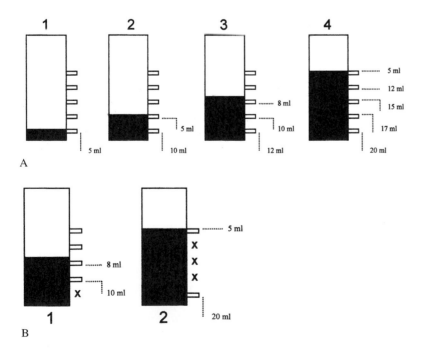

Figure 12.32 In (**B**), *X* represents the taps missing compared to (**A**) (i.e., loss of motor units). The flow rate corresponds to motor unit firing frequency.

through the first tap increases owing to higher water pressure in the tank. This corresponds to the increased MU firing rate with force. When the level reaches the second tap, water flows through it at a lower rate (see Figures 12.16B and 12.32A-2). As the level is raised again, the rate of flow through the first and second taps increases. This illustrates the recruitment of the second MU and so on (see Figures 12.16C and 12.32A-3,4). If the flow of water is stopped, the water level drops. The flow through the second tap stops and then the flow from the first tap (see Figure 12.16D–F). Note that the flow rate in all taps increases or decreases in parallel when the water level in the tank changes. This is analogous to the central drive.

Number of Motor Units

With increased force, additional MUs are recruited, and the firing rate of discharging MUs increases. The increased number of MUAPs in the signal gives higher values for NT in quantitative IP analysis.[62] As the MUAPs superimpose and summate, the resulting potential has fewer turns than the sum of turns in individual MUAPs. Therefore, at high force levels the NT may increase only slightly or may even decrease (see Figure 12.23B). This also affects the audio component of the EMG signal that is often a little duller at maximum effort compared to the signal at moderate activation.

IP amplitude increases with force. This, however, does not reflect the size principle of MU recruitment.[91] Remember that MUAP amplitude depends on the distance and size of the MFs closest to the recording electrode. If the MFs of the second recruited MU are distant compared to the first MU, then the second MUP will have a smaller amplitude compared to the first MUAP. Therefore, the inherent size of the MU is subsumed in importance to the position of that MU relative to the recording electrode. As force is increased, some recruited MUs have MFs close to the electrode and produce larger amplitude MUAPs. This makes it easy to recognize their recruitment in clinical recordings.

Computer simulations[62] indicate that high-amplitude spikes in the EMG signal are rarely generated by summation of several different MUAPs. The rise time of an MU is less than 1 millisecond. Therefore, the MUAPs must occur within a few hundred microseconds for constructive summation. If the peaks of two MUAPs are separated by even a 1-millisecond difference, the rising edge of one MUAP coincides with the falling edge of the second. In effect, concurrently discharging MUAPs tend to cancel each other rather than summate. Based on this argument, the envelope amplitude of the IP reflects the amplitude of the largest MUAPs in the signal.

PUTTING IT TOGETHER

The EMG signal can be quantified using a variety of techniques and measurements. Each measurement gives information about a specific aspect of the MU and, hence, different diagnostic sensitivity and specificity.[92–94] When all of these pieces of information are put together, we get a better understanding of the underlying pathophysiology. It also helps us to interpret the unexpected or apparently inconsistent findings (e.g., fast firing and high-amplitude MUAPs in myopathy).

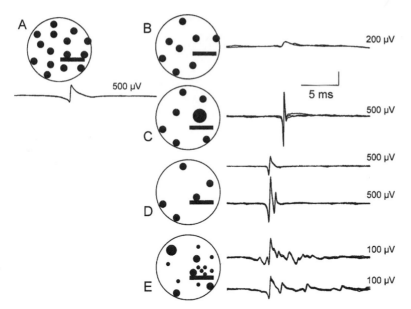

Figure 12.33 The motor unit in myopathy. Normal motor unit architecture and motor unit action potential are shown in (**A**). Motor unit architecture and corresponding motor unit action potential waveforms are shown in (**B–E**). Amplitude calibration is indicated next to each motor unit action potential.

Myopathy

In myopathy, the primary disease process is the loss of MFs and increased variability in fiber diameter. Hypertrophic MFs may split into several smaller fibers. Some MFs may be generated from satellite cells. MFs may undergo necrosis to produce denervated fibers. Such MFs may receive reinnervation. These processes give focal grouping of MFs in myopathy.[95,96] The overall MU architecture is shown in Figure 12.27C.

If the needle electrode is located in an area of MF loss, one would record a very-low-amplitude MUAP (Figure 12.33B). On many occasions, we may fail to recognize such MUAPs. If the MF is close to a hypertrophic fiber, the MUAP may have increased amplitude (see Figure 12.33C). However, it will have a thin waveform that gives reduced values of area to amplitude ratio and duration. If the needle is close to a normal MF, the MUAP will have normal amplitude but short duration (see Figure 12.33D). Sometimes the polyphasic MUAPs may also have reduced duration. If the electrode is in an area with regeneration, the MUAP has a complex waveform with long duration (see Figure 12.33E). The MUAP waveform is unstable, indicating immature end plates of regenerated MFs undergoing reinnervation (see Figure 12.15).

Due to fiber loss, an MU generates less force than a normal MU. Hence, even a mild contraction is perceived as a relatively higher force for the affected muscle. This activates more MUs than anticipated (see Figure 12.24A). Furthermore, the MU discharge rate is higher. Note that the recruitment is detected mainly by the spike component of the MUAP. This is, in turn, defined by MFs very close to the needle tip (Figure 12.34A). If an MU has lost all of its MFs near the needle tip, its MUAP is not recognized (see Figure 12.34C). In essence, the recording looks similar to that after a loss of MUs (see Figure 12.34B)—that is, fast firing MUs (see Figure 12.15). It is for this reason that we get "neurogenic" findings in severely affected muscles of

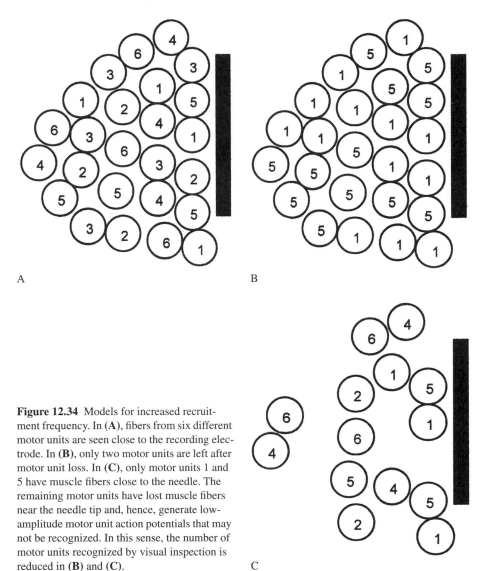

Figure 12.34 Models for increased recruitment frequency. In (**A**), fibers from six different motor units are seen close to the recording electrode. In (**B**), only two motor units are left after motor unit loss. In (**C**), only motor units 1 and 5 have muscle fibers close to the needle. The remaining motor units have lost muscle fibers near the needle tip and, hence, generate low-amplitude motor unit action potentials that may not be recognized. In this sense, the number of motor units recognized by visual inspection is reduced in (**B**) and (**C**).

patients with myopathy. It should not be misinterpreted as evidence of neurogenic involvement.

The number of MUs is relatively normal in patients with myopathy. Therefore, one obtains a full pattern even in a weak or wasted muscle (see Figures 12.18 and 12.24A). The amplitude is reduced due to many factors. Atrophic MFs generate smaller-amplitude APs. If an MU has lost MFs near the needle tip, the MUAP amplitude is low (see Figure 12.33B). Fibrotic tissue also attenuates signal amplitude. In contrast, hypertrophic MFs should give high amplitude to the signal (see Figure 12.33C). Indeed, one can see this bimodal amplitude distribution in the IP recordings (Figure 12.35A). The high-amplitude spikes are thin by visual assessment. Therefore, they are consistent with myopathy, although they appear to dis-

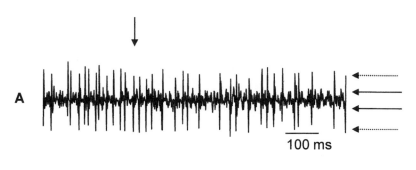

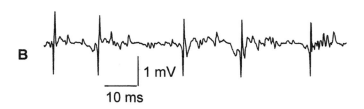

Figure 12.35 A. Interference pattern recording in severe myopathy. The signal shows bimodal distribution of amplitude spikes (*solid* and *dotted horizontal lines*). The amplitude should be measured using the solid horizontal arrows to exclude the large motor unit action potential. **B.** A portion of the signal around the vertical arrow is shown with faster sweep. The high-amplitude thin motor unit action potential is firing at approximately 50 Hz.

charge at a high rate (see Figure 12.35B). In automated analysis methods, discharges of one such MUAP may give high values of envelope amplitude as seen on the upper side of the normal cloud in Figure 12.26. Again, one must use the overall distribution of data points to assess abnormalities. Relying solely on the automated envelope amplitude measurements can be misleading.

Neuropathy: Partial Lesions

In patients with neuropathy, the primary disease process is loss of MUs. The surviving MUs generate collateral sprouts to innervate the denervated MFs from the lost MUs. This gives increased local density of MFs in the MU territory. The reinnervation occurs only in the area where the territories of the surviving and lost MUs overlap. As a result, the MF distribution may be normal in some portions of MU territory, whereas it may show MF-type grouping in other parts (Figure 12.36B). The MU size is increased mainly due to increased density of fibers, and the MU territory remains relatively constant.

Due to increased density of MFs, the MUAP amplitude is increased. If the APs of the MFs are dispersed, they generate a polyphasic potential (see Figure 12.36B). This dispersion can be increased due to slow conduction in newly formed axons, MF hypertrophy, atrophy of newly reinnervated MFs during their denervated state, and increased end-plate zone, among other causes. An increased number of MFs also gives higher values of MUAP duration. During reinnervation, the newly formed axon sprouts, and end plates are immature and may fail to propagate and transmit AP in a reliable manner.[97] This produces unstable MUAPs.

Due to loss of MUs, we expect to observe increased recruitment frequency and recruitment ratio. Review of reference values shows a rather wide range for the recruitment frequency. Referring to Figure 12.32B-2, the change in recruitment frequency is seen quite easily if MUs 2, 3, and 4 are lost. However, if MU 1 were lost, the recruitment frequency would be normal (see Figure 12.32B-1). It is our opinion that these measurements are not sensitive in detecting loss of a few MUs. Reduced

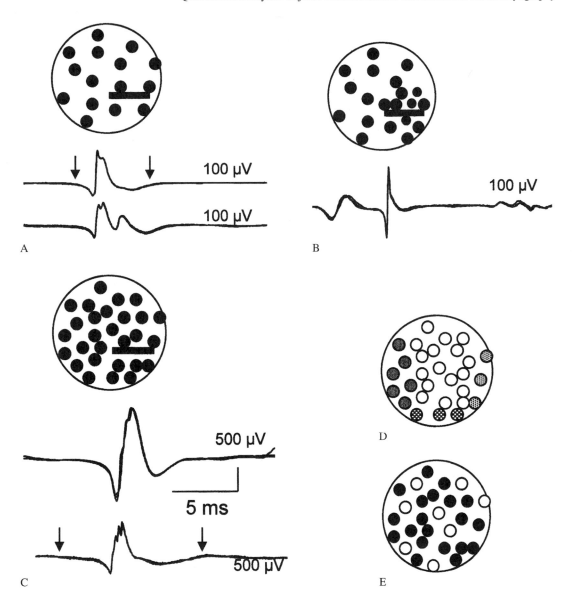

Figure 12.36 Motor unit (MU) architecture in neuropathy. In (**A**), the MU architecture and motor unit action potentials (MUAPs) are normal. The arrows indicate the beginning and end of the MUAP. Occasional polyphasic MUAPs are also found in normal muscles. In the early stages of reinnervation (**B**), the MUAPs are polyphasic. The amplitude and duration are normal. The reinnervation is patchy within the MU territory. After chronic reinnervation, as shown in (**C**), the MU size is increased. The MUAP amplitude and duration are increased. The arrows indicate the beginning and end of the MUAP. In (**D**), the large reinnervated MU in (**C**) is lost. Fibers at the periphery that are innervated by other MUs are shown by circles with a different shade pattern. Unfilled circles at the center indicate denervated fibers that are too far away to receive axonal branches and are not reinnervated. In (**E**), the large reinnervated MU has lost only some of its fibers. The lost fibers are also indicated by unfilled circles. Circles without shading represent denervated muscle fibers. This is called *fractionation*. Amplitude calibration is indicated next to each trace.

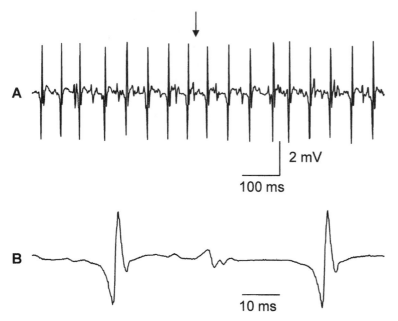

Figure 12.37 Discrete interference pattern in neuropathy is shown at slow **(A)** sweep speeds. A portion of this signal near the arrow is shown at fast sweep speed in **(B)**. At maximal effort, the interference pattern contains discharges of one large motor unit. The other potentials seen in **(B)** are from distant motor units.

recruitment is reported when two MUs are discharging at a higher rate than 15 Hz. This usually requires an extensive MU loss (see Figure 12.24B; Figure 12.37).

We expect a reduced IP due to loss of MUs; however, IP is also not a sensitive measurement. In a normal muscle, the IP is generated by more than 20 MUs that are in the immediate vicinity of the electrode. If half of them were lost, we still would have 10 surviving MUs. Assuming a spike duration of 5 milliseconds and a firing rate of 20 Hz, the discharges of the remaining MUs can completely obscure the baseline (200 MU discharges × 5 milliseconds = 1,000 milliseconds of spike component) (see Figure 12.21). As a corollary, a reduced pattern at maximal effort indicates a significant MU loss (see Figure 12.24B).

In early stages of reinnervation, the MUAP amplitude and duration are relatively normal. This gives a normal pattern on QA. The increased incidence of polyphasic MUAPs may give a high-pitched sound that is unexpected in a patient with neuropathy.

It is quite possible for reinnervation to fully compensate the denervation process. When reinnervation is complete, MUAPs are stable. Thus, stability is an important feature to assess the response of the neuromuscular system after nerve injury.[98] Unstable MUAPs are a good sign because they indicate ongoing MU reinnervation. Thus, recovery is not yet complete. Stable MUAPs indicate no ongoing reinnervation.

A patient may have no clinical weakness even when half of the MUs are lost. The MU may continue to reinnervate until it is approximately 20 times its normal size (see Figure 12.36C).[99] Such MUAPs have very high amplitude and duration. Furthermore, they can be seen quite easily as giant MUAPs discharging at a high rate in a reduced pattern (see Figures 12.15 and 12.37). The discharge rate may be 25–30 Hz, but it should not be considered as abnormal or as an increased excitation of the motor neuron. Precision decomposition shows similar rates even in normal muscles. It is, however, not possible to appreciate these rates in normal muscle due to the concurrent full IP.

Giant MUAPs are seen in slowly progressive diseases in which reinnervation can compensate for MU loss. Nevertheless, some loss of MUs will continue to occur. Hence, one may find unstable MUAPs even several years after the initial insult to the nervous system (e.g., patients with polio).[100] If a large MU dies, it leaves behind a large pool of denervated MFs. If there is no overlapping MU, the MFs at the center of the territory may not get collateral axon branches. The MFs at the periphery may receive reinnervation. In Figure 12.36D, the open circles at the center indicate denervated fibers. Filled circles are reinnervated MFs. Different patterns are used to indicate different MUs.

It is also possible that the large reinnervated MUs may not be able to maintain the large pool of MFs. Hence, several years after reinnervation, the MUs may lose some of their fibers. The loss may occur randomly within the MU territory (see Figure 12.36E); this process is called *MU fractionation*. The MUAP's amplitude and duration reduce, but they are still increased compared to normal.[101]

In rapidly progressing degenerative disease (e.g., amyotrophic lateral sclerosis), the reinnervation cannot keep up with denervation. Furthermore, the reinnervated MUs also die from the disease process. Therefore, the MUAPs may have only a moderate increase in amplitude and duration. They are markedly unstable compared to the slow progressive disease.[32]

Neuropathy: Complete Lesion

A severe trauma to the nerve may affect every axon innervating a muscle (e.g., nerve transection in an injury). As a result, none of the MUs in the muscle can be activated. The muscle is completely paralyzed. The needle EMG in the tested muscle records no voluntary activity. In fact, the presence of a single voluntarily activated MU provides hope by indicating continuity of at least one axon.

As the nerve is regenerated via axonal regrowth, new MUs are formed. However, these MUs start out with very few MFs packed within a very small territory. Their MUAPs have a low-amplitude, short-duration, polyphasic, and unstable waveform (Figure 12.38). They are sometimes called *nascent MUAPs* to denote their special origin from axonal regrowth as opposed to collateral sprouting. Except for its pronounced instability and firing rate, the MUAP resembles the waveforms seen in myopathic disorders. In addition, the reduced number of MUs at maximal effort indicates that these MUAPs do not reflect a myopathy. Further formation of MUs restores the muscle's function. As these MUs mature, they increase in size, and their MUAPs appear similar to those seen in other patients with neuropathic disorders with partial lesions.

Motor Unit Control Abnormalities

In diseases of the upper motor neuron, excitation to the lower motor neuron is reduced or lost. This makes it difficult for patients with such disorders to activate MUs. When these MUs do discharge, they fire at much lower and erratic rates. The IP at maximal effort is reduced. It does not, however, imply a structural MU loss. Because the structure of the MU is not affected, individual MUAP waveforms may be normal. The sequential IDI plot in a normal subject shows a negative correlation.

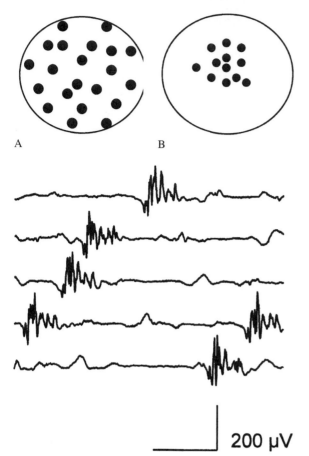

Figure 12.38 Motor unit after complete nerve lesion. **A.** Normal motor unit. **B.** After nerve growth, the motor unit architectures show groups of atrophic muscle fibers. The nascent motor unit action potential is shown in (**C**).

When the force of contraction is maintained, a long IDI is followed by a short IDI. In upper motor neuron diseases, this pattern is disrupted.

The reduced pattern of recruitment is quite different from other conditions. In normal subjects, reduced IP at submaximal effort shows a normal MUAP firing rate at minimal effort. Patients with lower motor neuron disorders show increased recruitment frequency, and the MUAPs also demonstrate abnormalities in waveform.

Many muscular activities involve control of two muscles: agonist and antagonist. When this control is disturbed, tremor may result. Several MUs may be activated almost simultaneously. As a result, one records a summation of many MUAPs (Figure 12.39). The waveforms are complex and do not repeat. This is easily recognized by the characteristic burst-like patterns ranging from approximately 5 Hz in extrapyramidal disorders to higher frequencies as seen in essential tremor (10–15 Hz). These bursts should not be confused with complex unstable MUAPs or abnormal spontaneous activity (e.g., myokymia).

Figure 12.39 Electromyography recording in tremor. In (**A**), the tremor is recognized from a 1-second sweep speed. Two bursts, indicated by arrows 1 and 2, are shown in (**B**) and (**C**), respectively. They demonstrate complex, high-amplitude, and long-duration waveforms that do not repeat.

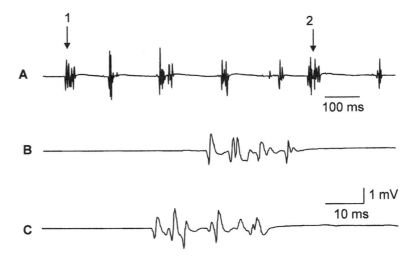

Neuromuscular Junction Diseases

Abnormalities of the neuromuscular junction affect the efficacy of AP transmission from the nerve terminal to the muscle end plate. In affected end plates, the time of AP transmission varies significantly from one discharge to another. In some discharges, the AP may fail to transmit (i.e., the APs are blocked). The shape of the MUAPs are not constant; they are variable. These are seen as unstable MUAPs. The degree of instability should be roughly proportionate to the degree of weakness.

Clues to a disorder of neuromuscular transmission are reduced amplitudes of the compound muscle action potentials (CMAPs), particularly in presynaptic disorders. If ACh receptors are being destroyed as in acquired autoimmune myasthenia gravis, the MF no longer belongs to the MU until functional neuromuscular transmission is restored by regeneration of the ACh receptors. If this destruction outpaces regeneration, then the MUs are functionally reduced in size. The resulting MUAP waveforms typically show reduced MUAP duration as may occur in myopathic disorders. Occasionally, complexity is increased. Although functionally denervated with respect to the ACh receptors, fibrillation potentials are typically not prominent. This is presumably due to maintained trophic influence on the MF by the presynaptic nerve terminal despite loss of normal Ach receptor (i.e., neuromuscular transmission) function.

Disorders of neuromuscular transmission are probably among the most elusive to diagnose, mainly because they are not suspected. A recent case we evaluated involved a patient urgently referred for treatment of what was diagnosed on three different electrodiagnostic studies as multifocal motor neuropathy. Although areflexic, the patient's weakness was proximal. The nerve conductions showed progressively reduced CMAP amplitude without evidence for dispersion. The values of the motor conductions were not remarkable. All prior studies described normal MUAPs. The latter was true if the analysis of the MUAPs were confined to amplitude, duration, and complexity. But even on free run mode, the MUAPs showed marked variability[102]; on later inspection with the 500-Hz low-frequency filter, instability and blocking were profuse. Repeat assessment of the CMAPs showed facilitation from 100% to 300%.

The message is that incomplete data were used to interpret the findings. The additional data needed to cinch the diagnosis of a presynaptic disorder (later confirmed by antibody testing to be Lambert-Eaton myasthenic syndrome) were a simple matter of more objectively analyzing the stability of the MUAPs seen on routine analysis. This was readily achieved by minimal interaction with the electromyograph (i.e., changing the low-frequency filter). To epitomize, anyone with unexplained proximal weakness and normal routine studies should be particularly scrutinized for a disorder of neuromuscular transmission.

CONCLUSIONS

QA has evolved over the last five decades, providing a foundation for our understanding of the routine needle EMG examination. QA demonstrates that there is no generic myopathic or neurogenic abnormality. Rather, each MUAP parameter in the setting of other electrophysiologic data gives specific information about the structure, number, and control of the MUs. By evaluating the changes in these individual features, one may construct a reasonably accurate picture of the underlying disease processes (e.g., the electrophysiologic biopsy). This not only facilitates diagnosis, but it also adds much more information about the disease duration, progression, and, perhaps, prognosis. Therefore, it is important to understand the principles of QA and incorporate the techniques in the routine EMG assessment. We hope that this chapter encourages the reader to be transformed from a passive observer to a more objective observer of the signal, someone who will interact with his or her instrumentation.

Acknowledgments

The first author (S.D.N.) would like to thank Oxford Instruments for its support in this project. Mr. Desh Nandedkar prepared and edited the figures in digital format. Most figures are reproduced by permission from CASA Engineering (http://www.casaengineering.com).

REFERENCES

1. Engel WK, Warmolts JR. The Motor Unit. Diseases Affecting It In Toto or In Portio. In J Desmedt (ed), New Developments in Electromyography and Clinical Neurophysiology, Vol 1. Basel, Switzerland: Karger, 1973;141–177.
2. Daube JR. The description of motor unit action potentials in electromyography. Neurology 1978;28:623–625.
3. Daube J. Needle examination in clinical electromyography. Muscle Nerve 1991;14:685–700.
4. Bertorini TE, Stålberg EV, Yuson CP, Engel WK. Single-fiber electromyography in neuromuscular disorders: correlation of muscle histochemistry, single-fiber electromyography and clinical findings. Muscle Nerve 1994;17:345–353.
5. Stålberg E, Trontelj JV. Single Fiber Electromyography in Healthy and Diseased Muscle (2nd ed). New York: Raven Press, 1994.
6. Barkhaus PE, Nandedkar SD. Electronic Atlas of EMG Waveforms. In SD Nandedkar (ed), EMG on CD, Vol 2. Hopewell Junction, NY: CASA Engineering, 1999.
7. Nandedkar S. "Objective EMG": Quantitation and Documentation in the Routine Needle Electromyographic Examination. In E Johnson (ed), Practical Electromyography (3rd ed). Baltimore: Williams & Wilkins, 1997:41–61.

8. Stålberg EV, Bischoff C, Falck B. Outliers: a way to detect abnormality in quantitative EMG. Muscle Nerve 1994;17:392–399.

9. Engstrom JW, Olney RK. Quantitative motor unit analysis: the effect of sample size. Muscle Nerve 1992;15:277–281.

10. Buchthal F, Guld C, Rosenfalck P. Action potential parameters in normal human muscles and their dependence on physical variables. Acta Physiol Scand 1954;32:200–218.

11. Buchthal F, Kamieniecka Z. The diagnostic yield of quantified electromyography and quantified muscle biopsy in neuromuscular disorders. Muscle Nerve 1982;2:265–280.

12. Buchthal F. Electrophysiological signs of myopathy as related with muscle biopsy. Acta Neurol (Napoli) 1977;32:1–29.

13. Buchthal F. Electromyography in the Evaluation of Muscle Diseases. In A Fuglsang-Frederiksen (ed), Methods in Clinical Neurophysiology, Vol 2. Skovlunde, Denmark: DANTEC Elektronik, 1991.

14. Rosenfalck P, Rosenfalck A. Electromyography and Sensory/Motor Conduction: Findings in Normal Subjects. Copenhagen: Laboratory of Clinical Neurophysiology, Rigshospitale, 1975.

15. Andreassen S. Methods for computer-aided measurement of motor unit parameters. Electroencephalogr Clin Neurophysiol Suppl 1987;39:13–20.

16. Czekajewski OJ, Ekstedt J, Stålberg E. Oscilloscopic recording of muscle fiber action potentials. The window trigger and the delay unit. Electroencephalogr Clin Neurophysiol 1969;27:536–539.

17. Stewart C, Nandedkar SD, Massey JM, et al. Evaluation of an automatic method of measuring features of motor unit action potentials. Muscle Nerve 1989;12:141–148.

18. Nandedkar S, Barkhaus P, Sanders D, Stålberg E. Analysis of the amplitude and area of the concentric needle EMG motor unit action potentials. Electroencephalogr Clin Neurophysiol 1988;69:561–567.

19. Nandedkar SD, Barkhaus PE, Charles A. Multi-motor unit action potential analysis (MMA). Muscle Nerve 1995;18:1155–1166.

20. Stålberg E, Falck B, Sonoo M, et al. Multi-MUP EMG analysis—a two year experience with quantitative method in daily routine. Electroencephalogr Clin Neurophysiol 1995;97:145–154.

21. Barkhaus PE, Periquet MI, Nandedkar SD. Quantitative motor unit action potential analysis in paraspinal muscles. Muscle Nerve 1997;20:272–275.

22. Bischoff C, Stålberg E, Falck B, Eeg-Olofsson K. Reference values of motor unit action potentials obtained with multi-MUAP analysis. Muscle Nerve 1994;17:842–851.

23. Bischoff C, Machetanz J, Conrad B. Is there age-dependent continuous increase in the duration of the motor unit potential? Electroencephalogr Clin Neurophysiol 1991;81:304–311.

24. Sonoo M, Stålberg E. The ability of MUAP parameters to discriminate between normal and neurogenic MUAPs in concentric EMG: analysis of MUAP "thickness" and the proposal of "size index." Electroencephalogr Clin Neurophysiol 1993;89:291–303.

25. Barkhaus PE, Nandedkar SD. On the selection of concentric needle electromyogram motor unit action potentials: is the rise time criterion too restrictive? Muscle Nerve 1996;19:1554–1560.

26. McGill KC, Dorfman LJ. Automatic Decomposition Electromyography (ADEMG). Methodologic and Technical Considerations. In JE Desmedt (ed), Computer-Aided Electromyography and Expert Systems. Clinical Neurophysiology Updates. Amsterdam: Elsevier, 1989;91–101.

27. Howard JE, McGill KC, Dorfman LJ. Properties of motor unit action potentials recorded with concentric and monopolar needle electrodes: ADEMG analysis. Muscle Nerve 1988;11:1051–1055.

28. Nandedkar SD, Sanders DB. Recording characteristics of monopolar EMG electrodes. Muscle Nerve 1991;14:108–112.

29. Chan RC, Hsu TC. Quantitative comparison of motor unit potential parameters between monopolar and concentric needles. Muscle Nerve 1991;14:1028–1032.

30. Stålberg E. Macro EMG, a new recording technique. J Neurol Neurosurg Psychiatry 1980;43:475–482.

31. King JC, Dumitru D, Nandedkar S. Concentric and single fiber electrode spatial recording characteristics. Muscle Nerve 1997;20:1525–1533.

32. Stålberg E, Sanders D. The Motor Unit in ALS Studies with Different Electrophysiological Techniques. In C Rose (ed), Progress in Motor Neuron Disease. London: Pitman Books, 1983.

33. Payan J. The blanket principle: a technical note. Muscle Nerve 1978;1:423–426.

34. Stålberg E, Sonoo M. Assessment of variability in the shape of the motor unit action potential, the "jiggle" at consecutive discharges. Muscle Nerve 1994;17:1135–1144.

35. Petajan JH, Phillips BA. Frequency control of motor unit action potentials. Electroencephalogr Clin Neurophysiol 1969;27:66–72.

36. Daube J. Clinical Neurophysiology. Philadelphia: FA Davis, 1996.

37. Petajan J. Antigravity posture for analysis of motor unit recruitment: the 45 degree test. Muscle Nerve 1990;13:355–359.
38. Yan K, Fang J. Motor unit behavior in stroke patients. Muscle Nerve 1998;21:1502–1506.
39. Freund H, Hefter H, Homberg V. Motor Unit Activity in Motor Disorders. In BT Shahani (ed), Electromyography in CNS Disorders: Central EMG. Boston: Butterworth Publishers, 1984.
40. Walton JN. The electromyogram in myopathy: analysis with the audio-frequency spectrometer. J Neurol Neurosurg Psychiatry 1952;15:219–226.
41. Jackson L. Digital Filters and Signal Processing. Boston: Kluwer, 1986.
42. Cenkovich FS, Gersten JW. Fourier analysis of the normal human electromyogram. Am J Phys Med 1963;42:192–204.
43. Cenkovich F, Hsu SF, Gersten JW. A quantitative electromyographic index that is independent of force of contraction. Electroencephalogr Clin Neurophysiol 1982;54:79–86.
44. Christensen H, Fuglsang-Frederiksen A. Power spectrum and turns analysis of EMG at different voluntary effort in normal subjects. Electroencephalogr Clin Neurophysiol 1984;64:528–535.
45. Lindstrom L, Magnusson R, Petersen I. Muscular fatigue and action potential conduction velocity changes studied with frequency analysis of EMG signals. Electromyography 1970;4:341–356.
46. Yarr I, Niles L. Muscle fiber conduction velocity and mean power spectrum frequency in neuromuscular disorders and fatigue. Muscle Nerve 1992;15:780–787.
47. Sandstedt P, Henriksson KG, Larsson LE. Quantitative electromyography in polymyositis and dermatomyositis. Acta Neurol Scand 1982;65:110–121.
48. Willison RG. Analysis of electrical activity in healthy and dystrophic muscle in man. J Neurol Neurosurg Psychiatry 1964;27:386–394.
49. Fuglsang-Frederiksen A, Mansson A. Analysis of electrical activity of normal muscle in man at different degrees of voluntary effort. J Neurol Neurosurg Psychiatry 1975;38:683–694.
50. Rose AL, Willison RG. Quantitative electromyography using automatic analysis: studies in healthy subjects and patients with primary muscle disease. J Neurol Neurosurg Psychiatry 1967;30:403–410.
51. Hayward M. Automatic analysis of the electromyogram in healthy subjects of different ages. J Neurol Sci 1977;33:397–413.
52. Hayward M, Willison RG. Automatic analysis of the electromyogram in patients with chronic partial denervation. J Neurol Sci 1977;33:415–423.
53. Fuglsang-Frederiksen A, Scheel U, Buchthal F. Diagnostic yield of the analysis of the pattern of electrical activity and of individual motor unit potentials in myopathy. J Neurol Neurosurg Psychiatry 1976;39:742–750.
54. Fuglsang-Frederiksen A, Scheel U, Buchthal F. Diagnostic yield of the analysis of the pattern of electrical activity and of individual motor unit potentials in neurogenic involvement. J Neurol Neurosurg Psychiatry 1977;40:544–554.
55. Smyth DP. Quantitative electromyography in babies and young children with primary muscle disease and neurogenic lesions. J Neurol Sci 1982;56:199–207.
56. Smyth DP, Willison RG. Quantitative electromyography in babies and young children with no evidence of neuromuscular disease. J Neurol Sci 1982;56:209–217.
57. Gilchrist JM, Nandedkar SD, Stewart CS, et al. Automatic analysis of the electromyographic interference pattern using turns: amplitude ratio. Electroencephalogr Clin Neurophysiol 1988;70:534–540.
58. Liguori R, Dahl K, Fuglsang-Frederiksen A. Turns-amplitude analysis of the electromyographic recruitment pattern disregarding force measurement. I: method and reference values in healthy subjects. Muscle Nerve 1992a;15:1314–1318.
59. Liguori R, Dahl K, Fuglsang-Frederiksen A, Trojaborg W. Turns-amplitude analysis of the electromyographic recruitment pattern disregarding force measurement. II: findings in patients with neuromuscular disorders. Muscle Nerve 1992b;15:1319–1324.
60. Stålberg E, Chu J, Bril V, et al. Automatic analysis of the EMG interference pattern. Electroencephalogr Clin Neurophysiol 1983;56:672–681.
61. Nandedkar SD, Sanders DB, Stålberg EV. On the shape of the normal turns-amplitude cloud. Muscle Nerve 1991;14:8–13.
62. Nandedkar SD, Sanders DB, Stålberg EV. Simulation and analysis of the electromyographic interference pattern. Part I: turns and amplitude measurements. Muscle Nerve 1986a;9:419–426.
63. Nandedkar SD, Sanders DB. Measurement of the amplitude of the EMG envelope. Muscle Nerve 1990;13:933–938.

64. Nandedkar SD, Sanders DB, Stålberg EV. Automatic analysis of the electromyographic interference pattern. Part II: findings in control subjects and in some patients with neuromuscular diseases. Muscle Nerve 1986b;9:491–500.

65. Dorfman L, Howard J, McGill K. Clinical Studies Using Automatic Decomposition Electromyography (ADEMG) in Needle and Surface EMG. In JE Desmedt (ed), Computer Aided Electromyography and Expert Systems. Clinical Neurophysiology Updates. Amsterdam: Elsevier, 1989;189–204.

66. Kopec J, Hausmanowa-Petrusewicz I. On-line computer application in clinical quantitative electromyography. Electroencephalogr Clin Neurophysiol 1976;31:404–406.

67. Sica REP, McComas AJ, Ferreira JC. Evaluation of an automated method of analysing the electromyogram. Can J Neurol Sci 1978;5:275–281.

68. Barkhaus PE, Nandedkar SD, Sanders D. Quantitative EMG in inflammatory myopathy. Muscle Nerve 1990;13:247–253.

69. Barkhaus PE, Periquet MI, Nandedkar SD. Quantitative electrophysiologic studies in sporadic inclusion body myositis. Muscle Nerve 1999;22:480–487.

70. Trojaborg W. Quantitative electromyography in polymyositis. A reappraisal. Muscle Nerve 1990;13:964–971.

71. Uncini A, Lange DJ, Lovelace RE, et al. Long duration polyphasic motor unit potentials in myopathies: a quantitative study with physiologic correlation. Muscle Nerve 1990;13:263–267.

72. Shahani BT, Wierzbicka MN, Parker SW. Abnormal single motor unit behavior in the upper motor neuron syndrome. Muscle Nerve 1991;14:64–69.

73. Feinstein B, Lindegard B, Nyman E, Wohlfart. Morphological studies of motor units in normal human muscles. Acta Anat 1955;23:127–142.

74. Stålberg E, Antoni L. Electrophysiological cross section of the motor unit. J Neurol Neurosurg Psychiatry 1980;43:469–474.

75. Stålberg EV, Dioszeghy P. Scanning EMG in normal muscle and in neuromuscular disorders. Electroencephalogr Clin Neurophysiol 1991;81:403–416.

76. Dubowitz V, Brooke M. Muscle Biopsy: A Modern Approach. Philadelphia: Saunders, 1973.

77. Stålberg E. Propagation velocity in single human muscle fibers. Acta Physiol Scand 1966; 287(Suppl):1–112.

78. Aquilonius SM, Askmark H, Gillberg PG, et al. Topographic localization of motor endplates in cryosections of whole human muscles. Muscle Nerve 1984;7:287–293.

79. Nandedkar S, Sanders D, Stålberg E, Andreassen S. Simulation of concentric needle EMG motor unit action potentials. Muscle Nerve 1988;2:151–159.

80. Thiele B, Bohle A. Anzahl der Spike-Komponenten im Motor Unit Potential. Elektroenzephalogr Elektromyogr Verwandte Geb 1978;9:125–130.

81. Nandedkar SD, Sanders DB. Simulation of myopathic motor unit action potentials. Muscle Nerve 1989;12:197–202.

82. Nandedkar SD, Dumitru D, King JC. Concentric needle electrode duration measurement and uptake area. Muscle Nerve 1997;20:1225–1228.

83. Falck B, Stålberg E, Bischoff C. Influence of recording site within the muscle on motor unit potentials. Muscle Nerve 1995;18:1385–1389.

84. Dumitru D, King JC, Rodgers WE. Motor unit action potential components and physiologic duration. Muscle Nerve 1999;22:733–741.

85. Stålberg E, Andreassen S, Falck B, et al. Quantitative analysis of individual motor unit potentials—a proposition for standardized terminology and criteria for measurement. J Clin Neurophysiol 1986;3:313–348.

86. Burke RE. Motor Unit Recruitment: What Are the Critical Factors? In JE Desmedt (ed), Motor Unit Types, Recruitment and Plasticity in Health and Disease. Progress in Clinical Neurophysiology, Vol 9. Basel, Switzerland: Karger, 1981.

87. Henneman E, Clamann HP, Gillus JD, Skinner RD. Rank order of motor neurons within a pool: law of combination. J Neurophysiol 1974;37:1338–1347.

88. Milner-Brown HS, Stein RB , Yemm R. The orderly recruitment of human motor units during voluntary isometric contractions. J Physiol 1973;230:359–370.

89. LeFever RS, DeLuca CJ. A procedure for decomposing the myoelectric signal into its constituent action potentials. I: technique, theory and implementation. IEEE Trans Biomed Eng 1982;29:149–157.

90. Stashuk D, Deluca CJ. Update on the Decomposition and Analysis of EMG Signals. In JE Desmedt (ed), Computer Aided Electromyography and Expert Systems. Clinical Neurophysiology Updates. Basel, Switzerland: Karger, 1989;39–53.

91. Ertas M, Stålberg EV, Falck B. Can the size principle be detected in conventional EMG recordings? Muscle Nerve 1995;18:435–439.

92. Sanders DB, Stålberg EV, Nandedkar SD. Analysis of electromyographic interference pattern. J Clin Neurophysiol 1996;13:385–400.

93. Stålberg E, Nandedkar SD, Sanders DB, Falck B. Quantitative motor unit potential analysis. J Clin Neurophysiol 1996;13:401–422.

94. Yu Y, Murray N. A comparison of concentric needle electromyography, quantitative EMG and single fiber EMG in the diagnosis of neuromuscular diseases. J Neurol Neurosurg Psychiatry 1984;58:220–223.

95. Hilton-Brown P, Stålberg EV. The motor unit in muscular dystrophy, single fiber EMG and scanning EMG study. J Neurol Neurosurg Psychiatry 1983;46:981–995.

96. Stålberg E. Electrogenesis in Human Dystrophic Muscle. In LP Rowland (ed), Pathogenesis of Human Muscular Dystrophies. Amsterdam: Excerpta Medica, 1977;570–587.

97. Stålberg E, Thiele B. Transmission block in terminal nerve twigs: a single fiber electromyographic finding in man. J Neurol Neurosurg Psychiatry 1972;35:52–59.

98. Stålberg EV. Electrodiagnostic assessment and monitoring of motor unit changes in disease. Muscle Nerve 1991;14:293–303.

99. Stålberg E, Grimby G. Dynamic electromyography and muscle biopsy changes in a 4-year follow up: study of patients with history of polio. Muscle Nerve 1995;18:699–707.

100. Weichers DO, Hubbell SL. Late changes in motor unit after acute poliomyelitis. Muscle Nerve 1981;4:524–528.

101. Grimby G, Stålberg EV. An 8 year longitudinal study of muscle strength, muscle fiber size and dynamic electromyogram in individuals with late polio. Muscle Nerve 1998;21:1428–1437.

102. Harvey AM, Masland RL. The electromyogram in myasthenia gravis. Bull Johns Hopkins Hosp 1941;48:1–13.

13

Single-Fiber and Macro Electromyography

Jože V. Trontelj and Erik Stålberg

SINGLE-FIBER ELECTROMYOGRAPHY

Introduction

Single-fiber electromyography (SFEMG) is an electrodiagnostic test that has been in clinical use for nearly four decades, since Ekstedt and Stålberg demonstrated that consecutive discharges of smooth biphasic action potentials (APs) of highly constant shape, when recorded with special high input impedance electrodes, belong to the single muscle fibers.[1–3] This was partly based on the observation that when two such potentials fired in a time-locked succession, the intervals between them showed slight instability from discharge to discharge. The variability was attributed to variation of the neuromuscular transmission (NMT) time. This was found to be excessively large in myasthenia gravis (MG), and it was associated with intermittent blocking according to the all-or-none principle. Soon afterward, SFEMG became recognized as a highly sensitive method to diagnose NMT disorders. The technique made it possible to use accurate and prolonged recordings from single muscle fibers and, thus, individual motor neurons in various conditions of their activation. In this way, SFEMG has also contributed to present knowledge of motor unit physiology and has helped in elucidating several phenomena in the electrophysiology of normal, diseased, and denervated muscle observed with conventional types of electrodes.[4] In this chapter, the main characteristics of SFEMG and its clinical uses are described.

Selective Recording of Single-Fiber Electromyography

To record single-fiber action potentials (SFAPs) of satisfactory amplitude, undisturbed by APs of neighboring muscle fibers from other motor units, it is essential to ensure high selectivity (i.e., to use an electrode with a small uptake radius). This requirement is most conveniently met with a standard SFEMG electrode (Figure 13.1). This consists of a needle cannula with a side port, in which a 25-μm platinum wire is exposed as the active electrode. The cannula serves as the reference; in some applications, the reference electrode can be a remote needle or a surface electrode. The electrical properties of the 25-μm leading-off surface are

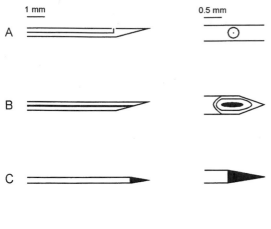

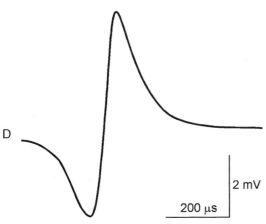

Figure 13.1 The single-fiber electromyography electrode (**A**) compared to a standard concentric electrode (**B**) and a monopolar electromyography electrode (**C**). Note the small active surface in the single-fiber electromyography electrode. **D.** A single-fiber action potential. (Reproduced with permission from E Stålberg, JV Trontelj. Single Fiber Electromyography. Studies in Healthy and Diseased Muscle [2nd ed]. New York: Raven Press, 1994;1–291.)

close to those of a point-size electrode, owing to its high input impedance and minimal shunting effect (Figure 13.2). Consequently, the amplitude of the recorded APs (compared to that obtained with a concentric electrode) is considerably higher when the source—the active muscle fiber—is close to the electrode, but it falls with a much steeper gradient with increasing distance.[4,5] Both of these properties enhance the recording selectivity. The size of the recording territory of the electrode depends on the power of the electrical generator and the volume conduction properties of the tissues between the generator and the electrode. In an adult normal limb muscle, the mean size of the recording territory of the SFEMG electrode (defined as the distance over which the AP amplitude declines to 5% of that recorded close to the muscle fiber) is approximately 300 μm. On the other hand, the sufficiently large size of the electrode and its position in a side port opposite to the needle bevel (which avoids recording from mechanically compressed, injured, and deformed muscle fibers) allow the recording of largely undistorted AP shape.

Another requirement for selective recording is a relatively low level of muscle activity. At stronger degrees of activation, APs of neighboring muscle fibers belonging to different motor units may overlap in the tracing, making reliable recognition and time measurements difficult or impossible.

Figure 13.2 The amplitude (ordinate in arbitrary units) versus recording distance for simulated action potentials recorded with different types of leading-off surfaces. Note the low amplitude obtained with large electrodes for short electrode-fiber distance. The curves for point-shaped and 25-μm electrodes practically overlap. (Reproduced with permission from J Ekstedt, E Stålberg. How the size of the needle electrode leading-off surface influences the shape of the single muscle fibre action potential in electromyography. Comput Programs Biomed 1973;3:204–212.)

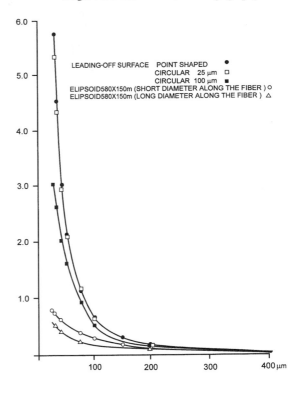

Fiber Density

Change in architecture of the motor unit—distribution of its muscle fibers within its territory—is often an early occurrence in progressive neuromuscular disorders, both in neurogenic diseases and in myopathy. In muscle biopsy, this is evident as loss of the normal mosaic pattern and its replacement by more or less pronounced fiber-type grouping. Increased fiber density (FD) is an electrophysiologic counterpart of the same phenomenon. FD, expressed quantitatively, is equivalent to the mean number of time-locked APs of different muscle fibers recorded with the use of random insertions of the SFEMG electrode during voluntary contraction (Figures 13.3 and 13.4).

Procedure

The patient is instructed to maintain slight voluntary contraction of the muscle under study. A SFEMG needle is inserted, and a position is found from which a SFAP is recorded. The electrode position is finely adjusted so that the selected SFAP is recorded with a maximum amplitude. Then other time-locked SFAPs, if any, are counted, and the number is recorded (including the SFAP selected). To be accepted, an AP must have an amplitude of more than 0.2 mV and a rise time of less than 0.3 millisecond. Partly superimposed SFAPs are counted if a distinct notch is seen on the AP (Figure 13.5). Care should be taken to exclude false SFAPs (injury potentials, often produced by a hook on a needle tip)[4] (Figure 13.6). Also, unrecognized extra discharges from the same muscle fiber may occasionally give rise to a false impression of increased FD (Figure 13.7).[4] For the next site, the needle is moved sufficiently to avoid recording from previously recorded muscle fibers. Thus, for the usual 20 recordings, there should be five

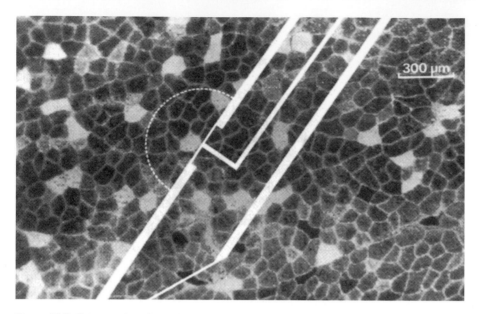

Figure 13.3 Cross-section of muscle stained for glycogen after stimulating an isolated motor axon to show one motor unit. A single-fiber electromyography electrode is superimposed to show the uptake area (*dashed semicircle*). (Reproduced with permission from E Kugelberg. Properties of the Rat Hind-Limb Motor Units. In JE Desmedt [ed], New Developments in Electromyography and Clinical Neurophysiology. Basel, Switzerland: Karger, 1973;1:2–13.)

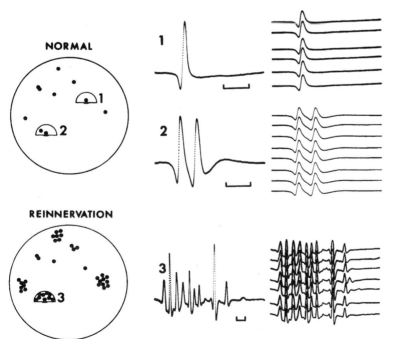

Figure 13.4 Single-fiber electromyography recordings in normal and reinnervated muscle. The diagram illustrates the number of muscle fibers of one motor unit recorded from one site. The uptake area of the electrode is represented as half-circles. In normal muscle (1,2), only one or two fibers are recorded. In reinnervation (3), many fibers are recorded due to increased fiber density in the motor unit. (Reproduced with permission from E Stålberg, JV Trontelj. Single Fiber Electromyography. Studies in Healthy and Diseased Muscle [2nd ed]. New York: Raven Press, 1994;1–291.)

Figure 13.5 Different single-fiber electromyography recordings indicated to represent one (1) or two (2) fibers in fiber density measurement. The fourth trace (*left*) contains a false (injury) potential. (Reproduced with permission from E Stålberg, JV Trontelj. Single Fiber Electromyography. Studies in Healthy and Diseased Muscle [2nd ed]. New York: Raven Press, 1994;1–291.)

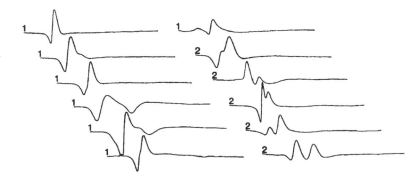

new skin penetrations oriented transversely to the muscle axis, each with recordings from several depths.

Normal values differ slightly between muscles and start to increase, especially in some muscles, after age 65 (Figure 13.8 and Table 13.1).[6] In disorders associated with collateral sprouting of motor axons, such as neurogenic disease with reinnervation, even very mild changes may be detected as an increase in FD. This parameter is more sensitive than histochemical fiber-type grouping (clusters of fibers of the same histochemical type may still belong to more than one motor unit), even when refined techniques such as enclosed fiber count are used. However, it should be noted that with FD measurement there is a bias towards low threshold motor units. At stronger contraction, the individual motor units cannot be well separated.

Figure 13.6 False action potentials (APs) recorded with raster (**A**) and superimposed (**B**) modes. The second AP is generated by the same fiber as the leading AP ("injury potential"). (Reproduced with permission from E Stålberg, JV Trontelj. Single Fiber Electromyography. Studies in Healthy and Diseased Muscle [2nd ed]. New York: Raven Press, 1994;1–291.)

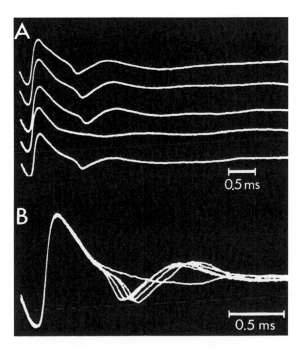

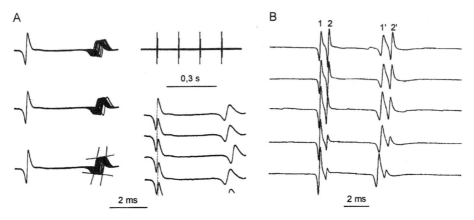

Figure 13.7. **A.** The second action potential (AP) is an extra discharge of the muscle fiber generating the first AP. On superimposed recording, the extra discharge is seen to have lower amplitude when the interval to the primary discharge is shorter, due to more pronounced partial subnormality of the membrane, which helps in identification. (Reproduced with permission from E Stålberg, JV Trontelj. Single Fiber Electromyography. Studies in Healthy and Diseased Muscle [2nd ed]. New York: Raven Press, 1994;1–291.) **B.** Another way to discriminate between an extra discharge and a genuine discharge of another muscle fiber from the same motor unit is to slightly move the recording needle; parallel change of both amplitudes proves that both APs originate in the same fiber. In the case illustrated, a pair of muscle fibers produces extra discharges. (Reproduced from E Stålberg, JV Trontelj. Clinical Neurophysiology: The Motor Unit in Myopathy. In LP Rowland, S DiMauro [eds], Diseases of Muscle. In Vinken PJ, Bruyn GW, Klawans HL [eds], Handbook of Clinical Neurology, Revised Series 18, Vol. 62. New York: North-Holland, 1992;49–84.)

In myopathy, there is an increased FD, which seems to be in contradiction with the known loss of muscle fibers from the motor units. The finding is explained by fiber-packing owing to nonuniform atrophy, fiber splitting, reinnervation after denervation, new innervation after regeneration or segmental necrosis, and, possibly, other mechanisms.[4]

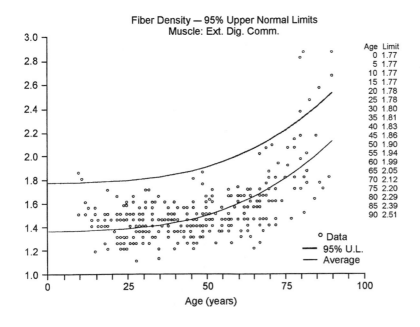

Figure 13.8 Fiber density in extensor digitorum communis (Ext. Dig. Comm.) of normal subjects of different ages. The 95% upper confidence limit (U.L.) is indicated by the upper line. There is an increase after the age of 65. (Reproduced with permission from JM Gilchrist and Ad Hoc Committee. Single fiber EMG reference values: a collaborative effort. Muscle Nerve 1992;15:151–161.)

Table 13.1 Upper Reference Limits (95% Confidence) of Fiber Density for Different Muscles and Ages as Suggested by the Collaborative Study

Muscle/ Age (yrs)	Frontalis	Deltoid	Biceps Brachii	Extensor Digitorum Communis	Quadriceps	Tibialis Anterior
10	—	—	1.52	1.77	1.93	1.94
20	1.67	1.56	1.52	1.78	1.94	1.94
30	1.68	1.57	1.53	1.80	1.96	1.96
40	1.69	1.57	1.54	1.83	1.99	1.98
50	1.70	1.58	1.57	1.90	2.05	2.02
60	1.73	1.59	1.60	1.99	2.14	2.07
70	1.76	1.60	1.65	2.02	2.26	2.15
80	—	1.62	1.72	2.29	2.34	2.26
90	—	—	1.80	2.51	—	—

Source: Reprinted with permission from JM Gilchrist and Ad Hoc Committee. Single fiber EMG reference values: a collaborative effort. Muscle Nerve 1992;15:151–161.

It should be understood that increased FD is seen in neurogenic disease and myopathy. For this reason, it is not specific for reinnervation and should be taken in the context of other electrophysiologic tests.

Duration of Multiple Potentials and Mean Interspike Interval

The duration of an AP's complex is measured between the peaks of the first and the last AP fulfilling the SFAP criteria: an amplitude greater than 0.2 mV and a rise time less than 0.3 millisecond. The delay of later SFAPs may be due to the longer time taken for conduction in the terminal axonal twig, greater delay at the neuromuscular junction (NMJ), or the longer time of SFAP propagation from the NMJ to the electrode. The latter can be due to the greater length of the muscle fiber segment between the end plate and the electrode (scatter of end plates), or slower conduction (small or split fibers in myopathy and/or recently reinnervated, still atrophic muscle fibers). The chance of recording long complexes increases with insertions far outside the motor end-plate zone.

Mean interspike interval (MISI) is calculated by dividing the sum of durations of all multiple potentials by the sum of the number of intervals (i.e., number of APs minus 1). Increased fiber size variation is an early finding in some myopathies, such as muscular dystrophies; this is readily detected as increased MISI in SFEMG. Mean values range between 0.42 and 0.65 millisecond (standard deviation, 0.2–0.3 millisecond) for limb muscles (Table 13.2).[4]

Jitter

The main use of SFEMG is in the assessment of jitter for the diagnosis of NMT disorders. The jitter phenomenon is manifested as the variability of interpotential intervals (IPIs) between two SFAPs, recorded from a consecutively discharging pair of neighboring muscle fibers of the same motor unit during voluntary contraction. It

Table 13.2 Mean Interspike Interval Values in Muscles of Normal Subjects Aged 10–75 Years*

Frontalis	Deltoid	Biceps Brachii	Extensor Digitorum Communis	First Dorsal Interosseus	Rectus Femoris	Tibialis Anterior	Extensor Digitorum Brevis
1.02	0.46	0.42	0.64	0.42	0.60	0.52	0.53
0.92	0.17	0.18	0.30	0.18	0.34	0.13	0.14

*Means (upper row) and standard deviation (lower row).
Source: Reprinted with permission from E Stålberg, JV Trontelj. Single Fiber Electromyography. Studies in Healthy and Diseased Muscle (2nd ed). New York: Raven Press, 1994;1–291.

has been shown that the main component of the jitter originates at the NMJ and that its magnitude is related to the safety factor of NMT.[7] The details of the phenomenon and its physiologic background are discussed elsewhere[4] (see Chapter 9); a brief description is given here for the situation with electrical stimulation of the motor axon (Figure 13.9).

When repetitive stimuli are delivered via an intramuscular needle electrode to a preterminal motor axon, consecutive responses of the muscle fiber show variation in latency, which in a normal case is in the range of a few tens of microseconds. The

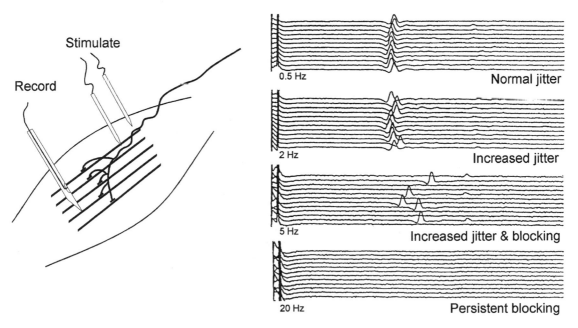

Figure 13.9 Jitter study with axonal stimulation technique. The jitter is measured between the stimulus and small-fiber action potentials from one muscle fiber. Different degrees of jitter at the same myasthenic neuromuscular junction, produced in this case by changing stimulation rate. (Reproduced with permission from Trontelj JV, Sanders DB, Stålberg E. Electrophysiological Methods for Assessing Neuromuscular Transmission. In W Brown, M Aminoff, C Bolton [eds], Clinical Neurophysiology and Neuromuscular Diseases. Philadelphia: Saunders, 2002.)

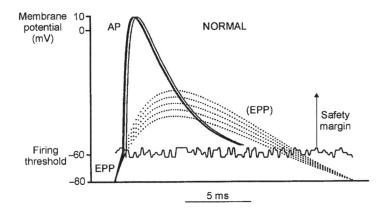

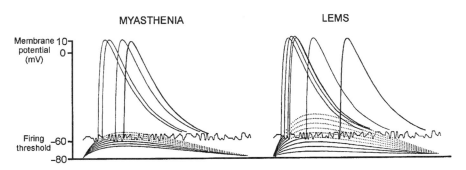

Figure 13.10 The mechanisms of jitter. **Top:** Normal neuromuscular junction (NMJ). Arrival of the nerve impulse to the terminal triggers a postsynaptic end-plate potential (EPP). When the EPP reaches the firing threshold of the muscle fiber, an action potential (AP) is generated. There is small variability of the delay of the APs (the jitter), mainly due to the oscillation of the firing threshold. **Bottom left:** At a myasthenic NMJ, increased jitter is mainly due to low EPPs, which reach the oscillating firing threshold with less steep slopes. Blocking occurs when EPPs fail to reach the firing threshold. In Lambert-Eaton myasthenic syndrome (LEMS) (**bottom right**), the EPPs have both abnormally low and excessively variable amplitudes. (Reproduced with permission from Trontelj JV, Sanders DB, Stålberg E. Electrophysiological Methods for Assessing Neuromuscular Transmission. In W Brown, M Aminoff, C Bolton [eds], Clinical Neurophysiology and Neuromuscular Diseases. Philadelphia: Saunders, 2002.)

variation in time needed to initiate an impulse in the motor axon is estimated to be less than 2 microseconds in most cases, provided that the stimulus is suprathreshold.[8] There is practically no variability in conduction time along the axon or in the muscle fiber from the NMJ to the recording electrode, provided that the interdischarge intervals are constant.[9] Thus, in normal muscle, nearly all latency variability is due to changes in NMT time.

At the normal NMJ, the jitter is due largely to small oscillations of the firing threshold of the muscle fiber, and, hence, variation of time taken for the end-plate potential (EPP) to reach the threshold and trigger a SFAP. In part, the variability is due to the variable amplitude, and, hence, the slope of the EPP (Figure 13.10, top). This latter factor becomes more important in pathology in which the EPPs have lower amplitude due to pre- or postsynaptic abnormality.

In MG, reduced postsynaptic sensitivity lowers the amplitude of the EPPs and thus increases the time they take to reach the firing threshold. Moreover, some EPPs do not reach the firing threshold, which results in failure to discharge the muscle fiber APs (blocking). The slowly rising EPP slope increases the effect of firing threshold oscillations and, consequently, the jitter (see Figure 13.10, bottom left). In Lambert-Eaton myasthenic syndrome (LEMS), the mean EPP amplitude is also reduced, although due to another cause—the decreased number of acetylcholine quanta released. In LEMS, an additional mechanism makes a significant contribution to the abnormal jitter: The number of quanta and, consequently, the EPP amplitudes vary greatly from discharge to discharge (see Figure 13.10, bottom right). For this reason, when clinically similarly affected muscles are compared, the jitter is more increased in LEMS than in MG.[10]

Jitter Study in Voluntarily Contracting Muscle

Jitter study in voluntarily contracting muscle is the originally described method, and it is still preferred in many laboratories. A detailed description can be found in several texts.[4,11] An SFEMG electrode is introduced into a muscle during slight voluntary activation. A limb muscle (e.g., extensor digitorum communis [EDC], biceps brachii, deltoid) or a facial muscle (e.g., frontalis, orbicularis oculi) is commonly used. A position is found from which time-locked SFAPs are recorded from a pair of muscle fibers. One of the SFAPs is used to trigger the sweeps of the oscilloscope, and the jitter is displayed on the other SFAP. Mild abnormality is seen as moderately increased jitter, and more severe results are seen in a further increase in jitter associated with intermittent blocking of one or the other SFAP, or both (Figure 13.11). The interpotential interval is measured on a selected point of the other SFAP, usually on the main positive-negative slope, or, in some equipment, on the SFAP peak determined by an algorithm. The jitter is then the combined result of the variations of synaptic delay at both NMJs. Usually 50 or 100 consecutive discharges are analyzed for each potential pair, and the jitter is calculated as MCD (i.e., *m*ean of absolute *c*onsecutive *d*ifferences of IPIs).

Normal Values. At normal NMJs of most muscles, the jitter ranges between 5 and 55 microseconds. Approximately 20 pairs are obtained in a full study, and the number of those outside the reference range, as well as the mean value of MCDs of all pairs, is recorded. One out of 20 MCD values may exceed the upper reference limit and the study still be accepted as normal. In the EDC, 52 microseconds is the upper reference limit for individual pairs, whereas 36 microseconds is the normal upper limit for the mean of 20 pairs. The corresponding values for the frontalis muscle are 45 and 30 microseconds, respectively (Table 13.3).

Abnormal Jitter and Blocking. The great sensitivity of SFEMG in detecting NMT disorders stems from the fact that abnormal jitter may be recorded before there is any weakness or fatigue due to NMT block. Indeed, in some patients with mild MG, there may be no NMJs with blocking, whereas the mean jitter of the whole sample may be clearly increased. Such muscles might not show any clinical weakness or fatigue. Thus SFEMG, in contrast to the repetitive nerve stimulation (RNS) test, can detect a disturbed NMT even before there is any loss of function.

Figure 13.11 Examples of recordings (individual and superimposed discharges) of jitter in voluntarily activated muscle. The jitter is measured between two single-fiber action potentials from the same motor unit. **A.** Normal. **B.** Moderately increased jitter. **C.** Greatly increased jitter with intermittent blocking (*arrows*). **B** and **C** are recordings from patients with myasthenia gravis. (Reproduced from E Stålberg, JV Trontelj. The study of normal and abnormal neuromuscular transmission with single fibre electromyography. J Neurosci Meth 1997;74:145–154, with permission from Elsevier Science.)

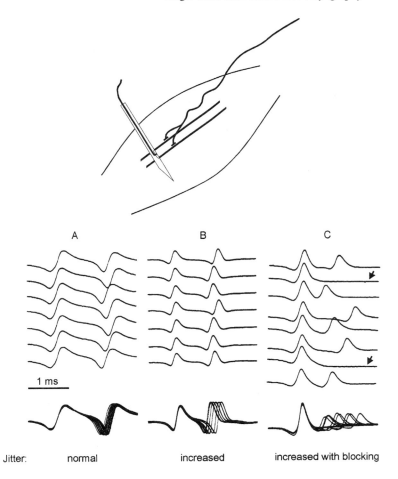

Jitter larger than 70 microseconds (e.g., as in MG or LEMS) is associated with intermittent blocking of NMT; with progressively larger jitter, the frequency of blocking increases.

Sources of Error in Jitter Studies in Voluntarily Contracting Muscle. Jitter measurement requires some experience, in particular to avoid acquiring invalid data. The following are common sources of error.

INTERFERING ACTION POTENTIALS FROM OTHER FIBERS FROM THE SAME OR DIFFERENT MOTOR UNITS. The pair of SFAPs studied should be undisturbed by other fibers' APs. When several SFAPs overlap partially or superimpose, the measured jitter is affected by vertical and horizontal AP shifts caused by variable degrees of summation and cancellation of amplitudes (Figure 13.12). Such disturbances may increase or decrease the calculated jitter of the individual components. The components with the largest jitter have their calculated MCD reduced, often quite significantly.

IRREGULAR DISCHARGE RATE. The propagation velocity of a SFAP usually varies from discharge to discharge as a function of the preceding interdischarge interval. With interdischarge intervals between approximately 5 milliseconds and 1 second, the muscle fibers show different degrees of supernormal conduction velocity. This is called the velocity recovery function (VRF).[3,9,12] When, as a result of VRF, SFAP

Table 13.3 Reference Values for Jitter (Mean of Consecutive Differences) in Different Muscles[a]

| Muscle | Upper Reference Limit: Individual NMJ[b] | | Upper Reference Limit: Mean Per Study | |
	Voluntary[c]	Axonal Stimulation	Voluntary[c]	Axonal Stimulation
Extensor digitorum communis	52/55	40	36/38	25
Frontalis	45	35	30	23
Orbicularis oculi	55/56	30	41/43	20
Orbicularis oris	57/65	—	36/38	—
Deltoid	45/46	32	33/33	24
Sternocleidomastoid	60	40	36	25

NMJ = neuromuscular junction.

[a]Ninety-fifth percentile for voluntary technique; ninety-seventh percentile for axonal stimulation technique.

[b]One out of 20 NMJs (voluntary technique) or one out of 40 NMJs (axonal stimulation technique) exceeding the given limit for the individual NMJs is accepted as normal.

[c]Data for voluntary technique are given for two age groups: below and above 60 years.

Source: The values for jitter studies with axonal stimulation are from JV Trontelj, M Mihelin, JM Fernández, E Stålberg. Axonal stimulation for end-plate jitter studies. J Neurol Neurosurg Psychiatry 1986;49: 677–685; JV Trontelj, A Khuraibet, M Mihelin. The jitter in stimulated orbicularis oculi muscle: technique and normal values. J Neurol Neurosurg Psychiatry 1988;51:814–819; JM Fernández, J Valls, AJ Khuraibet, et al. Axonal stimulation for jitter studies in the frontalis muscle. Electroencephalogr Clin Neurophysiol 1998;106(Suppl 1001):19; and from unpublished material.

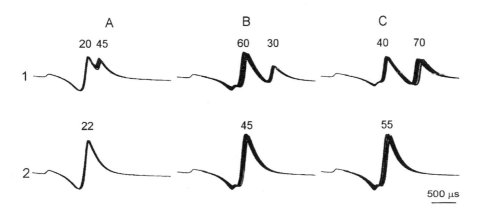

Figure 13.12 Computer simulation to show effect on jitter when the action potentials of two muscle fibers are superimposed. Each recording represents two muscle fibers activated by an electrical stimulus through their own motor axons. **1.** Partial (**A, B**) or complete separation of the single-fiber action potentials (SFAPs) (**C**), each having its own jitter as indicated. **2.** The latency of the second SFAP is made shorter so as to result in a close superimposition of the two SFAPs. The jitter value of the resulting composite spike is larger than that of the SFAP with the smaller jitter and smaller than that of the SFAP with the larger jitter. The common jitter depends not only on the amount of jitter, but also on the relative amplitude of each of the two components. In actual recordings, measurement of jitter from composite spikes tends to obscure abnormalities. (Reproduced with permission from E Stålberg, JV Trontelj. Single Fiber Electromyography. Studies in Healthy and Diseased Muscle [2nd ed]. New York: Raven Press, 1994;1–291.)

conduction time from the NMJ to the recording electrode changes to different degrees in the two muscle fibers, there is an effect on the measured jitter. The extrajunctional, myogenic contribution to the jitter may become significant with uneven discharge rates, particularly when the mean IPI exceeds 4 milliseconds. This is relatively uncommon in normal muscle but is frequent in myopathy. Intermittent blocking of either of the two SFAPs doubles the interval to the next unblocked discharge, which may produce a particularly large extrajunctional contribution to the jitter.

SPLIT MUSCLE FIBERS.   Occasionally, the jitter between a pair of SFAPs is quite low: 5 microseconds or less. A jitter of less than 4 microseconds is not seen at human NMJs. Most of these cases are believed to represent recordings from two branches of a split muscle fiber, which occur particularly in myopathies.[13] Rarely, in cases of pathologic hyperexcitability of muscle fibers, low jitter may occur as a result of ephaptic transmission between adjacent muscle fibers.[4]

Single-Fiber Electromyography with the Concentric Electrode. When an electromyography (EMG) signal recorded with a concentric (or the standard monopolar) electrode is subjected to extreme filtering, with the low-pass setting at 1 or 2 kHz, the contribution of distant muscle fibers is greatly attenuated. The recordings roughly resemble those made by a SFEMG electrode, and peaks looking like SFAPs can be isolated, although generally with a lower amplitude (see Figure 13.2). The jiggle of an unstable complex motor unit potential (MUP) is then seen as increased jitter and blocking of individual single-fiber components in a multispike potential. This has been described as the "blanket principle."[4,14] The reasons for trying this kind of recording are the convenience of switching between the conventional and SFEMG at the same session, just by changing the low-pass filter setting, and the use of the conventional electrodes instead of the expensive SFEMG needles.[15,16] Although qualitative impression can be obtained, the milder degrees of abnormality are likely to be missed, because the common jitter of composite APs is smaller than that of the most abnormal components (see the section Interfering Action Potentials from Other Fibers from the Same or Different Motor Units). The reference values collected for SFEMG (this also applies to FD) cannot be used.

Jitter Study with Axonal Microstimulation

Jitter study with axonal microstimulation has certain advantages compared to the classic technique of using voluntary muscle contraction. First of all, it is easier to learn and to use, as searching for muscle fiber pairs is not needed. It requires less patient cooperation and can be used in children. It has been experimentally applied in the rat[17] and in the mouse.[18] Individual NMJs are studied one at a time; their function can be accurately explored through a greater range of discharge rates, allowing the assessment of pre- and postsynaptic aspects. Some sources of error with the classic technique are not present (discharge rate irregularity), but some others need careful attention (e.g., inadvertent threshold stimulation). The following sections suggest some practical guidelines for jitter studies using intra- or extramuscular axonal microstimulation.[19]

Stimulation. The stimulating cathode is a simple needle insulated almost to the tip, such as the monopolar needle electrodes used in routine EMG. The cathode is inserted into the muscle near the motor point. The anode may be a similar needle placed subcutaneously or intramuscularly approximately 2–3 cm away at the right angle to the direction of the muscle fibers or a surface electrode (see Figure 13.9).

Brief rectangular pulses (10–50 microseconds) are used to increase selectivity of stimulation and make fine adjustments of stimulus strength easier. Amplitudes of less than 1–10 mA suffice in nearly all cases.

A position of the stimulating cathode is found from which a relatively weak stimulus elicits minute twitches in a small portion of muscle. The stimulation is usually only weakly felt or is not perceived at all. In cases of stimulation of a facial nerve branch in the face, the sensation of pain usually indicates proximity of a trigeminal nerve branch. With slight change of the electrode position, pain disappears.

A stimulation rate of 10 Hz is commonly used, as this is inside the range of physiologic discharge rates at which jitter is estimated in voluntarily activated muscle (the latter is usually between 8 Hz and 15 Hz). Furthermore, this is close to an optimum rate for demonstration of mildly impaired transmission in myasthenia. Significantly higher rates—30 Hz and above—may be used less easily because of cumulative local refractoriness of the stimulated axon and an increasing subnormality of the muscle fibers, evident as progressive lengthening of the latency owing to slowing of propagation velocity, decreasing AP amplitude, and occasionally even disintegration of its shape.

Assessment of an abnormal NMJ at several rates (e.g., 0.5, 5.0, 10.0, and 15.0 or 20.0 Hz) may provide valuable information regarding the type of the NMT disturbance. Postsynaptic abnormality tends to be most prominent at rates between 5 Hz and 10 Hz, and it often decreases at 15–20 Hz. Transmission is least impaired at very low rates (e.g., 0.5 Hz). Presynaptic dysfunction, on the other hand, tends to produce the largest jitter and the most frequent blocking at lower rates (e.g., 1 or 2 Hz), and this may improve dramatically at 15–30 Hz.[10]

When intermittent blocking is present, regardless of its mechanism, stimulation rates of more than 1 Hz may produce significant additional jitter owing to the effects of VRF in the muscle fiber.[9] At rates less than or equal to 1 Hz, the effect does not appear.

At approximately 10 Hz, the differences in stimulation thresholds between the adjacent axons often are larger than at lower rates, making selective activation slightly easier.

Recording. A recording SFEMG needle is inserted into the twitching part of the muscle (located by palpation), usually approximately 20 mm away from the stimulating cathode, either proximal or distal along the presumed direction of the muscle fibers. The position is adjusted until satisfactory recordings are obtained. The SFAPs from which jitter measurements are made should satisfy the SFAP criteria (see the section Fiber Density). They should appear and disappear according to the all-or-none principle when stimulus is at threshold and should not overlap with APs from other fibers. The low amplitude SFAPs from distant fibers giving rise to an unstable baseline can be attenuated by using a high-pass filter setting of 1 kHz. Once satisfactory needle position is reached, fine adjustments to improve the quality of the recording even further may be made by manipulating the cable rather than the needle holder.

Latency Measurement and Data Acquisition. With the stimulation technique, the *jitter* is defined as variation of latencies of consecutive responses (i.e., time measurement is made between the stimulus and a selected SFAP [see Figure

13.12]). This means that only a single NMJ is assessed at a time. Pairs or multiple potentials from the same motor unit are not required as they are in the case of jitter study in voluntarily activated muscle, in which one SFAP is needed as a time reference for the others.

The latency reading point is selected manually on the steep part of the rising slope of the SFAP. In some equipment, the time reading is performed automatically on SFAPs' peaks, which are detected by a mathematical algorithm. Again, the jitter is expressed as MCD, *m*ean of absolute *c*onsecutive latency *d*ifferences.

MCD is usually computed from a series of 50 responses. A full study in a muscle should include MCD values for 30–40 different SFAPs (it should be borne in mind that the recommended sample of 20 AP pairs in the voluntarily activated muscle[4] actually represents 40 NMJs). However, if the task of the study is just to *confirm* (rather than *exclude*) disturbed NMT, a sample of less than 30 NMJs—demonstrating abnormal readings in the first two or three—may suffice.

To exclude wrong data—if not too numerous (e.g., due to occasional interfering discharges)—the algorithms of most EMG equipment automatically eliminate individual consecutive difference values exceeding four standard deviations.

At the beginning of a series of stimuli at rates higher than 1 Hz, the first few responses tend to show progressive shortening of latency owing to increasing propagation velocity along the muscle fiber (cumulative effect of VRF). The shortening is more pronounced at higher rates (e.g., 20 Hz). Data acquisition should only be started after a steady state is reached, usually after 1 second of stimulation.

Sources of Error in Jitter Studies with Axonal Stimulation. Compared to the classic technique using voluntary activation, the stimulation technique is easier for the examiner and for the patient but is fraught with additional pitfalls. Care must be exercised to avoid errors due to the causes described in the following sections.[17]

OVERLAPPING SINGLE-FIBER ACTION POTENTIALS AND UNSATISFACTORY QUALITY OF RECORDING. As with the classic method, the SFAP selected should be undisturbed by other fibers' APs. As discussed in the section Interfering Action Potentials from Other Fibers from the Same or Different Motor Units, the error in jitter measurement due to superimposing SFAPs can occur in both directions, so that the calculated jitter value is either increased or decreased. The likely overall result, however, is that moderate abnormality is obscured.

Potentials that do not satisfy the SFAP criteria should also be rejected; this includes APs with prolonged rise time generated by distant muscle fibers and the monophasic positive waves ("injury potentials"; see Figure 13.6). The superimposing activity of distant fibers as well as the mains noise (noise from the main power lines) may be reduced by high setting of the high-pass filter (1 kHz). Recording of consistently low-amplitude APs suggests that the SFEMG electrode may need cleaning to restore its input impedance.

THRESHOLD STIMULATION AND SPURIOUS BLOCKING. It has been shown that, compared to well-suprathreshold stimulation, near-liminal stimulation may result in a small additional jitter of approximately 5 microseconds originating in the motor axon when there is no blocking.[20] This "jitter of the stimulated Ranvier nodes" is actually rarely seen, because it occurs at a rather narrow interval of stimulus values.

The perfect regularity of the electrical stimulation is an advantage of the axonal stimulation technique, as it removes the myogenic contribution to the measured jitter sometimes present in the technique with voluntary activation. However, the regularity is lost at threshold stimulation, when the responses are

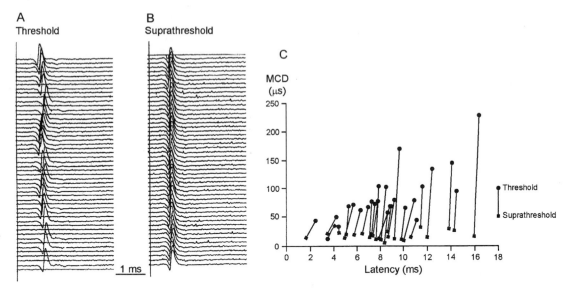

Figure 13.13 A, B. Jitter at threshold stimulation (demonstrated by intermittent spurious blocking) is significantly larger compared to that on suprathreshold stimulation. **C.** The difference between jitter on threshold and suprathreshold stimulation for a number of muscle fibers plotted against their respective latencies. The added jitter on threshold stimulation arises in the muscle fiber and results from changing muscle fiber conduction velocity due to disrupted rhythmicity of firing. The effect is more pronounced in fibers with longer latencies and presumably longer distances between the neuromuscular junction and the recording electrode. (MCD = mean of consecutive differences.)

interspersed with intermittent (spurious) blockings. Then, a much larger additional jitter may arise in the muscle fiber due to uneven activation rate, as a result of the VRF of the muscle fiber.[3,9] The magnitude of this "myogenic jitter" varies considerably, depending on the length of the muscle fiber segment between the NMJ and the SFEMG electrode and on the strength of the VRF of the particular muscle fiber. This additional jitter may be negligible when the SFEMG electrode happens to be close to the NMJ but may run into hundreds of microseconds with more remote positions (Figure 13.13). In addition, it obviously depends on the frequency and temporal pattern of blocking.

Therefore, it is important to keep the stimulus well above the threshold, bearing in mind the possibility that its efficacy may change during the acquisition of responses. To make the stimulus sufficiently suprathreshold, its amplitude is raised by approximately 10–15% or 2–3 mA beyond the value at which no further blocking is seen. It is helpful to visually monitor not only the actual SFEMG recording but also the sequential histogram of latencies and particularly the sudden onset or increased frequency of blocking.

When large jitter with or without blocking is seen, one should always exclude the possibility of inadequate stimulus strength before pronouncing it abnormal. An increase in stimulus strength of 1–3 mA distinguishes between the two possibilities. Stability of recording should be carefully monitored, because the efficacy of an initially adequate stimulus may change as a result of minor displacement of the stimulating cathode and either approach the threshold (the jitter and the latency increase and some blocking may appear, or, if present before, it may become more frequent) or the stimulus may become effectively stronger, and some new SFAPs may be recruited, possibly interfering with the measured potential. Occasionally, the margin between the adequate stimulus for the studied muscle fiber and the threshold for other interfering muscle fibers may be narrow; it is then best to change the position of the stimulating or the recording needle, or both.

In cases of multiple potential recordings, the different SFAPs often belong to more than one motor axon. This can be proved by smoothly lowering stimulus amplitude; as a result, the individual axons with their muscle fibers drop out one by one. Therefore, stimulus must be made supraliminal for each of the SFAPs before it is accepted for analysis.

LARGE JITTER WITH GENUINE BLOCKING. The presence of any intermittent blocking, whether spurious or genuine, introduces great irregularity in the activation rate and may cause additional jitter due to changing propagation velocity in the muscle fiber. When a blocking NMJ is studied quantitatively, the proportion of blocks is used instead of the jitter value to describe the degree of NMT failure.

AXON REFLEXES. Occasionally, the SFAPs of a muscle fiber are seen to alternate randomly between two latency positions. When the stimulus amplitude is slightly raised, responses with the shorter latency are obtained exclusively. Conversely, after the stimulus intensity is lowered, all the responses occur at the longer latency. The muscle fiber in this case is activated through an axon reflex, and the nerve AP takes a longer pathway than via the direct route (Figure 13.14).[21] Separate jitter measurements from either of the two latency positions may be acceptable, provided that the stimulus is supraliminal for the position used. There is normally no additional jitter in the axon reflex.

"LOW" JITTER DUE TO DIRECT MUSCLE STIMULATION. Jitter of 4 microseconds or less is considered to indicate direct activation of the muscle fibers (i.e., not via their motor axons and across NMJs). Such responses are commonly elicited with intramuscular stimulation and have to be distinguished from those with normal endplate jitter. During direct stimulation of muscle fibers at threshold stimulus strength, the jitter tends to be larger than when the motor axon is stimulated at the threshold. On increasing the stimulus gradually, the latency shortens and the jitter becomes small. With further increasing of the stimulus, additional SFAPs are recruited one by one in the same fashion, initially with a long latency and large jitter, after which they often superimpose on the previously recruited SFAPs, producing composite potentials without any visible mutual jitter, often looking like SFAPs. When the stimulus strength is reduced, the same characteristic sequence of events is seen to occur in the reverse order. Although direct muscle responses tend to have somewhat shorter latency compared to those of axonal stimulation, the latencies of the two types of responses definitely overlap. Moreover, even the stimulation threshold of the muscle fibers is similar to that of the motor axons, and both types of responses may (infrequently) occur in one and the same tracing (Figure 13.15). Direct muscle fiber stimulation may not be recognized when the recording conditions are not good (due to noise or interfering potentials) and when stimulation is near threshold. The jitter values may then be slightly more than 4 microseconds. Failure to recognize low jitter results in an underestimated mean MCD value for the whole study.

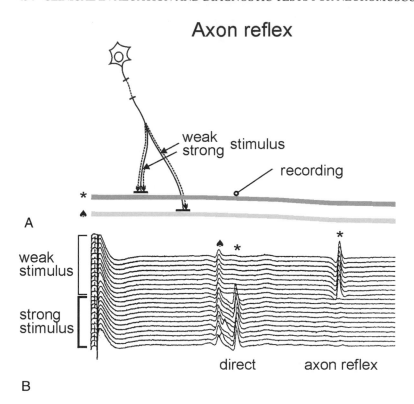

Axon reflex

A

B

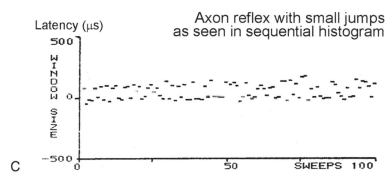

Figure 13.14 A. A muscle fiber (∗) activated through its own axonal twig (with a stronger stimulus) or indirectly through a twig to another muscle fiber (♠) and an axon reflex (with a weaker stimulus). **B.** At a critical stimulus strength, there is random alternation between the two latency positions. When latency jumps are small, they may be overlooked and will then increase the measured jitter. They can be detected as having a bimodal distribution in a sequential latency histogram (**C**). (Reproduced with permission from Trontelj JV, Sanders DB, Stålberg E. Electrophysiological Methods for Assessing Neuromuscular Transmission. In W Brown, M Aminoff, C Bolton [eds], Clinical Neurophysiology and Neuromuscular Diseases. Philadelphia: Saunders, 2002.)

Extramuscular nerve stimulation is free from this pitfall. A practical approach is to use muscles whose nerves divide in small branches proximal to their entry points, such as muscles of the face.[22] The needle stimulation cathode is positioned near one such branch outside the muscle.

Normal Values. Normal jitter values are available for the EDC, sternocleidomastoideus, orbicularis oculi, and frontalis. In the EDC and sternocleidomastoideus, the upper normal limit is 40 microseconds for the individual NMJs and 25 microseconds for the mean MCD of 20–30 NMJs. In the orbicularis oculi and

Figure 13.15. Occasionally, responses to axonal and direct (*arrows*) muscle fiber stimulation (belonging to different muscle fibers) may occur in the same traces. In most cases, the latter occur at somewhat shorter latencies (*top*), exceptionally longer than those to axonal stimulation (*bottom*). Both recordings are from patients with myasthenia.

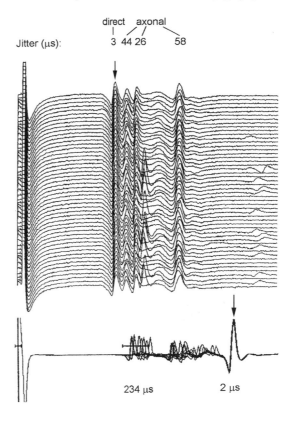

frontalis muscles, the upper reference limits are 30 and 35 microseconds (for individual NMJs) and 20 and 23 microseconds (for a mean MCD of 20 NMJs), respectively. Limited material exists for the deltoid (32 and 24 microseconds, respectively) (see Table 13.3).

Compared to jitter measured in voluntarily activated muscle fiber pairs, the jitter of stimulated single NMJs should, theoretically, be lower by a factor of $\sqrt{2}$ on the average. This relationship has been confirmed experimentally.[23] Therefore, for any muscle in which normal jitter values have been established for voluntary activation, multiplying those by 0.8 gives provisional normal limits.

As in jitter studies using voluntary activation, one out of 20 readings exceeding the individual upper normal limit is accepted as normal.

In the EDC and the orbicularis oculi, normal jitter values on axonal stimulation do not seem to increase with age; therefore, the same reference limits are used even after 70 or 80 years of age.

The narrow distribution of normal values makes the stimulation technique particularly sensitive to detect mild NMT disturbances. Thus, there is virtually no overlap of normal values (mean MCD per subject) with results obtained in myasthenia even when the symptoms are mild or confined to the extraocular muscles (Figure 13.16).

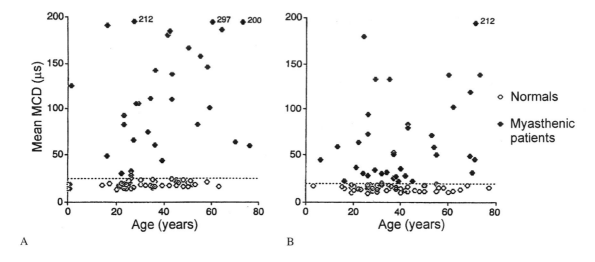

Figure 13.16 Mean jitter values in 78 patients with myasthenia gravis on their first presentation, plotted against age and in comparison to normal material. Either extensor digitorum communis (**A**) or orbicularis oculi (**B**) was studied (37 and 41 patients, respectively), depending on distribution of symptoms. There is virtually no overlap between the normal and patient population. Even patients with very mild ocular disease usually have convincingly abnormal jitter. (MCD = mean of consecutive differences.) (Reproduced with permission from E Stålberg, JV Trontelj. Single Fiber Electromyography. Studies in Healthy and Diseased Muscle [2nd ed]. New York: Raven Press, 1994;1–291.)

Jitter Findings in Myasthenia Gravis and Lambert-Eaton Myasthenic Syndrome

The main clinical use of SFEMG is in the diagnosis of NMJ disorders such as myasthenia and LEMS.

Moderately increased jitter is the first sign of low safety margin of NMT. Larger jitter (MCD >70 microseconds, occasionally >55 microseconds with the axonal stimulation technique) is associated with intermittent transmission blocking. With increasing jitter values, blocking becomes progressively more frequent and may more or less persist at a proportion of the NMJs.

The proportion of potentials with blocks correlates with clinical weakness and fatigue in that muscle. Moreover, the degree of SFEMG abnormality reflects the functional status of the patient, and serial jitter studies have been used in MG to monitor the effects of treatment.[24]

The recording of jitter and blocking, whether performed in the classic way or with axonal stimulation, has been shown to be currently the most sensitive method in the diagnosis of MG and LEMS. SFEMG reveals increased jitter in virtually all patients with MG. In a series of 550 patients, 99% of patients with generalized MG and 97% of those with the ocular form had abnormal jitter in at least one muscle.[25] In two series of patients with LEMS—50 and 73, respectively—the jitter study was abnormal in all.[26,27]

Both SFEMG techniques owe their high sensitivity to the fact that already mild involvement of a NMJ is manifested as increased jitter before there is any actual NMT dysfunction, and hence, before such dysfunction is detectable by other methods. Thus, clearly abnormal jitter may be seen in very mildly involved muscles with no demonstrable clinical weakness and with a normal RNS test. When decrement is present, there is a correlation with the degree of SFEMG abnormalities in the same muscle. However, SFEMG may also detect blocking NMJs even when decrement studies are normal. Conversely, a decremental response seen during RNS is only seen in muscles that also show blocking on SFEMG.[28]

No single muscle is more frequently abnormal than other muscles in MG patients. However, either the EDC or a facial muscle (frontalis or orbicularis oculi) is most often examined first. In ocular myasthenia, a facial muscle is more likely to be abnormal than the EDC. In one of our laboratories (J.V.T.'s), axonal stimulation technique is used almost exclusively, and the orbicularis oculi is usually examined first, even in the generalized disease. If this muscle is normal, which may happen in very mild and new-onset cases, the EDC or the deltoid muscle is also examined. If this also is normal and a NMT disorder is still suspected, a follow-up SFEMG is done after a few weeks. It should be added that a normal jitter study in a symptomatic muscle practically excludes MG or LEMS. Even when a complete remission is achieved, approximately one-half of patients still have abnormal jitter studies. In symptomatic muscles, the degree of abnormality (frequency of increased jitter and blocking) correlates with severity of fatigability and weakness. The RNS test is optionally added as a baseline to follow up the effect of treatment.

MG and LEMS give rise to increased jitter and intermittent impulse blocking but at different stimulation rates; the degree of abnormality usually changes in different ways. Many myasthenic NMJs are normal or mildly abnormal at 0.5–1.0 Hz, but they markedly deteriorate as the rate increases. Most often, the jitter and blocking are most pronounced at 5–10 Hz. When stimulation rate is increased further to 15–20 Hz, the jitter and blocking increase even more at some NMJs, but the majority shows improvement owing to tetanic facilitation (Figure 13.17).

In an occasional case of a very sick myasthenic NMJ, a stimulation rate of less than 2 Hz may be needed to produce more than just a few initial responses; at higher rates, such NMJs may be pushed into persistent NMT block. These NMJs can be studied at 1 Hz.

In contrast, in LEMS the jitter tends to be most abnormal and blocking most frequent at low stimulation rates, whereas transmission may improve dramatically with higher rates (Figure 13.18). In a suspected LEMS patient, it is advisable to explore every new stimulation and recording site with a frequency of 15 or 20 Hz, because in this condition up to one-third of NMJs in a muscle have been seen to be completely inexcitable at rates lower than this. The finding of muscle fibers that start to respond only at higher stimulation rates provides strong support to the diagnosis of LEMS. Similar observations may be made in botulism (Figure 13.19).

It should be pointed out, however, that in each of the three conditions, one can find individual (or even many) NMJs that depart from the previously described patterns.[25]

As could be expected, abnormal jitter is also seen in patients with congenital myasthenic syndromes, such as congenital myasthenia, familial infantile myasthenia, slow channel syndrome, and congenital acetylcholinesterase deficiency.[29]

Specificity of Abnormal Jitter in Neuromuscular Transmission Disorders. It must be emphasized that abnormal jitter and blocking are not specific for MG, LEMS, and other NMT diseases but may be seen as manifestations of weak NMJs in a variety of neuromuscular disorders, both neurogenic and myopathic. In recent reinnervation, this may also be caused by abnormal conduction along the terminal nerve twigs. The muscle fiber is not a source of increased jitter, unless the activation rate is irregular.[9]

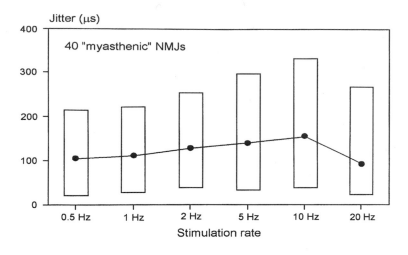

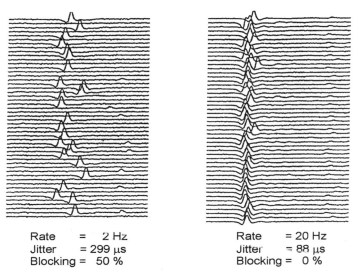

Figure 13.17 In myasthenia gravis, the jitter tends to be most abnormal at stimulation rates of 5–10 Hz (*top*) at a majority of neuromuscular junctions (NMJs). At 20 Hz (*bottom right*), transmission improves at many myasthenic NMJs due to tetanic facilitation. (Reproduced with permission from E Stålberg, JV Trontelj. Single Fiber Electromyography. Studies in Healthy and Diseased Muscle [2nd ed]. New York: Raven Press, 1994;1–291.)

Most often, large jitter is caused by low safety margin of NMT. When large jitter is found in a patient with suspected NMT disorder, not only the sensitivity but also the specificity of the findings is high.

SFEMG can be helpful in distinguishing MG from fatigability of nonorganic (psychogenic) or central causes (e.g., some cases of multiple sclerosis). In ocular myopathy, the jitter in the orbicularis oculi or frontalis is usually normal, but FD and MISI may be increased. On the other hand, in mitochondrial cytopathy with chronic progressive ophthalmoplegia, the jitter may be increased.[30] Polymyositis, thyroid myopathy, and steroid myopathy may also have to be considered in the differential diagnosis. However, the clinical picture, conventional EMG, and other tests help in resolving possible dilemmas.[4] As in any case of a neuromuscular disorder, the results of electrophysiologic studies have to be carefully interpreted in light of the clinical picture and other laboratory data.

Figure 13.18 In Lambert-Eaton myasthenic syndrome (LEMS), abnormal jitter (*top*) and blocking are usually most pronounced at the lowest activation rates. Improvement with higher rates is often quite marked (*bottom*). (NMJs = neuromuscular junctions.) (Reproduced with permission from E Stålberg, JV Trontelj. Single Fiber Electromyography. Studies in Healthy and Diseased Muscle [2nd ed]. New York: Raven Press, 1994;1–291.)

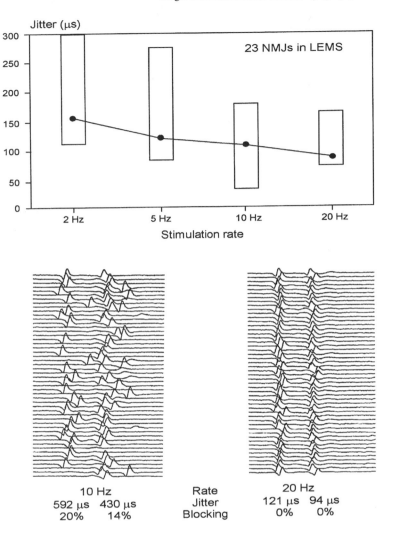

	10 Hz		Rate	20 Hz	
	592 μs	430 μs	Jitter	121 μs	94 μs
	20%	14%	Blocking	0%	0%

MACRO ELECTROMYOGRAPHY

Introduction

The pathologic changes within a motor unit are often unevenly distributed, particularly in neurogenic diseases, but also in myopathies. Thus, the information obtained by the conventional needle EMG from individual recording sites is often not representative. Macro EMG was created with the purpose of obtaining a global view of the motor unit, in particular an estimate of the whole motor unit size. In addition, the technique offers simultaneous SFEMG recording that provides information on narrowly focused details within the same motor unit, such as FD. Such combined information is not obtained with the conventional needle EMG or SFEMG, nor with other electrodiagnostic methods. Macro EMG thus provides a valuable new look at the motor unit.[31]

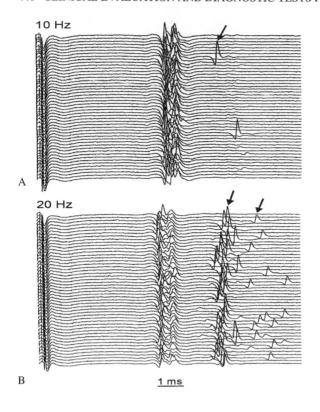

Figure 13.19 A recording from a patient in acute stage of botulism, showing improved transmission as the stimulation rate is raised from 10 (**A**) to 20 Hz (**B**). Blocking is dramatically reduced in one fiber (*arrow, top*; *left arrow, bottom*), and another fiber emerges from previously persistent block (*right arrow, bottom*). Such recordings are also common in Lambert-Eaton myasthenic syndrome. (Reproduced with permission from E Stålberg, JV Trontelj. Single Fiber Electromyography. Studies in Healthy and Diseased Muscle [2nd ed]. New York: Raven Press, 1994;1–291.)

Method

The recording electrode consists of a modified SFEMG electrode with the cannula insulated except for the distal 15 mm. The SFEMG recording surface is exposed 7.5 mm from the tip. These values were chosen with the knowledge that a normal motor unit has a diameter of 5–10 mm. Recording is made on two channels; one recording from the cannula with a remote reference, and the other one recording SFEMG for triggering (Table 13.4 and Figure 13.20).

The SFEMG signal is used to trigger the display and the averaging process. The signal from the cannula is fed to the averager. The electrode is inserted into voluntarily activated muscle, and a position is found where an acceptable SFAP is recorded. The averaging process is started and is continued until a smooth baseline and a constant macro MUP are obtained on the "cannula" channel. At the same time, the number of SFAPs time-locked to the triggering SFAP is counted for FD determination.

Table 13.4 Two-Channel Recording in Macro Electromyography

	Recording Electrode	Reference Electrode	Filters	Function
Channel 1	Cannula	Remote surface	5–10,000 Hz	Obtains averaged macro motor unit potential
Channel 2	Single-fiber electromyography	Cannula	500–10,000 Hz	Triggers the averager and gives fiber density

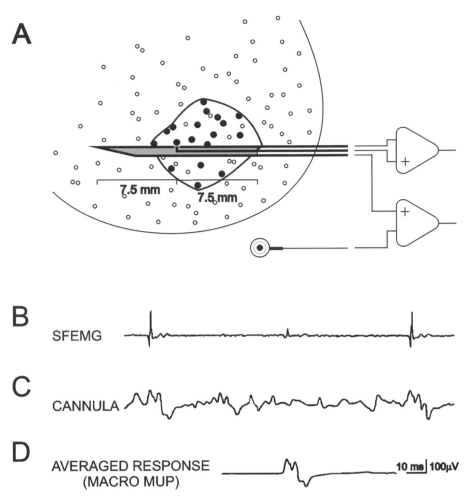

Figure 13.20 Macro electromyography. Schematic description of recording principle. **A.** The modified single-fiber electromyographic (SFEMG) electrode with distal 15-mm bare cannula inserted into the muscle. One motor unit territory is encircled. **B.** SFEMG signals (derived between SFEMG surface and the cannula) obtained during voluntary contraction, used to trigger the sweep and the averager. **C.** Macro electromyography derived between the cannula and a remote surface electrode. The sweep is triggered from the SFEMG channel. **D.** The macro motor unit potential (MUP) extracted after averaging the cannula signal. (Reproduced with permission from E Stålberg. Macro EMG and Scanning EMG. In EW Johnson, WS Pease [eds], Practical Electromyography [3rd ed]. Baltimore: Williams & Wilkins, 1997.)

The macro recording is nonselective because of the large recording surface. A majority of fibers from the entire motor unit contribute to the signal. Due to the shunting effect, the APs from immediately adjacent muscle fibers are recorded with low amplitudes and therefore contribute much less to the final signal than they do with the use of conventional needle electrodes. Owing to the filtering effect of the tissue, APs from remote muscle fibers contain a larger proportion of low frequency components, which are well detected by the electrode. Nevertheless, the remote fibers are recorded with an amplitude approximately one-half of that of the closest fibers.

The peak-to-peak amplitude and area of the macro EMG signal are positively correlated to the number and size of muscle fibers in the entire motor unit.[32] Studies with live recordings as well as computer simulations suggest that the macro MUP parameters reflect the size of the motor unit much better than the amplitude or duration of MUPs recorded with conventional techniques. One of the reasons for this is that in the latter case, individual muscle fiber APs are recorded with shorter duration, resulting in a more pronounced cancellation effect.

An estimate of the number of motor units in a muscle can be obtained by dividing the response to supramaximal nerve stimulation (M response) obtained from the cannula with the mean macro MUP size (amplitude or area).

Normal Muscle

Normal values regarding shape, amplitude, and area have been collected for some muscles.[31] There is a great variation of individual macro MUP amplitudes in normal muscle. Normal values, given for low degree of activity (i.e., low-threshold motor units), vary for different muscles. In some muscles, the values increase with age; the increase is more pronounced in the tibialis anterior muscle than in the biceps brachii or vastus lateralis muscles. This change is probably due to collateral sprouting after the physiologic loss of motor neurons.

In the biceps brachii muscle, the ratio between the largest and the smallest macro MUP may be 1–10 in individuals younger than the age of 60 and up to 1–20 in those older than 60 years. Later recruited motor units have larger macro MUPs than those recruited earlier, reflecting the so-called size principle. The mean macro MUP amplitude of motor units recruited at 20% of maximal force may be five times larger than that of motor units recruited at lower force. Thus, it is important to establish reference values for given ranges of contraction levels and to perform patient investigation within the same level.

Myopathies

As expected, the electrical size of the motor unit reflected by the macro MUP is decreased in myopathies as a group. In individual cases, however, values are often within normal limits. Large mean amplitude macro MUPs have been found in muscles of some patients with facioscapulohumeral and limb-girdle muscular dystrophy with slight or no weakness.[33] This finding may indicate a compensatory hypertrophy. Thus, macro MUP parameters themselves are not sensitive in detecting early myopathic changes. The possible reasons for the normal or nearly normal amplitudes may include fiber regeneration, fiber splitting, occasional fiber hypertrophy, and general packing of fibers owing to atrophy. These changes cause increase in the FD value, however. Therefore, the finding of increased FD values obtained from the SFEMG channel during the macro EMG study, combined with normal or slightly reduced macro MUP value, is a useful indicator of myopathy. These findings can be used to differentiate myopathy from neuropathy in questionable cases.

Reinnervation

During reinnervation by collateral sprouting, the most common type of compensation in neurogenic conditions, the number of muscle fibers in a given motor unit increases. This is seen as increased macro MUP amplitude.[34-36] Macro EMG offers the possibility to follow reinnervation quantitatively.

The individual macro MUPs in reinnervation can have amplitudes exceeding the normal mean by a factor of 10. In patients with amyotrophic lateral sclerosis, the picture is variable.[34,37,38] In some patients with rapid progression, the macro MUP amplitudes are increased only slightly, and FD is only moderately increased. In cases of slow progression, the macro MUPs increase considerably more, with individual macro MUPs reaching values 10–20 times larger than the upper reference limit for the normal mean, in parallel with a pronounced increase in FD, indicating a homogeneous and effective reinnervation. In later stages, the mean macro MUP amplitude may start to decline, although the FD remains high. This has been interpreted as fragmentation of large motor units or an effect of selective dropout of the largest motor units, leaving the smaller ones preserved.

In patients with a history of poliomyelitis, the macro EMG amplitudes are usually increased dramatically with individual values more than 20 times the normal mean value. In a study of patients with examinations 8 years apart, macro EMG and biopsy were performed in the vastus lateralis muscle.[36] The macro MUP amplitude increased with time even in strong muscles. After 4–8 years the amplitudes may have increased to 10–20 times the normal mean. This progressive increase was felt to be due to an increase in the number of fibers per motor unit due to continuing collateral sprouting. In patients with initially very large macro MUPs, exceeding 20 times the normal, follow-up studies sometimes showed a decline in values, associated with loss of force of knee extension. At a stage of fully used reinnervation capacity, further loss of motor units cannot be compensated. Continued loss of motor units then presents clinically as a new or accelerating development of weakness.

Figure 13.21 shows macro MUPs in the tibialis anterior muscle of a healthy subject, a patient with polymyositis, and a patient with a history of poliomyelitis.

Uses of Macro Electromyography

As a complement to conventional EMG, macro EMG offers additional insight into the motor unit in health and disease. The combination with the FD parameter and the macro MUP amplitude may provide clinically relevant information on individual motor units (Table 13.5). The technique may be useful in estimating motor unit size and in normal muscle, as well as in studies of recruitment order in which information regarding the motor unit size is of interest. It can be applied in diagnostic evaluation of neurogenic conditions and follow-up studies of reinnervation processes. It may also be valuable in evaluation of myopathic conditions.

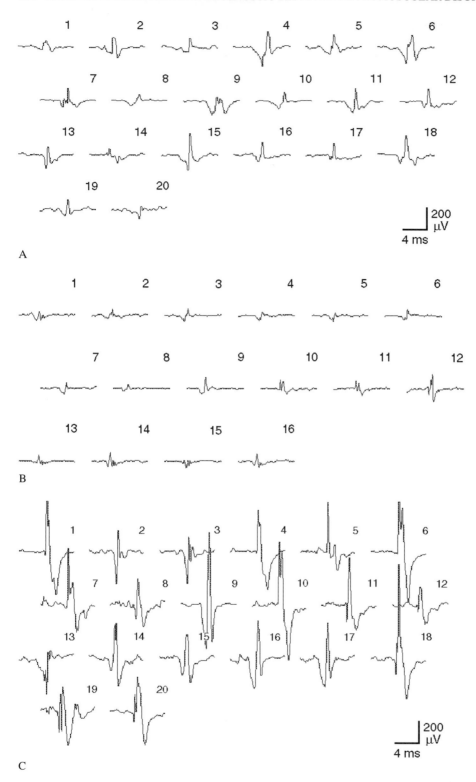

Figure 13.21 Examples of macro electromyography recordings from the tibialis anterior muscle of a healthy subject (**A**), a patient with polymyositis (**B**), and a patient with history of polio (**C**).

Table 13.5. Relationship between Macro Electromyography Amplitude and Fiber Density

	Macro Motor Unit Potential Amplitude			Fiber Density	
	Decreased	Normal	Increased	Normal	Increased
Small normal motor unit	+			+	
Average motor unit		+		+	
Large normal motor unit			+	+	
Neuropathy			+		+
Myopathy	(+)	+			+

+ = definite association; (+) = occasional association.

CONCLUSIONS

The two needle EMG techniques described in this chapter offer two grossly different perspectives in examination of the motor unit, much like two widely different microscope magnifications. SFEMG focuses on small structural and functional details at the level of single NMJs and single muscle fibers. Macro EMG remains selective in the sense that it studies individual motor units; however, unlike other needle EMG methods, the aim of this technique is to grasp the global view of the whole motor unit.

With SFEMG, the recording territory has a hemisphere with a radius of approximately 300 μm, equivalent to approximately five to six breadths of an average muscle fiber. Owing to the highly constant shape of the recorded SFAPs, time measurements with an accuracy of 1 microsecond or, exceptionally, even 0.1 microsecond in certain research applications, may make sense in terms of showing physiologic details; this time resolution, in fact, may be close to the limits of biological relevance in neurophysiology.

On the other hand, the recording territory of the macro EMG electrode is a cylinder of 15 × 7 mm—a volume that is approximately 25,000 times larger than that of the SFEMG electrode. The meaningful time resolution is reduced to 0.1 millisecond, which is 1,000 times coarser than with the SFEMG recordings.

The two techniques described here have provided valuable information in studies of important physiologic and clinical questions. Moreover, SFEMG has become part of the standard diagnostic armamentarium in many EMG laboratories and is routinely applied in the diagnostic assessment and follow-up of patients with NMT disorders. In addition, the technique can be useful in evaluation of patients with on-going denervation and reinnervation, as it reveals early changes and allows sequential studies for the assessment of disease progression. It can be helpful in the prediction of the course of the disease. In myopathy, SFEMG can detect early abnormality in terms of increased fiber size variation and focally increased FD.

The mainstay of indications for SFEMG is in diagnosis of NMT disorders, particularly MG, for which it is the most sensitive electrophysiologic test. Its results naturally have to be taken in the context of the clinical picture and of other electrodiagnostic tests, as abnormal jitter can also occur in other diseases. However, differentiation can most often be easily made.

On the other hand, macro EMG has not been extensively used in clinical routine. As a complement to conventional EMG, the macro MUP amplitude in combination with information on FD offers additional insight into the motor unit and often provides clinically relevant information about its changes in disease. The technique may be useful in estimating motor unit size, as well as in studies of recruitment order.

In clinical medicine, macro EMG examination can be applied in the diagnosis of neurogenic conditions and in the evaluation and follow-up of the reinnervation process. The technique may also be valuable in the assessment of primary muscle disorders.

REFERENCES

1. Ekstedt J, Stålberg E. A method of recording extracellular action potentials of single muscle fibers and measuring their propagation velocity in voluntarily activated human muscle. Bull Am Assoc EMG Electrodiagn 1963;10:16.
2. Ekstedt J. Human single muscle fiber action potentials. Acta Physiol Scand 1964;61(Suppl 226):1–96.
3. Stålberg E. Propagation velocity in human single muscle fibers in situ. Acta Physiol Scand 1966;70(Suppl 287):1–112.
4. Stålberg E, Trontelj JV. Single Fiber Electromyography. Studies in Healthy and Diseased Muscle (2nd ed). New York: Raven Press, 1994;1–291.
5. Ekstedt J, Stålberg E. How the size of the needle electrode leading-off surface influences the shape of the single muscle fibre action potential in electromyography. Comput Programs Biomed 1973;3:204–212.
6. Gilchrist JM and Ad Hoc Committee. Single fiber EMG reference values: a collaborative effort. Muscle Nerve 1992;15:151–161.
7. Schiller H, Stålberg E, Schwartz M. Regional curare for the reduction of safety factor in human motor end-plates studied with single fibre electromyography. J Neurol Neurosurg Psychiatry 1975;38:805–809.
8. Trontelj JV, Stålberg E, Mihelin M, Khuraibet A. Jitter of the stimulated motor axon. Muscle Nerve 1992;15:449–454.
9. Trontelj JV, Stålberg E, Mihelin M. Jitter in the muscle fibre. J Neurol Neurosurg Psychiatry 1990;53:49–54.
10. Trontelj JV, Stålberg E. The function of single motor end plates in myasthenia gravis and Lambert-Eaton syndrome. Muscle Nerve 1991;14:226–232.
11. Sanders DB, Stålberg EV. AAEE minimonograph #25: single-fiber electromyography. Muscle Nerve 1996;19:1069–1083.
12. Mihelin M, Trontelj JV, Stålberg E. Muscle fiber recovery functions studied with double pulse stimulation. Muscle Nerve 1991;14:739–747.
13. Hilton-Brown P, Stålberg E, Trontelj J, Mihelin M. Causes of the increased fibre density in muscular dystrophies studied with single fibre EMG during electrical stimulation. Muscle Nerve 1985;8:383–388.
14. Pajan J. The blanket principle: a technical note. Muscle Nerve 1978;1:423–426.
15. Ertas M, Baslo B, Yildiz N, et al. Concentric needle electrode for neuromuscular jitter analysis. Muscle Nerve 2000;23:715–719.
16. Wiechers DO. Single fiber electromyography with a standard monopolar electrode. Arch Phys Med Rehabil 1985;66:47–48.
17. Lin TS, Cheng TJ. Stimulated single fiber electromyography in the rat. Muscle Nerve 1998; 21:482–489.
18. Gooch CL, Mosier DR. Stimulated single fiber electromyography in the mouse: technique and normative data. Muscle Nerve 2001;24:941–945.
19. Trontelj JV, Stålberg E. Jitter measurements by axonal stimulation. Guidelines and technical notes. Electroencephalogr Clin Neurophysiol 1992;85:30–37.
20. Stålberg E, Trontelj JV. Clinical Neurophysiology: The Motor Unit in Myopathy. In LP Rowland, S DiMauro (eds), Diseases of Muscle. In Vinken PJ, Bruyn GW, Klawans HL (eds), Handbook of Clinical Neurology, Revised Series 18, Vol. 62. New York: North-Holland, 1992;49–84.
21. Stålberg E, Trontelj JV. Demonstration of axon reflexes in human motor nerve fibers. J Neurol Neurosurg Psychiatry 1970;33:571–579.

22. Trontelj JV, Khuraibet A, Mihelin M. The jitter in stimulated orbicularis oculi muscle: technique and normal values. J Neurol Neurosurg Psychiatry 1988;51:814–819.
23. Trontelj JV, Mihelin M, Fernández JM, Stålberg E. Axonal stimulation for end-plate jitter studies. J Neurol Neurosurg Psychiatry 1986;49:677–685.
24. Sanders DB, Howard JF Jr. Single-fiber electromyography in myasthenia gravis. Muscle Nerve 1986;9:809–819.
25. Sanders DB, Massey JM, Howard JF Jr, 2001, in preparation.
26. O'Neill JH, Murray NMF, Newsom-Davies J. The Lambert-Eaton myasthenic syndrome. A review of 50 cases. Brain 1988;111:577–596.
27. Tim RW, Massey JM, Sanders DB. Lambert-Eaton myasthenic syndrome: electrodiagnostic findings and response to treatment. Neurology 2000;54(11):2176–2178.
28. Gilchrist JM, Massey JM, Sanders DB. Single fiber EMG and repetitive nerve stimulation of the same muscle in myasthenia gravis. Muscle Nerve 1994;17:171–175.
29. Sanders DB, Trontelj JV, Stålberg E. Diseases Associated with Disorders of Neuromuscular Transmission. In W Brown, M Aminoff, C Bolton (eds), Clinical Neurophysiology and Neuromuscular Diseases. Philadelphia: Saunders, 2002.
30. Krendel DA, Sanders DB, Massey JM. Single fiber electromyography in chronic progressive external ophthalmoplegia. Muscle Nerve 1985;8:624.
31. Stålberg E, Fawcett PRW. Macro EMG changes in healthy subjects of different ages. J Neurol Neurosurg Psychiatry 1982;45:870–878.
32. Nandedkar SD, Stålberg E. Simulation of macro EMG motor unit potentials. Electroencephalogr Clin Neurophysiol 1983;56:52–62.
33. Hilton-Brown P, Stålberg E. Motor unit size in muscular dystrophy; a macro EMG and scanning EMG study. J Neurol Neurosurg Psychiatry 1983;46:996–1005.
34. Dengler R, Konstanzer A, Kuther G, et al. Amyotrophic lateral sclerosis: macro-EMG and twitch forces of single motor units. Muscle Nerve 1990;13:545–550.
35. Tollbäck A, Borg J, Borg K, Knutsson E. Isokinetic strength, macro EMG and muscle biopsy of paretic foot dorsiflexors in chronic neurogenic paresis. Scand J Rehab Med 1993;25:183–187.
36. Grimby G, Stålberg E, Sandberg A, Stibrant-Sunnerhagen K. An 8-year longitudinal study of muscle strength, muscle fiber size, and dynamic electromyogram in individuals with late polio. Muscle Nerve 1998;21:1428–1437.
37. Stålberg E. Single fiber EMG, macro EMG, and scanning EMG. New ways of looking at the motor unit. CRC Crit Rev Clin Neurobiol 1986;2:125–167.
38. Tackmann W, Vogel P. Fiber density, amplitude of macro-EMG motor unit potentials and conventional EMG recordings from the anterior tibial muscle in patients with amyotrophic lateral sclerosis. Acta Physiol Scand 1988;235:149–154.

14

Motor Unit Number Estimates

Catherine Lomen-Hoerth

Motor unit number estimation (MUNE) refers to a group of electrophysiologic techniques that estimate the number of lower motor neurons innervating a muscle.[1,2] A *motor unit* refers to one motor neuron and all of the muscle fibers innervated by that neuron. The *number* of motor units is the number of functioning motor neurons innervating a muscle. The motor unit number must be estimated, because there is no method to count the actual number of functioning lower motor neurons innervating a given muscle.

Determining the motor unit number is important in neurogenic diseases in which there is lower motor neuron loss. The size of the compound muscle action potential (CMAP) may not be an accurate measure of the degree of lower motor neuron loss because of compensatory reinnervation. Furthermore, the decreased CMAP is not even specific for neurogenic processes, as it may be seen in myopathies.[3]

In neurogenic disorders, collateral reinnervation enables the CMAP amplitude to be maintained until the degree of motor neuron loss is too great for the remaining motor units to fully compensate. In this setting, weakness occurs when reinnervation does not compensate for the degree of motor unit loss.

MUNE assesses the loss of lower motor neurons separately from reinnervation, and for this reason, MUNE studies have potential value for following patients with neurogenic disorders over time. MUNE is more sensitive at detecting change over time than is isometric strength testing, measurement of the CMAP area, or forced vital capacity in amyotrophic lateral sclerosis (ALS) patients, and MUNE is important for prognosis.[4–6] Additionally, it may be valuable in drug studies to determine the effectiveness of the drug on slowing the rate of motor unit loss and is being used in current drug trials for ALS.

Needle electromyography (EMG) is sensitive to the presence of denervation and reinnervation; however, it is not a substitute for MUNE. EMG is important for distinguishing neuropathic and myopathic disorders, showing how widespread the disease is, and localizing the lesion to peripheral nerve, plexus, or roots.

The features of EMG in neurogenic processes include reduced motor unit recruitment, increased motor unit size, and abnormal spontaneous activity (e.g., fibrillation potentials, which are not specific for neurogenic processes). These measurements are not quantitative to determine change over time. However, they may be more sensitive than MUNE for an earlier diagnosis of ALS.[5]

MUNE is obtained by dividing the size of the maximal CMAP by the size of the mean surface-recorded motor unit potential (SMUP). MUNE techniques differ in the ways in which they obtain samples of SMUPs from which the mean size is determined. All methods are quite reproducible, and the reliability improves as the number of motor units reduces. This review covers the most commonly used techniques of MUNE: incremental stimulation, multiple-point stimulation, the F-wave method, spike-triggered averaging, and the statistical method. There are several assumptions inherent in every technique of MUNE,[7] including the following:

1. Sampling a limited number of motor units in a muscle is representative of the entire population of motor units in the muscle.
2. All motor units are of similar size.
3. Motor units are the same size with each activation.
4. All motor axons are activated by maximal stimulation.

Violations of these assumptions occur with neurogenic disease because motor units are different sizes, axons may have different thresholds to stimulation, and it may be more difficult to obtain representation of all the motor units by testing a small area. However, the reliability and use of the MUNE count in clinical studies of ALS patients and controls are excellent, which supports its continued use.[5]

The choice of the MUNE method for use depends on several factors. For proximal muscles, spike-triggered averaging is the best choice. With limitations in equipment choices, multiple-point stimulation is easy to perform using any EMG equipment. If speed is desired, incremental stimulation and the statistical method are automated and quick. The advantages and disadvantages of each technique are discussed below, along with suggestions for performing each study and clinical applications.

INCREMENTAL STIMULATION

The first technique of MUNE was developed by McComas and colleagues in 1971.[8] This technique is termed *incremental stimulation* and is based on surface nerve stimulation of single motor unit action potentials by gradually increasing the intensity of electrical stimulation in steps so that the mean SMUP can be calculated. A single all-or-none motor unit is the first response generated, gradually increasing in a stepwise manner until 10 or more individual responses are obtained. With increasing steps, it is difficult to distinguish additional SMUPs, so an average SMUP is determined by dividing the amplitude of the last step by the number of steps (Figure 14.1).

The advantages of incremental stimulation include its speed and patient comfort. Its disadvantages include the requirement for small distal muscles, its difficulty to use, superficial nerves, and alternation. *Alternation* refers to the problems that occur when two motor units are capable of being activated at the same stimulus level. One or the other (or both) motor units may be recruited at any given time. Computer processing during data acquisition has helped to alleviate this problem.[9] New motor units are difficult to distinguish with increasing stimulus level because of the need to increase the gain to accommodate the increasing CMAP on the screen and because

Figure 14.1 Incremental responses of extensor digitorum brevis in a 30-year-old man after excitation of deep peroneal nerve with threshold and slightly suprathreshold stimuli (**A**) and maximal stimuli (**B**). In (**A**), several traces have been superimposed for each size of response. In the lowest trace (**C**), surface electrodes on the dorsum of the foot were used to excite selectively the first dorsal interosseus muscle, and the electrotonically conducted potentials were recorded by the standard electrodes over the extensor digitorum brevis and the sole. The earth electrode was situated between the stimulating and recording electrodes. (Reprinted with permission from AJ McComas, PR Fawcett, MJ Campbell, RE Sica. Electrophysiological estimation of the number of motor units within a human muscle. J Neurol Neurosurg Psychiatry 1971;34:121–131.)

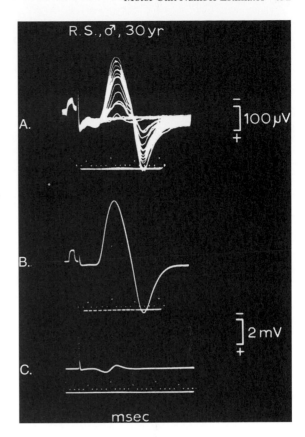

of stimulus artifact.[10] Small-amplitude motor units may be missed with this technique, resulting in an overestimate of the mean SMUP size and an underestimate of MUNE. Several modifications have been developed to minimize these errors.[9,11,12] Incremental stimulation MUNE has been applied to super dioxide dismutase (SOD1) transgenic knockout mice and familial ALS mice. The motor unit number in the distal hind limb declined even before weakness was observed, and the SMUP increased accordingly.[13]

Methodology

Surface recording electrodes are used, and the active electrode is placed over the motor point of the muscle of interest with the reference electrode appropriately placed, as in routine motor nerve conduction studies. The stimulating disk electrodes are placed over the motor nerve, and incremental responses are evoked (in small steps to stimulate individual axons progressively) at approximately 1 Hz. The responses are amplified and displayed on an oscilloscope.[14] The average SMUP is estimated from the average CMAP increment. Modifications include automated computer measurement of the steps and increasing the stimulus size. A software program can control the stimulus intensity, and detection of new response increments is achieved by fast Fourier analysis. Individual motor unit potentials are derived by the subtraction of templates in the computer memory, and the areas rather than the amplitudes of the responses are used in the calculations. A separate algorithm detects and rejects instances of alternation. Largely because of the elimination of alternation, the MUNEs tend to be lower than those obtained by the manual method.[9]

Application in Control Subjects

In healthy controls, 79 subjects aged 20–98 years underwent MUNE on the thenar, biceps, and extensor digitorum brevis muscles. MUNE was noted to decrease significantly with age in the distal muscles but appeared to remain constant in the biceps muscles. The test-retest coefficient of variation was reported at 20%[9] and 11–32%.[14] MUNE values ranged from 31 to 421 for the thenar muscle, 33 to 316 for the biceps brachii muscle, and 22 to 253 for the extensor digitorum brevis muscle, with statistically significant differences occurring in MUNE in subjects between ages 20 and 39 years and older than age 60 years, except for the biceps brachii muscle, in which there was no decline with aging.[9]

Application in Disease

Application of incremental stimulation to acute motor axonal neuropathy syndrome showed that MUNE was decreased at the peak of the illness and recovered more slowly with time than did the CMAP amplitude, suggesting that early recovery in acute motor axonal neuropathy may be due to collateral reinnervation and later recovery due to nerve regeneration.[15] MUNE was used to assess 18 patients with congenital brachial palsy recording from the thenar and biceps brachii muscles, along with hypothenar MUNE in 11 of the subjects. MUNE was approximately half of the control value for affected arms, and the mean MUNE was reduced in unaffected arms but was not significantly different from the control mean.[16]

Motor unit numbers measured with the manual incremental method were correlated with the maximal discharge rate in concentric needle EMG recordings. There was a strong correlation between the number of motor units and the maximal discharge rate, with the rate increasing with denervation in patients having a variety of underlying causes. There was no change in the discharge rate or motor unit number in patients with myopathies.[17]

Incremental stimulation has been applied in several studies of motor neuron disease. Incremental stimulation was used in 76 patients with prior polio, showing a 13% reduction in motor unit number, which was twice that occurring from normal aging in healthy subjects aged older than 60 years.[18] Survival was predicted in ALS using the thenar, hypothenar, and extensor digitorum brevis muscles and correlating them with isometric grip, foot dorsiflexion strength, and forced vital capacity in 34 patients. The change in MUNE was highly predictive of survival from time of disease onset as compared to other measures.[19] A longitudinal analysis of 123 patients with ALS showed that all tested muscles had motor unit loss. The MUNE value typically dropped by 50% over a 6-month period and then more slowly thereafter.[20] Finally, a combination of incremental stimulation and the statistical method was used to compare the abductor pollicis brevis and abductor digiti minimi muscles in ALS patients, and it was noticed that the extent of motor unit loss was greater in the abductor pollicis brevis than in the abductor digiti minimi muscle. This ratio was

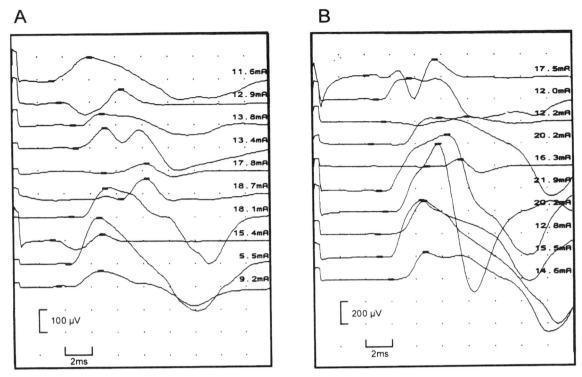

Figure 14.2 Samples of hypothenar surface-recorded motor unit potentials collected by the multiple-point method in a control subject (**A**) and in an amyotrophic lateral sclerosis patient (**B**). Recordings were initially made using a gain of 100–200 μV per division; however, if individual surface-recorded motor unit potentials blocked the amplifier, then lower gains (e.g., 500 μV/division) were used. Notice the differences in gain between the control and amyotrophic lateral sclerosis patient. (Reprinted with permission from C Lomen-Hoerth, RK Olney. Comparison of multiple point and statistical motor unit number estimation. Muscle Nerve 2000;23:1525–1533.)

smaller than that found in healthy subjects, patients with cervical spondylotic amyotrophy, Kennedy's syndrome, or peripheral neuropathy.[21]

MULTIPLE-POINT STIMULATION

Kadrie et al. first described multiple-point stimulation.[22] Doherty et al. applied multiple-point stimulation to motor unit number estimation to avoid the problem of alternation with the incremental stimulation method.[12] Samples of SMUPs are collected based on an all-or-none response to ensure that only one motor axon has been activated. Stimulation intensity is set low enough to only activate one motor axon, and different motor axons are obtained by moving up or down the motor nerve. An average of 10 SMUPs are used to calculate the MUNE value (Figure 14.2).

This technique is relatively easy to learn and is not painful for the patient. Long superficial nerves are needed for stimulation, and it samples only 10–20 SMUPs to compute the mean SMUP. The main concern with this technique is the possibility that these units do not adequately represent all the motor units of different sizes contributing to the CMAP. It is critical to make sure the SMUP represents an all-or-none result by increasing and decreasing the stimulus intensity slightly to confirm. This method is more time consuming than the previous method of incremental stimulation, but computerized software for acquisition has helped to speed up this technique.[1]

Methodology

Recording electrodes are set up as for a motor nerve conduction study, with the active electrode over the motor point and the reference appropriately placed. A maximum CMAP is generated and then the stimulating electrode is moved up and down the nerve with low-intensity stimulation (only as much as is needed to generate one all-or-none response). The current is then increased and decreased slightly to ensure an all-or-none response. Multiple-point stimulation uses low-intensity stimulation that activates only one SMUP at each point along the motor nerve. The stimulating electrode is moved to obtain different SMUPs at different sites. Ten or more responses are recorded from different stimulation sites and averaged together. The MUNE is calculated as described earlier.

Application in Control Subjects

Young and old subjects were compared using multiple-point stimulation, showing that the MUNE value declines nearly 50% with aging for the thenar muscle, similar to the results found for incremental stimulation. The test-retest reproducibility was excellent, with a correlation coefficient of 0.88. MUNE values averaged 288 ± 95 for subjects 20–40 years of age and 139 ± 68 for subjects older than 63 years of age.[23] Other investigators found similar results with aging for the thenar muscle group, showing progressive decline with age that correlated with the decline in the maximal single thenar motor unit F-wave velocities.[24,25] Finally, studying the thenar muscle in 16 controls, the test-retest correlation coefficient was 0.85, with a mean difference between test-retest values of 17% for healthy subjects, and the number of motor units ranged from 122 to 386.[26]

Application in Disease

In a cross-sectional study, maximal voluntary isometric contraction, CMAP, and MUNE were recorded in the intrinsic hand muscles of 10 subjects with ALS/motor neuron disease. Test-retest correlations were excellent for all measures; however, MUNE did not correlate well with grip, perhaps owing to the fact that MUNE does not reflect reinnervation.[27] In a longitudinal study over 1 year, the change in MUNE was the most sensitive measure of ALS progression, compared to CMAP amplitude, isometric hand grip strength, Medical Research Council manual muscle testing score, Appel ALS functional rating scale, and forced vital capacity.[4] Felice also reported reproducibility in 20 ALS patients and demonstrated greater reproducibility in ALS patients than in controls 43 ± 36 (range, 6–145), r = 0.99 (p <.001).[26]

F-RESPONSE METHOD

Analysis of F waves is an alternative method to measure the SMUP. F waves that are reproducibly the same size and shape are likely to be single SMUPs and can be used to determine an average SMUP size.[28,29] An automated computer-based technique for

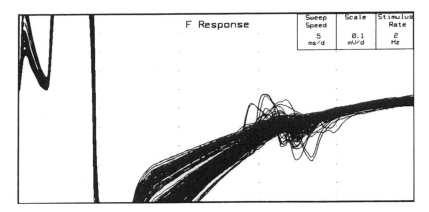

Figure 14.3 Drawn superimposed in a 50-millisecond sweep with 5 millisecond per division are 300 typical M potentials and their related F responses. The M potentials are clipped at the amplitude scale used (0.1 mV/division). The range of F-response onset latencies (27–32 milliseconds) and magnitudes (up to 450 μV peak-to-peak) can be approximated. The variability of the M potential after positivity can also be seen. F responses can then be analyzed in individual raster sweeps. (Reprinted with permission from DW Stashuk, TJ Doherty, A Kassam, WF Brown. Motor unit number estimates based on the automated analysis of F-responses. Muscle Nerve 1994;17:881–890.)

analysis of F waves has been developed to isolate the responses representing single SMUPs.[29]

This technique is well tolerated because low-intensity stimulation is used and provides information about the conduction velocities of motor units at the same time. As for the other techniques discussed thus far, distal muscles with superficial nerves are required for analysis. There may be a problem with activation of multiple rather than single motor units. This can result in overestimating the SMUP, which then underestimates the MUNE. Automated correction of these drawbacks by template-matching software has helped to correct this problem.[29] Finally, only a small percentage of the stimuli generate an F wave, which may theoretically bias the size of SMUP, but, practically, there does not appear to be a clear selection bias[28] (Figure 14.3).

Methodology

Surface electrodes are positioned over the motor end plate of the respective muscle, and the reference electrode is placed appropriately, as in conventional F-wave latency measurements. The nerve is stimulated with disk electrodes at 10–50% of the maximum needed to obtain a supramaximal CMAP. Three hundred stimuli are applied at 2 Hz. To qualify, the waveform needs to be repeated and show the identical shape, size, and latency. The program then stores all F waves that meet these criteria. The stimulator may need to be adjusted to collect more F waves if the first site does not provide the numbers needed.[29]

Application in Control Subjects

Young and old subjects were compared using the SMUP of the thenar muscle, and the older subjects had a 39% higher SMUP than younger subjects, resulting in a lower MUNE.[28,29] The MUNE values in 33 subjects ranged from 101 to 457 with manual collection and from 83 to 493 with automated selection, with a test-retest correlation coefficient of 0.71.[29]

Applications in Disease

The F-response method has been applied to patients with stroke, comparing the motor unit numbers between the affected and unaffected sites. There was no difference between motor unit numbers on either side and between test and retest values on the same side in healthy subjects. Among stroke patients, the motor unit number was lower on the affected side. This was hypothesized to be due to the transsynaptic degeneration secondary to an upper motor neuron lesion.[30]

A cross-sectional study of 10 ALS patients comparing MUNE, CMAP amplitude, fiber density, macro EMG amplitude, and maximal isometric strength demonstrated no significant correlations among these measures.[31] The F-response method was applied in ALS patients and compared to control subjects using the thenar muscle. There were significant differences between MUNE of patients and controls.[32]

SPIKE-TRIGGERED AVERAGING

The spike-triggered averaging technique is the only technique that does not rely on stimulation of the motor nerve to obtain SMUP but, instead, uses voluntary activation of motor units.[33] It requires placement of an EMG electrode into the muscle, allowing additional electrophysiologic information to be recorded simultaneously with the collection of SMUP. Using a single-fiber, concentric, or monopolar EMG needle electrode and a two-channel EMG machine, SMUP sizes are averaged from a second channel that is recording the surface EMG, triggered by a motor unit potential isolated on the first channel. Several SMUPs are recorded and averaged to determine the mean SMUP (Figure 14.4).

This method is the only method that can record from more proximal muscles or muscles with deep nerves. It can be performed with any electromyographic equipment that has signal-averaging capacities. It is, however, invasive and does require cooperation from the subject during testing. There is a risk that the single-fiber triggering electrode may pick up temporally distributed potentials arising from fibers of the same motor unit and also different motor units, disrupting the triggering process. In diseased muscle, there may be variations in conduction and jitter and in terminal nerve twigs; thus, the single-fiber potential is no longer a stable trigger source. Spike-triggered averaging assumes that voluntary activation recruits the full range of sizes of motor units, and because the smaller, most readily recruited units are recorded, there may be a bias toward higher MUNE values.[34] The spike-triggered technique has been improved by the addition of automated decomposition software that simultaneously identifies several motor units that can be used as trigger sources to extract several SMUPs at the same time, shortening the time required to perform this technique.[29]

Methodology

A strip electrode is placed on the motor point of the muscle of interest with an appropriately placed reference electrode to record SMUPs from a triggering motor unit. The triggering spikes are recorded from different depths and different

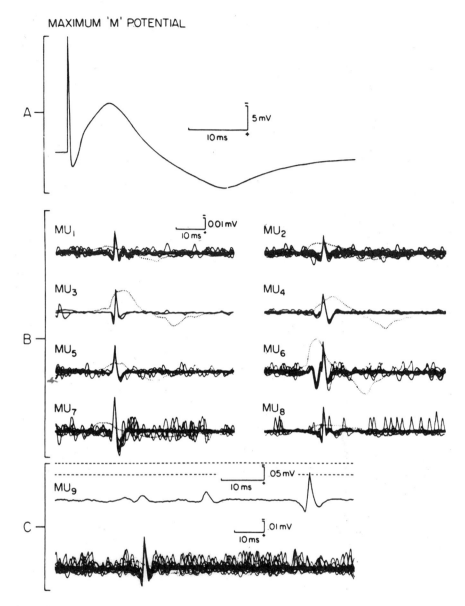

Figure 14.4 Studies from one representative control subject (36 years of age). **A.** The maximum biceps-brachialis M potential in response to supramaximal stimulation of the musculocutaneous nerve. **B.** Eight of 10 surface-recorded and electronically averaged motor unit potentials (*dotted traces*) are shown superimposed on their corresponding intramuscularly recorded triggering potentials—successive potential triggered sweeps of which, delayed by a constant period set by the operator, are superimposed and stored. The surface-recorded motor unit potentials were all biphasic and, in every case, shorter than 40 milliseconds in duration. The amplitude calibration refers to the surface-recorded motor unit potentials and not to the intramuscular recordings, which were carried out at various gains differing by up to 10-fold. **C.** The ninth of 10 motor units selected in this study. At the top are shown the upper and lower window levels set by the operator to help select one spike potential from among the several spikes of differing size corresponding to the recruitment of other motor units. Below are shown the corresponding superimposed and stored successive spike-triggered and delayed sweeps on which are imposed the averaged surface-recorded motor unit potential that was time locked to the chosen spike. The subject in this case was asked to make a steady isometric contraction of moderate intensity. (Reprinted with permission from WF Brown, MJ Strong, R Snow. Methods for estimating numbers of motor units in biceps-brachialis muscles and losses of motor units with aging. Muscle Nerve 1988;11:423–432.)

parts of the muscle. A single-fiber macro-EMG recording electrode is introduced into the muscle 3–5 cm distal to the recording electrode. The triggering motor unit spike potentials are generated by weak voluntary muscle contractions, and the SMUP is recorded by the strip electrode.[35] A variation of this technique involving decomposition of the EMG signal has helped to shorten the time of the study and of subject cooperation.[36]

Application in Control Subjects

Spike-triggered averaging was tested in the biceps brachii of 40 healthy subjects, showing a 50% drop in MUNE with aging by comparing subjects younger than 60 years of age to those older than 60 years of age. The results for subjects younger than 60 years of age was 911 ± 254 and 479 ± 220 for those older than 60 years of age.[33] These values differ from the results for incremental stimulation for the same muscle, which showed no decline with aging.[9]

Applications in Disease

The spike-triggered averaging technique was applied to the elbow flexor muscles in 31 patients with ALS, comparing MUNE with isometric strength, CMAP, SMUP amplitude, and fiber density. The results showed excellent test-retest reproducibility with a correlation coefficient of 0.54. EMG values and MUNE were similarly correlated with isometric strength. Isometric strength and MUNE were the only independent measures reaching statistical significance.[27]

STATISTICAL METHOD

Daube developed a statistical method for MUNE based on the observation that when a nerve is stimulated at a given current level, the responses naturally tend to form a Poisson distribution, as do other phenomena in nature, such as quanta release at the neuromuscular junction.[37] A Poisson distribution has decreased numbers at higher values, forming a right skew (named for the direction of the long tail). The variance among a series of values that have a Poisson distribution is equal to the mean size of the varying units. This technique analyzes the variance of submaximal CMAP sizes that have a Poisson distribution to determine the mean size of motor units at that stimulus intensity, thus eliminating the need for potentials associated with individual units to be identified. Because the statistical method measures only the variance of the CMAP and does not require identification of individual components, it can be used when the sizes of single motor unit potentials are too small to be isolated, and it can also measure the variance of high-amplitude CMAPs.

In contrast to other techniques, the statistical method is useful to determine the size of the mean SMUP at stimulus intensities at which many SMUPs are activated, sampling at least 30% of the total population of SMUPs. This method examines both high threshold and low threshold units. Furthermore, the size of the mean SMUP is usually determined at more than one stimulus intensity. In one study, the statistical method is quicker than the multiple-point technique and has excellent reproducibility.[38] The main difficulty with the technique is accepting the validity of the Poisson statistics as applied to this situation. With reinnervation, the motor units do not remain the same size—a requirement of Poisson statistics. The MUNE must be done showing a display of the histogram of the responses to ensure that the responses form a Poisson distribution for the calculation to be valid. A normal or right-skewed distribution (Poisson) results in an accurate calculation of the MUNE; however, a left-skewed distribution (the opposite of a Poisson distribution) produces significant errors and results in an artificially high MUNE. The statistical method is more complicated to learn than the other methods, but it has excellent test-retest reproducibility and is quick once the user is familiar with the technique.

Methodology

Motor electrodes are placed over the motor point, and the reference electrode is placed appropriately, as in routine motor nerve conduction studies. Stimulating electrodes are taped over the nerve to obtain a maximal CMAP and for submaximal stimulation. For best reproducibility, each MUNE submaximal stimulation should be recorded at four standardized stimulation current levels in control subjects and two to four stimulation current levels in disease subjects.[38] Using nomenclature in which 0% equals the highest stimulus intensity that does not activate the initial threshold SMUP and 100% is the lowest stimulus intensity that activates all SMUP, these standardized recording windows are 10–20%, 25–35%, 40–50%, and 55–65%. Within each recording window, series of 30 submaximal CMAPs were recorded continuously until the standard deviation was less than 10% of the mean, and recording was then stopped. For best reproducibility, before recording begins in each window, the stimulation current is set in the lower quarter of the window and not varied during testing.[39] A Poisson distribution is reliably observed the majority of the time.

For ALS patients, standardized recording window levels are not used if there is a greater than 15% gap on the scan that was confirmed by recording 30 submaximal CMAPs in a recording window set to contain the gap and the first submaximal CMAP above and below the gap. The recording windows often need to be expanded if there is no submaximal CMAP variation within the 10% recording window owing to loss of motor units. When more than 50% of the responses fall outside of the recording window, the recording window is expanded. MUNE is calculated with the number-weighted statistical method, in which the mean SMUP amplitude at each level is multiplied by the number of motor units estimated at each level, the products are added, and the result is divided by the sum of the number of motor units determined at each level.[40] The maximum CMAP amplitude for each test is divided by this modified mean SMUP amplitude to calculate the MUNE. For ALS patients in whom a single SMUP was demonstrated to account for greater than or equal to 15% of the entire CMAP range by itself, the calculations are modified. The size of this SMUP is then measured as a percent of the CMAP range, and it is counted as one toward the MUNE; then, the corresponding percentage is subtracted from 100% before calculating the remaining number of motor units[38] (Figure 14.5).

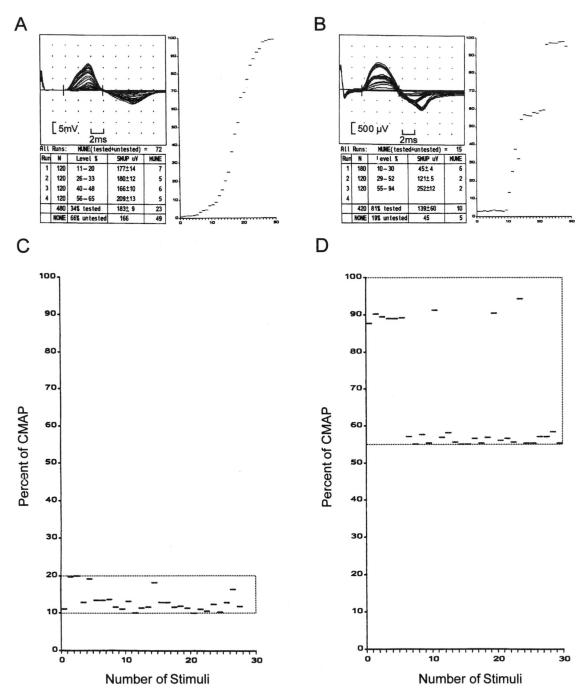

Figure 14.5 Samples of scans spanning from 0% to 100% stimulus (**A,B**) and recording windows spanning an individual testing range (**C,D**) performed by the statistical method in a control subject (**A,C**) and in an amyotrophic lateral sclerosis patient (**B,D**). For controls, 30 submaximal stimulations at 2–3 Hz were recorded (one group demonstrated in **C**), and the process was repeated at each of the above stimulus ranges until the standard error of the mean surface-recorded motor unit potential (SMUP) was less than 10% or 10 trials were completed (one run). For controls, the four standard levels were chosen for all four runs. For the amyotrophic lateral sclerosis patient, (**D**) demonstrates a single large SMUP that was counted visually and manually calculated into the total motor unit number estimation (MUNE) using the modified statistical method. This resulted in a value nearly identical to the program-determined value and higher than the weighted statistical values. (CMAP = compound muscle action potential.) (Reprinted with permission from C Lomen-Hoerth, RK Olney. Comparison of multiple point and statistical motor unit number estimation. Muscle Nerve 2000;23:1525–1533.)

Application in Control Subjects

The first data regarding MUNE in control subjects were reported in an abstract form in 1988 by Daube, who developed the statistical method technique, briefly discussed the methodology, and described the values in control ALS and polio subjects.[37] Control subjects had an average thenar MUNE of 315 ± 48 and an extensor digitorum brevis MUNE of 185 ± 48. In a review article, Daube reports a standard deviation of less than 10% for SMUPs with repeated measurement of groups of 30 stimuli in control subjects.[2] Excellent reproducibility has been shown by a variety of investigators. In a study by Simmons and colleagues,[41] 48 healthy subjects were analyzed with the statistical method, and the intrasubject coefficient of variation was measured. Averaging two MUNE observations for each determination brought the intrasubject coefficient of variation from 16.48% to 8.77%. MUNE reproducibility was found to improve when a new method of calculation was used. Instead of estimating what the untested units would be by assigning a motor unit size equal to the smallest size estimate made at any stimulus strength, the motor unit size estimates were weighted according to the number of motor units estimated at any given response level. This variation produced improvements in test-retest reliability and a reduction in the total MUNE with an average of 143 ± 26 for the hypothenar muscle group.[40] Further modifications in performing the technique (as described in the section Methodology above) resulted in a coefficient of variation of 7% for a single test in both control and ALS subjects.[39]

Application in Disease

Reproducibility studies in ALS patients demonstrate excellent test-retest reproducibility for the MUNE in hypothenar muscle groups.[42] Reproducibility in ALS was studied in 16 ALS patients tested on 52 occasions, with coefficients of variation of 19% and correlation coefficients from 0.75 to 0.86.[42] Using the new methods outlined above, the coefficient of variation was reduced to 7% for a single test.[39]

Even in the absence of significant change in clinical weakness of CMAP amplitude, there is a significant decrease in the number of motor units in ALS patients over time.[3] Thus, MUNE changes are more sensitive measures of ALS progression than are isometric hand-grip strength or the size of the CMAP and should be helpful to measure rate of progression in experimental studies and change of rate in response in drug trials.[2,6]

COMPARISON OF TECHNIQUES

There have been few studies directly comparing these MUNE techniques to one another. One study compares multiple-point and statistical methods in the same subject population.[38] Twenty controls and 10 ALS patients underwent left hypothenar muscle group MUNE with both techniques. For controls, the mean of two MUNE (± standard deviation) was 60 (±5) for the statistical method and 108 (±38) for multiple point. For ALS patients, these values were 21 (±16) for the statistical method and 55 (±39) for multiple point. Test-retest correlation coefficients and coefficients of variation for the mean of two MUNE were 0.98 and 7% for the statistical method and 0.90 and 12% for multiple point, respectively. The statistical method was more reproducible and faster than multiple point, supporting its use in monitoring rates of MUNE change.[38]

The other published study comparing MUNE techniques in the same patient population included multiple-point stimulation with spike-triggered averaging in control subjects.[12] Fourteen healthy subjects were studied with both techniques on the thenar muscle, and the results showed excellent correlation between the techniques, with a correlation coefficient of 0.82 ($p < .001$). The MUNE values were 160 ± 78 for the spike-triggered averaging technique and 160 ± 70 for the multiple-point stimulation technique. Both techniques gave identical values for MUNE and were similar in reproducibility.

CORRELATION WITH PATHOLOGY

No one knows what the real number of functioning motor units to a muscle is to compare these techniques, but work by Santo and others[43] used histologic methods to estimate the number and size of human flexor digiti minimi muscle motor units from 10 fresh cadavers aged 33–74 years. An assumption was made that 60% of all large-sized myelinated nerve fibers were alpha motor neurons. Results showed an average number of 130 motor units, fitting with the range of MUNE values determined from all of the different techniques outlined above except for the statistical method. The number of motor units did not decrease in subjects older than 70 years compared to those younger than 70 years.[43] Practically, the actual number may not matter as much as its reproducibility, because there is a wide range of normal values, and change over time may be the only way to document disease progression.

CONCLUSIONS

Motor unit number estimates may be useful in monitoring the progression of neurogenic diseases for research and clinical purposes. There are several well-studied methods for MUNE that are reproducible and have been applied successfully to neurogenic diseases. The choice of method depends on several factors, including proximal versus distal muscles, the equipment available, speed, the ability of the patient to cooperate with the study, and the experience of the examiner performing the studies. Currently, there is no consensus on the best method of study, given the advantages and disadvantages of each method. However, at least one of these techniques should be taught as a part of electrodiagnostic training, given its use in monitoring change and application in drug trials for neurogenic diseases.

REFERENCES

1. McComas AJ. Motor unit estimation: anxieties and achievements. Muscle Nerve 1995;18:369–379.
2. Daube JR. Estimating the number of motor units in a muscle. J Clin Neurophysiol 1995;12: 585–594.
3. Shefner JM. Motor unit number estimation in human neurological diseases and animal models. Clin Neurophysiol 2001;112(6):955–964.
4. Felice KJ. A longitudinal study comparing thenar motor unit number estimates to other quantitative tests in patients with amyotrophic lateral sclerosis. Muscle Nerve 1997;20:179–185.

5. Olney RK, Lomen-Hoerth C. Motor unit number estimation: how may it contribute to the diagnosis of ALS? Amyotroph Lateral Scler Other Motor Neuron Disord 2000;23:S41–S49.

6. Yuen EC, Olney RK. Longitudinal study of fiber density and motor unit number estimate in patients with amyotrophic lateral sclerosis. Neurology 1997;49:573–578.

7. Slawnych MP, Laszlo CA, Hershler C. A review of techniques employed to estimate the number of motor units in a muscle. Muscle Nerve 1990;13:1050–1064.

8. McComas AJ, Fawcett PR, Campbell MJ, Sica RE. Electrophysiological estimation of the number of motor units within a human muscle. J Neurol Neurosurg Psychiatry 1971;34:121–131.

9. Galea V, de Bruin H, Cavasin R, McComas AJ. The numbers and relative sizes of motor units estimated by computer. Muscle Nerve 1991;14:1123–1130.

10. Milner-Brown HS, Brown WF. New methods of estimating the number of motor units in a muscle. J Neurol Neurosurg Psychiatry 1976;39:258–265.

11. Ballantyne JP, Hansen S. New method for the estimation of the number of motor units in a muscle. 2. Duchenne, limb-girdle and facioscapulohumeral, and myotonic muscular dystrophies. J Neurol Neurosurg Psychiatry 1974;37:1195–1201.

12. Doherty TJ, Stashuk DW, Brown WF. Determinants of mean motor unit size: impact on estimates of motor unit number. Muscle Nerve 1993;16:1326–1331.

13. Shefner JM, Reaume AG, Flood DG, et al. Mice lacking cytosolic copper/zinc superoxide dismutase display a distinctive motor axonopathy. Neurology 1999;53:1239–1246.

14. McComas AJ. Invited review: motor unit estimation: methods, results, and present status. Muscle Nerve 1991;14:585–597.

15. Kuwabara S, Ogawara K, Mizobuchi K, et al. Mechanisms of early and late recovery in acute motor axonal neuropathy. Muscle Nerve 2001;24:288–291.

16. Scarfone H, McComas AJ, Pape K, Newberry R. Denervation and reinnervation in congenital brachial palsy. Muscle Nerve 1999;22:600–607.

17. Schulte-Mattler WJ, Georgiadis D, Tietze K, Zierz S. Relation between maximum discharge rates on electromyography and motor unit number estimates. Muscle Nerve 2000;23:231–238.

18. McComas AJ, Quartly C, Griggs RC. Early and late losses of motor units after poliomyelitis. Brain 1997;120:1415–1421.

19. Armon C, Brandstater ME. Motor unit number estimate-based rates of progression of ALS predict patient survival. Muscle Nerve 1999;22:1571–1575.

20. Dantes M, McComas A. The extent and time course of motoneuron involvement in amyotrophic lateral sclerosis. Muscle Nerve 1991;14:416–421.

21. Kuwabara S, Mizobuchi K, Ogawara K, Hattori T. Dissociated small hand muscle involvement in amyotrophic lateral sclerosis detected by motor unit number estimates. Muscle Nerve 1999; 22:870–873.

22. Kadrie HYS, Milner-Brown WF. Multiple point electrical stimulation of ulnar and median nerves. J Neurol Neurosurg Psychiatry 1976;39:973–985.

23. Doherty TJ, Brown WF. The estimated numbers and relative sizes of thenar motor units as selected by multiple point stimulation in young and older adults. Muscle Nerve 1993;16:355–366.

24. Wang FC, de Pasqua V, Delwaide PJ. Age-related changes in fastest and slowest conducting axons of thenar motor units. Muscle Nerve 1999;22:1022–1029.

25. Wang FC, Delwaide PJ. Number and relative size of thenar motor units estimated by an adapted multiple point stimulation method. Muscle Nerve 1995;18:969–979.

26. Felice KJ. Thenar motor unit number estimates using the multiple point stimulation technique: reproducibility studies in ALS patients and normal subjects. Muscle Nerve 1995;18:1412–1416.

27. Bromberg MB, Larson WL. Relationships between motor-unit number estimates and isometric strength in distal muscles in ALS/MND. J Neurol Sci 1996;139(Suppl):38–42.

28. Doherty TJ, Komori T, Stashuk DW, et al. Physiological properties of single thenar motor units in the F-response of younger and older adults. Muscle Nerve 1994;17:860–872.

29. Stashuk D, Qu Y. Adaptive motor unit action potential clustering using shape and temporal information. Med Biol Eng Comput 1996;34:41–49.

30. Hara Y, Akaboshi K, Masakado Y, Chino N. Physiologic decrease of single thenar motor units in the F-response in stroke patients. Arch Phys Med Rehabil 2000;81:418–423.

31. Bromberg MB, Forshew DA, Nau KL, et al. Motor unit number estimation, isometric strength, and electromyographic measures in amyotrophic lateral sclerosis. Muscle Nerve 1993;16:1213–1219.

32. Felice KJ. Nerve conduction velocities of single thenar motor axons based on the automated analysis of F waves in amyotrophic lateral sclerosis. Muscle Nerve 1998;21:756–761.

33. Brown WF, Strong MJ, Snow R. Methods for estimating numbers of motor units in biceps-brachialis muscles and losses of motor units with aging. Muscle Nerve 1988;11:423–432.

34. Bromberg MB, Abrams JL. Sources of error in the spike-triggered averaging method of motor unit number estimation (MUNE). Muscle Nerve 1995;18:1139–1146.

35. Bromberg MB. Motor unit estimation: reproducibility of the spike-triggered averaging technique in normal and ALS subjects. Muscle Nerve 1993;16:466–471.

36. Stashuk DW, Doherty TJ, Kassam A, Brown WF. Motor unit number estimates based on the automated analysis of F-responses. Muscle Nerve 1994;17:881–890.

37. Daube JR. Statistical estimates of number of motor units in the thenar and foot muscles in patients with amyotrophic lateral sclerosis of the residual of polymyositis. Muscle Nerve 1988;11:957–958.

38. Lomen-Hoerth C, Olney RK. Comparison of multiple point and statistical motor unit number estimation. Muscle Nerve 2000;23:1525–1533.

39. Lomen-Hoerth C, Olney RK. Effect of recording window and stimulation variables on the statistical technique of motor unit number estimation. Muscle Nerve 2001;24(12):1659–1664.

40. Shefner JM, Jillapalli D, Bradshaw DY. Reducing intersubject variability in motor unit number estimation. Muscle Nerve 1999;22:1457–1460.

41. Simmons Z, Epstein DK, Borg B, et al. Reproducibility of motor unit number estimation in individual subjects. Muscle Nerve 2001;24:467–473.

42. Olney RK, Yuen EC, Engstrom JW. Statistical motor unit number estimation: reproducibility and sources of error in patients with amyotrophic lateral sclerosis. Muscle Nerve 2000;23:193–197.

43. Santo Neto H, de Carvalho VC, Marques MJ. Estimation of the number and size of human flexor digiti minimi muscle motor units using histological methods. Muscle Nerve 1998;21:112–114.

15

Quantitative Assessment of Muscle Strength and Mechanical Performance: Dynamometry, Ergometry, and Muscle Contraction Analysis Techniques

Judy W. Griffin and Mary L. O'Toole

Weakness and fatigue, classic symptoms in persons with neuromuscular disorders, are essentially problems of voluntary muscle force generation and maintenance.[1] Impaired ability to generate muscular force may occur long before the patient recognizes a change in function.[2,3] However, progressive weakness eventually leads to loss of ability to perform activities of daily living (ADL) and may ultimately result in disability and reduced quality of life.[4]

Measurement of strength (i.e., force generated by a muscle group) is the most direct way to assess impaired muscle function.[2] Change in strength is a key sign of deterioration or improvement in many neuromuscular diseases, and strength measurements are regarded as direct measures of disease status.[5] Objective, reliable, accurate measurements of strength are needed to document the extent of neuromuscular deficit, disease progression, and the effect of therapeutic intervention.[6–9] Measurements should be valid for the specific disease or problem and sensitive enough to monitor strong and weak ends of the strength spectrum.[7,10]

In the evaluation of neuromuscular diseases, assessment of muscle strength and fatigue and the analysis of the metabolic effects of exercise can be used to monitor performance and determine disease progression. Clinical assessments require the patient's maximal voluntary cooperation. However, other assessments that do not require voluntary motor response also provide valuable information. Electrophysiologic studies done routinely in neuromuscular disorders include analysis of electrical activity of nerve and muscle. Analysis of the mechanical properties of muscle contraction, such as measurements of twitch tension, relaxation times, and fatigue, is also valuable. In vitro analysis of muscle contractions is being used in the diagnosing of conditions such as channelopathies. In this chapter, we review the various aspects of muscle performance during isometric and isokinetic testing and ergometry. We also discuss in vivo and in vitro muscle contraction tests and their clinical applications.

STRENGTH TESTING OF PERSONS WITH NEUROMUSCULAR DISORDERS

Terminology and Definitions for Strength Testing

Strength and Weakness

Strength, for the purposes of this chapter, is defined as the force recorded during a maximal voluntary muscular action, when the type of muscle action, limb velocity, and joint angles are specified.[11] *Weakness* is defined as lack of strength. Strength is dependent on factors such as amount of muscle mass, ability to activate motor units, and motivation.[4]

Quantitative and Qualitative Strength Testing

Strength testing is qualitative when examiner judgment determines the force value for the subject's maximal effort; qualitative measurements are recorded on ordinal or nominal scales. *Manual muscle testing* (MMT) is the qualitative strength system most commonly applied in clinical medical contexts. Functional rating scales are another qualitative test frequently used in management of patients with neuromuscular disease; a discussion of functional tests is beyond the scope of this chapter.

Quantitative implies that an instrument is used to determine the value for the subject's maximal voluntary muscular effort. Measurements are objective (not influenced by examiner judgment) and are recorded on an interval scale, usually as force or torque. Units of force (e.g., pounds, kilograms, Newtons) are recorded from the instrument's sensor applied to the body segment being tested. Torque (moment), obtained by multiplying force by the distance of the instrument moment arm, is recorded in units of foot-pounds or Newton-meters. Thus, torque produced by the muscle group being tested is estimated by the instrument; that is, the actual muscle tension force and muscle moment arm are not directly measured.

The types of quantitative muscle testing to be described in this section are strain gauge isometric testing, isokinetic testing, and handheld dynamometry. Advantages and limitations of these methods are listed in Table 15.1. Quantitative strength measurements are now considered an essential component of clinical trials in many neuromuscular diseases[3,10,12,13] and are increasingly being used for documentation in clinical practice.[6]

Reliability and Validity

Reliability refers to consistency and reproducibility of measurements when other conditions are constant.[14] Reliability of measurements for each strength-testing method is included with the related disease category. *Validity* concerns how closely measurements reflect the element to be measured and how the measurements are used.[14,15] Validity of strength measurements is a complex issue. Qualitative and quantitative strength measurements certainly have "face" validity, because they represent records of force exerted by a subject during a maximal voluntary muscular effort. Because no method currently available can exactly measure "true" deficit in voluntary muscle capacity, there is, unhappily, no gold standard against which to compare isometric, isokinetic, and MMT measurements. However, some evidence for validity can be found in studies comparing these measurements with other inde-

Table 15.1 Advantages and Limitations of Strength Tests

Factor	Manual Muscle Test	Isometric (Maximal Voluntary Isometric Contraction)	Isokinetic	Handheld Dynamometer
Cost of instrument	None	Moderate	High	Low
Dedicated space required	No	Yes	Yes	No
Documented reliability of measurements	Yes	Yes	Yes	Yes
Feasibility for exam of multiple muscle groups in single session	Yes	Yes	No	Yes
Useful for measuring strong (MRC score, 4–5) muscle groups	No	Yes	Yes	No
Useful for measuring weak (MRC score, 0–2) muscle groups	Yes	Yes, but further studies needed	Further studies needed	Further studies needed
Standardized testing protocols for neuromuscular disorders	Yes	Yes	No	No

MRC = Medical Research Council.

pendent analyses of muscle function and in studies comparing isometric, isokinetic, and MMT measurements with each other. Reliability and validity are included in discussions of strength measurements.

Impairment, Functional Limitation, and Disability

Health professionals use impairment, functional limitation, and disability when referring to the disablement resulting from disease.[16–18] Strength measurements are measurements of *impairment.* Clinicians consider objective, reliable, and valid measurements of impairment necessary for diagnosis and management of patients with neuromuscular disorders. However, patients (and increasingly those who pay for health care) are concerned with functional limitation and disability, rather than amount of impairment. *Functional limitation* refers to inability to perform usual ADL (e.g., walking, dressing, using public transportation, shopping). *Disability* is the inability to maintain normal role performance within home, work, play, or community sociocultural contexts.[18] Impairments do not necessarily lead to functional limitation or to disability. A patient assessed as having 50% of normal isometric leg strength has an impairment but may not necessarily be unable to walk or to function as parent, spouse, and worker. Yet, all too familiar is the patient with progressive neuromuscular disease who, having exhibited slow, steady deterioration in strength with time, suddenly loses functional ability and becomes disabled.

Critical levels of strength seem to be necessary for performance of specific functional abilities[19]; that is, functional ability can remain unaffected until strength falls below an impairment threshold, at which time an abrupt loss in function occurs. The relationship between strength impairment and functional disability is not linear, however, and it is an area of much needed research.[4] Little evidence indicates what proportion of maximal force is required to perform a functional activity such as walking or rising from a chair.[20] Therefore, how much strength a patient can lose before functional loss is near is unknown. Greater research is needed to identify the critical levels of strength needed in the critical muscle groups to perform specific functional activities. When possible in this discussion of strength impairment measurement, any links to functional limitation or disability are included.

Types of Strength Assessments

Qualitative Strength Measurements: Manual Muscle Testing

The standard clinical test of strength is MMT. The examiner judges strength of the patient's maximal voluntary effort, based on the patient's ability to move a body segment against gravity and then to hold against manual resistance applied by the examiner (Figure 15.1A). The examiner rates strength based on the amount of force applied before the subject "gives" to the examiner's overcoming force. If the subject is unable to move the body segment against gravity, the segment is placed in a gravity-eliminated position, and the examiner rates strength by judging the quantity of active motion present. Strength grades range from 0 to 5 (Medical Research Council [MRC] scale),[21] or the scale can be expanded from 0 to 10 (see Chapter 2).[22,23]

Advantages of Manual Muscle Testing. Muscles can be examined quickly, with little to no equipment required. Thus, severity of weakness in a large number of muscle groups can be determined, which is important for diagnostic purposes.[2] MMT can be conducted in any environment; thus, the patient does not have to be moved to a special area. Testing is relatively inexpensive, with cost primarily related to examiner expertise and time. Testing requires close personal interaction with the patient, and may create more patient cooperation and motivation than is possible when tests interface the patient with a machine. MMT measurements have documented sensitivity and reliability for testing very weak (grade, 0–2) muscles.[24]

Limitations of Manual Muscle Testing. MMT measurements are not objective. Grades are recorded on an ordinal scale, so that categories are ordered from high to low, but intervals are not equally spaced.[9] Ordinal scale data limit statistical data manipulation to nonparametric statistics, which are less powerful and require a greater number of subjects to demonstrate significance in clinical trials.[9,10,19] Reliability studies and natural history studies using MMT have been based on the average score of multiple muscle groups; therefore, MMT would be inappropriate for a therapeutic trial assessing response of a single muscle group.[23]

A major limitation of MMT is its insensitivity at stronger grades (MRC 4 and 5).[2,3,10,12] In a classic study, Beasley[25] confirmed Lovett and Martin's early report[26] of MMT insensitivity in assessing strength of postpolio patients. Beasley documented that knee extensor isometric force measurements for 752 patients that had been graded "normal" by MMT actually averaged 54% of the reference norm (based on measurements from 2,728 knees of healthy subjects). Findings for hip extensor and plantar flexor muscle groups were similar.[25] Thus, patients might lose up to one-half of normal strength before weakness is detectable by

Figure 15.1 Four methods of measuring strength of knee extensor muscle group. Arrows represent direction of external resistance to subject's maximal voluntary knee extension effort. **A.** Manual muscle testing. **B.** Fixed isometric strain-gauge system. **C.** Isokinetic dynamometer. Motion from position 1 to 2 is concentric; motion from 2 to 1 is eccentric contraction of knee extensors. **D.** Handheld dynamometer.

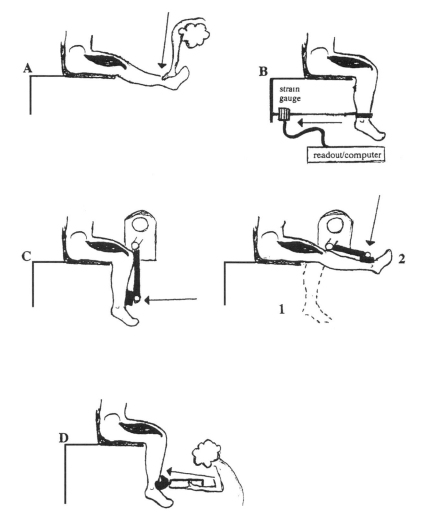

MMT.[25,27] Andres reported that MMT grades in patients with amyotrophic lateral sclerosis (ALS) often remained normal until up to 50% of strength was lost by isometric measurements.[12]

MMT grades recorded for strong subjects (MRC 4 and 5) are influenced by the strength of the examiner[28] and have not been found to correspond well with quantitative measurements.[10,25,29,30] Aitkens et al. compared MMT with isometric force measurements from patients with various chronic neuromuscular diseases, measuring flexor and extensor muscle groups of elbow, hip, and knee. Isometric force values from muscle groups graded as 4 (good) and 5 (normal) were not significantly different.[10] Similar findings were reported for isokinetic versus MMT measurements in patients with ALS (i.e., isokinetic torque values for patients with MMT grades of 3, 4, and 5 overlapped and were indistinguishable).[29,30] Thus, large changes in quantitative strength measurements might occur before change would be detectable with MMT.

Such insensitivity is a great disadvantage in assessment and follow-up of patients with minor degrees of weakness, such as presymptomatic ALS patients[7] or patients recovering from inflammatory myopathy. Longitudinal studies have reported that MMT was less sensitive than isometric measurements in documenting strength change in children with dermatomyositis (DM)[31] and in patients with ALS.[3,12,19] MMT has also been reported to be less sensitive than isokinetic measurements in monitoring strength changes over time in patients with ALS[29,30] and other neuromuscular diseases.[32,33] A serial study of one patient with polymyositis illustrates that isokinetic torque (expressed as percentage of a matched control subject's torque) was much more reflective of her strength changes over time than were MMT measurements (Figure 15.2).[34]

Manual Muscle Testing in Patients with Duchenne's Muscular Dystrophy and Other Neuromuscular Disorders. In a longitudinal study of 23 boys with Duchenne's muscular dystrophy (DMD), Ziter et al. reported a linear decrease in total MMT scores over 8 years, with rates of decline varying among patients.[35] Similar findings were reported by Allsop[36] and Cohen,[37] but reliability of MMT measurements was not assessed in any of those studies. Substantial credibility for MMT as an instrument to detect change in DMD resulted from the pioneering work of Brooke et al.,[38] who included MMT as one element of a standardized protocol. MMT measurements (scored on a transformed scale and averaged over 17 muscle groups) demonstrated high intra- and inter-rater reliability.[24,39,40] Their MMT protocol was used to describe the natural history of DMD and established the amount of strength change expected per unit of time.[22,41–44] Such fundamental research indicated that MMT could be a reliable and sensitive index of DMD disease progression. MMT scores reportedly differentiated a benign form of DMD demonstrated by "outliers," who were only partially deficient in dystrophin, from severe DMD.[23] MMT has now been used as an outcome measure in many clinical trials assessing efficacy of therapeutic agents for DMD.[45–50]

Finding a significant correlation between upper-extremity MMT scores and upper-extremity functional grades in patients with DMD, Lord et al. theorized that MMT of shoulder abductor and elbow flexor muscle groups could be used to predict upper-extremity functional ability.[51] Scott and colleagues reported a significant correlation between total MMT score and the Motor Ability Score of function and concluded that physical performance in DMD depended on strength.[52] Heckmatt et al. noted that walking time and Motor Ability Scores remained fairly steady until boys with DMD abruptly lost ambulatory ability, whereas MMT measurements showed more linear decreases; they concluded that strength change was independent of the functional loss of ambulation.[53]

In longitudinal studies of strength and functional ability in children with DMD, a dominant feature reported was sudden loss of milestone activities such as the ability to stand up from a supine position and walk; MMT measurements during this period showed a constant rate of strength decrease. Apparently, declines in strength did not result in deterioration of function until weakness reached a critical level in key muscle groups.[35,36,51] Allsop reported that the functional task most closely reflecting total MMT strength was standing from a supine position; at the time DMD patients lost this ability, strength loss by MMT was 50% (of total possible score).[36] Loss of independent ambulation in DMD occurred when MMT strength reached 50% (of total possible score).[52,54] Weakness of specific muscle groups could not be related to loss of an ability, such as walking, in patients with DMD.[36,55] However, clinical reports have linked knee extensor and hip abductor groups[52] and hip extensor and knee extensor groups[54,56] to loss of ambulation in DMD.

Figure 15.2 Manual muscle testing (MMT) compared with isokinetic testing values in a patient with polymyositis, for elbow flexion (**A**), knee extension (**B**), and knee flexion (**C**). The patient had two disease exacerbations during time of study, at 6 months and 19 months after initial diagnosis. Relative strength for isokinetic testing is expressed as percent patient torque of the patient's matched control (her sister), given for eccentric (ECC) and concentric (CONC) testing at 30 degrees per second angular velocity. (dx = diagnosis; Mo. = months.)

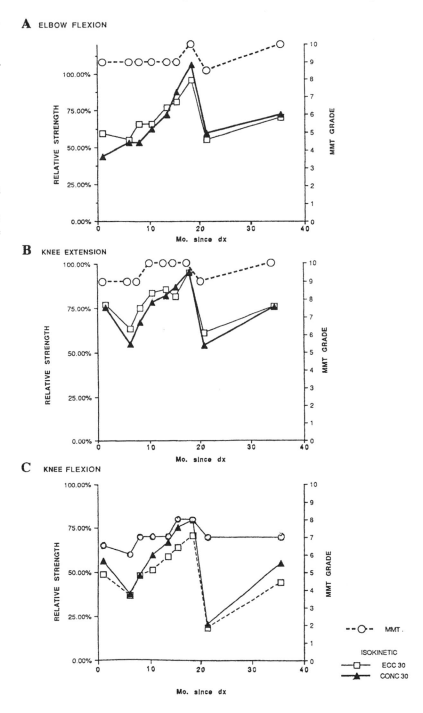

In other muscular dystrophies, such as facioscapulohumeral muscular dystrophy (FSHD), high intra- and inter-rater reliability for MMT measurements have been reported,[57] and MMT has been used in conjunction with quantitative strength testing for natural history studies of this disease.[58,59] MMT has been one of the outcome measures for clinical trials of therapeutic agents for FSHD.[60,61]

In patients with ALS, MMT measurements have some documented reliability; however, the sensitivity to change is reportedly less than with isometric measurements.[8,12] MMT has been used for some natural history studies[62] and clinical trials in ALS.[63,64] Muscle strength (measured by MMT before death) and numbers of large motor neurons (measured at autopsy) werc highly correlated in patients with ALS.[65,66]

Quantitative Strength Tests: Isometric Testing, Isokinetic Testing, and Handheld Dynamometry

Isometric Testing. Force data can be recorded from a subject's maximal voluntary isometric contraction (MVIC) or from dynamic (concentric or eccentric) muscle actions, depending on the biomechanical instrumentation used. In an isometric muscle action, the muscle generates tension, muscle length remains unchanged, and there is no joint motion. Instrumentation for measuring an MVIC has generally been the strain gauge or cable tensiometer (for a review of instrumentation, see Mayhew and Rothstein[20]). Strain gauges have been the most prevalently used instrument in assessing patients with neuromuscular disorders. In the typical fixed isometric testing system, the patient is asked to contract a muscle group maximally against an immovable resistance, provided by a strap attached to the limb. The strap, connected to a strain gauge, is attached to a rigid frame (see Figure 15.1B). Force is transduced with the strain gauge, amplified, and recorded; computerized systems permit calculation of torque and comparisons with stored norms. Hand MVIC can be measured with handgrip and pinch dynamometers; these are not covered in this chapter. Quantitative measurements of respiratory and bulbar function and timed tests of function likewise are not covered.

Early in 1900, Lovett and Martin used isometric strength testing to demonstrate that patients classified as "partly paralyzed" were not equally affected, and they emphasized the necessity for an objective, quantitative method to differentiate levels of weakness.[26] MVIC is by far the oldest and most widely used quantitative strength measurement for patients with neuromuscular disease. Strain-gaugc isometric measurements based on the pioneering studies of Munsat and Andres[8,67,68] with the Tufts Quantitative Neuromuscular Examination (TQNE) and Edwards[1,69] have been rigorously investigated for a variety of neuromuscular diseases (see the section Maximal Voluntary Isometric Contraction Measurements in Patients with Motor Neuron Disease).

ADVANTAGES OF ISOMETRIC TESTING. In isometric and isokinetic testing, examiner strength and judgment are eliminated as error factors, and objective, interval-level data are produced. The fixed strain-gauge MVIC testing system is applicable for patients at mild and severe stages of disease—that is, when patients are asymptomatic (strong) and when weakness exists.[8,57] Multiple muscle groups can be measured with minimal changes of body position required from the patient; thus, isometric testing may be less fatiguing to the patient than isokinetic testing. Weaker muscle groups can be tested in gravity-eliminated or gravity-neutral positions. Standardized protocols for measuring MVIC have been established for disease-specific conditions such as ALS,[8,70] FSHD,[57] and DMD.[71] Testing is fairly cost and time efficient.

LIMITATIONS OF ISOMETRIC MEASUREMENTS. Cost of the isometric testing system is moderate. A dedicated space is required for the rigid testing frame and equipment. The system is not portable, requiring the patient to come to a testing area for strength assessment. The sensitivity for measuring very weak (MRC 2 or lower) muscles may be low.[57] Brussock et al. reported an inability to measure hip extension, adduction, and abduction in boys with DMD because of weakness severity and difficulty preventing substitution patterns.[71]

True for all quantitative measurements (MVIC, isokinetic, and handheld dynamometer [HHD]), torque should preferably be calculated instead of force to account for changes in limb mass or length that occur with growth or disease.[71,72] The capacity for rapid calculation of torque depends on the computer interface available for the strain-gauge testing system.

Also true for any strength test is the fact that measurements can be affected by patient cooperation, understanding, effort, and motivation. Children younger than 5 years generally do not cooperate well with tests of strength impairment.

Isokinetic Testing. Isokinetic dynamometers are used to measure force generated during maximal voluntary dynamic (concentric or eccentric) muscle actions (see Figure 15.1C). In a *dynamic* muscle action, changes occur in muscle length and joint angle as the limb moves through an arc of motion. Dynamic muscle actions can be concentric (muscle shortens while generating tension) or eccentric (muscle lengthens while generating tension). *Isokinetic* refers to the fact that the angular velocity of the limb is held constant and does not refer to a constant velocity of muscle contraction.[73] The patient is asked to move as hard and fast as possible against the lever attached to his extremity. Regardless of the magnitude of force generated by the patient, the velocity of limb motion is constrained to the preset speed (available ranges usually are 0–400 degrees per second). As the patient exerts increased force, resistance to limb motion proportionally increases (accommodating resistance).[74] Most protocols test at a relatively slow (30 or 60 degrees per second) and a relatively fast (120 or 180 degrees per second) angular velocity. An isokinetic dynamometer set at zero velocity can be used to measure MVIC.

ADVANTAGES OF ISOKINETIC TESTING. Isokinetic dynamometer technology enables study of in vivo dynamic muscle capacity.[75] Computerized isokinetic dynamometry provides a record of force, torque, work, or power produced throughout a movement, with the variable of velocity controlled. Isokinetic measurements in patients with neuromuscular disorders may thus provide information about weakness during motion that is not apparent from static MVIC testing. Theoretically, measurement of dynamic muscle capacity might provide a more functional measurement than MVIC; however, no evidence exists that dynamic testing is a better predictor of functional ability than isometric testing.[20]

Isokinetic testing is particularly useful for strong subjects, because the dynamometer cannot be overpowered by the subject.[76] Knee, ankle, and elbow muscle groups are the easiest to test in patient populations.

LIMITATIONS OF ISOKINETIC TESTING. The cost of an isokinetic dynamometer is considerable. A dedicated space is required for equipment and patient testing, similar to that required for a fixed computerized MVIC testing system. Isokinetic testing is time consuming for patient and examiner and may be more fatiguing to the patient than MVIC testing, because each muscle group is usually tested at more than one velocity (if both concentric and eccentric efforts are assessed, more potential fatigue for the patient exists). Isokinetic testing of upper- and lower-extremity or bilateral measurements, or all of these, can require multiple position changes and transfers; this may be difficult for very weak patients.[29] Respiratory compromise of ALS patients in the supine position was a shortcoming reported during upper-extremity testing.[29]

Presence of contractures limits the range of motion available for testing. Patients too weak to move against gravity may be unable to generate enough force to move the extremity plus dynamometer arm at the preset velocity.[29,32] Such problems may be somewhat circumvented if the dynamometer has a robotic (passive mode) capacity.[33] However, reliability of measurements from patients too weak to move actively against gravity using such a protocol has not been reported.

Testing of hip and shoulder muscle groups may be time consuming because special attachments and patient repositioning are usually required, and stabilization of trunk and pelvis for testing of these joints in patients weakened by neuromuscular disease is difficult.[76]

Gravitational forces must be accounted for in isokinetic torque or force calculations. Errors caused by failure to correct for gravity reportedly can reach 500% for knee flexor testing.[77] The amount of error caused by not correcting for gravity increases in weaker patients who generate low torque values.[77,78]

Handheld Dynamometer Testing. HHDs were developed to quantify MMT measurements (i.e., to remove examiner judgment and to assign numeric values [kilogram, pound, Newton] to the forces exerted by the patient). The dynamometer is placed between the examiner's hand and the patient's limb (see Figure 15.1D). For MMT and HHD testing, the examiner usually uses a "break" test to score muscle force. In a break test, the examiner exerts enough force to overcome the maximal voluntary effort of the subject to hold the test position; the examiner stops resisting at the moment the extremity gives way, essentially producing an eccentric contraction.[79] This is essentially the same maneuver used in MMT. Some clinicians prefer to use "make" tests with the HHD. For a make test, the subject exerts maximal force against the HHD while the examiner acts as an immovable external resistance; this theoretically is equivalent to an MVIC.[79]

ADVANTAGES OF HANDHELD DYNAMOMETER TESTING. HHDs are fairly inexpensive. No additional equipment is required for testing. HHDs are portable and lightweight, so they can be brought to the patient, whether in a hospital room or home setting. HHDs are usually simple to operate, and testing can be done quickly. Some HHDs provide a hard copy of test results, and some electronic units can be interfaced with a computer. Precautions to be taken to enhance accuracy and reliability of HHD measurements have been described.[5,80]

LIMITATIONS OF HANDHELD DYNAMOMETER TESTING. Standardized testing protocols have not been universally accepted. Considerable measurement error can be introduced unless consistent routines are used for joint testing angle, placement of the unit on the tested limb, and positioning of limb in reference to gravity. For patients who are (or are anticipated to become) very weak, gravity-eliminated or gravity-neutral testing positions should be selected.[5,72] If the test position requires a muscle group to act against gravity or with gravity assisting the motion, gravity-compensation calculations must be performed to add or subtract the weight of the limb to the force or torque measurement.[5,80]

Some investigators use "make"[72,81,82] and others use "break"[5,52,80,83–85] techniques for HHD measurements. Make and break force readings from the same subject may not be equivalent.[79] Also, different examiners may not have the same concept of "break," leading to poor inter-rater reliability of measurements.[86]

The HHD is limited in measuring force from large muscle groups in adults or healthy children. This can be due to examiner weakness relative to the patient and to insensitivity of the HHD.[5,72,79,81,83,84,87] To obtain a break or a make measurement, the examiner must be able to exert more force than the patient, as well as to stabilize both the patient and the HHD.[80,88] Otherwise, the HHD reading underestimates muscle force and leads to unreliable measurements.[89,90] Wikhold and Bohannon found that a strong examiner recorded significantly greater forces than a weak examiner for the same muscle group in healthy subjects. The effect of examiner strength was greater in a strong muscle group (knee extensors) than a weaker muscle group (shoulder external rotators).[90] Some muscle groups may just be too strong to be reasonably measured with an HHD held by an average examiner.[2] The extent to which the HHD can produce reliable, accurate measurements of minor degrees of weakness in large muscle groups of adults and children remains unknown.[19] This deficiency (shared with MMT) limits use of the HHD for sequential monitoring of patients with mild weakness.

A variety of HHDs are commercially available, but little evidence exists about the extent to which they can be used interchangeably. In one study, two dynamometers of the same brand did not give consistent readings with each other; this may indicate that the same examiner should test a patient every time with the same device.[82] Some spring dynamometers may lose elasticity over time.

Normative data concerning what range of values is normal for specific muscle groups tested by specific protocols are needed; normative values should be recorded in torque, rather than force units, to encompass consideration of limb length differences.[72]

Validity of Quantitative Strength Measurements. Quantitative strength measurements have been related to muscle cross-sectional area (CSA). In 50 patients with various muscular dystrophies, knee extensor MVIC was proportional to quadriceps muscle CSA (measured by computerized tomography); all patients with more than 22% fat replacement of quadriceps had knee extension force below 35% of normal values.[91] In healthy subjects, a significant correlation was reported between torque (isokinetic measurement) and muscle CSA in knee and elbow muscle groups.[92]

A maximal muscle contraction evoked by tetanic electrical stimulation elicits forces no greater than the force produced during an MVIC.[3] This has been reported for healthy subjects [69,93,94] and for subjects with muscular dystrophy,[55,95,96] indicating that muscle can be activated as fully during voluntary effort as during an externally induced maximal contraction. Additionally, a similar rate of rise in muscle temperature was reported during MVIC and supramaximal tetanic electrically stimulated contractions of quadriceps muscle.[97] Metabolic demand of maximally activated forearm muscles, measured by phosphorous nuclear magnetic spectroscopy, was found to be similar under MVIC, supramaximal tetanic electrical stimulation, and isokinetic (15 degrees per second) testing conditions.[98]

Electrophysiologically based estimates of the number of motor neurons in a muscle, which are conducted without need for patient voluntary effort,[99] were reported to be highly correlated with MVIC measurements.[100,101]

A significant correlation between MVIC and HHD knee extensor measurements has been noted in patients with muscular dystrophy[53,83] and ALS.[102] MVIC and MMT measurements have been reported to be significantly related in patients with ALS,[12,103] FSHD,[57] and patients with varied neuromusculoskeletal problems.[10,104] Such findings indicate that MVIC, HHD, and MMT measurements are probably all measuring the common variable strength.

Use of Quantitative Strength Tests in Neuromuscular Disease

Muscular Dystrophy

Maximal Voluntary Isometric Contraction Measurements in Patients with Muscular Dystrophy. In 1967, Fowler and Gardner reported MVIC measurements from 43 patients with DMD and 32 patients with other types of muscular dystrophy, using a cable tensiometer to measure MVIC from 13 muscle groups and a handgrip dynamometer to measure hand strength. Acceptable test-retest reliability of measurements was reported. Patient MVIC measurements were compared with those of healthy subjects, and some patients were followed over a 3-year period. Differential involvement of proximal versus distal muscle groups was documented, and the investigators advocated increased use of quantitative muscle testing to establish the natural history of neuromuscular diseases.[105]

Edwards used a strain-gauge method originally described by Tornvall[106] to study knee extensor MVIC in healthy subjects[69] and later in patients with muscular dystrophy.[55,107] Other investigators used this method to measure knee extensor MVIC in patients with DMD[52,84,85] and other peripheral neuromuscular disorders.[5] High test-retest reliability for MVIC measurements was reported by each group. Reliability of knee extensor MVIC measurements in DMD patients tested with an isokinetic dynamometer also has been reported.[108]

Muscle groups other than knee extensors have also been assessed using strain-gauge methodology in patients with varied neuromuscular diseases. Reliability of elbow and wrist MVIC was reported by deBoer and colleagues, who compared patients with controls and documented changes over time in 11 patients.[109] Aitkens found good reliability of strain-gauge measurements for hip, knee, and elbow muscle groups in patients.[10] Brussock and colleagues reported good intra- and inter-rater reliability of MVIC measurements from seven muscle groups for patients with DMD and for control subjects.[71]

MVIC measurements accurately distinguished muscle force values of healthy control subjects from those of DMD patients in two studies.[71,84] In another report, MVIC measurements detected strength differences between weak DMD patients that were not apparent from MMT measurements.[110] Strain-gauge MVIC of specific muscle groups has been used to assess the effects of myoblast transplant procedures[96,111] and medication intervention[95] in boys with DMD. A measurement system similar to the one used in the TQNE (see the section Maximal Voluntary Isometric Contraction Measurements in Patients with Motor Neuron Disease) can be adapted for the evaluation of DMD in children (see Figure 15.4B).

In natural history studies of FSHD, MVIC testing was used in combination with MMT and functional testing. The MVIC from nine muscle groups (six upper- and three lower-extremity groups) was measured. Excellent intrarater and inter-rater reliability of MVIC measurements was reported for both patients and controls.[57] Longitudinal MVIC measurements have now been reported for FSHD natural history,[58,59] and MVIC has been used in clinical trials of medications with FSHD patients.[60,61]

Isokinetic Measurements in Muscular Dystrophy. deLateur used isokinetic measurements to demonstrate that resistive exercise had neither a detrimental nor beneficial effect on knee extensor strength in four boys with DMD.[112] In a case report of a patient with scapuloperoneal muscular dystrophy, Wagner et al. used isokinetic testing to document the effect of attempts to reverse signs of overwork weakness.[113] Subsequently, others documented reliability of isokinetic measurements on patients with muscular dystrophy.[33,114]

Isokinetic measurements have been used to document changes in strength over time in children and adults with a variety of neuromuscular diseases.[32,33] In one of the cases described by Merlini et al., isokinetic testing documented differential strength between left and right knee extension, confirming the pattern of muscle involvement indicated by a thigh computed tomography scan; however, the patient's MMT measurements showed equal grades for left and right knees.[33] Two early isokinetic studies of relative dynamic endurance in knee extensor muscles of patients with neuromuscular disease have noted a pattern of fatigue different from that exhibited by healthy subjects.[33,115]

Handheld Dynamometer Measurements in Muscular Dystrophy. Edwards and McDonnell introduced the Hammersmith HHD as a clinical tool for quantifying MMT ratings of force from patients with neuromuscular disease.[83] Hosking et al. reported reliability of measurements using this device to measure six muscle groups in 19 healthy children and 16 children with muscle disease.[84] DMD children younger than 5 years were noted to be unable to cooperate well enough to produce reliable readings with the Hammersmith HHD.[116]

Use of the Hammersmith HHD apparently was limited for measuring weak children, and a more sensitive device, the Penny-Giles electronic myometer, was developed for this purpose.[85] Hyde et al. reported intra- and inter-rater reliability of measurements using this HHD with six muscle groups of 12 children with neuromuscular disease.[85] Scott reported highly reproducible measurements for eight muscle groups using the Penny-Giles HHD in 61 boys with DMD.[52] Myometry measurements were combined with MMT scores, strain-gauge knee extensor force measurements, and functional ability tests to describe the natural history of DMD.[52] Edwards et al. reported reliability of measurements with the Penny-Giles HHD in a longitudinal study of 21 boys with DMD over a 2-year period; HHD measurements of 10 muscle groups were used to chart the differential rate of loss of strength in upper- and lower-extremity muscle groups.[55]

Stuberg and Metcalf used a Spark HHD to measure four muscle groups in 14 boys with DMD who were matched with healthy controls. High intrarater reliability for measurements was reported; however, the hip and knee extensor muscle groups could not be measured in the healthy controls because their force exceeded the HHD capacity.[72] Reliability of measurements was reported by Mendell and Florence using the Penny-Giles HHD to measure four muscle groups in 30 boys with DMD; however, only 62 of the 84 boys were able to cooperate with testing.[23] The Penny-Giles HHD, in conjunction with MMT, was used as an outcome measure in DMD clinical trials with prednisone[117] and isaxonine.[53] HHD force measurements were used in a clinical trial of myoblast transfer in DMD.[118]

Bohannon reported high intrarater reliability using a Spark dynamometer to measure 18 muscle groups in 30 patients with various neuromuscular disorders.[81] In later studies, Bohannon and Andrews used the Chatillon HHD to measure six muscle groups in 30 patients with varied neurologic and neuromuscular disorders; they reported good to high reliability of measurements, with intrarater reliability being greater than inter-rater reliability.[119] Greater intra- rather than inter-rater reliability for HHD has also been reported by others for patients with neuromuscular disease[80] and for healthy subjects.[86]

Inflammatory Myopathy

Maximal Voluntary Isometric Contraction Measurements in Patients with Inflammatory Myopathy. The first reports using MVIC measurements to monitor patients with inflammatory myopathy were conducted on distal (hand and ankle) muscle groups. Dinsdale and colleagues reported serial MVIC measurements in a patient with DM over a 15-month period of treatment with prednisone and exercise; increases in plantar flexor MVIC (strain-gauge) and grip-strength force measurements reflected level of DM disease activity.[120] Using the same protocol in longitudinal studies of DM patients, Resnik et al.[121] (six cases) and Miller et al.[31] (16 cases) noted that isometric tests of plantar flexion and hand-grip strength provided a sensitive index of patient response to therapy.

Use of knee extensor MVIC (strain-gauge) measurements to monitor inflammatory myopathy was first reported by Edwards.[122,123] In a case study describing deterioration and subsequent recovery of a patient with polymyositis (PM), Edwards et al. found that changes in MVIC measurements were paralleled by changes in muscle mass (estimated from metabolic balance studies).[122] Kroll and colleagues monitored changes in MVIC from knee flexor and extensor muscle groups in 14 patients with PM/DM. The investigators found that changes over time in serum enzyme level did not correlate well with MVIC measurements and emphasized the importance of quantitative strength measurements for assessing disease activity.[124]

Kroll et al. later used the same strain-gauge testing method to document that knee extensor MVIC was significantly more impaired than knee flexor MVIC in 45 patients with PM/DM.[125] Wiesinger found that knee extensor MVIC was significantly lower in 22 patients with PM/DM than in control subjects.[126] Although different instrumentation was used to measure MVIC (Wiesinger used a Cybex dynamometer), knee extensor MVIC relative to control values was similar in the two studies; Wiesinger et al. found that patient knee extensor MVIC was 57% of control values, compared with 59% of control values in the Kroll et al. study.

To examine potential effects of resistive exercise during rehabilitation of patients with PM/DM, several investigators have used isokinetic dynamometers to measure MVIC. Using a Lido dynamometer, Escalante et al. reported that MVIC of hip and knee muscle groups increased in concert with patients' ADL scores; no evidence of adverse effects from exercise was noted.[127] In a case report, Hicks et al. used a Cybex dynamometer to provide resistive isometric exercise and to measure MVIC of elbow flexor and knee extensor groups; they reported an increase in torque with no rise in creatine phosphokinase over the patient's trial period of resistive exercise.[128] Wiesenger et al. reported that significant increases in MVIC (measured with a Cybex unit) from hip flexor and knee extensor groups were one of the beneficial effects of a 6-month training program for eight patients with chronic PM/DM; other outcomes that improved significantly more than the control group were ADL scores and aerobic capacity.[129]

Isokinetic Measurements in Inflammatory Myopathy. Eccentric and concentric isokinetic measurements in 22 patients having PM/DM were reported by Griffin et al. using a Kin-Com dynamometer; excellent reliability for torque measurements from elbow and knee muscle groups was reported.[34] Patients' relative strength (patient torque expressed as percentage of a matched control torque) did not differ among muscle groups, indicating that knee extensors did not exhibit greater deficits than the other two muscle groups (Figure 15.3). Patients able to perform the task of squatting down and standing up unassisted had significantly greater knee extensor and flexor torque than the patients who were unable to perform these tasks. Eccentric and concentric capacity appeared equally affected in all muscle groups, possibly indicating that, for this diagnostic group, either eccentric or concentric testing would provide comparable information.[34]

Figure 15.3 Relative strength (plus one standard deviation) of 22 patients with polymyositis/dermatomyositis from isokinetic testing of elbow flexor (EF), knee extensor (KE), and knee flexor (KF) muscle groups. Relative strength is patient torque as percentage of matched control torque. Because patients' relative strength did not differ by test velocity (30 or 120 degrees per second) or type of muscle action (concentric or eccentric), values were averaged to obtain one overall relative strength for each muscle group.

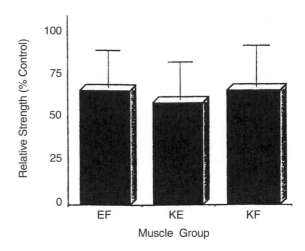

PM/DM is reportedly a disease predominantly affecting proximal (hip/shoulder) muscles; however, no studies comparing quantitative strength of proximal muscle groups relative to intermediate (knee/elbow) and distal (foot/hand) muscle groups are available. Greater research is needed to document relative involvement of proximal to distal muscles in PM/DM and the rate of recovery of strength in different muscle groups during treatment.

Handheld Dynamometer Measurements in Inflammatory Myopathy. Wiles and Karni used the Penny-Giles HHD to measure 12 adult patients having clinical weakness due to peripheral neuromuscular disease. Satisfactory reproducibility of HHD measurements from nine muscle groups was reported, and reliability for HHD knee extensor measurements was comparable to that of strain-gauge MVIC.[5] Wiles et al. later presented sequential studies of 17 patients with PM/DM, using HHD measurements from 30 healthy adults as reference values. They reported that in many cases HHD measurements were a more sensitive indication of patient progress than serum muscle enzymes or functional performance criteria.[80] Those investigators also noted that the point at which large changes in function occurred was when average strength dropped below 40% of the normal range for age and gender.[80]

Motor Neuron Disorders

Maximal Voluntary Isometric Contraction Measurements in Patients with Motor Neuron Disease. MVIC measurements are considered a valid and sensitive index of ALS disease severity and progression[8] and are one of the most useful primary endpoints for a therapeutic trial.[13,70] The TQNE was developed to assess neuromuscular deficit and disease rate in patients with ALS.[8,67,68,130] A central element of the TQNE consists of MVIC of nine muscle groups (measured bilaterally with a computerized fixed strain-gauge system) (Figure 15.4) and handgrip strength (using a Jamar dynamometer). High intra- and inter-rater reliability of MVIC measurements using the TQNE protocol was reported for both strong and weak muscles in ALS patients.[8,12,68,103,131,132] The TQNE and its subsequent modifications have been used in natural history studies to document a linear rate of strength loss in some stages of ALS.[67,133–138] The MVIC-TQNE protocol has also been used to examine effects of various therapeutic agents in ALS[103,131,139–141] and postpolio syndrome.[142]

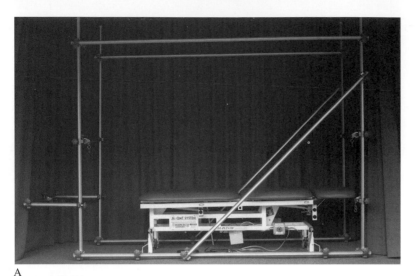

A

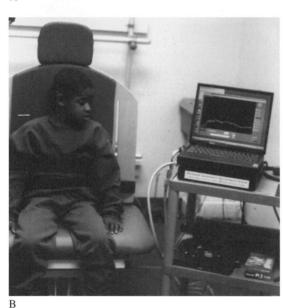

B

Figure 15.4 **A.** Table and frame for the quantitative muscle testing (QMT) by Biomech Designs Ltd., Edmonton, Alberta, Canada. **B.** QMT table adapted for children in clinical trials. Provided by Richmond Quantitative Measurement Systems (Richmond, VA).

Some investigations of patients with ALS have related progressive strength impairment to functional limitations. A statistically significant relationship between MVIC strength (modified TQNE protocol) and functional disability or quality of life, or both, as measured by the Sickness Impact Profile, was reported both initially and over a 3-month interval.[143,144] Total muscle MVIC measurements (TQNE protocol) were highly correlated with functional ability measured by the ALS Functional Rating Scale both cross-sectionally and longitudinally.[145–147]

In one longitudinal study of 20 patients with ALS, MMT, MVIC, and functional ability (Norris functional rating scale) were measured monthly; although all measurements declined over the 9-month assessment period, MVIC was noted to deteriorate steadily, whereas functional ability and MMT showed slower decline with plateau periods (Figure 15.5).[3,12] This was interpreted as reduced sensitivity of func-

Figure 15.5 Plot of averaged arm manual muscle testing (MMT), maximal voluntary isometric contraction (MVIC), and arm (functional) score, expressed as percent of normal, for an individual patient with amyotrophic lateral sclerosis followed for 10 months. (Reproduced with permission from PL Andres, LM Skerry, B Thornell, et al. A comparison of three measures of disease progression in ALS. J Neurol Sci 1996; 139[Suppl]:54–70.)

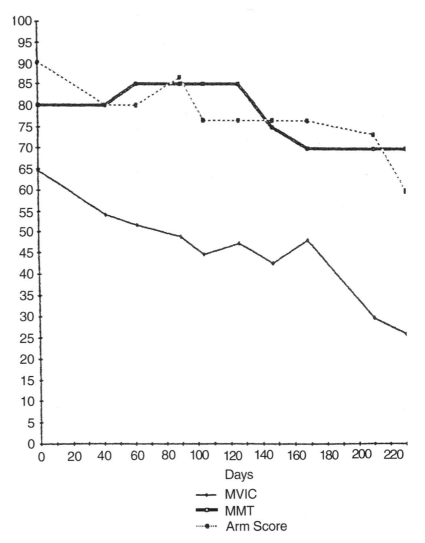

tional and MMT measurements to the rate of ALS disease progression. Focusing solely on change in functional ability as an index of disease would have produced an erroneous conclusion of a long period of disease latency, followed by disease exacerbation; in fact, steady decrease in strength was occurring.[3,12] This example also illustrates the phenomenon of "crash effect" in patients with ALS—that is, the abrupt loss of a functional ability when the number of functioning motor units falls below the critical level.[7] What percentage of normal MVIC this critical level represents remains undocumented. Clinical reports of ALS patients suggest that functional limitation may escalate when MVIC strength falls below 20% of normal,[12] and that weakness becomes obvious to the patient with ALS when 80% of motor neurons to the functional group are lost.[135]

In patients with ALS, deterioration in upper-extremity MVIC scores was a predictor of early death,[103] but deterioration in combined upper- and lower-extremity MVIC scores was not.[148] Linear estimates of ALS disease progression, which were based on isometric measurements, were found to be a good predictor of survival.[149]

Spinal muscular atrophy is a hereditary motor neuron disease that is being investigated with MVIC methodology in a multicenter study of spinal muscular atrophy natural history; MVIC testing of 12 muscle groups using a fixed Chatillon tensiometer is part of the measurement protocol.[150,151] Reliability of measurements was acceptable,[152,153] and longitudinal data have been reported.[154]

Isokinetic Measurements in Motor Neuron Disease. Longitudinal isokinetic studies in patients having ALS were reported by Sufit[29] and Brooks and colleagues,[30] who used a Cybex unit to measure peak torque from knee and elbow muscle groups at six angular velocities. Reliability of measurements was not reported. Those investigators reported that decreases in concentric torque over the 16-month study period were greater in muscle groups that were initially stronger, and that during the first 8 months of study, decrease in torque of the stronger muscles at the fast (180 degrees per second) angular velocity was significantly greater than the decrease in isometric torque.[29,30] Such findings implied that such isokinetic testing might be more sensitive to early changes in presymptomatic ALS patients than isometric testing.[135] Those investigators hypothesized that the deficit they observed in ALS patients during fast-velocity concentric isokinetic testing was related to upper motor neuron deficit.[29,30] Others have documented particular deficits at fast concentric isokinetic testing in patients with hypertonia due to hereditary ataxia,[155] multiple sclerosis,[156] and hereditary spastic paresis.[157]

Combining eccentric with concentric isokinetic measurements may yield greater information about the influence of upper motor neuron deficit on dynamic motor capacity. Knutsson documented in patients with hereditary spastic paresis that their ability to generate torque during eccentric testing was relatively well preserved, relative to a very impaired ability to generate torque during concentric testing.[158,159] Ponichtera et al. documented that patients with multiple sclerosis exhibited a percentage difference between eccentric and concentric capacity that was twice as large as non–multiple sclerosis patients.[160] Patients with spastic paresis due to ALS have been found to exhibit a similar pattern with eccentric and concentric isokinetic testing.[161] A Kin-Com dynamometer was used to test knee flexor and extensor muscle groups in spastic ALS patients, nonspastic patients, and matched controls; high reliability of measurements was documented. ALS patients with spastic paresis exhibited a larger difference between eccentric and concentric torque at the fast (120 degrees per second) velocity than either nonspastic patients or controls (see Figure 15.5). Disparity between eccentric and concentric capacity continued to be a prominent feature over time, as demonstrated by serial tests of one patient (Figure 15.6).[161] Further research is needed to investigate how isokinetic testing of eccentric and concentric ability may complement isometric testing in assessing early motor deficit in ALS.

Isokinetic torque measurements have been related to functional ability in some studies of patients with motor neuron disease. Sufit[29] and Brooks and colleagues[30] reported a significant correlation in ALS patients between walk velocity and knee flexor peak torque at 180 degrees per second test velocity; no correlation was found between knee extensor isokinetic measurements and walking velocity. Griffin et al. reported that in ALS patients with spastic paresis, ambulatory ability was related to knee flexor eccentric and concentric torque ratios—that is, patients with the most abnormal ratios demonstrated greatest difficulty with ambulation.[161]

Figure 15.6 Knee flexor (KF) relative strength over time for a patient with amyotrophic lateral sclerosis (**A**), a patient with primary lateral sclerosis (**B**), and a patient with progressive muscular atrophy (**C**). Relative strength is patient torque as percentage of matched control. The patients in (**A**) and (**B**), who had clinical evidence of spasticity, demonstrated large differences between eccentric (ECC) and concentric (CONC) relative strength that were not exhibited by patients with nonspastic conditions, such as the patient in **C**. (MO = months.) (Reproduced with permission from JW Griffin, RE Tooms, R Vander Zwaag, et al. Eccentric and concentric muscle performance in patients with spastic paresis secondary to motor neuron disease. A preliminary report. Neuromusc Disord 1994;4:131–135.)

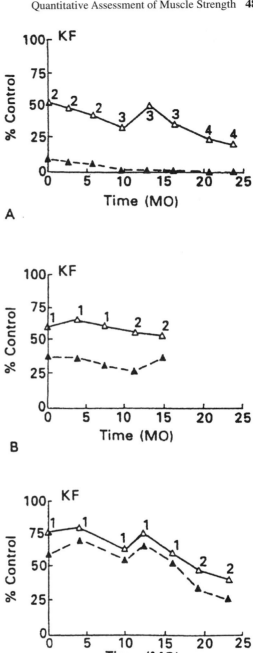

Handheld Dynamometer Measurements in Motor Neuron Disorders. Goonetil-like et al. investigated the reliability and accuracy of the Penny-Giles HHD in patients having motor neuron disorders.[162] Intrarater was better than inter-rater reliability, and poorer reproducibility was found for weaker muscles. The investigators reported reliability was improved by using a composite score of eight muscle groups rather than individual muscles and by using a single rater. Bohannon used HHD measurements (Chatillon unit) to study the effect of a resistive exercise program in a patient with ALS; large increases in HHD measurements (40–64%) were noted in 14 of 18 muscles tested; conversely, MMT of the same groups reflected no change in strength.[163]

ERGOMETRY TESTING OF PERSONS WITH NEUROMUSCULAR DISORDERS

Technically, an *ergometer* is any device that provides external resistance to exercise. Ideally, an ergometer should have the capability to be calibrated to provide a range of constant and known rates of work in an activity mode that is familiar to most individuals. Within the context of this broad definition, all devices providing resistance, including various types of dynamometers (see the sections Handheld Dynamometer Testing and Isokinetic Measurements in Inflammatory Myopathy), are classified as ergometers. In the following section (Types of Ergometers), the definition of ergometry is narrowed to include only those devices that require the performance of *dynamic exercise* by large muscle groups and rely on the integration of cardiorespiratory and neuromuscular input. These ergometers are used to measure whole-body aerobic or anaerobic capacities and may be used with or without gas exchange measurements (see all following sections).

Types of Ergometers

Ergometers can be broadly categorized as those requiring weight-bearing activity and those that are independent of body weight. Examples of commonly used ergometers are motor-driven treadmills, mechanically braked arm or leg cycle ergometers, combined arm and leg ergometers, rowing machines, or stepping machines. Each has its own advantages and disadvantages.

Weight-Bearing Ergometers

Motor-driven treadmills are the most common ergometers using weight-bearing exercise. The main advantage of treadmill testing is that it provides a familiar type of exercise stress (i.e., walking or running). Treadmills can be used for individuals with marked differences in age or fitness levels because of the wide range of walking and running speeds available. When assessment of maximal aerobic capacity is of interest, treadmill testing results in attainment of the highest values in comparison with other types of ergometry. Several disadvantages are also associated with treadmill testing. Good balance and locomotor skills are necessary for accurate testing. Although most treadmills have a front and at least one side rail for individuals to steady themselves, accurate measurements result only when the test is performed without holding the handrails. For this reason, many individuals require practice walking on the treadmill before any meaningful testing can be done. Many patients with neuromuscular disease may have poor balance and may not be able to walk independently on a treadmill. Other disadvantages of using a treadmill for ergometry testing include the expense of a treadmill, inability to move it easily, and difficulty in making some measurements (e.g., taking exercise blood pressures [BPs]). Stepping machines are an alternative weight-bearing ergometer, but are they are difficult to use without holding handrails and, therefore, may result in poor standardization of resistance.

Non–Weight-Bearing Ergometers

Cycle ergometers provide the option for non–weight-bearing exercise that may be useful in testing patients with neuromuscular disease. Resistance can be easily adjusted in small increments. Although older mechanically braked ergometers (e.g., Monark) require that proper pedal rate be maintained to obtain the desired resistance, many of the newer models (electronically braked) are pedal-rate independent so that appropriate resistance results across a wide range of pedal rates. Physiologic monitoring is considerably easier than during treadmill testing because there is much less arm and chest movement. For example, electrocardiograms (ECGs), BP, and even periodic blood sampling are easily accomplished during a leg cycle ergometer test. Cycle ergometers are relatively inexpensive, require little space, and are easily transportable. Semirecumbent leg cycle ergometers are a good alternative for patients with poor sitting balance. The major disadvantage of leg-cycle ergometry is that most individuals in the United States (and Canada) are unfamiliar with this type of exercise and may experience local (particularly quadriceps) muscle fatigue that prematurely limits test performance before adequate stress has been placed on the cardiorespiratory systems. Arm ergometers may be used for individuals with limited lower-body function. An arm ergometer may be purchased or a leg cycle ergometer adapted by replacing the pedals with handles and mounting the unit on a table at shoulder height. As with leg ergometry, resistance may be crank-rate dependent (mechanical braking) or crank-rate independent (electronic braking). For best results, arm ergometry should be performed with the exerciser in a seated position and the fulcrum of the handle on the ergometer adjusted to shoulder height. Arm ergometry has several disadvantages. During arm ergometry, a small muscle mass is used, and local arm and shoulder fatigue tends to be even more limiting than leg ergometry. Another major disadvantage of arm ergometry is that use of the arms to exercise precludes measurement of exercise BP. BPs can be measured during brief rests between stages but may under- or overestimate true BPs. If ECG monitoring is desired, electrodes should be placed to minimize muscle artifact. For individuals with hemiparesis or hemiplegia, combination arm and leg ergometers, such as the Schwinn Air-Dyne, may be used. Rowing machines may also be used, but they are less useful for ergometry testing because resistance is usually controlled by voluntary effort of the exerciser.

Metabolic Cost from Gas Exchange Measurements

During ergometry, the metabolic cost of each exercise intensity can be estimated from work rate (i.e., watts [W] or speed and grade). However, for any given individual, the estimate of metabolic cost may be quite different from actual energy expenditure. When more precise metabolic information is desired, open-circuit spirometry may be used to measure oxygen uptake. In this procedure, the test subject (patient) breathes through a low-resistance valve, which causes a sample of expired air to be routed through analyzers that measure oxygen and carbon dioxide fractions as well as minute volumes. From these three variables, oxygen uptake ($\dot{V}o_2$) and carbon dioxide production (Vco_2) are calculated. Oxygen uptake is directly related to metabolic equivalents (METs) such that one MET is defined as resting energy expenditure and is equivalent to 3.5 ml per kg per minute oxygen uptake. Thus, by measuring oxygen uptake, an accurate MET level can be determined. Additionally, the ratio of V_{CO_2} to $\dot{V}_{O_2}$ used gives an estimate of the relative proportions of carbohydrate and fat being used for substrate. This information may be of interest for patients with metabolic myopathies (see the section Metabolic Myopathies). Gas exchange measurements can also be useful in noninvasive monitoring of anaerobic thresholds. Several methods are accepted for this determination. Automated systems are available that are easy to use and provide a detailed printout of test results.[164] The V-slope method and the ventilatory equivalent of oxygen ($VE/\dot{V}_{O_2}$) versus the ventilatory equivalent of carbon dioxide (VE/V_{CO_2}) comparison are commonly used and programmed into most metabolic carts.

Types and Uses of Ergometry Tests

The most common uses of ergometry testing for healthy individuals are to acquire information with which to develop an individualized exercise prescription and to monitor progress in response to an exercise training program. For patient populations, including neuromuscular disease patients, additional uses are to evaluate suspected deficits in cardiovascular or metabolic function and to monitor disease-related decreases in physical function. Ergometry may be used to assess cardiorespiratory fitness by measuring maximal aerobic capacity ($\dot{V}_{O_2}$max). These tests are typically incremental, with work rates starting at low intensity and progressing up to maximal effort. Ergometry may also be used to measure physiologic variables at several incremental, but submaximal, exercise intensities. These variables, such as heart rate (HR) or energy cost, can be monitored over time and used (similar to the use of maximal values) to measure increases or decreases in physical functioning. Submaximal variables are less useful for developing individualized exercise prescriptions. Ergometry tests may also be used to monitor substrate use and hormonal, cardiovascular, or pulmonary responses over a prolonged period of time to exercise at a single submaximal intensity (see the section Submaximal Exercise Tests). Ergometry tests are also available to measure anaerobic capacity (see the section Wingate Test for Anaerobic Power and Capacity).

Ergometry Protocols

Specific ergometry protocols are chosen in accord with the purpose of the test, the outcome measures of interest, and the individual being tested.

Maximal Exercise Tests

When cardiorespiratory fitness ($\dot{V}_{O_2}$max) is of interest, a test to maximal effort is the gold standard.

Multistage Protocols. Ergometry tests to maximal effort have traditionally been multistage graded exercise tests (GXTs). Although the specifics of individual protocols may differ from one another, all follow a similar basic pattern. Stages are set for a determined period of time (usually 1–3 minutes) and follow an incremental pattern. The size of the increments is usually between 1 and 3 METs. Initial stages are at a relatively low intensity, but exercise intensity increases with each subsequent stage until maximal effort is reached. In the absence of signs or symptoms of exercise intolerance,[165] the test continues until the person being tested requests to stop. If there are indications for terminating the exercise test, the test is stopped before maximal subjective effort. Ending values from such a test are referred to as "peak" rather than "maximal." Tests are most commonly continuous, with no rest between stages. However, if excessive neuromuscular fatigue is expected to interfere with attainment of adequate stress on the cardiorespiratory system, tests may be discontinuous with 1- to 3-minute rest periods interspersed between each exercise stage. Usual monitoring during testing includes 12-lead ECG, HR, BP, and rating of perceived exertion.

Energy expenditure at each stage can be estimated from work rate or it can be measured from the direct measurement of expired gases. Because of the inaccuracies associated with estimating energy expenditure from work rate, particularly for neuromuscular disease patients (see the section Use of Ergometry for Selected Neuromuscular Diseases), gas exchange measurements are recommended when information about energy expenditure, substrate use, or pulmonary function is of interest.

Many standardized GXT protocols are available for treadmill and leg cycle ergometry testing.[165] For treadmill protocols, intensity is increased by an increase in treadmill speed, grade, or some combination of each. The Bruce protocol[165] is probably the most well known and the most commonly used. However, this protocol may not be suitable for many individuals because the increments between stages are relatively large (approximately 3 METs). Protocols with large increments or high treadmill speeds such as this are better suited to young, active individuals than to older or less functionally capable individuals such as neuromuscular disease patients. Protocols with much lower increments (e.g., 1 MET/stage) are available[165] and more suitable for this latter group. Multistage protocols of a similar format are available for cycle ergometry.[165] Exercise intensity is increased by adjusting the resistance to pedaling either mechanically or electronically in 2- to 3-minute stages. Leg ergometry increments are frequently 25–50 W, whereas 10-W resistance increments have been used during arm ergometry for a variety of patient populations.[166]

Ramping Protocols. An alternative to a multistage protocol is a ramp protocol, in which intensity is increased in a constant and continuous manner.[167,168] Ramp protocols have been available for many years for use with electronically controlled cycle ergometers. Ramping rates of 15–20 W per minute are common, with higher rates used for younger, well-conditioned individuals. Only recently have treadmill manufacturers developed controllers for ramping speed and grade. For patient populations, increases in treadmill grade of 1–3% per minute are appropriate. Reported advantages to using a ramp protocol include the avoidance of large or unequal (or both) increments in intensity, more accurate estimates of exercise capacity, facilitation of individualizing the test by an individualized ramp rate, and a better control of test duration. Ideally, protocols are chosen so that maximal effort is reached between 8 and 12 minutes.

Submaximal Exercise Tests

Multistage or ramp tests can also be used for submaximal testing. During submaximal testing, the endpoint is predetermined. A common endpoint for a submaximal test is some percentage (e.g., 75% or 85%) of age-predicted maximal HR or a predetermined work rate such as 150 W. Submaximal tests may have 1- to 3-minute stages similar to maximal tests, or they may incorporate longer stages (4–6 minutes) to monitor steady-state responses. Steady-state responses reflect homeostatic adjustment to a submaximal exercise level and can be used to develop exercise prescriptions or to assess appropriateness of cardiovascular, pulmonary, or metabolic responses. Either of these two submaximal protocol types can be used in a manner similar to maximal responses to monitor changes in fitness or disease progression with less reliance on volitional effort. Additionally, responses to submaximal exercise intensities can be extrapolated to estimate maximal exercise capacity. However, because individual variation may exist in actual maximal HRs and particularly in mechanical efficiency, submaximal testing to estimate maximal exercise capacity is not very accurate for neuromuscular disease patients.

A single-stage ergometry test may also be used. During a single-stage test, the participant exercises on an ergometer (e.g., treadmill, leg cycle ergometer) for a prolonged period of time at a single, submaximal exercise intensity. Endpoints are either a set period of time or until the patient can no longer keep pace with the ergometer. Measures of cardiovascular variables such as HR and BP are the mainstays of single-stage tests and are assessed over time. Other uses include tracking substrates, (e.g., glucose, lactate, fatty acids), electrolytes (e.g., sodium, potassium), hormones (e.g., insulin, epinephrine), or a combination of these for a prolonged period of time. Single-stage tests may also be used to measure energy expenditure (caloric cost) of a specific exercise intensity. They may also be used to assess the relative contribution of carbohydrate and fat as substrate during that exercise intensity and may be particularly useful in quantifying caloric expenditure of an activity.

Wingate Test for Anaerobic Power and Capacity

The ergometry tests discussed above stress and allow assessment of systems involved in aerobic metabolism and reflect the interaction between the cardiorespiratory, metabolic, and neuromuscular systems. Ergometry can also be used to assess anaerobic energy systems—use of adenosine triphosphate (ATP), phosphocreatine (PC), and anaerobic glycolysis. The most common of these tests is the Wingate anaerobic test. This test requires a cycle ergometer specifically equipped and interfaced with a computer program. These are commercially available. The test requires fast pedaling against a resistance based on weight and gender. Peak power (measured during the first 5 seconds of the test) reflects ATP-PC energy release; mean power (averaged over 30 seconds of the test) reflects ATP-PC and anaerobic glycolytic capacities. This ergometry test has been used to assess children with a neuromuscular disease[169] and may be appropriate for adults with neuromuscular disease as well.

Use of Ergometry for Selected Neuromuscular Diseases

Ergometry with or without gas exchange measurement is potentially useful in the assessment and treatment of a variety of neuromuscular diseases. The following section addresses the potential uses, suggested protocols, and recommended monitoring for several common neuromuscular diseases.

Amyotrophic Lateral Sclerosis

Little information is available regarding the use of ergometry for patients with ALS.[170] Although use of a specific ergometry protocol for ALS patients has not been reported, the choice of ergometry testing mode and protocol should be dependent on the stage of disease and the anticipated rate of disease progression. In early stages, responses to ergometry testing may be near normal. At that time, any testing mode (i.e., treadmill, upright leg cycle ergometer, combined arm and leg ergometer, semi-recumbent cycle ergometer) may be acceptable. However, because of increasing balance and coordination problems as disease progresses and because exercise responses may differ among ergometry testing modes, sequential testing using a semirecumbent cycle ergometer or a combined arm and leg ergometer is recommended. Choice of initial work rate and amount of increments should be governed by estimates of the degree of disease involvement so that maximal effort is reached within 8–12 minutes. If gas exchange capability is available, additional important information on actual energy costs for submaximal intensities is helpful in estimating what functional activities the patient can still perform. METs estimated from work rates can be used but are likely to be much less accurate. Use of gas exchange also provides information about ventilatory response to submaximal exercise intensities and provides an indication of the degree of limitation caused by dyspnea. A dyspnea index, such as is used with chronic obstructive pulmonary disease patients, may also be of use. As disease progresses, ergometry may have to be adapted to accommodate balance or coordination problems. No evidence is available to suggest that exercise training affects disease progression or prognosis. However, aerobic exercise training may have a positive effect on daily functional ability by maximizing efficiency in those fibers that remain innervated. No research is available regarding aerobic exercise training for individuals with ALS. Activity requiring 30–50% of maximal capacity has been recommended to maintain functional capacity for as long as possible. Training goals should be very short-term and should be based on rate of disease progression and readjusted frequently to avoid patient frustration.

Polymyositis/Dermatomyositis

Recently, the measurement of peak aerobic exercise capacity (peak $\dot{V}O_2$) has been reported to be of value in assessing patients with PM/DM. Wiesinger et al.[129] used peak $\dot{V}O_2$ along with $\dot{V}O_2$ at anaerobic threshold and isometric torque measurements to assess the effects of a 6-month training program consisting of stationary cycling and step aerobics. Peak $\dot{V}O_2$ was increased by an average of 28% in eight patients who exercised and was unchanged in five control patients. The authors concluded that stationary cycling and step aerobics could be undertaken by patients with chronic inflammatory myopathy without exacerbation of inflammatory activity. Improvements in fitness from these training programs were documented by improvements in oxygen uptake during cycle ergometry testing. Wiesinger et al.[126] also used a case-control study to examine differences in peak $\dot{V}O_2$ between eight outpatients with chronic DM, three outpatients with chronic PM, and 11 healthy controls. Controls were healthy individuals matched by age (±3 years) and gender. Peak $\dot{V}O_2$ was measured using a symptom-limited, incremental cycle ergometer protocol. Cardiorespiratory capacity (peak $\dot{V}o_2$) for patients was 53% of matched-control values. In patients, peak $\dot{V}o_2$ correlated well (r = 0.763) with peak isometric torque but was unrelated (r = 0.056) to serum creatine phosphokinase. The authors concluded that aerobic ergometry testing may be a useful assessment tool in patients with PM/DM. More data are necessary to determine whether information gained from aerobic ergometry contributes significantly above that gained from isometric muscle testing.

Muscular Dystrophy

Ergometry testing can best be of use for individuals with muscular dystrophy by assessing peak mechanical power and the oxygen cost of movement (i.e., efficiency at submaximal exercise intensities).[171] Maximal aerobic capacity is less important because it is seldom a limiting factor for the performance of everyday activities. The Wingate anaerobic test has been found to be feasible and reliable for these measurements in individuals with Duchenne's or Becker's muscular dystrophy.[169,172] This test appears to be sensitive to both training-related changes and changes due to natural deterioration. Either the upper or lower limbs can be tested, and very low peak power (e.g., 10–20 W) is to be expected. Therefore, ergometers must allow for very small increments in power (e.g., 2–3 W). Because many commercial ergometers require muscle power greater than 10 W to initiate movement, they may need to be adapted. Submaximal tests with 4- to 6-minute stages or a single-stage ergometry test can provide useful information about movement efficiency. Ideally, these tests should be done on a treadmill because the effects of a distorted gait pattern on oxygen uptake may be of interest. The treadmill protocol should employ very small increments (0.5–1.0 MET) between stages. Oxygen uptake, HR, and perceived exertion may theoretically be used to monitor disease progression or training-related improvements. No data are available regarding the clinical use of monitoring changes in submaximal oxygen uptake in muscular dystrophy patients. Aerobic capacity can also be measured during treadmill protocols (0.5–1.0 MET increments per stage), leg cycle ergometers (2–3 W per 3-minute stage), or arm ergometers. HR, ECG, BP, and rating of perceived exertion should always be monitored under physician supervision during tests of aerobic capacity. Peak HRs are usually low (120–140 beats per minute) despite an all-out effort. The usefulness of these measurements is unknown.[173]

Metabolic Myopathies

Patients with metabolic myopathies have impaired muscle oxidative capacity. This may be manifest as a marked limitation in maximal aerobic capacity during a treadmill or cycle ergometry test.[174] However, a maximal ergometry test may not be useful for diagnosing metabolic myopathy because there are many other potential causes of reduced maximal aerobic capacity, including general deconditioning. Recently, there has been interest in measuring serum lactate levels during moderate ergometry exercise as a tool to aid in the diagnosis. Finsterer et al.[175] reported significantly elevated lactate levels during a 15-minute cycle ergometer test at 30 W for patients in comparison to healthy controls. They reported a 69% sensitivity for this test and suggested that it may be useful in complementing electrophysiologic and bioptic findings. Siciliano et al.[176] also reported elevated lactate levels and were able to document that these increased lactate levels were independent of the catecholaminergic response to increasing exercise intensity. Other exercise tests may include ischemic forearm exercise, aerobic cycle exercise, and phosphorus 31 magnetic resonance spectroscopy, discussed in Chapter 16.[177] Near-infrared spectroscopy is another method used in the evaluation of metabolic myopathies to measure mean oxygenation of blood hemoglobin and muscle myoglobin and determining arterial-venous O_2 differences.[178] Taivassalo and colleagues[179,180] have demonstrated that patients with mitochondrial myopathies do benefit from aerobic exercise training. Not only were peak aerobic capacities improved (30%), but blood lactate responses were reduced by a similar amount.[179] They have concluded, as have others regarding many neuromuscular diseases, that chronic deconditioning exacerbates the primary mitochondrial dysfunction.

Postpolio Syndrome

Combined arm and leg ergometry (e.g., Schwinn Air-Dyne) is recommended for testing patients with postpolio syndrome to take advantage of as large a muscle mass as possible.[181] Treadmill protocols are not recommended because weakened lower-extremity musculature fatigues before an adequate challenge of the cardiovascular system. Some experts recommend a single-stage submaximal intensity test to avoid excessive residual fatigue.[182] During the single-stage test, an efficiency index (HR or $\dot{V}O_2$ at a given submaximal intensity) can be calculated and used to monitor training effects or disease progression. As with other neuromuscular diseases, estimated MET values may be inaccurate because of extra energy needed to maintain balance or correct other inefficiencies of movement. A multistage protocol with small increments per stage may be used to measure maximal capacity if coronary artery disease is suspected or diagnosed. Measurement of energy expenditure by gas exchange is useful to predict the type or amount of daily living tasks possible for a given individual. The individuals may have labile BPs that should be carefully monitored before, during, and after ergometry testing. Peripheral fatigue may be a limiting factor and cause premature termination of a GXT. It is not unusual to record maximal HRs that are 20–30 beats per minute less than expected. Increased fatigue, weakness, or pain as a result of either ergometry or aerobic training is a clear signal to decrease the amount or intensity, or both, of exercise.

IN VIVO AND IN VITRO MUSCLE CONTRACTION TESTS USING EXTERNAL STIMULATION

In Vivo Analysis of Muscle Contraction

The mechanical characteristics of muscle contractions can be analyzed not only by voluntary activity, but also during electrical or magnetic nerve stimulation. These studies started with the initial observation of Erb[182] on the difference of contractions between normal and denervated muscles. Later studies using strength-duration curves were based on the relative sensitivity of denervated muscle to long and short duration stimuli.[183] In 1985, Jolly noticed the decreased amplitude of muscle contractions during repetitive nerve stimulation in myasthenia gravis.[184] Clinical electrodiagnostic tests subsequently evolved to analyze the electrical responses of compound muscle action potential (CMAP) during electrical stimulation. Measurements of nerve conduction velocity and changes of CMAP amplitude during repetitive stimulation are now used routinely in the diagnosis of neuromuscular diseases.

The mechanical characteristics of muscle contractions are not analyzed routinely, but their study could be helpful in the evaluation of some neuromuscular conditions,[185–188] particularly in Brody's disease[189–191] and in the assessment of the origin of neuromuscular fatigue.[192–196]

The characteristics of muscle twitch can be studied in individual motor units[197] as well as in muscle groups during electrical[194–196] or magnetic stimulation.[198] Muscle performance and fatigue can be analyzed to determine the origin and possible causes of fatigue with measurement of the muscle twitch and CMAP, as well as surface electromyogram.[199] For example, in disorders of neuromuscular transmission, fatigue is accompanied by reduction of the CMAP as well as muscle twitch, whereas in myopathies muscle twitch is primarily affected. In central nervous system causes of fatigue, there is evidence that there is greater decrease in muscle force during repetitive muscle contraction than during electrical stimulation; with the addition of single stimuli or trains of stimuli during maximal voluntary contractions, there is evidence of increased muscle tension using the technique of twitch interpolation.[200,201]

The following are the characteristics of muscle contractions that can be analyzed to assess neuromuscular function. The maximal force produced by a single supramaximal nerve stimulation is called *twitch tension* or *torque*. During repetitive stimulation, the twitch responses begin to fuse after 10 Hz to produce a persistent contraction (tetanic contraction), which is usually tested at approximately 20 Hz. *Contraction time* is defined as the time that it takes from the beginning of the response to the peak of the contraction after a single stimulus. The *half-relaxation time* is the time that it takes from the peak to half the time that the response takes to return to the baseline. The slope of the relaxation is the slope of the curve from peak to baseline (Figure 15.7). The half-relaxation time can also be measured during tetanic contraction.

Slow rate of stimulation produces changes in the twitch response called *staircase phenomena*. For example, with stimulation at 1 Hz there is a shortening of the contraction time during the first five to six stimuli, and a reduction in amplitude of approximately 10% that occurs during the first 20 stimuli. This is called the *negative staircase*. Continuous stimulation after 20 stimuli to 5 minutes produces an increment in amplitude called the *positive staircase*. The causes of the staircase changes are not

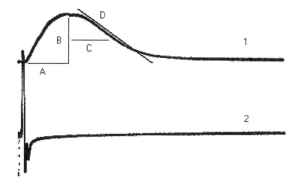

Figure 15.7 1. Analysis of contraction of the abductor pollicis muscle during ulnar nerve stimulation using a TECA-TE42. Contraction time (A), peak twitch (B), half-relaxation time (C), and relaxation slope (1 N/cm, 100 msec/cm) (D). 2. Compound muscle action potential recording during the same stimulation (2 mV/cm, 100 milliseconds/cm).

clearly understood and might be related to the activity-induced electrical-contraction coupling.[186]

Observations of muscle contraction and relaxation can help in the diagnosis of Brody's disease and in the evaluation of myotonia and hypothyroidism, conditions that have a prolonged half-relaxation time. In Brody's disease, there is also shortening of contraction time and a lack of shortening of the relaxation time that occur during the staircase phenomena. Assessment of the CMAP during exercise has also been used in the diagnosis of channelopathies (see the section Hand Exercise Testing in Chapter 2).

In summary, the combined analyses of electrical stimulation and voluntary action are used to analyze muscle contraction, force, relaxation, and fatigue and are becoming an increasingly valuable tool in evaluation of neuromuscular disorders.

In Vitro Study of Muscle Contracture of Small Muscle Fascicles

In vitro study of contracture of small muscle fascicles can be analyzed in animals and humans during exposure to various compounds for the diagnosis of malignant hyperthermia (MH) and other neuromuscular diseases.

Malignant Hyperthermia

MH is a hereditary condition characterized by anesthesia-induced rigidity and myoglobinuria, caused by abnormalities of calcium release channels.[202–205] Muscles of patients at risk for MH have a lower threshold and increased intensity of contraction during electrical stimulation when exposed to either caffeine or halothane. For this reason, in vitro studies are used to identify individuals at risk for MH (Figure 15.8).

In the contracture test, small strips of muscle (approximately 2.0–2.5 cm) are stimulated at one end, and the response is measured with a strain gauge at the other end. During stimulation, the segments are maintained in Krebs-Ringer biological solution, properly oxygenated with 95% O_2 and 5% CO_2 at a standard temperature of 37°C. During this test, the muscle strip is stimulated at various rates, and contractions are recorded during exposure to varying concentrations of halothane and caf-

Figure 15.8 Twitch response of muscle fascicles during electrical stimulation before and after halothane in a patient with malignant hyperthermia (MH+) and a normal control (MH–). Arrows indicate the points at which halothane was administered.

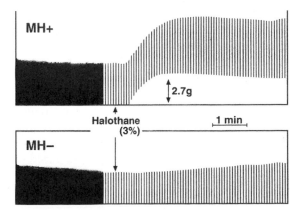

feine.[206–210] More recently, ryanodine[205,211] and chlorocresol[212] have also been used for screening.

Guidelines for performing this test have been published,[213] but because of variation in the techniques, groups of European[214] and North American[215] investigators have standardized protocols to provide similar sensitivities in the detection of individuals at risk.[216]

Other Myopathies

Physiologic studies of muscle segments during routine biopsies are valuable in the study of miniature end-plate potentials, end-plate potentials, muscle twitch, and calcium concentrations in neuromuscular disorders.[217] In vitro studies have aided the analysis of the electrical characteristics of myotonic muscle[218] and have been applied recently in the diagnosis of hyperkalemic and hypokalemic periodic paralysis.[219] In hypokalemic periodic paralysis, the exposure of muscle to low potassium concentrations, particularly with the addition of adrenaline or insulin, causes decreased twitch force, whereas increasing potassium concentration produces weaker contractions in hyperkalemic periodic paralysis.

An advantage of these techniques is that they can be performed in vitro with pieces of muscle obtained during routine biopsies, without exposing the patient to other, sometimes risky, challenging tests used for diagnosis of channelopathies.

CONCLUSIONS

We present here the various methods of analyzing muscle strength. For all these, thorough training and clinical experience of examiners is essential, as is documentation of measurement reliability for the specific patient population. A standardized testing protocol must be consistently followed, because inconsistency in testing method can produce large variations in force or torque measurements. Normal values for each specific testing protocol are needed to interpret patient measurements. Patients with neuromuscular disease can exhibit great day-to-day variability in strength measurements.[5,55] Edwards documented that such variability can be independent of voluntary effort and may be physiologic.[55] Thus, there may be need for making several sets of initial measurements for individual patients, to demonstrate a trend and to increase likelihood of detecting true changes in force over time.[5]

A single strength-testing method is not appropriate for every neuromuscular disorder. In many cases a combination is appropriate, based on the known natural history and the specific physical problems of interest. Strength measurements alone are appropriate when weakness is the major impairment.[2] Although used much less frequently than muscle strength testing, ergometry assessments have the potential to complement more traditional strength and other physiologic findings. This chapter has described methodology used in ergometry testing and summarized what little is known about ergometry testing of persons with neuromuscular disorders. Because of the paucity of knowledge regarding ergometry testing in persons with neuromuscular disorders, it is hoped that this chapter stimulates clinicians to investigate the use of ergometry testing as a means to better evaluate and assess treatment of these patients.

Strength, ergometry, or both types of assessment should be accompanied by a functional assessment to interpret clinical relevance of measured impairments.

Although all studies of natural history for specific disorders have included these, much more is known about the rate of change of specific strength and ergometry measurements than about how such change is related to functional ability and disability. The future challenge for those realizing the importance of quantitative assessment of neuromuscular function is to document the link between measured impairment and functional limitation.

Finally, assessment of the characteristics of muscle twitch during voluntary and electrical stimulation and the in vitro muscle contraction tests are also valuable in the study of neuromuscular disorders.

REFERENCES

1. Edwards RHT, Hyde S. Methods of measuring muscle strength and fatigue. Physiother 1977;63:51–55.
2. Wiles CM, Mills KR, Edwards RHT. Quantitation of Muscle Contraction and Strength. In P Dyck (ed), Peripheral Neuropathy. Philadelphia: Saunders, 1993;698–705.
3. Munsat TL, Hollander D, Andres P, Finison L. Clinical Trials in ALS: Measurement and Natural History. In LP Rowland (ed), Advances in Neurology, Vol 56. Amyotrophic Lateral Sclerosis and Other Motor Neuron Diseases. New York: Raven Press, 1991;515–519.
4. Lexell J. Muscle structure and function in chronic neurological disorders: the potential of exercise to improve activities of daily living. Exerc Sport Sci Rev 2000;28:80–84.
5. Wiles CM, Karni Y. The measurement of strength in patients with peripheral neuromuscular disorders. J Neurol Neurosurg Psychiatry 1983;46:1006–1013.
6. Munsat TL. Preface. In TL Munsat (ed), Quantification of Neurological Deficit. Boston: Butterworths, 1989;xv–xvi.
7. Munsat TL. Clinical trials in neuromuscular disease. Muscle Nerve 1990;13(Suppl):S3–S6.
8. Andres PL, Skerry LM, Munsat TL. Measurement of Strength in Neuromuscular Diseases. In TL Munsat (ed), Quantification of Neurological Deficit. Boston: Butterworths, 1989;87–100.
9. Cook JD, Glass DS. Strength evaluation in neuromuscular disease. Neurol Clin 1987;5:101–122.
10. Aitkens S, Lord J, Bernauer E, et al. Relationship of manual muscle testing to objective strength measurements. Muscle Nerve 1989;12:173–177.
11. Knuttgen HG (ed), Neuromuscular Mechanisms for Therapeutic and Conditioning Exercise. Baltimore: University Park Press, 1976;xi.
12. Andres PL, Skerry LM, Thornell B, et al. A comparison of three measures of disease progression in ALS. J Neurol Sci 1996;139(Suppl):54–70.
13. Miller RG, Munsat TL, Swash M, et al. Consensus guidelines for design and implementation of clinical trials in ALS. J Neurol Sci 1999;147:97–111.
14. Kerlinger FN. Foundations of Behavioral Research (2nd ed). New York: Rinehart and Winston, 1973.
15. Rothstein J. Measurement and Clinical Practice: Theory and Application. In JM Rothstein (ed), Measurement in Physical Therapy. New York: Churchill Livingstone, 1985;1–46.
16. National Advisory Board on Medical Rehabilitation Research. Draft V: Report and Plan for Medical Rehabilitation Research. Bethesda, MD: National Institutes of Health, 1992.
17. Defining Primary Care: An Interim Report. Washington, DC: Institute of Medicine, National Academy Press, 1995.
18. American Physical Therapy Association. Guide to Physical Therapist Practice. Phys Ther 2001;81:1–768.
19. Andres PL, Thibodeau LM, Finison LJ, et al. Quantitative assessment of neuromuscular deficit in ALS. Neurol Clin 1987;5:125–141.
20. Mayhew TP, Rothstein JM. Measurement of Muscle Performance with Instruments. In JM Rothstein (ed), Measurement in Physical Therapy. New York: Churchill Livingstone, 1985;57–102.
21. Medical Research Council. Aids to the Investigation of Peripheral Nerve Injuries. London: Her Majesty's Stationery Office, 1976.
22. Brooke MH, Fenichel GM, Griggs RC, et al. Clinical investigation in Duchenne dystrophy, II. Determination of the "power" of therapeutic trials based on the natural history. Muscle Nerve 1983;6:91–103.

23. Mendell JR, Florence J. Manual muscle testing. Muscle Nerve 1990;13(Suppl):S16–S20.
24. Florence JM, Pandya S, King W, et al. Intrarater reliability of MMT (MRC scale) grades in Duchenne's muscular dystrophy. Phys Ther 1992;72:115–122.
25. Beasley WC. Quantitative muscle testing: principles and applications to research and clinical services. Arch Phys Med Rehabil 1961;42:398–425.
26. Lovett RW, Martin EG. The spring balance muscle test. Am J Orthop Surg 1916;14:415.
27. Beasley WC. Influence of method on estimates of normal knee extensor force among normal and postpolio children. Phys Ther Rev 1956;36:21–41.
28. Nicholas JA, Sapega A, Kraus H, et al. Factors influencing manual muscle tests in physical therapy: the magnitude and duration of force applied. J Bone Joint Surg 1978;60:186–190.
29. Sufit R, Clough JA, Schram M, et al. Isokinetic assessment in ALS. Neurol Clin 1987;5:197–212.
30. Brooks BR, Sufit RL, Clough JA, et al. Isokinetic and Functional Evaluation of Muscle Strength over Time in Amyotrophic Lateral Sclerosis. In TL Munsat (ed), Quantification of Neurological Deficit. Boston: Butterworths, 1989;143–154.
31. Miller LC, Michael AF, Baxter TL, Kim Y. Quantitative muscle testing in childhood dermatomyositis. Arch Phys Med Rehabil 1988;69:610–613.
32. Griffin JW, McClure MH, Bertorini TE. Sequential isokinetic and muscle testing in patients with neuromuscular disease. Phys Ther 1986;66:32–35.
33. Merlini L, Dell'Accio D, Holzl A, et al. Isokinetic muscle testing (IMT) in neuromuscular diseases. Preliminary report. Neuromuscul Disord 1992;2:201–207.
34. Griffin JE, Bertorini TE, O'Toole ML, et al. Isokinetic assessment of muscle performance in patients with inflammatory myopathy. Phys Ther 1994;74:SS118(abst).
35. Ziter FA, Allsop KG, Tyler FH. Assessment of muscle strength in DMD. Neurology 1977;27: 981–984.
36. Allsop KG, Ziter FA. Longitudinal strength and functional decline in Duchenne muscular dystrophy. Arch Neurol 1981;38:406–411.
37. Cohen L, Morgan J, Babbs R, et al. A statistical analysis of the loss of muscle strength in Duchenne muscular dystrophy. Res Commun Chem Pathol Pharmacol 1982;37:123–137.
38. Brooke MH, Griggs RC, Mendell JR, et al. Clinical trial in Duchenne dystrophy. I. The design of the protocol. Muscle Nerve 1981;4:186–197.
39. Florence JM, Pandya S, King W, et al. Clinical trials in Duchenne dystrophy. Standardization and reliability of evaluation procedures. Phys Ther 1984;64:41–45.
40. Barr AE, Diamond BE, Wade CK, et al. Reliability of testing measures in Duchenne or Becker muscular dystrophy. Arch Phys Med Rehabil 1991;72:315–319.
41. Mendell JR, Province MA, Moxley RT, et al. Clinical investigation of Duchenne muscular dystrophy: a methodology for therapeutic trials based on natural history controls. Arch Neurol 1987;44:808–811.
42. Brooke MH, Fenichel GM, Griggs RC, et al. Duchenne muscular dystrophy; pattern of clinical progression and effects of supportive therapy. Neurology 1989;39:475–481.
43. Brooke MH. A Clinician's View of Neuromuscular Diseases (2nd ed). Baltimore: Williams & Wilkins, 1986.
44. Kilmer DD, Abresch RT, Fowwler WM, et al. Serial manual muscle testing in Duchenne muscular dystrophy. Arch Phys Med Rehabil 1993;74:1168–1171.
45. Mendell JR, Moxley RT, Griggs RC, et al. Randomized double-blind six-month trial of prednisone in Duchenne's muscular dystrophy. N Engl J Med 1989;320:1592–1597.
46. Brooke MH, Fenichel GM, Griggs RC, et al. Clinical investigation of Duchenne muscular dystrophy. Arch Neurol 1987;44:812–817.
47. Fenichel GM, Mendell JR, Moxlley RT, et al. A comparison of daily and alternate-day prednisone therapy in the treatment of Duchenne muscular dystrophy. Arch Neurol 1991;48:575–579.
48. Griggs RC, Moxley RT, Mendell JR, et al. Randomized double-blind trial of mazindol in Duchenne dystrophy. Muscle Nerve 1990;13:1169–1173.
49. Griggs RC, Moxley RT, Mendell JR, et al. Prednisone in Duchenne dystrophy: a randomized controlled trial defining the time course and dose response. Arch Neurol 1991;48:383–388.
50. Bonifati MD, Ruzza G, Bonometto P, et al. A multicenter, double-blind, randomized trial of deflazacort versus prednisone in Duchenne muscular dystrophy. Muscle Nerve 2000;9:1344–1347.
51. Lord JP, Portwood MM, Lieberman JS, et al. Upper extremity functional rating for patients with Duchenne muscular dystrophy. Arch Phys Med Rehabil 1987;68:151–154.
52. Scott OM, Goddard C, Dubowitz V, et al. The quantification of muscle function in children: a prospective study in DMD. Muscle Nerve 1982;5:291–301.

53. Heckmatt JZ, Hyde SA, Gabain A. Therapeutic trial of isaxonine in Duchenne muscular dystrophy. Muscle Nerve 1988;11:836–847.
54. Vignos PJ, Archibald KC. Maintenance of ambulation in childhood muscular dystrophy. J Chronic Dis 1960;12:273–290.
55. Edwards RHT, Chapman SJ, Newham DJ, et al. Practical analysis of variability of muscle function measurements in Duchenne muscular dystrophy. Muscle Nerve 1987;10:6–14.
56. Siegel IM. Pathomechanics of stance in Duchenne muscular dystrophy. Arch Phys Med Rehabil 1972;53:403–406.
57. Personius KE, Pandya S, King W, et al. Facioscapulohumeral dystrophy natural history study; standardization of testing procedures and reliability of measurements. Phys Ther 1994;74:253–263.
58. Tawil R, McDermott MP, Mendell JR, et al. Facioscapulohumeral muscular dystrophy (FSHD): design of natural history study and results of baseline testing. Neurology 1994;44:442–446.
59. FSH-Dy Group. A prospective, quantitative study of the natural history of facioscapulohumeral muscular dystrophy (FSHD): implications for therapeutic trials. Neurology 1997;48:38–46.
60. Tawil R, McDermott MP, Pandya S, et al. A pilot trial of prednisone in facioscapulohumeral muscular dystrophy (FSHD). Neurology 1997;48:46–49.
61. Kissei JT, McDermott MP, Natarajan MA, et al. Pilot trial of albuterol in facioscapulohumeral muscular dystrophy. Neurology 1998;50:1402–1406.
62. Caroscio JT, Mulvihill MN, Sterling R, et al. Amyotrophic lateral sclerosis: its national history. Neurol Clin 1987;5:1–8.
63. Lacomblez L, Bensimon G, Leigh PN. Riluzole in amyotrophic lateral sclerosis. Lancet 1996;347: 1425–1431.
64. Beghi E, Chio A, Inghilleri M, et al. A randomized controlled trial of recombinant interferon beta-1a in ALS: Italian group. Neurology 2000;54:469–474.
65. Sobue G, Matsuoka Y, Mukai E, et al. Pathology of myelinated fibers in cervical and lumbar ventral spinal roots in amyotrophic lateral sclerosis. J Neurol Sci 1981;50:413–421.
66. Sobue G, Sahashi K, Takahashi A, et al. Degenerating compartment and functioning compartment of motor neurons in ALS: possible process of motor neuron loss. Neurology 1983;33:654–657.
67. Munsat TL, Andres P, Skerry. The Use of Quantitative Techniques to Define ALS. In TL Munsat (ed), Quantification of Neurological Deficit. Boston: Butterworths, 1989.
68. Andres PL, Hedlund W, Finison L, et al. Quantitative motor assessment in amyotrophic lateral sclerosis. Neurology 1986;36:937–941.
69. Edwards RHT, Young A. Human skeletal muscle function. Clin Sci Mol Med 1977;52:283–290.
70. Brinkmann JR, Andres P, Mendoza M, et al. Guidelines for use and performance of quantitative outcome measures in ALS clinical trials. J Neurol Sci 1997;147:97–111.
71. Brussock CM, Haley SM, Munsat TL, et al. Measurement of isometric force in children with and without Duchenne's muscular dystrophy. Phys Ther 1992;72:105–114.
72. Stuberg WA, Metcalf WK. Reliability of quantitative muscle testing in healthy children and in children with Duchenne muscular dystrophy using a hand-held dynamometer. Phys Ther 1988; 68:977–982.
73. Osternig LR. Isokinetic dynamometry: implications for muscle testing and rehabilitation. Exerc Sport Sci Rev 1986;14:45–80.
74. Perrine JJ. Isokinetic exercise and mechanical energy potential of muscle. J Health Phys Educ Rec 1968;39:40–44.
75. Kramer JF, MacDerrmid J. Isokinetic measures during concentric-eccentric cycles of the knee extensors. Austral J Physiother 1989;35:9–14.
76. Delitto A. Isokinetic dynamometry. Muscle Nerve 1990;13(Suppl):S53–S57.
77. Winter DA, Wells RP, Orr GW. Errors in the use of isokinetic dynamometers. Eur J Appl Physiol 1981;46:398–408.
78. Westing SH, Seger JY. Eccentric and concentric torque-velocity characteristics, torque output comparisons and gravity effect corrections for quadriceps and hamstring muscles in females. Int J Sports Med 1989;10:175–180.
79. van der Ploeg RJO, Fidler V, Osterhius HJGH. The "make/break" test as a diagnostic tool in functional weakness. J Neurol Neurosurg Psychiatry 1991;54:248–251.
80. Wiles CM, Karni Y, Niclin J. Laboratory testing of muscle function in the management of neuromuscular disease. J Neurol Neurosurg Psychiatry 1990;53:384–387.
81. Bohannon R. Test-retest reliability of hand-held dynamometry during a single session of strength assessment. Phys Ther 1986;66:206–209.
82. Trudelle-Jackson E, Jackson AW, Frnakowski CM, et al. Interdevice reliability and validity assessment of the Nicholas hand-held dynamometer. J Orth Sport Phys Ther 1994;20:302–306.

83. Edwards RHT, McDonnell M. Hand-held dynamometry for evaluating voluntary muscle function. Lancet 1974;2:757–758.

84. Hosking GP, Bhat US, Dubowitz V, et al. Measurements of muscle strength and performance in children with normal and diseased muscle. Arch Dis Child 1976;51:957–963.

85. Hyde SA, Scott OM, Goddard CM. The myometer: the development of a clinical tool. Physiotherapy 1983;69:424–427.

86. Rheault JR, Beal JL, Kubik KR, et al. Intertester reliability of the hand-held dynamometer for wrist flexion and extension. Arch Phys Med Rehabil 1989;70;907–910.

87. van der Ploeg RJ, Oosterhuis HJ, Reuvekamp J. Measuring muscle strength. J Neurol 1984;231: 200–203.

88. Byl NN, Richards S, Asturias J. Intrarater and interrater reliability of strength measurements of the biceps and deltoid using a hand-held dynamometer. J Orthop Sports Phys Ther 1988;9:399–405.

89. Deones VL, Wiley SC, Worrell T. Assessment of quadriceps muscle performance by a hand-held dynamometer and an isokinetic dynamometer. J Orthop Sports Phys Ther 1994;20:296–301.

90. Wikhold JB, Bohannon RW. Hand-held dynamometer measurements: tester strength makes a difference. J Orthop Sports Phys Ther 1991;13:191–198.

91. Grinrod S, Tofts P, Edwards R. Investigation of human skeletal muscle strength and composition by X-ray computerized tomography. Eur J Clin Invest 1983;13:465–468.

92. Schantz P, Randall-Fox E, Hutchison W, et al. Muscle fiber type distribution, muscle cross-sectional area and maximal voluntary strength in humans. Acta Physiol Scand 1983;117:219–226.

93. Bigland B, Lippold OCJ. Motor unit activity in the voluntary contraction of human muscle. J Physiol (Lond) 1954;125:322–335.

94. Jones DA, Bigland-Ritchie B, Edwards RHT. Excitation frequency and muscle fatigue: mechanical responses during voluntary and stimulated contractions. Exp Neurol 1979;64:401–413.

95. Sharma KR, Mynhier MA, Miller RG. Cyclosporin increases muscular force generation in Duchenne muscular dystrophy. Neurology 1993;42:527–532.

96. Miller RG, Sharma KR, Pavlah GK, et al. Myoblast implantation in Duchenne muscular dystrophy. Muscle Nerve 1997;20:469–478.

97. Edwards RHT. Muscle fatigue. Postgrad Med J 1975;51:137–143.

98. Shenton DW, Heppenstall RB, Chance B. Electrical stimulation of muscle studied using ^{31}P-nuclear magnetic resonance spectroscopy. J Orthop Res 1986;4:204–211.

99. McComas AJ. Invited review: motor unit estimation: methods, results and present status. Muscle Nerve 1991;14:585–597.

100. Armon C, Brandstater ME. Motor unit number estimates and quantitative strength testing: a validation study. Muscle Nerve 1997;20:1072–1073.

101. Armon C, Brandstater ME, Peterson GW. Motor unit number estimates and quantitative strength measurements of distal muscles in patients with amyotrophic lateral sclerosis. Muscle Nerve 1997;20:499–501.

102. Beck M, Giess R, Warffel W, et al. Comparison of maximal voluntary isometric contraction and Drachman's hand held dynamometry in evaluating patients with amyotrophic lateral sclerosis. Muscle Nerve 1999;22:1265–1270.

103. Smith RA, Melmed S, Sherman B, et al. Recombinant growth hormone treatment of amyotrophic lateral sclerosis. Muscle Nerve 1993;16:624–633.

104. Bohannon RW. Manual muscle test and dynamometer scores of knee extensors. Arch Phys Med Rehabil 1986;67:390–392.

105. Fowler WM, Gardner GW. Quantitative strength measurements in muscular dystrophy. Arch Phys Med Rehabil 1967;48:629–644.

106. Tornvall G. Assessment of physical capabilities. Acta Physiol Scand 1963;58(Suppl 201):1–102.

107. Edwards RHT. Studies of muscular performance in normal and dystrophic subjects. Br Med Bull 1980;36:159–164.

108. Filusch E, Burnett C. Reliability of Cybex II dynamometer strength measurements in dystrophic children. Phys Ther 1989;69:70(abst).

109. deBoer A, Boukes RJ, Sterk JC. Reliability of dynamometry in patients with neuromuscular disorders. Eng Med 1982;11:169–174.

110. Russman BS, Iannaccone ST, Cook JD, et al. Sensitivity of the DCN-SMA study group methodology. Muscle Nerve 1990;13(Suppl):S13–S15.

111. Mendell JR, Kissell JT, Amato AA, et al. Myoblast transfer in the treatment of Duchenne's muscular dystrophy. New Engl J Med 1995;333:832–838.

112. deLateur BJ, Giaconi RM. Effect on maximum strength of submaximal exercise in Duchenne muscular dystrophy. Am J Phys Med 1979;58:26–36.

113. Wagner MB, Vignos PJ, Fonow DC. Serial isokinetic evaluation used for a patient with scapuloperoneal muscular dystrophy: a case report. Phys Ther 1986;66:1110–1113.

114. Florence J, Scheirbecker J. The use of LidoActive isokinetic system in Duchenne muscular dystrophy. Phys Ther 1989;69:370–371(abst).

115. Bohannon RW. Relative dynamic muscular endurance of patients with neuromuscular disorders and of healthy matched control subjects. Phys Ther 1987;67:18–22.

116. Smith RA, Newcombe RG, Sibert JR, et al. Assessment of locomotor function in young boys with Duchenne muscular dystrophy. Muscle Nerve 1991;14:462–469.

117. Griggs RC, Moxley RT, Mendell JR, et al. Duchenne dystrophy: randomized controlled trial of prednisone (18 months) and azathioprine (12 months). Neurology 1993;43:520–527.

118. Karpati F, Ajukovic D, Arnold D, et al. Myoblast transfer in Duchenne muscular dystrophy. Ann Neurol 1993;34:8–17.

119. Bohannon RW, Andrews W. Interrater reliability of hand-held dynamometry. Phys Ther 1987;67:931–933.

120. Dinsdale SM, Cole TM, Zaki FG, Awad EA. Measurements of disease activity in dermatomyositis. Arch Phys Med Rehabil 1971;52:201–206.

121. Resnick JS, Mammel M. Muscular strength as an index of response to therapy in childhood dermatomyositis. Arch Phys Med Rehabil 1981;62:12–19.

122. Edwards RHT, Wiles CM, Round JM, et al. Muscle breakdown and repair in polymyositis: a case study. Muscle Nerve 1979;2:223–228.

123. Edwards RHT, Isenberg DA, Wiles CM, et al. The investigation of inflammatory myopathy. J Roy Coll Phys Lond 1981;15:19–24.

124. Kroll M, Otis J, Kagen L. Serum enzyme, myoglobin and muscle strength: relationships in polymyositis and dermatomyositis. J Rheumatol 1986;13:349–355.

125. Kroll M, Otis JC, Kagen LJ. Abnormalities in quadriceps-hamstring strength. Relationships in polymyositis and dermatomyositis. J Rheumatol 1988;15:1782–1788.

126. Wiesinger GF, Ouittan M, Nuhr M, et al. Aerobic capacity in adult dermatomyositis/polymyositis patients and healthy subjects. Arch Phys Med Rehabil 2000;81:1–5.

127. Escalante A, Miller L, Beardmore TD. Resistive exercise in the rehabilitation of polymyositis/dermatomyositis. J Rheumatol 1993;20:1340–1344.

128. Hicks JE, Miller F, Plotz P, et al. Isometric exercise increases with strength and does not produce sustained creatine phosphokinase increases in a patient with polymyositis. J Rheumatol 1993;20:1399–1401.

129. Wiesinger GF, Ouittan M, Ganinger M, et al. Benefit of 6 months long-term physical training in polymyositis/dermatomyositis. Br J Rheumatol 1998;37:1338–1342.

130. Andres P, Finison LJ, Conlon T, et al. Use of composite scores (megascores) to measure deficit in amyotrophic lateral sclerosis. Neurology 1988;38:405–408.

131. Miller RG, Moore D, Young LA, et al. Placebo-controlled trial of gabapentin in patients with amyotrophic lateral sclerosis. Neurology 1996;39:256–260.

132. Hoagland RJ, Mendoza A, Armon C, et al. Reliability of maximal voluntary isometric contractions testing in a multicenter study of patients with amyotrophic lateral sclerosis. Muscle Nerve 1997;20:691–695.

133. Munsat TL, Andres PL, Burnside S, et al. The natural history of ALS. Ann Neurol 1985;18:157.

134. Munsat TL, Andres PL, Finison L, et al. The natural history of motoneuron loss in ALS. Neurology 1988;38:452–458.

135. Brooks BR, Sufit RL, DePaul R, et al. Design of Clinical Therapeutic Trials in Amyotrophic Lateral Sclerosis. In LP Rowland (ed), Advances in Neurology, Vol 56. Amyotrophic Lateral Sclerosis and Other Motor Neuron Diseases. New York: Raven Press, 1991;521–546.

136. Ringel SP, Murphy JR, Alderson MK, et al. The natural history of ALS. Neurology 1993;43:1316–1322.

137. Pradas J, Finison L, Andres PL, et al. The natural history of amyotrophic lateral sclerosis and the use of natural history controls in therapeutic trials. Neurology 1993;43:751–755.

138. Brooks BR. Natural history of ALS: symptoms, strength, pulmonary function and disability. Neurology 1996;47(Suppl 2):571–582.

139. ALS CNTF Treatment Study Group. A double-blind, placebo-controlled trial of subcutaneous recombinant ciliary neurotrophic factor in ALS. Neurology 1996;46:1244–1249.

140. Miller RG, Petajan JH, Bryan WW, et al. A placebo-controlled trial of recombinant human ciliary neurotrophic (rh CNTF) factor in amyotrophic lateral sclerosis. Ann Neurol 1996;39:256–260.

141. Miller RG, Smith SA, Murphy JR, et al. A clinical trial of Verapamil in ALS. Muscle Nerve 1996;19:511–515.

142. Trojan DA, Collet JP, Shapiro S, et al. A multicenter, randomized double blinded trial of pyridostigmine in postpolio syndrome. Neurology 2000;55:899–901.

143. McGuire D, Garrison L, Armon C, et al. Relationship of the Tufts Quantitative Neuromuscular Exam (TQNE) and the Sickness Impact Profile (SIP) in measuring progression of ALS. Neurology 1996;46:1442–1444.

144. McGuire D, Garrison L, Armon C, et al. A brief quality of life measure for ALS clinical trials based on a subset of items from the SIP. J Neurol Sci 1997;152(Suppl):S18–S22.

145. The ALS CNTF Treatment Study (ACTS) Phase I-II Study Group. The amyotrophic lateral sclerosis functional rating scale. Arch Neurol 1996;53:141–147.

146. Cedarbaum JM, Wittes J, Brittain E, et al. Correlation between rates of change in functional rating scales and muscle strength measures in amyotrophic lateral sclerosis. Neurology 1994;44(Suppl 2):A256–A257.

147. Cedarbaum JM, Stambler N. Performance of the amyotrophic lateral sclerosis functional rating scale (ALSFRS) in multicenter clinical trials. J Neurol Sci 1997;152(Suppl 1):S1–S9.

148. Stambler N, Charatan M, Cedarbaum JM. Prognostic indicators of survival in ALS. Neurology 1998;50:66–72.

149. Armon C, Graves MC, Moses D, et al. Linear estimates of disease progression predict survival in patients with amyotrophic lateral sclerosis. Muscle Nerve 2000;23:874–882.

150. Cook JD, Iannaccone ST, Russman BS, et al. Cooperative study for the assessment of therapeutic trials for the SMAs: a methodology to measure the strength of SMA patients. DCN-SMA Study Group. Muscle Nerve 1990;13(Suppl):S7–S10.

151. Samaha F, Cook JD, Iannaccone ST, et al. Cooperative study for the assessment of therapeutic trials for the SMAs: preliminary observations on the reliability of the DCN-SMA Study Group methodology. Muscle Nerve 1990;13(Suppl):S11–S12.

152. Samaha F, Cook JD, Iannoccone ST. Preliminary observations on the reliability of the DCN-SMA study group methodology. DCN-SMA study group. Muscle Nerve 1990;13(Suppl):S11–S12.

153. Barker L, Smith C, Perkus B, et al. Clinical trials in spinal muscular atrophy: protocol development and reliability of quantitative strength assessment methods. J Neurol Rehabil 1992;6:175–183.

154. Iannaccone ST, Russman BS, Browne RH, et al. A prospective analysis of strength in spinal muscular atrophy. J Child Neurol 2000;15:97–101.

155. Richards C, Bouchard JP, Bouchard R, et al. A preliminary study of dynamic muscle function in hereditary ataxia. Can J Neurol Sci 1980;7;367–377.

156. Armstrong LE, Winant DM, Swasey PR, et al. Using isokinetic dynamometry to test ambulatory patients with multiple sclerosis. Phys Ther 1983;63:1274–1279.

157. Knutsson E, Martensson A. Dynamic motor capacity in spastic paresis and its relation to prime mover dysfunction, spastic reflexes and antagonist co-activation. Scand J Rehabil Med 1980;12:93–106.

158. Knutsson E, Gransberg L, Martensson A. Facilitation and inhibition of maximal voluntary contractions by the activation of muscle strength reflexes in patients with spastic paresis. Electroencephalogr Clin Neurophysiol 1988;70:37.

159. Knutsson E, Martensson A, Gransberg L. Influences of muscle stretch reflexes on voluntary, velocity-controlled movements in spastic paraparesis. Brain 1997;120:1621–1633.

160. Ponichtera JA, Rodgers MM, Glaster RM. Concentric and eccentric isokinetic loser extremity strength in MS and able bodies. J Orthop Sports Phys Ther 1992;16:114–122.

161. Griffin JW, Tooms RE, Vander Zwaag R, et al. Eccentric and concentric muscle performance in patients with spastic paresis secondary to motor neuron disease. A preliminary report. Neuromusc Disord 1994;4:131–135.

162. Goonetilleke A, Modanes-Sadeghi H, Guiloff R. Accuracy, reproducibility and variability of hand held dynamometry in motor neuron disease. J Neurol Neurosurg Psychiatry 1994;57:326–332.

163. Bohannon R. Results of resistance exercise on a patient with amyotrophic lateral sclerosis. Phys Ther 1983;63:965–968.

164. Davis JA. Direct Determination of Aerobic Power. In PJ Maud, C Foster (eds), Physiological Assessment of Human Fitness. Champaign, IL: Human Kinetics, 1995;9–17.

165. ACSM's Guidelines for Exercise Testing and Prescription (6th ed). Philadelphia: Lippincott Williams & Wilkins, 2000.

166. Balady GJ, Weiner DA, Rose L, et al. Physiologic responses to arm ergometry exercise relative to age and gender. J Am Coll Cardiol 1990;16:130–135.

167. Myers J, Buchanan N, Smith D, et al. Individualized ramp treadmill: observations on a new protocol. Chest 1992;101:236S–241S.
168. Kaminsky LA, Whaley MH. Evaluation of a new standardized ramp protocol: the BSU/Bruce ramp protocol. J Cardiopulm Rehabil 1998;18:438–443.
169. Van Mil E, Schoeber N, Calvert RE, Bar-Or O. Optimization of force in the Wingate Test for children with a neuromuscular disease. Med Sci Sports Exerc 1996;28:1087–1092.
170. Nau KL. Amyotrophic Lateral Sclerosis. In ACSM's Exercise Management for Persons with Chronic Diseases and Disabilities. Champaign, IL: Human Kinetics, 1997;200–205.
171. Bar-Or O. Role of exercise in the assessment and management of neuromuscular disease in children. Med Sci Sports Exerc 1996;28:421–427.
172. Tirosh E, Bar-Or O, Rosenbaum P. New muscle power test in neuromuscular disease. Feasibility and reliability. Am J Dis Child 1990;144:1083–1087.
173. Bar-Or O. Muscular Dystrophy. In ACSM's Exercise Management for Persons with Chronic Diseases and Disabilities. Champaign, IL: Human Kinetics, 1997;180–184.
174. Elliot DL, Buist NR, Goldberg L, et al. Metabolic myopathies: evaluation by graded exercise testing. Medicine (Baltimore) 1989;68:163–172.
175. Finsterer J, Eichberger H, Jarius C. Lactate-stress testing in 54 patients with mitochondriopathy. Eur Arch Psychiatry Clin Neurosci 2000;250:36–39.
176. Siciliano G, Renna M, Manca ML, et al. The relationship of plasma catecholamine and lactate during anaerobic threshold exercise in mitochondrial myopathies. Neuromuscul Disord 1999;9: 411–416.
177. Martin A, Haller RG, Barohn R. Metabolic myopathies. Curr Opin Rheumatol 1994;6:552–558.
178. Bank WJ, Chance B. A oxidative defect in metabolic myopathies. Diagnosis by tissue oximetry. Ann Neurol 1999;36:850–857.
179. Taivassalo T, DeStefano N, Argov Z, et al. Effects of aerobic training in patients with mitochondrial myopathies. Neurology 1998;50:1055–1060.
180. Taivassalo T, DeStefano N, Chen J, et al. Short-term aerobic training response in chronic myopathies. Muscle Nerve 1999;22:1239–1243.
181. Birk TJ. Polio and Post-Polio Syndrome. In ACSM's Exercise Management for Persons with Chronic Diseases and Disabilities. Champaign, IL: Human Kinetics, 1997;206–211.
182. Erb W. Handbook of Electrotherapeutics. Translated by L. Pertzel. New York: William Wood, 1883.
183. Lambert E. Neurophysiological techniques useful in the study of neuromuscular diseases. Neuromuscul Disord 1958;9:247–273.
184. Jolly F. Uber myasthenia gravis pseudoparalytica. Berl Klin Wschr 1895;32:1–7.
185. Sharma A, Miller RG. Electrical and mechanical properties of skeletal muscle underlying increased fatigue in patients with amyotrophic lateral sclerosis. Muscle Nerve 1996;19:1391–1400.
186. Quinlan J, Iaizzo PA, Lambert EH, Gronert GA. Ankle dorsiflexion twitch properties in malignant hyperthermia. Muscle Nerve 1989;12:119–125.
187. Takamori M, Gutman L, Shane SR. Contractile properties of human skeletal muscle normal and thyroid disease. Arch Neurol 1971;25:535–546.
188. Sharma KR, Mynhier MA, Miller RG. Muscular fatigue in Duchenne muscular dystrophy. Neurology 1995;45:306–310.
189. Quinlan J, Iaizzo PA, Gronert GA, Lambert EH. Twitch response in a myopathy with impaired relaxation, but no myotonia. Muscle Nerve 1990;13:326–329.
190. Brody TA. Muscle contracture induced by exercise. New Engl J Med 1968;281:187–192.
191. De Ruiter CJ, Wevers RA, Baziel GM, et al. Muscle function in a patient with Brody's disease. Muscle Nerve 1999;22:704–711.
192. Shields R. Fatigability, relaxation properties in and electromyographic response of the human paralyzed soleus muscle. J Neurophysiol 1995;73(6);2195–2206.
193. Kent-Braun JA, Le Blanc R. Quantitation of central activation failure during maximal voluntary contractions in humans. Muscle Nerve 1996;19:861–869.
194. Kent-Braun JA. Noninvasive measure of central and peripheral activation in human muscle fatigue. Muscle Nerve 1997;5:S98–S101.
195. Binder-Macleod SA, Lee S, Baadte SA. Reduction of the fatigue-induced force decline in human skeletal muscle by optimized stimulation trains. Arch Phys Med Rehabil 1997;78:1129–1137.
196. Newton JP, Yemm R. Changes in the contractile properties of the human first dorsal interosseous muscle with age. Gerontology 1986;32:98–104.
197. Westling G, Johansson RS, Thomas CK, Bigland-Ritchie B. Measurement of contractile and electrical properties of single human thenar motor units in response to intraneural motor-axon stimulation. J Neurophysiol 1990;64(4);1331–1338.

198. Polkey MI, Kyroussis D, Hamnegard C, et al. Quadriceps strength and fatigue assessed by magnetic stimulation of the femoral nerve in man. Muscle Nerve 1996;19:549–555.

199. Lind AR, Petrofsky JS. Amplitude of the surface electromyogram during fatiguing isometric contractions. Muscle Nerve 1979;2:257–264.

200. Allen GM, Gandevia SC, McKenzie DK. Reliability of measurements of muscle strength and voluntary activation using twitch interpolation. Muscle Nerve 1995;18:593–600.

201. Miller M, Downhan D, Lexell J. Superimposed single impulse and pulse train electrical stimulation: a quantitative assessment during submaximal isometric knee extension in young, healthy men. Muscle Nerve 1999;22:1038–1046.

202. Britt BA. Malignant hyperthermia. Can J Anesth 1985;72:666–677.

203. Kaus SJ, Rockoff MA. Malignant hyperthermia. Pediatr Clin North Am 1994;41(1):221–237.

204. Bertorini T. Myoglobinuria, malignant hyperthermia, neuroleptic malignant syndrome and serotonin syndrome. Neurol Clin 1997;15(3):649–671.

205. Hopkins PM. Malignant hyperthermia: advances in clinical management and diagnosis. Br J Anaesth 2000;85:118–128.

206. Kalow W, Britt BA, Richter A. The caffeine test of isolated human muscle in relation to malignant hyperthermia. Can Anaesth Soc J 1977;24(6):678–694.

207. Britt B, Scott E, Frodis W, et al. Dantrolene—in vitro studies in malignant hyperthermia susceptible (MHS) and normal skeletal muscle. Can Anaesth Soc J 1984;31(2):130–154.

208. Ording H. Diagnosis of susceptibility to malignant hyperthermia. Br J Anesth 1988;60:287–302.

209. Iaizzo PA, Lehmann-Horn F. In vitro determination of susceptibility to malignant hyperthermia. Muscle Nerve 1989;12:184–190.

210. Iaizzo P, Wedel D, Gallagher W. In vitro contracture testing for determination of susceptibility to malignant hyperthermia: a methodologic update. Mayo Clin Proc 1991;66:998–1004.

211. Hopkins PM, Hartung E, Wappler F. The European Malignant Hyperthermia Group. Multicenter evaluation of ryanodine contracture testing in malignant hyperthermia. Br J Anaesth 1998;80:389–394.

212. Ording H, Slahn K, Sara T, et al. 4-chloro-m-cresol test, a possible supplementary test for diagnosis of malignant hyperthermia susceptibility. Acta Anaesthesiol Scand 1997;41:967–972.

213. Ellis FR, Harriman DGF, Currie S, Cain PA. Screening for Malignant Hyperthermia in Susceptible Patients. In JA Aldrete, BA Britt (eds), Second International Symposium on Malignant Hyperthermia. New York: Grune & Stratton, 1978;273–285.

214. European Malignant Hyperpyrexia Group. A protocol for the investigation of malignant hyperpyrexia (MH) susceptibility. Br J Anaesth 1984;56:1267–1269.

215. Larach MG. Standardization of the caffeine halothane muscle contraction test. North American Malignant Hyperthermia Group. Anesth Analg 1989;69:511–515.

216. Fletcher JE, Rosenberg H, Aggarwal M. Comparison of European and North American malignant hyperthermia diagnostic protocol outcomes for use in genetic studies. Anesthesiology 1999;90(3): 654–661.

217. Lehmann-Horn F, Iaizzo PA. Resealed fiber segments for the study of the pathophysiology of human skeletal muscle. Muscle Nerve 1990;13:222–231.

218. Iaizzo PA, Lehmann-Horn F. The correlation between electrical after-activity and slowed relaxation in myotonia. Muscle Nerve 1990;13:240–246.

219. Iaizzo PA, Quasthoff S, Lehmann-Horn F. Differential diagnosis of periodic paralysis aided by in vitro myography. Neuromuscul Disord 1995;5(2):115–124.

16

Phosphorus Magnetic Resonance Spectroscopy in the Clinical Investigation of Muscle Disorders

Raffaele Lodi and Tanja Taivassalo

Phosphorus (phosphorus 31 [^{31}P]) magnetic resonance (MR) spectroscopy (^{31}P MRS) has been used to study skeletal muscle energy metabolism in vivo in both health and disease since 1981.[1–3] In the past two decades, the use of ^{31}P MRS in the detection of human muscle pathology has been concurrent with its development and technical refinement, making it a powerful, noninvasive probe of tissue biochemistry and physiology. It has also found a unique role as a marker of treatment response in various clinical trials owing to capabilities of continuous metabolic monitoring and ease of repetitive assessments. The study of other biologically important nuclei, such as hydrogen (^{1}H) for creatine, lactate, and lipid assessment, and naturally abundant carbon (^{13}C) for glycogen assessment, has more recently been applied to the investigation of human muscle. However, the use of ^{1}H and ^{13}C MRS with respect to myopathies is still limited. This chapter presents the use of ^{31}P MRS as a clinical and research tool in the evaluation of patients with muscle disorders.

OVERVIEW OF CELLULAR ENERGY METABOLISM

The understanding of cellular energy metabolism in healthy skeletal muscle is necessary for the interpretation of spectroscopic findings in the various disease states presented later. ^{31}P MRS has the capacity to evaluate energy metabolism in a resting state as well as during dynamic processes related to skeletal muscle activity and resultant metabolic stress. Metabolic stress is particularly valuable in detecting abnormalities of energy metabolism that are often not apparent at rest, when demand for energy is low.

Energy Sources and Metabolic Pathways

The hydrolysis of adenosine triphosphate (ATP) to adenosine diphosphate (ADP) and inorganic phosphate (Pi) provides the immediate source of energy for muscle

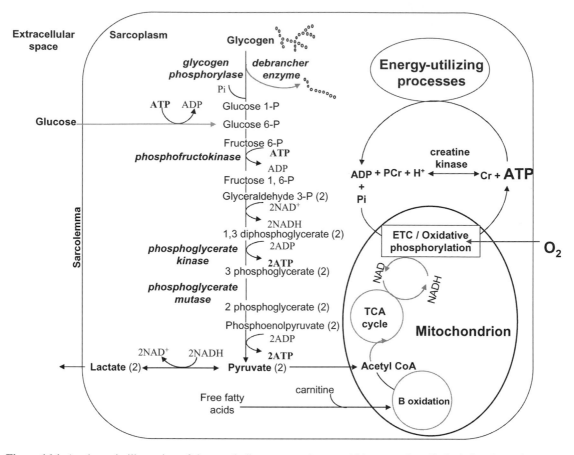

Figure 16.1 A schematic illustration of the metabolic energy pathways within a muscle cell, depicting the various enzymatic reactions involved in adenosine triphosphate (ATP) generation (phosphocreatine hydrolysis, anaerobic glycolysis, and mitochondrial oxidative phosphorylation). Only sites of enzymatic glycogenolytic/glycolytic deficiencies discussed in the chapter are illustrated. (ADP = adenosine monophosphate; CoA = coenzyme A; Cr = creatine; ETC = electron transfer chain; NAD$^+$ = oxidized form of nicotinamide adenine dinucleotide; NADH = nicotinamide adenine dinucleotide [reduced form]; PCr = phosphocreatine; Pi = inorganic phosphate; TCA = tricarboxylic acid cycle.)

contraction and relaxation. Concentrations of endogenous ATP in muscle are limited and capable of supplying energy for only a few seconds of maximal exercise.[4] Thus, sustaining exercise requires the ability of muscle to resynthesize ATP, which is accomplished through three primary metabolic processes: phosphoryl transfer, anaerobic glycolysis, and oxidative phosphorylation (Figure 16.1). Each metabolic process is uniquely important in supplying cellular energy demands at various points and intensities of exercise.

ATP in the cytoplasm is in chemical equilibrium with phosphocreatine (PCr), another high-energy compound, through the reaction catalyzed by creatine kinase (CK). By means of the CK equilibrium reaction (PCr + ADP + H$^+$ $\rightleftarrows$ ATP + Cr), the hydrolysis of PCr and phosphoryl transfer to ADP during exercise provides a rapid source of energy and buffers ATP concentrations near resting levels.[4] This near-equilibrium reaction limits increases in ADP concentration as energy use exceeds ATP synthesis rates. It is only after PCr concentrations are nearly depleted that a significant proportion of the energy for contraction is supplied by net hydrolysis of endogenous ATP.[5] The adenylate kinase reaction (2 ADP $\rightleftarrows$ ATP + AMP [adenosine monophosphate]) also helps to maintain low concentrations of ADP, whereas PCr is depleted.

Anaerobic glycolysis involves a series of enzymatic reactions in the cellular cytoplasm (see Figure 16.1) allowing for rapid formation of ATP by substrate-level phosphorylation with concomitant production of lactate and decrease in muscle pH. Muscle glycogen and blood glucose serve as substrates for this pathway. Oxidative phosphorylation, a process that couples electron transfer to the phosphorylation of ADP within the mitochondria (see Figure 16.1), is the dominant source of ATP for the cell. Carbon-containing substrates in the form of pyruvate and fatty acids serve as substrates in this oxidative process.

Pattern of Energy Transfer

Energy for basal metabolism in resting skeletal muscle is supplied primarily through mitochondrial oxidative phosphorylation. In exercising muscle, the immediate demand for ATP to allow for muscle contraction is supplied by PCr hydrolysis and glycogenolysis. Delivery of oxygen and substrate to mitochondria allows oxidative phosphorylation to become the dominant energy-yielding pathway for sustained exercise. The recovery from exercise involves restoration to the resting state after the metabolically stressful perturbation of muscle contraction. In this phase, the only source of ATP production is oxidative phosphorylation, which continues at an accelerated rate to replenish high-energy phosphate stores.[6]

PHOSPHORUS MAGNETIC RESONANCE SPECTROSCOPY INVESTIGATION IN HEALTHY MUSCLE

The phenomenon of nuclear MR can be induced in the naturally occurring isotope of phosphorus, making it ideal for studying key phosphate-containing compounds associated with skeletal muscle bioenergetics. The technique allows for measurement of Pi, PCr, three resonances of phosphorus nuclei in ATP (gamma, alpha, beta), phosphomonoesters (PME, phospholipid precursors, and sugar phosphates), and phosphodiesters (PDE, membrane phospholipids). A typical MR spectrum obtained from a healthy muscle at rest is shown in Figure 16.2A. The spectral peaks are distinguished by their molecular configurations and characteristic spin-spin coupling patterns and identified based on chemical shift distances in the frequency domain expressed in parts per million of the field strength. Peak intensities (or areas) are proportional to the number of nuclei belonging to the corresponding molecule within the sensitive region of the signal-acquiring surface coil. This coil, typically placed on or under the muscle of interest, receives a signal from an approximate volume that corresponds to a disk with a diameter equal to that of the coil and depth equal to the radius of the coil (see Figure 16.2B). Given the various sizes of surface coils, volumes may be on the order of tens of cubic centimeters, where the signal strength from tissue closest to the coil is stronger than the signal farther away. Therefore, the spectrum represents an average of the energy state of all muscle fibers within the sensitive area of the coil. Metabolite peak intensities are usually converted to concentrations relative to ATP, an internal standard believed to remain constant in normal working muscle at approximately 8 mM.[7,8]

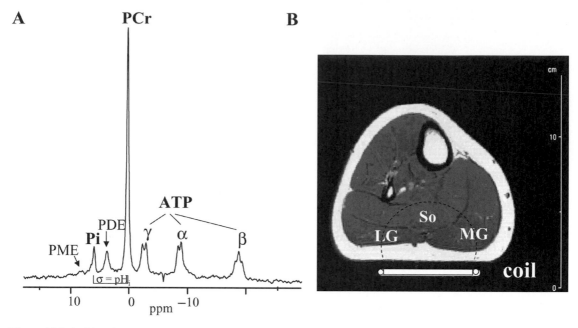

Figure 16.2 A. Phosphorus magnetic resonance spectroscopy spectrum of muscle at rest in a healthy subject. Spectral peaks arise from inorganic phosphate (Pi) and phosphocreatine (PCr), and the positions of the three phosphate atoms of adenosine triphosphate (ATP) are marked as α, β, and γ. Signals from the phosphomonoesters (PME) and phosphodiesters (PDE) may also be detected. The chemical shift, σ, between PCr and Pi is used for pH determination. Spectral distances are presented in parts per million (ppm). **B.** T1-weighted spin echo magnetic resonance image showing muscles of the lower limb (axial plane) at the level of the center of the phosphorus coil of a healthy individual obtained during phosphorus magnetic resonance spectroscopy examination of the calf muscle. The dashed line indicates the approximate volume of signal acquisition using a 6-cm surface coil. (LG = lateral head of gastrocnemius; MG = medial head of gastrocnemius; pH_i = intracellular pH; So = soleus.)

The relative simplicity of the ^{31}P spectrum stems from the fact that not all phosphorus-containing compounds present in living human muscle produce visible, narrow signals. Compounds must be present in concentrations in the millimolar range and not bound to give rise to distinct resonances. Accordingly, much of the signal stems from phosphates in the cytosolic rather than mitochondrial compartments within the cell. Furthermore, membrane phospholipids and the majority of ADP are not spectroscopically detectable. The concentration of "free," metabolically active ADP however, can be derived from the CK equation, with the knowledge that $K_{CK} = 1.66 \times 10^9 M^{-1}$ and total creatine ([TCr], the sum of PCr and free creatine) remains constant at 42.5 mM,[7] as [ADP] = ([ATP][Cr])/([PCr][H$^+$]K_{CK}). Another calculated variable indicating energy reserve within resting muscle is the phosphorylation potential (PP).[9]

$$PP = \frac{[ATP]}{[ADP] \times [Pi]}$$

The chemical shift of Pi from PCr (σ, in parts per million) provides distinctive information on muscle pH.[10] ^{31}P MRS is the only noninvasive method for measuring muscle intracellular pH (pH_i)[2] in vivo, calculated as

$$pH_i = 6.77 + \log\left[\frac{\sigma - 3.27}{5.69 - \sigma}\right]$$

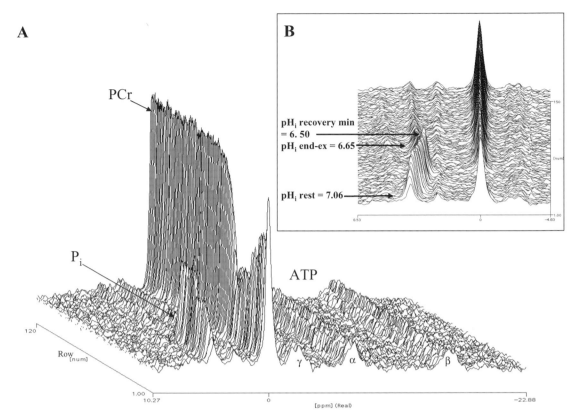

Figure 16.3 A. Stack plot showing serial phosphorus spectra (120 rows) during rest (*first row*), exercise (approximately 2 minutes in duration), and recovery (16 minutes) in the vastus lateralis muscle of a healthy subject. Each spectrum is a signal average of four free-induction decays with a time resolution of 8 seconds between each row. Note the fall in phosphocreatine (PCr) with concomitant increase in inorganic phosphate (P_i) during exercise with recovery to baseline values proceeding rapidly after exercise has stopped (within 1 minute after exercise). Adenosine triphosphate (ATP) peak areas remain stable during exercise and recovery. **B.** The inset displays changes in chemical shift of P_i with respect to PCr during exercise and recovery. At the end of exercise (pH_i end-ex), a further decrease in pH occurs in response to PCr resynthesis and reaches a minimum value during initial recovery (pH_i recovery min) and gradually returns to its pre-exercise state. (pH_i = intracellular pH.)

The acquisition of ^{31}P MR spectra is relatively routine, and good-quality spectra can be obtained within minutes. The time resolution, currently as low as 1 second, allows for detailed evaluation of the dynamic processes relating to energy metabolism during exercise and recovery.

^{31}P MR spectra obtained during exercise show that the concentration of PCr falls, whereas the concentration of Pi is stoichiometrically increased (Figure 16.3A), the magnitude of these changes corresponding to the pattern and extent of muscle work. Intracellular pH becomes acidic as lactate accumulates in the cell with increasing exercise intensity (see Figure 16.3B). The calculated cytosolic free ADP rises with exercise, and ATP remains constant. There is large variability in metabolite and pH response during exercise owing to various physiologic factors (glycolytic flux, oxidative ATP synthesis, blood flow, fiber type).

When muscle contraction stops, the rate of ATP turnover is immediately and dramatically reduced, and as previously mentioned, ATP synthesis through oxidative phosphorylation continues to restore high-energy phosphate stores to pre-exercise levels. Commonly assessed indices to quantify this recovery process include PCr recovery, ADP recovery, and rates of mitochondrial capacity.

Phosphocreatine Recovery

The rate of PCr repletion after exercise reflects precisely the rate of mitochondrial ATP synthesis.[7,11,12] The total oxidative phosphorylation dependence of PCr resynthesis has been demonstrated in human subjects during recovery from ischemic exercise during which time no resynthesis of PCr occurs.[13,14] As no work is done during the recovery phase, the absolute rate of PCr resynthesis is an estimate of the oxidative ATP synthesis rate (less a small component of basal ATP turnover).[14,15] The resynthesis of PCr is directly visible in a recovery spectrum (see Figure 16.3A) and is typically quantified as the time taken to replenish half the difference in [PCr] between the end of exercise and rest (PCr $t_{1/2}$). The recovery of PCr has been the most commonly used index of mitochondrial phosphorylation.

The resynthesis of PCr generates protons during recovery, according to the CK reaction. These protons, as well as those generated during exercise, are effluxed from the cell during recovery. These processes can be seen in the recovery spectrum as an initial shift of Pi towards PCr (reflecting an immediate increase in acidosis owing to PCr resynthesis after the end of exercise) followed by its return to baseline position (see Figure 16.3B). No method of quantification of this biphasic recovery of pH to resting levels has been reported to date. Only the initial rate of proton efflux has been calculated.[16]

Adenosine Diphosphate Recovery

The calculation of cytosolic free ADP recovery has been proposed as a sensitive measure of in vivo mitochondrial function.[17] High end-exercise ADP concentrations recover to concentrations found in muscle at rest, in which the initial recovery phase represents a transition from the active mitochondrial state to the resting state.[18] Rephosphorylation of ADP is commonly expressed as the time required for [ADP] to reach the halfway recovery point (ADP $t_{1/2}$) and reflects the initial rate of oxidative phosphorylation. ADP has been observed to transiently decrease below resting levels during recovery.[18] A second-order step response recovery model has recently been proposed to better reflect this in vivo behavior.[19]

Rates of Mitochondrial Capacity

Kemp and colleagues[15,20] have derived two valuable quantitative indices of mitochondrial function from ^{31}P MRS–measured metabolites. To normalize for the amount of PCr depletion, the initial rate of postexercise PCr resynthesis can be used,[20] given as

$$V = ([PCr]_{rest} - [PCr]_{end-exercise}) \times \frac{0.693}{PCrt_{1/2}}$$

A hyperbolic relationship exists between rate of PCr resynthesis and [ADP].[20] Using this hyperbolic relationship, Kemp et al.[20] have estimated the apparent maximum rate of oxidative ATP synthesis (V_{max}) under the assumption that K_m is normally equal to 30 μM and estimating the end-exercise rate of mitochondrial ATP synthesis by V.

$$V_{max} = V\left(1 + \left[\frac{K_m}{ADP_{end-exercise}}\right]\right)$$

V_{max} provides a quantitative index of mitochondrial function that can be directly related to tissue respiratory rates and has been found to agree reasonably well with enzyme analysis.[21] These recovery indices of oxidative phosphorylation rates are functions of the density and capacity of working mitochondria as well as the supply of substrate and oxygen and are independent of muscle mass.[21]

The study of in vivo skeletal muscle bioenergetics using ^{31}P MRS–derived indices of metabolic recovery requires an appropriate exercise ergometer to allow for sufficient metabolic stress. The relatively small bore diameter of standard MR magnets limits the range of motion and restricts the muscles involved. Consequently, most exercise devices have been designed to examine small muscle groups, and traditionally distal muscles (e.g., forearm finger flexors, wrist flexors, calf muscles) have been studied. There have been fewer ^{31}P MRS studies on quadriceps muscles (either medial or lateral vastus). The spectroscopic study of the quadriceps affords advantages of assessing a larger muscle mass (improving data analysis owing to better signal to noise ratio) and allows for meaningful comparison to the more traditional modalities of assessing muscle function (biopsy, electromyography, bicycle ergometer testing) that are often performed on the quadriceps.

PHOSPHORUS MAGNETIC RESONANCE SPECTROSCOPY: INTERPRETATION AND ASSUMPTIONS

Various physiologic input affects metabolite concentrations and the rate of metabolic recovery in healthy muscle, which may lead to a broad range of control values. In the interpretation of results, it is important to take into account the amount of metabolic work performed, age, and physical conditioning.

Metabolic Work

The relative intensity of exercise can influence the rate of metabolic recovery, owing to the effects of acidosis on PCr resynthesis. End-exercise pH, or the minimum pH reached during recovery from exercise, has been shown to be strongly correlated to the rate of PCr resynthesis.[7,22–24] PCr recovery rate is slower when the pH is more acidotic. Intracellular acidosis occurs to different degrees in each subject during exercise, and PCr recovery rates cannot be compared unless corrections for pH are introduced.[22–24] Unlike the half-time for PCr recovery, half-time of initial ADP recovery, and the maximal rate of mitochondrial ATP synthesis, V_{max} in normal controls is not affected by the instantaneous values of cytosolic pH or [ADP] at the end of exercise.[7,18,24]

Age

Muscle oxidative capacity has been reported to differ in children and adults, with children demonstrating a faster PCr $t_{1/2}$ and V_{max} compared to adults, with no differences in adults of varying ages.[25] Age-related effects on ^{31}P MRS indices at rest have also been reported as lower [PCr] in children (younger than 12 years of age) and the elderly (older than 70 years of age) when compared to young adults (ages 20–29 years). [PDE] was also found to increase with age, which is suggestive of fiber atrophy or accumulated damage to sarcolemma and other membranes.

Physical Conditioning

Perhaps the greatest influence on metabolic recovery in healthy individuals is the state of physical conditioning. ^{31}P MRS recovery indices have proven useful in identifying a range of skeletal muscle oxidative capacities in healthy subjects and trained athletes. Numerous studies have shown endurance athletes to demonstrate enhanced recovery kinetics compared to healthy sedentary individuals, consistent with increased mitochondrial content and oxidative enzyme activity in trained muscle.[26–28] Likewise, deconditioning is expected to affect metabolic recovery and demonstrate changes in skeletal muscle oxidative capacity opposite to those observed with endurance training. Only recently has this been demonstrated in a ^{31}P MRS study[29] in which healthy individuals with low levels of physical activity had slower ^{31}P MRS recovery kinetic indices of oxidative energy metabolism than more conditioned subjects. Physical activity levels, therefore, need to be considered in the ^{31}P MRS evaluation of patients with chronic diseases in which muscle physical activity is reduced.

Assumptions

The quantitation of ^{31}P MRS indices is based on a few assumptions that are routinely made in the interpretation of results and deserve mention: (1) Cytosolic [ATP] does not change significantly during exercise or recovery; (2) [ATP] is similar in healthy as well as diseased muscle; and (3) the observed metabolic system is a closed one with no loss of phosphate metabolites or TCr during exercise and recovery. The first assumption can be confirmed by comparison of the acquired ATP signal at each time point to the rest spectra as a reference value and by calculation of metabolite concentrations during recovery using the ATP value from the same spectrum, thus correcting for any possible change in ATP signal due to technical factors. With respect to the second assumption, total adenine nucleotides and TCr in biopsied specimens were found to be similar to those of healthy subjects in most patients with mitochondrial cytopathies[17,30] but were reduced in muscle biopsies of patients with inflammatory myopathy and muscular dystrophy (MD).[30] This could account for errors in ^{31}P MRS–derived calculations of resting metabolite concentrations but would not affect the recovery kinetics. The third assumption can be verified by calculating the total sum of phosphate metabolites in the spectra.

PHOSPHORUS MAGNETIC RESONANCE SPECTROSCOPY IN PRIMARY METABOLIC MUSCLE DISEASES

Primary metabolic myopathies include inherited disorders of glycogen and glucose metabolism, lipid metabolism, and defects affecting mitochondrial oxidative phosphorylation. In most forms of metabolic myopathies, there is impairment of anaerobic or aerobic metabolism (or both) that can be assessed precisely by ^{31}P MRS.

Disorders of Carbohydrate Metabolism

Deficiency of glycogenolytic or glycolytic enzymes leads to impaired anaerobic synthesis of ATP in association with reduced production of lactate (see Figure 16.1). The insufficient production of reducing mitochondrial equivalents (nicotinamide adenine dinucleotide [NADH]) and pyruvate during aerobic exercise can also result in impaired mitochondrial ATP production. This represents the biochemical basis for a distinctive muscle ^{31}P MRS pattern in glycogenolytic or glycolytic enzyme defects, characterized by a rapid depletion of PCr, appearance of cytosolic alkalosis, or reduced acidification during muscle exercise and slow rate of PCr resynthesis during recovery after exercise. The abnormal relationship between pH_i and PCr during ischemic and, in most cases, aerobic exercise forms the basis of a sensitive diagnostic test that can be an alternative to the ischemic lactate test (Figure 16.4). The investigator can monitor the level of PCr depletion to ensure that an adequate amount of work is performed, in which the rate of change in pH_i is a measure of lactic acid synthesis.

Myophosphorylase Deficiency (McArdle's Disease)

The first clinical ^{31}P MRS study was carried out in 1981 on a patient with myophosphorylase deficiency.[3] The findings of rapid PCr depletion and paradoxic increase in muscle pH (due to proton consumption by PCr hydrolysis) during exercise (Figure 16.5), which were later confirmed by others,[31,32] correlated with clinical aspects of myophosphorylase deficiency disorder. The characteristic cramps experienced by these patients were found to coincide with particularly high concentrations of ADP—a situation that develops as PCr concentration decreases, but pH_i does not fall. In the "second-wind" phenomenon, cramps

Figure 16.4 Flow diagram indicating the utility of phosphorus magnetic resonance spectroscopy (^{31}P MRS) testing in the clinical evaluation of patients with suspected metabolic myopathies. (EMG = electromyography.)

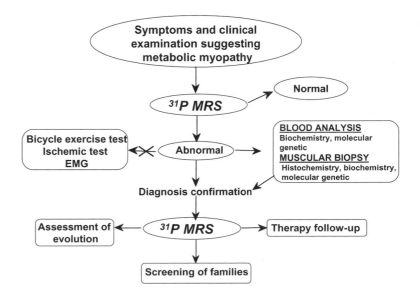

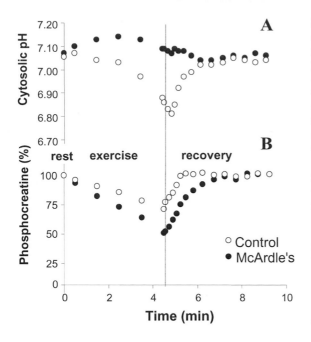

Figure 16.5 Time-dependent changes in cytosolic pH (**A**) and phosphocreatine (**B**) expressed as percentage of resting phosphocreatine content from the calf muscle of a patient with McArdle's disease and a gender- and age-matched control. The data were acquired at rest during an aerobic incremental exercise of plantar flexion and the following recovery phase. Lack of lactate production during exercise is indicated in the patient by an intracellular pH more alkaline than that at rest. Impairment of oxidative phosphorylation in the patient is indicated by a faster phosphocreatine consumption during exercise and a slower phosphocreatine recovery rate than that in the control subject.

diminish, and the ability to exercise is restored as delivery to muscle of blood glucose and fatty acids increases, and pH_i and metabolite concentrations return to normal levels.[33] Exercise protocols must be designed carefully to elicit these diagnostic features, as use of short and intense exercise protocols do not bring forth the second-wind phenomenon.[34,35]

Myophosphorylase releases the distal glucose residues from glycogen molecules. In the muscles of patients with McArdle's disease, there is no synthesis of glucose-6-phosphate or other sugar phosphates of the glycolytic pathway (see Figure 16.1), so there is no increase in the PME peak.[32,34,35] Infusion of glucose bypasses the block in glycogenolysis, thereby reducing net PCr depletion, generating pyruvate, and reducing the mitochondrial equivalents that serve as mitochondrial substrates.[31] The slow recovery of PCr[32,34,35] and ADP[36] after exercise in myophosphorylase deficiency suggests that oxidative phosphorylation is inhibited owing to lack of substrates and may not be delayed if the second wind has been reached. In spite of the evidence for reduced ATP synthesis by both glycolysis and oxidative phosphorylation, there is no simple correlation between symptoms and muscle ATP concentration. The high PCr/ATP ratio found in resting muscle is consistent with a reduced ATP concentration, but neither aerobic[31] nor ischemic exercise,[31,35] nor sustained muscular contracture has been found to lead to a further decrease in muscle ATP content.

Debrancher Enzyme Deficiency

The debrancher enzyme, which releases glucose at branching points, is essential for the complete degradation of glycogen. ^{31}P MRS findings in muscles of patients lacking debrancher activity are qualitatively similar to those of myophosphorylase deficiency. Muscle glycogen can be broken down by myophosphorylase but only until the branch points are reached, which is the reason a mild degree of acidification can be achieved with exercise.[32]

Phosphofructokinase Deficiency

Patients with muscle involvement due to mutations affecting the M subunit of phosphofructokinase (PFK) fall into two broad groups: patients with purely exercise-induced symptoms (typical presentation) and patients with early- or late-presentation myopathy. In typical[37] and early presentation cases,[38] PFK activity is absent, whereas in late presentation myopathy, PFK activity has been reported as either absent or partially reduced.[39,40] The latter group includes patients with progressive proximal muscle weakness but generally no exercise intolerance,[39,40] although exercise intolerance has be reported in one case.[41] PFK is a key regulatory enzyme of glycolysis, and in the absence of enzyme activity, glycolytic ATP production from both glycogen and glucose is prevented.

The typical ^{31}P MRS features include a lack of pH_i decrease during either aerobic or ischemic exercise and a striking increase in the PME peak owing to accumulation of hexose phosphates.[32,42,43] As with myophosphorylase deficiency, PCr/ATP at rest has been reported to increase and represent a decrease in muscle ATP content of up to 30% (Figure 16.6A); however, in contrast with myophosphorylase deficiency,

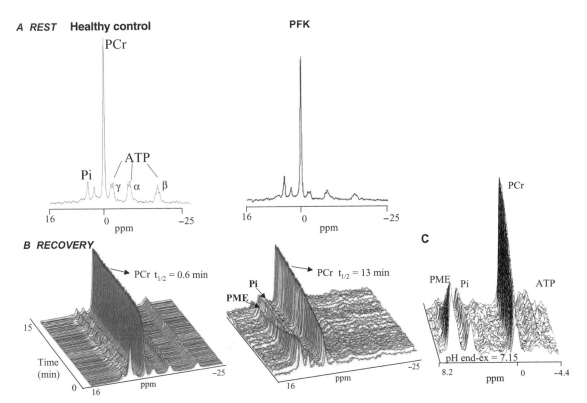

Figure 16.6 A. Phosphorus magnetic resonance spectroscopy (^{31}P MRS) spectra obtained at rest in a healthy control and patient with phosphofructokinase (PFK) deficiency. Note the decrease in signal intensity in the three spectral peaks (γ, α, β) composing adenosine triphosphate (ATP) in the spectrum of the patient as compared to the control. **B.** The ^{31}P MRS spectra obtained during recovery after exercise in the patient with PFK deficiency (*right*) demonstrates delayed resynthesis of phosphocreatine (PCr) and slow decrease in the phosphomonoester (PME) signal, which is not elevated after exercise in the healthy control (*left*). Also evident is the very low signal in ATP throughout recovery in the PFK-deficient patient, whereas it remains stable in the control. The decrease in inorganic phosphate (Pi) typically associated with increasing PCr during recovery is not observed in PFK disease, which is clearly demonstrated in **(C)**. This relates to slow continual release of Pi from PME. (End-ex = end exercise.)

ATP concentration during either aerobic or ischemic exercise has been found to drop dramatically (by as much as half).[42,44] Increased PCr consumption[44,45] and slow PCr recovery[32,44] are also commonly found. The Pi within muscle cells, which is required for ATP synthesis, becomes effectively trapped in the sugar phosphate intermediate, contributing to ATP depletion and slow PCr recovery (see Figures 16.6B and 16.6C). Compatible with the site of the biochemical defect and the absence of the second-wind phenomenon, intravenous glucose administration during exercise does not improve exercise kinetics,[42] but lactate infusion is able to bypass the enzymatic block and decrease the rate of PCr depletion.[45]

Only three patients with late-onset disease have been investigated by ^{31}P MRS. Two patients showed a rapid depletion of PCr and a modest increase in PME, consistent with partial PFK deficiency (in vitro activity in one of the subjects was reported to be 33% of normal).[41] In the third patient (showing 4% of normal PFK activity in vitro), the only abnormality revealed by ^{31}P MRS was a mildly decreased acidification during exercise.[39] This discrepancy could rely on enzyme instability rather than its absence, and this situation might be common in other late-onset cases of PFK deficit.[46]

Deficiencies of the Distal Glycolytic Pathway

The ^{31}P MRS pattern of abnormality in phosphoglycerate kinase (PGK) and phosphoglycerate mutase (PGM) is similar to that in PFK deficiency and is characterized by PME accumulation and reduced acidification during exercise. The only patient with PGK deficiency investigated by ^{31}P MRS[32] presented a striking accumulation of PME during exercise associated with some degree of acidification.[32] This is probably due to H$^+$ production by the synthesis of 1-3 diphosphoglycerate, which accumulates because of the enzymatic block and may help to differentiate PGK from PFK deficit. A deficit in oxidative metabolism was demonstrated in this patient as a slow PCr recovery rate. Muscle metabolism has been investigated using ^{31}P MRS in two patients with residual PGM activities of 6%[47] and 8%.[48] The patient with the lower residual PGM activity showed a mildly reduced PCr recovery rate, whereas the patient with the higher residual PGM activity showed a small drop in pH$_i$ as the only abnormality during mild aerobic exercise and a small PME accumulation during more intense aerobic exercise.

Phosphorus Magnetic Resonance Spectroscopy in Therapeutic Monitoring

Various treatments aimed to improve muscle energy availability in patients with McArdle's disease have given unsatisfactory results.[49,50] Dietary creatine supplementation monitored using ^{31}P MRS resulted in an increase in work capacity associated with increased PCr breakdown.[51] These findings were small and present only when ischemic exercise was performed. Higher PCr consumption and enhanced exercise performance suggest that the effect of creatine supplementation affected the ability to exercise longer rather than improving energy availability.[51]

Deficit of Oxidative Phosphorylation Due to Mitochondrial DNA Mutations

Mitochondrial disorders comprise a heterogeneous group of diseases caused by molecular defects affecting one or more of the many biochemical steps in the oxidation of substrates: substrate transport into mitochondria, tricarboxylic acid cycle, electron transport chain, and oxidation and phosphorylation coupling (see Chapter 17). Electron transport chain defects due to mutations in mitochondrial DNA (mtDNA) (either rearrangements or point mutations) make up the majority of adult cases of mitochondrial disorders and have been the ones studied most often using this noninvasive technique.

Phosphorus Magnetic Resonance Spectroscopy Diagnostic Patterns

^{31}P MRS has been extensively used to investigate patients with and without clinical involvement of skeletal muscle. Despite the diversity of biochemical lesions and clinical presentations, mtDNA-related disorders share a characteristic pattern of ^{31}P MRS–detectable abnormality, which reflects the common deficit of mitochondrial ATP synthesis. In comparison with other functional evaluations (e.g., testing for increased blood lactate), ^{31}P MRS has demonstrated high sensitivity in the detection of abnormal oxidative metabolism. In specialized centers where it is available, evaluation by ^{31}P MRS may precede muscle biopsy and genetic analysis in the diagnostic protocols of mitochondrial myopathy and mtDNA defects (see Figure 16.4).

Various studies have reported that from 43%[11] to greater than 80%[12,17,52] of patients with different forms of mitochondrial encephalomyopathies show abnormal ^{31}P MRS at rest. Typically, PCr/ATP is reduced, and Pi/ATP is increased. Results from a single patient illustrating common findings are shown in Figure 16.7. The limited data on biochemical analyses of ATP concentration in mitochondrial myopathy suggest that it remains unaffected by the disease.[12,17] The low PCr/ATP and increased Pi/ATP thus imply that the absolute concentration of PCr is decreased and Pi is high in these patients. Some studies indicate that an elevation in Pi is the most prominent feature,[11,52] whereas others suggest that a reduction in PCr concentration is the most prominent feature.[12,53] These differences are unexplained and do not seem to relate to the muscle group investigated[12] or the clinical, biochemical, or molecular phenotype. These abnormalities have been detected at rest in the absence of any muscle symptoms or signs in Leber's hereditary optic neuropathy (LHON) patients[54,55] and symptom-free carriers of primary LHON mutations.[55] In cases in which ADP concentration has been calculated, it was abnormally increased in approximately two-thirds of patients.[12,17,55] Not surprisingly, the PP at rest has been reported to be low in the majority of patients and, in some studies, has been the most frequently detected abnormality. PP was low in the finger flexor digitorum in 20 out of 24 mitochondrial patients (most of them with chronic progressive ophthalmoplegia, Kearns-Sayre syndrome, and mitochondrial encephalomyopathy with lactic acidosis and stroke-like episodes [MELAS][12]) and in the calf muscle of all 10 subjects carrying one of the primary LHON mutations.[55] There is no consistent finding with respect to pH$_i$ at rest. Although in most cases it is within the normal range, in a small percentage of patients' muscle cytosolic pH has been found to be abnormally alkaline[12] (see Figure 16.7), even in the presence of elevated resting blood lactate.[17,52] Although resting abnormalities are common in patients with mtDNA defects, low PCr and high Pi cannot be considered specific indices of defective mitochondrial respiration per se. Similar changes have been described in sporadic inclusion body myositis (s-IBM)[53,56] and Becker's muscular dystrophy (BMD),[57–59] conditions associated with normal mitochondrial respiration as shown by normal PCr and ADP recovery rate or V$_{max}$.[53,56,59]

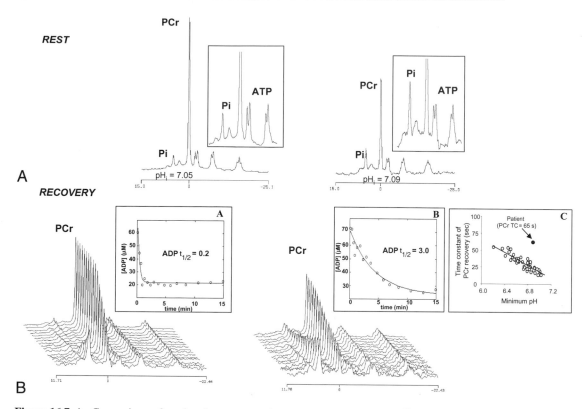

Figure 16.7 A. Comparison of a phosphorus magnetic resonance spectroscopy (^{31}P MRS) spectrum obtained at rest between a healthy control (*left*) and a patient harboring the mitochondrial encephalomyopathy with lactic acidosis and stroke-like episodes (MELAS) A3243G mitochondrial DNA mutation (*right*), demonstrating lower signal intensity in phosphocreatine (PCr) and higher signal intensity in inorganic phosphate (Pi) (*inset*) in skeletal muscle. **B.** ^{31}P MRS spectra obtained during 16 minutes of recovery from brief ischemic exercise in the healthy control and patient. Consecutive ^{31}P MRS spectra are shown, and the resulting calculated curve of intracellular adenosine diphosphate (ADP) recovery is drawn in the inset for both subjects, whereas the patient (**B**) demonstrates a markedly slower recovery (ADP $t_{1/2}$) compared to that of the healthy control (**A**). Note that although the degree of end-exercise PCr depletion is comparable between the two scans (first spectra), the time for recovery of the PCr peak to resting levels is markedly slower in the patient with mitochondrial myopathy. This is more evident in inset (**C**) where, in view of the influence of the degree of acidification on the rate of PCr resynthesis,[22,23] the rate of PCr recovery expressed as a time constant (TC) is plotted versus the minimum pH reached during the recovery phase in a group of healthy subjects (*open circles*) and in the patient with mitochondrial myopathy (*closed circle*). (ATP = adenosine triphosphate; pH$_i$ = intracellular pH.) (Data from R Lodi, GJ Kemp, S Iotti, et al. Influence of cytosolic pH on in vivo assessment of human muscle mitochondrial respiration by phosphorus magnetic resonance spectroscopy. MAGMA 1997;5:165–171.)

The consequence of a deficit in mitochondrial ATP production during exercise is an increase in nonoxidative energy production (i.e., increased PCr consumption and glycolytic activity).[11,12,17] Thus, patients with mitochondrial myopathies tend to exhibit a more rapid rate of PCr depletion per unit work than healthy individuals during exercise, consistent with decreased exercise tolerance that is characteristic of these disorders. Noteworthy is the fact that this rapid decline in energy state occurs without an accompanying severe intracellular acidosis.[11,12,17] This small decrease in pH relative to the degree of PCr depletion in patients with mtDNA defects is a somewhat paradoxic finding given the increased lactic acid production associated with increased anaerobic glycolysis supplying the necessary energy for ATP synthesis. This finding has been attributed to stimulated buffering systems,[11] or enhanced lactic acid extrusion from the cell[17] in response to chronic overproduction of lactate. Standardization of muscle exercise is an unresolved problem, making it somewhat difficult to define specific ^{31}P MRS diagnostic criteria during the exercise state. Exercise changes similar to those found in patients with mitochondrial myopathies (short exercise duration, increased PCr consumption, high [ADP]) can be present in patients affected by a pathologic process leading to muscle fiber degeneration but with normal mitochondrial respiration rate, such as in BMD and s-IBM.[53,59]

The analysis of recovery from exercise increases the sensitivity and specificity of the ^{31}P MRS examination in detecting mitochondrial dysfunction, as oxidative metabolism is markedly activated during recovery. Measures of postexercise high-energy phosphate recovery have been particularly useful in the quantitative assessment of the presence as well as extent of dysfunction. A large majority of patients with mtDNA defects shows abnormalities during this process, reflecting a reduced rate of mitochondrial ATP production (see Figure 16.7).[11,12] The recovery rates of PCr and ADP (or PCr $t_{1/2}$ and ADP $t_{1/2}$) as well as the maximum rate of mitochondrial ATP production, V_{max}—all of which are independent of muscle mass or muscle fiber content in the volume studied by ^{31}P MRS—are typically low (slow) in mitochondrial patients when compared to healthy subjects.

A unique characteristic of the recovery spectrum in mitochondrial myopathies relates to proton handling, whereas on cessation of exercise, there is an increased rate of pH recovery[17] and of calculated apparent proton efflux during the initial phase of recovery.[16] Arnold et al.[17] first reported this phenomenon in five mitochondrial patients who demonstrated a faster return of cytosolic pH to resting values after exercise than healthy subjects in the flexor digitorum superficialis muscle, despite having high resting blood lactate levels.[17] This was confirmed later in a larger series of patients.[12] Taylor et al.[12] have suggested that this rapid return of pH to resting levels may be due to an upregulation of sodium-proton antiporters. Kemp and Radda[21] have proposed that an adaptive increase in proton efflux leads to faster recovery of pH, allowing for a slower recovery of [ADP], thereby providing a prolonged mitochondrial drive for PCr resynthesis.

However, in a small proportion of patients with identified mtDNA mutations, abnormalities in recovery indices may not be detected. Metabolic heterogeneity owing to the focal distribution of metabolically compromised mitochondria or subthreshold levels of mutant mtDNA within the MRS-studied muscle could theoretically account for normal findings. ^{31}P MRS measures an averaged response of a large number of muscle fibers; therefore, small groups of metabolically different cells may not affect the overall MR observation. It is the general notion, however, that the more severe clinical presentations and biochemical deficiencies result in abnormal ^{31}P MRS recovery indices.

Relationship between Genotype and In Vivo Biochemical Expression

^{31}P MRS has been used in studies attempting to gain insight into the complex genotype and biochemical phenotype relationships, and a few such studies are mentioned. It is important to remember that ^{31}P MRS measures overall mitochondrial ATP generation by the mitochondrial respiratory chain, whereas in vitro enzymatic

assays reveal information regarding individual respiratory chain complex capacities. In patients with mtDNA defects, the nature of the mutation, the degree to which a certain enzyme complex is compromised, the level of control that enzyme exerts on the rate of mitochondrial respiration, and the influence of other genetic (mitochondrial or nuclear) factors may lead to disparity between the two modes of measurement. Therefore, enzyme activities measured in vitro do not always correspond to the results obtained in vivo.

For example, LHON patients carrying a primary mtDNA point mutation at one of three nucleotide positions (11778, 14484, or 3460) in genes coding for different subunits of complex I of the respiratory chain showed slow PCr recovery rate and low V_{max} for mitochondrial ATP synthesis.[54,55,60] In vitro, the specific activity of complex I was markedly decreased for 3460 and normal for 11778, but in vivo, mitochondrial activity was lowest in subjects homoplasmic for 11778, higher for 14484, and just within the normal range for 3460 (V_{max}, 27%, 53%, and 65% of the normal mean, respectively).[55] The controversial issue of the pathogenic role of "secondary" mtDNA point mutations, when occurring in association with "primary" mutations in patients with LHON, has also been addressed using ^{31}P MRS.[61] Ten patients homoplasmic for the 11778/ND4 mtDNA mutation and ten patients homoplasmic for the same mutation occurring in the presence of the secondary LHON mtDNA mutations, 4216/ND1 and 13708/ND5, were studied. The degree of impairment of brain and skeletal muscle bioenergetics measured during recovery from exercise was comparable in the two groups of patients, not supporting a "synergistic" role of the 4216/ND1 and 13708/ND5 secondary mutations with the 11778/ND4 primary mutation in determining the deficit of energy metabolism in LHON.[61]

The A3243G mtDNA mutation, one of the most common pathogenic mtDNA point mutations classically associated with the MELAS phenotype,[62] is usually heteroplasmic. In cybrid cell lines (human cell lines completely devoid of their original mtDNA and harboring the mutant mtDNA under study), the mutation load must exceed a critical threshold level (approximately 85%) before a biochemical defect is expressed.[63] However, patients carrying lower proportions of mutant mtDNA often have clinical features of mtDNA disease.[64] ^{31}P MRS demonstrated a markedly reduced V_{max} (35% of the normal mean) in the calf muscle of a patient complaining of mild exercise intolerance with only 6% of A3243G mutation load in the same muscle.[65] This indicates that low levels of the A3243G mutation can cause mitochondrial dysfunction and that there may not be a clear mutation threshold effect in vivo. A larger study showed lack of correlation between A3243G mutation load in muscle and PCr/Pi at rest and V_{max} after exercise in individuals from different pedigrees.[66] These findings suggest that the nuclear genetic background may modulate the extent of mitochondrial dysfunction in vivo for a given mtDNA mutation load. This interpretation is supported by the influence of the nuclear background demonstrated in the biochemical expression of the A3243G mutation in cybrid cell lines.[67] A similar influence has also been found in cybrid cell clones homoplasmic for the LHON 3460/ND1 mutations displaying either normal or reduced complex I activity depending on nuclear background.[68] A tissue-specific distribution of the biochemical expression of the A3460G was found in vivo in subjects homoplasmic for this mutation that presented abnormal brain ^{31}P MRS in association with normal muscle oxidative phosphorylation as measured during recovery from exercise.[69]

Phosphorus Magnetic Resonance Spectroscopy in Therapeutic Monitoring

^{31}P MRS of skeletal muscle has been widely used to objectively evaluate the response to specific treatments in different forms of mitochondrial myopathies since the beginning of its application to studies of in vivo human muscle bioenergetics. Classically, therapeutic approaches have been pharmacologic in nature and focused on supplementation with large doses of vitamins and cofactors to bypass the biochemical defect and augment respiratory chain flux and mitochondrial energy production. Administration of vitamins K_3 and C to a patient with complex III deficit resulted in clinical improvement in association with dramatic improvements of ^{31}P MRS indices.[70] Similarly, coadministration with riboflavin and nicotinamide in a MELAS patient with complex I deficiency showed evidence of improved muscle oxidative metabolism, which paralleled the clinical response.[71] The evidence was made more compelling, as both clinical and spectroscopic responses paralleled an off-treatment washout phase followed by readministration. Coenzyme Q_{10} administration has yielded the most inconclusive results (likely owing to the fact that it has been the most widely used agent) and has been found to enhance oxidative metabolism in some cases[72,73] but not in others.[74] Dichloroacetate is an agent that was shown to stimulate pyruvate dehydrogenase activity, reduce blood lactate levels, and improve indices of brain oxidative metabolism but not improve ^{31}P MRS–assessed recovery indices of mitochondrial ATP production.[75] However, the administration of dichloroacetate after 8 weeks of aerobic training resulted in a further improvement of ^{31}P MRS recovery indices of oxidative metabolism in a single patient with severe cytochrome oxidase deficiency.[76]

The positive effect of moderately intense aerobic training alone for 8 weeks on muscle oxidative metabolism was confirmed in 10 patients with various mtDNA abnormalities, in whom improvements in exercise performance and blood lactate concentrations (both 30%) were associated with an even greater (60%) improvement in ^{31}P MRS–assessed ADP recovery rate.[77] In contrast, ADP recovery did not improve after a similar training regimen in patients with various forms of MDs or in sedentary control subjects.[78] More recently, the enzymatic (respiratory chain enzyme activities) and genetic (proportion of mutant and wild-type genomes) basis of the oxidative capacity increase with aerobic training was investigated in 10 different patients carrying heteroplasmic mtDNA mutations.[79] Improvements in ^{31}P MRS recovery indices reflecting ATP production obtained from the vastus lateralis muscle (35% for V_{max}) were associated with increased activities of deficient respiratory chain enzymes assessed from muscle biopsies of the same muscle in patients with complex I (36%) and complex IV (25%) defects. However, genetic analysis showed that the proportion of wild-type mtDNA was unchanged in three patients and fell in six patients, suggesting a trend toward preferential proliferation of mutant genomes.[79] Despite positive physiologic and biochemical effects of aerobic training, the long-term implications of training-induced increases in mutant relative to wild-type mtDNA need to be assessed before training can be proposed as a general treatment option in patients with defects of mtDNA.

A clinically effective therapy for mtDNA disorders has yet to be identified. ^{31}P MRS is certainly an ideal tool to assess any new treatment approach, including the monitoring of patients undergoing a novel and promising "gene shifting" therapy, which is based on the proliferation and incorporation of satellite cells with normal mtDNA into existing myofibers.[80,81]

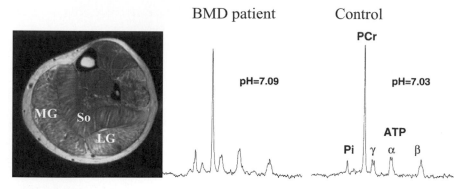

Figure 16.8 T1-weighted leg axial images (TR = 600 msec; TE = 20 msec), at the level of the center of the phosphorus coil placed underneath the calf muscle in a patient with Becker's muscular dystrophy (BMD), depicting fatty replacement of muscle fibers. The phosphorus magnetic resonance spectroscopy spectrum obtained from the calf muscle at rest shows increased intracellular pH and inorganic phosphate (Pi) and reduced phosphocreatine (PCr) compared to that of a healthy subject. (ATP = adenosine triphosphate; LG = lateral head of gastrocnemius; MG = medial head of gastrocnemius; So = soleus.)

MUSCULAR DYSTROPHIES

MDs comprise a large and heterogeneous group of inherited disorders characterized by progressive muscle weakness and wasting. Structural alterations, caused by fiber atrophy, necrosis, and fatty replacement of muscle tissue, are easily detectable by computed tomography or MR imaging (Figure 16.8). MRS can detect some of the biochemical abnormalities that arise from the individual genetic defects and that underlie structural changes. MDs associated with dystrophin-glycoprotein complex (DGC) defects and myotonic MDs have been extensively investigated by MRS.

Muscular Dystrophies Due to Dystrophin-Glycoprotein Complex Defects

In striated muscle cells, the DGC provides a link between the extracellular basal lamina and the intracellular cytoskeleton. *Dystrophin* is a subsarcolemmal protein connecting F-actin to a large group of proteins and glycoprotein, which includes the dystroglycan, sarcoglycan, and syntrophyn complexes. The extracellular component of the dystroglycan complex binds to laminin, one of the main components of the basal lamina.[82]

Duchenne's and Becker's Muscular Dystrophies

Duchenne's muscular dystrophy (DMD) and Becker's muscular dystrophy (BMD) are X-linked recessive allelic disorders caused by mutations of the dystrophin gene.[83] Dystrophin is usually absent in DMD but is present in reduced amounts or smaller molecular weight (or both) in the milder BMD phenotype. Immunohistochemical studies have revealed a reduction in all dystrophin-associated proteins proportional to the dystrophin deficit in DMD and BMD.[82] Although the structure and localization of dystrophin are well defined, the functional role of this protein and the biochemical mechanisms leading to muscle necrosis in DMD and BMD are still unknown. A large number of ^{31}P MRS studies have investigated muscle metabolism in DMD and BMD patients as well as in female carriers. In all three groups, the muscle at rest shows an increase in pH_i and Pi and reduced PCr (see Figure 16.8). As a result, the calculated sarcolemmal free ADP concentration is increased, and the PP is low with less energy available from ATP hydrolysis. These abnormalities are more pronounced in DMD than in BMD patients and carriers and tend to increase with age and disease progression.[57,58,84–87] Early ^{31}P MRS investigations of DMD patients have also revealed high concentrations of PDE in skeletal muscle, consistent with cell necrosis and membrane breakdown.[87] The increase in resting-muscle pH_i found in dystrophinopathies, but also in other forms of MDs (e.g., oculopharyngeal MD),[88] is thought to arise from changes in the membrane-bound system that maintains the intracellular proton content of resting muscle, the Na^+ and H^+ antiporter.[89] The altered energetic state found at rest and, in particular, the high resting [ADP] are not necessarily indexes of abnormal mitochondrial control but could point to increased ATP turnover. In dystrophin-deficient muscle, high proton content is associated with a number of other ionic changes,[90,91] which may require increased basal ATP consumption.

During exercise, a rapid depletion of energy reserves has been demonstrated in BMD patients,[57–59] consistent with low muscle mass and low PP. ADP concentration is high not only at rest but throughout exercise.[15,58,59] ADP is an important regulator of ATP synthesis, so maintaining a high concentration helps to increase ATP production as the progressively decreasing muscle mass struggles to cope with the relative increase in energy demand. There is evidence that the integrity of the cytoskeleton is necessary for the proper functioning of glycolysis and the tricarboxylic acid cycle,[92,93] and this suggests a possible role for defective energy metabolism in muscle fiber degeneration. However, it is clear from quantitative analysis of ^{31}P MRS recovery data that in dystrophinopathies, the rate of mitochondrial ATP production is not reduced.[15,58,59] This would seem to rule out any major role for impaired oxidative energy production in the progressive fiber necrosis in dystrophinopathies. On the other hand, the evaluation of muscle cytosolic pH in BMD patients during an incremental exercise showed reduced acidification in the later stages[59] (Figure 16.9). This was associated with an unchanged rate of proton efflux from muscle fibers, providing evidence that there may be reduced glucose availability to dystrophin-deficient muscles during exercise.[59] Consistently, myocardial glucose transport during insulin stimulation was reduced to less than half of normal in the hearts of mdx mice.[94] It is glycolytically produced ATP that is thought to be used preferentially to provide energy for the ion pumps of the cell membrane, and in dystrophin deficiency, there is a general imbalance of ionic homeostasis involving Na^+, Mg^{2+}, K^+, and Ca^{2+}.[90,91] Whether this deficit in glycolytic ATP production due to decreased glucose availability is severe enough to compromise ion transport has not been resolved. Delayed recovery of Pi after exercise has been reported in BMD patients and DMD and BMD carriers and interpreted as an effect of altered ionic equilibrium.[57,85]

The recent development of the new utr-dys mouse model for dystrophinopathies, which lacks in both dystrophin and utrophin and exhibits many of the pathophysiologic features that are present in DMD and BMD but absent in mdx

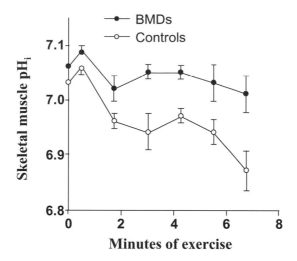

Figure 16.9 Calf muscle pH changes from rest to exercise in a group of patients with Becker's muscular dystrophy (BMD) and healthy controls. The magnitude of pH changes is similar during the first 2 minutes of aerobic incremental exercise in BMDs and controls. In later phases of exercise, a reduced acidification in BMDs is clearly evident when compared to controls. (pH_i = intracellular pH.) (Reprinted with permission from R Lodi, GJ Kemp, F Muntoni, et al. Reduced cytosolic acidification during exercise suggests defective glycolytic activity in skeletal muscle of patients with Becker muscular dystrophy. An in vivo ^{31}P magnetic resonance spectroscopy study. Brain 1999;122:121–130.)

mice,[95] certainly helps to better understand the mechanisms leading to progressive muscle necrosis. The first in vivo ^{31}P MRS study of utr-dys mice[96] has shown metabolic abnormalities in skeletal muscle at rest, during exercise, and during recovery similar to those present in DMD and BMD patients and more severe than those found in the muscles of mdx mice.[90,97]

Sarcoglycan-Deficient Limb-Girdle Muscular Dystrophy

Deficits in sarcoglycan glycoproteins are responsible for four subtypes of autosomal recessive limb-girdle MDs that share several common features with DMD. The primary deficiency of one of the four sarcoglycans almost invariably causes a secondary reduction in the expression of the others. The general pattern of ^{31}P MRS–detectable abnormality in sarcoglycan-deficient muscles is similar to that present in DMD and BMD. However, some important differences have been described. A ^{31}P MRS study of seven patients, all with substantial muscle wasting, showed increased cytosolic pH at rest and normal PCr and Pi content relative to ATP.[98] This finding led to speculation that the normal dystrophin expression in sarcoglycan-deficient muscles may prevent changes in phosphorylated compound concentrations. As found in BMD patients,[59] muscle mitochondrial ATP production assessed during recovery from incremental exercise was normal in sarcoglycan-deficient patients.[98] These observations indicate that in MDs due to defects of the DGC, mitochondrial dysfunction is not a prominent feature and likely does not play a role in initiating muscle fiber necrosis.

Phosphorus Magnetic Resonance Spectroscopy in Therapeutic Monitoring

As for many other muscle disorders, therapy with a clear influence on the natural course of various forms of MDs is not yet available. The success of genetic therapies is under investigation in animal models of DMD. ^{31}P MRS abnormalities present in the skeletal muscle of mdx mice[90,97] display a near-normalization in mdx mice in which expression of a truncated form of utrophin is obtained transgenetically.[99]

Myotonic Dystrophy

Myotonic dystrophy type 1 is a dominantly inherited multisystem disorder caused by an unstable expansion of a CTG triplet repeat in the gene (on chromosome 19q13.3) encoding for myotonin, a cyclic AMP–dependent serinethreonine protein kinase of unknown function. Skeletal and cardiac muscle, nervous tissues, and other organ systems are usually affected. In addition to the myotonia, the skeletal muscle exhibits weakness that may be out of proportion to the degree of wasting. At the sarcolemmal level, abnormal Na^+ channel activity and altered intracellular concentrations of Na^+, K^+, Cl^-, and Ca^{2+} have been reported.[89] In myotonic dystrophy type 1, as in many other muscle diseases, the extent of biochemical abnormalities detected by ^{31}P MRS increases with clinical severity. The ^{31}P MRS results provide evidence that some of the clinical weakness and fatigue experienced by patients may indeed be due to defects in energy supply. The general findings include a decrease in PP, high free ADP concentration, and higher than normal ATP turnover during exercise.[89,100] Differences have been found between muscle groups, with the calf showing a pattern similar to dystrophin deficiency but the forearm maintaining a normal pH_i at rest regardless of clinical state. Recovery kinetics point to a small but significant reduction in mitochondrial function, and ischemic exercise in the forearm provides evidence of a relative reduction in the use of glycogen for ATP production. These findings may account for the reduced acidification seen during exercise in both limbs. The question remains as to how much of the abnormal bioenergetics is due directly to the product of the affected gene. The relationship between muscle metabolic abnormalities and genetics has not been investigated. However, neurochemical alterations observed in the brain of myotonic dystrophy patients with proton MRS are proportional to the size of the CTG expansion.[101]

IDIOPATHIC INFLAMMATORY MYOPATHIES

Idiopathic inflammatory myopathies (IIMs) form a heterogeneous group of acquired muscle disorders characterized by muscle weakness and chronic inflammatory infiltrates within the skeletal muscle. For the three major forms, polymyositis (PM), dermatomyositis (DM), and s-IBM, different pathogenic mechanisms have been proposed.[102] In DM, there is a complement-dependent humoral attack against muscle capillaries and secondary muscle fiber necrosis. In PM, the endomysial cell infiltrate contains abundant CD8T cells with invasion of non-necrotic muscle fibers by the same cells and macrophages. In s-IBM, characterized by inflammatory infiltrates, partial invasion of non-necrotic fibers, rimmed vacuoles, amyloid deposits, and 15- to 18-nm tubulofilaments, the immunopathologic factors are less understood. ^{31}P MRS has been used in IIM to investigate different aspects of muscle bioenergetics and to assess the rate of proton efflux from muscle fibers, which is an indirect measurement of muscle blood flow.

Dermatomyositis and Polymyositis

Despite the fact that clinical and imaging abnormalities tend to be mostly proximal in DM and PM patients, ^{31}P MRS has detected bioenergetic abnormalities in proximal and distal limb muscles.[103–108] ^{31}P MRS changes in DM tend to correlate with the severity of patients' symptoms and clinical findings. Quadriceps of amyopathic (without weakness) patients were normal at rest, but myopathic subjects had low PCr and ATP concentrations.[105] In patients with muscle weakness, PCr concentration was lower in those with more severe strength deficit.[103] Similar resting changes are also reported in children with the juvenile variant of DM[107] and, less pronounced, in the muscle of PM patients.[108] These in vivo findings have been recently confirmed in muscle biopsies of PM and DM patients, demonstrating reductions in [ATP] (23%) and in [PCr] (29%).[30] In all forms of DM, a metabolic dysfunction is detected during exercise, but in the amyopathic patients, these abnormalities are unmasked only at a high workload.[105,107] Greater decreases in [PCr] and pH have been found during incremental aerobic exercise in both PM and DM patients.[105,107,108] Quantitative analysis of recovery from exercise in DM and PM patients has shown an association between slow PCr resynthesis rate,[103,108] reduced V_{max} (Figure 16.10), and reduced rate of proton extrusion from muscle fibers into the extracellular space.[108] A reduced oxidative phosphorylation rate is typically associated with low pH during exercise and slow proton efflux in healthy subjects exercising in ischemic conditions[14] and in patients with peripheral vascular disease.[109] Exercise and recovery muscle abnormalities reported in PM and DM are consistent with a deficit of

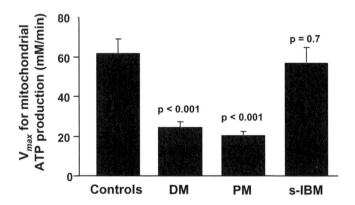

Figure 16.10 Decreased maximal rate of mitochondrial adenosine triphosphate (ATP) production, V_{max}, in skeletal muscle of patients with dermatomyositis (DM) and polymyositis (PM). In contrast, muscle V_{max} in patients with sporadic inclusion body myositis (s-IBM) is similar to control subjects. (Data from R Lodi, DJ Taylor, SJ Tabrizi, et al. Normal in vivo skeletal muscle oxidative metabolism in sporadic inclusion body myositis assessed by ^{31}P-magnetic resonance spectroscopy. Brain 1998;121:2119–2126; and G Cea, D Bendahan, D Manners, et al. Reduced oxidative phosphorylation and proton efflux suggest reduced capillary blood supply in skeletal muscle of patients with dermatomyositis and polymyositis: a quantitative ^{31}P MRS and MRI study. Brain, *in press*.)

oxidative phosphorylation secondary to impaired blood supply and suggest that the mitochondrial abnormalities reported in some DM and PM biopsy studies[110–112] are probably secondary to the inflammatory process. This interpretation is supported by the findings of reduced capillary density and damage not only in DM[113,114] but also in PM.[115]

Phosphorus Magnetic Resonance Spectroscopy in Therapy Monitoring

Longitudinal follow-up of DM patients shows a good correlation between ^{31}P MRS data, severity of clinical features, and response to steroids and immunosuppressant therapy, demonstrating the value of muscle ^{31}P MRS in guiding therapy strategies.[106,116] ^{31}P MRS is highly sensitive, and assessment of muscle bioenergetic abnormalities is particularly useful in patients with normal levels of serum creatine phosphokinase, muscle strength, and muscle MRI.[104,116]

Sporadic Inclusion Body Myositis

The clinical pattern of s-IBM differs from PM and DM by (1) the high frequency of weakness and atrophy affecting both proximal and distal muscle groups, (2) characteristic early involvement of the quadriceps and deep finger flexors, and (3) slow progression and unresponsiveness to steroid and immunosuppressant treatment.[102,117]

Reports of increased frequency in cytochrome oxidase-deficient fibers and ragged red fibers in association with multiple deletions of mtDNA in skeletal muscle of s-IBM patients[118,119] raised the possibility that a defect of oxidative metabolism might play a role in the pathogenesis of s-IBM and might be involved in the progressive skeletal muscle degeneration. This question has been addressed in two ^{31}P MRS studies,[53,56] both of which showed that the calf muscle mitochondrial ATP production rate as measured from postexercise recovery data is normal in s-IBM (see Figure 16.10). The conclusions were that the accumulation of mtDNA deletions and the presence of other mitochondrial abnormalities are secondary processes and do not contribute to the pathogenesis of the muscle weakness and atrophy. In contrast to the finding of normal oxidative metabolism, resting muscle in most s-IBM patients shows abnormalities in the concentrations of the phosphorus-containing metabolites and an increased pH_i. In our experience, the degree of ^{31}P MRS abnormality at rest in a particular muscle correlates positively with the degree of signal intensity increase on the T1-weighted image. This suggests that the ^{31}P MRS-detectable changes are nonspecific indices of muscle damage and disease progression in s-IBM.

MUSCLE PHOSPHORUS MAGNETIC RESONANCE SPECTROSCOPY STUDY OF OTHER DISORDERS

Malignant Hyperthermia

Malignant hyperthermia, which may occur in association with or without other musculoskeletal defects, is a genetically heterogeneous disorder that, in over 50% of families, is associated with autosomal dominant inherited mutations in the ryanodine receptor gene on chromosome 19.[120] The gene product, RYR1, is a large calcium release channel protein situated in the membrane of the sarcoplasmic reticulum. In malignant hyperthermia–susceptible (MHS) subjects, exposure to certain halogenated and nonhalogenated anesthetics and depolarizing muscle relaxants leads to excessive release of free Ca^{2+} from the sarcoplasmic reticulum through the ryanodine receptor into the myoplasm. The resulting high cytoplasmic Ca^{2+} concentration is thought to be responsible for symptoms characterized by muscle contractures and hypermetabolism. The standard method of identifying MHS individuals is based on exposing a large fresh muscle biopsy to caffeine and halothane.[121]

^{31}P MRS investigations of MHS subjects have identified a consistently high rate of ATP use during exercise, as shown by a rapid depletion of PCr and excessive degree of acidification.[122–124] These findings are consistent with increased glycolytic activity to supply the increased demand for ATP. Analysis of ^{31}P MRS recovery indices suggests that mitochondrial oxidative metabolism is not impaired in MHS individuals. The slower PCr recovery rate reported by some studies is, as suggested by Bendahan et al., a consequence of increased acidification rather than of a primary defect of oxidative phosphorylation.[122–124] There is no definitive explanation, however, for the finding in some,[125,126] but not all,[122,123] laboratories of abnormal phosphorus metabolite concentrations in resting muscle. In vitro assays have established that the increase in PDE peak at rest observed in vivo[126] is due to an increase in glycerophosphorylcholine, although the mechanism responsible remains unidentified.[127]

The abnormal ^{31}P MRS profiles of MHS subjects have been compared to results from the in vitro contracture test and have been found to be diagnostically reliable both retrospectively and prospectively. Sensitivity and specificity, greater than 90% when only ^{31}P MRS resting parameters were used,[126] increased to 100% when resting, exercise, and recovery ^{31}P MRS parameters were combined.[122] It may, however, be difficult to establish whether all genetic variations of the disease are detected equally reliably, and larger prospective ^{31}P MRS studies are certainly needed before using this method alone for diagnosis.

Chronic Fatigue Syndrome

Controversies over chronic fatigue syndrome (CFS) pathogenesis are reflected in the inconsistent muscle ^{31}P MRS results that followed the first case report of a patient studied using this technique. The patient showed an excessive acidification in his forearm muscles during aerobic exercise but normal mitochondrial oxidative metabolism.[128] Excessive glycolytic activity was postulated to account for this finding, which was supported by predominance of type II fibers on biopsy analysis. Subsequent larger studies, however, showed that such a ^{31}P MRS pattern is not a consistent finding in CFS patients. Most of these studies have shown that ^{31}P MRS abnormalities, such as excessive acidification during exercise[129] and reduced rate of mitochondrial ATP production,[130,131] are present only in a small proportion of CFS patients. Taken together, these studies point to CFS as a heterogeneous disorder. This notion has been confirmed in studying CFS patients with normal (SATET –ve) and increased lactate production (SATET +ve) in the subanaerobic threshold exercise test (SATET).[132] In SATET +ve CFS patients, pH_i was significantly lower and the mitochondrial ATP synthesis rate was slower than in controls and SATET –ve patients. In addition, the proportion of type I fibers (which have the greatest oxidative capacity) was lower in the SATET +ve than in the SATET –ve group.[132] These findings indicate that in a subpopulation of patients with CFS syndrome, there is a deficit of oxidative phosphorylation and a relatively higher glycolytic capacity, suggesting that there is a peripheral component to fatigue in some cases of CFS.

Fibromyalgia

There is no established pathophysiology for fibromyalgia, which is generally defined by widespread musculoskeletal or soft tissue pain and multiple tender points. Despite the occasional description of mitochondrial abnormalities (i.e., ragged red and cytochrome oxidase–negative fibers) in muscle biopsies from patients with fibromyalgia,[133] most of the ^{31}P MRS results seem to rule out a role for a deficit of oxidative phosphorylation in the pathophysiology of this disorder.[134,135] ^{31}P MRS findings were negative even when the data were collected at tender sites.[136] In one ^{31}P MRS study, it was concluded that the greater changes in PCr and Pi relative to work performed that were observed in the muscles of fibromyalgia patients were due to a deficit of oxidative phosphorylation.[137] However, deconditioning and reduced muscle mass in the patient group could well explain this result.

CONCLUSIONS

^{31}P MRS is sensitive in detecting abnormalities in energy metabolism and should be considered in the clinical workup of patients with suspected muscle disorders, particularly if a metabolic dysfunction is suspected. The assessment of intracellular pH and phosphorylated compound kinetics during exercise and recovery from exercise provides criteria for distinction of the various muscle disorders. As summarized in Table 16.1, ^{31}P MRS can distinguish between glycolytic and mitochondrial defects and between glycogenolytic and glycolytic defects, as well as help in differentiating the site of enzymatic block along the glycolytic pathway (PFK-PGM). Impaired mitochondrial oxidative capacity is a common feature in many metabolic myopathies, although oxidative disorders related to lipid metabolism (e.g., carnitine palmitoyl transferase II deficiency) are more difficult to unmask using standard exercise protocols and, therefore, often show no ^{31}P MRS–distinguishable pattern. Delayed recovery of high-energy phosphates after exercise is common to many muscle disorders and suggests either primary mitochondrial disease or secondary mitochondrial dysfunction owing to a lack of substrate or oxygen availability, as well as the effects of chronic physical inactivity. ^{31}P MRS investigations of various forms of MDs and IIMs have also provided important clues to their pathophysiology.

In addition to its value in the diagnostic screening of patients with muscle disorders, the ability of ^{31}P MRS to evaluate dynamic biochemical processes in vivo has provided insight into the complex relationship between genotype and functional expression in intact tissues in various metabolic defects. Finally, the ability of ^{31}P MRS to provide for noninvasive, repetitive assessment makes it a powerful monitoring tool of therapeutic efficacy. Particularly in an era in which molecular medicine holds great promise in identifying or advancing therapies for muscle disorders, such a tool is necessary for the functional evaluation of these treatment effects.

Table 16.1 Summary of Abnormal Phosphorus Magnetic Resonance Spectroscopy (^{31}P MRS) Findings in Muscle Disorders

Muscle Disorder	Nonspecific ^{31}P MRS Abnormalities	Distinguishing ^{31}P MRS Features
Metabolic disorders		
Myophosphorylase deficiency	REST: high PCr/ATP (low ATP); EX: rapid PCr depletion; REC: slow PCr resynthesis, slow ADP recovery	pH$_i$ alkalosis with moderate exercise; no PME peak increase during exercise
Debrancher deficiency	Same as myophosphorylase deficiency	Mild degree of acidification with exercise compared to myophosphorylase deficiency; no PME peak during exercise
Phosphofructokinase deficiency	REST: same as myophosphorylase deficiency; EX: same as myophosphorylase deficiency; REC: slow recovery of PCr, ADP, and Pi	Alkalosis or lack of acidification, marked increase in PME peak, and loss of ATP during exercise; slow recovery of PME peak
Phosphoglycerate kinase/ mutase deficiency	Same as phosphofructokinase deficiency	Mild acidification and increase in PME peak during moderate exercise
Mitochondrial electron transport chain defects	REST: reduced PCr/ATP, increased Pi, low PP; EX: rapid PCr depletion	Rapid decline in PCr without accompanying acidosis during exercise; slow PCr and ADP recovery; increased rate of pH$_i$ recovery
Muscular dystrophies		
Duchenne's and Becker's	REST: reduced PCr, increased Pi, ADP, PDE, and pH$_i$; EX: rapid PCr depletion and reduced acidification; REC: delayed Pi recovery	REC: normal PCr and ADP recovery rates and V$_{max}$; low signal to noise ratio
Sarcoglycan-deficient limb-girdle muscular dystrophy	REST: high pH$_i$	Normal PCr and ADP recovery rates and V$_{max}$; low signal to noise ratio
Myotonic dystrophy	REST: high Pi and ADP, low PCr and PP; EX: excessive PCr depletion and reduced acidification	Slow PCr recovery; low signal to noise ratio
Idiopathic inflammatory myopathies		
Dermatomyositis and polymyositis	REST: low PCr, ATP, high Pi; EX: excessive PCr depletion and acidification	REC: slow PCr recovery associated with reduced rate of proton extrusion (secondary mitochondrial dysfunction)
Sporadic inclusion body myositis	REST: Low PCr and PP, high Pi, ADP, and pH	Normal PCr and ADP recovery rates and V$_{max}$; low signal to noise ratio
Miscellaneous		
Malignant hyperthermia	REST: high PDE; EX: exaggerated PCr depletion and acidification	—
Chronic fatigue syndrome	EX: excessive acidification in some cases; REC: slow PCr and recovery and low V$_{max}$ in some cases	—
Fibromyalgia	Exaggerated PCr depletion	—

ADP = adenosine diphosphate; ATP = adenosine triphosphate; EX = exercise; PCr = phosphocreatine; PDE = phosphodiesters; pH$_i$ = intracellular pH; Pi = inorganic phosphate; PME = phosphomonoesters; PP = phosphorylation potential; REC = recovery; REST = resting; V$_{max}$ = maximum rate of oxidative ATP synthesis.

Acknowledgments

Raffaele Lodi would like to thank Bruno Barbiroli, Doris Taylor, and Peter Styles for their valuable help and advice in discussing many of the clinical studies reported here. Tanja Taivassalo is indebted to Douglas Arnold for his invaluable mentorship and guidance in the area of ^{31}P MRS, to Jacqueline Chen for assistance in data analysis and output, and to Ronald Haller for providing exceptional support and the opportunity to study many of these interesting patients.

REFERENCES

1. Chance B, Eleff S, Leigh JS Jr, et al. Mitochondrial regulation of phosphocreatine/inorganic phosphate ratios in exercising human muscle: a gated ^{31}P NMR study. Proc Natl Acad Sci U S A 1981;78:6714–6718.
2. Gadian DG, Radda GK, Dawson MJ, Wilkie DR. pHi measurements of cardiac and skeletal muscle using ^{31}P-Nmr. Kroc Found Ser 1981;15:61–77.
3. Ross BD, Radda GK, Gadian DG, et al. Examination of a case of suspected McArdle's syndrome by ^{31}P nuclear magnetic resonance. N Engl J Med 1981;304:1338–1342.
4. Sahlin K. Metabolic Changes Limiting Muscle Performance. In B Saltin (ed), Biochemistry of Exercise VI. Champaign, IL: Human Kinetics Publishers, 1986;323.
5. Meyer RA, Foley JM. Cellular Processes Integrating the Metabolic Response to Exercise. In LB Rowell, JT Shepherd (eds), Handbook of Physiology, Section 12, Exercise: Regulation and Integration of Multiple Systems. New York: Oxford University Press, 1996;841–869.
6. Taylor DJ, Bore PJ, Styles P, et al. Bioenergetics of intact human muscle. A ^{31}P nuclear magnetic resonance study. Mol Biol Med 1983;1:77–94.
7. Arnold DL, Matthews PM, Radda GK. Metabolic recovery after exercise and the assessment of mitochondrial function in vivo in human skeletal muscle by means of ^{31}P NMR. Magn Reson Med 1984;1:307–315.
8. Harris R, Hultman E, Nordesjo L-O. Glycogen, glycolytic intermediates and high energy phosphates determined in biopsy samples of musculus quadriceps femoris of man at rest. Methods and variance of values. Scand J Clin Lab Invest 1974;33:109–120.
9. Veech R, Lawson J, Cornell N, Krebs H. Cytosolic phosphorylation potential. J Biol Chem 1979;254:6538–6547.
10. Bore P, Chan L, Gadian D, et al. Non-invasive pH measurements of human tissue using 31-P NMR. In R Nuccitelli, DW Deamer (eds), Intracellular pH: Its Measurement, Regulation, and Utilizations in Cellular Functions. New York: Alan R. Liss, 1982;527–535.
11. Argov Z, Bank WJ, Maris J, et al. Bioenergetic heterogeneity of human mitochondrial myopathies: phosphorus magnetic resonance spectroscopy study. Neurology 1987;37:257–262.
12. Taylor DJ, Kemp GJ, Radda GK. Bioenergetics of skeletal muscle in mitochondrial myopathy. J Neurol Sci 1994;127:198–206.
13. Quistorff B, Johansen L, Sahlin K. Absence of phosphocreatine resynthesis in human calf muscle during ischaemic recovery. Biochem J 1992;291:681–686.
14. Kemp GJ, Thompson CH, Barnes PR, Radda GK. Comparisons of ATP turnover in human muscle during ischemic and aerobic exercise using ^{31}P magnetic resonance spectroscopy. Magn Reson Med 1994;31:248–258.
15. Kemp GJ, Taylor DJ, Thompson CH, et al. Quantitative analysis by ^{31}P magnetic resonance spectroscopy of abnormal mitochondrial oxidation in skeletal muscle during recovery from exercise. NMR Biomed 1993;6:302–310.
16. Kemp GJ, Taylor DJ, Styles P, Radda GK. The production, buffering and efflux of protons in human skeletal muscle during exercise and recovery. NMR Biomed 1993;6:73–83.
17. Arnold DL, Taylor DJ, Radda GK. Investigation of human mitochondrial myopathies by phosphorus magnetic resonance spectroscopy. Ann Neurol 1985;18:189–196.
18. Argov Z, De Stefano N, Arnold DL. ADP recovery after a brief ischemic exercise in normal and diseased human muscle—a ^{31}P MRS study. NMR Biomed 1996;9:165–172.
19. Chen JT, Argov Z, Kearney RE, Arnold DL. Fitting cytosolic ADP recovery after exercise with a step response function. Magn Reson Med 1999;41:926–932.

20. Kemp GJ, Taylor DJ, Radda GK. Control of phosphocreatine resynthesis during recovery from exercise in human skeletal muscle. NMR Biomed 1993;6:66–72.

21. Kemp GJ, Radda GK. Quantitative interpretation of bioenergetic data from ^{31}P and 1H magnetic resonance spectroscopic studies of skeletal muscle: an analytical review. Magn Reson Q 1994; 10:43–63.

22. Bendahan D, Confort-Gouny S, Kozak-Reiss G, Cozzone PJ. Heterogeneity of metabolic response to muscular exercise in humans. New criteria of invariance defined by in vivo phosphorus-31 NMR spectroscopy. FEBS Lett 1990;272:155–158.

23. Iotti S, Lodi R, Frassineti C, et al. In vivo assessment of mitochondrial functionality in human gastrocnemius muscle by ^{31}P MRS. The role of pH in the evaluation of phosphocreatine and inorganic phosphate recoveries from exercise. NMR Biomed 1993;6:248–253.

24. Lodi R, Kemp GJ, Iotti S, et al. Influence of cytosolic pH on in vivo assessment of human muscle mitochondrial respiration by phosphorus magnetic resonance spectroscopy. MAGMA 1997; 5:165–171.

25. Taylor DJ, Kemp GJ, Thompson CH, Radda GK. Ageing: effects on oxidative function of skeletal muscle in vivo. Mol Cell Biochem 1997;174:321–324.

26. Laurent D, Bernus G, Alonso J, et al. Effect of training on the calf muscle energy metabolism. A ^{31}P-NMR study on four elite downhill skiers challenged with a standardized exercise protocol. Int J Sports Med 1992;13:313–318.

27. McCully KK, Boden BP, Tuchler M, et al. Wrist flexor muscles of elite rowers measured with magnetic resonance spectroscopy. J Appl Physiol 1989;67:926–932.

28. Yoshida T, Watari H. Metabolic consequences of repeated exercise in long distance runners. Eur J Appl Physiol Occup Physiol 1993;67:261–265.

29. Tartaglia MC, Chen JT, Caramanos Z, et al. Muscle phosphorus magnetic resonance spectroscopy oxidative indices correlate with physical activity. Muscle Nerve 2000;23:175–181.

30. Tarnopolsky MA, Parise G. Direct measurement of high-energy phosphate compounds in patients with neuromuscular disease. Muscle Nerve 1999;22:1228–1233.

31. Argov Z, Bank WJ, Maris J, Chance B. Muscle energy metabolism in McArdle's syndrome by in vivo phosphorus magnetic resonance spectroscopy. Neurology 1987;37:1720–1724.

32. Duboc D, Jehenson P, Tran-Dinh S, et al. Phosphorus NMR spectroscopy study of muscular enzyme deficiencies involving glycogenolysis and glycolysis. Neurology 1987;37:663–671.

33. Radda GK, Rajagopalan B, Taylor DJ. Biochemistry in vivo: an appraisal of clinical magnetic resonance spectroscopy. Magn Reson Q 1989;5:122–151.

34. Bendahan D, Confort-Gouny S, Kozak-Ribbens G, Cozzone PJ. 31-P characterization of the metabolic anomalies associated with the lack of glycogen phosphorylase activity in human forearm muscle. Biochem Biophys Res Comm 1992;185:16–21.

35. Siciliano G, Rossi B, Martini A, et al. Myophosphorylase deficiency affects muscle mitochondrial respiration as shown by 31 P-MR spectroscopy in a case with associated multifocal encephalopathy. J Neurol Sci 1995;128:84–91.

36. De Stefano N, Argov Z, Matthews PM, et al. Impairment of muscle mitochondrial oxidative metabolism in McArdle's disease. Muscle Nerve 1996;19:764–769.

37. Rowland LP, DiMauro S, Layzer RB. Phosphofructokinase Deficiency. In AG Engel, BQ Banker (eds), Myology. New York: McGraw-Hill, 1986;1603–1617.

38. Servidei S, Bonilla E, Diedrich RG, et al. Fatal infantile form of muscle phosphofructokinase deficiency. Neurology 1986;36:1465–1470.

39. Massa R, Lodi R, Barbiroli B, et al. Partial block of glycolysis in late-onset phosphofructokinase deficiency myopathy. Acta Neuropathol 1996;91:322–329.

40. Danon MJ, Servidei S, DiMauro S, Vora S. Late-onset muscle phosphofructokinase deficiency. Neurology 1988;38:956–960.

41. Sivakumar K, Vasconcelos O, Goldfarb L, Dalakas MC. Late-onset muscle weakness in partial phosphofructokinase deficiency: a unique myopathy with vacuoles, abnormal mitochondria, and absence of the common exon 5/intron 5 junction point mutation. Neurology 1996;46:1337–1342.

42. Argov Z, Bank WJ, Maris J, et al. Muscle energy metabolism in human phosphofructokinase deficiency as recorded by ^{31}P nuclear magnetic resonance spectroscopy. Ann Neurol 1987;22: 46–51.

43. Edwards RHT, Dawson MJ, Wilkie DR, et al. Clinical use of nuclear magnetic resonance in the investigation of myopathy. Lancet 1982;1:725–731.

44. Grehl T, Muller K, Vorgerd M, et al. Impaired aerobic glycolysis in muscle phosphofructokinase deficiency results in biphasic post-exercise phosphocreatine recovery in ^{31}P magnetic resonance spectroscopy. Neuromuscul Disord 1998;8:480–488.

45. Bertocci LA, Haller RG, Lewis SF. Muscle metabolism during lactate infusion in human phospho-fructokinase deficiency. J Appl Physiol 1993;74:1342–1347.

46. Vora S, DiMauro S, Spear D, et al. Characterization of the enzymatic defect in late-onset muscle phosphofructokinase deficiency. New subtype of glycogen storage disease type VII. J Clin Invest 1987;80:1479–1485.

47. Argov Z, Bank WJ, Boden B, et al. Phosphorus magnetic resonance spectroscopy of partially blocked muscle glycolysis. An in vivo study of phosphoglycerate mutase deficiency. Arch Neurol 1987;44:614–617.

48. Vita G, Toscano A, Bresolin N, et al. Muscle phosphoglycerate mutase (PGAM) deficiency in the first Caucasian patient: biochemistry, muscle culture and ^{31}P-MR spectroscopy. J Neurol 1994;241:289–294.

49. Steele IC, Patterson VH, Nicholls DP. A double blind, placebo controlled, crossover trial of D-ribose in McArdle's disease. J Neurol Sci 1996;136:174–177.

50. MacLean D, Vissing J, Vissing SF, Haller RG. Oral branched-chain amino acids do not improve exercise capacity in McArdle disease. Neurology 1998;51:1456–1459.

51. Vorgerd M, Grehl T, Jager M, et al. Creatine therapy in myophosphorylase deficiency (McArdle disease): a placebo-controlled crossover trial. Arch Neurol 2000;57:956–963.

52. Matthews PM, Allaire C, Shoubridge EA, et al. In vivo muscle magnetic resonance spectroscopy in the clinical investigation of mitochondrial disease. Neurology 1991;41:114–120.

53. Lodi R, Taylor DJ, Tabrizi SJ, et al. Normal in vivo skeletal muscle oxidative metabolism in sporadic inclusion body myositis assessed by ^{31}P-magnetic resonance spectroscopy. Brain 1998;121:2119–2126.

54. Cortelli P, Montagna P, Avoni P, et al. Leber's hereditary optic neuropathy: genetic, biochemical, and phosphorus magnetic resonance spectroscopy study in an Italian family. Neurology 1991;41:1211–1215.

55. Lodi R, Taylor DJ, Tabrizi SJ, et al. In vivo skeletal muscle mitochondrial function in Leber's hereditary optic neuropathy assessed by ^{31}P magnetic resonance spectroscopy. Ann Neurol 1997;42:573–579.

56. Argov Z, Taivassalo T, De Stefano N, et al. Intracellular phosphates in inclusion body myositis—a ^{31}P magnetic resonance spectroscopy study. Muscle Nerve 1998;21:1523–1525.

57. Barbiroli B, Funicello R, Iotti S, et al. ^{31}P-NMR spectroscopy of skeletal muscle in Becker dystrophy and DMD/BMD carriers. Altered rate of phosphate transport. J Neurol Sci 1992;109:188–195.

58. Kemp GJ, Taylor DJ, Dunn JF, et al. Cellular energetics of dystrophic muscle. J Neurol Sci 1993;116:201–206.

59. Lodi R, Kemp GJ, Muntoni F, et al. Reduced cytosolic acidification during exercise suggests defective glycolytic activity in skeletal muscle of patients with Becker muscular dystrophy. An in vivo ^{31}P magnetic resonance spectroscopy study. Brain 1999;122:121–130.

60. Barbiroli B, Montagna P, Cortelli P, et al. Defective brain and muscle energy metabolism shown by in vivo ^{31}P magnetic resonance spectroscopy in nonaffected carriers of 11778 mtDNA mutation. Neurology 1995;45:1364–1369.

61. Lodi R, Montagna P, Cortelli P, et al. Secondary 4216/ND1 and 13708/ND5 Leber's hereditary optic neuropathy mitochondrial DNA mutations do not further impair in vivo mitochondrial oxidative metabolism when associated with the 11778/ND4 mitochondrial DNA mutation. Brain 2000;123:1896–1902.

62. Goto Y, Nonaka I, Horai S. A mutation in the tRNA(Leu)(UUR) gene associated with the MELAS subgroup of mitochondrial encephalomyopathies. Nature 1990;348:651–653.

63. Taylor RW, Turnbull DM. Laboratory Diagnosis of Mitochondrial Disease. In DA Applegarth, J Dimmick, JG Hall (eds), Organelle Diseases. London: Chapman & Hall, 1997.

64. Chinnery PF, Howell N, Lightowlers RN, Turnbull DM. Molecular pathology of MELAS and MERRF. The relationship between mutation load and clinical phenotypes. Brain 1997;120:1713–1721.

65. Chinnery PF, Taylor DJ, Brown DT, et al. Very low levels of the mtDNA A3243G mutation associated with mitochondrial dysfunction in vivo. Ann Neurol 2000;47:381–384.

66. Chinnery PF, Taylor DJ, Brown DT, et al. No correlation between muscle A3243G mutation load and mitochondrial function in vivo. Neurology 2001;56(8):1101–1104.

67. Dunbar DR, Moonie PA, Jacobs HT, Holt IJ. Different cellular backgrounds confer a marked advantage to either mutant or wild-type mitochondrial genomes. Proc Natl Acad Sci U S A 1995;92:6562–6566.

68. Cock H, Tabrizi S, Cooper J, Schapira A. The influence of nuclear background on the biochemical expression of 3460 Leber's hereditary optic neuropathy. Ann Neurol 1998;44:187–193.

69. Lodi R, Carelli V, Cortelli P, et al. Phosphorus MR spectroscopy demonstrates a tissue specific distribution of the in vivo biochemical expression of G3460A Leber's Hereditary Optic Neuropathy mtDNA mutation. J Neurol Neurosurg Psychiatry, *in press*.

70. Eleff S, Kennaway N, Buist N, et al. ^{31}P NMR study of improvement in oxidative phosphorylation by vitamins K3 and C in a patient with a defect in electron transports at complex III in skeletal muscle. Proc Natl Acad Sci U S A 1984;81:3529–3533.

71. Penn AM, Lee JW, Thuillier P, et al. MELAS syndrome with mitochondrial tRNA(Leu)(UUR) mutation: correlation of clinical state, nerve conduction, and muscle ^{31}P magnetic resonance spectroscopy during treatment with nicotinamide and riboflavin. Neurology 1992;42:2147–2152.

72. Bendahan D, Desnuelle C, Vanuxem D, et al. ^{31}P NMR spectroscopy and ergometer exercise test as evidence for muscle oxidative performance improvement with coenzyme Q in mitochondrial myopathies. Neurology 1992;42:1203–1208.

73. Barbiroli B, Frassineti C, Martinelli P, et al. Coenzyme Q10 improves mitochondrial respiration in patients with mitochondrial cytopathies. An in vivo study on brain and skeletal muscle by phosphorous magnetic resonance spectroscopy. Cell Mol Biol 1997;43:741–749.

74. Matthews PM, Ford B, Dandurand RJ, et al. Coenzyme Q10 with multiple vitamins is generally ineffective in treatment of mitochondrial disease. Neurology 1993;43:884–890.

75. De Stefano N, Matthews PM, Ford B, et al. Short-term dichloroacetate treatment improves indices of cerebral metabolism in patients with mitochondrial disorders. Neurology 1995;45:1193–1198.

76. Taivassalo T, Matthews P, De Stefano N, et al. Combined aerobic training and dichloroacetate improve exercise capacity and indices of aerobic metabolism in muscle cytochrome oxidase deficiency. Neurology 1996;47:529–534.

77. Taivassalo T, De Stefano N, Argov Z, et al. Effects of aerobic training in patients with mitochondrial myopathies. Neurology 1998;50:1055–1060.

78. Taivassalo T, Stefano ND, Chen J, et al. Short-term aerobic training response in chronic myopathies. Muscle Nerve 1999;22:1239–1243.

79. Taivassalo T, Shoubridge EA, Chen J, et al. Aerobic conditioning in patients with mitochondrial myopathies: physiological, biochemical, and genetic effects. Ann Neurol 2001;50(2):133–141.

80. Clark KM, Bindoff LA, Lightowlers RN, et al. Reversal of a mitochondrial DNA defect in human skeletal muscle. Nat Genet 1997;16:222–224.

81. Taivassalo T, Fu K, Johns T, Arnold D, et al. Gene shifting: a novel therapy for mitochondrial myopathy. Hum Mol Genet 1999;8:1047–1052.

82. Campbell KP. Three muscular dystrophies: loss of cytoskeleton-extracellular matrix linkage. Cell 1995;80:675–679.

83. Hoffman EP, Brown RH, Kunkel LM. Dystrophin: the protein product of the DMD locus. Cell 1987;51:919–928.

84. Edwards RH, Griffiths RD, Cady EB. Topical magnetic resonance for the study of muscle metabolism in human myopathy. Clin Physiol 1985;5:93–109.

85. Barbiroli B, McCully KK, Iotti S, et al. Further impairment of muscle phosphate kinetics by lengthening exercise in DMD/BMD carriers. An in vivo ^{31}P-NMR spectroscopy study. J Neurol Sci 1993;119:65–73.

86. Newman RJ, Bore PJ, Chan L, et al. Nuclear magnetic resonance studies of forearm muscle in Duchenne dystrophy. BMJ 1982;284:1072–1074.

87. Younkin DP, Berman P, Sladky J, et al. ^{31}P NMR studies in Duchenne muscular dystrophy: age-related metabolic changes. Neurology 1987;37:165–169.

88. Zochodne DW, Koopman WJ, Witt NJ, et al. Forearm P-31 nuclear magnetic resonance spectroscopy studies in oculopharyngeal muscular dystrophy. Can J Neurol Sci 1992;19:174–179.

89. Barnes PR, Kemp GJ, Taylor DJ, Radda GK. Skeletal muscle metabolism in myotonic dystrophy A ^{31}P magnetic resonance spectroscopy study. Brain 1997;120:1699–1711.

90. Dunn J, Frostick S, Brown G, Radda G. Energy status of cells lacking dystrophin an in vivo/in vitro study of mdx mouse skeletal muscle. Biochim Biophys Acta 1991;1906:115–120.

91. Dunn J, Radda G. Total ion content of skeletal and cardiac muscle in the mdx mouse dystrophy: Ca2+ is elevated at all ages. J Neurol Sci 1991;103:226–231.

92. Letellier T, Malgat M, Mazat JP. Control of oxidative phosphorylation in rat muscle mitochondria: implications for mitochondrial myopathies. Biochim Biophys Acta 1993;1141:58–64.

93. Pagliaro L. Glycolysis revisited. News Physiol Sci 1993;8:219–223.

94. Hopkins JC, Bia BL, Crilley JG, et al. Muscular dystrophy: from gene to patient. MAGMA 2000;11:7–9.

95. Deconinck AE, Rafael JA, Skinner JA, et al. Utrophin-dystrophin-deficient mice as a model for Duchenne muscular dystrophy. Cell 1997;90:717–727.
96. Cole ME, Rafael JA, Carr M, et al. A quantitative study of bioenergetics in skeletal muscle lacking utrophin and dystrophin. Neuromuscul Disord 2002;12:247–257.
97. Dunn J, Tracey I, Radda G. A 31 P-NMR study of muscle exercise metabolism in mdx mice: evidence for abnormal pH regulation. J Neurol Sci 1992;113:108–113.
98. Lodi R, Muntoni F, Taylor J, et al. Correlative MR imaging and ^{31}P-MR spectroscopy study in sarcoglycan deficient limb girdle muscular dystrophy. Neuromuscul Disord 1997;7:505–511.
99. Goudemant JF, Deconinck N, Tinsley JM, et al. Expression of truncated utrophin improves pH recovery in exercising muscles of dystrophic mdx mice: a ^{31}P NMR study. Neuromuscul Disord 1998;8:371–379.
100. Taylor DJ, Kemp GJ, Woods CG, et al. Skeletal muscle bioenergetics in myotonic dystrophy. J Neurol Sci 1993;116:193–200.
101. Chang L, Ernst T, Osborn D, et al. Proton spectroscopy in myotonic dystrophy. Correlation with CTG repeats. Arch Neurol 1998;55:305–311.
102. Dalakas MC. Polymyositis, dermatomyositis, and inclusion-body myositis. N Engl J Med 1991; 325:1487–1498.
103. Park JH, Vansant JP, Kumar NG, et al. Dermatomyositis: correlative MR imaging and P-31 MR spectroscopy for quantitative characterization of inflammatory disease. Radiology 1990;177: 473–479.
104. Park J, Vital T, Ryder N, et al. Magnetic resonance imaging and P-31 magnetic resonance spectroscopy provide unique quantitative data useful in the longitudinal management of patients with dermatomyositis. Arthritis Rheum 1994;37:736–746.
105. Park JH, Olsen NJ, King L, et al. Use of magnetic resonance imaging and P-31 magnetic resonance spectroscopy to detect and quantify muscle dysfunction in the amyopathic and myopathic variants of dermatomyositis. Arthritis Rheum 1995;38:68–77.
106. Park JH, Kari S, King LE, Olsen NJ. Analysis of ^{31}P MR spectroscopy data using artificial neural networks for longitudinal evaluation of muscle diseases: dermatomyositis. NMR Biomed 1998;11:245–256.
107. Park JH, Niermann KJ, Ryder NM, et al. Muscle abnormalities in juvenile dermatomyositis patients: P–31 magnetic resonance spectroscopy studies. Arthritis Rheum 2000;43:2359–2367.
108. Cea G, Bendahan D, Manners D, et al. Reduced oxidative phosphorylation and proton efflux suggest reduced capillary blood supply in skeletal muscle of patients with dermatomyositis and polymyositis: a quantitative ^{31}P MRS and MRI study. Brain, *in press*.
109. Kemp GJ, Hands LJ, Ramaswami G, et al. Calf muscle mitochondrial and glycogenolytic ATP synthesis in patients with claudication due to peripheral vascular disease analysed using ^{31}P magnetic resonance spectroscopy. Clin Sci 1995;89:581–590.
110. Chariot P, Ruet E, Authier FJ, et al. Cytochrome c oxidase deficiencies in the muscle of patients with inflammatory myopathies. Acta Neuropathol (Berl) 1996;91:530–536.
111. Blume G, Pestronk A, Frank B, Johns DR. Polymyositis with cytochrome oxidase negative fibres. Early quadriceps weakness and poor response to immunosuppressive therapy. Brain 1997;120:39–45.
112. Campos Y, Arenas J, Cabello A, Gomez-Reino JJ. Respiratory chain enzyme defects in patients with idiopathic inflammatory myopathy. Ann Rheum Dis 1995;54:491–493.
113. Emslie-Smith AM, Engel AG. Microvascular changes in early and advanced dermatomyositis: a quantitative study. Ann Neurol 1990;27:343–356.
114. DeVisser M, Emslie-Smith AM, Engel AG. Early ultrastructural alterations in adult dermatomyositis. Capillary abnormalities precede other structural changes in muscle. J Neurol Sci 1989;94:181–192.
115. Carry MR, Ringel SP, Starcevich JM. Distribution of capillaries in normal and diseased human skeletal muscle. Muscle Nerve 1986;9:445–454.
116. King LE, Park JH, Adams LB, Olsen NJ. Phosphorus 31 magnetic resonance spectroscopy for quantitative evaluation of therapeutic regimens in dermatomyositis. Arch Dermatol 1995;131: 522–524.
117. Griggs RC, Askanas V, DiMauro S, et al. Inclusion body myositis and myopathies. Ann Neurol 1995;38:705–713.
118. Oldfors A, Larsson NG, Lindberg C, Holme E. Mitochondrial DNA deletions in inclusion body myositis. Brain 1993;116:325–336.
119. Santorelli FM, Sciacco M, Tanji K, et al. Multiple mitochondrial DNA deletions in sporadic inclusion body myositis: a study of 56 patients. Ann Neurol 1996;39:789–795.

120. Jurkat-Rott K, McCarthy T, Lehmann-Horn F. Genetics and pathogenesis of malignant hyperthermia. Muscle Nerve 2000;23:4−17.

121. Larach M. Standardization of the caffeine halothane muscle contracture test. North American Malignant Hyperthermia Group. Anesth Analg 1989;69:511−515.

122. Bendahan D, Kozak-Ribbens G, Rodet L, et al. ^{31}Phosphorus magnetic resonance spectroscopy characterization of muscular metabolic anomalies in patients with malignant hyperthermia: application to diagnosis. Anesthesiology 1998;88:96−107.

123. Monsieurs K, Heytens L, Kloeck C, et al. Slower recovery of muscle phosphocreatine in malignant hyperthermia-susceptible individuals assessed by ^{31}P-MR spectroscopy. J Neurol 1997; 244:651−656.

124. Webster DW, Thompson RT, Gravelle DR, et al. Metabolic response to exercise in malignant hyperthermia-sensitive patients measured by ^{31}P magnetic resonance spectroscopy. Magn Reson Med 1990;15:81−89.

125. Olgin J, Rosenberg H, Allen G, et al. A blinded comparison of noninvasive, in vivo phosphorus nuclear magnetic resonance spectroscopy and the in vitro halothane/caffeine contracture test in the evaluation of malignant hyperthermia susceptibility. Anesth Analg 1991;72:36−47.

126. Payen JF, Bosson JL, Bourdon L, et al. Improved noninvasive diagnostic testing for malignant hyperthermia susceptibility from a combination of metabolites determined in vivo with ^{31}P-magnetic resonance spectroscopy. Anesthesiology 1993;78:848−855.

127. Payen JF, Fouilhe N, Sam-Lai E, et al. In vitro ^{31}P-magnetic resonance spectroscopy of muscle extracts in malignant hyperthermia-susceptible patients. Anesthesiology 1996;84:1077−1082.

128. Arnold DL, Bore PJ, Radda GK, et al. Excessive intracellular acidosis of skeletal muscle on exercise in a patient with a post-viral exhaustion/fatigue syndrome. A ^{31}P nuclear magnetic resonance study. Lancet 1984;1:1367−1369.

129. Barnes PR, Taylor DJ, Kemp GJ, Radda GK. Skeletal muscle bioenergetics in the chronic fatigue syndrome. J Neurol Neurosurg Psychiatry 1993;56:679−683.

130. Lodi R, Taylor DJ, Radda GK. Chronic fatigue syndrome and skeletal muscle mitochondrial function. Muscle Nerve 1997;20:765−766.

131. McCully KK, Natelson BH, Iotti S, et al. Reduced oxidative muscle metabolism in chronic fatigue syndrome. Muscle Nerve 1996;19:621−625.

132. Lane RJ, Barrett MC, Taylor DJ, et al. Heterogeneity in chronic fatigue syndrome: evidence from magnetic resonance spectroscopy of muscle. Neuromuscul Disord 1998;8:204−209.

133. Pongratz DE, Spath M. Morphologic aspects of fibromyalgia. Z Rheumatol 1998;57:47−51.

134. Simms R, Roy S, Hrovat M, et al. Lack of association between fibromyalgia syndrome and abnormalities in muscle energy metabolism. Arthritis Rheum 1994;37:794−800.

135. Vestergaard-Poulsen P, Thomsen C, Norregaard J, et al. ^{31}P NMR spectroscopy and electromyography during exercise and recovery in patients with fibromyalgia. J Rheumatol 1995;22:1544−1551.

136. de Blecourt AC, Wolf RF, van Rijswijk MH, et al. In vivo ^{31}P magnetic resonance spectroscopy (MRS) of tender points in patients with primary fibromyalgia syndrome. Rheumatol Int 1991;11:51−54.

137. Park JH, Phothimat P, Oates CT, et al. Use of P-31 magnetic resonance spectroscopy to detect metabolic abnormalities in muscles of patients with fibromyalgia. Arthritis Rheum 1998;41:406−413.

17

Biochemical Evaluation of Metabolic Myopathies

Salvatore DiMauro, Sara Shanske, Ali Naini, and Sindu Krishna

Metabolic myopathies encompass a large group of hereditary disorders resulting in impaired energy provision for muscle contraction. Metabolic myopathies are conveniently classified into three major groups: disorders of glycogen metabolism, disorders of lipid metabolism, and disorders of the mitochondrial respiratory chain (Figure 17.1). The first two groups reflect the importance of carbohydrate and long-chain fatty acids as major "fuels" of the "muscle motor." The third group reflects the crucial role of oxidative phosphorylation for the terminal combustion of acetyl-coenzyme A (CoA), the common product of carbohydrate and lipid metabolism, to form adenosine triphosphate (ATP), the energy "currency" of muscle.

Defects of substrate utilization in muscle cause two main clinical presentations: (1) acute, recurrent, reversible muscle dysfunction manifesting as exercise intolerance or myalgia with or without painful cramps and often culminating in muscle breakdown and myoglobinuria; or (2) fixed (often progressive) weakness sometimes simulating dystrophic or neurogenic processes (see Figure 17.1). In general, there is a good correlation between the circumstances leading to exercise intolerance and the different roles of glycogen and lipid metabolism in the provision of energy to contracting muscles. For example, in agreement with the concept that glycogen metabolism is crucial for anaerobic or intense aerobic exercise, the symptoms in patients with glycogenoses are almost invariably related to strenuous bouts of exercise, and the muscles that hurt or cramp are those that have been exercised.

In contrast, patients with disorders of lipid metabolism, such as carnitine palmitoyl transferase (CPT) II deficiency, usually have no difficulty with short-term intense exercise, and their muscle symptoms follow prolonged moderate exercise, especially when associated with fasting. Impending myoglobinuria in these patients may be heralded by aching of exercising muscles but is not accompanied by actual shortening of muscles in the painful cramps that are typical of muscle glycogenolytic or glycolytic defects. In addition, prolonged fasting in and of itself may cause myoglobinuria—in which case, any muscle

535

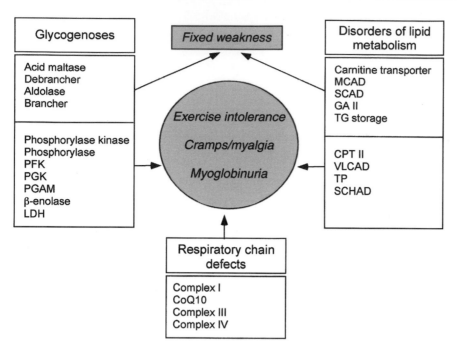

Figure 17.1 The two major syndromes associated with hereditary metabolic myopathies. (CoQ10 = coenzyme Q10; CPT = carnitine palmitoyl transferase; GA II = glutaric aciduria type II; LDH = lactate dehydrogenase; MCAD = medium-chain acyl-coenzyme A dehydrogenase; PFK = phosphofructokinase; PGAM = phosphoglycerate mutase; PGK = phosphoglycerate kinase; SCAD = short-chain acyl-coenzyme A dehydrogenase; SCHAD = short-chain 3-hydroxy-acyl-coenzyme A dehydrogenase; TG = triglyceride; TP = trifunctional protein; VLCAD = very-long-chain acyl-coenzyme A dehydrogenase.) (Modified from S DiMauro, RG Haller. Metabolic Myopathies: Substrate Use Defects. In AHV Schapira, RC Griggs [eds], Muscle Diseases. Boston: Butterworth–Heinemann, 1999;225–249.)

groups, including respiratory muscles, can be affected.[1] The deleterious effect of fasting in CPT II deficiency is easily explained by the increased dependence of muscle on free fatty acid (FFA) oxidation, which is virtually blocked. Conversely, some patients with myophosphorylase deficiency (McArdle's disease) note a beneficial effect of fasting on their exercise ability: The mobilization of FFA triggered by fasting probably facilitates the physiologic switch from glycogen utilization (which is impeded) to lipid utilization.

Figure 17.2 illustrates schematically glycogen metabolism and mitochondrial energy metabolism. Note how glycogenolysis and glycolysis take place in the cytoplasm, whereas most of the steps involved in lipid utilization are intramitochondrial. Pyruvate, the terminal product of aerobic glycolysis, is transported across the inner mitochondrial membrane through a symport system "in the wake" of hydrogen ions flowing inward down their electrochemical gradient. Transport of FFA requires a more complex system, which includes two enzymes (CPT I and CPT II), a carrier molecule (L-carnitine), and a translocase (carnitine-acylcarnitine translocase). After oxidation of pyruvate through the pyruvate dehydrogenase complex and oxidation of fatty acyl-CoAs through β-oxidation, carbohydrate and lipid fuels converge into a common central metabolite, acetyl-CoA, which is further oxidized in the Krebs cycle.

BIOCHEMICAL ANALYSIS OF MUSCLE: GENERAL CONSIDERATIONS

Although it is fair to state that biochemical assays in muscle biopsies are still a mainstay in the diagnosis of metabolic myopathies, several considerations should be kept in mind.

Alternative Tissues

Some of the metabolic myopathies are due to defects of muscle-specific isozymes or enzyme subunits (e.g., myophosphorylase deficiency in McArdle's disease and phosphofructokinase [PFK] muscle [M] deficiency in Tarui disease); other myopathies are due to mutations in mitochondrial DNA (mtDNA) that are confined to skeletal muscle (e.g., many mutations in the cytochrome-*b* gene).[2] In these cases, muscle is obviously indispensable for biochemical assays. However, in several metabolic myopathies, the enzyme defect is not confined to muscle but involves some or all nonmuscle tissues. For example, phosphoglycerate kinase (PGK) deficiency affects all tissues except sperm; CPT II deficiency is expressed in lymphocytes and fibroblasts. In these cases, biochemical diagnosis can be established in tissues, such as blood cells or cultured skin fibroblasts, which are more easily accessible than muscle. Mitochondrial encephalomyopathies due to mutations in mtDNA present a special problem in that respiratory chain enzyme defects are invariably partial and may be especially difficult to detect in tissues that are less rich in mitochondria than muscle, such as fibroblasts.

Histochemistry

One glycogenolytic enzyme (phosphorylase) and one glycolytic enzyme (PFK) can be evaluated by histochemical assays. Adenylate deaminase, an enzyme of the purine nucleotide cycle, can also be assessed histochemically. These assays are usually reliable diagnostic tools, but they are qualitative, and we think that they should be confirmed by quantitative biochemical tests. In addition, histochemistry can sometimes be deceiving: For example, biopsies taken from patients with McArdle's disease shortly after an episode of myoglobinuria may contain abundant regenerating fibers,[3] which stain positive for phosphorylase because they express transiently the brain isozyme.[4] An indirect histochemical clue to the diagnosis of acid maltase deficiency is a positive reaction for acid phosphatase. This stain, which is usually undetectable owing to the scarcity of lysosomes in normal human muscle, becomes prominent in acid maltase deficiency because of the proliferation of glycogen-laden lysosomes.

Molecular Analysis

Biochemical defect hunters have been followed by molecular defect hunters, and our molecular knowledge of metabolic myopathies has advanced so rapidly that it is sometimes possible to bypass biochemistry and go directly to molecular analysis of blood cells. Although this approach often spares the patient the discomfort and expense of a muscle biopsy, it requires at least two conditions: (1) The clinical diag-

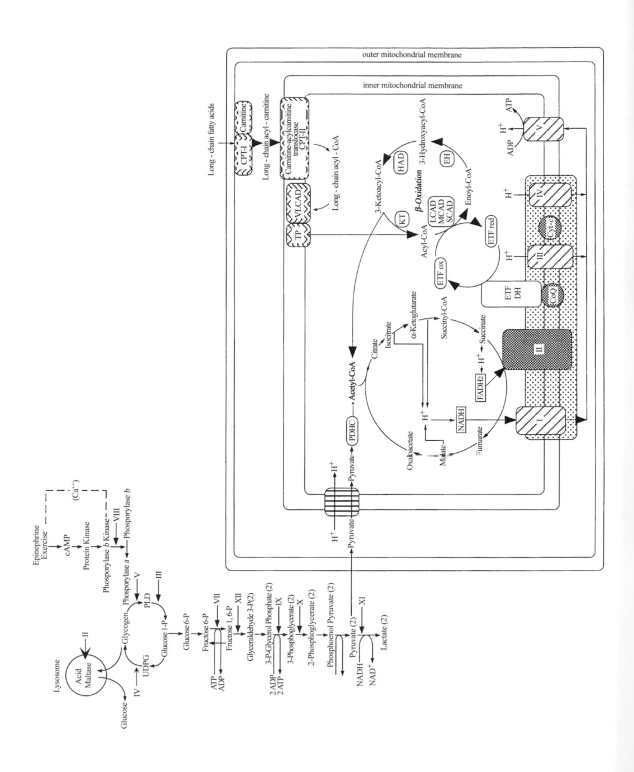

nosis has to be convincing, and (2) the disease in question must be caused by one—or a few—common mutations. A white patient with suspected myophosphorylase deficiency—especially if he or she is of Anglo-Saxon descent—can be tested for the Arg49Stop mutation in genomic DNA extracted from blood with good probability of success, because this mutation is present in 81% of the alleles in British patients[5] and in 63% of the alleles in American patients.[6] Similarly, European or American patients with suspected CPT deficiency can be tested for the common Ser113Leu mutation.[7] However, negative results do not exclude the diagnosis in either condition and make biochemical studies of muscle the next logical step.

Again, the situation is different in mitochondrial encephalomyopathies due to point mutations in mtDNA, such as mitochondrial encephalomyopathy with lactic acidosis and stroke-like episode (MELAS), myoclonus epilepsy with ragged red fibers (MERFF), and neuropathy, ataxia, and retinitis pigmentosa (NARP). In patients with strongly suggestive clinical phenotypes and evidence of maternal inheritance, looking for the common mutations (A3243G for MELAS, A8344G for MERRF, and T8993G for NARP) in blood cells, hair follicles, or urinary sediment is the logical first diagnostic step.

Biochemical Analysis in Its Proper Context

It is clear from the items mentioned previously that biochemical studies of muscle, which are often time consuming and expensive, should not be conducted in isolation but should be part of a logical diagnostic sequence. This starts with a detailed clinical and electrophysiologic evaluation followed by careful morphologic analysis of the muscle biopsy. For example, a young adult with lifelong exercise intolerance and recurrent episodes of myoglobinuria could have a defect in glycogen metabolism, lipid metabolism, or the respiratory chain. The type of exercise that triggers symptoms, the presence of other precipitating factors (e.g., fasting), the resting and postexercise levels of blood creatine kinase

◀ **Figure 17.2** General scheme of muscle metabolism. On the left, outside the mitochondrion, is a representation of glycogen metabolism and glycolysis. Roman numerals in this area of the figure (II–XII) indicate enzymes whose deficiencies are associated with muscle glycogenoses. (II = acid maltase; III = debrancher; IV = brancher; V = myophosphorylase; VII = phosphofructokinase; VIII = phosphorylase b kinase; IX = phosphoglycerate kinase; X = phosphoglycerate mutase; XI = lactate dehydrogenase; XII = aldolase A.) On the right, in the mitochondrial respiratory chain, components or complexes (I–V) encoded exclusively by nuclear DNA are solid; complexes containing some subunits encoded by nuclear DNA and others encoded by mitochondrial DNA are crosshatched. (ADP = adenosine diphosphate; AMP = adenosine monophosphate; ATP = adenosine triphosphate; CoA = coenzyme A; CoQ = coenzyme Q; CPT = carnitine palmitoyl transferase; Cyt c = cytochrome-c; ETF = electron-transfer flavoprotein; ETF DH = ETF-CoQ oxidoreductase; ETF ox = oxidized form of ETF; ETF red = reduced form of ETF; $FADH_2$ = flavin adenine dinucleotide; H^+ = hydrogen ion; HAD = hydroxyacyl dehydrogenases; KT = 3-ketothiolase; LCAD = long-chain acyl-CoA dehydrogenase; MCAD = medium-chain acyl-CoA dehydrogenase; NAD^+ = oxidized form of nicotinamide adenine dinucleotide; NADH = nicotinamide adenine dinucleotide; P = phosphate; PDHC = pyruvate dehydrogenase complex; PLD = phosphorylase-limit dextrin; SCAD = short-chain acyl-CoA dehydrogenase; TCA = tricarboxylic acid; TP = trifunctional protein; UDPG = uridine diphosphate glucose; VLCAD = very-long-chain acyl-CoA dehydrogenase.) (Modified from S DiMauro, RG Haller. Metabolic Myopathies: Substrate Use Defects. In AHV Schapira, RC Griggs [eds], Muscle Diseases. Boston: Butterworth–Heinemann, 1999;225–249.)

(CK) and lactate, and the occurrence (or not) of electrically silent contractures are all clues pointing to problems in one or another metabolic pathway. Muscle biopsy may show accumulation of glycogen, which can be relatively abundant (as in myophosphorylase or PFK deficiency) or scant (as in defects of terminal glycolysis). The coexistence of normal glycogen and diastase-resistant polysaccharide staining intensely with iodine (polyglucosan) suggests PFK deficiency. Histochemical stains can suggest a specific diagnosis (myophosphorylase or PFK deficiency). If the biopsy is completely normal, the more likely diagnosis is CPT II deficiency or a defect of β-oxidation. If the Gomori trichrome or the succinate dehydrogenase (SDH) stain suggest abnormal mitochondrial proliferation or frank ragged red fibers (RRFs), a defect in the respiratory chain is likely. If the RRFs are associated with lipid storage, a primary defect of coenzyme Q10 (CoQ10) ought to be considered, especially because patients with this condition respond to CoQ10 supplementation. The staining of RRFs with the cytochrome-*c* oxidase (COX) histochemical reaction offers important clues. If RRFs are COX-positive, mutations (possibly a de novo somatic mutation in myogenic stem cells) in mtDNA genes encoding complex I or complex III subunits have to be considered. If the RRFs (or non-RRFs) are COX-negative, then mutations in one of the three mtDNA genes encoding COX subunits are likely. At this point, biochemical studies of muscle become crucial to confirm the diagnosis and to plan molecular analysis.

With these general principles as background, we now briefly review individual disorders in the three pathways, with special emphasis on the importance and limitations of biochemical testing.

DISORDERS OF GLYCOGEN METABOLISM

Tissue Preparation

Muscle specimens for biochemical analysis should be flash-frozen at the time of biopsy, stored in liquid nitrogen or in a freezer at −130°C, and shipped to the diagnostic laboratory in dry ice. Any delay in the initial freezing or any subsequent thawing may result in loss of activity of some or all enzymes. PFK is notoriously labile, and interpretation of low activities becomes difficult if these conditions are not adhered to. In fact, we often use PFK activity as a marker of tissue viability to validate low activities of other enzymes.

Enzymes of glycogen metabolism and glycolysis are in the cytoplasm, either free or bound to glycogen particles. Therefore, we measure them in 10,000-g supernatants of 10% muscle homogenates in appropriate media. We follow the Roman numeric order of the glycogenoses, as indicated in Figure 17.2.

Glycogenosis Type II, Acid Maltase Deficiency

Clinical Features

There are two major clinical presentations of glycogenosis type II: a generalized form (Pompe's disease) and a myopathic form. Pompe's disease starts at or near birth and is characterized by profound weakness ("floppy child" or "rag doll" appearance), massive cardiomegaly, lesser hepatomegaly, and occasionally macroglossia. These children rarely survive more than one year. The myopathic form of acid maltase deficiency (AMD) comes in three varieties (depending on age at onset): infantile, childhood, and adult. Patients with infantile AMD resemble children with Pompe's disease but have no cardiopathy and tend to live longer.[8] Childhood AMD may mimic Duchenne's muscular dystrophy or other forms of muscular dystrophy: These patients die in the second or third decade of respiratory insufficiency. Adult-onset AMD mimics limb-girdle muscular dystrophy or polymyositis; truncal and respiratory muscles are especially affected. Serum CK is markedly elevated in all forms of AMD, and electromyography shows myopathic features together with fibrillation potentials and bizarre, high-frequency, myotonic discharges.

Muscle Biopsy

In Pompe's disease and in the infantile and childhood variants of myopathic AMD, there is massive accumulation of both intralysosomal and free glycogen, distorting the contractile system. In adult AMD, glycogen accumulation is milder and may be difficult to detect in some muscles. There is no histochemical stain for acid maltase, but intense staining for acid phosphatase (another lysosomal enzyme) provides an indirect clue to the diagnosis.

Biochemistry

The defective enzyme is an acid α-1,4-glucosidase and α-1,6-glucosidase, capable of digesting glycogen all the way to glucose. This lysosomal enzyme is a single polypeptide encoded by a gene on chromosome 17 and expressed in all tissues. A sensitive biochemical test commonly used for diagnostic analysis is based on the hydrolysis (at a pH of 4.0) of an artificial substrate, 4-methyl-umbelliferyl α-D-glucoside (MUαG). Liberation of umbelliferone, which is fluorescent, can be measured in a fluorometer.

Because the acid maltase enzyme is present in all tissues, the biochemical analysis can be conducted in tissues other than muscle, and cultured amniocytes have been used reliably for prenatal diagnosis. However, caution must be used in interpreting data obtained from mixed white blood cells (WBCs) because granulocytes contain a "renal" α-glucosidase isoform active at acid pH, which may mask the enzyme defect in AMD patients. If WBCs have to be used, then isolated lymphocytes are the cells of choice.[9]

Although there is no evidence that use of the artificial substrate may result in false-negative results (i.e., that some mutations may allow the enzyme to hydrolyze MUαG but not glycogen), assays can be run with glycogen or maltose as substrates, in which glucose is measured as the reaction product.

Until recently, a biochemical puzzle was represented by an X-linked disorder characterized by cardiomyopathy, mental retardation, and autophagic vacuolar myopathy. Muscle biopsy was often reminiscent of AMD, and the disease was also called "lysosomal glycogen storage disease with normal acid maltase."[10] We now know that this is due to mutations in lysosome-associated membrane protein–2 (LAMP-2), which is not directly involved in glycogen metabolism.[11]

Molecular Genetics

Although more than 50 mutations have been identified in the gene encoding α-glucosidase, and this has simplified prenatal diagnosis, biochemical tests in muscle biopsies remain the mainstay of diagnosis.

Glycogenosis Type III (Debrancher Deficiency)

Clinical Features

The typical presentation of glycogenosis type III is that of a benign hepatopathy of infancy or childhood, with hepatomegaly, growth retardation, and fasting hypoglycemia. Clinical myopathy often manifests in adult life with weakness and wasting of distal leg and intrinsic hand muscles, sometimes suggesting motor neuron disease or peripheral neuropathy.[12] Subclinical cardiac involvement is revealed by laboratory tests in most patients. Serum CK is variably increased, and electromyography shows myopathic features associated with fibrillations, positive sharp waves, and myotonic discharges. Nerve conduction studies may be abnormal, reflecting peripheral nerve involvement.

Muscle Biopsy

There is severe vacuolar myopathy with deposits of periodic acid-Schiff (PAS)–positive material under the sarcolemma and between myofibrils. Ultrastructurally, the vacuoles correspond to large pools of free, normal-looking glycogen β-particles.

Biochemistry

The *debranching enzyme* is a single polypeptide encoded by a gene on chromosome 1, which possesses two distinct catalytic functions, oligo-1,4-1,4-glucantransferase and amylo-1,6-glucosidase. After phosphorylase has shortened the peripheral chains of glycogen to approximately 4 glucosyl units (this partially "chewed up" glycogen is called *phosphorylase-limit-dextrin* [PLD]), the transferase activity of the debrancher enzyme removes a maltotriosyl unit, leaving behind a single glucosyl unit in an α-1,6-glucosidic link. This glucosyl unit is then hydrolyzed by the amylo-1,6-glucosidic activity of the debrancher. Patients with debrancher deficiency are classified into three groups: IIIa, lacking both enzymatic activities in both liver and muscle; IIIb, also lacking both activities in liver, whereas heart and muscle are spared; IIIc, lacking only the amylo-1,6-glucosidase activity; and IIId, lacking only the transferase activity in both liver and muscle.[13,14] Most patients belong to group IIIa.

The most common enzyme assay is based on the reverse amylo-1,6-glucosidase reaction and uses uniformly labeled ^{14}C-glucose and glycogen as substrates[15]: Incorporation of labeled glucose is measured in a scintillation counter after precipitating glycogen on filter paper disks. We prefer a spectrophotometric assay, which measures both enzyme activities and is based on the release of glucose-1-phosphate (G-1-P) from PLD (the physiologic substrate for the debranching enzyme).[12] An indirect way of documenting debrancher deficiency in muscle is to reveal the abnormal structure of glycogen through the absorption spectrum of the glycogen-iodine complex. The rate of absorption at two wavelengths (A460/A390) for abnormally short-chained glycogen (PLD) is lower than for normal glycogen.[12] Because the enzyme defect is generalized, at least in patients belonging to the IIIa group, biochemical assays can be performed in erythrocytes, WBCs, or cultured fibroblasts.

Molecular Genetics

Several mutations have been identified in both type IIIa and IIIb patients and can be used for prenatal diagnosis. Spectrophotometric determination of debrancher activity in muscle is the keystone of diagnosis in patients with myopathy.

Glycogenosis Type IV (Branching Enzyme Deficiency)

Clinical Features

Typically, glycogenosis type IV is a rapidly progressive disease of early childhood, with hepatosplenomegaly, cirrhosis, hepatic failure, and death before 4 years of age. However, clinical presentations vary widely, with predominant involvement of muscle, heart, or brain in different patients. Brain involvement (adult polyglucosan body disease [APBD]) is manifested by late-onset progressive upper and lower motor neuron disease, sensory loss, sphincter dysfunction, and dementia.

Muscle Biopsy

The hallmark of glycogenosis type IV is the presence of basophilic, intensely PAS-positive polysaccharide deposits, which are partially resistant to diastase digestion and which, ultrastructurally, consist of filamentous and finely granular material. The abnormal polysaccharide, called *polyglucosan*, has been documented in skin, liver, muscle, heart, and brain, but the amount varies widely in different tissues from different patients. In APBD, polyglucosan bodies are seen in processes (but not in perikarya) of neurons and astrocytes in both gray and white matter.[16]

Biochemistry

The branching enzyme catalyzes the last step in glycogen biosynthesis by adding short glucosyl chains (approximately 7 glucosyl units long) to linear peripheral chains of glycogen in α-1,6-glucosidic bonds. The newly added stubs are then elongated by glycogen synthetase. The enzyme is a monomeric protein encoded by a gene on chromosome 3 and expressed in all tissues.

Because no specific substrate for branching enzyme is available, activity is measured by an indirect method based on the stimulation of the incorporation of ^{14}C-labeled G-1-P into glycogen by phosphorylase in the absence of exogenous glycogen primer. Nonspecific incorporation into endogenous glycogen is measured with boiled tissue and subtracted.[17] As the enzyme defect is generalized, tissues other than muscle can be used for diagnosis. For example, Lossos et al.[18] first documented branching enzyme deficiency in leukocytes from patients with APBD. We confirmed the biochemical defect in leukocytes and peripheral nerve of Ashkenazi Jewish patients, whereas non-Jewish patients with APBD had normal brancher activities in the same tissues.[19] The reason for this discrepancy remains unknown.

The polysaccharide stored in brancher deficiency (polyglucosan) has longer than normal peripheral linear chains and fewer branching points, thus resembling amylopectin. The abnormal structure of polyglucosan is reflected by the abnormal absorption spectrum of the iodine complex, with a shift of the peak toward higher wavelengths.[17] However, this cannot be used as a diagnostic tool per se, because polyglucosan accumulates in other conditions such as PFK deficiency and Lafora's disease (see below).

Molecular Genetics

Mutations have been identified in patients with different clinical phenotypes, including myopathy[20] and APBD.[21]

Glycogenosis Type V (Myophosphorylase Deficiency; McArdle's Disease)

Clinical Features

Elegantly described by Brian McArdle in 1951,[22] glycogenosis type V is characterized by exercise intolerance with premature fatigue, myalgia, and cramps in exercising muscles, relieved by rest. Symptoms are more likely to occur with intense isometric exercise, such as lifting weights, or with less intense but sustained dynamic exercise, such as walking uphill. Approximately half of the patients have acute muscle necrosis and myoglobinuria after exercise. Although exercise intolerance starts in childhood, cramps and myoglobinuria develop later, and the diagnosis is rarely established in children. The severity of symptoms varies considerably, from "poor stamina" to frequent and almost incapacitating cramps. A few patients have severe generalized weakness soon after birth, with respiratory insufficiency and death in infancy. Patients with typical symptoms may develop fixed weakness later in life.

Laboratory tests show increased serum CK levels even at rest. Electromyography is usually normal or compatible with mild myopathy. During cramps, however, shortened muscles are electrically silent, true "contractures." The forearm ischemic exercise shows no rise of venous lactate. This test, which is not specific for McArdle's disease and depends on the active cooperation of the patient, is less commonly used nowadays, because it is painful and may result in localized muscle necrosis. Especially in children, a semi-ischemic test may be preferable,[23] and molecular genetic analysis of blood cells may secure a diagnosis,[6] thus avoiding both forearm ischemic exercise and muscle biopsy, as previously discussed.

Muscle Biopsy

Typically, there are subsarcolemmal and intermyofibrillar vacuoles filled with glycogen, which are PAS-positive and digested by diastase. The histochemical reaction shows no staining of muscle fibers, whereas smooth muscle of intramuscular vessels stains normally. However, false-positive staining of regenerating fibers (which express a different isozyme) may occur, especially when the biopsy is taken soon after an episode of myoglobinuria.[3]

Biochemistry

Phosphorylase catalyzes the phosphorylytic stepwise removal of α-1,4-glucosyl residues from the outer branches of glycogen with liberation of G-1-P. This reaction goes on until the peripheral chains have been shortened to 4-glucosyl units, and the resulting PLD can be acted on by the debranching enzyme (see above). *Muscle phosphorylase* is a dimer of two identical subunits encoded by a gene on chromosome 11. The enzyme reaction is based on the liberation of G-1-P, which is converted to G-6-P by exogenous phosphoglucomutase. G-6-P is oxidized by exogenous G-6-P dehydrogenase, and the resulting reduced nicotinamide adenine dinucleotide (NAD) phosphate (NADPH) is measured spectrophotometrically.

Molecular Genetics

Approximately 30 mutations have been reported, but by far the most frequent among white (especially Anglo-Saxon) patients is R49X. The frequency of this nonsense mutation in the first exon of the gene explains why the enzyme protein is commonly absent in muscle. The high frequency of this mutation among white (and especially Anglo-Saxon) patients has also made it possible to diagnose McArdle's disease by molecular analysis of blood cells, thus making muscle biopsy unnecessary in some cases.[6]

Glycogenosis Type VII (Phosphofructokinase Deficiency; Tarui Disease)

Clinical Features

In its typical presentation, PFK deficiency is indistinguishable from myophosphorylase deficiency: intolerance to intense exercise and cramps of exercising muscles, relieved by rest. Myoglobinuria may be less frequent than in McArdle's disease. When present, jaundice (caused by mild hemolysis) and gouty arthritis are useful clues to the correct diagnosis. Helpful laboratory signs include reticulocytosis and increased serum bilirubin and uric acid. As in McArdle's disease, resting serum CK values are variably increased, and the forearm ischemic exercise causes no increase in venous lactate. Clinical variants include (1) late-onset weakness; and (2) fatal infantile myopathy, often accompanied by brain involvement.

Muscle Biopsy

There is excessive subsarcolemmal and intermyofibrillar normal-looking glycogen. However, a distinctive morphologic feature is the additional presence of polyglucosan deposit, especially in older patients.[24–26] The histochemical reaction is a useful diagnostic tool.[27]

Biochemistry

PFK is a tetrameric enzyme under the control of three genes encoding muscle (M), liver (L), and platelet (P) subunits.[28] Mature human muscle expresses only the M subunit and contains the homotetramer M4. Erythrocytes express both the M and the L subunits and contain five isoforms, the homotetramers M4 and L4, plus the three hybrid forms. In PFK deficiency, mutations in the PFKM-encoding gene (on chromosome 1) cause total lack of PFK activity in muscle and partial enzyme deficiency in erythrocytes (hence the hemolytic trait).

PFK catalyzes the phosphorylation of fructose-6-phosphate (F-6-P) to fructose-1,6-P (F-1,6-P), and PFK deficiency results in a marked accumulation of both F-6-P and its immediate glycolytic precursor, glucose-6-P (G-6-P). As G-6-P is a physiologic activator of glycogen synthetase, we proposed that an abnormally increased ratio of glycogen synthetase versus branching enzyme activity could be responsible for the deposit of polyglucosan.[24,25] This concept seems bolstered by recent studies of Lafora's disease, a severe autosomal recessive form of myoclonus epilepsy with generalized deposit of polyglucosan, which, in the brain, takes the shape of round PAS-positive structures called *Lafora's bodies*. The gene product, laforin, is a tyrosine phosphatase that may play a role in the cascade of reactions controlling the activity of glycogen synthetase. Mutations in the laforin gene probably result in an abnormal activation of synthetase and a skewed synthetase to brancher ratio.[29,30]

The biochemical assay for PFK is based on the conversion of F-6-P to F-1,6-P and the further breakdown of F-1,6-P to the two triose-phosphates (glyceraldehyde-3-P and dihydroxyacetone-P) in the presence of exogenous aldolase. In the presence of excess triose-phosphate isomerase and α-glycerophosphate-dehydrogenase, dihydroxyacetone is reduced to α-glycerol-P, and the oxidation of the reduced form of NAD (NADH) to NAD is recorded spectrophotometrically.

Molecular Genetics

Approximately 20 mutations have been identified in the PFKM gene on chromosome 1. Some of these are more common among Ashkenazi Jewish patients and can be screened in blood from patients with suspected PFK deficiency even before a muscle biopsy is performed.

Glycogenosis Type VIII (Phosphorylase b Kinase Deficiency)

Clinical Features

The myopathic form of phosphorylase *b* kinase (PhK) deficiency manifests as a milder version of myophosphorylase deficiency, with exercise intolerance, cramps, and occasional myoglobinuria.[31] Some patients, however, have fixed weakness, and others have combined muscle and liver involvement with static myopathy. Serum CK is variably increased, and the lactate response to ischemic exercise is often normal or blunted.

Muscle Biopsy

There is mild to moderate subsarcolemmal accumulation of glycogen, predominantly in type IIb fibers.

Biochemistry

PhK is a decahexamer of four different subunits, α, β, γ, and δ: $(\alpha\beta\gamma\delta)_4$. The γ subunit is catalytic, the α and β subunits are regulatory, and the δ subunit is identical to calmodulin and confers calcium sensitivity to the enzyme. There are two α subunits: one specific for muscle (α_M), the other specific for liver (α_L), encoded by two distinct genes on the X-chromosome. The PhK assay is based on the activation of purified phosphorylase *b* to phosphorylase *a* by a muscle extract and depends on the purity of commercially available phosphorylase *b*.[31]

Molecular Genetics

The prevalence of affected men is probably explained by the existence of an X-linked muscle-specific α gene; in fact, both mutations documented thus far in patients with myopathy have been in the α_M gene.[32,33]

Glycogenosis Type IX (Phosphoglycerate Kinase Deficiency)

Clinical Features

PGK deficiency usually causes hemolytic anemia, seizures, and mental retardation. However, isolated myopathy has been reported in half a dozen patients who had exercise intolerance, cramps, and myoglobinuria. Resting serum CK levels are inconsistently elevated, and the rise of venous lactate after ischemic exercise is absent or blunted.

Muscle Biopsy

The PAS stain may show diffuse glycogen storage.

Biochemistry

PGK is a single polypeptide encoded by a gene on the X-chromosome and expressed in all tissues except the testis. The enzyme is measured by a simple spectrophotometric assay based on the oxidation of the reaction product, 3-phosphoglyceraldehyde (3-P-glyceraldehyde), in the presence of exogenous 3-P-glyceraldehyde dehydrogenase.

Molecular Genetics

A few mutations have been identified in patients with isolated myopathy, but, in this disorder, biochemical documentation is the crucial first step.

Glycogenosis Type X (Phosphoglycerate Mutase Deficiency)

Clinical Features

All patients described (approximately a dozen) had exercise intolerance, cramps, and recurrent myoglobinuria. Forearm ischemic exercise causes abnormally low increase of venous lactate. An unusual number of heterozygous patients can be symptomatic.[34,35]

Muscle Biopsy

There is mild glycogen storage, which may difficult to detect in some patients.

Biochemistry

Phosphoglycerate mutase (PGAM) is a dimeric enzyme containing various proportions of a muscle (M) subunit and a brain (B) subunit. In normal mature human muscle, approximately 95% of total PGAM activity is accounted for by the MM homodimer. The small amount of residual PGAM activity found in muscle from patients is due to the BB homodimer. The enzyme reaction uses 3-phosphoglycerate as a substrate: 2-Phosphoglycerate formation is then measured spectrophotometrically in terms of NADH oxidized through three reactions catalyzed by exogenous enolase, pyruvate kinase, and lactate dehydrogenase (LDH).

Molecular Genetics

The M subunit of PGAM is encoded by a gene on chromosome 7. Mutations have been identified in the PGAM-M gene in all patients with myopathy, but biochemical analysis of muscle is needed for diagnosis.

Glycogenosis Type XI (*Lactate Dehydrogenase Deficiency*)

Clinical Features

Glycogenosis type XI disorder is also characterized by exercise intolerance, cramps, and myoglobinuria. One diagnostic clue is that the forearm ischemic exercise causes little or no increase of lactate but a large increase in pyruvate.

Muscle Biopsy

Histochemistry may show a mild increase of glycogen.

Biochemistry

LDH is a tetrameric enzyme composed of two subunits, one of which (LDH-M) predominates in skeletal muscle, whereas the other (LDH-H) predominates in cardiac muscle. Random tetramerization results in the formation of five isozymes, the two homotetramers (M4 and H4), and three heterotetramers. Muscle from patients contains only the H4 isoform. The enzyme assay is based on the reduction of pyruvate to lactate, resulting in the oxidation of NADH, which is followed spectrophotometrically.

Molecular Genetics

Mutations in the gene encoding LDH-M (which is on chromosome 11) have been identified in all patients with myopathy.

Glycogenosis Type XII (*Aldolase A Deficiency*)

Clinical Features

Aldolase A deficiency has been reported in a single patient with episodic exercise intolerance and weakness triggered by febrile illnesses.[36]

Biochemistry

Aldolase A is composed of four identical subunits encoded by a gene on chromosome 16. Enzyme activity is measured in the physiologic direction, with fructose-1,6-diphosphate as substrate. In the presence of exogenous triose-phosphate isomerase, dihydroxy-acetone-P is continuously converted to glyceraldehyde-3-P, which is reduced by exogenous glyceraldehyde-3-P dehydrogenase. The associated oxidation of NADH is measured spectrophotometrically.

Molecular Genetics

A mutation (E206K) has been identified in the patient.

Glycogenosis Type XIII (β-Enolase Deficiency)

Clinical Features

Glycogenosis type XIII been described in one man with adult-onset exercise intolerance and chronically elevated serum CK.[37]

Biochemistry

Enolase is a dimeric enzyme, and the muscle-specific isoform β-enolase is a homodimer of the β subunit, which is encoded by a gene on chromosome 17. The reaction measures the conversion of 2-phosphoglycerate to lactate in the presence of exogenous pyruvate kinase and LDH and is based on the spectrophotometric determination of NADH oxidation.

Molecular Genetics

The patient was a compound heterozygote harboring two missense mutations: G156D and G374R.

DISORDERS OF LIPID METABOLISM

Two major metabolic pathways are needed for long-chain fatty acid utilization: (1) transport and activation of fatty acids (the carnitine cycle); and (2) mitochondrial fatty acyl-CoA oxidation (β-oxidation). In this section, we review only those disorders that cause neuromuscular disease.

Tissue Preparation

As both metabolic pathways are within mitochondria and many enzymes are bound to the outer or inner mitochondrial membrane, we measure carnitine concentration and determine enzyme activities in whole muscle homogenate.

Defects of the Carnitine Cycle

The carnitine cycle consists of four steps mediated by a plasma membrane carnitine transporter, CPT I, a carnitine-acylcarnitine translocase, and CPT II (see Figure 17.2).

Primary Systemic Carnitine Deficiency

Clinical Features. Approximately 30 patients have been described, and almost half of them had a sibling who died of cardiopathy or sudden death. Mean age at onset is 2 years, ranging from 1 month to 7 years of age. Progressive cardiomyopathy is the most common presentation: Echocardiography and electrocardiogram show dilative cardiomyopathy, peaked T waves, and signs of ventricular hypertrophy. Myopathy is usually associated with cardiomyopathy and is manifested by mild motor delay, hypotonia, or slowly progressive proximal weakness. Some infants may present with acute encephalopathy together with hypoketotic hypoglycemia and hepatomegaly with liver steatosis. Cardiac dysfunction and muscle weakness respond dramatically to carnitine supplementation, and these patients, who would otherwise die of cardiac failure, can live normal lives with continued replacement therapy. Serum CK can be normal or slightly elevated.

Muscle Biopsy. There is severe lipid storage, which is best revealed by the oil-red-O or the Nile-blue stain for neutral lipids. Endomyocardial biopsies or postmortem studies also show massive lipid storage.

Biochemistry. Both total and free carnitine concentrations are extremely low (usually below 10% of normal) in skeletal muscle, and, when measured, carnitine concentration in the myocardium was less than 5% of normal. We measure free L-carnitine by a modification of the radioisotopic method of McGarry and Foster.[38] We incubate a neutralized perchloric acid extract of muscle homogenate with [1-^{14}C]acetyl-CoA and carnitine acetyltransferase: The labeled acetyl-carnitine formed in the reaction is measured in a scintillation counter after binding all unreacted acetyl-CoA to an anion exchange resin and separating the resin by centrifugation. Total carnitine is determined after alkaline hydrolysis to liberate carnitine from its acyl esters. Esterified carnitine is then calculated as the difference between total and free carnitine.

Molecular Genetics. Primary systemic carnitine deficiency, an autosomal recessive disorder, involves a genetic defect of the plasma membrane carnitine transporter in the kidney, intestine, muscle, heart, and fibroblasts, but not in the liver. Defective carnitine transport in the kidney causes defective carnitine reabsorption and excessive carnitine excretion. Deficient intestinal transport results in poor and delayed carnitine absorption. The combination of defective renal and intestinal carnitine handling causes carnitine levels to fall in blood. Hence, it is important to measure blood carnitine concentrations in all infants and young children with unexplained cardiomyopathy. Linkage analysis has localized the gene responsible for primary carnitine deficiency to chromosome 5q. The gene, which encodes one member of a family of organic cation transporters, has been isolated, and several pathogenic mutations have been identified in patients and their asymptomatic parents.[39,40]

Primary Myopathic Carnitine Deficiency

Clinical Features. Primary myopathic carnitine deficiency, characterized by decreased muscle carnitine vis-à-vis normal serum carnitine, was the first example of carnitine deficiency in a young woman with progressive proximal weakness and lipid storage myopathy responsive to corticosteroids.[41] The existence of this entity, however, is controversial because there is no definitive documentation of an isolated defect of carnitine uptake in muscle. It is possible that patients with the diagnosis of carnitine deficiency myopathy may have other fatty acid oxidation defects, either generalized or muscle-specific. In some of the patients described, symptoms appeared in the first years of life, but in most, onset was between the second and third decade. There was progressive and sometimes fluctuating weakness of proximal limb and axial muscles of variable severity. A few of these patients had associated cardiomyopathy.

Muscle Biopsy. In all patients, there was severe lipid storage, especially in type I fibers.

Biochemistry. Muscle carnitine levels were 20% of normal or less, whereas plasma carnitine levels were normal or slightly reduced. Some of the patients improved with carnitine administration.

Secondary Carnitine Deficiency

Secondary carnitine deficiency—characterized by decreased levels of carnitine in blood and, often, in tissues—can accompany diverse disorders, including inborn errors of metabolism, acquired medical conditions, and iatrogenic states.[42]

Examples of inborn errors of metabolism include numerous defects of fatty acid metabolism affecting both the carnitine cycle and β-oxidation, disorders of branched-chain amino acid metabolism, and defects of the mitochondrial respiratory chain.

Examples of acquired medical conditions include those causing decreased carnitine biosynthesis (e.g., hepatic cirrhosis or extreme prematurity), those causing decreased carnitine intake (e.g., malnutrition, chronic total parenteral nutrition, strict vegetarian diet, soy protein infant formula, malabsorption), those causing decreased body stores of carnitine in the face of increased requirements (e.g., pregnancy and lactation, extreme prematurity, infant of carnitine-deficient mother), and those causing increased carnitine loss (e.g., Fanconi syndrome).

Examples of iatrogenic factors include valproate therapy, hemodialysis, and zidovudine administration.

It is important to keep in mind these diverse causes of carnitine deficiency because carnitine replacement often results in marked improvement.

Carnitine Palmitoyl Transferase I Deficiency

After cytosolic long-chain fatty acids are activated to the corresponding acyl-CoAs thioesters by a long-chain acyl-CoA synthetase bound to the outer mitochondrial membrane, another enzyme of the outer mitochondrial membrane, CPT I, transfers acyl residues from CoA to carnitine. There are two isoforms of CPT I—a liver type and a muscle type—but only liver CPT I deficiency has been described.

Carnitine-Acylcarnitine Translocase Deficiency

Clinical Features. Patients with translocase deficiency present with life-threatening episodes in the neonatal period: There is generalized weakness, cardiac arrhythmia, hyperammonemia, and inconsistent hypoglycemia.

Biochemistry. An inner mitochondrial membrane translocase is needed to shuttle the acylcarnitines formed by CPT I across the inner membrane in exchange for carnitine. This 301 amino acid intramembranous protein is encoded by a gene on chromosome 3p21.31.

Carnitine Palmitoyl Transferase II Deficiency

Clinical Features. CPT II deficiency causes two distinct phenotypes, myopathic and hepatocardiomuscular. The more common, myopathic form usually presents in adolescents or young adults, predominantly males, with recurrent myoglobinuria after prolonged (although not necessarily strenuous) exercise, prolonged fasting, or a combination of the two conditions. Other precipitating factors include cold exposure, lack of sleep, and, especially in children, intercurrent illnesses with high fever. Between attacks, these patients have normal physical and neurologic examinations. Unlike what happens in the glycogenoses, the attacks of myoglobinuria are not heralded by painful cramps. In addition, exercising muscles are not necessarily the only ones undergoing acute necrosis, and a few patients have been admitted to the hospital in respiratory distress.[1] Another distinguishing feature from the glycogenoses is the normal level of serum CK between attacks of myoglobinuria. Plasma carnitine levels are usually normal. CPT II deficiency, first described in 1973,[43] appears to be the most common cause of hereditary myoglobinuria.[44]

Muscle Biopsy. When the biopsy is taken far enough from an episode of myoglobinuria, it can be completely normal. When present, lipid storage is much milder than in the primary or myopathic forms of carnitine deficiency.

Biochemistry. Once long-chain acylcarnitines are inside the inner mitochondrial membrane, they have to be reconverted to acyl-CoA esters to enter the β-oxidation spiral. This is done by CPT II, a single enzyme without tissue-specific isoforms, which is loosely bound to the inner mitochondrial membrane and is encoded by a gene on chromosome 1p32. The most common enzyme assay is based on the "isotope exchange" between methyl-^{14}C-carnitine and unlabeled palmitoyl carnitine: Labeled palmitoyl carnitine is extracted in L-butanol and counted.[45] Although this method measures predominantly CPT II activity in muscle homogenates (residual activities in patients are below 30%), it is not specific for CPT II, and false-negative (i.e., apparently normal) results may be seen in a few patients.

Molecular Genetics. Numerous mutations have been described, but one of them (Ser113Leu) is commonly encountered in both European and American patients.[7] The relative frequency of this disease and the special circumstances triggering myoglobinuria often suggest the diagnosis. In these cases, the more common mutations can be looked for in blood cells, thus potentially avoiding the need for a muscle biopsy.

The rarer and much more severe hepatocardiomuscular form can affect infants or children. Patients with the infantile form die within weeks, after presenting with hepatopathy, encephalopathy, cardiomegaly, and cardiac arrhythmia. Patients with later onset have fasting hypoketotic hypoglycemia, hepatopathy, cardiomyopathy, and mild myopathy. They are at risk for sudden death. In contrast to the myopathic form, plasma carnitine levels are severely decreased in the generalized form.

Defects of β-Oxidation

Once long-chain fatty acids have gained access to the mitochondrial matrix as acyl-CoAs, the second major pathway involved in their use is the multienzyme β-oxidation. This pathway is more complex than previously thought, as two new enzymes, both bound to the inner membrane, have been identified: very-long-chain acyl-CoA dehydrogenase (VLCAD) and mitochondrial trifunctional protein (TP) (see Figure 17.2). There are four sequential steps of β-oxidation, in which an acyl-CoA ester undergoes dehydrogenation, hydration, a second dehydrogenation, and thiolytic cleavage. First, three acyl-CoA dehydrogenases act on fatty acids of different chain lengths: long-chain acyl-CoA dehydrogenase (LCAD), medium-chain acyl-CoA dehydrogenase (MCAD), and short-chain acyl-CoA dehydrogenase (SCAD). Recent evidence suggests that long-chain acyl-CoA dehydrogenase has a minor role in the dehydrogenation of straight-chain acyl-CoAs, whereas this reaction is catalyzed by the membrane-bound VLCAD. The prosthetic group of VLCAD, MCAD, and SCAD is flavin adenine dinucleotide, which is reoxidized by the matrix enzyme electron-transferring flavoprotein (ETF). ETF, in turn, passes reducing equivalents to another flavoprotein bound to the inner mitochondrial membrane, ETF-dehydrogenase (ETFDH), from which electrons are fed to CoQ10, a component of the respiratory chain (see Figure 17.2). The second reaction in β-oxidation is catalyzed by two enoyl-CoA hydratases: Crotonase acts on short-chain substrates, whereas hydration of long-chain 2-trans-enoyl-CoAs is catalyzed by the membrane-bound TP. The third step of β-oxidation involves a long-chain 3-hydroxyacyl-CoA dehydrogenase (LCHAD) and a short-chain enzyme (SCHAD). The final step of β-oxidation requires two thiolases, a soluble medium-chain 3-ketoacyl-CoA thiolase, and a long-chain thiolase that is part of the membrane-bound TP.

Short-Chain Acyl-Coenzyme A Dehydrogenase Deficiency

A single adult case of lipid storage myopathy with SCAD deficiency confined to skeletal muscle[46] was probably due to a different primary metabolic defect, because there are no tissue-specific isoforms of SCAD. Most patients with generalized SCAD deficiency present in infancy with poor feeding, vomiting, failure to thrive, lethargy, and hypotonia. Psychomotor retardation, seizures, and hyperactivity have also been described. Myopathy was prominent only in a 13-year-old girl with congenital facial and neck weakness, which spread to limb, axial, and respiratory muscle.[47] She also had ptosis, progressive external ophthalmoplegia (PEO), and cataracts. Muscle biopsy showed type I fiber predominance, hypotrophy, and multicores.

Medium-Chain Acyl-Coenzyme A Dehydrogenase Deficiency

MCAD is a relatively common condition that presents in childhood as an episodic acute illness with hypoketotic hypoglycemia after intercurrent infection and fasting. The presenting symptoms and signs (in order of decreasing frequency) include lethargy, vomiting, encephalopathy, respiratory arrest, hepatomegaly, seizures, apnea, cardiac arrest, and sudden death. Myopathy is uncommon.

Very-Long-Chain Acyl-Coenzyme A Dehydrogenase Deficiency

There are three major clinical phenotypes of VLCAD: (1) a more common severe infantile form with hypertrophic cardiomyopathy and early death; (2) a less severe form with recurrent episodes of hypoketotic hypoglycemia, reminiscent of MCAD deficiency; (3) a myopathic form closely resembling CPT II deficiency and characterized by recurrent episodes of muscle breakdown and myoglobinuria after prolonged exercise, prolonged fasting, or both.[48–50] The abnormal profile of acylcarnitines in plasma is the laboratory test of choice.

Trifunctional Protein Deficiency

In the "typical" form, all three enzymatic functions of TP are defective. Presentation is in infancy, usually dominated by cardiomyopathy, with or without a previous episode of hypoketotic hypoglycemia. There is cardiomegaly, left ventricular hypertrophy, and, sometimes, pericardial effusion. Three patients had a milder presentation, with recurrent myoglobinuria (resembling CPT II deficiency) and chronic progressive polyneuropathy.[51]

Long-Chain 3-Hydroxyacyl-Coenzyme A Dehydrogenase Deficiency

LCHAD is a special case of the mitochondrial TP deficiency described above, because LCHAD is one of the functions of TP. In TP deficiency, all three enzymatic functions are affected, whereas in this case only the long-chain hydroxyacyl-CoA dehydrogenase activity is impaired. This disorder can present in infancy with episodic hypoketotic hypoglycemia after prolonged fasting due to intercurrent infections. Some infants succumb to rapidly progressive cardiomyopathy. Milder and later onset presentations include a myopathic form with exercise-induced episodic muscle breakdown and myoglobinuria, resembling CPT II deficiency. However, these patients often have additional features not seen in CPT II deficiency, including peripheral neuropathy and hepatomegaly with liver dysfunction. Still other patients had childhood-onset hypoglycemia, cardiomyopathy, hypotonia, hepatomegaly, lactic acidosis, and low plasma carnitine.

Short-Chain 3-Hydroxyacyl-Coenzyme A Dehydrogenase Deficiency

Of the three patients with SCHAD described thus far, two were infants with episodic vomiting, ketosis, and hypoglycemia induced by fasting. The third patient was a 16-year-old girl with hypoketotic hypoglycemic encephalopathy, cardiomyopathy, and recurrent myoglobinuria.[52] As SCHAD activity was normal in fibroblasts, it was suggested that the defect involved a muscle-specific isoform, but this remains to be proven.

Electron-Transferring Flavoprotein Deficiency and Electron-Transferring Flavoprotein–Dehydrogenase

ETF and ETFDH result in multiple acyl-CoA dehydrogenase deficiency (glutaric aciduria type II) and give rise to three major clinical phenotypes: (1) a severe neonatal disorder, with hypotonia, hepatomegaly, hypoglycemia, multiple congenital anomalies, and early death; (2) a milder disorder, without congenital anomalies and with longer survival, but frequently accompanied by cardiomyopathy; and (3) a later-onset form with vomiting, hypoglycemia, hepatomegaly, and weakness with lipid storage myopathy. An 8-year-old boy with ETFDH had a limb-girdle syndrome in addition to hepatomegaly and episodic hypoketotic hypoglycemia.[53] Postmortem examination showed severe lipid storage myopathy and muscle carnitine deficiency. Of considerable practical importance is the riboflavin-responsive form of glutaric aciduria type II, which has been seen in adults with lipid-storage myopathy. In these patients, riboflavin administration improved wasting and weakness within weeks.

DEFECTS OF THE MITOCHONDRIAL RESPIRATORY CHAIN

The reducing equivalents produced in the Krebs cycle and in the β-oxidation spirals are passed along a chain of proteins embedded in the inner mitochondrial membrane (the electron-transport chain). The electron-transport chain consists of four multi-meric complexes (I–IV) plus two small electron carriers, coenzyme Q (or ubiquinone) and cytochrome-*c*. The energy generated by these reactions is used to pump protons from the mitochondrial matrix into the space between the inner and outer mitochondrial membranes. This creates an electrochemical proton gradient across the inner membrane. A fifth multimeric complex (complex V or ATP synthase) converts the energy of the electrochemical proton gradient into ATP, in a process known as *oxidation/phosphorylation coupling*.

The *respiratory chain*, which includes all five complexes and catalyzes both electron transport and oxidative phosphorylation, is indeed the "business end" of mitochondrial metabolism, where the energy generated by carbohydrate and lipid oxidation is released as ATP. A unique characteristic of the respiratory chain is that this is the only metabolic pathway in the cell under dual genetic control. Of the approximately 80 proteins that make up the respiratory chain, 13 are encoded by mtDNA, and all the others are encoded by nuclear DNA (nDNA). As indicated by the different shadings in Figure 17.2, complex II, coenzyme Q, and cytochrome-*c* are entirely encoded by nDNA. In contrast, complexes I, III, IV, and V contain some subunits encoded by mtDNA: seven for complex I, one for complex III, three for complex IV, and two for complex V. Both inheritance and clinical expression of mutations in mtDNA are governed by the distinctive rules of mitochondrial genetics, which include maternal inheritance, heteroplasmy, and the threshold effect. A discussion of these features is beyond the scope of this chapter and can be found in recent reviews.[54] Suffice it to say that "mitochondrial medicine" has mushroomed in the 12 years since the discovery of the first mtDNA mutations. Over 100 pathogenic point mutations and innumerable rearrangements (deletions and duplications) have been associated with an impressive variety of clinical presentations, usually affecting multiple tissues (mitochondrial encephalomyopathies).

Tissue Preparation

There is some controversy as to whether frozen muscle biopsies are adequate or fresh tissue is needed for accurate biochemical analyses. Polarographic studies require fresh muscle in sufficient amount to allow isolation of functionally intact mitochondria.[55] Although these studies have contributed greatly to our understanding of respiratory chain defects in the first patients with mitochondrial myopathies, exemplified by Luft syndrome,[56,57] they have been largely replaced by assays of individual respiratory chain complexes in recent years.

A second question is whether frozen tissue allows the researcher to determine accurately the activity of large complexes, especially complex I. We cannot exclude the possibility that the sensitivity of our complex I assay may be compromised by the use of frozen tissue, and this may explain why we have identified few patients with Leigh syndrome and complex I deficiency. On the other hand, we have had no trouble in identifying complex I deficiency in patients with mutations in mtDNA complex I genes.[58,59]

The limitations of using frozen muscle are amply compensated, we think, by practical factors, especially by the possibility of studying samples shipped to us from all over the United States and many foreign countries.

Enzyme Assays

We perform routinely the following assays: NADH–cytochrome-c reductase (complexes I + III); NADH-dehydrogenase (complex I); succinate–cytochrome-c reductase (complex II + III); succinate dehydrogenase (complex II); cytochrome-c oxidase (complex IV); and citrate synthase (CS). In addition, we measure CoQ10 concentration whenever warranted. Complex I and complex III are not measured directly, but we have had no problems identifying complex III deficiency in numerous patients.[2] We refer enzyme activities both to wet tissue weight and to CS activity. CS is a matrix enzyme and a good marker of mitochondrial abundance; thus, reference to CS activity is essential to compensate for mitochondrial proliferation, which often occurs in mitochondrial myopathies or encephalomyopathies and is often reflected histochemically by RRF and by increased SDH activity ("ragged blue fibers").

Defects of the Respiratory Chain

From the genetic point of view, defects of the respiratory chain can be divided into two major groups: those due to mutations in mtDNA, and those due to mutations in nDNA. We consider separately the myopathies associated with each group.

Myopathies Due to Defects in Mitochondrial DNA

As the term *encephalomyopathy* implies, skeletal muscle is almost invariably affected in mitochondrial encephalomyopathies, although exercise intolerance and weakness may be overshadowed by brain dysfunction in these often devastating disorders. However, involvement of extraocular muscles, with ptosis and PEO, should always raise the question of mitochondrial dysfunction. PEO can be part of a purely myopathic disease or one of the manifestations of a multisystem disorder. This is best exemplified by two sporadic conditions, both due to single deletions in mtDNA: PEO with RRFs (a relatively benign disorder) and Kearns-Sayre syndrome (KSS; a devastating multisystem disorder characterized by PEO, pigmentary retinal degeneration, and heart block).

There are two main types of mtDNA mutations, those that affect mitochondrial protein synthesis in toto and those in protein-coding genes.

Mutations Affecting Mitochondrial Protein Synthesis. Mutations affecting protein synthesis include single deletions (which always encompass one or more transfer RNA [tRNA] genes) and point mutations in ribosomal RNA or in tRNA genes. Numerous clinical observations have suggested that these mutations are usually associated with multisystem disorders, lactic acidosis, and massive mitochondrial proliferation in muscle resulting in the "ragged red" appearance of fibers in the muscle biopsy.[60] Histochemical studies have shown that the RRFs in these conditions react intensely with the SDH stain but weakly or not at all with the COX stain.[61] This staining pattern is explained by the fact that SDH is entirely encoded by the nuclear genome (and therefore unaffected by mtDNA mutations), whereas three of the 13 subunits of COX are encoded by mtDNA.

Although mutations in tRNA genes are usually associated with multisystem disorders, in rare cases there is involvement of a single tissue, most commonly skeletal muscle. In some of these patients, the mutation is detectable in other tissues, such as blood or skin fibroblasts, implying that the selective muscle involvement is due to "skewed heteroplasmy," with preferential accumulation of the pathogenic mutation in skeletal muscle. In other patients, however, there is no evidence of the mutation in blood cells, cultured fibroblasts, or cultured muscle, suggesting a "somatic mutation" which arose during embryogenesis in myogenic stem cells after germ-layer differentiation.[54]

Mutations in Protein-Coding Genes. Generalizations regarding mutations in mtDNA protein-coding genes were based on the only two disorders of this type that were known until recently: Leber's hereditary optic neuropathy and NARP/maternally inherited Leigh syndrome (NARP/MILS). Leber's hereditary optic neuropathy is associated with three main mutations in complex I (NADH dehydrogenase [ND]) genes: G11778A in ND4,[62] G3460A in ND1,[63] and T14484C in ND6.[64] NARP/MILS is associated with the T8993G mutation in the ATPase 6 gene.[65] Because both conditions are multisystemic, maternally inherited, inconsistently accompanied by lactic acidosis, and never associated with RRF in muscle, the syllogistic conclusion was drawn that all mtDNA mutations in protein-coding genes would have the same characteristics. In fact, recent experience from patients with exercise intolerance has taught us that all three generalizations were incorrect.

We have come to appreciate that exercise intolerance, myalgia, or myoglobinuria can be the sole presentation of respiratory chain defects. These can affect complex I, complex III, or complex IV, although they seem to be more commonly associated with complex III deficiency.[2]

Exercise intolerance (without myoglobinuria) was the predominant clinical feature in two sporadic patients with complex I deficiency and COX-positive RRF in their muscle biopsies. One patient had a nonsense mutation (G11832A) in the ND4 gene,[59] whereas the other had an intragenic inversion of seven nucleotides within the ND1 gene, resulting in the alteration of three amino acids.[66]

Nine patients with isolated complex III deficiency in muscle complained of exercise intolerance, but only two had myoglobinuria.[67] All patients in whom muscle histochemistry was performed showed COX-positive RRF. The nine mutations in the cytochrome-*b* gene were different from one another, although except for a single deletion, they were all G-to-A transitions.

The first mtDNA molecular defect identified in a patient with complex IV (COX) deficiency was a 15-bp microdeletion in the COX III gene. The patient was a 16-

year-old girl with recurrent myoglobinuria triggered by prolonged exercise or viral illness.[68] Between attacks, both physical and neurologic exams were normal, as were routine laboratory tests, including serum CK and lactate. No tissue other than muscle was affected, and family history was entirely negative. Muscle biopsy showed many SDH-positive, COX-negative RRFs and marked isolated COX deficiency. We have identified a nonsense mutation (G5920A) in the COX I gene of muscle mtDNA in a 34-year-old man with lifelong exercise intolerance and recurrent myoglobinuria induced by intense or repetitive exercise.[69] His muscle biopsy showed scattered COX-negative RRFs, numerous COX-negative non-RRFs, and isolated COX deficiency. The mutation was not present in blood or fibroblasts from the patient nor in blood from his asymptomatic mother and sister.

Myopathies Due to Defects in Nuclear DNA

Coenzyme Q10 Deficiency. CLINICAL FEATURES. Isolated, presumably primary defects of CoQ10 in muscle have been identified in three clinical conditions: (1) a predominantly myopathic disorder, with exercise intolerance and myoglobinuria[70–72]; (2) a severe infantile syndrome dominated by encephalopathy and nephropathy[73]; and (3) a heterogeneous syndrome characterized by cerebellar ataxia, weakness, and cerebellar atrophy.[74,75] It is noteworthy that all patients responded to oral CoQ10 supplementation, although the degree of improvement varied from patient to patient. MUSCLE BIOPSY. In the myopathic variant, there is a characteristic association of RRFs and lipid storage. In the other variants, muscle biopsy shows rather nonspecific myopathic changes. BIOCHEMISTRY. CoQ10 concentration is markedly but variably decreased in muscle (4–35% of normal). CoQ10, or ubiquinone, is a lipophilic component of the electron-transport chain, which transfers to complex III electrons delivered from complex I and complex II (see Figure 17.2). CoQ10 also plays a role as a membrane stabilizer and an oxygen radical scavenger. We measure CoQ10 by reverse phase high-performance liquid chromatography after extraction from muscle in ethanol-*N*-hexane, evaporation of the solvent, and dissolution of the residue in an ethanol and methanol mixture.[75] GENETICS. All three clinical variants appear to be inherited as autosomal recessive traits. Given the complexity of the CoQ10 biosynthetic pathway and the heterogeneity of the clinical presentations, it is likely that different steps may be involved, but this remains to be documented.

Complex IV (Cytochrome-*c* Oxidase Deficiency). CLINICAL FEATURES. There are two main myopathic presentations of COX deficiency, both with onset at or soon after birth but with different outcomes. The first, fatal infantile COX-deficient myopathy, is characterized by generalized and progressive weakness, causing respiratory insufficiency and death before age one year.[76] The second, benign infantile COX-deficient myopathy, has similar onset, with profound, life-threatening weakness often requiring assisted ventilation. However, with appropriate support, these infants improve spontaneously and are usually completely healthy by three years of age.[77] There is lactic acidosis in both conditions, but blood lactate decreases gradually to normal levels in the benign form. MUSCLE BIOPSY. Initially, there are RRFs and generalized histochemical COX deficiency in both fatal and benign myopathies. However, in the benign form, increasing numbers of fibers reacquire normal COX reactivity, whereas RRFs gradually disappear, and later biopsies appear normal.

BIOCHEMISTRY. In both conditions, there is isolated, severe COX deficiency in early biopsies, but COX activity returns to normal within approximately one year in the benign form.

GENETICS. There is no evidence of maternal inheritance in either condition, both genders are equally affected, and there have been affected siblings, suggesting autosomal recessive inheritance. The molecular defects remain unknown in both fatal and benign COX-deficient myopathies.

How Does Biochemistry Help in the Diagnosis of Mitochondrial Encephalomyopathies?

Finding a severe defect in the activity of a single respiratory chain complex in muscle suggests three possibilities: (1) a defect in a nuclear-encoded subunit of that particular complex[78]; (2) a defect in a nuclear-encoded ancillary protein needed for the assembly of that particular complex[78]; and (3) a defect in a mtDNA-encoded subunit of that particular complex[54] (Figure 17.3A).

Finding partial defects in the activities of complex I, complex III, and complex IV in the face of normal SDH activity suggests a defect of mitochondrial protein synthesis in toto because all three complexes contain one or more subunits encoded by mtDNA (see Figure 17.3B). As discussed in the section Mutations Affecting Mitochondrial Protein Synthesis, this situation prevails when there are mutations in tRNA or ribosomal RNA genes, deletions, or depletion of mtDNA. However, this is just a "rule of thumb," as complex I activity may be preferentially decreased in muscle from patients with MELAS,[79–81] and COX activity may be especially affected in patients with MERRF.[82,83]

Although biochemical assays can provide valuable clues to the nature of the underlying molecular defect, it is fair to state that definitive diagnosis for most mitochondrial myopathies is based on documentation of a specific molecular defect and its pathogenic significance.

DEFECTS OF PURINE METABOLISM

Adenylate Deaminase Deficiency

Adenylate deaminase deficiency has variable manifestations. Some patients have no symptoms. Others complain of muscle cramping, stiffness, or pain after exercise. The serum CK concentration may be increased, but myoglobinuria is extremely rare. Muscle biopsy is usually normal, but a specific histochemical stain facilitates the diagnosis and shows that the enzyme defect is often encountered in virtually asymptomatic subjects. In agreement with this observation, molecular genetic analysis has shown that a common mutation in the adenylate deaminase–1 gene (Q12X), which encodes the muscle isozyme, can explain the 2% incidence of myoadenylate deficiency encountered in the general population.

CONCLUSIONS

Biochemical studies of muscle are clearly pivotal in the diagnostic evaluation of hereditary metabolic myopathies. Because these tend to cause two broad clinical syndromes (see Figure 17.1), it is not irrational to group enzyme assays into two

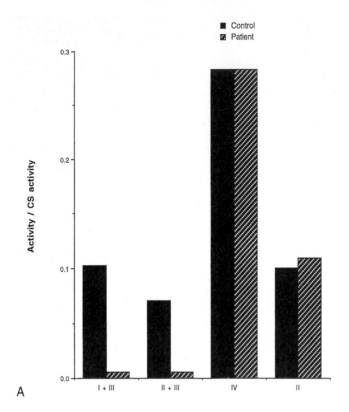

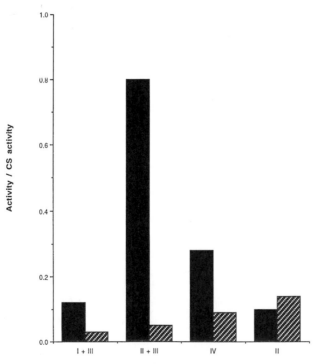

Figure 17.3 Comparison of mitochondrial respiratory chain activities (normalized to citrate synthase [CS]) in muscle from a patient with a point mutation (C3256T) in the transfer RNALeu(UUR) gene of mitochondrial DNA (**A**) and a patient with a mutation (G15168A) in the cytochrome-*b* gene of mitochondrial DNA (**B**). (I + III = nicotinamide adenine dinucleotide–cytochrome-*c* reductase; II + III = succinate–cytochrome-*c* reductase; II = succinate dehydrogenase; IV = cytochrome-*c* oxidase.)

"panels," one for each syndrome. Thus, the "exercise intolerance and myoglobinuria" panel would comprise PhK, phosphorylase, PFK, PGK, PGAM, β-enolase, and LDH among the enzyme of glycogen metabolism; CPT II, VLCAD, and SCHAD among the enzyme of lipid metabolism; and the respiratory chain complexes plus CoQ10 measurement. Conversely, the "progressive weakness" panel would include acid maltase, branching enzyme, debrancher, and aldolase; carnitine concentration; and, again, respiratory chain complexes.

However, it is also evident that such a mechanistic approach would be time consuming and expensive. It is important to reiterate that biochemistry is only one step in the diagnostic process. This starts with careful clinical assessment, because not all exercise intolerances are alike and not all weaknesses are alike. The type of exercise causing discomfort, the presence of contractures, the concurrence of other precipitating factors besides exercise, the occurrence and frequency of myoglobinuria, and routine or "provocative" laboratory tests can all orient toward one set of biochemical tests or another. Similarly, weakness is usually proximal but can be distal (as in debrancher deficiency), affect truncal and respiratory muscles preferentially (as in adult-onset AMD), or affect extraocular muscles (as in defects of the mitochondrial respiratory chain).

The importance of careful muscle histology and histochemistry cannot be overestimated: As a rule, we do not perform biochemical tests until we have discussed the results of morphology. Electron microscopy has lost much of its diagnostic importance, but it can be useful in special cases.

Standardized exercise physiology, nuclear magnetic resonance spectroscopy (phosphorus 31 magnetic resonance spectroscopy), and near-infrared spectroscopy can precede or follow biochemical evaluation and nicely complement it.

Finally, molecular genetic analyses are usually targeted on the basis of biochemical results, although sometimes (as in the cases of McArdle's disease, CPT II deficiency, and respiratory chain defects) we can "jump the gun" and go directly to nDNA or mtDNA for answers.

The recent discovery of yet another glycogenosis[37] (when this area of metabolism seemed pretty much dormant) and the description of new disorders associated with muscle CoQ10 deficiency[73,75] are testimony of the continuing vitality of muscle biochemistry.

Acknowledgments

Part of the work described here was supported by National Institutes of Health grants PO1 HD32062 and NS11766 and by grants from the Muscular Dystrophy Association. Dr. Naini is supported by a grant from the National Ataxia Foundation.

REFERENCES

1. Bertorini T, Yeh Y-Y, Trevisan C P, et al. Carnitine palmityltransferase deficiency: myoglobinuria and respiratory failure. Neurology 1980;30:263–271.
2. Andreu AL, Hanna MG, Reichmann H, et al. Exercise intolerance due to mutations in the cytochrome b gene of mitochondrial DNA. N Engl J Med 1999;341:1037–1044.
3. Mitsumoto H. McArdle disease: phosphorylase activity in regenerating muscle fibers. Neurology 1979;29:258–262.

4. DiMauro S, Arnold S, Miranda AF, Rowland LP. McArdle disease: the mystery of reappearing phosphorylase activity in muscle culture. A fetal isoenzyme. Ann Neurol 1978;3:60–66.

5. Bartram C, Edwards R, Clague J, Beynon R J. McArdle's disease: a nonsense mutation in exon 1 of the muscle glycogen phosphorylase gene explains some but not all cases. Hum Mol Genet 1993;2:1291–1293.

6. El-Schahawi M, Tsujino S, Shanske S, DiMauro S. Diagnosis of McArdle's disease by molecular genetic analysis of blood. Neurology 1996;47:579–580.

7. Kaufmann P, El-Schahawi M, DiMauro S. Carnitine palmitoyltransferase II deficiency: diagnosis by molecular analysis of blood. Mol Cell Biochem 1997;174:237–239.

8. Slonim AE, Balone L, Ritz S, et al. Identification of two subtypes of infantile acid maltase deficiency. J Pediatr 2000;137:283–285.

9. Shanske S, DiMauro S. Late-onset acid maltase deficiency. Biochemical studies of leukocytes. J Neurol Sci 1981;50:57–62.

10. Hart ZH, Servidei S, Peterson PL, et al. Cardiomyopathy, mental retardation, and autophagic vacuolar myopathy. Neurology 1987;37:1065–1068.

11. Nishino I, Fu J, Tanji K, Yamada T, et al. Primary LAMP-2 deficiency causes X-linked vacuolar cardiomyopathy and myopathy (Danon disease). Nature 2000;406:906–910.

12. DiMauro S, Hartwig GB, Hays AP, et al. Debrancher deficiency: neuromuscular disorder in five adults. Ann Neurol 1979;5:422–436.

13. Chen YT, He JK, Ding JH, Brown BI. Glycogen debranching enzyme: purification, antibody characterization, and immunoblot analysis of type III glycogen storage disease. Am J Hum Genet 1987;41:1002–1015.

14. Ding JH, DeBarsy T, Brown BI, et al. Immunoblot analysis of glycogen debranching enzyme in different subtypes of glycogen storage disease type III. J Pediatr 1990;116:95–100.

15. Hers HG, Verhue W, Van Hoof F. The determination of amylo-1,6-glucosidase. Eur J Biochem 1967;2:257–264.

16. Robitaille Y, Carpenter S, Karpati G, DiMauro S. A distinct form of adult polyglucosan body diseases with massive involvement of central and peripheral neuronal processes and astrocytes. Brain 1980;103:315–336.

17. Servidei S, Riepe RE, Langston C, et al. Severe cardiopathy in branching enzyme deficiency. J Pediatr 1987;111:51–56.

18. Lossos A, Barash V, Soffer D, et al. Hereditary branching enzyme dysfunction in adult polyglucosan body disease: a possible metabolic cause in two patients. Ann Neurol 1991;30:655–662.

19. Bruno C, Servidei S, Shanske S, et al. Glycogen branching enzyme deficiency in adult polyglucosan body disease. Ann Neurol 1993;33:88–93.

20. Bruno C, DiRocco M, Doria Lama L, et al. A novel missense mutation in the glycogen branching enzyme gene in a child with myopathy and hepatopathy. Neuromuscul Disord 1999;9:403–407.

21. Lossos A, Meiner Z, Barash V, et al. Adult polyglucosan body disease in Ashkenazi Jewish patients carrying the Tyr329 Ser mutation in the glycogen-branching enzyme gene. Ann Neurol 1998; 44:867–872.

22. McArdle B. Myopathy due to a defect in muscle glycogen breakdown. Clin Sci 1951;10:13–33.

23. Bruno C, Bado M, Minetti C, Cordone G. Forearm semi-ischemic exercise test in pediatric patients. J Child Neurol 1998;13:288–290.

24. Agamanolis DP, Askari AD, DiMauro S, et al. Muscle phosphofructokinase deficiency: two cases with unusual polysaccharide accumulation and immunologically active enzyme protein. Muscle Nerve 1980;3:456–467.

25. Hays AP, Hallett M, Delfs J, et al. Muscle phosphofructokinase deficiency: abnormal polysaccharide in a case of late-onset myopathy. Neurology 1981;31:1077–1086.

26. Danon MJ, Servidei S, DiMauro S, Vora S. Late-onset muscle phosphofructokinase deficiency. Neurology 1988;38:955–960.

27. Bonilla E, Schotland DL. Histochemical diagnosis of muscle phosphofructokinase deficiency. Arch Neurol 1970;22:8–12.

28. Vora S. Isozymes of phosphofructokinase. Curr Topics Biol Med 1982;6:119–167.

29. Minassian BA, Lee JR, Herbrick JA, et al. Mutations in a gene encoding a novel protein tyrosine phosphatase cause progressive myoclonus epilepsy. Nature Genet 1998;20:171–174.

30. Serratosa JM, Gomez-Garre P, Gallardo ME, et al. A novel protein tyrosine phosphatase gene is mutated in progressive myoclonus epilepsy of the Lafora type (EPM2). Hum Mol Genet 1999;8:345–352.

31. Wilkinson DA, Tonin P, Shanske S, et al. Clinical and biochemical features of 10 adult patients with muscle phosphorylase kinase deficiency. Neurology 1994;44:461–466.

32. Wehner M, Clemens PR, Engel AG, Kilimann MW. Human muscle glycogenosis due to phosphory-lase kinase deficiency associated with a nonsense mutation in the muscle isoform of the alpha sub-unit. Hum Mol Genet 1994;3:1983–1987.

33. Bruno C, Manfredi G, Andreu AL, et al. A splice junction mutation in the alpha-M gene of phos-phorylase kinase in a patient with myopathy. Biochem Biophys Res Comm 1998;249:648–651.

34. Tsujino S, Shanske S, Sakoda S, et al. The molecular genetic basis of muscle phosphoglycerate mutase (PGAM) deficiency. Am J Hum Genet 1993;52:472–477.

35. Hadjigeorgiou GM, Kawashima N, Bruno C, et al. Manifesting heterozygotes in a Japanese family with a novel mutation in the muscle-specific phosphoglycerate mutase (PGAM-M) gene. Neuro-muscul Disord 1999;9:399–402.

36. Kreuder J, Borkhardt A, Repp R, et al. Inherited metabolic myopathy and hemolysis due to a muta-tion in aldolase A. New Engl J Med 1996;334:1100–1104.

37. Comi GP, Fortunato F, Lucchiari S, et al. β-enolase deficiency, a new metabolic myopathy of distal glycolysis. Ann Neurol 2001;50(2):202–207.

38. McGarry JD, Foster D W. An improved and simplified radioisotopic assay for the determination of free and esterified carnitine. J Lipid Res 1976;17:277–281.

39. Lamhonwah AM, Tein I. Carnitine uptake defect: frameshift mutations in the human plasmalemmal carnitine transporter gene. Biochem Biophys Res Comm 1998;252:396–401.

40. Tang NLS, Ganapathy V, Wu X, et al. Mutations of OCTN2, an organic cation/carnitine transporter, lead to deficient cellular carnitine uptake in primary carnitine deficiency. Hum Mol Genet 1999;8:655–660.

41. Engel AG, Angelini C. Carnitine deficiency of human skeletal muscle with associated lipid storage myopathy: a new syndrome. Science 1973;179:899–902.

42. Pons R, DeVivo DC. Primary and secondary carnitine deficiency syndrome. J Child Neurol 1995.

43. DiMauro S, DiMauro-Melis PM. Muscle carnitine palmityltransferase deficiency and myoglobin-uria. Science 1973;182:929–931.

44. Tonin P, Lewis P, Servidei S, DiMauro S. Metabolic causes of myoglobinuria. Ann Neurol 1990; 27:181–185.

45. Norum KR. Pamityl-CoA: carnitine palmityltransferase: purification from calf liver mitochondria and some properties of the enzyme. Biochim Biophys Acta 1964;89:95–108.

46. Turnbull DM, Bartlett K, Stevens DL, et al. Short-chain acyl-CoA dehydrogenase deficiency associ-ated with a lipid-storage myopathy and secondary carnitine deficiency. N Engl J Med 1984;311:1232–1236.

47. Tein I, Haslam RHA, Rhead WJ, et al. Short-chain acyl-CoA dehydrogenase deficiency. A cause of ophthalmoplegia and multicore myopathy. Neurology 1999;52:366–372.

48. Straussberg R, Harel L, Varsano I, et al. Recurrent myoglobinuria as a presenting manifestation of very long chain acyl coenzyme A dehydrogenase deficiency. Pediatrics 1997;9:894–896.

49. Minetti C, Garavaglia B, Bado M, et al. Very-long-chain acyl-coenzyme A dehydrogenase defi-ciency in a child with recurrent myoglobinuria. Neuromuscul Disord 1998;8:3–6.

50. Smelt AH, Poorthuis BJ, Onkenhout W, et al. Very long chain acyl-coenzyme A dehydrogenase deficiency with adult onset. Ann Neurol 1998;43:540–544.

51. Schaefer J, Jackson S, Dick DJ, Turnbull DM. Trifunctional enzyme deficiency: adult presentation of a usually fatal β-oxidation defect. Ann Neurol 1996;40:597–602.

52. Tein I, De Vivo DC, Hale DE, et al. Short-chain L-3-hydroxyacyl-CoA dehydrogenase deficiency in muscle: a new cause for recurrent myoglobinuria and encephalopathy. Ann Neurol 1991; 30:415–419.

53. DiDonato S, Frerman FE, Rimoldi M, et al. Systemic carnitine deficiency due to lack of electron transfer flavoprotein: ubiquinone oxidoreductase. Neurology 1986;36:957–963.

54. DiMauro S, Andreu AL. Mutations in mtDNA: are we scraping the bottom of the barrel? Brain Pathol 2000;10:431–441.

55. Makinen MW, Lee CP. Biochemical studies of skeletal muscle mitochondria. I. Microanalysis of cytochrome content, oxidative and phosphorylative activities of mammalian skeletal muscle mito-chondria. Arch Biochem Biophys 1968;126:75–82.

56. Luft R, Ikkos D, Palmieri G, et al. A case of severe hypermetabolism of nonthyroid origin with a defect in the maintenance of mitochondrial respiratory control: a correlated clinical, biochemical, and morphological study. J Clin Invest 1962;41:1776–1804.

57. DiMauro S, Bonilla E, Lee CP, et al. Luft's disease. Further biochemical and ultrastructural studies of skeletal muscle in the second case. J Neurol Sci 1976;27:217–232.

58. Santorelli FM, Tanji K, Kulikova R, et al. Identification of a novel mutation in the mtDNA ND5 gene associated with MELAS. Biochem Biophys Res Comm 1997;238(2):326–328.

59. Andreu AL, Tanji K, Bruno C, et al. Exercise intolerance due to a nonsense mutation in the mtDNA ND4 gene. Ann Neurol 1999;45:820–823.

60. Engel AG, Cunningham CG. Rapid examination of muscle tissue: an improved trichome stain method for fresh-frozen biopsy sections. Neurology 1963;13:919–923.

61. DiMauro S, Bonilla E. Mitochondrial Encephalomyopathies. In RN Rosenberg, SB Prusiner, S DiMauro, RL Barchi (eds), The Molecular and Genetic Basis of Neurological Disease (2nd ed). Boston: Butterworth–Heinemann, 1997;201–235.

62. Wallace DC, Singh G, Lott MT, et al. Mitochondrial DNA mutation associated with Leber's hereditary optic neuropathy. Science 1988;242:1427–1430.

63. Huoponen K, Vilkki J, Aula P, et al. A new mtDNA mutation associated with Leber hereditary optic neuroretinopathy. Am J Hum Genet 1991;48:1147–1153.

64. Johns DR, Neufeld MJ, Park RD. An ND-6 mitochondrial DNA mutation associated with Leber hereditary optic neuropathy. Biochem Biophys Res Comm 1992;187:1551–1557.

65. Holt IJ, Harding AE, Petty RK, Morgan Hughes JA. A new mitochondrial disease associated with mitochondrial DNA heteroplasmy. Am J Hum Genet 1990;46:428–433.

66. Musumeci O, Andreu AL, Shanske S, et al. Intragenic inversion of mtDNA: a new type of pathogenic mutation in a patient with mitochondrial myopathy. Am J Hum Genet 2000;66:1900–1904.

67. DiMauro S. Exercise intolerance and the mitochondrial respiratory chain. Ital J Neurol Sci 1999;20:387–393.

68. Keightley JA, Hoffbuhr KC, Burton MD, et al. A microdeletion in cytochrome c oxidase (COX) subunit III associated with COX deficiency and recurrent myoglobinuria. Nature Genet 1996;12:410–415.

69. Karadimas CL, Greenstein P, Sue CM, et al. Recurrent myoglobinuria due to a nonsense mutation in the COX I gene of mtDNA. Neurology 2000;55:644–649.

70. Ogasahara S, Engel AG, Frens D, Mack D. Muscle coenzyme Q deficiency in familial mitochondrial encephalomyopathy. Proc Natl Acad Sci U S A 1989;86:2379–2382.

71. Servidei S, Spinazzola A, Crociani P, et al. Replacement therapy is effective in familial mitochondrial encephalomyopathy with muscle CoQ10 deficiency. Neurology 1996;46:A420.

72. Sobreira C, Hirano M, Shanske S, et al. Mitochondrial encephalomyopathy with coenzyme Q10 deficiency. Neurology 1997;48:1238–1243.

73. Rotig A, Appelkvist E-L, Geromel V, et al. Quinone-responsive multiple respiratory-chain dysfunction due to widespread coenzyme Q10 deficiency. Lancet 2000;356:391–395.

74. Boitier E, Degoul F, Desguerre I, et al. A case of mitochondrial encephalomyopathy associated with a muscle coenzyme Q10 deficiency. J Neurol Sci 1998;156:41–46.

75. Musumeci O, Naini A, Slonim AE, et al. Familial cerebellar ataxia with muscle coenzyme Q10 deficiency. Neurology 2001;56(12).1739–1745.

76. DiMauro S, Mendell JR, Sahenk Z, et al. Fatal infantile mitochondrial myopathy and renal dysfunction due to cytochrome-c-oxidase deficiency. Neurology 1980;30:795–804.

77. DiMauro S, Nicholson JF, Hays AP, et al. Benign infantile mitochondrial myopathy due to reversible cytochrome c oxidase deficiency. Trans Am Neurol Assoc 1981;106:205–207.

78. Sue CM, Schon EA. Mitochondrial respiratory chain diseases and mutations in nuclear DNA: a promising start? Brain Pathol 2000;10:442–450.

79. Kobayashi M, Morishita H, Sugiyama N, et al. Two cases of NADH-coenzyme Q reductase deficiency: relationship to MELAS syndrome. J Pediatr 1987;110:223–227.

80. Ichiki T, Tanaka M, Nishikimi M, et al. Deficiency of subunits of complex I and mitochondrial encephalomyopathy. Ann Neurol 1988;23:287–294.

81. Ichiki T, Tanaka M, Kobayashi M, et al. Disproportionate deficiency of iron-sulfur clusters and subunits of complex I in mitochondrial encephalomyopathy. Pediatr Res 1989;25:194–201.

82. Silvestri G, Ciafaloni E, Santorelli F, et al. Clinical features associated with the AÆG transition at nucleotide 8344 of mtDNA ("MERRF mutation"). Neurology 1993;43:1200–1206.

83. Lombes A, Mendell JR, Nakase H, et al. Myoclonic epilepsy and ragged-red fibers with cytochrome oxidase deficiency: neuropathology, biochemistry, and molecular genetics. Ann Neurol 1989;26:20–33.

18

Imaging Techniques

Hollis Halford and Alan Graves

Imaging techniques play important roles in the diagnosis and management of patients with neuromuscular diseases; imaging techniques can also evaluate disease progression as well as response to treatment. Radionuclide imaging techniques can assess the extent and severity of inflammatory myopathies, and ultrasound techniques not only assess the degree of muscle involvement but also help in the determination of the best site for muscle biopsy. Newer ultrasound techniques give an excellent anatomic resolution of peripheral nerves.

Cross-sectional imaging procedures including ultrasound, computed tomography (CT), and magnetic resonance (MR) imaging provide excellent spatial resolution. MR is the method that provides the best soft tissue contrast and anatomic resolution of any cross-sectional imaging method. This, along with the fact that there is no ionizing radiation, usually makes MR the imaging procedure of choice. MR neurography, a newer imaging technique, can help in the assessment of focal nerve injury.

This chapter covers the imaging techniques used in evaluation of neuromuscular disease, and because clinicians are also called on to assess segmental disorders (e.g., root lesions or disk disease), we also briefly cover the use of MR and CT in evaluating spinal disorders.

NUCLEAR MEDICINE

Nuclear medicine offers a noninvasive way to evaluate the whole body or large groups of muscles in a single examination. Imaging agents include technetium-labeled phosphates, indium-labeled antibodies, and gallium-67 citrate. Each of these agents allows whole-body imaging with abnormal areas showing increased uptake.

Technetium-99m pyrophosphate (Tc-PYP) accumulates in diseased muscle secondary to increased binding from the higher concentration of calcium in necrotic cells and from crystals of hydroxyapatite and calcium phosphate in ischemic tissue. Patients with muscular dystrophies and inflammatory myopathies usually present with symmetric and diffuse uptake, but patchy and asymmetric activity often occurs (Figure 18.1).[1] Infectious myositis is usually focal and asymmetric. The sensitivity of Tc-PYP is approximately 90% in inflammatory muscle disease.[2]

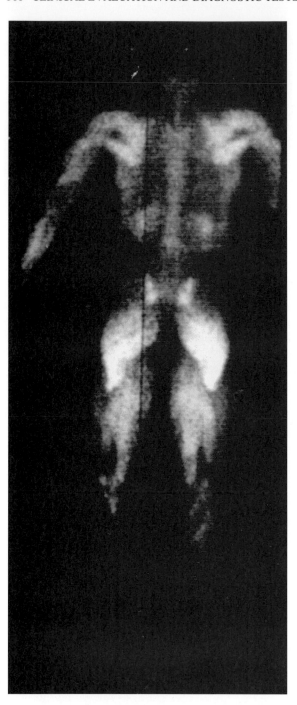

Figure 18.1 Posterior view of a whole-body bone scan, using technetium 99m–medronate diphosphate in a patient with active polymyositis. There is diffuse symmetric abnormal activity.

Another method of muscle evaluation is indium-labeled antimyosin monoclonal antibodies. This agent binds to the exposed myosin sites in muscle damaged by the loss of skeletal muscle plasma membrane integrity.

Muscular dystrophies have a primary defect in the sarcoplasmic membrane, and myositis causes inflammation and destruction of skeletal muscle cells; both lead to

Figure 18.2 Anterior (*left*) and posterior (*right*) whole-body images from a gallium scan. There are multiple areas of abnormal increased activity (*arrows*), indicating active muscle inflammation in this patient with rhabdomyolysis.

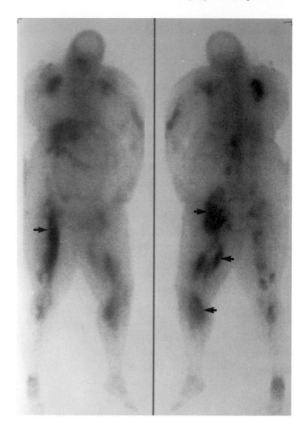

increased muscular uptake or activity.[3] The increased uptake tends to be diffuse in most patients and usually most prominent in the lower extremities. In patients with muscular dystrophy, the greatest intensity is usually in the calves, which may be owing to the preserved muscle bulk in the calves relative to the atrophic musculature in the thigh in these patients.[4] The intensity is greater in areas of active inflammation and is less prominent in areas of atrophy. Studies have shown that the intensity of activity correlates with areas of edema on T2-weighted MR scans.

Gallium is an agent commonly used in the imaging of inflammatory myopathies. The mechanism of uptake is complex. Adequate blood supply and increased vascular permeability allow localization of gallium-bound iron-binding molecules.[5] Areas of active inflammation show increased uptake (Figure 18.2). In inflammatory myopathies, the sensitivity of gallium is approximately 90%.[2]

Radionuclide scintigraphy easily images the whole body or large muscle groups, and because scintigraphy provides physiologic information, it may be more useful for assessing the severity of inflammation.[4] Scintigraphy may be beneficial in selecting an appropriate site for biopsy due to the sometimes patchy nature of muscle involvement. This could help to avoid false-negative results in patients with focal asymmetric disease.[1] Disadvantages include radiation exposure and lack of resolution to define individual muscle groups, which is better detailed with cross-sectional imaging.

ULTRASOUND

Ultrasound is a widely available modality that offers rapid imaging with relatively short examination times. This makes ultrasound very useful in younger children and in patients who cannot tolerate longer imaging times and are unable to remain still.

Imaging is best performed with a high-frequency linear array transducer, usually 7–12 MHz.[6] Obese patients may require a 5-MHz transducer to achieve adequate depth of penetration.[7] The patient should be imaged in a relaxed, comfortable position, typically seated. Images are obtained in the transverse and longitudinal planes over the muscle groups of interest.

Normal muscle has a hypoechoic appearance. Multiple hyperechoic septa are present within the muscle from the fascial planes. These septa have a pinnate arrangement on longitudinal images and appear as multiple punctate foci on transverse images. Bone cortex has a well-defined hyperechoic surface with posterior shadowing (Figure 18.3). Muscle contraction shows an apparent increase in muscle mass due to thickening of muscle bundles and causes an overall decrease in muscle echogenicity.[7]

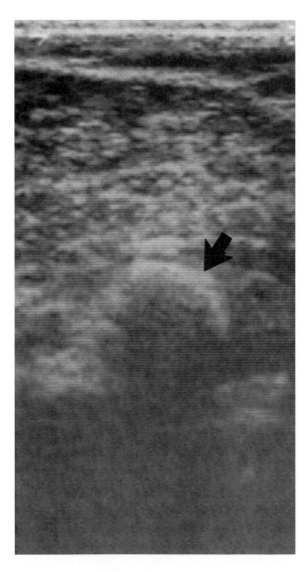

Figure 18.3 Transverse ultrasound image of normal biceps muscle. Multiple punctate echogenic foci are seen. The humerus is well demarcated with distal acoustic shadowing (*arrow*). Ultrasound is performed using 75-MHz liner array probe, Hitachi EUB 310. (Courtesy of Francis Walker, Bowman Gray University. Reprinted with permission from H Halford, A Graves, T Bertorini. Muscle and nerve imaging techniques in neuromuscular diseases. J Clin Neuromuscul Dis 2000;2[1]:41–51.)

Figure 18.4 Transverse images from biceps muscle. Image on left is from a patient with polymyositis and muscle atrophy. Note increased muscle echogenicity and loss of bone shadowing. The muscle is also small. The biceps on the right is from a healthy control. (Courtesy of Francis Walker, Bowman Gray University. Reprinted with permission from H Halford, A Graves, T Bertorini. Muscle and nerve imaging techniques in neuromuscular diseases. J Clin Neuromuscul Dis 2000;2[1]:41–51.)

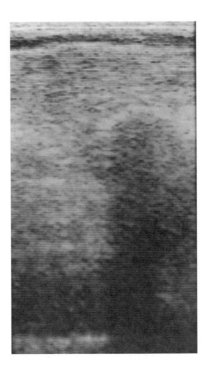 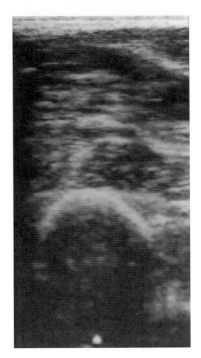

Abnormal muscle typically shows increased echogenicity. This is owing to pathologic changes that disrupt the normal muscle architecture and increase the number of reflective surfaces within the muscle.[8–10] Some neuromuscular disorders are associated with a reduced volume of muscle fascicles, which leads to an increased number of septa and increased echointensity.[11] Acute processes may increase muscle thickness, and chronic processes lead to muscle thinning and atrophy. As the echogenicity of muscle increases, there is decreased visualization of the underlying bone (Figure 18.4). In the most severe disease, the distinction of bone from muscle may be absent. Color and power Doppler can be used to show the degree of vascularity in inflammatory processes.[12] The extended field of view function available on some machines allows visualization of large continuous sections of anatomy without disturbing anatomic relationships[13] (Figure 18.5). This test can be used in the assessment of focal nerve lesions; in addition, standard ultrasonography can be helpful in the evaluation of patients with carpal tunnel syndrome.

Several methods have been developed to quantify the degree of muscle involvement. Heckmatt's criteria grade the muscle echogenicity and the distinctness of underlying bone shadow, giving a score from I (normal) to IV (severe).[8,14] A second method described by Dock et al.[11] involves counting the number of hyperechoic septa within a muscle thickness of 1 cm measured in the thigh. Healthy subjects showed values ranging from 8 to 13 septa per centimeter, but never greater than 13. Muscular dystrophy patients showed an increased number of septa per centimeter with some overlap with the control group.

The sensitivity of ultrasound for muscle involvement ranges from 78% to 83%, and specificity ranges from 91% to 96%.[8,15] Positive predictive values are relatively high, ranging from 95% to 100%. Sensitivity and specificity improve in patients older than 3 years of age, likely because pathologic changes may not have progressed enough in younger children to be adequately visualized by ultrasound. No specific patterns of muscle involvement have been found to differentiate the types of neuromuscular disease.

Advantages of ultrasound include lack of ionizing radiation, low cost, quick scan time, multiplanar capability, and dynamic real-time imaging. Drawbacks include the

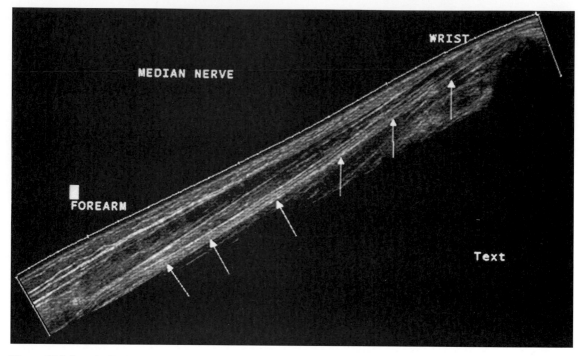

Figure 18.5 Longitudinal image in a healthy subject of the median nerve (*arrows*), which is seen superficially. The image is obtained from the wrist to the antecubital fossa and reconstructed from gradual movement of the transducer up the forearm using technology that displays an extended field of view with a 13.5-MHz phased array probe on a Sonoline Elegra (Seimens, Greensboro, NC). (Courtesy of Francis Walker, Bowman Gray University. Reprinted with permission from H Halford, A Graves, T Bertorini. Muscle and nerve imaging techniques in neuromuscular diseases. J Clin Neuromuscul Dis 2000;2[1]:41–51.)

operator's dependency on the technique and the need for specialized training. The quality and consistency of the examination rely on the expertise of the examiner. Ultrasound can be used to guide electromyographic needle sites in focal disease and to direct sites for muscle biopsy, particularly in children.[6,8]

DUAL ENERGY X-RAY ABSORPTIOMETRY

Dual energy x-ray absorptiometry (DEXA) is a radiographic method that assesses total body mineral composition. The DEXA technique uses a scanner with an x-ray tube with K-edge filtration to produce x-rays with two different peaks of energy. Body tissues have varying x-ray absorption ratios depending on density, and because of this property, it is possible to differentiate the three major body components. These components are bone mineral content (BMC), lean body mass (LBM) mainly formed by skeletal muscle, and total fat body mass (FBM) under stimulation of the body lipid content.[16]

The DEXA method is used in the assessment of osteopenia and has been applied in the evaluation of neuromuscular diseases to determine the amount of lean muscle mass and fat. The technique has great potential in the follow-up evaluation of clinical therapeutic trials in patients with neuromuscular diseases. The accuracy of the determinations is established by the fact that the sum of the three components (LBM + BMC + FBM) is within 1% of the actual total body mass.[17]

Using this technique, Kanda et al.[18] reported a decrease in LBM and an increase in FBM in patients with various myopathies, and studies in our center demonstrated a significant correlation between muscle function (as assessed by manual muscle testing) and LBM.[19] DEXA has also been useful in assessing LBM in a clinical trial.[20]

The DEXA technique can be used not only to determine muscle mass but also to assess the effects of medications, such as corticosteroids, on the degree of osteopenia. DEXA was useful in preliminary studies in the evaluation and follow-up of patients with polymyositis.[21]

COMPUTED TOMOGRAPHY

The introduction of CT in the mid-1970s opened a new era in muscle and nerve imaging, allowing the evaluation of normal muscle anatomy as well as evaluation of changes produced by disease.[22,23] CT measures the x-ray attenuation of tissues, which is based on the electron density of the tissue. This density measurement is expressed quantitatively in *Hounsfield units* (HU), which is a relative scale based on the density, or x-ray attenuation values, of water and air, which are 0 HU and –1,000 HU, respectively. The density measurements for normal muscle range from 30 HU to 80 HU[24] (Figure 18.6).

In neuromuscular disease, particularly in long-standing or more severe cases, there is muscle atrophy and replacement of normal muscle with fat. This causes decreased attenuation on CT (Figure 18.7), because fat cells are smaller and less dense than muscle cells.[22]

CT images can be interpreted quantitatively or qualitatively. The degree of muscle fiber loss and fat tissue replacement can be quantified using indices of percent of cross-sectional area of muscle and fat.[25] These indices correlate with muscle strength clinically and can be used in assessing the efficacy of therapeutic interventions. The reliability of qualitative analysis (i.e., of simple inspection) is fairly good with acceptable intraobserver and interobserver variance.[22]

CT can be helpful in differentiating muscular dystrophy from spinal muscular atrophy. In general, muscular dystrophies reveal focal areas of decreased attenua-

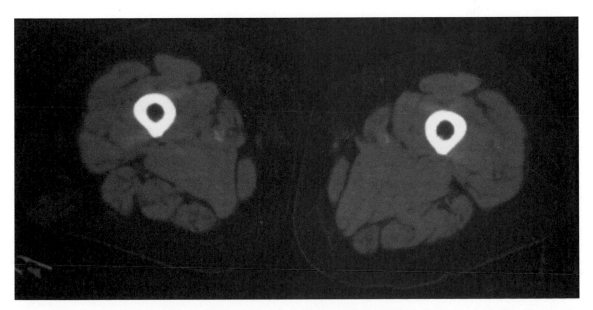

Figure 18.6 Computed tomography mid-thigh in a healthy volunteer. Muscle density is uniform and intermediate when compared with the lower density of the subcutaneous fat and the denser bone cortex.

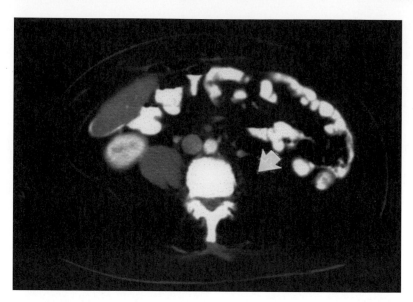

Figure 18.7 Computed tomography of the abdomen in a patient with limb-girdle muscular dystrophy. There is marked atrophy of the left psoas muscle (*arrow*), which is diminished in size and of decreased attenuation when compared to the contralateral psoas muscle. There is also severe symmetric atrophy of paraspinous muscles. (Reprinted with permission from H Halford, A Graves, T Bertorini. Muscle and nerve imaging techniques in neuromuscular diseases. J Clin Neuromuscul Dis 2000;2[1]:41–51.)

tion in individual muscles. As the diseases progress, the entire muscle is gradually replaced by fat. In the majority of patients with neurogenic diseases, such as spinal muscular atrophy, the muscles become diffusely atrophic.

CT is reliable for the diagnosis of neuromuscular disorders with an overall accuracy of nearly 85%.[26] CT can also be used to determine specific muscle involvement and to localize the best site for muscle biopsy. Serial CT studies using computerized analysis have also been applied to determine the effect of training on the size of muscle mass in neuromuscular disorders.[27]

The practical usefulness of CT in routine clinical practice is now limited mainly to the diagnosis of focal lesions or tumors. Because CT provides no advantage over MR except its higher sensitivity in the detection of calcifications, and because this advantage CT offers does not justify the exposure to ionizing radiation, MR is usually used for muscle imaging.

MAGNETIC RESONANCE

MR provides not only the best soft tissue contrast but also the best anatomic detail of any of the available imaging modalities. MR creates images by first exposing the tissues to a static magnetic field. Commercially available MR systems are proton imagers. The magnetic field causes protons to precess or spin at a particular frequency, which is determined by the field strength of the magnet. A radio frequency pulse is then applied, which causes the protons to spin at the same frequency but at a higher energy level. When the radio frequency pulse is turned off, the protons release this energy and "relax" back to their original energy state. This release of energy is measured in relaxation times (i.e., T1 and T2). *T1 relaxation time* (T1) is a time constant, related to the time it takes the protons to realign themselves with the main magnetic field. The *T2 relaxation time* (T2) is a time constant, related to the time it takes the protons to lose their precession or spin in a plane 90 degrees to the main magnetic field.

The signal intensity or brightness of the tissue is dependent on the T1 and T2 relaxation times, as well as the proton density (PD) of the tissue. The tissue type and presence of disease affect the T1, T2, and PD of the tissue, which determine the brightness or appearance of the tissue on the image. By varying scanning parameters, images are generated so that the appearance is due primarily to T1 relaxation time, T2 relaxation time, or PD. These images are referred to as being *T1-weighted*, *T2-weighted*, or *PD-weighted* images, respectively.

The signal intensity of normal skeletal muscle is higher than that of water, much lower than that of fat on T1-weighted images, and much lower than that of both fat and water on T2-weighted images (Figure 18.8). Disease states can cause alterations

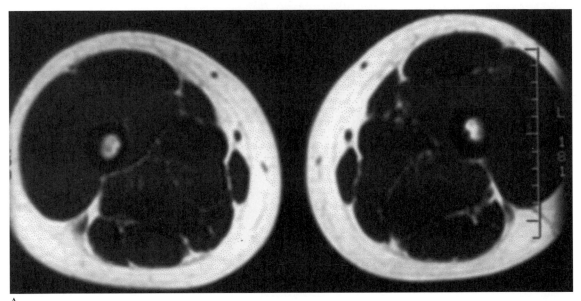

A

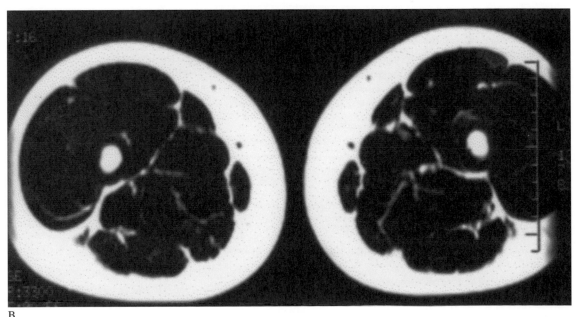

B

Figure 18.8 A. Axial T1-weighted (TR/TE = 500/14) spin echo image of the thigh in a healthy volunteer. The signal intensity of the healthy muscle is lower than that of the subcutaneous fat. **B.** Axial T2-weighted (TR/TE = 3,300/90) fast spin echo image of same patient. The muscle signal is much lower than that of the fat.

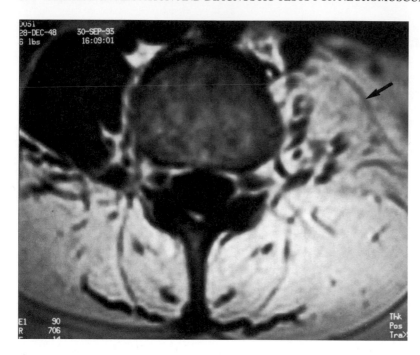

Figure 18.9 T1-weighted axial spin echo image (TR/TE = 706/14) in a patient with limb-girdle muscular dystrophy. There is fatty replacement of the left psoas muscle (*arrow*), which is hyperintense on this T1-weighted image when compared to the more normal right psoas muscle. There is also fatty replacement of the paraspinous muscles (same patient as in Figure 18.8).

in the T1 and T2 of muscle, changing the signal intensity of the muscle. Pathologic conditions can also affect muscle size with either muscle atrophy or hypertrophy. As opposed to CT, MR can be performed in any imaging plane, which aids in the evaluation of individual muscles. In addition, MR does not use ionizing radiation and has no known biological hazards.

Muscle Atrophy

Muscle atrophy causes muscles to be decreased in size, usually with areas of fatty replacement of normal muscle fiber. The areas of fatty replacement appear hyperintense on T1-weighted images compared to normal muscle[28] (Figure 18.9). Because the signal intensity difference between fat and muscle is so great and the spatial resolution is so good, even thin intermuscular fat planes can be easily demonstrated, and early or minimal fatty replacement can be detected.

Myopathies generally present in their early stages as focal areas of fatty infiltration, gradually spreading to involve the entire muscle as the disease progresses (Figure 18.10). The different myopathies tend to involve certain muscles and muscle groups predominantly.

Duchenne's muscular dystrophy and Becker's muscular dystrophy tend to involve the biceps femoris, adductor magnus, gluteus, and medial head of the gastrocnemius early in the disease.[29,30] As the disease progresses, the vastus lateralis, paravertebral, anterior leg compartment, and iliopsoas muscles become involved (Figure 18.11). Limb-girdle muscular dystrophy involves muscles in a similar distribution to Duchenne's muscular dystrophy and Becker's muscular dystrophy. In facioscapulohumeral dystrophy, there is prominent involvement of the shoulder and

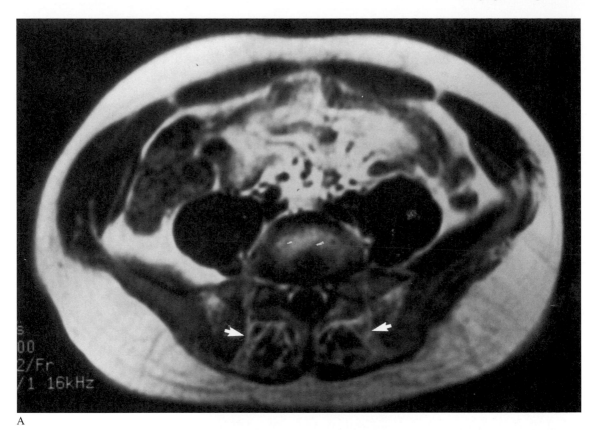

A

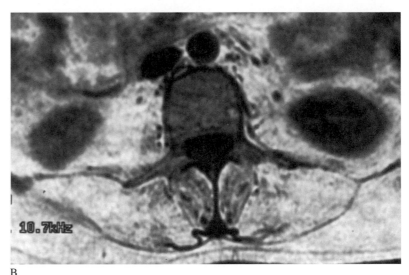

Figure 18.10 A. Axial T1-weighted (TR/TE = 500/12) spin echo image of a patient with mild (early) involvement with Becker's muscular dystrophy. There is minimal fatty infiltration as noted by the prominent intermuscular fat planes (*arrows*). **B.** Axial T1-weighted (TR/TE = 550/20) spin echo image of another patient with Becker's muscular dystrophy. There is more severe (long-standing) involvement with near-complete fatty replacement of both psoas muscles as well as paraspinous musculature.

B

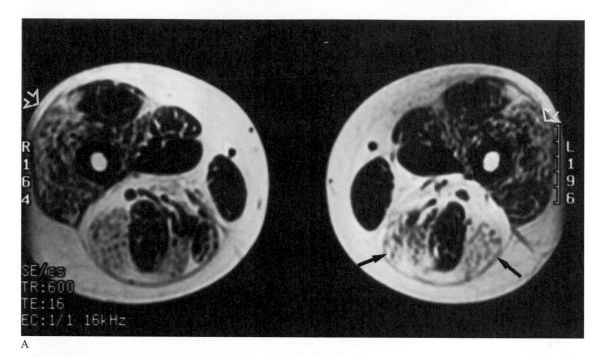

A

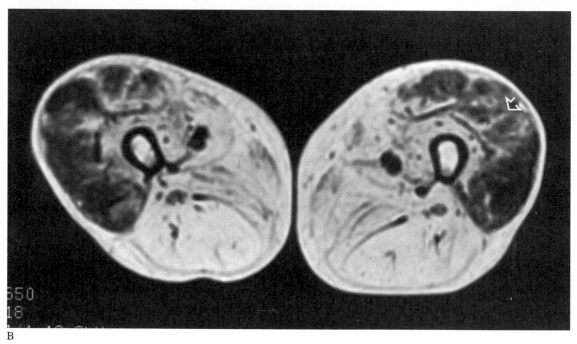

B

Figure 18.11 Axial T1-weighted spin echo images in two different patients with Becker's muscular dystrophy with moderate (**A**) and severe (**B**) involvement. In both patients, there is more involvement of the hamstrings (*arrows* in **A**) and relatively less involvement of the vastus lateralis muscles (*open arrows* in **A** and **B**).

Figure 18.12 Axial T1-weighted spin echo image demonstrating small atrophic sternocleidomastoid muscles (*arrows*). Patient has myotonic muscular dystrophy.

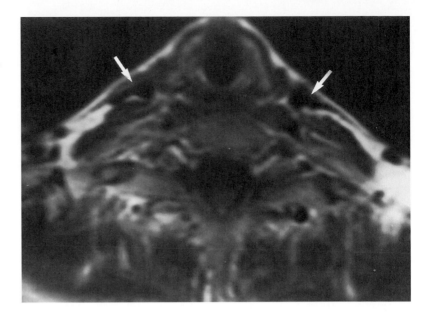

upper arm muscles.[31] There is early, prominent involvement of the sternocleidomastoid muscle with myotonic dystrophy[32] (Figure 18.12). Muscle atrophy with associated fatty infiltration can also be seen with chronic muscle diseases, including those caused by denervation[33] and as a result of corticosteroid use.

Muscle Edema

MR is particularly useful in evaluating conditions that cause muscle edema.[34] Muscle edema due to increased intracellular or extracellular free water[33] causes increased signal intensity on T2-weighted images compared to the normal low signal intensity of muscle. This can be focal or may involve the entire muscle or multiple muscles.

The increased signal of edema can be quite subtle on routine spin echo or fast spin echo T2-weighted images. Fat-suppressed T2-weighted images are much more sensitive in detecting subtle muscle edema. Fat-suppressed images can be performed by using short tau inversion recovery techniques or by using a presaturation pulse to suppress the fat signal[35–37] (Figure 18.13).

Muscle edema can be seen in inflammatory myopathies, such as polymyositis, dermatomyositis, inclusion body myositis, muscle injuries,[38–41] infectious myositis,[42] compartment syndrome,[43] and rhabdomyolysis,[44] and as a physiologic finding after exercise.[45,46]

The inflammatory myopathies are a heterogeneous group of muscle diseases, which includes polymyositis, dermatomyositis, and inclusion body myositis.[47–51] All three forms are characterized by proximal and often symmetric muscle weakness that develops relatively quickly over weeks to months.[52,53]

Typical MR findings early in the course of polymyositis and dermatomyositis are bilateral and symmetric muscle edema involving the pelvic and thigh muscula-

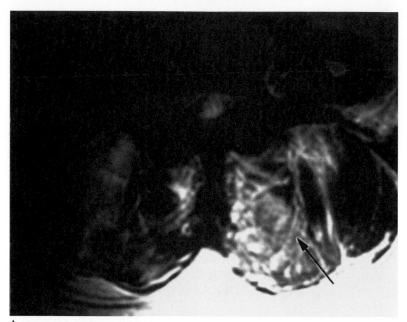

A

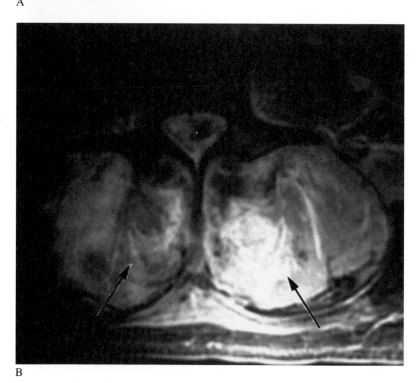

B

Figure 18.13 A. Axial fast spin echo T2-weighted (TR/TE = 3,500/106 effective echo). **B.** Axial fast spin echo T2-weighted image with same parameters as **(A)** but also with fat suppression using selective chemical shift saturation pulse. Patient has infectious myositis secondary to streptococcus infection. There is edema involving the paraspinous muscles seen as areas of hyperintensity on both images (*arrows* in **A** and **B**). The edema is better seen and the extent better appreciated on the fat-suppressed image.

ture (Figure 18.14), especially the vastus lateralis and vastus intermedius muscles.[54,55] Over months to years, there is progression to atrophy with associated fatty infiltration.

Muscle injuries, such as muscle contusions and muscle strains, cause muscle edema. Muscle strains are most frequent in muscles that cross joints and contract dur-

Figure 18.14 Axial (**A**) and coronal (**B**) fast spin echo T2-weighted fat-suppressed images in a patient with active polymyositis. Fat suppression was performed using a short tau inversion recovery technique. (TR/TE = 3,500/45 milliseconds inversion time = 160 milliseconds.) There is diffuse extensive abnormal signal involving all muscle groups in the thigh. This increased signal is due to muscle edema.

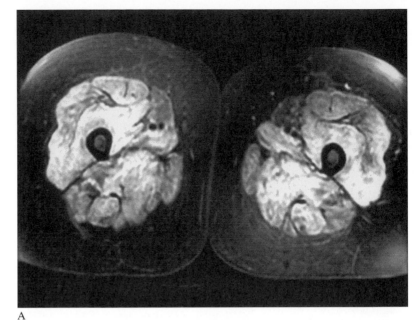

A

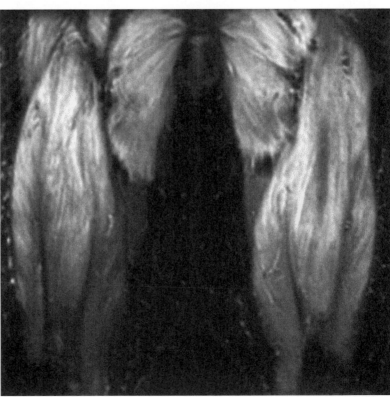

B

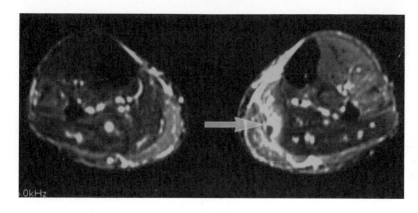

Figure 18.15 Axial T2-weighted (TR/TE = 3,500/55 effective echo) fast spin echo image with fat suppression showing abnormal hyperintensity involving the left soleus muscle (*arrow*) in the mid-calf in this patient with pain associated with jumping. This is edema secondary to muscle strain.

ing elongation, such as the hamstrings, gastrocnemius, and biceps brachii.[56] Muscle strains may only show edema at the musculotendinous junction, whereas more severe strains may reveal hematomas and demonstrate torn muscle fibers[41] (Figure 18.15).

Muscle infection (myositis) produces muscle edema and may be associated with abscess or osteomyelitis. MR is particularly useful in determining the extent of the infection as well as the presence or absence of associated abscess or bone involvement.

Compartment syndrome is caused by increased pressure in a confined, nondistensible space. This causes venous occlusion and muscle edema, which further increase the pressure, eventually leading to arterial occlusion and tissue necrosis. This muscle edema can be accessed with MR.

Rhabdomyolysis is a severe form of muscle injury caused by loss of cell membrane integrity. It can be the result of trauma, muscle ischemia, burns, and exposure to toxins. MR is particularly useful in diagnosing and defining the extent of muscle involvement in cases of rhabdomyolysis[57] (Figure 18.16). Assessing the extent of

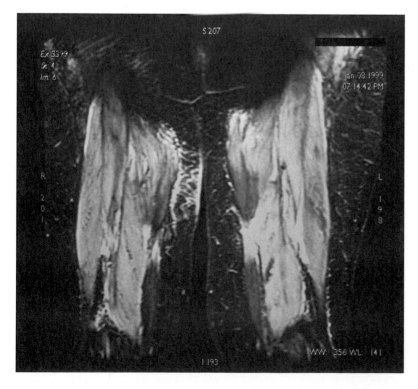

Figure 18.16 Coronal T2-weighted (TR/TE = 3,500/52 effective echo) image in a patient with rhabdomyolysis showing abnormal increased signal involving thigh muscles. (Reprinted with permission from H Halford, A Graves, T Bertorini. Muscle and nerve imaging techniques in neuromuscular diseases. J Clin Neuromuscul Dis 2000;2[1]:41–51.)

involvement is important, because life-threatening sequelae (including metabolic disorders) are likely with more extensive muscle involvement. MR provides greater anatomic detail as to the muscles involved and the extent of involvement than does Tc-PYP radionuclide imaging.

The increased signal on T2-weighted images that represents muscle edema or edema-like signal can also be seen as a transient finding following vigorous muscle exercise.[58]

Mass Lesions

Because of its greater tissue characterization, MR is the procedure of choice for evaluating mass lesions. Mass lesions may be secondary to neoplasm, abscess formation, focal hematoma, and myositis ossificans[59] (Figure 18.17). The size and extent of the mass can be determined as well as the presence or absence of bone involvement. An appropriate site for biopsy can be localized for percutaneous biopsy when necessary.

On routine T1- and T2-weighted imaging, it may be difficult to distinguish a mass, such as local neoplasm or abscess, from associated muscle edema. Contrast enhancement often can identify the exact size and extent of the mass itself, because these masses frequently enhance intensely. Postcontrast, fat-suppressed T1-weighted images can be particularly sensitive for evaluating enhancing mass lesions (Figure 18.18).

Attention to the signal intensity characteristics of the mass on the different pulse sequences can help to narrow the differential diagnosis and give a clue as to the etiology of the mass. Also, administration of intravenous gadolinium often aids in evaluating mass lesions (Figures 18.19 and 18.20). The enhancement pattern of the lesion helps to establish the correct diagnosis. Peripheral enhancement can indicate central necrosis or cystic nature of the mass, whereas central enhancement indicates that central necrosis is unlikely. Lack of enhancement is also helpful, indicating a very avascular tumor or possibly a benign mass, such as a hematoma.

Magnetic Resonance Neurography

MR neurography is a method of generating a tissue-specific image of nerves. Nerves are rendered in isolation, much like a vessel appears in a subtraction angiogram.[60] An image is obtained by using a heavily T2-weighted, fat-suppressed sequence. This pulse sequence effectively suppresses the signal from non-neural structures. A region of interest is then selected that encompasses the nerve. Projectional images are then obtained by using a maximum-intensity projection algorithm (Figure 18.21).

The MR neurography technique is designed to exploit differences in water content and connective tissue structures of the fascicles and perineurium versus the surrounding epineurium and to allow the fascicular pattern to be visualized.[61] In the setting of trauma or tumors, increased endoneurial free water alters the signal characteristics of the nerve. An abnormal nerve becomes increasingly hyperintense to muscle on T2-weighted images. The nerve may be enlarged with fascicular distortion.[62]

This technique can be useful in the diagnosis of focal root or nerve lesions, inflammation, and edema. MR and MR neurography have also been applied in the

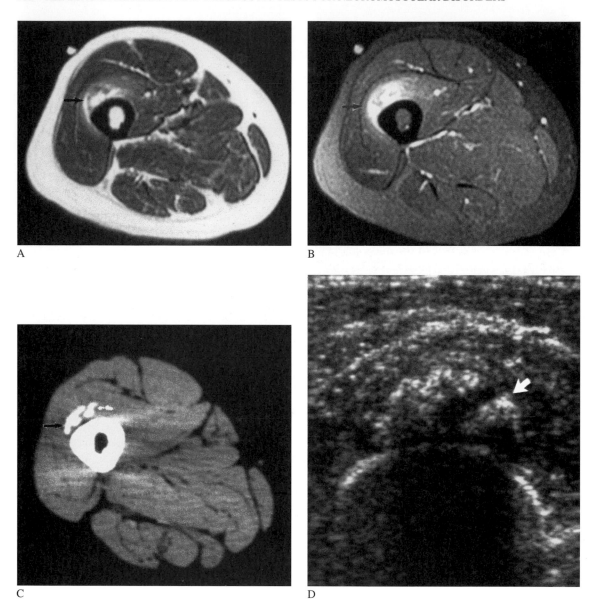

Figure 18.17 Axial T1-weighted spin echo image (TR/TE = 500/15) before (**A**) and after (**B**) contrast enhancement with fat suppression shows hyperintense mass (*arrows* in **A** and **B**) adjacent to the femur. There is very little enhancement and no bone involvement. Computed tomography (**C**) at this same level performed at the time of biopsy demonstrates associated dystrophic calcification (*arrow*) indicating the nature of this mass, which was biopsy-proven myositis ossificans. Axial ultrasound (**D**) at this same level demonstrates hyperechoic mass (*arrow*) with distal shadowing consistent with calcifications.

diagnosis of compression neuropathies, such as carpal tunnel syndrome (CTS).[63] Electrodiagnostic studies are more sensitive, specific, and cost effective than MR in the routine evaluation of CTS. MR may be useful in evaluating patients with convincing symptoms but normal electrodiagnostic studies. MR may also be useful in identifying a rare anatomic lesion as the cause of CTS.

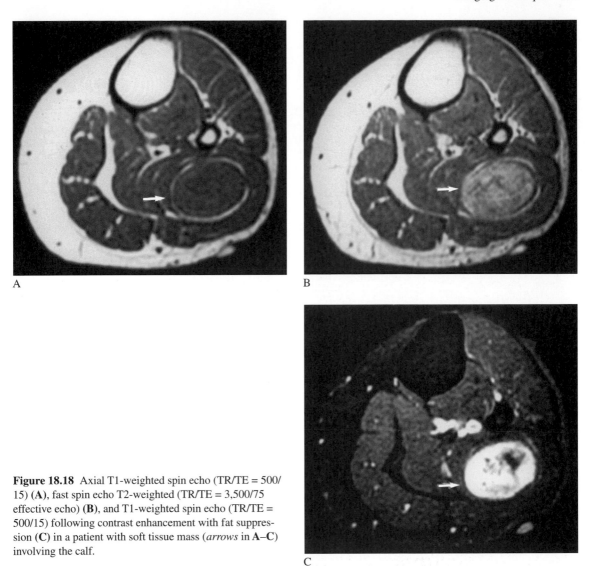

A

B

C

Figure 18.18 Axial T1-weighted spin echo (TR/TE = 500/15) (**A**), fast spin echo T2-weighted (TR/TE = 3,500/75 effective echo) (**B**), and T1-weighted spin echo (TR/TE = 500/15) following contrast enhancement with fat suppression (**C**) in a patient with soft tissue mass (*arrows* in **A–C**) involving the calf.

Magnetic Resonance Imaging in Spinal Canal Disease

Neuromuscular specialists are often involved in the diagnosis of nerve root compression. Spinal canal stenosis and disk disease can mimic focal nerve disorders. Lumbar spinal canal stenosis is often due to a combination of diffuse disk bulging, facet hypertrophy, and ligamentous thickening. Lumbar spinal canal stenosis is most common at the L3, L4, and L5 disk levels and causes lower extremity claudication or focal radiculopathy (Figure 18.22). Patients who have congenital spinal stenosis due to "short pedicles" develop symptoms with less severe superimposed acquired disease. Symptoms of lumbar canal stenosis usually occur with an anteroposterior diameter of less than 11.5 mm.[64] Spinal canal stenosis in the cervical spine is usually

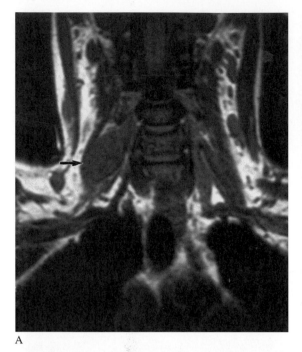

A

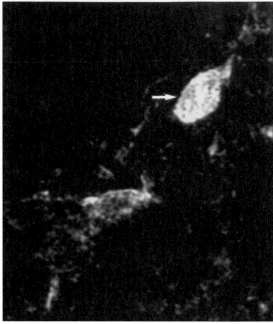

B

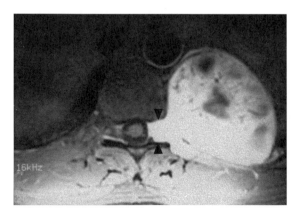

C

Figure 18.19 Coronal T1-weighted spin echo (TR/TE = 500/15) (**A**), coronal T2-weighted fast spin echo (TR/TE = 3,500/75 effective echo) with fat suppression (**B**), and axial T1-weighted spin echo following contrast showing a mass (*arrows* in **A–C**) in the right neck that extends to a cervical neuroforamen. This mass is isointense to muscle on T1-weighted image (**A**) and is hyperintense on T2-weighted image (**B**). This mass enhances with contrast (**C**). This is consistent with a nerve sheath tumor in this biopsy-proven schwannoma.

Figure 18.20 Another patient with schwannoma involving lumbar nerve. This mass demonstrates intense enhancement with several small areas of nonenhancement consistent with areas of necrosis. There is widening of the neuroforamen (*arrowheads*) from this slow-growing mass T1-weighted spin echo image (TR/TE = 500/15).

Figure 18.21 Neurogram of the lumbar spine at the L5 disk level performed using a heavily T2-weighted fat-suppressed sequence (**A**) and projectional image obtained using a maximum intensity projection algorithm (**B**) in a patient with neuropraxic injury. There is enlargement and increased signal intensity involving the left L4 (*large arrows*) and L3 (*small arrows*) nerve roots owing to nerve root swelling.

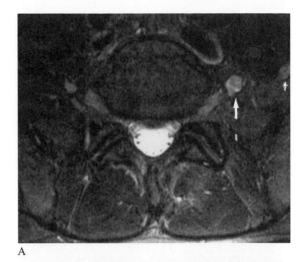

A

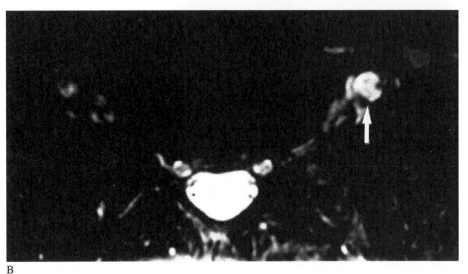

B

due to spondylosis and ligamentous thickening (Figures 18.23 and 18.24). Patients are at risk for myelopathy or radiculopathy if the anteroposterior diameter of the cervical spine is less than 11 mm.

Focal disk herniation often causes radiculopathy with sensory deficits or muscle weakness. Referred pain is often in the dermatomal distribution of the affected nerve root or disk level. Extruded disk fragments can be subligamentous or posterior to the longitudinal ligament. Midline disk herniations are more common in the cervical spine than in the lumbar region (Figures 18.25 and 18.26). Posterolateral disk herniations are more common in the lumbar spine but also occur in the cervical spine (Figure 18.27). Far lateral disk herniations are not uncommon in the lumbar spine but are rare in the cervical spine. CT with intradural contrast and MR are both excellent for diagnosing patients with nerve root compression due to spinal disease (Figure 18.28).

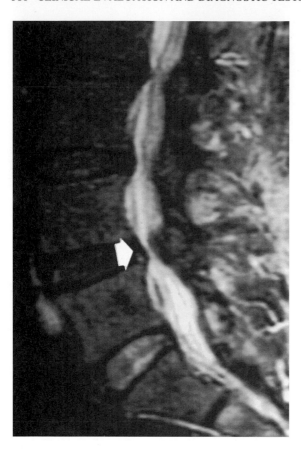

Figure 18.22 Sagittal T2-weighted image using a fat-suppressed fast spin echo inversion recovery technique (TR/TE/TI = 3,500/30 effective echo/150). There is spinal canal stenosis at multiple disk levels that is worse at L4-5 (*arrow*). This is due to disk bulging anteriorly and ligamentous hypertrophy posteriorly.

MR imaging is generally considered the test of choice for evaluating the spinal canal and nerve roots. It is the single most sensitive, specific, and versatile examination. MR has proved effective in identifying a surgical lesion caused by spondylosis or disk herniation in more than 90% of patients.[65] MR can also aid in diagnosing causes of nerve root edema. Enhancement of the lumbosacral roots, which is usually not seen in other neuropathies, can be seen in inflammatory demyelinating neuropathy.[66] This root enhancement can also be seen in Guillain-Barré syndrome.

CONCLUSIONS

The definite diagnosis of most neuromuscular disorders is made by muscle and nerve histology, biochemistry, and molecular genetics and frequently by electromyography. Imaging techniques are also valuable in the assessment of the characteristics and distribution of muscle involvement, and they serve to localize the most ideal areas for biopsy, particularly with MR and ultrasound. MR can also be used to assess the response to therapy in inflammatory myopathies in

Figure 18.23 A. Sagittal T2-weighted gradient echo image (TR/TE/θ = 500/7.9/20°). **B.** Axial T2-weighted gradient echo image (TR/TE/θ = 1,046/17.9/40°) at C4 disk level. There is mild spinal canal stenosis at multiple levels with narrowing of anterior-posterior dimension of canal. Axial image (**B**) also demonstrates narrowing of both neuorforamina—worse on the right (*arrow*).

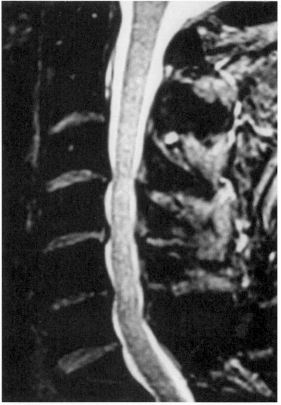

A

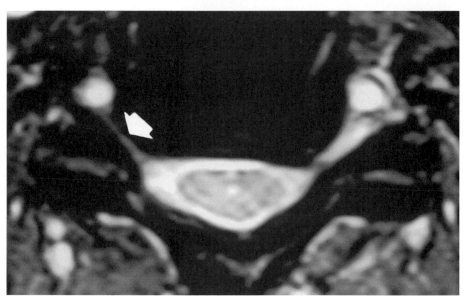

B

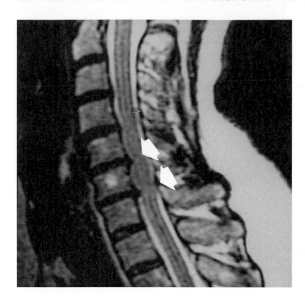

Figure 18.24 Sagittal T2-weighted fast spin echo image (TR/TE = 3,200/104 effective echo) showing mild canal stenosis at C5 and C6 disk levels due to posterior spondylosis at both levels (*arrows*).

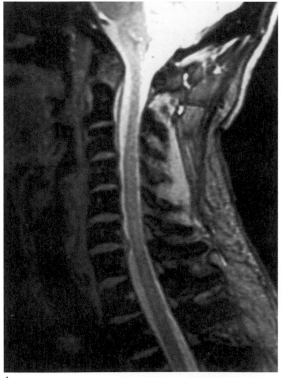

A

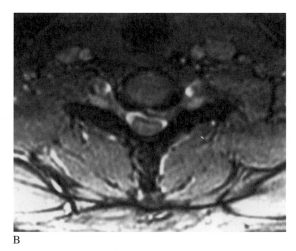

B

Figure 18.25 Sagittal (**A**) and axial (**B**) T2-weighted gradient echo images showing a focal left paracentral disk herniation.

Figure 18.26 A. Sagittal T2-weighted fast spin echo image (TR/TE = 3,566/106 effective echo). **B.** Axial T2-weighted gradient echo (TR/TE/θ = 517/15/20°). There is a large central (*slightly right*) paracentral disk herniation at C5 disk level (*arrow*).

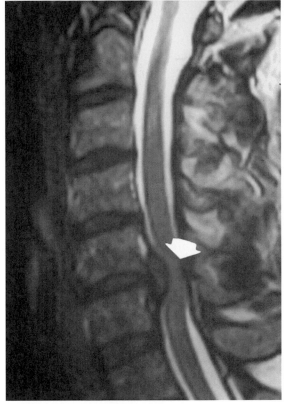

A

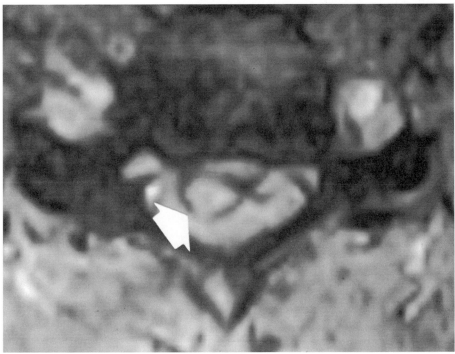

B

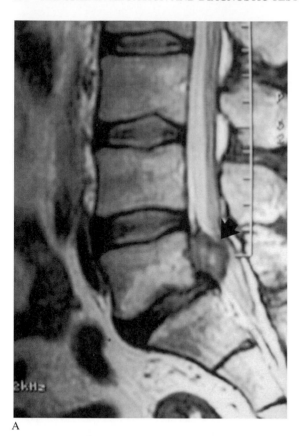

A

Figure 18.27 Sagittal (**A**) and axial (**B**) T2-weighted fast spin echo images (TR/TE = 2,300/99 effective echo) showing large recurrent disk herniation at L5 disk level (*arrows*). This effaces dural sac-right paracentral.

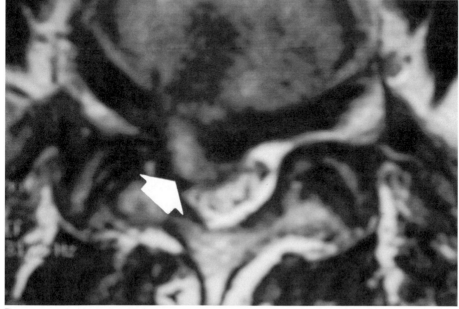

B

Figure 18.28 Axial computed tomography at the C5 disk level with intradural contrast (following cervical myelogram). There is a focal left paracentral disk herniation, which effaces the dural sac and causes mild compression on the cervical cord.

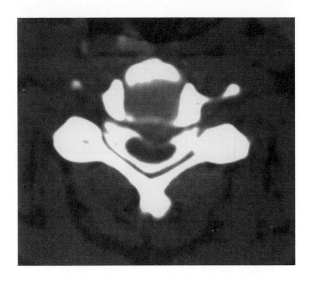

which the increased signals on T2-weighted imaging correlate well with the presence and severity of edema and necrosis. DEXA is a radiographic computerized method that allows the assessment of muscle and fat content as well as determination of the degree of osteopenia, an important complication of therapy in these disorders. MR neurography is a newer technique applied to the assessment of nerve anatomy and to the determination of focal pathology and entrapments in nerves. Imaging of the spine is most useful in the evaluation of radiculopathies and in ruling out spinal cord diseases that can mimic some muscular diseases.

REFERENCES

1. Von Kempis J, Kalden P, Gutfleisch J, et al. Diagnosis of idiopathic myositis: value of 99m technetium pyrophosphate muscle scintigraphy and magnetic resonance imaging in targeted muscle biopsy. Rheumatol Int 1998;17:207–213.
2. Fleckstein JL, Reimers CD. Inflammatory myopathies: radiologic evaluation. Radio Clin North Am 1996;34:427–439.
3. Lofberg M, Liewendahl K, Savolainen S, et al. Antimyosin scintigraphy in patients with acquired and hereditary muscular disorders. Eur J Nucl Med 1994;21:1098–1105.
4. Lofberg M, Liewendahl K, Lamminem A, et al. Antimyosin scintigraphy compared with magnetic resonance imaging in inflammatory myopathies. Arch Neurol 1998;55:987–993.
5. Thrall JH, Ziessman HA (eds), Nuclear Medicine: The Requisites. St. Louis: Mosby-Year Book Inc., 1995;149–170.
6. Lin J, Fessell DP, Jacobson JA, et al. An illustrated tutorial of musculoskeletal sonography: part 1, introduction and general principles. AJR Am J Roentgenol 2000;175:637–645.
7. Holsbeck MV (ed), Musculoskeletal Ultrasound. St. Louis: Mosby-Year Book Inc., 1991;13–56.
8. Zuberi SM, Matta N, Nawaz S, et al. Muscle ultrasound in the assessment of suspected neuromuscular disease in childhood. Neuromuscul Disord 1999;9:203–207.
9. Heckmatt J, Rodillo E, Doherty M, et al. Quantitative sonography of muscle. J Child Neurol 1989;4:S101–S106.
10. Topaloglu H, Gucuyener K, Yalaz K, et al. Selective involvement of the quadriceps muscle in congenital muscular dystrophies: an ultrasound study. Brain Dev 1992;14:84–87.

11. Dock W, Happak W, Grabenwoger F, et al. Neuromuscular diseases: evaluation with high-frequency sonography. Radiology 1990;177:825–828.
12. Newman JS, Adler RS, Bude RO, et al. Detection of soft-tissue hyperemia: value of power Doppler sonography. AJR Am J Roentgenol 1994;163:385–389.
13. Barberie JE, Wong ADW, Cooperberg PL, et al. Extended field of view sonography in musculoskeletal disorders. AJR Am J Roentgenol 1998;171:751–757.
14. Heckmatt JZ, Leeman S, Dubowitz V. Ultrasound imaging in the diagnosis of muscle disease. J Pediatr 1982;101:656–660.
15. Reimers CD, Fleckenstein JL, Witt TN, et al. Muscular ultrasound in idiopathic inflammatory myopathies of adults. J Neurol Sci 1993;116:82–92.
16. Jensen MD, Kanley JA, Roust LR, et al. Assessment of body composition with use of Dual-Energy X-ray Absorptiometry: evaluation and comparison with other methods. Mayo Clin Proc 1993;68:867–873.
17. Brodie D, Moscrip V, Hutcheon R. Body composition measurement: a review of hydrodensitometry, anthropometry and impedance methods. Nutrition 1998;14:296–310.
18. Kanda F, Fujii Y, Takahashi K, Fujita T. Dual-Energy X-ray absorptiometry in neuromuscular diseases. Muscle Nerve 1994;17:431–435.
19. Palmieri GMA, Bertorini TE, Griffin JW, et al. Assessment of whole body composition with dual energy X-ray absorptiometry in Duchenne muscular dystrophy: correlation of lean body mass with muscle function. Muscle Nerve 1996;19:777–779.
20. Kissel JT, McDermott MP, Natarajan R, et al. Pilot trial of albuterol in facioscapulohumeral muscular dystrophy. Neurology 1998;50:1402–1406.
21. Narayanaswami P, Bertorini TE, Palmieri GMA, et al. Dual energy X-ray absorptiometry (DEXA) in the evaluation of patients with muscular diseases. Neurology 1999;52(6):382.
22. Termote JL, Baert A, Crolla D, et al. Computed tomography of the normal and pathologic muscle system. Radiology 1980;137:439–444.
23. Hawley RJ Jr, Schellinger D, O'Doherty DS. Computer tomographic patterns of muscles in neuromuscular disease. Arch Neurol 1984;41:383–387.
24. Bulcke JA, Termote JL, Palmers Y, Crolla D. Computed tomography of the human skeletal muscular system. Neurology 1979;17:127.
25. Liu M, Chino N, Ishihara T. Muscle damage progression in Duchenne muscular dystrophy evaluated by a new quantitative computed tomography method. Arch Phys Med Rehabil 1993; 74(5):507–514.
26. Van der Vliet AM, Thijssen HOM, Joosten E, Merx JL. CT in neuromuscular disorders: a comparison of CT and histology. Neuroradiology 1988;30:421.
27. McCartney N, Moroz D, Garner SLD, et al. The effects of strength training in patients with selected neuromuscular disorders. Med Sci Sports Exerc 1988;20:362–368.
28. Murphy WA, Tofty WA, Carrol JE. MRI of normal and pathologic skeletal muscle. AJR Am J Roentgenol 1986;146:565–574.
29. Lamminen AE. Magnetic resonance imaging of primary skeletal muscle diseases: Patterns of distribution and severity of involvement. Br J Radiol 1990;63:946.
30. DeVisser M, Verbeeten B Jr. Computed tomography of the skeletal musculature in Becker-type muscular dystrophy and benign infantile spinal muscular atrophy. Muscle Nerve 1985;8:435.
31. Jiddane M, Gastant JL, Pellissier JF, et al. CT of primary muscle disease. Am J Neuroradiol 1983;4:773.
32. Richards D, Isherwood J, Hutchinson R, et al. Computed tomography in dystrophia myotonia. Neuroradiology 1982;24:27.
33. Fleckenstein JL, Watamull D, Conner KE, et al. Denervated human skeletal muscle: MR imaging evaluation. Radiology 1993;187:213–218.
34. Halford H, Graves A, Bertorini T. Muscle and nerve imaging techniques in neuromuscular diseases. J Clin Neuromuscul Dis 2000;2(1):41–51.
35. Hernandez RJ, Keim DR, Chenevert TL, et al. Fat suppressed MR imaging of myositis. Radiology 1992;182:217–219.
36. Greco A, McNamara MT, Escher MB, et al. Spin echo and STIR MR imaging of sports related injuries at 1.5 T. J Comput Assist Tomogr 1991;15:994–999.
37. Fleckenstein JL, Archer BT, Barker BA, et al. Fast short-tau inversion-recovery MR imaging. Radiology 1991;179:499–504.
38. Remiers CD, Schedel H, Fleckenstein JL, et al. Magnetic resonance imaging of skeletal muscles in idiopathic inflammatory myopathies of adults. J Neurol 1994;241:306–314.

39. Fleckenstein JL, Weatherall PT, Parkey RW, et al. Sports related muscle injuries evaluation with MR imaging. Radiology 1989;172:793–798.
40. McCally K, Shellock FA, Bank WJ, Posner JD. The use of nuclear magnetic resonance to evaluate muscle injury. Med Sci Sports Exerc 1992;24:537–542.
41. De Smet AA. Magnetic resonance findings in skeletal muscle tears. Skeletal Radiol 1993;22:479–484.
42. Resnick D, Niwayama G. Osteomyelitis, Septic Arthritis and Soft Tissue Infection Mechanisms and Situations. In D Resnick (ed), Diagnosis of Bone and Joint Disorders (3rd ed). Philadelphia: Saunders, 1945;2375–2418.
43. Stoller DN, Ferkel RD. The Ankle and Foot. In DW Stoller (ed), Magnetic Resonance Imaging in Orthopaedics and Sports Medicine (2nd ed). Philadelphia: Lippincott–Raven, 1997;443–595.
44. Shurtani S, Shiigai T. Repeat MRI in acute rhabdomyolysis correlation with clinicopathological findings. J Comput Assist Tomogr 1993;17:786–791.
45. Fleckenstein JL, Weatherol PT, Parkey RW, et al. Acute effects of exercise on MR imaging of skeletal muscle in normal volunteers. AJR Am J Roentgenol 1988;151:231–237.
46. Saab G, Thompson RT, Marsh AD. Effects of exercise on muscle transverse relaxation. J Appl Physiol 2000;88:226–233.
47. Bohan A, Peter JB. Polymyositis and dermatomyositis: part 1. N Engl J Med 1975;292:344–347.
48. Bohan A, Peter JB. Polymyositis and dermatomyositis: part 2. N Engl J Med 1975;292:403–407.
49. Medsger TA Jr, Oddis CV. Classification and diagnostic criteria for polymyositis and dermatomyositis. J Rheumatol 1995;22:581–585.
50. Dalakas MC. Review article: polymyositis dermatomyositis and inclusion body myositis. N Engl J Med 1991;325:1487–1493.
51. Resnick D. Disorders Due to Medications and other Chemical Agents. In D Resnick (ed), Diagnosis of Bone and Joint Disorders (3rd ed). Philadelphia: Saunders, 1995;3309–3342.
52. Sayers ME, Chou SM, Calabrese LH. Inclusion body myositis: analysis of 32 cases. J Rheumotol 1992;19:1385–1389.
53. Calabrese LH, Chou SM. Inclusion body myositis. Rheum Dis Clin North Am 1994;20:955–972.
54. Chapman S, Southwood TR, Fowler J, et al. Rapid changes in magnetic resonance imaging of muscle during the treatment of juvenile dermatomyositis. Br J Rheumatol 1994;33:184–186.
55. Hernandez RJ, Sullivan DB, Chenevent TL, et al. MR imaging in children with dermatomyositis: musculoskeletal findings and correlation with clinical and laboratory findings. AJR Am J Roentgenol 1993;161:359–366.
56. Palmer WE, Kuong SJ, Elmadbough HM. MR imaging of myotendinous strain. AJR Am J Roentgenol 1999;173:703–709.
57. Zagoria RJ, Karstaedt N, Konbek TD. MR imaging of rhabdomyolysis. J Comput Assist Tomogr 1986;10:268–270.
58. Dister DG, Cohen MS, Krebs DE, et al. Dynamic evaluation of exercising leg muscle in healthy subjects with echo planar MR imaging: work rate and total work determine rate of T_2 change. J Magn Reson Imaging 1995;5:588–593.
59. Kransdorf MJ, Meis JM, Jalinek JS. Myositis ossificans: MR appearance with radiologic-pathologic correlation. AJR Am J Roentgenol 1990;157:243–248.
60. Filler AG, Howe FA, Hayes CE, et al. Magnetic resonance neurography. Lancet 1993;341:659–661.
61. Filler AG, Kliot M, Howe FA, et al. Application of magnetic resonance neurography in the evaluation of patients with peripheral nerve pathology. J Neurosurg 1996;85:299–309.
62. Maravilla KR, Aagaard BD, Kliot M. MR neurography. Magn Reson Imaging Clin N Am 1998;6(1):179–194.
63. Cosgrove J. Magnetic Resonance Imaging in the evaluation of carpal tunnel syndrome: A literature review. J Neuromuscul Dis 2000;1(4):175–180.
64. Ulrich CA, Binet EF, Sanecki MA, Kieffer SA. Quantitative assessment of the lumbar spinal canal by computed tomography. Radiology 1980;134:137–143.
65. Wilson DW, Pezzuti RT, Place JN. Magnetic resource imaging in the preoperative evaluation of cervical radiculopathy. Neurosurgery 1991;28:175–179.
66. Bertorini T, Halford H, Lawrence J, et al. Contrast-enhanced magnetic resonance imaging of the lumbosacral roots in the dysimmune inflammatory polyneuropathies. J Neuroimaging 1995;5:9–15.

19

Histology and Histochemistry of Muscle and Nerve

Tulio E. Bertorini and Linda H. Horner

Muscle and nerve biopsies are important diagnostic tools in the evaluation of neuromuscular disorders. Muscle biopsy is useful in patients with suspected myopathy, undiagnosed weakness, or muscle pain, and in the evaluation of neurogenic disease. The biopsy provides histologic information regarding the cause of these conditions, such as the presence of inflammation or vasculitis, dystrophy, or metabolic derangement. It also determines the presence of muscle atrophy or grouping from reinnervation as seen in neurogenic disorders. Immunohistochemical staining and Western blot analysis of muscle aid in diagnosing protein defects in some of the dystrophies,[1,2] and biochemical studies are used to detect enzyme deficiencies. DNA studies can also be performed in muscles for hereditary diseases.

Peripheral nerve biopsy is performed to provide a better understanding of the pathogenic mechanisms in neuropathies, including determination of abnormalities of vessels, as in vasculitis, and the presence of storage material, as in amyloidosis. Nerve biopsy also allows a morphologic analysis of myelinated and unmyelinated axons and the differentiation between the axon and its myelin sheath as the primary target of pathology, and it helps to demonstrate whether the process is secondary to axonal degeneration versus segmental demyelination. Nerve biopsies are done less frequently and should be reserved for selected cases. The nerve biopsy must be properly studied; otherwise, it might not be as informative and is a more traumatic procedure than a muscle biopsy.

Skin biopsy has also recently been recommended and applied to the study of terminal axons in sensory neuropathies.

MUSCLE BIOPSY

A muscle that is affected by the disease process, but not severely, is usually selected for biopsy. Normal or mildly affected and end-stage muscle are avoided because the pathology is useless for diagnosis. Frequently, the muscle chosen is contralateral to the one that shows abnormality on electromyography or those that appear abnormal on magnetic resonance imaging.

The biceps, deltoids, and quadriceps are the most frequently biopsied muscles; if others are selected, it is important that the pathologist is familiar with their histologic characteristics. Some muscles, like the gastrocnemius, are avoided because the findings of increased connective tissue and internalized nuclei can be misdiagnosed as myopathic in neuropathies or even in normals. Sometimes, however, specimens from this muscle are obtained with a sural nerve biopsy at the calf for the diagnosis of vasculitis. The intercostal and anconeus muscles can also be selected because they are rich in neuromuscular junctions, allowing microelectrode studies and electron microscopy (EM) analysis of the end plates. The peroneus brevis is sometimes obtained in conjunction with biopsy of the superficial peroneal nerve using a single incision.[3]

The procedure is generally performed with an open biopsy technique and may include the fascia to determine the presence of fasciitis. It is also helpful to obtain a skin specimen of affected areas in dermatomyositis (DM).

Some use a needle biopsy technique, especially in children, because it is less invasive or in research when multiple biopsy sites are necessary. This technique has the disadvantages of being performed blindly and of being as painful as an open biopsy. Also, the specimen obtained is small and may not be adequate for histochemical analysis of muscle fiber–type distribution or for special analyses, such as biochemistry. For descriptions of the actual surgical procedures, the reader is referred to excellent textbooks that are available.[4–7]

Characteristics of Normal Muscle

To understand the pathologic features of muscle, this section provides a brief overview of normal muscle fibers and their structure.

The entire muscle is surrounded by connective tissue, called the *epimysium* (Figure 19.1). The perimysium separates muscle fascicles, and the *endomysium* is the fine network of collagenous fibers around each muscle fiber or myofiber.

Medium-sized arterioles and vessels are located between muscle fascicles, whereas small capillaries are parallel and between muscle fibers. The muscle spindles appear as encapsulated formations with small intrafusal muscle fibers (see Color Plate B1).

The myofibers are polygonal in shape and normally have a diameter of approximately 40–80 µm in men and 30–70 µm in women.[8] Individual fibers are surrounded by a sarcolemma or muscle membrane. Their nuclei are located in the periphery, close to the sarcolemma, and normally less than 3% of fibers have internalized nuclei.

Muscle fibers are composed of myofibrils that are irregular polygons of approximately 1 µm in diameter in transverse sections on EM. Each myofibril consists of a bundle of myofilaments, the thick filaments of myosin and the thin filaments of actin. As seen on EM, the myofilaments are arranged in segments called *sarcomeres* that are repeated throughout the length of the fiber, giving the muscle its striated appearance. A sarcomere is the region between two *Z lines* with a span of approximately 3 µm. Within the sarcomere, there is a dark, central anisotropic *A band* that contains the myosin filaments in a regular, parallel arrangement, and in the middle of the A band is a dark line called the *M line* that forms cross bridges of these filaments. The M line is surrounded by a paler *H zone*[9] that is limited by the termination of the thin filaments and is, therefore, composed of only thick filaments (see Figure 19.1). This

Figure 19.1 Diagrammatic representation of muscle and myofibrils. (A = A band; H = H zone; I = I band; M = M line; Z = Z line.)

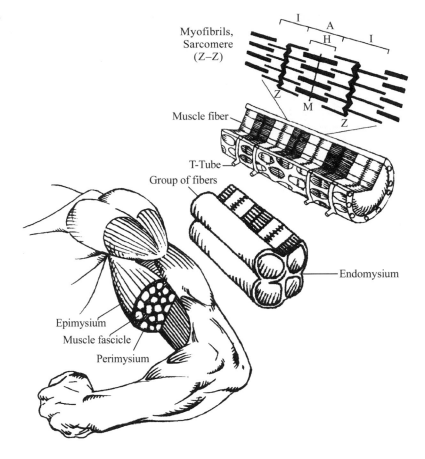

zone changes in size with muscle contraction. The pale *I* (isotropic) *band* is situated on either side of the A band and consists of parallel thin filaments composed mainly of actin but also of troponin and tropomyosin. This represents the area where thin filaments lie between two sarcomeres with the Z line in the center (Figure 19.2).

The cytoskeleton of the fiber is held together by filamentous proteins and microtubules. These include the microtubular protein *tubulin*; the microfilament proteins *severin, fragmin, gelsolin, profilin,* and α-*actinin*; and the intermediate filaments *vimentin, filamin,* and *desmin.* The accumulation of filamentous proteins, especially desmin, is associated with a form of myopathy with cardiomyopathy. Other proteins are those of the elastic filaments, such as the large protein nebulin, and titin (or conectin), which links thick myosin with the Z band and interacts with *telethonin,* a protein important in the assembly of the sarcomere. The gene that encodes telethonin is deficient in limb-girdle muscular dystrophy (LGMD) 2G.[10] In another form of muscular dystrophy, LGMD 2A, there is a deficiency of the cytosolic protease *calpain-3* that also interacts with *titin.*

Proteins of the plasma membrane include *vinculin,* which binds *actin* filaments; *spectrin; ankyrin;* and *dystrophin,* which is deficient in Duchenne's and Becker's muscular dystrophies. Dystrophin is linked to a glycoprotein complex that includes the *sarcoglycans;* deficiency of different sarcoglycans is associated with various forms of LGMD. Dystrophin is also linked to the *dystroglycans, sarcospan, syntrophins,* and *dystrobrevin* (Figure 19.3).[11]

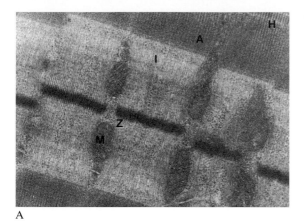

A

Figure 19.2 A. Electron micrograph of a muscle fiber in longitudinal orientation (original magnification ×58,680). **B.** Cross-section of muscle demonstrating the thick and thin filaments in the area of the A band (×79,920). (A = A band; H = H zone; I = I band; M = mitochondria; Z = Z line.)

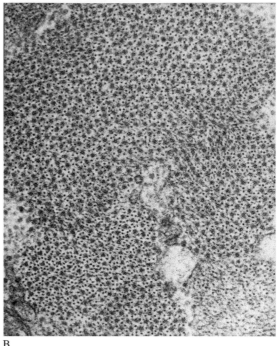

B

Other membrane proteins include *dysferlin*, which is deficient in Miyoshi myopathy and in LGMD 2B,[1,12,13] and *caveolin*, a protein of the membrane invaginations or caveola. Mutations of caveolin-3 have been reported in LGMD 1C.[14] *Laminin* together with *collagen IV*, nidogen, and *perlecan* form the backbone structure of the basement membrane, which also includes *fibronectin*, *proteoglycans*, and *cadherins*. Laminin α2 (*merosin*) links the sarcolemma with the extracellular matrix by binding to dystroglycan, which in turn binds dystrophin. Laminin α2 is deficient in a form of congenital muscular dystrophy,[15] whereas extracellular collagen VI mutations cause Bethlem

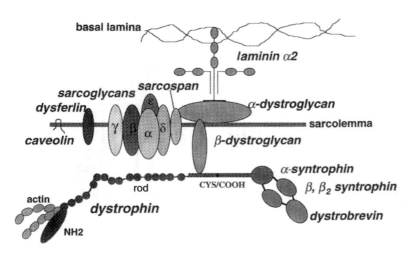

Figure 19.3 Dystrophin and other proteins of the muscle membrane. (Reproduced from T Bertorini. Muscular Dystrophies. In R Pourmand [ed], Neuromuscular Diseases: Expert Clinicians' Views, Boston: Butterworth–Heinemann, 2001;235.)

myopathy.[16] The gene that expresses the novel protein *fukutin*, which is likely located in the extracellular matrix, is affected in the Fukuyama type of muscular dystrophy.[17] The *integrins* are proteins that also serve as receptors for laminin $\alpha2$, and mutations of *integrin* $\alpha7$ have been reported to be associated in a form of congenital myopathy.[18]

The contractile proteins include *troponin, tropomyosin, actin*, and *myosin*. The latter is selectively damaged in the critical illness myopathy. In addition, other proteins such as utrophin and rapsyn are located predominantly in the neuromuscular junctions. Alterations of rapsyn and receptor proteins, as well as those in the ionic channels, are also associated with various other neuromuscular disorders.

The nuclei of muscle fibers are located beneath the sarcolemma, and the satellite cell lies between the basal lamina and the sarcolemma. The satellite cells have denser nuclei, and they divide to form myotubules during the process of regeneration. In adults, approximately 4% of the peripheral nuclei are from satellite cells.[19]

Nuclear membrane proteins may also be associated with neuromuscular disorders. For example, mutations of the gene for *emerin* and *lamin A/C* are associated with X-linked and autosomal dominant Emery-Dreifuss muscular dystrophy (EDMD), respectively.[20,21]

The mitochondria are located in the sarcoplasm, adjacent to I bands or beneath the sarcolemma. They are ovoid in shape, have a diameter of 0.1 nm, and are more abundant in type I muscle fibers. Alterations in the shape and number of the mitochondria can be observed in mitochondrial myopathies. The T-tubular system is a network of tubes continuous with muscle membrane in invaginations that connect throughout the muscle fibers. The sarcoplasmic reticulum consists of a series of sacs around the myofibers that terminate in the cisterna at either end of the junction between the A band and the I band. At this level, the sarcoplasmic reticulum cisterna come in proximity with the T-tubular system forming what is known as a *triad*. In those, the voltage-activated and the calcium-release channels are joined together. Important proteins in the sarcoplasmic reticulum include, among others, calsequestrin, triadin, calmodulin, and sarcolipin.

Other constituents of muscle include fine granules of glycogen, which are more abundant in type II fibers; lipid droplets or vacuoles of neutral lipids that are found predominantly in type I fibers; microtubules; ribosomes; Golgi complexes; and granules of lipofuscin. Enzymes of the energy metabolism located in the cytosol and mitochondria are fundamental to muscle function, and their deficiencies cause various metabolic myopathies discussed in Chapter 17 and in the section Metabolic Myopathies.

Neuromuscular junctions and intramuscular nerves can also be observed in muscle biopsies. The neuromuscular junctions are recognized by their dark staining with nonspecific esterase (see Color Plate B1) and their identification on EM by the characteristic invaginations in the muscle membrane that surround the associated axon, which is sometimes out of the plane of sectioning and not identified. The myotendinous junctions are areas in which muscle and connective tissue join (see Color Plate B2). In these areas, the muscle fibers are small and have increased internalized nuclei and increased esterase staining.

Muscle fibers are of two major types: *type I* and *type II*. The histochemical and physiologic characteristics of each type is determined by the firing rate of the innervating motor neuron (Table 19.1; Figure 19.4; see Color Plate B3).[8,22,23] A motor neuron, its axon, and all muscle fibers innervated by that axon form the motor unit. Muscle fibers of a motor unit are intermixed with fibers of other motor units. Subtypes of the two major types of fiber can be distinguished by special histochemical staining.[24,25]

Table 19.1 Major Skeletal Muscle Fiber Types

	Type I	Type II
Contraction time	Slow (tonic)	Fast (twitch)
Oxidative enzyme content (NADH-TR)	High	Low
Capillary supply	Rich	Poor
Myofibrillar adenosine triphosphatase (pH 9.4)	Low	High
Myofibrillar adenosine triphosphatase (pH 4.3)	High	Low
Glycolytic activity	Low	High
Lipid content	High	Low

NADH-TR = nicotinamide adenine dinucleotide-tetrazolium reductase.

Histologic Analysis of Muscle Biopsy

Muscle biopsies can be studied with several histologic techniques. Frozen sections of approximately 10 μm are stained with hematoxylin and eosin (H&E), modified trichrome, for fat and glycogen, and with histochemical techniques to detect and study, among others, adenosine triphosphatase (ATPase) and the various glycolytic and oxidative enzymes. Muscle biopsies are also useful in determining the presence of inflammation and in the assessment of structural abnormalities, fiber-type distribution, fiber atrophy, and fiber-type grouping. Immunofluorescence techniques can be performed on frozen sections to determine the presence of various muscle proteins and to characterize inflammatory cells.

The fine structure of muscle is analyzed by EM (e.g., the study of some congenital myopathies, such as central core disease [CCD] and rod myopathy, and the assessment of mitochondria and lipid and glycogen content in fibers). Semi-thin or thick sections stained with toluidine blue (see Color Plate B4) are useful to select areas for morphologic studies at the EM level and for quantifying the number of capillaries.

A portion of the muscle biopsy embedded in paraffin allows the analysis of a larger area of muscle within one section and provides a good method to identify

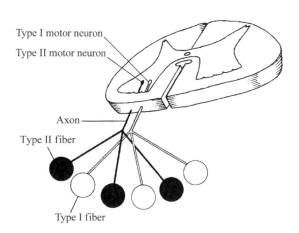

Figure 19.4 Diagram demonstrating motor units of the two major muscle fiber types innervated by different motor neurons. (See Color Plates B3, B11, and B12 for histologic appearance of normal fiber-type distribution.)

Figure 19.5 Myosin-stained section of muscle demonstrates a normal fiber-type distribution. Macrophages in necrotic fibers are also seen in a patient with rhabdomyolysis (original magnification ×200). (This and all other figures are original magnifications.)

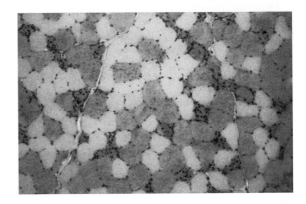

inflammatory cells. Paraffin sections can also be studied by immunohistochemistry to detect, for example, the presence of merosin, dystrophin, and the sarcoglycans, as their absence or deficiency is diagnostic of the various muscular dystrophies. When paraffin-embedded sections are stained with myosin antibodies, they provide excellent fiber-type differentiation (Figure 19.5) and are useful when frozen specimens are not available.[26,27]

Muscle specimens can also be analyzed biochemically to measure glycogen and lipid content and their enzymes and the enzymes of the mitochondrial respiratory chain.

Histologic Studies on Cryostat Sections

The methodology of staining and freezing muscle is not discussed in detail. For this, the reader is referred to excellent muscle histology textbooks.[7,28–30] The following sections detail commonly used stains.

Hematoxylin and Eosin. The H&E stain allows the study of the size and shape of fibers and the number of centrally located nuclei. The stain is also useful in the analysis of connective tissue proliferation or increase in fat between the muscle fibers.

With H&E staining, the muscle fibers appear pink and the nuclei blue (see Color Plate B5). The applications of this and the following stains are summarized in Table 19.2. Regenerating fibers are recognized by their bluish cytoplasm and their centrally located nuclei. Necrosis, phagocytosis, atrophy, hypertrophy, fiber splitting, perifascicular fiber atrophy, and the presence of inflammation, granulomas, or parasites can also be recognized with this stain. Vacuolization can be observed, including the subsarcolemmal vacuoles of glycogen storage disease, the tiny vacuoles of fat accumulation, the so-called empty vacuoles of hypokalemic paralysis, the "punched-out" vacuoles of inflammatory myopathies, and the *rimmed vacuoles* of inclusion-body myopathies and oculopharyngeal dystrophy (Table 19.3). Cores, targets, intramuscular nerves, encapsulated spindles, and myotendinous junctions may also be recognized with H&E.

Modified Gomori Trichrome. The modified trichrome of Engel and Cunningham[31] is also used to study the morphologic characteristics of muscle (see Color Plate B6). In this stain, the fibers are green and the nuclei are red to purple. The technique is particularly helpful in the recognition of *ragged red fibers*, nemaline or rod

Table 19.2 Common Stains for the Study of Muscle

Stain	Uses
Routine histologic stains	
Modified Gomori trichrome	Overall assessment: identification of ragged red fibers, rimmed vacuoles, inclusion bodies, vacuolar changes, tubular aggregates, inflammation, atrophy, degeneration, nemaline rods, cytoplasmic bodies, sarcoplasmic masses, and intramuscular nerves and vessels.
Hematoxylin and eosin	Overall assessment: vasculitis, inflammatory infiltrates, necrosis, regeneration, atrophy, splitting, pyknotic nuclei, vessels, and connective tissue.
Periodic acid–Schiff	Detection of carbohydrates for diagnosing glycogen storage, basement membrane, targets, and ring fibers; type II fibers stain darker.
Congo red	Detection of amyloid in amyloidosis and in the inclusion bodies of inclusion body myositis.
Oil red O and Sudan black B	Assessment of neutral lipids for lipid storage myopathies; type I fibers have more lipid content.
Toluidine blue	Study of muscle structure, counting capillaries, identification of cores, targets, mitochondrial accumulations, and vacuoles—rimmed and others; all fibers stain bluish.
Histochemical stains	
Adenosine triphosphatase	Fiber-type differentiation, fiber-type size and distribution, fiber-type grouping, selective group atrophy, fiber-type predominance; using alkaline pH, type II fibers stain darker; using acid pH type I, fibers stain darker.
Nicotinamide adenine dinucleotide-tetrazolium reductase	Fiber-type differentiation; intermyofibrillar pattern; mitochondrial, endoplasmic reticulum activity, or both; denervation; targets; targetoids; central cores; pale centers; moth-eaten and whorled fibers; tubular aggregates; and lobulated fibers; type I fibers stain dark, type II pale.
Succinic dehydrogenase	As above; specific for mitochondrial activity and for detecting mitochondrial myopathy (increased stain, particularly in ragged red fibers); type I fibers stain dark, type II pale.
Myophosphorylase	Determination of phosphorylase deficiency (McArdle's disease); identification of regenerating fibers and targets; type II fibers stain dark, type I pale.
Nonspecific esterase	Determination of denervation and lysosomal breakdown; identification of end plates; macrophages in necrotic fibers; angular atrophic fibers; type I fibers stain dark, type II pale.
Myoadenylate deaminase	Detection of deaminase deficiency; type I fibers stain dark blue, type II pale.
Menadione-linked α-glycerophosphate dehydrogenase	Detection of menadione deficiency (vitamin K_3); identification of reducing bodies and subtypes in type I predominance; type II fibers stain dark, type I pale.
Acid phosphatase	Detection of increased lysosomal activity (red) in acid maltase deficiency and macrophages in necrotic fibers; all normal fibers stain green.
Alkaline phosphatase	Detection of abnormalities in reactive blood vessels, regenerating capillaries, capillary proliferation, connective tissue, and regenerating myofibers (dark blue); all normal fibers stain yellow.
Phosphofructokinase	Detection of phosphofructokinase deficiency (Tarui's disease); type I fibers stain darker.
Cytochrome oxidase	Detection of cytochrome oxidase deficiency, cytochrome oxidase deficiency–negative ragged red fibers (has a prognostic value in increased numbers in inflammatory myopathy); type I fibers stain darker, type II paler.
Immunohistochemistry	Identification of inflammatory cell types; protein defects (i.e., merosin, dystrophin, and sarcoglycans).

Table 19.3 Muscle Vacuoles

Description	Associated Disease(s)
Subsarcolemmal, PAS+	Glycogen storage disease (especially phosphory-lase and phosphofructokinase) deficiencies
Large, diffuse, subsarcolemmal predilection, PAS+	Debrancher enzyme deficiency
Small, PAS+, diastase resistant or partially sensitive	Polyglucosan body disease (branching enzyme deficiency)
Single or few, membrane bound, in some fibers, empty appearing	Periodic paralysis
Multiple, small, empty, irregular	Sarcotubular myopathy (sarcotubular system dilatation)
Rimmed, basophilic border on hematoxylin and eosin stain, dark red or trichrome	Inclusion body myositis distal dystrophies (i.e., Welander, Nonaka types), oculopharyngeal dystrophy
Multiple, very small, mainly in type I fibers (lipid stains show lipid deposits in the vacuoles)	Lipid storage myopathy (i.e., carnitine deficiency), mitochondrial myopathies (these can also be seen in otherwise normal biopsies that do not have biochemical abnormalities)
Multiple irregular, PAS+, acid phosphatase+, glycogen in lysosomes and cytoplasm	Acid maltase deficiency
"Punched-out" appearance, dilatation of T-tubules	Dermatomyositis (perifascicular area), poly-myositis, T-tubular myopathy
Autophagic, irregular with cellular debris	Chloroquine myopathy, polymyositis, familial vacuolar myopathy
Central, around the nucleus	Adult-onset centronuclear myopathy

+ = positive; PAS = periodic acid–Schiff.
Source: Modified with permission from S Carpenter, G Karpati. Abnormal Organellar Structures in Skeletal Muscles. In Pathology of Skeletal Muscle (2nd ed). Oxford, UK: Oxford University Press, 2001;298.

bodies, rimmed vacuoles, intramuscular nerves, and aggregates of T tubules, all readily distinguished by their appearance and red staining.

Van Gieson's. Van Gieson's stain demonstrates collagen as deep red, whereas the muscle fibers appear yellow, and the nuclei are brown-black. The Verhoeff-Van Gieson modification is useful to demonstrate the elastic lamina in vessels and myelin in nerves.

Phosphotungstic-Acid Hematoxylin. The phosphotungstic-acid hematoxylin stain is another technique used to demonstrate the striation of muscle fibers and nemaline rods as shades of blue.

Oil Red O and Sudan Black B. Either the oil red O or Sudan black B methods are used in the detection of lipid accumulation in muscle fibers. The oil red O stain is based on the principle that the dye is more soluble in lipids, providing easily identifiable red lipid droplets (see Color Plates B7 and B8). The Sudan black B stains lipid a blue-black color.

Periodic Acid–Schiff. The periodic acid–Schiff (PAS) stain detects glycogen accumulation in various glycogen storage diseases (see Color Plate B9). This stain is based on the principle that glycol groups are oxidized by periodic acid to form aldehydes, allowing the colorless Schiff's reagent to impart a magenta color to glycogen. Diastase is added to differentiate glycogen from other PAS-positive substances, such as mucopolysaccharides, which are not digested by this enzyme, whereas glycogen is digested and no longer visible after exposure to diastase.

Congo Red and Crystal Violet. Amyloid accumulation can be detected in paraffin or frozen sections stained with Congo red, staining an apple-green color under a birefringent light or with fluorescent microscopy. Crystal violet stains amyloid a bright magenta color.

Alizarin Red S and von Kossa. Alizarin red S is used to demonstrate calcium within muscle or vessels with a red-orange color (see Color Plate B10). The von Kossa stains calcium accumulations black.

Myofibrillar Adenosine Triphosphatase. Fiber-type differentiation and distribution are best demonstrated with the myofibrillar ATPase (see Color Plates B3 and B11). This histochemical stain depends on a complex series of reactions. First, the section of tissue is incubated with adenosine triphosphate (ATP) and calcium. ATPase splits the terminal phosphate from ATP, which combines with calcium to form calcium phosphate. Then, the specimen is incubated with cobalt chloride, and cobalt is exchanged with calcium, forming cobaltous phosphate at the site of calcium deposition. The section is then placed in ammonium sulfide to form black cobaltous sulfide.

ATPase incubated at pH 9.4 allows the fixation of calcium, as Ca phosphate is insoluble at alkaline pH, and this is localized at the site of enzyme activity. The type I fibers appear pale, whereas type II fibers are dark. A more acidic incubation at pH 4.3 or 4.6 produces differentiation of the type II fibers into the subtypes due to the inhibitory influence of acid pH on ATPase activity (see Color Plate B11).[28–30]

Nicotinamide Adenine Dinucleotide-Tetrazolium Reductase. The nicotinamide adenine dinucleotide-tetrazolium reductase (NADH-TR) stain allows the demonstration of oxidative activity in the mitochondria and endoplasmic reticulum. NADH is a coenzyme that transfers hydrogen to an acceptor (insoluble tetrazolium salt) that turns dark blue when reduced. This reaction is catalyzed by the muscle flavin system.[32] The darker type I fibers have more oxidative capacity (see Color Plate B12). Increased oxidative staining is useful to demonstrate accumulations of mitochondria, tubular aggregates, target fibers, and cores.

Succinic Dehydrogenase. The succinic dehydrogenase (SDH) stain is specific for mitochondria and is useful in the detection of increased mitochondrial oxidative activity. This method is based on the ability of SDH to remove hydrogen from a substrate, succinate, which is converted to fumarate. The released hydrogen then reduces the tetrazolium salt, producing deposits at the site of the enzyme activity. The type I muscle fibers have more oxidative capacity and stain darker than the type II fibers (see Color Plate B13).

Cytochrome Oxidase. Cytochrome oxidase (COX) is an enzyme selective for cytochromes, which are proteins that transfer electrons in the respiratory chain in mitochondria. The histochemical method uses cytochrome-c and diaminobenzidine to produce brown staining at the site of enzyme activity, with type I fibers staining darker (see Color Plate B14).

Myoadenylate Deaminase. The myoadenylate deaminase technique is used to detect a deficiency of this enzyme that converts adenosine monophosphate (AMP) to inosine monophosphate, an alkylogenic hydrolytic reaction that reduces tetrazolium by dithiothreitol (see Color Plate B15). In normal tissue, the type I fibers appear blue, and the type II fibers are a pale pink.[33,34] Muscle deficient in this enzyme has no stain reaction and, therefore, no color or decreased staining.

Myophosphorylase. The myophosphorylase stain imparts a pale blue or a light brown coloration to type I fibers and a dark bluish-purple or brown to type II fibers, which have more glycogen and phosphorylase activity. The stain is useful in determining the absence of myophosphorylase in McArdle's disease. Necrotic fibers appear pale. The methods stain active and inactive phosphorylase by the addition of AMP. Phosphorylase catalyzes the hydrolysis and synthesis of amylase-type molecules and is based on the reaction (1,4-α–D-glucosyl) n + orthophosphate $\rightleftarrows$ (1,4-α-D-glucosyl) n_{-1} + D-glucose-1-phosphate. The equilibrium of this reaction is dependent on the pH. A low pH transfers glycosyl residues to the glucosyl chain, which stains with iodine, and its color increases with the length of the chain. The stain has the disadvantage of fading with storage (see Color Plates B16 and B17).[29,30,32]

Phosphofructokinase. Staining for phosphofructokinase allows the determination of the presence or absence of this enzyme. Fructose-6-phosphate is converted to lactic acid in the Embden-Meyerhof pathway, generating NADH. During incubation of the tissue with fructose-6-phosphate, NADH reduces the nitroblue tetrazolium to blue formazan, which stains type I muscle fibers a darker blue than type II fibers (see Color Plate B18).[29,30]

Acid Phosphatase and Alkaline Phosphatase. Acid phosphatase is localized mainly in lysosomes, and the stain detects the bright red color of increased activity of this enzyme in the lysosomes, as appreciated in some conditions such as acid maltase deficiency. Macrophages in necrotic fibers also stain positive. This is not present in normal muscle, which stains green with the methyl green counterstain. The staining is based on the hydrolysis of the substrate with naphthol (during the first reaction), which is then combined in a second reaction with a diazonium salt at the site of enzyme activity (see Color Plate B19).

Alkaline phosphatase is present in cell membranes, particularly the endothelium of vessels, and in the endoplasmic reticulum. The stain is based on the hydrolysis of naphthol to produce an insoluble naphthol that couples with a diazonium salt to impart a dark staining insoluble azo dye at the site of activity (see Color Plate B20). Normal muscle does not stain positive, but there is increased alkaline phosphatase activity in necrotic fibers and in regenerating capillaries.

Nonspecific Esterase and Acetylcholinesterase. The nonspecific esterase reaction occurs when esterases hydrolyze α-naphthyl acetate to form α-naphthol, which when combined with a diazonium salt produces an insoluble azo dye. The reaction is present as dark staining at the site of enzyme activity, such as the end plates (see Color Plate B1) and myotendinous junction. Atrophic denervated fibers appear dark with this stain (see Color Plate B21), differentiating them from atrophy due to other causes, such as disuse, in which the atrophic fibers do not stain dark. The acetylcholinesterase method stains neuromuscular junctions and is used in conjunction with methylene blue or silver stains to visualize the terminal axons also (see Color Plate B22).

Other Staining Methods

Methyl Green Pyronine. Methyl green pyronine can demonstrate increased RNA in regenerating fibers.

Lactate Dehydrogenase and Menadione-Mediated α-Glycerophosphate Dehydrogenase. Staining for lactate dehydrogenase (LDH) is useful in differentiating type I fiber subtypes and determining whether there is a deficiency of LDH. Staining with menadione-mediated α-glycerophosphate dehydrogenase is another method valuable in differentiating fiber types and type I fiber subtypes (see Color Plate B23).

Immunohistochemistry

With the ability to produce monoclonal antibodies against various muscle proteins, immunohistochemical techniques are now used routinely in the evaluation of various myopathies, particularly the muscular dystrophies, for which they have become the most important diagnostic tool. These methods also allow for the differentiation of inflammatory cells and complements. These techniques are reviewed in detail elsewhere.[35,36]

Immunohistochemical studies can be performed on cryostat sections or on paraffin-embedded specimens.[34] The techniques can also be applied to EM. Immunohistochemistry localizes the chosen antigens that react with their corresponding antibody (i.e., staining human muscle dystrophin with mouse antidystrophin primary Ig [immunoglobulin] G antibodies). Most staining methods use a secondary antibody against the primary antibody (indirect method), such as rabbit antimouse IgG antibodies conjugated with a visible marker such as a fluorochrome, a metal, or enzyme (e.g., peroxidase). Thus, the secondary antibody and its marker are localized at the site of the primary antibody deposition. In immunohistochemistry, two types of methods are used: immunofluorescence and those that use insoluble reactants like peroxidase (see Color Plate B24).

Immunofluorescence

Immunofluorescence uses fluorescent compounds (fluorescein, isothiocyanate, rhodamine conjugates, or Texas red) as markers of the antigen/antibody reaction.

These markers are very sensitive, but background fluorescence can be detected. They can be applied to frozen but not paraffin sections, and the reaction fades relatively easily.

Antibody-Enzyme Conjugates

Antibodies can be conjugated to enzymes, such as peroxidase, to produce insoluble reactions that can be applied to frozen and paraffin sections. These methods use diaminobenzidine for staining, and the intensity can be increased with the inclusion of imidazoles.[35] Glucose oxidase, galactosidase, and alkaline phosphatase can also be used.

Amplification

Amplification techniques are applied to enhance the intensity of weak staining (e.g., the avidin/biotin and the enzyme-antienzyme systems). The most widely used are the peroxidase-antiperoxidase and the gold-silver techniques.

The avidin/biotin method is based on the rapid conjugation of the egg-white avidin with the egg-yolk vitamin biotin.[37] The primary antibody is usually mouse IgG antibodies to the protein of interest (i.e., dystrophin, conjugated to avidin and then reacted with dystrophin in the specimen). The secondary antimouse antibody is tagged with biotin or "biotinylated" and reacted with the avidin to produce a large molecule that is visualized with a marker such as peroxidase.

The peroxidase-antiperoxidase method uses peroxidase with antibodies against peroxidase of the same species as the primary antibody.[35,38] Similar methods are used in conjunction with electron markers (colloidal gold) that produce an electron-dense product with osmium for EM studies.

Artifacts and Normal Structures Seen Infrequently in Muscle Biopsy

A common artifact in frozen sections occurs with slow freezing of muscle, which causes ice crystals to form in the myofibrils, making rounded holes that have a vacuolated appearance under the microscope (Figure 19.6A). This occurs particularly if the specimen is transported on regular ice, causing it to slowly freeze, or if the quick-freezing process is carried out too slowly by the technician. Stretching during surgery can produce an excessive number of over-contracted fibers and a distortion of fibers.

Another common artifact is caused by a blunt knife, which tears or splits and cracks the myofibrils (see Color Plate B10). Folding or "crusting" is also caused by improper drying, placing the specimen on the slide, or removing it from the knife (see Figure 19.6B). Uneven coloration with trichrome is produced by improper differentiation during staining or by the use of blunt knives.[6]

Artifacts on EM are commonly produced by mishandling of the specimen during biopsy or overhandling when preparing the biopsy for fixation. The traumatized muscle may show disruption of the myofibrils and the falsely apparent accumulations of glycogen in the periphery of the fibers owing to contraction. Contraction of the myofibrils can also cause abnormal appearance of the Z line and an inability to obtain true

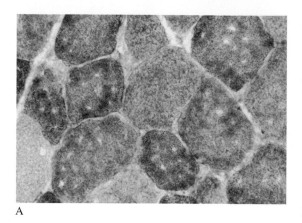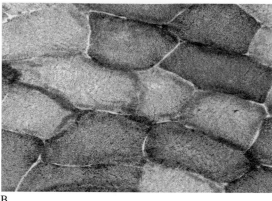

A   B

Figure 19.6 A. Freezing artifacts, appearing as irregular holes within fibers. **B.** "Crusting" or overlapping of fibers, an artifact that occurs during placement of the specimen on the slide **(A)** and **(B)** (×250, modified trichrome).

longitudinal or cross-sectional cuts of the muscle, inhibiting the proper analysis of EM organelles. Overfixation or dehydration of specimens can produce shrinkage artifacts.

The interpreter of a muscle biopsy should recognize not only artifacts but also normal structures (nerves, spindles) (see Color Plates B1, B3, and B6) that are not seen in all specimens. Also, normal morphologic variations should not be mistaken for pathologic abnormalities. One example is the increase in internalized nuclei, small fibers, and connective tissue at the myotendinous junction (see Color Plate B2).

MUSCLE BIOPSY FINDINGS IN NEUROGENIC DISEASES

The most characteristic change of neurogenic disease and denervation is the presence of atrophic angular fibers that have more intense staining with ATPase and oxidative techniques (Figure 19.7). These fibers also stain intensively positive with nonspecific esterase (see Color Plate B21); this could be caused by increased cholinesterase

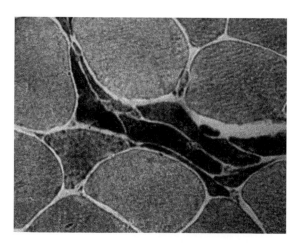

Figure 19.7 Dark-staining atrophic, angular denervated fibers of neurogenic disease (nicotinamide adenine dinucleotide-tetrazolium reductase, ×250).

Figure 19.8 Prominent pyknotic nuclei in a patient with a chronic motor neuron disease (hematoxylin and eosin, ×250).

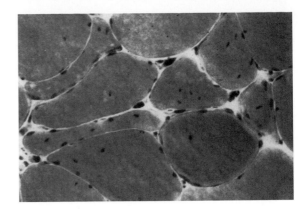

activity, which correlates with the diffuse, extrajunctional acetylcholine receptor found in denervated muscle.[39] These fibers maintain their ATPase-staining characteristics; they stain pale with PAs and phosphorylase and dark with oxidative stains.

Other changes include the presence of frequent pyknotic nuclei (Figure 19.8) and target fibers (Table 19.4). Target fibers have three concentric zones. A central pale zone is seen in the oxidative stains and ATPase. This is surrounded by a darkly stained area seen on oxidative stains; outside this is the normally staining portion of the muscle fiber. This is observed particularly well with the NADH-TR method (Figure 19.9).[40,41] Targets are also visible in the H&E, trichrome, ATPase, and phosphotungstic-acid hematoxylin stains. Target fibers occur mainly in type I muscle fibers. Targetoid fibers are similar to targets but do not have the distinct, dark-staining ring around the pale center; these are also sometimes seen in myopathies.

Reinnervation is recognized histologically as fiber-type grouping, which is characterized by clusters of both fiber types and a loss of the normal, almost checkerboard pattern of fiber distribution (Figure 19.10).[42] The presence of grouping is analyzed qualitatively by the experienced reader, but special methods can also be applied. Fiber-type grouping should be differentiated from fiber-type predominance,

Table 19.4 Histologic Changes in Muscle Biopsy Found Predominantly in Neurogenic Disease and Myopathies[a]

Neurogenic Disease	Myopathy
Atrophic, esterase-positive angular fibers	Necrosis, phagocytosis
Targets; targetoids	Regenerating fibers
Large fiber-type grouping	Round atrophic and hypertrophic fibers (variation in fiber size); fiber splitting
Group atrophy	Internalized nuclei and capillaries; lobulated fibers
Pyknotic nuclei[b]	Proliferation of endomysial connective tissue and fat
	Specific fiber abnormalities (e.g., ragged red fibers, storage, inflammation, vacuoles, protein deficiencies)

[a]Some of these can be seen in both myopathies and neurogenic diseases; the prominence of the findings would suggest one or the other in diagnosis.
[b]Can be prominent in some myopathies as well (e.g., myotonic dystrophy).

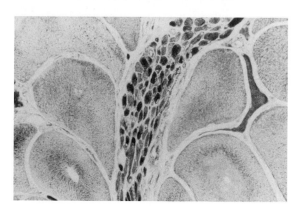

Figure 19.9 "Target" fibers and a group of very atrophic fibers. Notice also an angular, atrophic fiber (nicotinamide adenine dinucleotide-tetrazolium reductase, ×250).

which is seen in various chronic neuromuscular diseases, especially in congenital myopathies. In grouping, clusters of both types should be present.

Group atrophy is described as clustering of atrophic fibers of the same type (see Figure 19.9; Figure 19.11). This is probably due to denervation of a group of fibers of the same type that cluster together after reinnervation, but it can, however, also occur owing to denervation by dropout of several motor units simultaneously.

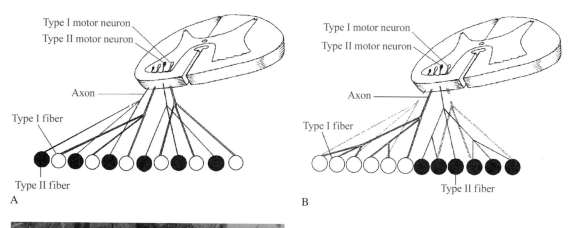

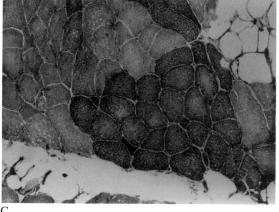

Figure 19.10 A. Diagram of the origin of fiber-type grouping. Normal innervation of type I and type II fibers. **B.** After damage of nerves or axons, the surviving nerves sprout and reinnervate the previously denervated fibers, causing grouping. **C.** Fiber grouping in nicotinamide adenine dinucleotide-tetrazolium reductase stain (×200).

Figure 19.11 Fiber-type grouping, group atrophy, and targets (adenosine triphosphatase, pH 9.4, ×200).

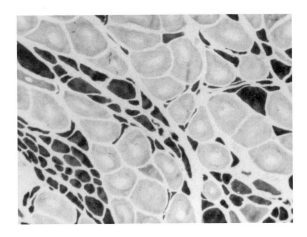

Selective atrophy of type II fibers (Figure 19.12), particularly of type IIb, which are not denervated and do not stain dark with esterase, is seen in steroid-induced muscle weakness or disuse. A selective type I atrophy is seen in several congenital myopathies and in myotonic dystrophy (Table 19.5).

"Myopathic" changes can also sometimes be seen in chronic denervated muscle. These include, for example, hypertrophy, fiber splitting, and internalized nuclei.

In infantile spinal muscular atrophy or Werdnig-Hoffman disease (see Color Plate B25), the denervated fibers do not appear angulated but are usually round. They stain dark with nonspecific esterase and are characteristically accompanied by hypertrophy, mostly of type I muscle fibers.[43]

Quantitation of Fiber Types and of Fiber-Type Distribution

As discussed, muscle fibers of the two major types are arranged in an almost checkerboard distribution with some variation and a predominance of one type in some muscles (Table 19.6).[44,45] There are also variations among individuals, some due to training as in weight lifting,[46] and there can be variation within the muscle in different layers.[47]

The type I fiber predominance observed in some neuromuscular disorders could be secondary to the change of activity of the muscle or to a paucity of type II motor

Figure 19.12 Type II fiber atrophy in a patient with steroid myopathy (adenosine triphosphatase, pH 9.4, ×200).

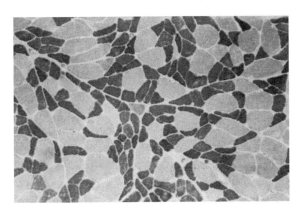

Table 19.5 Conditions Associated with Selective Atrophy by Muscle Fiber Types

Type I	Type II
Myotubular myopathy	Disuse atrophy and myasthenia gravis
Nemaline myopathy	Cachexia
Myotonic dystrophy	Steroid myopathy and Cushing's disease
Congenital fiber-type disproportion	Other endocrine abnormalities (i.e., hyperparathyroidism)

neurons. In some, the type I fiber predominance contains a normal distribution of the type I fiber subtypes, which are recognized by some stains such as the menadione-mediated α-glycerophosphate dehydrogenase.[24,25] Fiber predominance could also be secondary to reinnervation (e.g., after recovery from acute poliomyelitis in which single surviving motor neurons incorporate a larger number of fibers). Grouping can be assessed qualitatively or by quantitative methods using histochemical stains, particularly the ATPase.[48] These are described below.

Enclosed Fiber

The method of assessing the number of fibers enclosed by fibers of the same type is useful to determine whether there are clusters of either fiber type.[49,50] An enclosed fiber is a fiber surrounded by approximately seven fibers of the same type. This analysis is performed on ATPase stains at pH 9.4. This and other methods are discussed in detail elsewhere.[51]

"Runs" Method

Also using the ATPase stain, a line is drawn randomly across a photograph of the specimen, and then the number of fibers of the same type crossed by the line is determined. An increased number of muscle fibers of one type sequentially crossed by the line indicates grouping, which can be quantitated.[52]

Codispersion Index

In the codispersion index technique, a fiber is selected randomly and called the *index fiber*. A line is drawn from the center of this fiber to the adjacent fiber with the shortest distance to the index fiber. Then, a table is made of the number of connections of type I to type I, type I to type II, type II to type I, and type II to type II. Next, the

Table 19.6 Percentage of Fiber Types in Superficial Layers of Frequently Biopsied Muscles

Muscle	Type I (%)	95% Confidence Level (%)	Type II (%)	95% Confidence Level (%)
Biceps	42.3	33.9–50.7	57.7	49.3–66.2
Superficial deltoid	53.3	43.4–63.2	46.7	36.8–56.7
Vastus lateralis	37.8	19.6–45.8	67.3	52.1–72.3

Source: Summarized from MA Johnson, J Polgar, D Weightman, D Appleton. Data on the distribution of fiber types in thirty-six human muscles. An autopsy study. J Neurol Sci 1973;18:111–124.

codispersion index is calculated by chi square statistics. If more fibers of the same type are neighboring each other, this indicates clustering.[53,54]

Prop I (Type I), Prop II (Type II) Method

In the Prop I (Type I), Prop II (Type II) method,[47] the mean fiber diameter is assessed first. Then, circles of twice the mean diameter are drawn around all fibers. The number of fibers of the same type within the circle is calculated. Circles that contain more than four fibers of the same type of the center fiber are counted for both fiber types. This number is divided by the total number of circled fiber type and multiplied by 100 to calculate their percentage.

Point-Sommet Method

A point sommet, or triad, is a point where three fibers meet. This method determines how many triads of the same or different fiber type are present. An increased number of triads of both fiber types indicates fiber-type groupings.[55]

MUSCLE BIOPSY FINDINGS IN MYOPATHIES

The most distinctive finding of primary myopathy on muscle biopsy is the presence of necrotic fibers, also referred to as *degenerated fibers*. In histochemical preparations, these fibers appear pale (Figure 19.13; see Table 19.4). They may have decreased staining with ATPase and PAS, and may have a granular appearance in oxidative and calcium stains. These fibers also demonstrate increased alkaline and acid phosphatase activity. The necrotic fibers may be undergoing phagocytosis (Figure 19.14). The macrophages in these fibers are identified by their dark appearance with the nonspecific esterase stain (see Color Plate B26) and are easily recognized on EM.

Necrotic fibers can have autophagic vacuoles and show degenerative mitochondria with disruption of the Z lines on EM. They might also have gaps in the plasma membrane, with disrupted myofilaments in these areas.

Figure 19.13 Necrotic fibers appear pale on hematoxylin and eosin (×250).

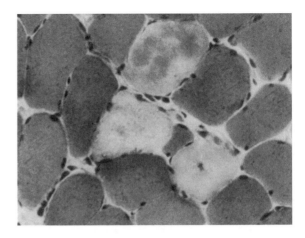

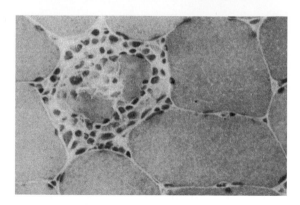

Figure 19.14 Phagocytosis of a necrotic fiber (modified trichrome, ×250).

Regenerating muscle fibers are recognized by their blue cytoplasm in the H&E and trichrome stains and by centrally located nuclei with prominent nucleoli (Figure 19.15; see Color Plate B27).

Opaque, "overcontracted," "hypercontracted," or hyaline fibers stain dark with most histochemical stains. These fibers are commonly seen in Duchenne's muscular dystrophy (DMD) but can be found in other myopathies, possibly representing a prenecrotic state. In myopathies, opaque fibers are distributed throughout the specimen; their presence only in the border of fascicles could be artifactual, caused by trauma during the biopsy.

Scattered, round atrophic fibers are also seen in myopathies, but most do not stain dark with nonspecific esterase. They are frequently accompanied by *fiber hypertrophy* and *fiber splitting*, which is seen first as a partial and then as a complete division of the myofiber, occurring mainly in hypertrophic fibers, accompanied by an increase in the number of internalized nuclei and capillaries (Figure 19.16).[56] Splitting can produce clusters of small fibers of the same type or "small fiber-type grouping."

Proliferation of endomysial connective tissue and fat is common in myopathies, especially in advanced cases (Figure 19.17). Other histologic features that can be seen in these diseases include *sarcoplasmic masses*, eosinophilic *cytoplasmic bodies* (Figure 19.18), *whorled* and *ring fibers* (Figure 19.19A,B; see Color Plate B28), *pale centers*, *moth-eaten fibers* (see Figure 19.19C), and *lobulated fibers*.

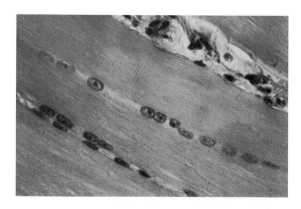

Figure 19.15 Longitudinal section of a basophilic regenerating muscle fiber with centrally located vesicular nuclei with prominent nucleoli (modified trichrome, ×400) (see Color Plate B27).

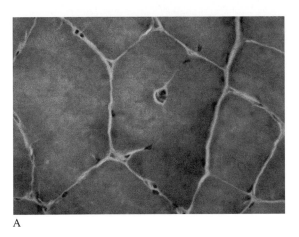
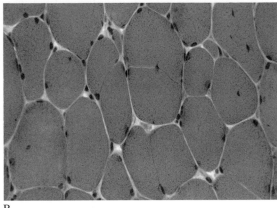

A   B

Figure 19.16 A. Fiber splitting and an internalized nucleus and capillary in a hypertrophic fiber (modified trichrome, ×400). **B.** Fiber splitting and internalized nuclei (hematoxylin and eosin, ×250).

Ring fibers are those in which the fiber's outer aspect loses its longitudinal orientation and wraps around the inner fibrils, forming a ring. Whorled fibers have a more disorganized pattern of the fibrils and are often large. *Moth-eaten fibers* are those that have patchy, decreased oxidative staining, whereas lobulated fibers have increased oxidative staining in the borders of the fibers. *Sarcoplasmic masses* are accumulations of sarcoplasm that have disorganized filaments on EM. *Cytoplasmic bodies* have an eosinophilic center and appear red on trichrome staining. EM shows this to be formed by accumulations of filaments. Myeloid bodies, degenerating mitochondria, honeycomb inclusions, duplication of basal lamina, and myofibril streaming can also be identified on EM in myopathies. Other findings are specific for certain diseases, such as glycogen or lipid accumulations, vacuoles, or ragged red fibers.

Mild fiber atrophy and hypertrophy of otherwise normal-appearing fibers are recognized as variation in fiber size, which is a pathologic feature of myopathy. However,

Figure 19.17 Hypertrophic muscle fiber with increased fat and connective tissue between the fibers in an end-stage muscle (modified trichrome, ×400).

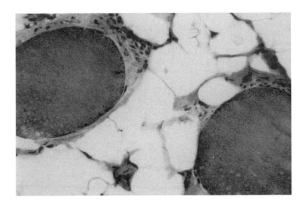

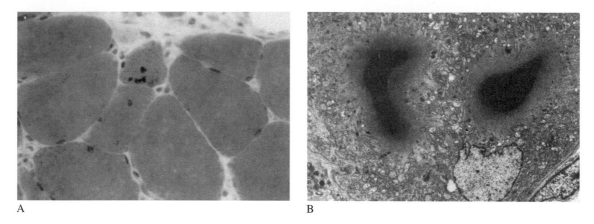

A   B

Figure 19.18 Small, dense areas within a fiber are nonspecific cytoplasmic bodies. **A.** Light level (modified trichrome-stained muscle, ×250) and **(B)** electron microscopy (×6,480).

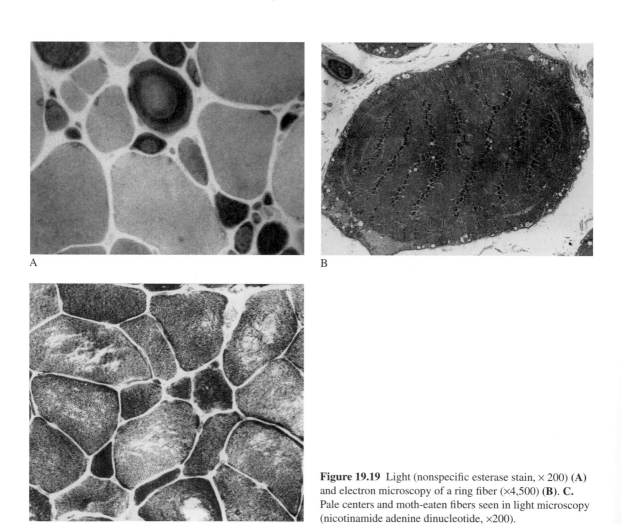

A   B

C

Figure 19.19 Light (nonspecific esterase stain, × 200) **(A)** and electron microscopy of a ring fiber (×4,500) **(B)**. **C.** Pale centers and moth-eaten fibers seen in light microscopy (nicotinamide adenine dinucleotide, ×200).

this terminology is not appropriate, because variation in fiber size can also be seen in neurogenic disease from atrophic, angular fibers. Table 19.4 outlines the prominent findings in the two groups of diseases in general terms. This is also an oversimplification, as "myopathic changes" can be seen in neuropathies, and "neurogenic changes," such as atrophic angular fibers and small groups, can be seen in myopathies.

Quantitation of Fiber Diameter

Evaluation of muscle fiber size is used to determine whether there is generalized atrophy or hypertrophy or whether it is selective for either fiber type (see Table 19.5). Routinely, this is done with qualitative assessment during biopsy reading or using more strict quantitative methods that are more important in clinical research studies (e.g., to determine the effect of training).

Muscle fiber size is best assessed by determining the fiber area using histographic techniques or by calculating fiber diameter with calibrated eye pieces in the microscope, with the use of a planimeter on projected images or by measuring directly from photographs. Fiber size varies according to age, gender, and the muscle studied.

Detailed measurements have been reported by various authors. Among them, Polgar et al.[57] studied 36 muscles of normal autopsies; Brooke and Engel[58] determined muscle fiber diameter in men and women; and Bell and Jacobs[59] found that type IIA fibers are larger in male body builders.

Fiber size is determined by measuring the maximum diameter across the lesser aspect of the muscle fiber,[60,61] which is the larger "minor axis" or second largest diameter of the fiber in a transverse section. With this information, a histogram of each fiber type can be made. To assess the severity of these abnormalities in each fiber type, determination of the degree of atrophy or hypertrophy and of the "atrophic" and "hypertrophic" factors is calculated as follows: If we consider, for example, that the normal type I fibers in men have a diameter of 40–80 μm, then the lower limit of normal is 40 μm, and fibers that measure from 30–40 μm are multiplied by 1 (lesser atrophy and lesser effect on the overall diameter); those that measure 20–30 μm are multiplied by 2; those that measure 10–20 microns are multiplied by 3; and those that measure less than 10 microns are multiplied by 4 (most atrophic). Then all products are added and divided by the number of fibers counted, and the results are multiplied by 1,000.[62]

The hypertrophic factor is determined similarly by multiplying the number of fibers from 80 to 90 μm by 1, 90–100 μm by 2, etc. Then the numbers are added and divided by the number of fibers counted, and this is multiplied by 1,000.

Statistical determination of the standard deviation (SD) of fiber size is another measure of variability (the normal SD is less than 10 μm). This is also determined by the variability coefficient, which is calculated by multiplying the SD by 1,000 and dividing the product by the mean diameter (SD × 1,000/fiber diameter). A variability coefficient of more than 250 indicates abnormal variation in fiber size.[4]

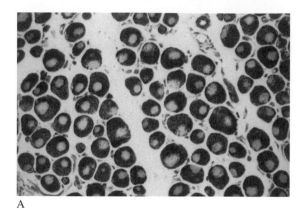

A

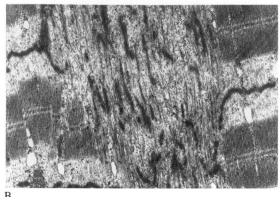

B

Figure 19.20 A. Central cores, the pale areas in the center of muscle fibers of a patient with central core disease (nicotinamide adenine dinucleotide-tetrazolium reductase, ×250). **B.** On electron microscopy, there is disorganization of the myofibrils and Z-band streaming (×34,580).

Histologic Findings in Specific Diseases

Congenital Myopathies

Congenital myopathies are disorders that are frequently hereditary and manifest at birth or in early infancy with floppy infants. The most important method for their diagnosis is to identify their specific characteristics on muscle biopsy.

Central Core Disease. CCD is an autosomal dominant myopathy that was initially described by Shy and Magee.[63] The disease manifests in early childhood with weakness and skeletal deformities and has a relatively benign course. Patients may be predisposed to malignant hyperthermia (MH), a disease that is allelic.[64,65]

Muscle biopsy in CCD shows areas devoid of oxidative staining, usually in the center or near the center of the fibers (core), giving the disease its name (Figure 19.20A). Cores differ from the targets of neurogenic disease in that cores have no variation in the staining pattern around the pale center. On EM studies, these pale areas lack mitochondria, and the myofilaments appear to be disorganized (unstructured cores) (see Figure 19.20B); in some cores, the myofilament pattern is not distorted (structured cores). Cores can be identified on the PAS and H&E stains, but are more prominent with NADH-TR and other oxidative stains.[66]

CCD frequently shows a type I fiber predominance on muscle biopsy, although there is no evidence of fiber-type grouping.[25] As the disease progresses, the variation in fiber size and the number of internalized nuclei may become more obvious and may be accompanied by increased connective tissue. Biopsy of the genetically affected parent, who can be asymptomatic, might reveal a type I fiber predominance, but cores may not be present. Details of the genetics of this and other hereditary diseases are discussed in Chapter 20.

Minicore or Multicore Disease. Minicore or multicore disease has a variable clinical presentation. Some affected children present as floppy babies, whereas others appear normal at birth. Delayed motor milestones with skeletal abnormal-

Figure 19.21 Multiple, small, pale areas (minicores) in a longitudinal section of muscle in minicore disease (plastic embedded, toluidine blue, ×400).

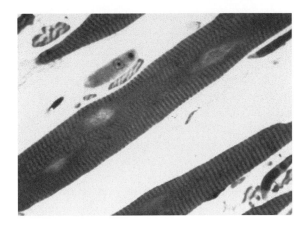

ities and somewhat slow progression are common. The disease is characterized on muscle biopsy by the presence of multiple, small areas that do not stain with oxidative methods (minicores), wherein the myofibrils are disrupted on EM (Figure 19.21).[67–69]

Nemaline or Rod Myopathy. Nemaline or rod myopathy is another congenital myopathy that was initially described by Shy et al.[70] These patients have weakness, hypotonia, elongated face, and skeletal abnormalities. In most cases, the disease has an autosomal dominant inheritance with low penetrance.[71,72] The name is derived from the Greek word *nema*, meaning *thread*, because of the presence of rod-like structures or "nemaline" bodies on muscle fibers that stain a dark red color with the modified trichrome stain (Figure 19.22A). These are difficult to see on H&E and oxidative stains and appear as pale areas with ATPase. The rods have no specific location within a fiber, although they are frequently found in subsarcolemmal areas

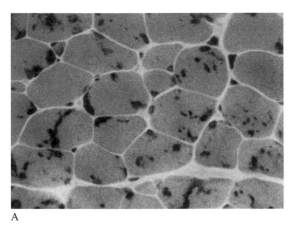

A

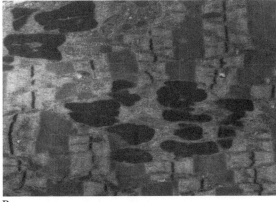

B

Figure 19.22 Dark-staining "rods" in a patient with nemaline or rod myopathy: modified trichrome (×250) **(A)**; electron microscopy (×9,120) **(B)**.

and might occur in the nuclei in severe cases. They appear refractile on phase contrast microscopy and, on EM, have a consistent periodicity. Their ultrastructure is similar to the Z line and may be continuous with the normal Z lines (see Figure 19.22B). The main protein constituent of the rods is α-actinin.[72]

Other histologic findings of nemaline myopathy are internalized nuclei, fiber atrophy, and type I fiber predominance. Central cores may occasionally be seen. Rods are found in the biopsies of adults who manifest with a slowly progressive myopathy called "adult rod myopathy"[73,74]; they are also seen after tenotomy and in thyroid myopathy, schizophrenia, and human immunodeficiency virus (HIV)–infected patients with myositis.

Centronuclear and Myotubular Myopathy. Myotubular myopathy, a disease initially described by Spiro et al.,[75] is characterized by distal and proximal weakness with dysmorphic features, accompanied by elongated face and ptosis. The disease manifests at birth, although late infantile, childhood, and adult forms have been described.[76–79] Some patients have ophthalmoplegia and facial diplegia.

The muscle biopsy is characterized by fiber atrophy, many with centrally located nuclei that resemble myotubes (Figure 19.23). There can be a type I fiber predominance. Oxidative staining shows decreased activity in the central zone around the nuclei. Other nonspecific changes are increased endomysial connective tissue and fiber necrosis.

A severe, X-linked form of myotubular myopathy manifests as the floppy infant syndrome with respiratory insufficiency.[80] The muscle biopsy shows fairly normal-appearing fibers with centrally located nuclei and central accumulations of glycogen and mitochondria. Some atrophic type I fibers may have areas of myofibril disruption. The disease is caused by a gene defect in chromosome Xp28 that expresses a protein called *myotubularin*.[81]

The use of the name *myotubular myopathy* has been questioned, as the atrophic fibers differ from the myotubes; thus, the term *centronuclear myopathy* is used.[78,82] In some cases, the abundant central nuclei can be seen mainly in the atrophic type I muscle fibers; for these, the descriptive name *type I fiber hypotrophy with central nuclei* has been proposed.[79] The term *myotubular myopathy* is usually reserved by others for the description of the X-linked infantile form of the disease.

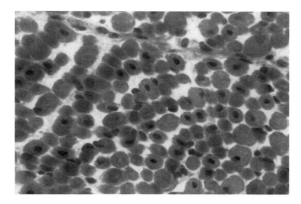

Figure 19.23 Muscle biopsy of an infant with X-linked recessive myotubular myopathy. Notice the tiny muscle fibers and the centrally located nuclei (modified trichrome, ×200).

Figure 19.24 Selective atrophy of type I muscle fibers in congenital fiber-type disproportion (nicotinamide adenine dinucleotide-tetrazolium reductase, ×250). Rare fibers have pale centers.

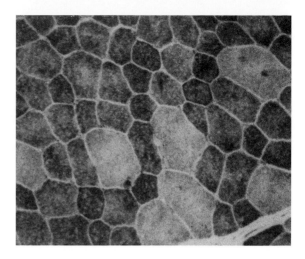

Congenital Fiber-Type Disproportion. Congenital fiber-type disproportion was reported in 1973 by Brooke[83] as a disease of children with elongated faces and "floppy" muscles, accompanied by contractures, generalized weakness, and respiratory insufficiency. The presentation is variable and often has a relatively benign course, but more severe and progressive forms occur. The mode of inheritance is unclear, although in some cases it appears to be autosomal dominant.[84,85]

The muscle biopsy of this condition shows type I fiber atrophy and a type I fiber predominance, without evidence of fiber-type grouping (Figure 19.24). Occasional fibers have internalized nuclei, but no other structural abnormalities, such as cores or rods. The histologic findings are similar to other neuromuscular disorders (i.e., myotonic dystrophy). Fiber-type disproportion might not represent a true separate disease entity, as the diagnosis of congenital fiber-type disproportion has been made in children that were later found to have other well-characterized myopathies.

Desmin Myopathy or Myofibrillar Myopathy. Desmin is a 50,000–molecular weight intermediate filament that forms a honeycomb network around myofibrils and Z disks. Desmin myopathies are those in which the main pathologic findings are structural changes and accumulations of myofilaments, particularly desmin, as determined by special staining for this protein. The clinical presentation is variable, and some patients also have cardiomyopathy and distal weakness. Genetic defects for desmin and α-B crystallin have been associated with the disease. Desmin can accumulate focally in myofibers in a number of pathologic muscle conditions, such as those with cytoplasmic bodies, and can even be found in atrophic fibers in spinal muscular atrophy. Thus, abnormal desmin accumulation in a muscle biopsy does not necessarily indicate an etiologic role.[86] Furthermore, because the biopsy may also show accumulations of other filamentous proteins, the disease may be better named *myofibrillar myopathy*.

Fingerprint Myopathy. Fingerprint myopathy is another disease of early childhood with a progressive course characterized by the presence on EM of concentric lamellae arranged in patterns resembling fingerprints that are localized in the subsarcolemmal areas and near the nucleus of muscles. These occur in more than 50% of fibers, appear eosinophilic on H&E and green on modified trichrome, and are found mainly in type I fibers.[87]

Sarcotubular Myopathy. Sarcotubular myopathy is an infantile myopathy, characterized histologically by the presence of membrane-bound vesicles only in type II muscle fibers. The membranes seem to represent dilated sarcoplasmic reticulum.[88]

Reducing Body Myopathy. Reducing body myopathy is a disease of variable presentation, but it manifests most frequently as floppy infants with delayed motor milestones. The muscle biopsy is characterized by purple areas on H&E that are pink on trichrome staining and are found in the subsarcolemmal areas or occupying large areas of the muscle fibers. These do not stain with routine oxidative or ATPase stains; they do, however, reduce the nitroblue tetrazolium and stain dark with the menadione stain.[89,90]

Cytoplasmic Body Myopathy. This condition may begin in early childhood with weakness that can be minimally progressive or severe. There is also a late onset presentation with distal weakness in the hands that later becomes generalized.[91,92]

Although cytoplasmic bodies can be found in rare muscle fibers in a variety of diseases, they are numerous in cytoplasmic body myopathy—thus the origin of the name. These structures are from 2 to 5 μm and usually appear in the subsarcolemmal area, staining red with trichrome. On EM, the bodies are dense, osmiophilic clusters surrounded by loosely packed proteins (see Figure 19.18),[92] and they are bound by osmiophilic material that might originate from the Z disk.

Spheroid bodies are numerous, small green masses on trichrome staining, which are similar to cytoplasmic bodies on EM but have a central area of osmiophilic material. A myopathy with abundant spheroid bodies has been reported.[93] These appear to represent accumulations of desmin; therefore, spheroid body myopathies could be considered desmin or myofibrillar myopathies, as discussed previously.

Hyaline Body Myopathy. Hyaline body myopathy[94] is a familial disease of relatively benign, nonprogressive course that presents as floppy infant syndrome. In the biopsy, the hyaline areas appear pale on trichrome and H&E staining. On enzymatic staining, the centers lack oxidative activity and are surrounded by an area of increased activity. On EM, these areas appear devoid of myofibrils and have granular and filamentous material of approximately 6–8 nm in diameter.

Zebra Body Myopathy. Zebra body myopathy also presents in early childhood with limb and facial weakness and delayed milestones. The zebra bodies are only seen on EM, in which they appear as osmiophilic striations approximately 2 nm in length, resembling Z lines.[95] On light microscopy, the biopsy shows nonspecific myopathic features.

Trilaminar Body Myopathy. Trilaminar body myopathy presents in newborns with severe rigidity that persists during sleep; symptoms improve during infancy. On EM, the trilaminar bodies consist of muscle fibers with three concentric zones of various densities. These areas have mitochondria, glycogen, and, in the middle, loosely packed spheroids.[96]

Myopathy with Tubular Aggregates. Aggregates of T-tubules can be found in a variety of neuromuscular conditions including, among others, periodic paralysis, myotonia congenita, and congenital myasthenic syndromes. The aggregates appear as dense red material in the trichrome stain and stain intensely dark blue with NADH-TR. They do not stain with ATPase, and on EM they are identified as areas of T-tubule accumulations (Figure 19.25).

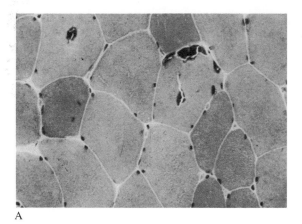
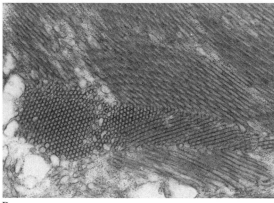

A   B

Figure 19.25 A. Biopsy of a patient with hyperkalemic periodic paralysis showing aggregates of T tubules, which are red on modified trichrome stain and appear as the darkest areas in the photograph (×200). **B.** On electron microscopy, these are accumulations of T tubules (×700).

A familial myopathy occurs with aberrant T-tubules as the main pathologic finding but without clinical features of the conditions mentioned in the previous paragraph. Of these, an autosomal dominant form begins in infancy[97]; an autosomal recessive, slowly progressive form begins in childhood[98]; and an adult-onset type usually presents with a history of exercise-induced muscle pain and stiffness.[99] The pathologic findings are similar in all forms.

Muscular Dystrophies

Muscular dystrophies are a heterogeneous group of hereditary progressive disorders that have traditionally been classified together because of the lack of known causes and the presence of progressive fiber degeneration. Because the specific protein deficiency has been identified in many of these disorders, newer classifications tend to group them according to their known protein or enzyme defect.

Most biopsies of muscular dystrophy have the histologic characteristics described previously for myopathies. These include fiber necrosis, variation in fiber size, internalized nuclei, fiber splitting, and proliferation of fat and connective tissue in the interstitium. In addition, there are known protein deficiencies associated with many of these diseases (i.e., dystrophin or sarcoglycans) that can be detected with immunohistochemical and Western blot analyses.[1,2]

Congenital Muscular Dystrophies. *Congenital muscular dystrophy* refers to diseases that manifest at birth and have biopsy features typical of muscular dystrophy.[11,100] Some are secondary to a deficiency of laminin α2, or merosin, and are recognized by a lack of staining for this protein (Figure 19.26),[101] whereas non–merosin-deficient forms have only the features of a chronic myopathy.[11] In the Fukuyama type of muscular dystrophy, patients have severe brain abnormalities, caused by a defect of the gene that expresses the protein fukutin.[17] The findings in muscle-eye-brain disease and Walker-Warburg syndrome are nonspecific.

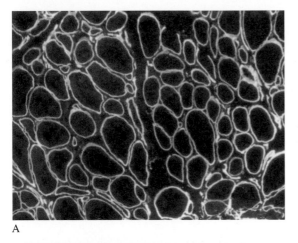

A

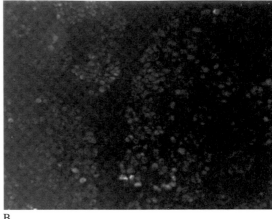

B

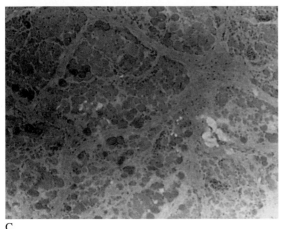

C

Figure 19.26 Immunofluorescent localization of merosin in the muscle of a normal patient (**A**), compared to the absence of antibody in a patient with merosin-deficient congenital muscular dystrophy (**B**). **C**. A hematoxylin and eosin–stained section of the merosin-deficient muscle biopsy showing increased connective tissue, a reduction in the number of fibers, and variability in fiber size (×100). (Reproduced from T Bertorini. Muscular Dystrophies. In R Pourmand [ed], Neuromuscular Diseases: Expert Clinicians' Views. Boston: Butterworth–Heinemann, 2001;229.)

Duchenne's and Becker's Muscular Dystrophies. DMD is a progressive, childhood-onset disease distinguished by prominent proximal weakness, hypertrophy of muscles (particularly of the calves), and cardiomyopathy. DMD has an X-linked recessive inheritance. There is a genetic defect resulting in an absence of the protein dystrophin, which is pathogenic. A partial deficiency of this protein results in Becker's muscular dystrophy (BMD), which is allelic to DMD.

The histologic findings in DMD were initially outlined by Erb in 1891.[102] These include degenerated fibers, some in clusters (especially in early cases), and many fibers undergoing phagocytosis.[103] In younger patients, there are many regenerating basophilic fibers and internalized nuclei, and there is rounding of most fibers. Endomysial connective tissue is increased early in the disease, and there are many opaque or overcontracted fibers that appear dark with most stains (Figure 19.27; see Color Plate B29). Mononuclear cells are sometimes identified that are mostly macrophages, but some are lymphocytes, particularly type T8.[104] In advanced stages of DMD, fiber atrophy and fat proliferation become prominent. On EM, there are scattered fibers with disruption of myofibrils, duplication of basal lamina, and discontinuity of the plasma membrane. Most characteristic of DMD is the absence of dystrophin in immunohistochemical studies (see Color Plates B30 and B31). Only small clusters

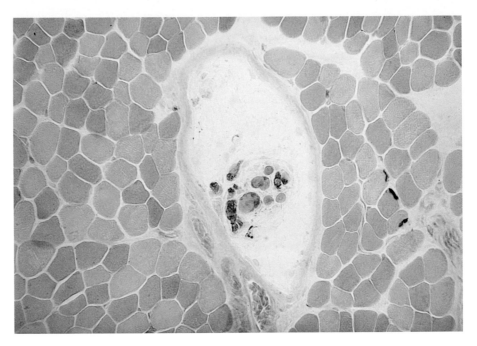

Color Plate B1 Muscle spindle with intrafusal muscle fiber and dark staining end plates in a non-specific esterase stain (100×).

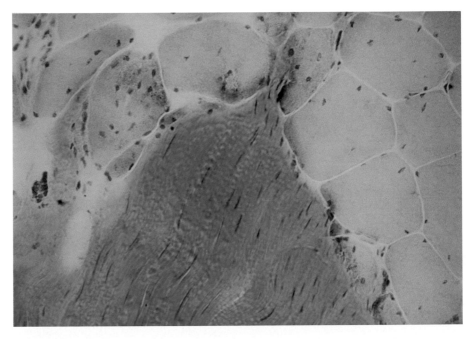

Color Plate B2 Modified trichrome-stained muscle at the myotendinous junction. Notice the pale green fibers, dark green connective tissue, atrophic fibers, and internalized nuclei (200×).

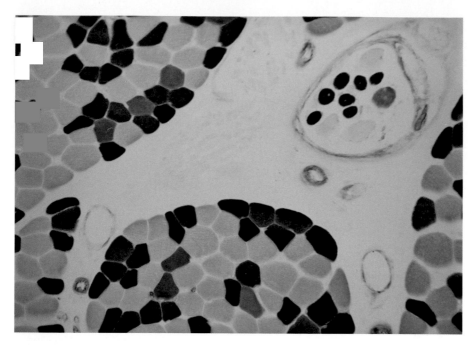

Color Plate B3 Adenosine triphosphatase stain at pH 9.4 of normal muscle. With the technique used in this specimen, type I fibers appear pale, type II fibers are dark, and type IIa fibers are intermediate. Notice that type differentiation is also present in the intrafusal fibers in the spindle (100×).

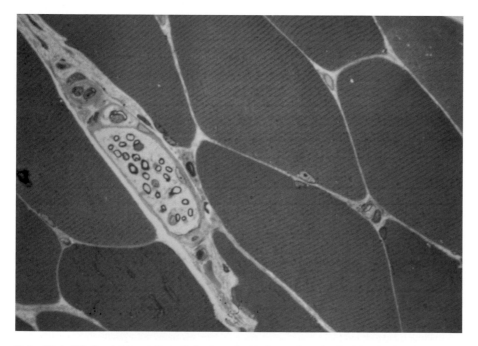

Color Plate B4 Semi-thin section of plastic-embedded muscle stained with toluidine blue shows the striation of the muscle fibers and an intramuscular nerve (400×).

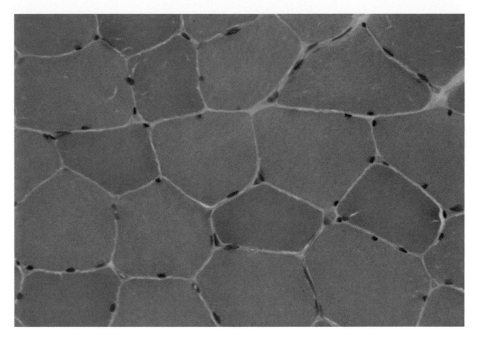

Color Plate B5 Hematoxylin and eosin stain of normal muscle. The muscle fibers are red and polygonal in shape, and the nuclei are darker (250×).

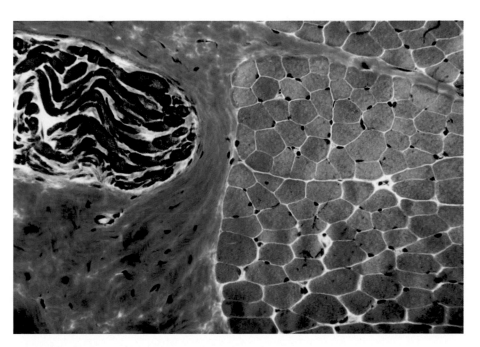

Color Plate B6 Normal muscle stained with the modified trichrome technique. Muscle fibers and connective tissue are green, and the muscle nuclei and myelin of an intramuscular nerve are red (100×).

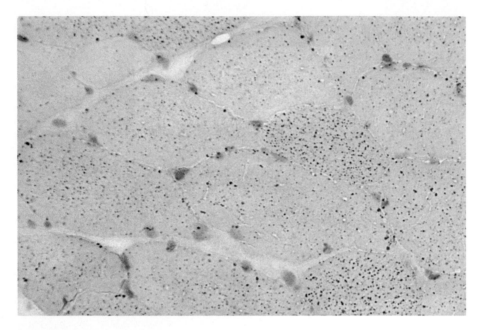

Color Plate B7 Oil red O lipid stain of normal muscle (400×).

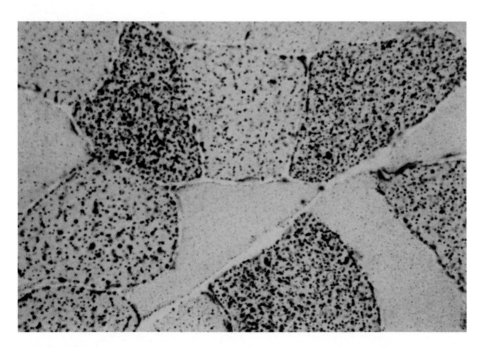

Color Plate B8 Increased staining in type I fibers in lipid storage myopathy (400×).

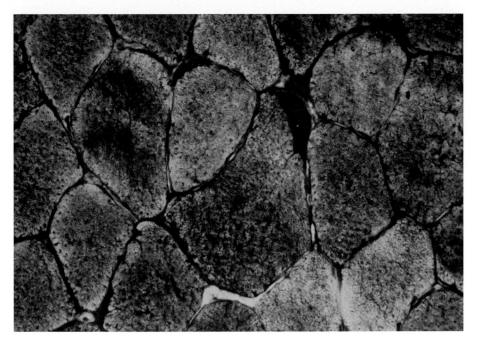

Color Plate B9 Periodic acid–Schiff stain of muscle in phosphorylase deficiency with more intense staining in a subsarcolemmal vacuole (400×).

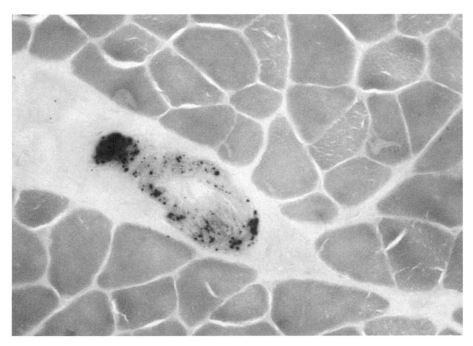

Color Plate B10 Alizarin red stain showing calcium accumulation in the vessel wall of a patient with hyperparathyroidism. Some fibers contain cracking artifacts (200×).

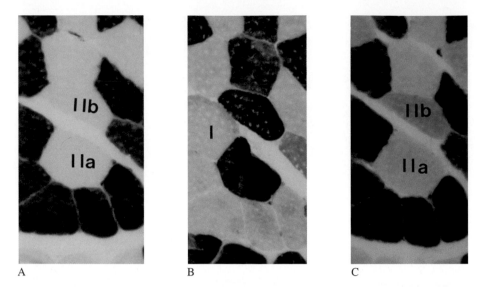

A   B   C

Color Plate B11 Adenosine triphosphatase–stained muscle at different pH. **A.** pH 4.3. **B.** pH 9.4. **C.** pH 4.6. The type I fibers are pale, and the type II fibers are dark at pH 9.4 but are pale at pH 4.3. Subtype IIb is intermediate in intensity at pH 4.6 (200×).

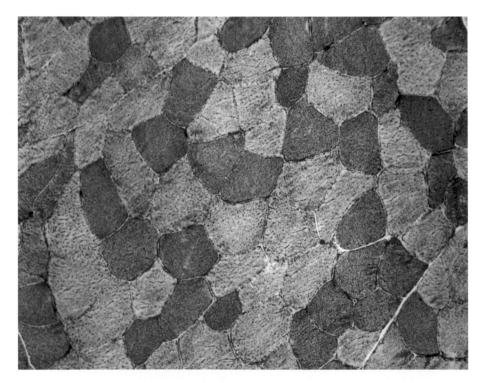

Color Plate B12 Nicotinamide adenine dinucleotide-tetrazolium reductase (NADH-TR)–stained normal muscle with dark type I fibers and pale type II fibers (200×).

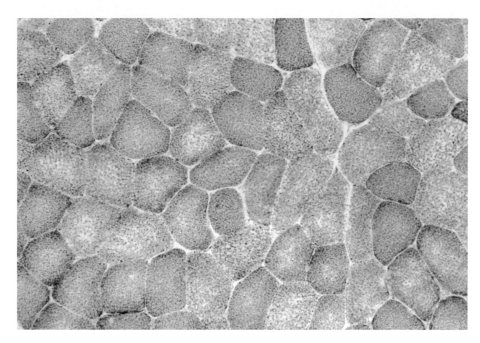

Color Plate B13 Type I fibers are dark and type II are pale in the succinic dehydrogenase staining of normal muscle (200×).

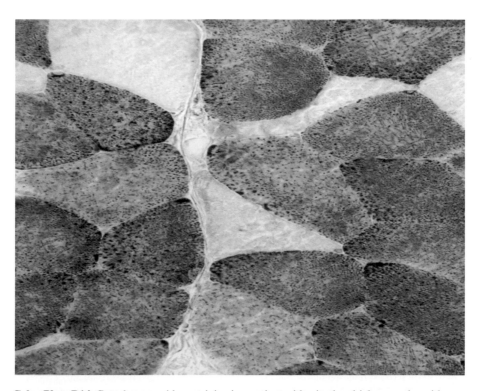

Color Plate B14 Cytochrome oxidase staining in a patient with mitochondrial myopathy with normal staining of most fibers, but there are some pale or cytochrome oxidase–negative fibers (200×).

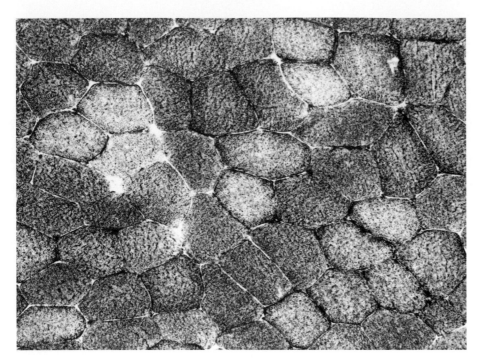

Color Plate B15 Myoadenylate deaminase staining of muscle showing darker type I and pale type II fibers (200×).

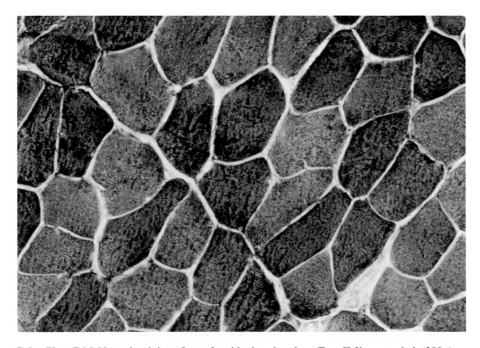

Color Plate B16 Normal staining of muscle with phosphorylase. Type II fibers are dark (200×).

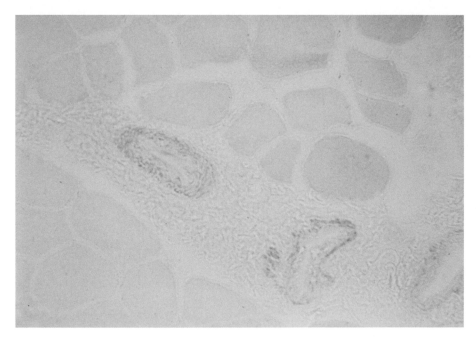

Color Plate B17 Negative staining with phosphorylase in myophosphorylase deficiency. Only the vessel wall stains positively (200×). Compare with normal staining in Color Plate B18.

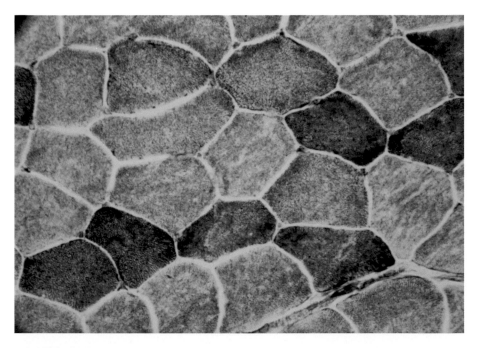

Color Plate B18 Normal phosphofructokinase stain. Type I fibers are dark (100×).

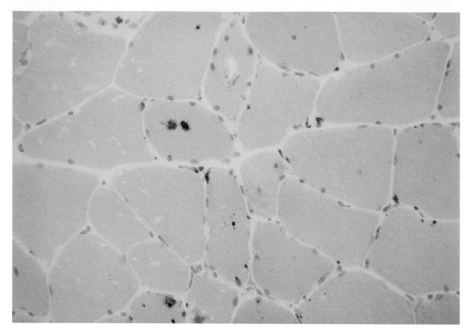

Color Plate B19 Acid phosphatase stain (200×). Notice the green fibers and darker green nuclei. The macrophages are red. This is a mildly abnormal muscle. Compare with the markedly increased acid phosphatase activity seen in acid maltase deficiency in Color Plate B34.

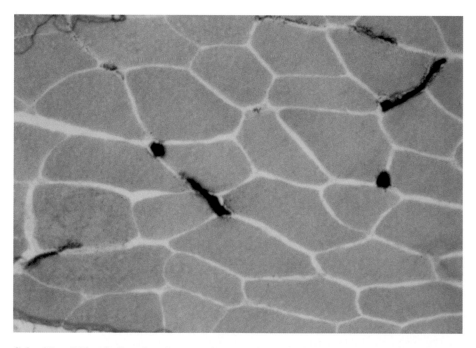

Color Plate B20 Alkaline phosphatase stains normal muscle fibers pale brown, and rare vessels are dark (200×).

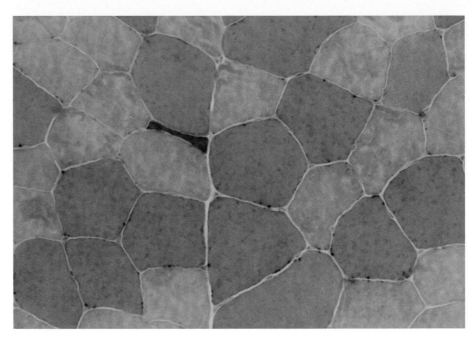

Color Plate B21 Nonspecific esterase stain showing dark type I and pale type II fibers and an intensely stained denervated fiber (200×).

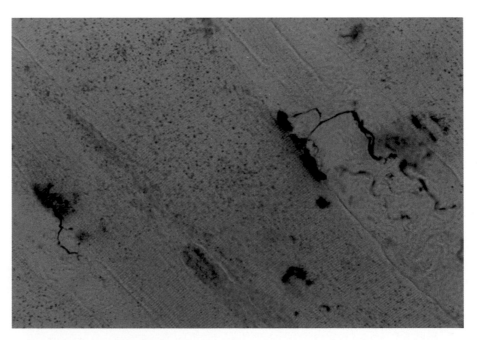

Color Plate B22 Acetylcholinesterase silver stain. Notice the black staining of intramuscular axons and blue staining of the end pates (400×).

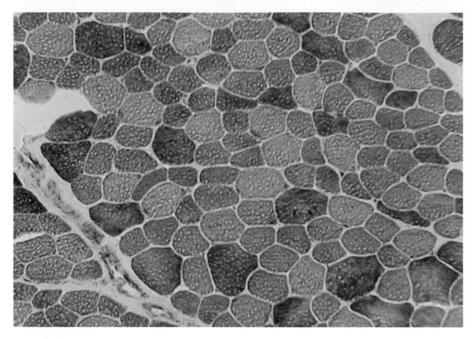

Color Plate B23 Menadione-mediated alpha glycerophosphate dehydrogenase defines two subtypes of type I fiber; type II fibers stain darker (100×).

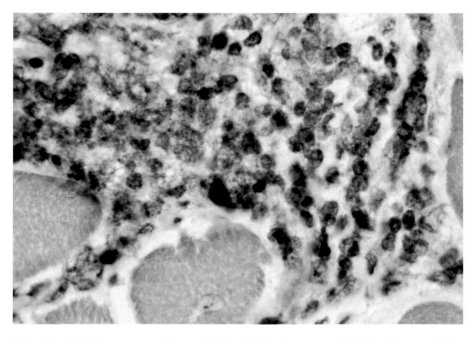

Color Plate B24 Immunoperoxidase stain. The CD4 lymphocytes are dark, invading muscle in a case of lymphoma (400×).

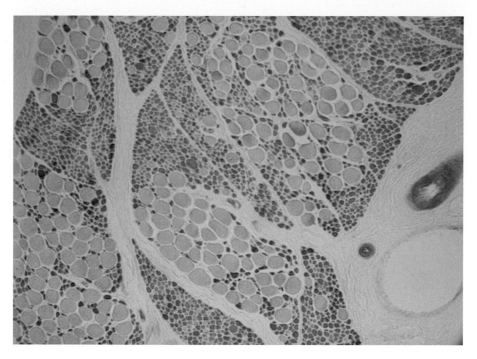

Color Plate B25 Muscle biopsy of infantile spinal muscular atrophy, showing groups of atrophic fibers and large type I fibers (adenosine triphosphatase, pH 9.4) (100×).

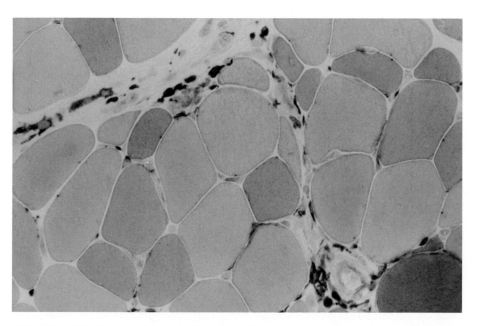

Color Plate B26 Macrophages are darkly stained with nonspecific esterase in a case of polymyositis (200×).

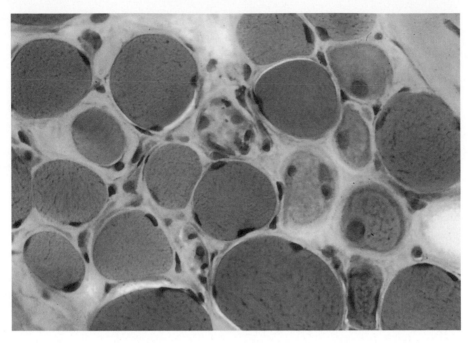

Color Plate B27 Muscle biopsy of polymyositis stained with hematoxylin and eosin, showing bluish coloration of regenerating fibers. Some fibers are undergoing phagocytosis (200×).

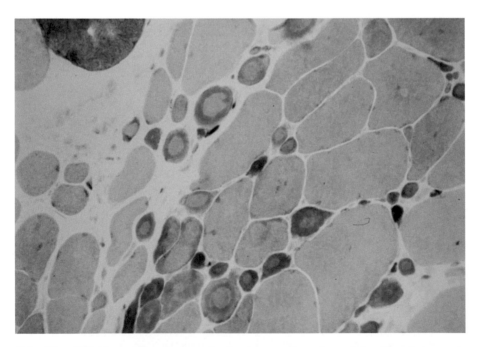

Color Plate B28 Nonspecific esterase stain showing type I atrophy and ring fibers in myotonic dystrophy (200×).

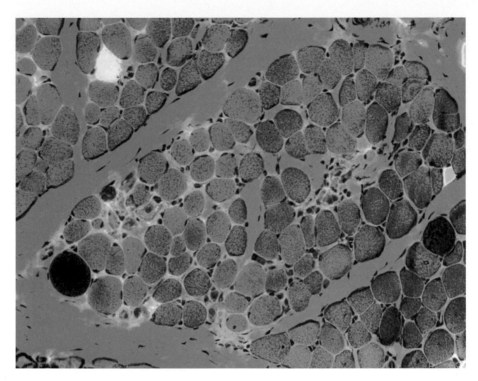

Color Plate B29 Modified trichrome stain of muscle in Duchenne's muscular dystrophy. Notice increased connective tissue, opaque fibers, and necrosis with phagocytosis and some regenerating muscle fibers (100×).

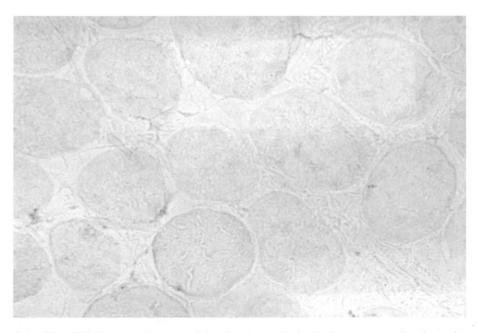

Color Plate B30 Negative immunostaining for dystrophin in Duchenne's muscular dystrophy (400×). Compare with normal staining in Color Plate B31.

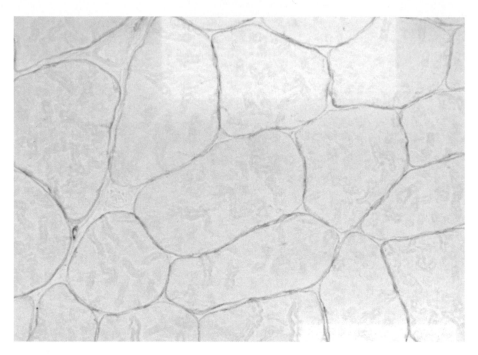

Color Plate B31 Immunoperoxidase staining for dystrophin in normal muscle is positive in the border of fibers (200×).

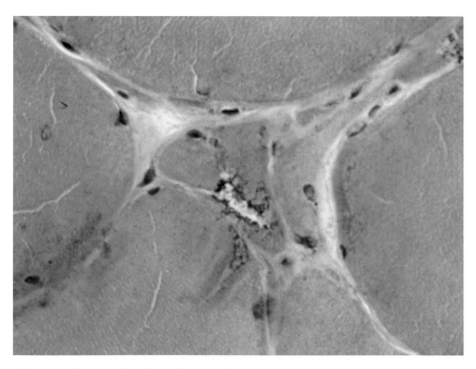

Color Plate B32 Atrophic fiber with a rimmed vacuole in oculopharyngeal dystrophy (trichrome stain, 400×).

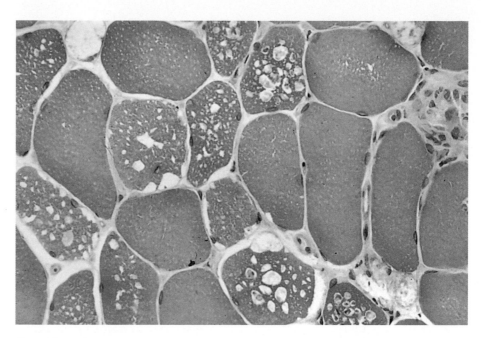

Color Plate B33 Hematoxylin and eosin stain shows irregular vacuoles and a necrotic fiber undergoing phagocytosis in adult acid maltase deficiency (250×).

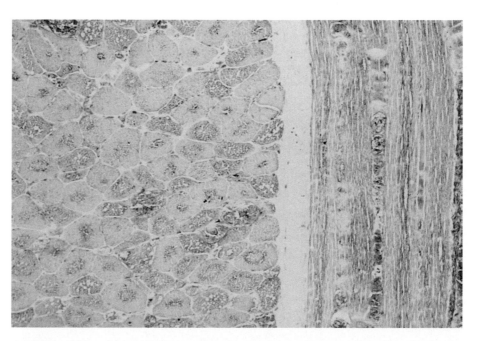

Color Plate B34 Acid phosphatase staining of acid maltase deficiency shows increased activity within vacuoles in cross- and longitudinal sections of muscle (100×).

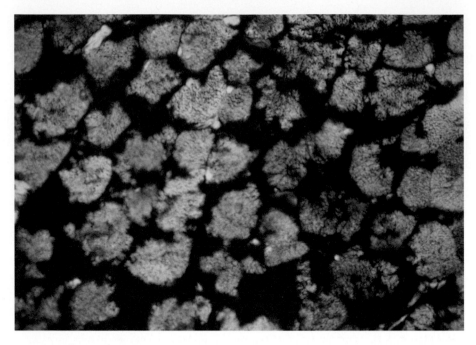

Color Plate B35 Periodic acid–Schiff stain demonstrates increased glycogen in debrancher enzyme deficiency (200×).

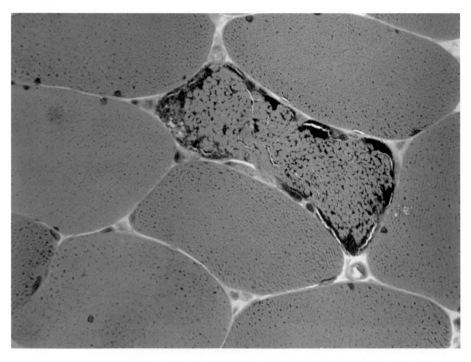

Color Plate B36 Ragged red fiber stained with modified trichrome in a case of mitochondrial myopathy (400×).

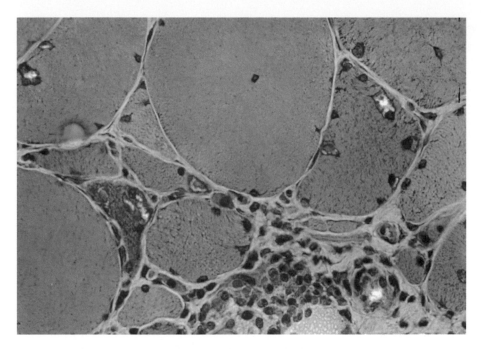

Color Plate B37 Trichrome-stained muscle biopsy of inclusion body myositis. Notice the rimmed vacuoles, atrophic fibers, and inflammatory infiltrate (400×).

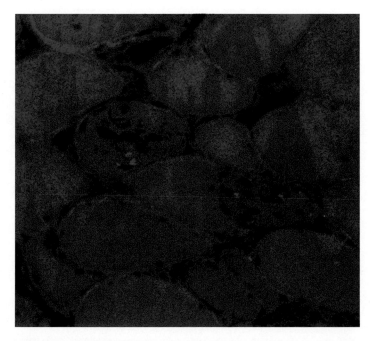

Color Plate B38 Congo red stain, studied with a focal laser scanning microscope. Notice the fluorescent inclusion bodies (250×).

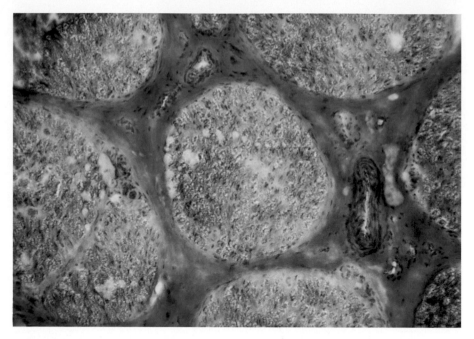

Color Plate B39 Modified trichrome-stained cross-section of a normal nerve stains the myelin red and the connective tissue blue-green (100×).

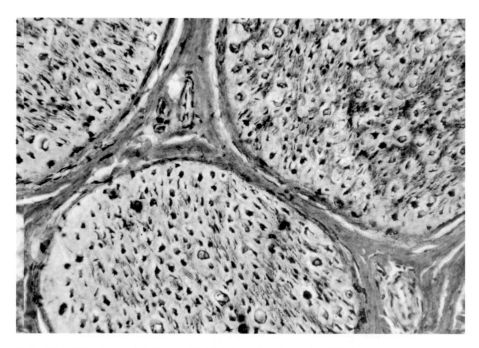

Color Plate B40 Axons stain black with Bielschowsky silver stain (200×).

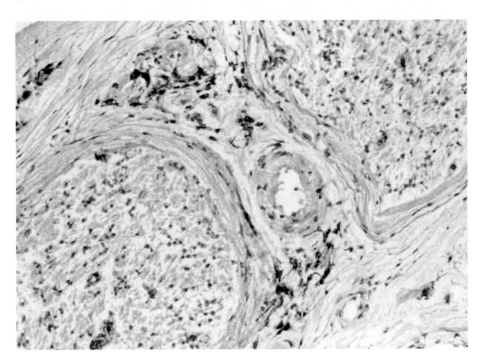

Color Plate B41 Immunoperoxidase staining for leukocyte-common antigen, showing positive-staining inflammatory cells in a case of chronic inflammatory demyelinating polyneuropathy (200×).

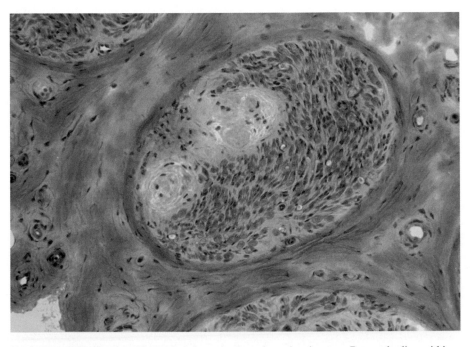

Color Plate B42 Hematoxylin and eosin–stained section, showing two Renaut bodies within a single fascicle (200×).

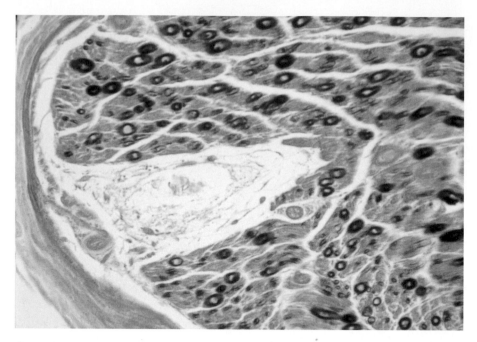

Color Plate B43 Renaut body on an osmium-fixed, paraffin-embedded section of nerve (400×).

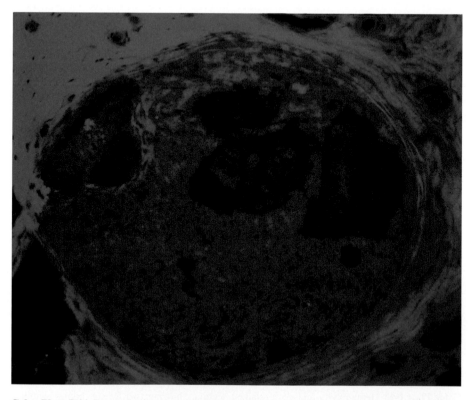

Color Plate B44 Renaut bodies do not fluoresce with Congo red in confocal microscopy (200×).

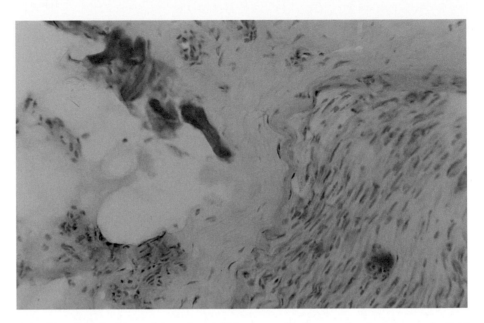

Color Plate B45 Positive staining of amyloid in nerve with Congo red stain under regular light microscopy (200×).

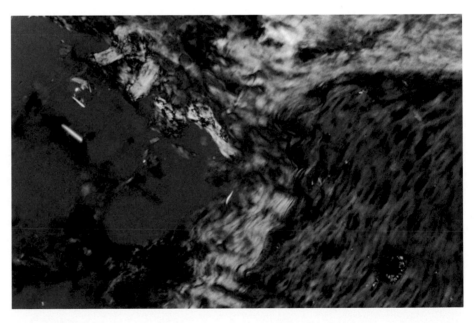

Color Plate B46 The apple-green birefringence of amyloid as viewed under polarized light (Congo red, 200×).

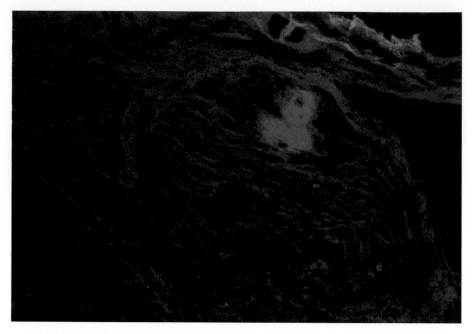

Color Plate B47 Fluorescence of amyloid using laser scanning confocal microscopy (200×).

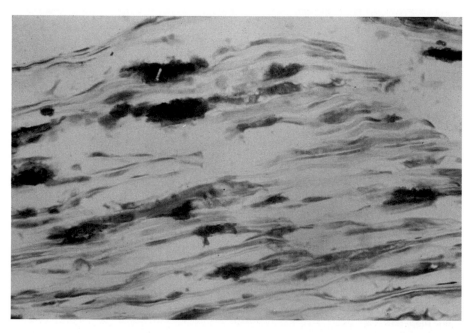

Color Plate B48 Positive staining with cresyl violet in metachromatic leukodystrophy (200×). (Courtesy of Dr. S. Shankar, National Institute of Mental Health and Neurosciences, Bangalore, India.)

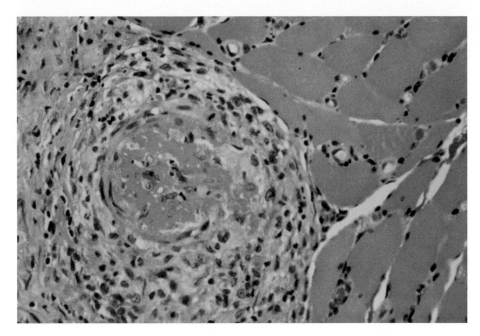

Color Plate B49 Muscle biopsy of a patient with periarteritis nodosa, stained with hematoxylin and eosin, showing an inflammatory infiltrate and fibrinoid necrosis in an occluded vessel (200×).

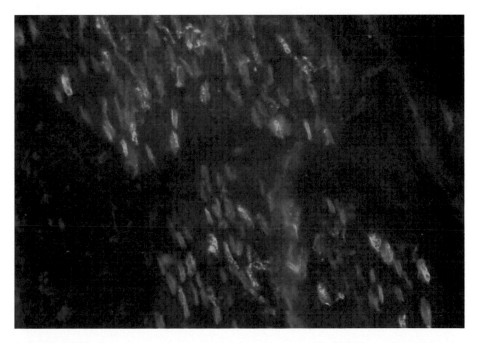

Color Plate B50 Green immunofluorescent staining of immunoglobulin M in a patient with a neuropathy with myelin-associated glycoprotein antibodies (400×). (This case was studied with the photographs provided by Dr. Thomas O'Brien with the Methodist Hospitals of Memphis, Tennessee.)

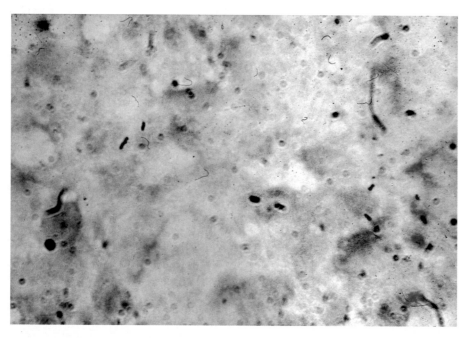

Color Plate B51 Red-staining, acid-fast bacilli of leprosy (Ziehl-Neelsen, 400×). (Courtesy of Dr. Adriana Ciudad, Lima, Peru.)

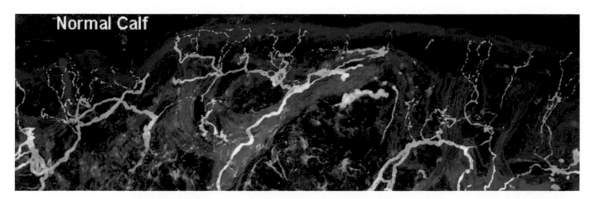

Color Plate B52 Laser scanning confocal microscope images of nerves in superficial skin localized by antibodies to PGP 9.5 and type IV collagen for the basement membrane. Vessels are labeled with ulex europaeus agglutinin type I. The intraepidermal nerve fibers appear aqua and lie within the blue epidermis. The subepidermal nerve plexus appears green or yellow. The dermal-epidermal junction is red, and capillaries are magenta. Numerous nerve fibers are seen crossing the basement membrane to innervate the epidermis. (Reproduced from WR Kennedy, G Wendelschafer-Crabb, D Walk. Use of skin biopsy and skin blister in neurological practice. J Clin Neuromuscular Disease 2000;1:196–204, with permission.)

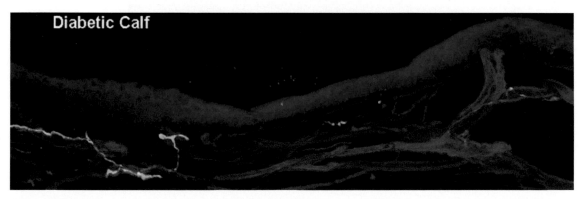

Color Plate B53 Diabetic subjects display a range of epidermal nerve fiber density, depending on the body location and degree of neuropathy. In this specimen, no epidermal nerve fibers are seen. A single nerve fiber is seen in the subepidermal plexus, but this does not cross into the epidermis. (Reproduced from WR Kennedy, G Wendelschafer-Crabb, D Walk. Use of skin biopsy and skin blister in neurological practice. J Clin Neuromuscular Disease 2000;1:196–204, with permission.)

Color Plate B54 An example of fluorescent in situ hybridization analysis of patient chromosomes. In this example, a woman with a history of recurrent pregnancy loss and a daughter with muscular dystrophy was studied with cloned human DNA from the telomeric region of the X chromosome (Xq28 yeast artificial chromosome [YAC 705] clone). The fluorescent signal corresponding to a normal, present Xq28 region in one of the woman's X chromosomes is shown (Xq28 YAC 705), whereas the second X chromosome fails to hybridize to the Xq28 probe [del(X)(q28)]. Thus, this woman has a deletion mutation of the Xq28 region on one of her X chromosomes, which is undetectable by light microscopy methods, but is detectable using fluorescent in situ hybridization methods. This deletion was shown to be responsible for the woman's recurrent spontaneous abortions, which were caused by a phenotypic trait cosegregating with the Xq28 deletion in her family. (Reprinted with permission from E Pegoraro, J Whitaker, P Mowery-Rushton, et al. Familial skewed X inactivation: a molecular trait associated with high spontaneous-abortion rate maps to Xq28. Am J Hum Genet 1997;61:160–170.)

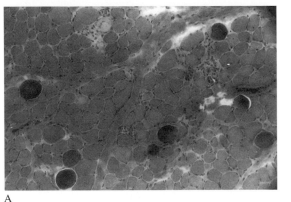
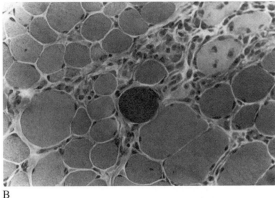

A   B

Figure 19.27 A. Trichrome-stained section of the muscle biopsy in Duchenne's muscular dystrophy showing necrosis, opaque fibers, mildly increased connective tissue, and variation in fiber size (×200). **B.** Higher magnification showing fiber atrophy, hypertrophy, necrosis, and interstitial mononuclear cells (×400). (Reproduced from T Bertorini. Muscular Dystrophies. In R Pourmand [ed], Neuromuscular Diseases: Expert Clinicians' Views. Boston: Butterworth–Heinemann, 2001;243.)

of so-called revertant fibers stain positively, indicating the presence of dystrophin in regenerating fibers (Figure 19.28).[11]

The histologic findings in BMD are internalized nuclei, fiber splitting, clusters of both fiber types, and the presence of some atrophic, angulated fibers.[105] The major differentiating factor between BMD and DMD is that BMD muscle does stain immunohistochemically for dystrophin, although in an attenuated and irregular pattern (Figure 19.29).[11]

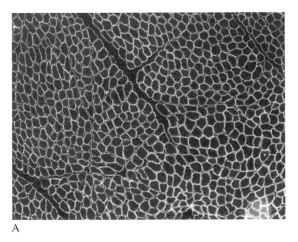
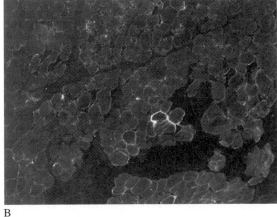

A   B

Figure 19.28 Immunofluorescent staining for dystrophin in a normal control (**A**) compared to absence of dystrophin staining except for a single positive fiber (revertant fiber) in a patient with Duchenne's muscular dystrophy (**B**). (Courtesy of Eric Hoffmann, Ph.D., Research Center for Genetic Medicine. Washington, D.C. Reproduced from T. Bertorini. Muscular Dystrophies. In R Pourmand [ed], Neuromuscular Diseases: Expert Clinicians' Views. Boston: Butterworth–Heinemann, 2001;244.)

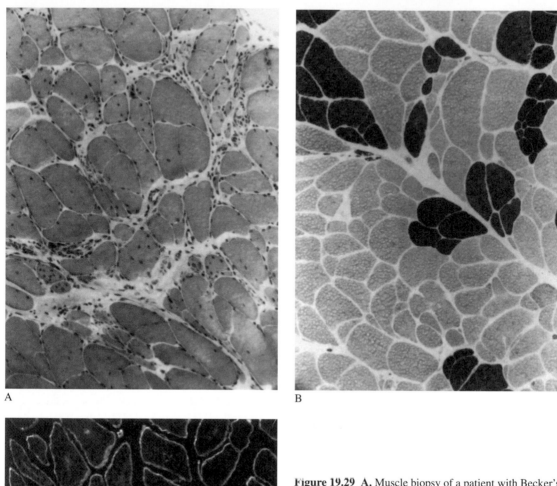

A

B

C

Figure 19.29 A. Muscle biopsy of a patient with Becker's muscular dystrophy shows internalized nuclei, hypertrophic fibers, and split fibers (×200). **B.** Muscle biopsy of the same patient stained with adenosine triphosphatase (pH 9.4) demonstrates type I fiber predominance and clusters of type II fibers (×200). **C.** Muscle biopsy fibers in Becker's muscular dystrophy show decreased intensity and attenuated staining with dystrophin immunofluorescence. (Reproduced from T Bertorini. Muscular Dystrophies. In R Pourmand [ed], Neuromuscular Diseases: Expert Clinicians' Views. Boston: Butterworth–Heinemann, 2001;251, 252.)

Emery-Dreifuss Muscular Dystrophy. EDMD is characterized by weakness, cardiomyopathy, and muscle contractures. The muscle biopsy shows variation in fiber size, internalized nuclei, some necrosis, and proliferation of connective tissue.[106,107] The X-linked recessive type of EDMD can be diagnosed by immunostaining for emerin,[11] the deficient protein in this disease. The gene defect of the autosomal dominant form of EDMD localizes to the region for the protein lamin A/C.[1]

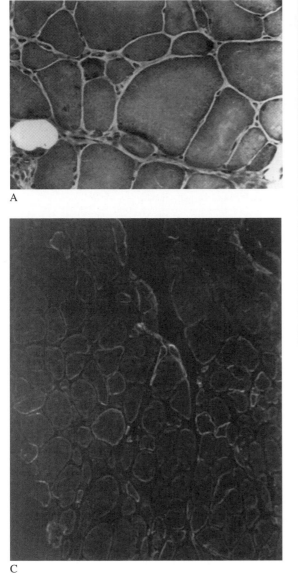

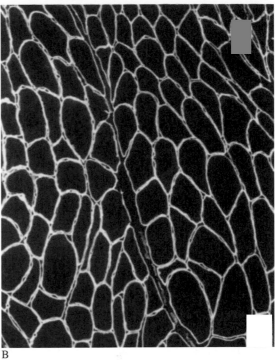

Figure 19.30 A. Muscle biopsy (from a patient with limb-girdle muscular dystrophy) stained with hematoxylin and eosin showing increased connective tissue, hypertrophy, and atrophy (×200). **B.** Normal immunofluorescent staining for α-sarcoglycan in a control patient, compared to the absence of immunofluorescent staining in a sarcoglycan-deficient patient (**C**). (Reproduced from T Bertorini. Muscular Dystrophies. In R Pourmand [ed], Neuromuscular Diseases: Expert Clinicians' Views Boston: Butterworth–Heinemann, 2001;261,262.) (Courtesy of Dr. Eric Hoffman.)

Limb-Girdle Muscular Dystrophies. LGMDs include several disorders with similar phenotypes but variable severity and course. They are either autosomal recessive or dominant and are caused by different protein deficiencies, such as the sarcoglycans, calpain, caveolin, and dysferlin.

Histologic changes in the LGMDs vary from minor myopathic findings to the severity of those observed in DMD. These include fiber atrophy, hypertrophy, splitting, internalized nuclei, and proliferation of connective tissue (Figure 19.30A), and fat infiltration; lobulated fibers can also be seen; in some cases, they are prominent.[108] Occasionally, there is a prominent necrotizing myopathy without, or with little, evidence of inflammation.

Immunostaining for dysferlin, calpain, and the various sarcoglycan proteins allows for the differentiation of some of the LGMDs (see Figure 19.30B,C). In a sarcoglycan deficiency, there is a secondary deficiency of the other sarcoglycans, making it ultimately impossible to histologically distinguish the different types.[2,11] However, in a recent report of a patient with partial α-sarcoglycan deficiency, the other sarcoglycans were normally present.[109]

Routinely, the biopsy of a patient with an apparent LGMD is initially stained for dystrophin and then for α-sarcoglycan. If dystrophin is normal, a deficiency of α-sarcoglycan is indicative of a sarcoglycanopathy, but DNA studies are necessary for further delineation of the type of sarcoglycanopathy. If sarcoglycan staining is normal, it is important to do Western blot analysis, DNA studies, or immunostaining, when possible, for the other proteins known to cause the various forms of LGMD, such as dysferlin, calpain, and caveolin, as well as merosin, because its deficiency rarely can also have this presentation.

Facioscapulohumeral Muscular Dystrophy. Facioscapulohumeral muscular dystrophy is an autosomal dominant, progressive disease that manifests with more severe weakness of the face, trapezius, biceps, and quadriceps muscles, accompanied by atrophy. The biopsy in facioscapulohumeral muscular dystrophy shows all the features of dystrophic muscle but can be normal in appearance if the muscle biopsied is not symptomatic. Other pathologic findings include the presence of lobulated fibers (Figure 19.31), which are recognized by their scalloped borders that stain dark with oxidative and trichrome stains. On EM, there are subsarcolemmal accumulations of mitochondria.[110] These are not pathogenic of the disease, as they also are in LGMD, as discussed previously. Foci of inflammatory cells can sometimes be found, especially in the childhood form of the disease. The genetic defect of fascioscapulohumeral muscular dystrophy is located in chromosome 4q35.

Oculopharyngeal Muscular Dystrophy. Oculopharyngeal muscular dystrophy is usually of late onset and is characterized by ptosis and dysphagia. Ophthalmoplegia and mild proximal weakness may occur later in the disease course.[111]

The muscle biopsy shows scattered, small atrophic fibers and rimmed vacuoles (Figure 19.32; see Color Plate B32). Filaments of 8.5 nm of external diameter can be

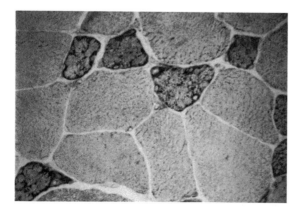

Figure 19.31 Lobulated fibers with scalloped borders in facioscapulohumeral dystrophy (nicotinamide adenine dinucleotide-tetrazolium reductase, ×400).

Figure 19.32 Fiber atrophy and a rimmed vacuole in oculopharyngeal dystrophy (modified trichrome, ×400). (Reproduced from T Bertorini. Muscular Dystrophies. In R Pourmand [ed], Neuromuscular Diseases: Expert Clinicians' Views. Boston: Butterworth–Heinemann, 2001;270.)

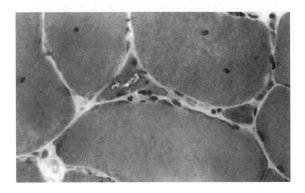

seen in the nuclei.[112] In advanced cases, there is increased connective tissue and fat with prominent fiber atrophy. Patients without significant limb weakness may have a normal-appearing muscle biopsy.

Distal Muscular Dystrophies. Several hereditary myopathies manifest with predominant distal weakness. Among these are the Welander, Markesberry-Griggs/Udd, and Nonaka types of muscular dystrophy, which have the biopsy findings of a chronic myopathy with frequent rimmed vacuoles (Figure 19.33).[113] In the early adult onset posterior compartment (Miyoshi type), the biopsy shows abundant muscle necrosis and stains negatively for dysferlin, similar to LGMD 2B, which is allelic.[2,13]

Myotonic Dystrophy. Myotonic dystrophy is an autosomal dominant disease that presents at variable ages with facial and neck weakness, as well as predominately distal weakness of the limbs, ptosis, myotonia, cataracts, and cardiomyopathy. The

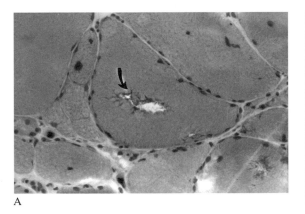

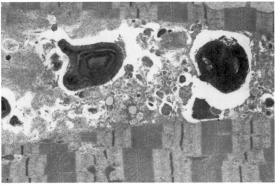

A   B

Figure 19.33 A. A rimmed vacuole (*arrow*) in Welander's distal dystrophy light microscopy (modified trichrome, ×400). **B.** Electron microscopy showing myeloid bodies within the vacuole (×9,120).

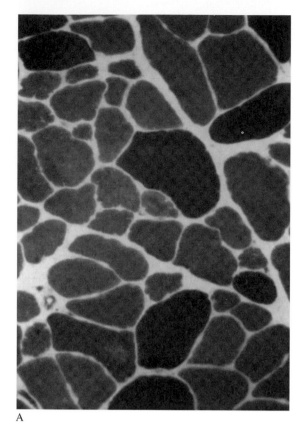

A

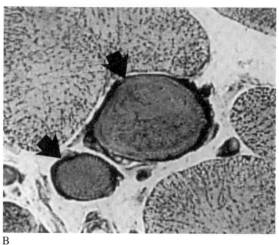

B

Figure 19.34 A. Muscle biopsy (from a patient with myotonic dystrophy) stained with adenosine triphosphatase at pH 9.4 shows the selective type I muscle atrophy. **B.** "Ring" fibers (*arrows*) (nicotinamide adenine dinucleotide-tetrazolium reductase stain). (Reproduced from T Bertorini. Muscular Dystrophies. In R Pourmand [ed], Neuromuscular Diseases: Expert Clinicians' Views. Boston: Butterworth–Heinemann, 2001;274.)

biopsy of these patients shows muscle fiber atrophy, particularly of type I fibers (Figure 19.34). There are scattered pale areas in muscle fibers on the oxidative stains and frequent internalized nuclei, often in chains. Other common findings are ring fibers ("ringbinden" or spiral annulets) (see Color Plate B28) and sarcoplasmic masses, which are homogeneous areas with disorganized myofibrillar material that stain bluish with H&E, red with trichrome, and dark with NADH-TR stains.[11,114] Later in the disease, the biopsy shows frequent pyknotic nuclei with more chronic changes, such as marked atrophy and proliferation of fat and connective tissue.

Proximal Myotonic Myopathy. Proximal myotonic myopathy is a disease similar to myotonic dystrophy but characterized by proximal, rather than distal, muscle weakness. The histologic findings are not specific for this condition but include variation in fiber size, internalized nuclei, and occasional sarcoplasmic masses.[11]

Metabolic Myopathies

The term *metabolic myopathies* encompasses a group of disorders that manifest primarily with muscle weakness or exercise intolerance. These are discussed in Chapter 17, which covers their clinical presentations, their genetic defect, and their diagnosis by biochemical analysis. To avoid repetition, only the histologic findings and representative illustrations are presented here.

Figure 19.35 Vacuolated fibers and a necrotic fiber undergoing phagocytosis in adult acid maltase deficiency (hematoxylin and eosin, ×250).

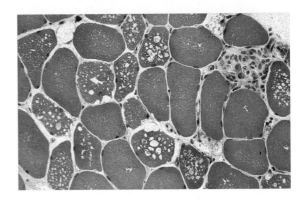

Glycogenosis

TYPE II: ACID MALTASE DEFICIENCY.   Muscle fibers in acid maltase deficiency have many small vacuoles on H&E (Figure 19.35; see Color Plate B33) and trichrome stains. These have granular accumulations of insoluble glycogen on PAS (Figure 19.36), intense acid phosphatase activity (Figure 19.37; see Color Plate B34), and abundant lysosomes on EM (Figure 19.38).[115,116] There are frequent internalized nuclei, ring fibers, and fiber atrophy, and, in advanced cases, there is fibrosis and type I fiber predominance.[117] More severe vacuolization is found in the infantile and juvenile forms of acid maltase deficiency.[118–121]

TYPE III: DEBRANCHING ENZYME DEFICIENCY.   In this disease, muscle fibers have large vacuoles (Figure 19.39A) filled with accumulations of glycogen (see Color Plate B35). These are easily demonstrated with frozen or paraffin-embedded sections and are seen on EM within and between myofibrils, spreading them widely in some areas (see Figure 19.39B).[122,123]

TYPE IV: BRANCHER ENZYME DEFICIENCY.   The muscle biopsy in brancher enzyme deficiency shows accumulations of fine granular material contained within vacuoles. These granules are intensely PAS-positive polysaccharides. They are present predominantly in atrophic fibers, are distributed unevenly throughout the muscle fiber, and are partially resistant to diastase digestion.[124]

TYPE V: MUSCLE PHOSPHORYLASE DEFICIENCY OR MCARDLE'S DISEASE.   The muscle biopsy in McArdle's disease shows subsarcolemmal vacuoles containing PAS-positive granules (Figure 19.40; see Color Plate B9) that have a fibrillar nature on EM. There is a lack of histochemical staining of fibers for phosphorylase, whereas

Figure 19.36 Periodic acid–Schiff staining of increased glycogen in some fibers in acid maltase deficiency (×200).

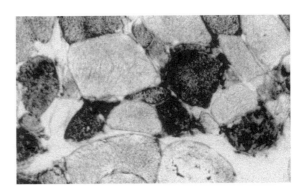

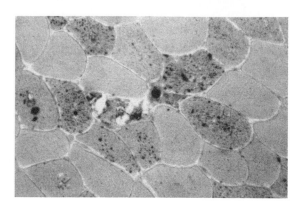

Figure 19.37 Increased acid phosphatase activity within the vacuolated fibers in the acid phosphatase stain in acid maltase deficiency (×200).

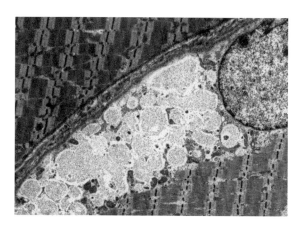

Figure 19.38 Electron microscopy of acid maltase deficiency showing accumulation of large lysosomes adjacent to the nucleus of a muscle fiber (×3,000).

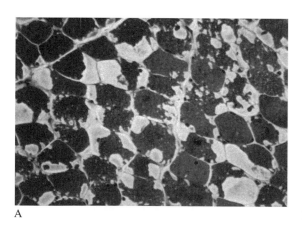

A

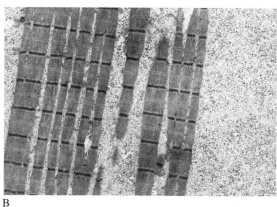

B

Figure 19.39 Multiple, vacuolated muscle fibers are rich in glycogen in debrancher enzyme deficiency. **A.** Modified trichrome stain (×200). **B.** Electron microscopy (×4,500).

Figure 19.40 Subsarcolemmal vacuoles in a patient with McArdle's disease (periodic acid–Schiff, ×200).

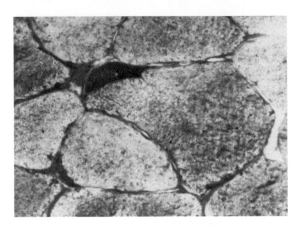

the vessel walls stain normally (see Color Plates B16 and B17).[125] Other histologic changes include internalized nuclei, regenerating fibers, and necrosis, which is especially evident in patients who have had a recent attack of myoglobinuria before biopsy. Regenerating fibers may show normal phosphorylase activity.[126]

TYPE VII: PHOSPHOFRUCTOKINASE DEFICIENCY OR TARUI'S DISEASE. The histologic findings in phosphofructokinase deficiency are characterized by the presence of vacuoles containing PAS-positive material that is partially digested with diastase. This material is seen as normal β-glycogen with EM. Degenerated and regenerating fibers and polyglucosan inclusions can also be seen.[127]

OTHER GLYCOGENOSES. In phosphoglycerate kinase deficiency, the muscle biopsy can appear normal, with only slight accumulations of glycogen. Necrosis is seen if there has been a recent attack of myoglobinuria.[128] In phosphoglycerate mutase deficiency, PAS-positive material is seen in subsarcolemmal areas, and tubular aggregates may also be present.[129] The muscle biopsy in phosphorylase *b* kinase deficiency shows nonspecific findings, but there may be some glycogen accumulation, mainly in type IIb fibers. In LDH and enolase deficiencies, the histologic findings are nonspecific.[130,131]

Lipid Storage Diseases

CARNITINE DEFICIENCY AND CARNITINE PALMITOYL TRANSFERASE DEFICIENCY. In carnitine deficiency, lipid stains demonstrate accumulations of neutral fat that appear as small vacuoles on H&E and trichrome stains (Figure 19.41A) and stain positive for fat with the oil red O (see Color Plate B8) and Sudan black. Lipid vacuoles are easily recognized by their rounded and empty appearance on EM (see Figure 19.41B). Later in the disease, fiber atrophy and myopathic features can be seen, sometimes with fiber necrosis.[132,133] In the myopathic form of carnitine palmitoyl transferase II deficiency, the muscle biopsy may appear normal histologically or may show lipid accumulation.[134,135] Fiber necrosis may be seen after a myoglobinuric attack.

Mitochondrial Myopathies. Mitochondrial myopathies can have variable clinical characteristics, but their most important histologic diagnostic feature is the presence of ragged red fibers, representative of accumulations of mitochondria. The ragged red fibers are easily recognized because of their ragged appearance and intense red staining, predominantly in the borders of fibers on the trichrome stain (Figure 19.42; see Color Plate B36). They are not obvious on H&E but can be distinguished by

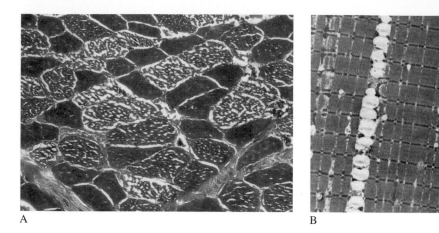

A   B

Figure 19.41 Fat accumulation in muscle fibers in lipid storage myopathy. **A.** Light microscopy shows small vacuoles (trichrome, ×200). (Courtesy of Dr. S. Shankar, National Institute of Mental Health and Neurosciences, Banglore, India.) **B.** Electron microscopy showing several lipid vacuoles (×3,000).

their basophilia in the subsarcolemmal area, whereas the oxidative stains, particularly SDH, show increased activity in these areas (Figure 19.43). At the EM level, many of the mitochondria have abnormal shapes with paracrystalline inclusions of differing patterns (Figure 19.44).[136–138]

Ragged red fibers stain negatively (see Color Plate B14), or only partially stain, with COX in most cases, but they could be COX-positive, as in patients with complex I and complex III deficiencies. Accumulations of fat can also be seen in ragged red fibers.

Ragged red fibers are not apparent in all mitochondrial myopathies. An example is complex IV or COX deficiency, which shows ragged red fibers that are COX-

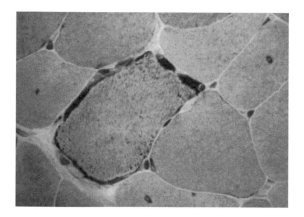

Figure 19.42 Ragged red fiber in mitochondrial myopathy (modified trichrome, ×400).

Figure 19.43 A succinic dehydrogenase–stained muscle in mitochondrial myopathy showing the dense staining from increased oxidative activity and accumulations of mitochondria in the border of two fibers (×200).

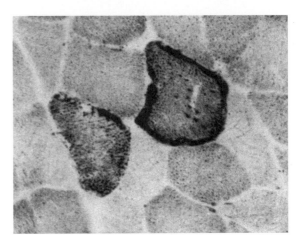

negative initially. In those with a more benign course, there is later a disappearance of the ragged red fibers and normal COX staining.[139]

Myoadenylate Deaminase Deficiency. Myoadenylate deaminase deficiency causes a myopathy in which patients present with muscle aches and pains. The muscle biopsy shows a lack of, or a decrease in, staining for this enzyme. Internalized nuclei and other mild myopathic features are also seen.[33,34] A nonspecific deficiency of this enzyme can also be seen in patients with other myopathies.

Brody's Disease or Sarcoplasmic Calcium–Adenosine Triphosphatase Deficiency. Brody's disease is characterized by muscle spasms, particularly during exercise.[140] The muscle biopsy might only demonstrate a type II fiber predominance, but on immunohistochemistry studies, there is a deficiency of sarcoplasmic calcium–ATPase, which is the cause of the symptoms.

Channelopathies

Hypokalemic Periodic Paralysis. Hypokalemic periodic paralysis is an autosomal dominant condition, characterized by attacks of paralysis after heavy meals or exercise. The muscle biopsy shows large vacuoles without lipid or glycogen on H&E and trichrome stains, and, thus, the vacuoles appear empty (Figure 19.45). Some fibers have glycogen accumulations. The vacuoles are usually single but can be multiple, and they are located in the central area of the fibers. In older patients who may develop a fixed weakness after recurrent episodes of paralysis, there is increased connective tissue and fiber atrophy. On EM, the vacuoles appear to be membrane-bound and empty, but some contain membranous profiles. There can also be tubular aggregates and dilatation of the tubular system and sarcoplasmic reticulum.[141–143]

Hyperkalemic Periodic Paralysis. Hyperkalemic periodic paralysis is characterized by attacks of paralysis or myotonia with cold exposure or exercise. The most characteristic histologic finding in this channelopathy is the abundance of tubular

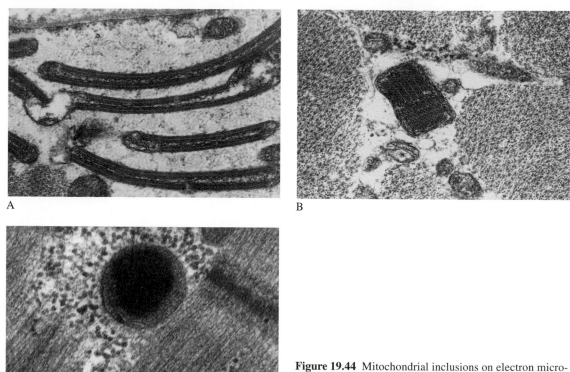

A

B

C

Figure 19.44 Mitochondrial inclusions on electron microscopy in mitochondrial myopathy. **A.** Longitudinal paracrystalline inclusions (×58,680). **B.** Another type of paracrystalline inclusion (×60,912). **C.** Dense, round inclusion (×95,300).

aggregates in muscle (see Figure 19.25A,B).[144] Vacuolization can also be present, as well as fiber atrophy and prominent internalized nuclei.[145]

Myotonia Congenita. Myotonia congenita manifests with myotonia as its main symptom, and the muscle biopsy can be normal or show only occasional internalized nuclei. Although absence of type IIb fibers has been reported, this is not a consistent finding.[146]

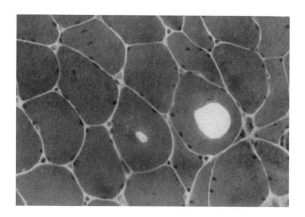

Figure 19.45 Large, empty vacuoles in the muscle of a patient with hypokalemic periodic paralysis (trichrome, ×200).

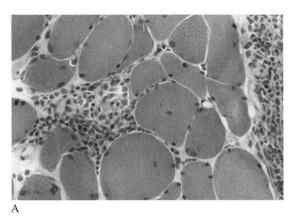
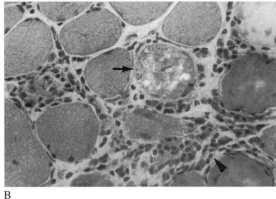

A   B

Figure 19.46 A. Inflammation, necrosis, and phagocytosis in the muscle of a patient with polymyositis (hematoxylin and eosin, ×200). **B.** Necrotic and vacuolated (*arrow*) fibers with interstitial inflammatory cells (*arrowhead*) in adult polymyositis (×295).

Malignant Hyperthermia. MH is distinguished by attacks of myoglobinuria during anesthesia, caused by a genetic defect in the calcium channel ryanodine receptor. The biopsy shows nonspecific findings of frequent pale centers and internalized nuclei. The condition is allelic to CCD, and the characteristic biopsy features of CCD can also be found in patients with MH, as discussed previously.[64,65]

Inflammatory Myopathies

Polymyositis and Dermatomyositis. Polymyositis (PM) and DM are acquired, autoimmune myopathies that cause prominent proximal muscle weakness with a characteristic skin rash in DM. They can be idiopathic, a manifestation of a systemic connective tissue disorder, or associated with malignancy. The muscle biopsy findings in PM/DM consist of fiber necrosis, phagocytosis, interstitial and perivascular inflammation (Figure 19.46), and basophilic regenerating fibers (see Color Plate B27).[145,146] Other changes are fiber atrophy, hypertrophy and splitting, internalized nuclei, and proliferation of connective tissue and fat, particularly in chronic cases.[147]

In children with DM, perifascicular atrophy and necrosis are frequently present (Figure 19.47),[147] accompanied by capillary abnormalities, including necrosis;[148–150] these findings may also be seen in adults with DM. In PM, fiber necrosis is scattered throughout the fascicle. In early stages, pale, necrotic fibers are seen with preservation of the muscle membrane, and these are frequently close to small arterioles.[147] The macrophages in necrotic fibers undergoing phagocytosis stain dark with nonspecific esterase (see Color Plate B26) and red with acid phosphatase. On EM, there is disorganization of the sarcomeres and streaming of the Z-line, and invading macrophages may be seen.[150–153] The increased number of necrotic fibers that do not stain with COX often suggests that there will be a poor response to therapy.[154]

Vacuolization in muscle fibers is noted in some cases. These appear as "punched-out" vacuoles and are often in the perifascicular area in childhood DM. With the trichrome stain, bluish-colored fibers may be present that seem to correspond to

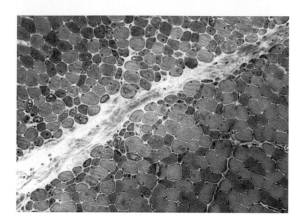

Figure 19.47 Perifascicular atrophy and some "punched out" vacuoles in childhood dermatomyositis (modified trichrome, ×100).

Z-line streaming on EM. Frequently, there is granular staining or pale centers in the NADH-TR stain.

Inflammatory infiltrates are the most important finding that distinguishes PM/DM from other necrotizing myopathies, but these may not always be obvious.[155] The inflammatory cells are mostly lymphocytes and macrophages, and there are some plasma cells. In acute cases, there are also polymorphonuclear cells. The lymphocytes in PM are mainly cytotoxic T8 cells, whereas in DM they are mainly T4 and B cells.[156–158] Inflammatory infiltrates are seen in perivascular areas, sometimes invading vessel walls. The vessels show duplication or disruption of the basal lamina with deposits of IgG and complement complexes in the walls, particularly in childhood DM. Histochemistry shows increased interstitial alkaline phosphatase activity, which correspond to the regenerating capillaries.

Skin biopsy of an affected area in DM shows epidermal atrophy, degeneration of the basal cell layer, hyperkeratosis, deposits of fibrinoid material, and inflammatory infiltrates. Biopsy of uninvolved skin may be normal.

Myositis in connective tissue disorders may have all the features of PM or show only small, scattered, inflammatory cell infiltrates around vessels.[159–161] The biopsy is usually normal or nonspecific in polymyalgia rheumatica.

Inclusion Body Myositis. Inclusion body myositis, the most common inflammatory myopathy in older persons, is characterized by weakness, affecting predominantly the quadriceps, biceps, forearm, and distal leg muscles. The biopsy shows variable interstitial inflammation, necrosis, and neurogenic-appearing fiber atrophy. The diagnosis is made by the presence of eosinophilic inclusions and rimmed vacuoles on light microscopy (Figure 19.48A,B; see Color Plate B37) and EM (see Figure 19.48C).[162,163]

The inclusion bodies reveal apple-green birefringence with Congo red, which is better demonstrated with fluorescence optics and special filters, such as rhodamine filter and confocal microscopy (see Color Plate B38). These bodies represent β-amyloid deposits. Staining for various proteins such as apolipoprotein E and ubiquitin has been reported.[163] Other findings include increased numbers of internalized nuclei and ragged red fibers. On EM, the rimmed vacuoles contain membranous myeloid whorls. The inclusion bodies are composed of tubular filaments that are 12–18 nm in diameter, and these sometimes occur in the nuclei.[164,165]

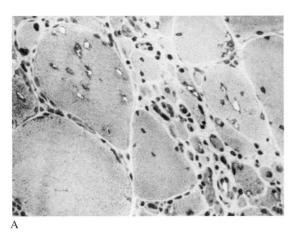

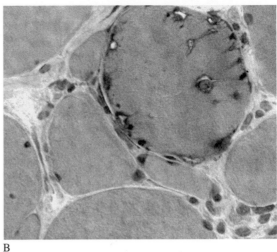

A   B

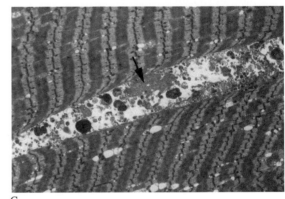

Figure 19.48 **A.** Modified trichrome-stained muscle in a patient with inclusion body myositis shows several fibers with rimmed vacuoles (×400). **B.** Multiple small vacuoles in one fiber (×400) (see Color Plates B37 and B38). **C.** Electron microscopy of a rimmed vacuole filled with myeloid debris and a small inclusion body (*arrow*) (×3,600).

C

Fasciitis. Muscle fascial inflammation occurs in eosinophilic fasciitis, as in the hypereosinophilic syndrome.[166,167] The biopsy can appear normal or show some necrosis. Inflammation of the fascia is characterized by infiltrates of mononuclear cells of various types, although eosinophils frequently predominate (Figure 19.49). Eosinophilic fasciitis can be seen with normal eosinophil count in the blood. This is sometimes found in patients with polymyalgia rheumatica or nonspecific muscle pains.[168] A fascial specimen during muscle biopsy is strongly recommended in these cases.

Sarcoidosis. Systemic sarcoidosis can present with a myopathy similar to PM or with various forms of neuropathy. Myopathy is sometimes the presenting symptom, even in those patients without weakness. The muscle biopsy is often helpful in the diagnosis of sarcoidosis to demonstrate the noncaseating granuloma with giant multinucleated cells, lymphocytes, and epithelioid cells, sometimes accompanied by fiber necrosis (Figure 19.50).[169–171]

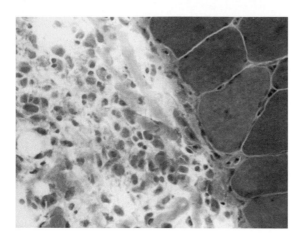

Figure 19.49 Inflammatory cells in the fascia of a patient with fascitis. The muscle fibers appear normal (hematoxylin and eosin, ×200).

Parasitic Myositis. Parasitic infestation can manifest with different muscle symptoms, such as weakness or hypertrophy. The histologic findings in parasitic myositis include fiber necrosis and inflammation. The larva of the parasite can sometimes be identified, particularly in trichinosis (Figure 19.51),[172] cysticercosis (Figure 19.52),[173] and toxoplasmosis.[174]

Viral Myositis. Acute viral infections such as influenza and coxsackie can manifest as an acute necrotizing myopathy. An inflammatory myopathy with frequent nemaline rods is seen in HIV-infected individuals.[175,176] Inflammatory myopathy is also seen in human T-cell lymphotrophic virus type I infections.[177]

Bacterial and Fungal Myositis. Bacterial and fungal muscle infections cause focal areas of muscle damage and abscesses with fiber necrosis and inflammatory cells. The responsible organisms are often identified.

Ischemic Myopathy. Ischemia of muscle from atherosclerosis, particularly in diabetics, can cause infarcts. Infarcts also occur after prolonged pressure in comatose patients and, rarely, in inflammatory myopathy. The biopsy shows muscle necrosis, prominent edema, and phagocytosis, particularly in the periphery of necrotic areas.

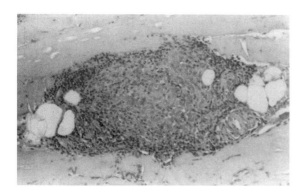

Figure 19.50 Sarcoid granuloma containing giant cells, lymphocytes, and epithelioid cells (hematoxylin and eosin, ×100).

Figure 19.51 Muscle fiber showing a parasite cyst in a case of trichinosis (hematoxylin and eosin, ×200).

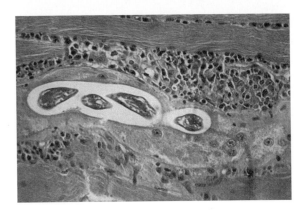

Toxic Myopathies

Toxins affect muscle by different pathologic mechanisms. A necrotizing myopathy with scattered pale necrotic fibers and some phagocytosis but no inflammation occurs with cholesterol-lowering drugs. This is also seen in severe drug-induced hypokalemia, alcoholism, and organophosphate poisoning and is sometimes caused by ε-aminocaproic acid.[178] Necrosis with inflammation can be caused by penicillamine, procainamide, phenytoin, and by ciguatera poisoning. A vacuolar myopathy with myeloid bodies and other cytoplasmic degradation products are seen in myopathies caused by chloroquine, amiodarone, perhexiline, colchicine, and vincristine.[178–180] A mitochondrial myopathy with frequent ragged red fibers can occur in patients receiving azidothymidine and germanium.

High doses of steroids and pharmacologic paralyzing agents can cause an acute quadriparesis in the "critical illness" myopathy, with disorganization of myofibrils and loss of thick filaments on EM and decreased staining for heavy chain myosin.[181]

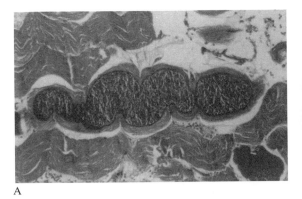

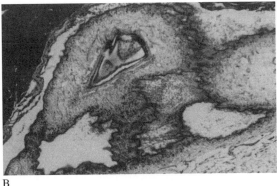

A   B

Figure 19.52 A. A cysticercosis larva inside a muscle fiber (hematoxylin and eosin, ×400). **B.** The scolex of a cysticercus (hematoxylin and eosin, ×200). (Courtesy of Dr. S. Shankar, National Institute of Health and Neurosciences, Bangalore, India.)

Endocrine Myopathies

Hypothyroidism and Hyperthyroidism. Patients with hypothyroidism may manifest with muscle spasms or weakness of variable severity. The muscle biopsy is usually minimally abnormal, showing nonspecific changes, even in those patients with marked elevation of serum creatine kinase. Hypertrophy of the mitochondria, dilatation of the transverse tubular system, and scattered glycogen accumulation can be seen at the EM level.[182] Patients with hyperthyroidism and weakness also have nonspecific or normal biopsy findings.

Hyperparathyroidism. In hyperparathyroidism, the muscle biopsy may show calcium accumulation in the capillaries and small vessels (see Color Plate B10) and scattered atrophic fibers, some of which stain positive with nonspecific esterase.[183,184]

Cushing's Disease and Steroid Myopathy. The myopathy of Cushing's disease is characterized by selective atrophy of type II muscle fibers, particularly of type IIb fibers, and frequent internalized nuclei. Most of the atrophic fibers do not stain dark with nonspecific esterase.[185,186]

Hyperpituitarism. The biopsy in hyperpituitarism can show fiber necrosis and atrophy of type II fibers.[187]

PERIPHERAL NERVE BIOPSY

General Aspects

Nerve biopsy is used in the diagnosis of some peripheral neuropathies, and for this, a sensory nerve is commonly biopsied, such as the sural nerve at the ankle. Other suitable nerves include the superficial peroneal, the sensory branch of the radial nerve, or a motor nerve, such as the one that innervates the peroneus brevis muscle.

For proper analysis, a cross-section of the entire nerve is preferred, although a fascicular biopsy can also be obtained.[188] Regardless of technique, it is best to remember that the longer the segment taken, the better the opportunity for adequate histologic studies, and usually 2–4 cm is sufficient. It is important that the surgeon and the laboratory personnel avoid excessive manipulation of the nerve to prevent stretching artifacts.

Complications of the procedure include loss of sensitivity in the dermatomal territory of the biopsied nerve and neuroma formation, causing chronic pain and infection. Vascular insufficiency with edema can occur, particularly if there is damage or sectioning of the adjacent lesser saphenous vein. The actual surgical procedure of the biopsy is not discussed here; for this, excellent textbooks that discuss this technique are recommended.[189–192]

Useful Histologic Techniques

Once excised, the nerve specimen is divided into several segments for submission to the laboratory. The longest length is submitted for frozen-section analysis or fixed in formalin for paraffin embedment and routine histology, or both. In this segment, staining is useful for the evaluation of vessels and for determining the presence of inflammation and granulomas. The modified Gomori trichrome stain is also helpful in detecting inflammatory cells. This stain (see Color Plate B39) and the Luxol fast blue provide better visualization of myelinated axons than the H&E. The frozen specimen is additionally stained with crystal violet and Congo red to detect amyloid deposits, whereas cresyl violet is used in the diagnosis of metachromatic leukodystrophy (MLD).

The Cajal, Bodian, and Bielschowsky silver stains are used to visualize axons in paraffin sections (see Color Plate B40), whereas the vessels are better studied with the elastic van Gieson method. The Heidenhain's hematoxylin technique improves visualization of myelin. Paraffin embedding of osmium-fixed specimens is used to study myelinated fibers and to determine whether there is a focal loss of fibers as occurs in vasculitis. Identification of inflammatory cells can be made with the use of immunoperoxidase staining for the leukocyte common antigen (see Color Plate B41) or specific lymphocyte markers.

Another segment of the nerve specimen is submitted for primary fixation in glutaraldehyde, followed by secondary fixation in osmium tetroxide for EM examination and teased nerve preparation. It is important that the fixatives are isosmolar, because hyperosmolar solutions alter normal fiber shape. Proper fixation is critical for these studies, as insufficient fixation can cause separation at the nodes of Ranvier or Schmidt-Lanterman incisures during handling, and excessive fixation can cause breakage of fibers during teasing.

The biopsy segment for teased nerve preparation is fixed overnight in osmium tetroxide to provide adequate visualization of myelinated axons. After a buffer rinse, the segment is placed in increasing percentages of aqueous glycerin, beginning with 66%, to a final solution of 90% over several days, until the individual myelinated axons can be separated. Some techniques use a final solution of 100% glycerin, but we find that this strength impairs the ability to grasp the fibers during separation or teasing.

Teased nerve preparations allow the evaluation of internodal length and the assessment of segmental demyelination, axonal degeneration, and abnormal myelin structures (e.g., tomaculi).

With teased nerve preparations, different types of myelinated fiber changes can be studied as proposed by P. J. Dyck.[188] Correlation of internodal length with fiber diameter is very useful in the evaluation. For example, when a regenerating axon is remyelinated, the internodal length becomes uniformly shortened, approximately 200–400 μm, depending on the diameter of the axon. In contrast, random demyelination results in long internodes mixed with short internodes.

Epoxy-embedded specimens are sectioned at approximately 1 μm and stained with toluidine blue (Figure 19.53) for light microscopic analysis of the vessels and of the myelinated fiber population. These sections are also useful in assessing axonal degeneration, the clustering of small myelinated axons in regeneration, and the onion-bulb formations in chronic demyelinating neuropathies. Morphometric analysis can be applied to these sections to fully define myelinated fiber density and population according to size and to determine whether there is a decrease in the number of myelinated fibers in a given area.

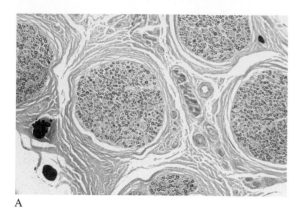
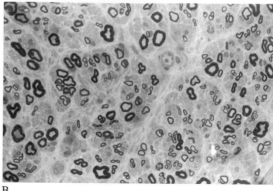

A   B

Figure 19.53 One-micron-thick plastic section of nerve shows several fascicles in cross-section in (**A**) and within a fascicle in (**B**). Notice the ability to make an overall assessment of the population of myelinated fibers in (**A**). In (**B**), the morphology and distribution of myelinated fibers can be assessed, helping to determine the presence of sprouting, onion-bulb formations, and degeneration (not seen here). (**A** = ×100; **B** = ×400.)

Unmyelinated axons are not visualized at the light level and are assessed by EM, which also allows the study of the basal laminae of vessels and the determination of degeneration, regeneration, and sprouting in both fiber types. EM is also useful in differentiating cell types to determine Schwann cell proliferation and to identify intracytoplasmic structures and storage material.

Components of Nerve

The principal components of nerve are the epineurium, the perineurium, and the endoneurium, the area in which nerve fibers and Schwann cells are located (Figure 19.54). The epineurium surrounds the entire fascicle and makes up one-half of the cross-sectional area of the nerve. This structure consists of connective tissue, capillaries, arterioles, and veins and contains fibroblasts, mast cells, and, occasionally, lymphocytes. Normal, but rarely seen, structures can sometimes be identified, such as a pacinian corpuscle (Figure 19.55).[193]

The sural nerve has approximately 6–15 fascicles and sometimes can have up to 20 fascicles.[189,193] The perineurium is the connective tissue layer surrounding each individual fascicle that has a network of collagen fibers in longitudinal and oblique orientations, particularly type III collagen.[194] Tangles of filaments that represent oxytalan, a precursor of elastic fibers, are seen. The Luse bodies are long-spacing collagen fibers that have the appearance of a raccoon's tail. Occasionally, calcifications are identified.

Small arterioles and venules are found in the epineurial and perineurial areas and are recognized by their lack of elastic laminae. Vessels are also sometimes seen in the perineurial septum, whereas in the endoneurium itself, there are mainly small capillaries.

The endoneurium is the region of the nerve fascicle internal to the perineurium. This has a cross-sectional area of 0.65–1.26 mm² and consists mainly of connective

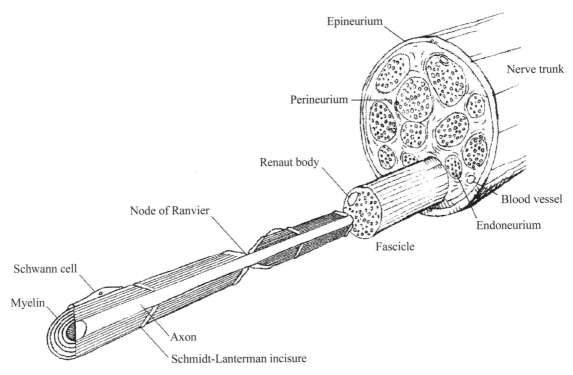

Figure 19.54 The components of nerve.

tissue, axons, and Schwann cells.[195] In this area, collagen runs longitudinally to the axons and is packed more closely, immediately in the area adjacent to the perineurium. Collagen in the endoneurium is mainly type I and type III collagen. Myelinated fibers and Schwann cells account for 24–36% of the total cross-sectional area; unmyelinated axons correspond to 11–12%; and dense, packed collagen is 35–45% of the endoneurial area.[193,196]

Figure 19.55 Pacinian corpuscle, a normal structure in nerve, in a cross-section embedded in paraffin and stained with hematoxylin and eosin (×40). The fascicles are artifactually distorted.

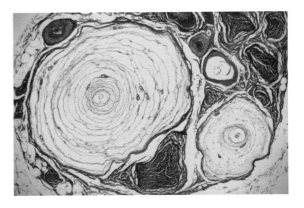

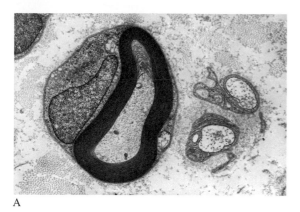

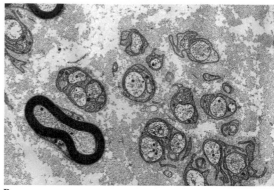

A

B

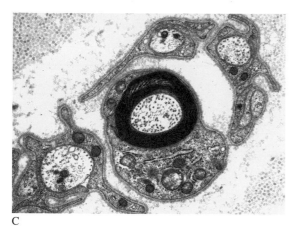

C

Figure 19.56 Electron micrographs of a Schwann cell and its associated single, myelinated axon (×9,000) **(A)** and a group of unmyelinated axons, several of which are associated with only one Schwann cell **(B)** (×6,000). The spreading of the myelin in **(C)** is a Schmidt-Lanterman incisure (×30,150).

Schwann cells surround both myelinated and unmyelinated axons. Each myelinated axon is associated with only one Schwann cell that provides its myelin (Figure 19.56). Several unmyelinated axons are contained within the cytoplasm of one Schwann cell. A Schwann cell profile surrounded by the same basal lamina and containing usually one to four unmyelinated axons is called a *Schwann cell subunit*, or *Remak fibers*. The cell processes have a basal lamina similar to endothelial and perineural cells, unlike fibroblasts, macrophages, lymphocytes, and plasma cells.

Capillaries and small venules, fibroblasts, pericytes, vascular endothelial cells, smooth muscle, and mast cells (Figure 19.57) can be seen in the endoneurium. An occasional lymphocyte is identified rarely in normals, but there are usually less than 10 leukocytes per mm^2.[197]

An eosinophilic structure sometimes identified in the endoneurium is the Renaut body, which consists of fibrous material that forms a whirled pattern close to the border of the endoneurium and adjacent to the perineurial membrane (see Color Plates B42 through B44). These can be mistaken for amyloid, but they are not congophilic. They differ in location, and, ultrastructurally, they are larger and less straight than amyloid fibrils. They do not contain axons, but do have fibroblasts,

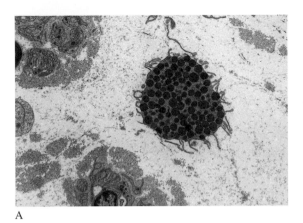
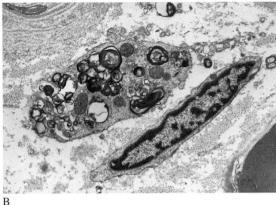

A   B

Figure 19.57 Electron micrographs of a mast cell (**A**) (×4,652) and a nucleated fibroblast adjacent to a macrophage within the endoneurium (**B**) (×12,000).

some small vessels, and, occasionally, mast cells. Although Renaut bodies are normal structures of no known significance, they may be increased with age or secondary to trauma and also in some peripheral neuropathies.

Axons

Nerve fibers within fascicles consist of large and small myelinated and unmyelinated fibers. Unmyelinated axons have an average diameter of 1.0–1.2 μm and have a unimodal distribution when diameters are plotted.

The normal sural nerve contains up to 9,400 evenly distributed myelinated fibers with a density of 5,200 to 8,000 per mm^2; this varies with age.[195] The unmyelinated fibers vary from 18,000–42,000 per mm^2.[195] The diameter of a myelinated axon is determined by measuring across the second largest diameter of the axon alone and including its myelin. A normal sural nerve has a bimodal distribution of myelinated fiber size when plotted. Thirty-two percent to 45% of myelinated axons are small, less than 7 μm in diameter[195]; 55–68% of the population is large, ranging from 7 μm to 14 μm in diameter. This and other morphometric details are discussed in detail elsewhere.[193,195]

The thickness of the myelin sheath is directly proportional to the axonal diameter. This comparison can be quantitated using the *G ratio*, which is the ratio of the diameter of the axon divided by the diameter of the axon plus its myelin. Normally, this ratio is 0.5 to 0.7.[195,198]

The axons contain primarily neurofilaments, which run parallel longitudinally to form a cytoskeleton. They are approximately 10 nm in diameter and are evenly distributed, with a density of 100–300 per μm^2.[198] They are the most abundant of the cytoplasmic organelles. The axonal microtubules are 25 nm in external diameter and 100–800 nm in length.[198] Other elements of the axon are the mitochondria, various membrane-bound structures, vesicles, and glycogen granules of approximately 30 μm.

An internode is the area of the axon myelinated by one Schwann cell. The internodal length can be measured on teased nerve preparations and is directly propor-

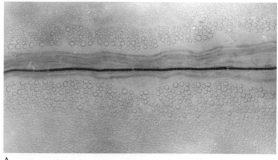

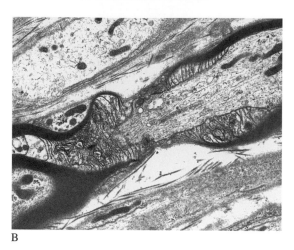

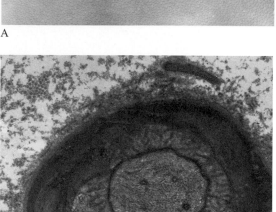

Figure 19.58 A. Teased nerve preparation of a myelinated axon and its equally spaced nodes of Ranvier, which are shortened (×100). **B.** Electron microscopy of a node of Ranvier in longitudinal section (×13,107) and in cross-section **(C)** (×7,600).

tional to the axonal diameter. In large axons, the internode is normally approximately 1.8 mm, and in small axons, it is 0.1 mm.[199]

The unmyelinated site at which two adjacent internodes meet is called the *node of Ranvier* (Figure 19.58). This region of the axon contains no myelin and, at this point, the membrane-bound organelles and microtubules are compact, whereas the neurofilaments are not significantly changed. The paranodal segment describes the area close to either side of the node. As the fiber approaches the node, it loses its rounded contour, creating a crenated cross-section of myelin around the axon (see Figure 19.58C).

Myelin

Myelin is a multilayer, laminated structure composed of layers of biochemically modified Schwann cell membrane, containing 45% water. Seventy-one percent of dehydrated myelin is lipid and 29% is protein.[200] There are normally 80–160 myelin lamella in each fiber, and this number increases with the axon's diameter. Important myelin lipids are phospholipids, glycolipids (e.g., gangliosides, cerebrosides, and sulfatides), and cholesterol. Important proteins include myelin-associated glycoprotein (MAG), which is a 100-kd transmembrane protein that makes up only 0.1% of myelin[201]; P0, P1, and P2 glycoproteins; and peripheral nerve myelin protein or PMP-22.[202]

Figure 19.59 Pi granules within Schwann cell cytoplasm (electron microscopy, ×12,000).

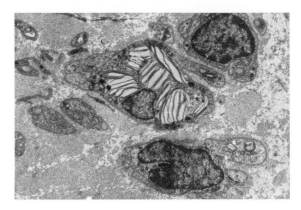

Myelin is transversed by the Schmidt-Lanterman clefts or incisures (see Figure 19.56). The clefts are uniform, and partial separations of myelin in this area represent interruption of the continuity of compact myelin. These are seen as oblique lines of noncompaction.[189] They can be mistaken for nodes of Ranvier on teased nerve preparations or for abnormal myelin separation on EM.[203]

Normal inclusions found in nerve include the granules of lipofuscin seen in Schwann cells and the Reich or Pi granules (Figure 19.59) that occur adjacent to the nucleus of Schwann cells of myelinated fibers. They are refractile under polarized light, stain positive with Sudan black B, and appear on EM as single, 1-μm membrane-bound organelles that have a lamellar pattern. The granules are nonspecific but can be more abundant in neuropathy. Other inclusions are Elzholz bodies or MU granules, which are round, osmiophilic bodies found in the cytoplasm of myelinating Schwann cells.

Artifacts of Nerve Electron Microscopy

Quality fixation of nerve for EM is difficult to achieve, and poor fixation makes it difficult to properly analyze the characteristics of myelin and neurofilaments within axons. Common EM artifacts include separation or disruption and swelling of myelin, swelling of neurofilaments, and separation of axons from myelin. These artifacts can also be produced by rough handling of the specimen before fixation. Excessive drying causes compaction of myelinated fibers, and, as discussed, in teased nerve preparations; this produces rupture of the fibers and separation of the nodes. These artifacts also occur with overfixation.

Pathologic Defects of Nerve

Wallerian Degeneration

Wallerian degeneration is the pathologic change that occurs distal to a nerve injury or transection and is named after the initial description by A. V. Waller.[204] During the first 12–24 hours after injury, the early pathologic changes observed in the axon are the abnormal accumulation of mitochondria, membranous organelles,

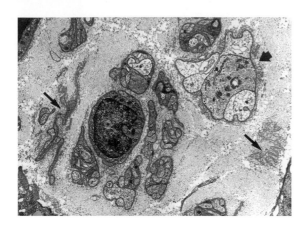

Figure 19.60 Sprouting of unmyelinated axons, bands of Büngner (*thick arrow*), many small unmyelinated axons, and empty Schwann cell subunits (*thin arrows*) on electron microscopy (×9,000).

glycogen, and lysosomes, with disorganization of microtubules and filaments in the node and paranodal region[205] and granular disintegration of the axon. Unmyelinated fibers show swelling distal to the injury, with accumulation of organelles and granular disintegration.

Myelin degradation begins after 24 hours with widening of the Schmidt-Lanterman incisures.[206] By 36 hours, it starts to form ovoids, beginning at the incisures and spreading throughout the internode. Three to 4 days after injury, macrophages begin to appear and contain myelin debris.

A week after transection, obvious increased cellularity is noted. *Bands of Büngner* are common (Figure 19.60); these are groups of Schwann cell processes that were previously associated with myelinated axons, and their presence indicates loss of myelinated axons. Axons regenerate within these bands. When unmyelinated axons degenerate and disappear, the Schwann cell processes encircling them become flattened.[207] These are called *denervated bands* or *denervated Schwann cell subunits* (Figure 19.61).[208]

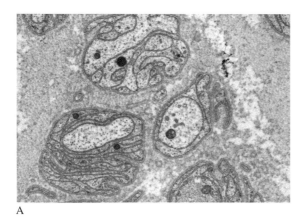

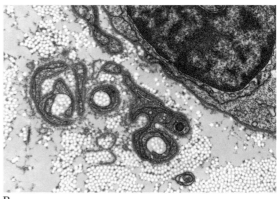

A   B

Figure 19.61 Electron micrographs of flattened axons and denervated Schwann cell processes (**A**) (×13,500) and collagen pockets (**B**) (×21,000).

AXONAL NEUROPATHY

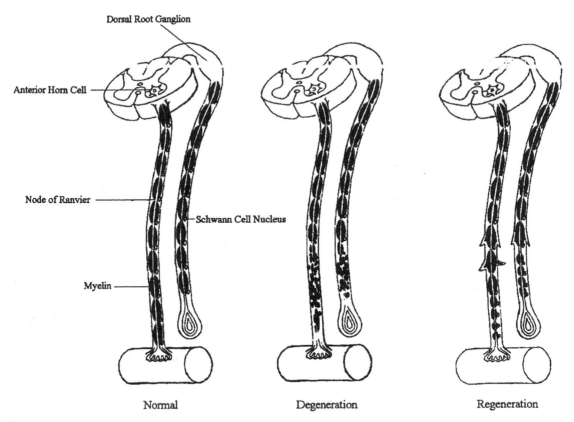

Figure 19.62 Diagrammatic representation of axonal degeneration and regeneration.

Axonal Degeneration

Axonal degeneration occurs primarily in diseases affecting the nerve cell, also called *axonopathies*. These affect the myelinated and the unmyelinated axons (Figure 19.62; see Table 5.7). The histologic findings are similar to wallerian degeneration, although more subtle, and are seen in isolated and scattered rather than in all axons. The degeneration is more chronic, occurring first in the distal nerve, secondary to the process of "dying back" of the axon.[209,210] Changes in the axon during degeneration include atrophy (Figure 19.63), swelling, formation of myelin ovoids (Figure 19.64; see Figure 5.9), paranodal retraction, and focal accumulations of abnormal mitochondria. In some neuropathies, there are accumulations of filamentous material (i.e., acrylamide toxicity). There are also tubular aggregates, vesicular formations, and evidence of nerve fiber loss. Unmyelinated fibers appear atrophic or flat, and empty Schwann cell processes are present. In chronic axonal neuropathy, the number of myelinated axons is usually decreased (Figure 19.65; Table 19.7; see Table 5.3).

Regeneration

Within 1 week after nerve damage, regeneration begins as growth cones in the tip of the damaged axon. The growth cone consists of terminal enlargement of the distal

Table 19.7 Biopsy Findings That Indicate Axonal Degeneration or Demyelination*

Axonal Degeneration	Demyelination
May affect myelinated and unmyelinated fibers	Affects primarily myelinated fibers
Axonal degeneration of myelinated fibers seen on thick plastic sections, teased nerve preparations (large ovoids)	Segmental demyelination
	Paranodal retraction, variation in internodal length
Axonal atrophy, inclusions	Large axons with thin myelin
Denervated Schwann cell subunits	Onion-bulb formations
Flattened, unmyelinated axons	Some tiny ovoids with variation in internodal length may be seen on teased nerve preparations
Bands of Büngner	
Regenerating clusters of myelinated fibers	—
Schwann cell processes with increased numbers of small unmyelinated axons	—

*These changes are not definitive for diagnosis and, in many neuropathies, could show evidence of both axonal degeneration and demyelination, with the diagnosis based on the predominance of one or the other to determine whether the process is primarily demyelinating or an axonopathy.

axon and contains numerous vesicular structures. During this period, there are giant axonal swellings, with central areas of filaments surrounded by vesicular organelles. Axonal regrowth occurs at a rate of 1–3 mm per day.[211]

During later stages of regeneration, there is axonal sprouting, which is identified histologically by the presence of several small myelinated axons occupying the space previously taken by a single myelinated fiber. These regenerated clusters are defined as three or more closely opposed, myelinated axons that are surrounded by a single basal lamina (Figure 19.66), which is not necessarily visualized in the plane of thin sectioning. On teased nerve preparations, the internodes of myelinated axons are shortened. Unmyelinated fibers also sprout, and the Schwann cell processes contain increased

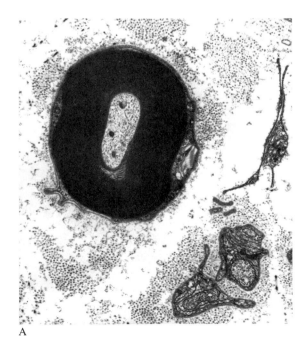

A

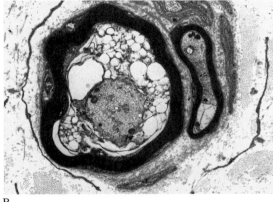

B

Figure 19.63 **A.** Electron micrograph of axonal atrophy (×13,500). The diameter of the axon is disproportionate to the diameter of the surrounding myelin. (Note the slender processes of a fibroblast.) **B.** An atrophic axon and early myelin degeneration (×9,000).

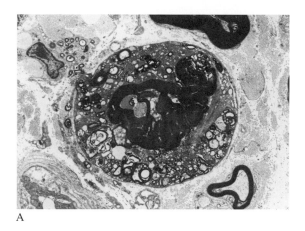

A

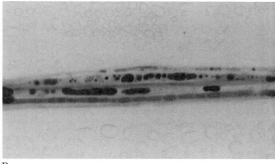

B

Figure 19.64 Degenerated axon on electron microscopy (×4,652) (**A**) and on teased nerve preparation (×100) (**B**). Myelin debris remains within the Schwann cell cytoplasm and appears as ovoids or balls in the teased nerve preparation.

numbers of axons, which can be very small, or the processes also surround connective tissue rather than axons to form "collagen pockets" (see Figure 19.61B).

Demyelination

The characteristic finding of primary demyelination is *segmental demyelination* (Figure 19.67), which can be initially observed on teased nerve preparations as a widening of the node of Ranvier, with paranodal retraction, and later, by a complete loss of myelin in the whole segment (Figures 19.68 and 19.69; see Figure 5.9). In this process, Schwann cell cytoplasm swells and may contain myelin debris. Large axons with thin myelin (Figure 19.70) or no myelin (Figure 19.71) and demyelinated or hypomyelinated internodal segments are also observed. Destructive stripping of myelin by macrophages is evident, mainly, but not exclusively, in inflammatory demyelinating neuropathies. Myelin degenerates first, forming vesicles, which appear between the myelin lamellae and in macrophages.

Secondary demyelination defines the demyelination that occurs in distal nerve secondary to axonal degeneration, as was elegantly demonstrated by Dyck and collaborators in uremic neuropathy.[209]

Figure 19.65 Thick plastic section of nerve showing marked dropout of myelinated axons (toluidine blue, ×200).

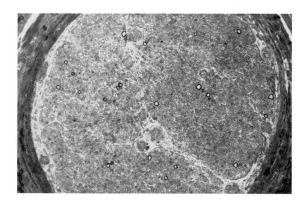

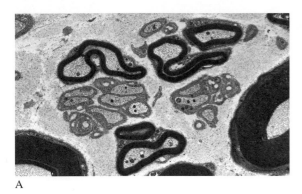

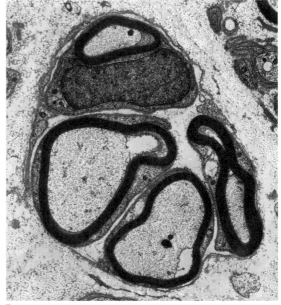

Figure 19.66 A. Clusters of small myelinated axons suggestive of sprouting (×9,000). **B.** Sprouting of small myelinated axons (×13,550).

B

DEMYELINATING NEUROPATHY

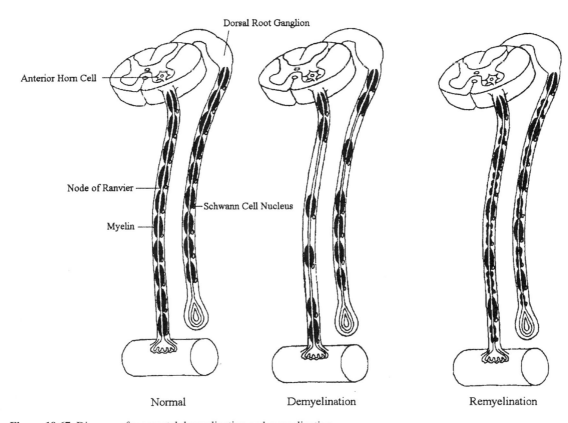

Figure 19.67 Diagram of segmental demyelination and remyelination.

Figure 19.68 Illustration of myelinated axons on teased nerve preparation: remyelination with shortened internodes (**A**), demyelination of a single segment or internode (**B**), and axonal degeneration with myelin ovoids (**C**).

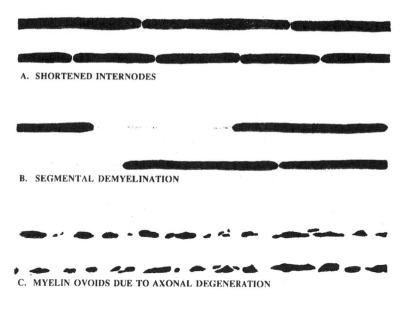

A. **SHORTENED INTERNODES**

B. **SEGMENTAL DEMYELINATION**

C. **MYELIN OVOIDS DUE TO AXONAL DEGENERATION**

Figure 19.69 Teased nerve preparation showing a single myelinated axon devoid of myelin in one internode (×100).

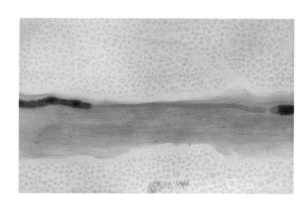

Figure 19.70 Electron micrograph of myelinated axons in cross-section shows disproportionate or thin myelin in the larger axons (×4,413).

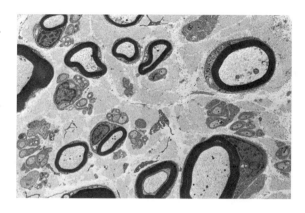

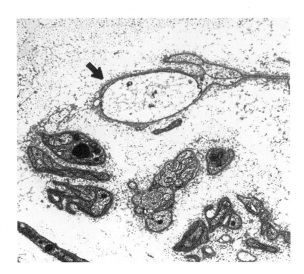

Figure 19.71 A large axon completely devoid of myelin (*arrow*) (×4,500). Also notice the many small unmyelinated axons.

Abnormalities in the periodicity of myelin are seen in some neuropathies. These include *uncompacted myelin*, in which the cytoplasmic aspect of the Schwann cell separates, does not attach, and appears on EM to have large amounts of cytoplasm between two layers of myelin. Uncompacted myelin can be seen in Guillain-Barré syndrome (GBS), chronic inflammatory demyelinating polyneuropathy (CIDP)

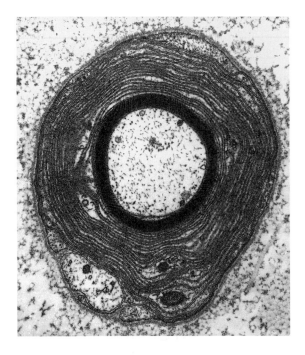

Figure 19.72 A myelinated axon with uncompacted myelin on electron microscopy (×45,360). This begins more frequently in the innermost areas but can also be seen in the periphery, as in this case of chronic inflammatory demyelinating polyneuropathy without gammopathy.

Figure 19.73 Widely spaced myelin. Typical appearance in a patient with circulating immunoglobulin M paraprotein and demyelinating neuropathy (×23,800). (Reproduced with permission from G Midroni, JM Bilbao. Schwann Cells and Myelin in the Peripheral Nervous System. In G Midroni, JM Bilbao, SM Cohen [eds], Biopsy Diagnosis of Peripheral Neuropathy. Boston: Butterworth–Heinemann, 1995;93.)

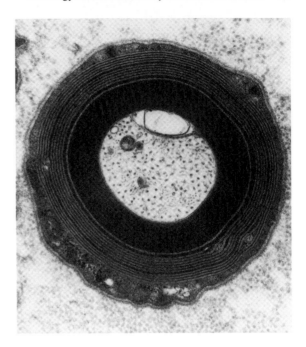

(Figure 19.72),[212] POEMS (*p*olyneuropathy, *o*rganomegaly, *e*ndocrinopathy, *m*onoclonal gammopathy, and *s*kin changes) syndrome, and in some hereditary neuropathies, such as hereditary neuropathy with liability to pressure palsy (HNPP).[213] Another alteration of the myelin sheath is *widely spaced myelin* (Figure 19.73), caused by separation of the interperiod lines of myelin, which appears as very regular separations, mainly in the outermost areas of myelin lamellae. This occurs most often in dysproteinemic neuropathies, particularly those caused by antibodies against MAGs, in which deposits of IgM are evident in these areas by immunofluorescence.[214] *Loose myelin* describes focal areas of slightly spaced lamellae that can be seen in various demyelinating neuropathies.

Tomaculous alterations are segmentally thickened myelin sheaths, either circumferentially or eccentrically (Figure 19.74), that on teased nerve preparations have a resemblance to sausages. They appear in the paranodal area but can occupy the whole internode and occur most often in HNPP. Less conspicuous, isolated segments with tomaculi are sometimes seen in other demyelinating neuropathies. Some biopsies of the Charcot-Marie-Tooth (CMT) disease type 4 have prominent myelin outfoldings.[215]

During the process of remyelination, there is proliferation of Schwann cells, and single axons can be surrounded by several Schwann cells. With regeneration, the new remyelinating Schwann cell appears close to the axon, and the others are displaced outward. The myelin lamellae are thin, and the Schwann cells and their processes surround the myelinated axon to form the characteristic *onion bulbs* of chronic demyelination and remyelination (Figure 19.75). The remyelinating Schwann cells have an abundance of rough endoplasmic reticulum and mitochondria, and the remyelinated axon may show redundant basal laminae. On teased nerve preparations, remyelinated axons have shortened internodes (see Figures 19.68 and 19.69).

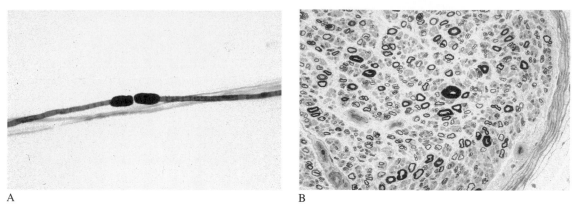

A   B

Figure 19.74 A. Teased nerve preparation of a paranodal tomaculous formation (×400). **B.** Toluidine blue–stained thick section of the same case showing the thickened myelin of a tomacula in cross-section (×400).

Nerve Biopsy in Specific Neuropathies

The nerve biopsy provides specific diagnosis only in some neuropathies, and those findings are described here. In many others, the findings are nonspecific and only show variations of the severity of the basic pathologic changes discussed previously. When describing specific disease entities, these findings should be correlated with those of the clinical and laboratory studies. For this reason, we include not only their histologic findings but also a brief description of the disease.

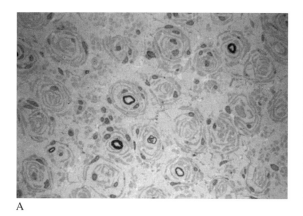

A

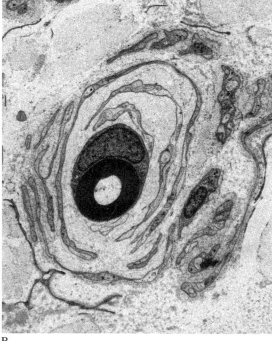

Figure 19.75 Onion-bulb formation on light (**A**) and electron (**B**) microscopy are composed of Schwann cell processes that wrap around the myelinated axon. (**A** = toluidine blue, ×400; **B** = ×6,075.)

B

Hereditary Neuropathies

A number of genetically determined disorders can be recognized by their clinical characteristics and biopsy findings. The exact pathogenesis of these is not clear, but in some, it is associated with defects of genes that express important nerve proteins. The most commonly recognized conditions are described.

Demyelinating Charcot-Marie-Tooth Disease. Demyelinating CMT (type 1 and type X) has also been classified as hereditary motor-sensory neuropathy type 1 (HMSN-I).[216] They are characterized by progressive weakness, with only mild sensory deficit, mainly affecting vibration and position sense, areflexia, high arches, hammer toes, enlarged nerves, and slow nerve conduction velocities. CMT 1 is autosomal dominant, and CMT X is X-linked recessive.

Most of the dominant forms are caused by mutations of the PMP-22 (CMT 1A)[202,217] and P0 protein genes (CMT 1B),[218] and some have defects of the gene that expresses early growth response protein (i.e., EGR2).[219] The X-linked recessive type is caused by defects of the gene for the gap protein connexin 32.[220] Histologically, these conditions show chronic demyelinating changes of variable severity; these include enlargement of fascicles, prominent onion-bulb formations (see Figure 19.75), a reduction in the number of myelinated fibers, and frequent axons with thin myelin, which is disproportionate for the axonal diameter. Axonal degeneration is rare, but regenerated clusters are sometimes seen. There is also prominent endoneurial connective tissue. Teased nerve preparations demonstrate segmental demyelination, variation in the internodal length, and, some, short internodes.[221,222]

Hereditary Neuropathy with Liability to Pressure Palsy. HNPP is an autosomal dominant disease caused by deletions of chromosome 17p 11.2-12[223,224] and, therefore is allelic to CMT 1A, which is associated with duplications of this gene. HNPP manifests by recurrent mononeuropathies caused by compression, although some patients may have a more severe phenotype that resembles CMT.

The most characteristic pathologic finding in this disease is the presence of *tomaculi* (Figure 19.76), which were described previously and are recognized most easily on teased nerve preparations.[225,226] There is also evidence of demyelination, and EM shows large axons with thickened myelin and some onion-bulb formations.

Axonal Charcot-Marie-Tooth Disease. CMT 2 is an axonal form of the disease and is also referred to as HMSN-II. CMT 2 usually has an autosomal dominant inheritance and may appear somewhat later in life than type 1, with distal weakness, sometimes normal proximal reflexes, fairly normal nerve conduction velocities, and evidence of denervation changes that can be prominent on EMG examination.[227,228] Histologic findings include a decreased number of myelinated fibers with only rare degenerated axons, some atrophic axons, and regenerating clusters.[228]

Dejerine-Sottas Disease (Charcot-Marie-Tooth Type 3 or Hereditary Motor-Sensory Neuropathy Type III). This disease usually has a more severe phenotype and can appear in early childhood with weakness and areflexia. Electrophysiologic

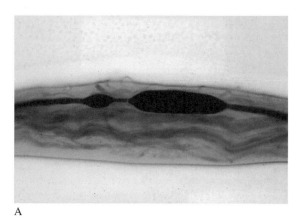
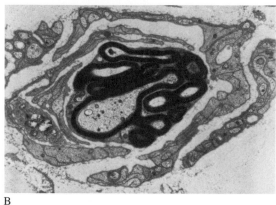

A   B

Figure 19.76 A. Tomaculous formation on teased nerve preparation from a case of hereditary neuropathy with liability to pressure palsy (×400). (This case was studied with Dr. Thomas O'Brien, the Methodist Hospitals of Memphis, who provided the photograph.) **B.** Myelin foldings or redundant loops of myelin (Charcot-Marie-Tooth type 4B). (Reproduced with permission from G Midroni, JM Bilbao, SM Cohen [eds], Biopsy Diagnosis of Peripheral Neuropathy. Boston: Butterworth–Heinemann, 1995;374.)

studies show marked slowing of nerve conduction. The genetic defects are similar to those of CMT 1,[217] although some have mutations of the periaxin gene. Pathologically, nerve biopsies show prominent onion bulbs and large axons with thin myelin. Axonal degeneration is rare.[216] In some cases, hypomyelination can occur, and many axons lacking myelin can be seen on biopsy.[229,230]

Charcot-Marie-Tooth Type 4. CMT 4 represents a group with autosomal recessive inheritance caused by different genetic defects, usually presenting in childhood with severe phenotypes caused by various genetic defects including those of myotubularin-related protein-2, ERG2, and periaxin. The nerve biopsy shows evidence of onion bulbs, demyelination, and, in some cases, prominent focal folded myelin (CMT 4B) (see Figure 19.76B).[215]

Hereditary-Sensory and Autonomic Neuropathies. Hereditary-sensory and autonomic neuropathies (HSAN) are a group of disorders of heterogeneous presentation with sensory or autonomic manifestations, or both, that have diffemrent inheritances.[231,232] HSAN type I is autosomal dominant and is associated with a defect in chromosome 9. It presents in adulthood with loss of sensation, pain, and skin ulcerations. Pathologically, there is a severe loss of unmyelinated and small myelinated fibers with axonal atrophy and degeneration.[231]

HSAN type II has an autosomal recessive inheritance and manifests in childhood with some sensory deficits and mutilation of the hands and feet. Pathologically, there is marked fascicular atrophy with an almost complete loss of myelinated fibers and some loss of unmyelinated fibers. In the Riley-Day syndrome (HSAN-III), myelinated fibers appear small, and there is a marked reduction in the number of unmyelinated fibers. The autonomic and the dorsal root ganglia show a decreased number of neurons. In HSAN-IV, there is a decreased number of small myelinated fibers with an absence of unmyelinated fibers. The unmyelinated fibers appear normal in type VI and are mildly reduced in HSAN type V, which also shows a reduced number of myelinated fibers. The pathologic findings in all of these disorders are otherwise nonspecific,[233] and the diagnosis should be made by correlating these with the history and clinical findings.

Giant Axonal Neuropathy. Giant axonal neuropathy is an autosomal recessive neuropathy of childhood onset that manifests by feeding and breathing difficulties, inability to walk, and clinical signs of neuropathy, but it also presents signs of central nervous system dysfunction, with profound mental retardation, ataxia, and facial weakness. Some patients may have seizures and characteristically tightly curled hair.[234,235] The disease affects the intermediate filaments and is linked to chromosome 16q24. Pathologically, large axons are scattered within fascicles, and these measure up to 50 μm, with thin myelin or no myelin, and the number of myelinated fibers may be decreased. The large axons have densely packed filaments that can also be seen in endothelial cells, Schwann cells, and fibroblasts.[235–237]

Infantile Neuronal Axonal Atrophy. Infantile neuronal axonal atrophy is an autosomal recessive disease of newborns, with mental and motor impairment. Pathologically, the changes occur in isolated fascicles and consist of atrophic or swollen axons with thin myelin and PAS-positive granular accumulations in the axoplasma with vesicular profiles.[238] Axonal degeneration and demyelination are not prominent.

Peripheral Neuropathies in Spinocerebellar Degeneration. The various types of spinocerebellar degenerations may present with variable sensory or motor symptoms of peripheral neuropathy. The most commonly recognized is Friedreich's ataxia, characterized by ataxia, dysarthria, areflexia, Babinski sign, and proprioceptive deficits, with a neuropathy affecting large myelinated axons, and other manifestations, such as cardiomyopathy and scoliosis. The nerve biopsy shows a decreased number of myelinated fibers with little evidence of axonal degeneration. There is some fibrosis and onion-bulb formation.[239,240]

Adult Polyglucosan Body Disease. Adult polyglucosan body disease may present with gait disturbance and cognitive impairment or features of a motor neuron disease with an axonal neuropathy. The characteristic histologic finding is the presence of deposits of PAS-positive inclusions in axons and sweat glands.[241]

Familial Amyloidosis. The amyloidoses are a group of conditions characterized by deposits of Congo red–positive proteins in tissues. *Primary amyloidosis* refers to a form of disease that is not inherited, which is described later. *Secondary amyloidosis* is associated with chronic inflammatory disorders. The *familial amyloidoses* have autosomal dominant inheritance.

The *transthyretin* type of familial amyloidosis is caused by a mutation of the transthyretin gene on chromosome 18,[242] which causes deposits of transthyretin, a protein that normally transports thyroxine and retinol. The disease presents in adulthood with predominantly sensory and autonomic neuropathy and cardiomyopathy.[243] *Apolipoprotein A1* amyloidosis has a presentation that begins in the 20s with a sensorimotor neuropathy, renal failure, endocrinopathy, and peptic ulcer disease. The gene defect has been mapped to chromosome 11.[244] *Gelsolin* familial amyloidosis presents with a mild neuropathy with corneal lattice atrophy, skin abnormalities,

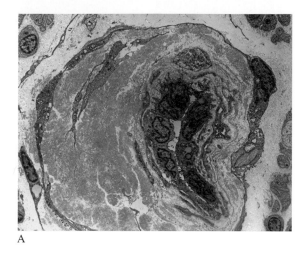

A

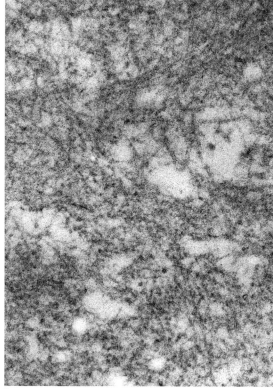

Figure 19.77 Amyloid in nerve around a vessel on electron microscopy (**A**) (×6,000) and at higher magnification (**B**) to show the organization of the amyloid fibers (×90,000).

B

and prominent cranial neuropathy.[245,246] The disease is linked to chromosome 9q32-34.[247]

As discussed above, the pathologic hallmark of these neuropathies is the presence of Congo red–positive material in nerves. This can be recognized by polarized light or immunofluorescence (Figure 19.77; see Color Plates B45 through B47). Amyloid is present mainly in vessels or in clumps in the endoneurial area, with a preferential involvement of the unmyelinated fibers with prominent axonal degeneration in some cases. The diagnosis can also be made by skin biopsy and, in the transthyretin type, can be recognized by immunofluorescence with antibodies against this protein.

Neuropathy in Hereditary Metabolic Disorders

Porphyrias. The porphyrias are a group of familial disorders caused by several hereditary enzyme deficiencies that result in abnormalities in heme synthesis. Those associated with peripheral neuropathy include *acute intermittent porphyria, δ-aminolevulinic acid dehydratase deficiency,*[248] and *hereditary coproporphyria* and *variegata porphyria*, both of which usually manifest with a skin disease.

Acute intermittent porphyria is caused by a deficiency of porphobilinogen deaminase from a genetic defect on chromosome 11q.[249] Coproporphyria is caused by a deficiency of coproporphyrinogen oxidase, expressed by a gene in chromosome

3q12,[250] and variegata porphyria by a deficiency of protoporphyrinogen oxidase, caused by missense mutations in chromosome 1q21-23.[251]

All are autosomal dominant, except for aminolevulinic acid dehydratase deficiency, which is an autosomal recessive disease of infancy caused by a defect on chromosome 9q34.[252]

Patients with porphyria present with sensory symptoms, autonomic dysfunction, areflexia, and weakness that may be prominent. Occasionally, the disease can manifest as a severe, acute, predominantly motor neuropathy with weakness, resembling GBS. The common pathologic finding in porphyria is that of axonal degeneration of unmyelinated and small myelinated fibers,[253,254] with some involvement of the large myelinated fibers; in some, there is also segmental demyelination,[255,256] which is believed to be secondary.[257]

Storage Diseases

SPHINGOLIPIDOSIS. Sphingolipidoses are disorders caused by accumulations of sphingolipids, which are lipids in which sphingosine replaces glycerol as the main component. These include important membrane constituents, such as gangliosides, cerebrosides, and sulfatides. Many of the sphingolipidoses manifest by central nervous system dysfunctions. Among the ones also presenting with neuropathy are MLD, Krabbe's and Fabry's diseases.

METACHROMATIC LEUKODYSTROPHY. MLD is an autosomal recessive disease caused by a deficiency of arylsulfatase A that is expressed in chromosome 22,[258] causing an accumulation of sulfatides. MLD is characterized by dementia, ataxia, visual loss, and a prominent demyelinating neuropathy, which can be the presenting symptom in some cases. The pathologic finding on peripheral nerve biopsy is the presence of PAS-positive granules that are brown, with cresyl violet stain (see Color Plate B48). There is also prominent demyelination.[259] Characteristic "tuffstone" inclusions are seen on EM in the cytoplasm of Schwann cells.[260] Also, there are other inclusions, such as the so-called herringbone or prismatic, the zebra bodies, and other osmiophilic inclusions (Figure 19.78).

GLOBOID CELL LEUKODYSTROPHY OR KRABBE'S DISEASE. This autosomal recessive disease is due to a gene defect on chromosome 14q24-32 that causes galactosylceramide-β-galactosidase deficiency. Patients manifest prominent and progressive central nervous system disease, with regression of milestones, spasticity, blindness, deafness, and a peripheral neuropathy, in which there is histologic evidence of

Figure 19.78 An osmiophilic inclusion in the cytoplasm of a Schwann cell of a myelinated fiber in metachromatic leukodystrophy (electron microscopy, ×30,000). (Courtesy of Dr. S. Shankar, National Institute of Mental Health and Neurosciences, Bangalore, India.)

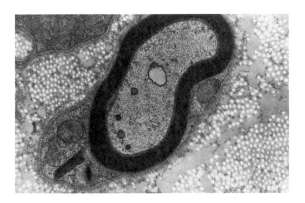

demyelination, accompanied by prominent onion bulbs and needle-like, or tubular, inclusions in Schwann cells and macrophages.[261]

FABRY'S DISEASE OR ANGIOKERATOMA CORPORIS DIFFUSUM. Fabry's disease is an X-linked recessive disorder with a genetic defect on chromosome Xq22, resulting in a deficiency of α-galactosidase A. The disease presents with skin lesions or angiokeratomas, renal dysfunction, and peripheral neuropathy.[262] The diagnosis is made by chemical analysis or skin biopsy.[263] A nerve biopsy is not always necessary for the diagnosis, but shows selective loss of small myelinated and unmyelinated fibers and osmiophilic storage material in all cell types in the nerve.[264,265] The inclusions are visible by EM and can be seen with light microscopy with birefringence that are used to detect the Maltese-cross pattern inclusions. These are also PAS- and oil red O–positive.

Lipoprotein Disorders. Lipoproteins are particles composed of lipids and proteins. Their lipid composition consists primarily of triglycerides, cholesterol, and phospholipids. They are molecules of various sizes that include very-low-density lipoproteins, low-density lipoproteins, intermediate density lipoproteins, high-density lipoproteins, and chylomicrons. Apolipoproteins are molecules situated on the surface of these particles that provide their structural stability. This is altered in the various lipoprotein diseases.

A-β lipoproteinemia and hypobetalipoproteinemia manifest with malabsorption, vitamin E deficiency, peripheral neuropathy, acanthocytosis, retinopathy, and ataxia. The pathologic changes in peripheral nerve are nonspecific and consist of axonal degeneration that affects mainly myelinated fibers, with secondary demyelination.[266] The gene for A-β lipoproteinemia expresses the microsomal triglyceride transfer protein in chromosome 4q22-24. The genetic effect causes the absence of apoprotein B–containing lipoproteins in plasma. A partial deficiency causes hypobetalipoproteinemia.

Tangier disease is caused by a genetic defect on chromosome 9q31 and is characterized by a deficiency of high-density lipoprotein–cholesterol in plasma. The predominant manifestation is a peripheral neuropathy of various presentations, such as mononeuropathy, mononeuritis multiplex, or polyneuropathy. The age of onset is variable.[267,268] The pathologic findings are nonspecific and include axonal degeneration, a reduced number of myelinated and unmyelinated fibers, and membrane-bound lipid accumulations in Schwann cells.

Peroxisomal Disorders. Peroxisomes are membrane-bound organelles that catalyze the β oxidation of fatty acids, such as the very-long-chain fatty acids, and peroxisomal disorders are caused by defects in their assembly from enzyme deficiencies that might manifest as a variety of neurologic disorders. In *Refsum's disease*, there is an accumulation of the 20-carbon, branched-chain fatty acid called *phytanic acid*, which is present in green vegetables.[269] Phytanic acid is normally metabolized by the enzyme phytanoyl coenzyme A hydroxylase, which is expressed on chromosome 10p. Its defect causes phytanic acid accumulation.

This autosomal recessive disorder is characterized by retinitis pigmentosa and other ocular manifestations, such as cataracts, glaucoma, and subluxation of the lenses. Patients also have hearing loss, anemia, ichthyosis, skeletal abnormalities, cardiac dysfunction, sensorimotor deficits, and ataxic peripheral neuropathy.[270,271] The pathologic findings in nerve are demyelination and accumulation of noncharacteristic osmiophilic material in Schwann cells with occasional onion-bulb formations.[272]

Adrenomyeloneuropathy is an X-linked recessive disorder caused by a defect of β oxidation of saturated unbranched very-long-chain fatty acids. It has various presentations, including adrenal insufficiency, intellectual deterioration, myelopathy, and a demyelinating neuropathy.[273,274] The disease is caused by a genetic defect on Xp22 in a gene that encodes a protein of the peroxisomal membrane. The neuropathy in this disease can be prominent and may exhibit not only demyelination but also axonal degeneration. An increased number of Pi granules in Schwann cells has been reported,[275] but this is likely a nonspecific finding.

Autoimmune Inflammatory Neuropathies

Acute Inflammatory Demyelinating Polyneuropathy (Guillain-Barré Syndrome)

GBS presents with an acute ascending paralysis, preceded by an infectious process in approximately 50% of the patients. They usually have areflexia, electrophysiologic evidence of demyelination, and albuminocytological dissociation of the spinal fluid.

The pathology of GBS is multifocal,[276] and sural nerve biopsy is usually unnecessary for the diagnosis. The biopsy may appear normal[277,278] or may show nonspecific changes. The most characteristic findings are the presence of demyelination with early vesicular degeneration of myelin, myelin breakdown, and macrophages with myelin debris and endoneurial lymphocytic infiltrates,[278,279] although they are not always present.[276] Axonal degeneration can occur and is prominent in severe cases. Immunohistochemistry shows evidence of deposits of C3d and terminal complement membrane attack complexes in the surface of myelinated fibers.[280]

Acute Motor Sensory Axonal Neuropathy

Acute motor sensory axonal neuropathy (AMSAN) is an axonal variant of GBS that usually presents with a rapidly developing, severe quadriparesis[281] and respiratory failure, often preceded by *Campylobacter jejuni* infection. It has a poorer prognosis than acute inflammatory demyelinating polyneuropathy, with slow recovery. Electrophysiologic studies demonstrate signs of axonal degeneration, confirmed by biopsy showing loss of myelinated and unmyelinated fibers, with prominent axonal degeneration.[282] On autopsy, these findings are prominent in the dorsal and ventral roots with many macrophages adjacent to the axons, which are displaced in some areas, but with little evidence of lymphocytic infiltrates.

Acute Motor Axonal Neuropathy

Acute motor axonal neuropathy (AMAN) is an acute, purely motor variant of GBS that is also usually preceded by *C. jejuni* infection. It is mainly reported in, but not limited to, Chinese children.[283,284] The condition develops rapidly, but usually has a very good recovery. The pathologic changes in AMAN occur mainly in the myelinated fibers of the ventral roots, where there is lengthening of the node of Ranvier and accumulation of filaments and dense bodies in the axolemma. Macrophages are seen in the perinodal region, and the perinodal myelin can be distorted and degenerated. On EM, the macrophages appear to be invading the Schwann cell basal lamina with minimal or no axonal degeneration. Lymphocytes are usually not identified.[283,285]

It appears that AMAN is initiated by deposits of IgG and complement in the node with recruitment of macrophages, which separate the myelin from its axon. The lack of significant axonal damage explains the relatively good recovery, despite the signs of denervation on electromyography.

Miller-Fisher Variant of Guillain-Barré Syndrome

The Miller-Fisher variant of GBS is characterized by ophthalmoplegia, ataxia, and areflexia, with little or no weakness and good prognosis for recovery. Pathologic findings have not been well delineated but may show patchy demyelination.[285]

Acute Pandysautonomic Neuropathy

Acute pandysautonomic neuropathy is an acute disease characterized primarily by autonomic manifestations, such as heat intolerance, orthostatic hypotension, sphincter dysfunction, areflexia, and, in some cases, sensory deficit. Nerve conduction studies are usually normal, whereas autonomic tests show evidence of autonomic failure.[286,287] Pathologic findings are nonspecific and can be normal or show scattered axonal degeneration with some foci of perivascular inflammatory cells.[288]

Sensory Guillain-Barré Syndrome

Purely sensory GBS, an acute sensory variant of GBS that is characterized by significant sensory deficit with areflexia, but no weakness, has been described.[289] In these patients, electrophysiologic studies show evidence of demyelination.[290] The pathology is not well characterized. Inflammation can be seen in the posterior root ganglia.

Another group of patients presents with an acute sensory ataxic neuropathy or ganglioneuritis.[291] The pathology of these syndromes is not well characterized. In one case with muscle weakness, there were lymphocytic infiltrates in nerve and posterior roots and demyelination.[292]

Chronic Inflammatory Demyelinating Polyneuropathy

CIDP is an acquired, subacute, or slowly progressive neuropathy with proximal and distal weakness and predominantly large fiber sensory loss, areflexia, elevation of spinal fluid protein, and electrophysiologic evidence of demyelination.[293,294] The disease has a variable presentation. Diagnostic criteria have been set for research purposes.[295]

Some patients with CIDP can manifest evidence of central demyelination or systemic disorders, such as diabetes and monoclonal gammopathies. Others can have a more distal sensory-motor deficit (distal autoimmune demyelinating polyneuropathy). Many of those patients have an IgM monoclonal gammopathy and have antibodies against MAG, which is discussed in the section Neuropathy and Monoclonal Gammopathy. A purely sensory form of CIDP has also been reported.[296]

The sural nerve findings in CIDP include demyelination and Schwann cell proliferation. These, however, are not always seen because the disease is multifocal and patchy. Lymphocytic infiltrates can be present (Figure 19.79A; see Color Plate B41) but are not commonly found.[297,298] Other abnormalities include endoneurial and subperineurial edema (see Figure 19.79B), myelin stripping by macrophages, and the presence of thinly myelinated axons, regenerating axons, and onion bulbs.

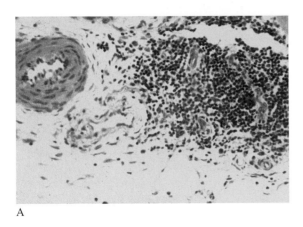
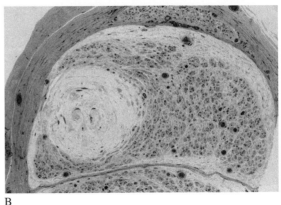

A   B

Figure 19.79 A. Nerve biopsy, chronic inflammatory demyelinating polyneuropathy showing perivascular inflammation on hematoxylin and eosin (×200). **B.** Subperineural edema in a fascicle of nerve, containing a Renaut body, in a case of chronic inflammatory demyelinating polyneuropathy (×200). There is also a decreased number of myelinated fibers.

Axonal degeneration can be present; this usually is not prominent but, in rare cases, can be severe.[299]

It should be stressed that none of these pathologic findings is diagnostic of CIDP and should be interpreted together with the clinical presentation, electrophysiologic findings, and the results of spinal fluid analysis. In this regard, Molenaar et al.,[298] in a study of 64 patients with CIDP, found that sural nerve biopsy did not provide additional diagnostic value, and Stewart et al.[300] found that sural nerve biopsy did not aid in the diagnosis of CIDP in patients with diabetes, as the findings could not be separated from those with classic diabetic polyneuropathy. In a retrospective study, however, Haaq et al.[301] found specificity of more than 80% in the diagnosis of CIDP using EM and teased nerve preparations of 24 patients with CIDP and 12 with diabetes.

Multifocal Motor Neuropathy and Multifocal Motor Sensory Neuropathy

Multifocal motor neuropathy (MMN) is a slowly progressive, asymmetric neuropathy involving mainly the upper extremities and resembling a motor neuron disorder. Often, there is electrophysiologic evidence of conduction block and the presence of antibodies against GM-1 gangliosides.[302,303] The nerve biopsy shows mild, nonspecific abnormalities, which include large axons with thin myelin, no inflammation or edema, and occasional onion-bulb formations.

Another group, initially described by Lewis and Sumner,[304] has evidence of sensory deficit and is called *multifocal motor sensory neuropathy* (MMSN). Pathologic studies in two cases of multifocal motor sensory neuropathy revealed changes that are not distinguishable from CIDP.[305]

Sarcoidosis

Sarcoidosis is an inflammatory disease characterized by the presence in various organs of noncaseating granulomas with giant cells, epithelial cells, and lymphocytes. Sarcoidosis might cause different types of neuropathies, such as mononeuropathy multiplex, radiculopathy, cranial neuropathy, and a demyelinating acute or chronic polyradiculoneuropathy. In these, sarcoid granulomas are similar to those seen in other organ systems. The granulomas can be identified in different layers of the nerve with variable axonal degeneration and demyelination.[306–308]

Vasculitis

Vasculitis is caused by a variety of infectious processes and frequently is idiopathic or autoimmune. It may be a manifestation of systemic disease, or it may affect only the peripheral nervous system. The various vasculitides often cause a peripheral neuropathy. Because peripheral nerve involvement is rare in giant cell arteritis, this is not discussed here.

Periarteritis nodosa (PA) is a systemic vasculitis that affects the peripheral nervous system in up to 60% of cases, usually manifesting as a mononeuritis multiplex.[309] Sometimes the process is so diffuse and severe that is resembles a polyneuropathy. The pathologic alterations may be present in muscle (see Color Plate B49) and nerve biopsies[310]; therefore, it is advisable to biopsy both to increase the diagnostic yield.

The histologic features of this disease are those clinically seen in all of the vasculitides. These are characterized by inflammatory infiltrates invading the endothelium and most of the vessel layers with necrosis (Figure 19.80). A typical finding in PA, but which could also be present in other vasculitides, is the fibrinoid necrosis (see Color Plate B49). The inflammatory cells in PA are more prominent in the epineurial vessels. Hemorrhage of the wall with thrombosis can also be seen. In more chronic cases, there is recanalization and hemosiderin deposits, but inflammation might not be visualized.[311,312] There is usually prominent axonal degeneration and focal nerve fiber loss.

Peripheral neuropathy is also seen in the vasculitides associated with antineutrophil cytoplasmic antibodies, such as *microscopic polyangiitis*, which affects small capillaries, arterioles, and venules. In the *Churg-Strauss syndrome*, the vasculitis primarily affects pulmonary vessels with prominent eosinophilic infiltrates. The peripheral neuropathy is similar to PA. A polyneuropathy also

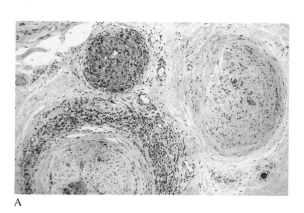

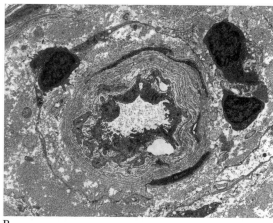

A   B

Figure 19.80 A. Perifascicular and perivascular inflammation (hematoxylin and eosin, ×100). **B.** Lymphocytes around a vessel with duplication of the basal lamina on electron microscopy in vasculitis (×6,059).

occurs in *Wegener's granulomatosis*, although this disease primarily affects the respiratory system and kidneys.

Connective tissue disorders sometimes cause a small vessel vasculitis. This can occur, for example, in rheumatoid arthritis, lupus erythematosus, systemic sclerosis, and mixed connective tissue disorders; this vasculitis could cause a mononeuritis, a mononeuritis multiplex, or a diffuse sensorimotor polyneuropathy.

Isolated vasculitis of the peripheral nervous system or *nonsystemic vasculitic neuropathy* affects primarily the small vessels and manifests as a mononeuritis multiplex or a diffuse polyneuropathy without evidence of systemic disease.[313,314] The histologic findings are those common to all vasculitides.

Ganglioneuritis

Patients with *Sjögren's syndrome* may present with an ataxic sensory neuropathy with a loss of large myelinated fibers without inflammation on sural nerve biopsy, whereas biopsy of the dorsal root ganglia shows neuronal loss with lymphocytic infiltrates.[315] A similar condition also occurs as a remote effect of cancer.[316]

Neuropathy and Monoclonal Gammopathy

A monoclonal gammopathy occurs in approximately 10% of patients with idiopathic polyneuropathy.[317,318] In most patients, the gammopathy is benign, although up to one-third of cases might eventually develop a malignancy.[319] The term *monoclonal gammopathy of undetermined significance* (MGUS) describes those patients without an apparent malignancy, and *nonmalignant dysglobulinemic polyneuropathy* describes those who also have neuropathy.

The most common peripheral neuropathy of patients with MGUS is a slowly progressive distal sensorimotor polyneuropathy, usually associated with IgM κ light chains, and, less frequently, with monoclonal IgG and IgA. Up to 65% of patients with IgM gammopathy are older persons with a distal demyelinating neuropathy and antibodies against MAG. The disease has a relatively benign course. The pathologic findings include myelinated fiber loss with segmental demyelination and, as discussed in the section Demyelination, wide spacing of the myelin lamellae (see Figure 19.73), which contain IgM deposits, demonstrated by immunohistochemistry (see Color Plate B50).[320–322] In patients with IgA and IgG MGUS, the pathologic findings are nonspecific, but some nerve biopsies have amyloid deposits.

Primary systemic amyloidosis is also associated with a monoclonal protein (mainly IgG, but also IgA and primarily λ light chain) and can be detected in serum and urine. Most cases are idiopathic and not associated in the other diseases, but some patients with primary acquired amyloidosis might develop multiple myeloma. Secondary or acquired amyloidoses are those associated with a chronic infectious process. All these manifest by a predominantly sensory distal or sensorimotor neuropathy, with autonomic dysfunction.[323,324] A nerve biopsy shows axonal degeneration, a decreased number of myelinated and unmyelinated fibers, and deposits of amyloid in the endoneurial areas and in vessels.

Waldenström's macroglobulinemia is a multisystemic condition that may have elevation of IgM κ light chain monoclonal protein. Some of these patients have a MAG-related neuropathy.[325]

Cryoglobulinemia may be associated with monoclonal or polyclonal gammopathies with a diffuse polyneuropathy or mononeuritis multiplex. The nerve biopsy in these patients usually shows evidence of vasculitis.[326,327]

Osteosclerotic myeloma is a form of localized myeloma that manifests by a neuropathy indistinguishable from CIDP, with a λ light chain and IgG or IgA monoclonal gammopathy. The nerve biopsy shows evidence of axonal degeneration with demyelination.[328,329] Some patients may manifest with the so-called Crow-Fukase syndrome or POEMS syndrome. Others have Castleman's disease or benign giant cell lymphoma.[330] Patients with multiple myeloma may present with a sensory or sensorimotor axonal polyneuropathy associated with an IgG or IgM κ light chain gammopathy.

Infectious Neuropathies

A number of infectious processes can manifest with peripheral nerve dysfunction; the most common are reviewed here.

Human Immunodeficiency Virus–Associated Neuropathy

HIV can cause diverse forms of peripheral neuropathy. A symmetric sensorimotor neuropathy usually occurs during the intermediate to late stages of the disease and has pathologic findings of axonal degeneration and atrophy, accompanied by foci of inflammatory cells.[331,332]

An acute or chronic demyelinating neuropathy resembling GBS and CIDP also occurs during seroconversion or early infection, usually accompanied by cerebrospinal fluid pleocytosis. Pathologically, there is evidence of inflammation and demyelination.[333,334] HIV-infected individuals may also present with a mononeuritis multiplex, showing varying degrees of axonal degeneration and inflammation[335]; a ganglioneuritis; or, in some patients, a necrotizing vasculitis.[336]

Cytomegalic virus infection in HIV patients may manifest with paralysis, low-back pain, and a lumbosacral radiculopathy. These are associated with characteristic nodular enhancing lesions on magnetic resonance imaging in the lumbosacral roots and spinal fluid pleocytosis. The pathologic findings on nerve biopsy consist mainly of diffuse lymphocytic infiltrates.

Diffuse infiltrating lymphocytosis is present with CD8 infiltrates in different organs and enlarged salivary glands, and sicca syndrome. This occurs in HIV patients and can manifest by a sensory peripheral neuropathy with histologic features of axonal degeneration and inflammation with many CD8 cells.[337] An axonal neuropathy is also seen in individuals infected by human T-cell lymphotrophic virus type I.[338]

Leprosy

Leprosy is caused by the acid-fast bacillus *Mycobacterium leprae*. The disease is an uncommon cause of neuropathy in North America and Europe, but it is prevalent in Africa, Asia, and South America.

Leprosy has two major presentations, lepromatous and tuberculoid,[339] with some intermediate forms. Lepromatous leprosy manifests by multiple, disseminated anes-

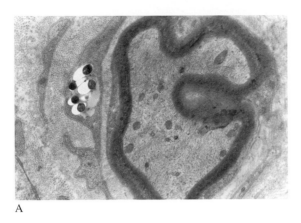
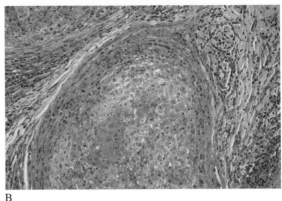

A   B

Figure 19.81 A. Lepra bacilli in Schwann cell cytoplasm on electron microscopy (×9,000.) **B.** Granuloma formation in leprosy (×900). (Courtesy of Dr. S. Shankar, National Institute of Mental Health and Neurosciences, Bangalore, India.)

thetic maculae and nodules, saddle-nose deformity, a leonine facies, ocular dysfunction, sensory loss in the cold areas of the body, especially the distal extremities and ears, and nerve enlargement. This form is seen in patients with poorly developed cell-mediated immunity. Tuberculoid leprosy occurs in patients with well-developed cell-mediated immunity and presents with well-delineated, hyperpigmented or hypopigmented maculae, which can be solitary or multiple, and with alopecia and anhidrosis over the maculae.

The neuropathy of leprosy is usually a mononeuritis multiplex, and a purely neuritic form of the disease without skin changes may occur that can be difficult to diagnose if leprosy is not considered. The pathologic findings in lepromatous leprosy consist of an inflammatory neuropathy with uneven involvement of various fascicles. The macrophages and Schwann cells are filled with organisms, which are easily recognized by the acid fast stains (see Color Plate B51). On EM, there are foamy inclusions in Schwann cells and macrophages. The inclusions contain membrane-bound, osmiophilic organisms surrounded by a clear halo (see Figure 19.81A). Mononuclear cell infiltrates, axonal degeneration, and segmental demyelination are also seen.[340,341]

In tuberculoid leprosy, there is an inflammatory reaction with prominent granuloma formation (see Figure 19.81B). The granuloma may be caseating. The epineurium is thickened, and there is axonal degeneration. The bacilli are sparse and may be difficult to identify.[342,343]

Diphtheria

Diphtheria, which has become very rare, has a characteristic presentation with paralysis of the palate and pharyngeal muscles that spreads to the diaphragm and produces respiratory failure accompanied by a sensorimotor neuropathy. The neuropathy may be the initial manifestation in some cases.[344] Pathologically, there is evidence of an inflammatory ganglioradiculoneuritis with segmental demyelination.[345]

Lyme Disease

Lyme disease is caused by the spirochete *Borrelia burgdorferi*, which is transmitted through a tick bite. It is clinically characterized by the presence of erythema migrans, myocarditis, and a mononeuritis multiplex, which may present with multiple cervical radiculopathies and cranial nerve dysfunction, most commonly affecting the facial nerve.[346] Histologic findings include mononuclear cell inflammation, mainly in the epineurial layer, but also affecting all components of the fascicles with axonal damage.[347,348]

Acquired Metabolic, Endocrine, and Nutritional Neuropathies

Diabetic Polyneuropathy

Peripheral nerve disease is the most common complication of diabetes and usually manifests as a sensory-motor neuropathy.[349,350] Other neuropathies include mononeuritis, mononeuritis multiplex, thoracic radiculopathy, and, among others, lumbosacral radiculoplexus neuropathy, also called *diabetic amyotrophy*.[349,350]

The pathologic findings in diabetic polyneuropathy include thickening of the endothelium and the basal laminae, reduplication of the basal laminae (Figure 19.82),[351] a decreased number of myelinated fibers, and axonal degeneration, accompanied by some onion-bulb formations.[352,353] There are also alterations of the unmyelinated fibers with denervated subunits and flattened axons.

It has been documented that focal neuropathies of diabetes are caused by a vasculopathy, and there can be evidence of nerve infarcts.[354–356] The findings of mononuclear cell infiltrates and microvasculitis in some cases raise the possibility of an autoimmune process.[357] Similarly, as discussed previously, a prominent neuropathy identical to CIDP may occur in diabetes and could have an autoimmune pathogenesis.[300]

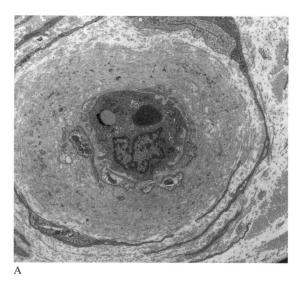
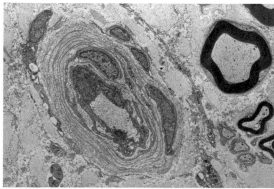

A   B

Figure 19.82 A. Electron micrograph of a thickened vessel (×9,000). **B.** A vessel with reduplicated basal lamina in diabetes (×4,401).

Hypothyroidism and Acromegaly

Hypothyroidism can cause a neuropathy in which the pathologic findings are non-specific, characterized mainly by axonal loss of large myelinated fibers, and, sometimes, excessive accumulations of glycogen in the various cell types.[358] The findings in acromegaly are nonspecific but with more prominent demyelination.[359]

Uremic Polyneuropathy

Uremic neuropathy is a distal symmetric sensorimotor neuropathy. However, patients affected by it are also predisposed to entrapment and focal, compressive neuropathies. The pathology consists of axonal degeneration affecting both myelinated fiber types but mainly the large fibers, with demyelination in some distal segments that is believed to be secondary.[209]

Vitamin Deficiency

Thiamine and pyridoxine deficiencies cause a predominantly sensory and sensorimotor neuropathy, with axonal degeneration that affects myelinated and unmyelinated fibers. In pernicious anemia or cobalamine deficiency from other causes, there is a decreased number of large myelinated fibers with some evidence of axonal degeneration and segmental demyelination.[360] Vitamin E deficiency can be caused by intestinal malabsorption. There is also a familial isolated vitamin E deficiency,[361] presenting with ataxia, blindness, ophthalmoplegia, and a predominantly large fiber sensory neuropathy. These cases have a loss of myelinated fibers, and electron-dense bodies are present in Schwann cells and endothelial cells in nerve biopsies. Patients undergoing gastric bypass procedures develop a predominantly axonal neuropathy, which can sometimes be present even in the absence of clinically well-defined malnutrition.[362]

Toxic Neuropathies

Toxic neuropathies include a very extensive group in which there are no significant characteristic pathologic features. The diagnosis is usually made by the history of exposure or the associated findings. The most common feature of most toxic neuropathies is axonal degeneration with some secondary demyelination. In some, however, there is a primary demyelinating neuropathy (see below). Toxins include substances such as lead, thallium, or arsenic, as well as some medications.

Medications

Amphiphilic cationic drugs, particularly the antiarrhythmic amiodarone, cause a predominantly demyelinating neuropathy, characterized by loss of myelinated fibers, axonal degeneration, and some segmental demyelination and regenerated clusters. Lysosomal inclusions are seen in vessels and in endoneurial cells (Figure 19.83). These consist of membrane-bound, osmiophilic material and might take on a reticular or lamellar appearance.[363] Perhexiline and the antimalarial chloroquine can cause similar pathologic findings, but the effects are less severe.[364,365]

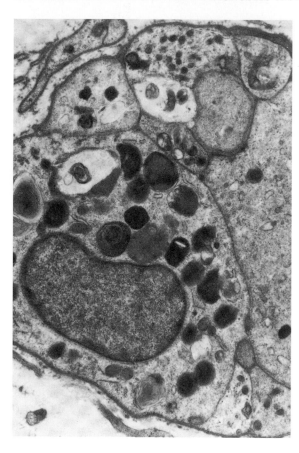

Figure 19.83 Amiodarone neuropathy: Schwann cells of the denervated band show lysosomal inclusions of varying morphologies (×14,560). (Reproduced with permission from G Midroni, JM Bilbao, SM Cohen [eds], Biopsy Diagnosis of Peripheral Neuropathy. Boston: Butterworth–Heinemann, 1995;336.)

Vincristine, a chemotherapeutic agent, is a vinca alkaloid that can cause a sensorimotor neuropathy with degeneration of the myelinated and unmyelinated axons.[366]

Cisplatin, another chemotherapeutic agent, causes a predominantly sensory neuropathy with axonal degeneration of myelinated fibers and relative sparing of the unmyelinated fibers. The neuropathy of paclitaxel (Taxol) affects predominantly sensory and autonomic fibers with axonal degeneration of myelinated and unmyelinated fibers and secondary demyelination.[367]

Pyridoxine taken in excessive quantities can result in a sensory neuropathy in which the nerve biopsy shows axonal degeneration of small and large myelinated fibers.[368,369]

A number of antibiotics might cause a sensory neuropathy, mainly affecting the large myelinated fibers. Examples of these are the antileprosy drug dapsone,[370] metronidazole,[371] nitrofurantoin,[372] and ethambutol.[373] Isoniazid, on the other hand, equally affects the myelinated and unmyelinated fibers.[374,375] A mild and indolent, predominantly sensory neuropathy that affects mainly large myelinated fibers, they appear decreased in number and show evidence of axonal atrophy, is seen with the chronic use of the anticonvulsant phenytoin.[376] Colchicine, which is used to treat autoimmune disorders, produces a myopathy and a neuropathy, whereas disulfiram can produce a sensory neuropathy with loss of myelinated fibers and swelling of axons with accumulations of dense membranous organelles.[377] A rare demyelinating neuropathy similar to CIDP, and that, apparently, is immune mediated can occur in patients receiving procainamide.[378] Tacrolimus, which is used as an immunosuppressant, also causes a demyelinating neuropathy.[379]

Alcoholic Neuropathy

A predominantly sensory or sensorimotor neuropathy is seen with chronic excessive use of alcohol; weakness and areflexia can develop later. The neuropathy is frequently associated with malnutrition, particularly from thiamine deficiency,[380] but it is likely that alcohol has a toxic effect on peripheral nerve.[381] Nerve biopsy shows axonal degeneration of myelinated and unmyelinated fibers and various degrees of secondary segmental demyelination.[382,383]

Lead Intoxication

Chronic lead intoxication in adults produces a predominantly motor neuropathy, with a predilection for the radial nerve, causing a characteristic wrist drop.[384] The pathology of this neuropathy is characterized by prominent axonal degeneration,[384] whereas it appears to be mainly demyelinating in animals.[385]

Arsenic

Arsenic, which is used as a wood preservative and as a pesticide, has a long history of being a homicidal instrument. In acute intoxication, patients develop nausea, vomiting, and, sometimes, encephalopathy. Chronic exposure causes a motor and sensory neuropathy. Sometimes, an acute neuropathy resembling GBS can also occur.[386] Pathologic findings in arsenic poisoning include axonal degeneration with some evidence of demyelination.[387]

Critical Illness Neuropathy

Gravely ill individuals can develop a predominantly axonal neuropathy. This is likely caused by hypoxia and ischemia, secondary to the systemic inflammatory response.[388] Nerve biopsy of these individuals shows a severe axonal degeneration.

Neoplasms

Peripheral neuropathy can occur in patients in the terminal stages of cancer. However, some cancer patients can also have a paraneoplastic syndrome from antibodies associated with a localized tumor (e.g., small cell carcinoma). In other cases, particularly with hematologic neoplasms, and, especially, lymphoma, the tumor cells may invade peripheral nerves. This lymphomatous polyneuropathy occurs more often in non-Hodgkin's lymphoma of the B-cell type. These patients usually present with a sensorimotor polyneuropathy but sometimes also with a mononeuritis multiplex. Pathologically, there is evidence of infiltrates of lymphomatous cells in all nerve compartments; these are more prominent in the perivascular area and can have an angiocentric appearance. This is accompanied by axonal degeneration and segmental demyelination (Figure 19.84).[389,390]

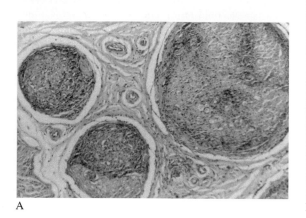
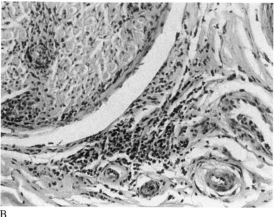

A   B

Figure 19.84 **A.** Tumor cells invading the nerve fascicles in a case of lymphoma (hematoxylin and eosin, ×100). **B.** Perineurial and endoneurial invasion of lymphocytes in lymphoma (hematoxylin and eosin, ×200).

SKIN BIOPSY IN THE EVALUATION OF PERIPHERAL NEUROPATHY

Punch skin biopsies have been studied for a long time in the evaluation of the nerve terminals, especially the Meissner's corpuscles using acetyl-cholinesterase and silver stains,[391,392] but were not routinely used in clinical practice.

More recently, epidermal fibers have been studied by immunohistochemistry with antibodies against nerve components, particularly to PGP9.5—a cytoplasmic marker that is used to identify nerve fibers in the epidermis and dermis. Other markers can also be used, such as substance P. These studies apply immunoperoxidase and immunofluorescence techniques and are analyzed by regular light microscopy and by confocal microscopy (see Color Plates B52 and B53),[393,394] allowing quantitation of the nerve terminals. With the use of simultaneous antibody markers against collagen IV, the basal lamina is also visualized, providing the opportunity to determine the localization of small axons. Skin biopsies are now being used in the evaluation of small-fiber neuropathies.

CONCLUSIONS

Histologic analysis of muscle remains an important tool in the evaluation of neuromuscular disorders—for example, to determine the presence of inflammation in PM and to diagnose vasculitis, inclusion body myositis, and congenital myopathies. Recognition of characteristic pathologic findings, such as the atrophic angular fibers, targets and grouping of neurogenic disease, and the abnormalities of the different metabolic diseases, is pertinent for their diagnosis.

Immunohistochemistry plays an important role in detecting protein deficiencies, which leads to the identification of specific diseases. Although many disorders can now be diagnosed with DNA analysis of lymphocytes, these techniques are useful only in some diseases and are not applicable to all cases, leaving histology as the alternative method of evaluation.

Nerve biopsy not only provides a valuable assessment of various conditions, such as amyloidosis and inflammatory processes, but it also is useful in determining if the target of the disease is the Schwann cell and its myelin or the axon. Skin biopsy is a technique that is less traumatic to the patient and aids in the assessment of axonal loss in some neuropathies.

Histology of muscle and nerve also provides the necessary knowledge to further understand the electrophysiologic abnormalities that are seen in neuromuscular disorders. Hopefully, this chapter helps the reader to acquire a basic knowledge in diagnostic interpretation of biopsies from patients with neuromuscular diseases.

Acknowledgments

We want to extend our appreciation to Dr. S. K. Shankar, Professor and Head of the Institute of Mental Health and Neurosciences, Bangalore, India, for sharing his material; Dr. Thomas O'Brien, with whom we have worked at Methodist Hospital Pathology Department, for sharing some cases and photographs; Dr. Curtis Dohan, Jr., for helping with some cases and for his continuous support; and Dr. Harry Jarret for his valuable comments. We also wish to thank Greg Campbell from the photography department at Baptist Memorial Hospital, Memphis.

We particularly want to thank Lou Grubbs, Adriana Nance, and Mari Alan Shadle who, over the years, have helped us with excellent histologic technology, and Dr. Maria Castillo-Bale for her valuable collaboration. A special thanks goes to the Integrated Microscopy Department at the University of Memphis, particularly Sharon Frase, Coordinator, and Dr. Lewis Coons, Director, for opening their doors and lending their support.

REFERENCES

1. Cohn RD, Campbell KP. Molecular basis of muscular dystrophies. Muscle Nerve 2000;23:1456–1471.
2. Sewry CA. Immunocytochemical analysis of human muscular dystrophy. Microsc Res Tech 2000;48:142–154.
3. Collins MP, Mendell JR, Periquet MI, et al. Superficial peroneal nerve/peroneus brevis muscle biopsy in vasculitic neuropathy. Neurology 2000;55:636–643.
4. Dubowitz V. The Procedure of Muscle Biopsy. In Muscle Biopsy. A Practical Approach (2nd ed). London: Bailliere Tindall, 1985;3–18.
5. Loughlin M. Muscle Biopsy Procedures. In Muscle Biopsy: A Laboratory Investigation. Oxford: Butterworth–Heinemann, 1993;25–37.
6. Cumming K, Fulthorpe J, Hudgson P, Mahon M. Preparation of the Biopsy. In Color Atlas of Muscle Pathology. London: Mosby-Wolfe, 1994;3–19.
7. Carpenter S, Karpati G. Methods of Tissue Removal and Preparation. In Pathology of Skeletal Muscle (2nd ed). New York: Oxford University Press, 2001;8–27.
8. Dubowitz V. Normal Muscle. In Muscle Biopsy. A Practical Approach (2nd ed). London: Bailliere Tindall, 1985;41–81.
9. Loughlin M. Muscle Structure, Function and Distribution. In Muscle Biopsy: A Laboratory Investigation. Oxford: Butterworth–Heinemann, 1993;6–24.
10. Moriera ES, Wiltshire TJ, Faulkner G, et al. Limb-girdle muscular dystrophy type 2G is caused by mutations in the gene encoding the sarcomeric protein telethonin. Nat Genet 2000;24:163–166.
11. Bertorini TE. Muscular Dystrophies. In R Pourmand (ed), Neuromuscular Diseases: Expert Clinician's Views. Boston: Butterworth–Heinemann, 2001;227–294.
12. Matsuda C, Aoki M, Hayashi YK, et al. Dysferlin is a surface membrane-associated protein that is absent in Miyoshi myopathy. Neurology 1999;53:1119–1122.
13. Saperstein DS, Amato AA, Barohn RJ. Clinical and genetic aspects of distal myopathies. Muscle Nerve 2001;24:1440–1441.

14. Minetti C, Sotgia F, Bruno C, et al. Mutations in the caveolin-3 gene cause autosomal dominant limb-girdle muscular dystrophy. Nat Genet 1998;4:365–368.
15. Voit T. Congenital muscular dystrophy: 1997 update. Brain Develop 1998;20:65–74.
16. Jobsis GJ, Keizers H, Vreijling JP, et al. Type VI collagen mutations in Bethlem myopathy, an autosomal dominant myopathy with contractures. Nat Genet 1996;14:113–115.
17. Kobayashi K, Nakahori Y, Miyaka M, et al. An ancient retrotransposal insertion causes Fukuyama-type congenital muscular dystrophy. Nature 1998;394:388–392.
18. Hayashi YK, Chou FL, Engvall E, et al. Mutations in the integrin alpha 7 gene cause congenital myopathy. Nat Genet 1998;19:94–97.
19. Schmalbruch H, Helhammer U. The number of satellite cells in normal human muscle. Anat Rec 1976;185:279–287.
20. Bonne G, Di Barletta MR, Varnovus S, et al. Mutations in the gene encoding lamin A/C cause autosomal dominant Emery-Dreifuss muscular dystrophy. Nat Genet 1999;21:285–288.
21. Manidal S, Pecan D, Sewry CA, et al. Mutations in Emery-Dreifuss muscular dystrophy and their effects on emerin protein expression. Hum Mol Genet 1998;7:855–864.
22. Brooke MH, Kaiser KK. Muscle fiber types: how many and what kind? Arch Neurol 1970;23:369–379.
23. Engel WK. Fiber-type nomenclature of human skeletal muscle for histochemical purposes. Neurology 1974;24:344–348.
24. Askanas V, Engel WK. Distinct subtypes of type I fibers of human skeletal muscle. Neurology 1975;25:879–887.
25. Bertorini TE, Stalberg E, Yuson CP, Engel WK. Single-fiber electromyography in neuromuscular disorders: correlation of muscle histochemistry, single-fiber electromyography, and clinical findings. Muscle Nerve 1994;17:345–353.
26. Billeter R, Weber H, Lutz H, et al. Myosin types in human skeletal muscle fiber. Histochemistry 1980;65:249–259.
27. Bertorini TE, Horner LH. Myosin-stained paraffin sections in the evaluation of neuromuscular disease (Abstr). Muscle Nerve 1997;20:1067.
28. Loughlin M. Preparation of Muscle Specimens. In Muscle Biopsy: A Laboratory Investigation. Oxford: Butterworth–Heinemann, 1993;38–64.
29. Schochet S Jr. Normal Muscle and General Techniques. In Diagnostic Pathology of Skeletal Muscle and Nerve. Norwalk, Connecticut: Appleton-Century Crofts, 1980;1–28.
30. Dubowitz V. Histological and Histochemical Reactions. In Muscle Biopsy. A Practical Approach. London: Bailliere Tindall, 1993;19–40.
31. Engel WK, Cunningham G. Rapid examination of muscle tissue: an improved trichrome method for fresh-frozen biopsy sections. Neurology 1963;13:919 923.
32. Loughlin M. Staining and Histochemical Methods. In Muscle Biopsy: A Laboratory Investigation. London: Mosby-Wolfe, 1994;65–111.
33. Fishbein WN, Griffin JL, Armbrustmacher VW. Stain for skeletal muscle adenylate deaminase. An effective tetrazolium stain for frozen biopsy specimens. Arch Pathol Lab Med 1980;104:462–466.
34. Fishbein WN, Armbrustmacher VW, Griffin JL. Myoadenylate deaminase deficiency: a new disease of muscle. Science 1978;200:545–548.
35. Fitzsimmons R, Sewry CA. Immunocytochemistry. In V Dubowitz (ed), Muscle Biopsy. A Practical Approach. London: Bailliere Tindall, 1985;184–207.
36. Polack JM, Van Noorden J (eds), Immunocytochemistry: Modern Methods and Applications. Bristol, UK: Wright, 1986.
37. Hsu SM, Raine L, Faunger H. Use of avidin-biotin-peroxidase complex (ABC) in immunoperoxidase techniques: a comparison between ABC and unlabeled antibody (PAP) procedures. J Histochem Cytochem 1981;29:577–580.
38. Vacca LL, Abrahams SJ, Naftchi NT. A modified peroxidase—antiperoxidase procedure for improved localization of tissue antigens: localization of substance P in rat spinal cord. J Histochem Cytochem 1980;28:297–307.
39. Ringel SP, Bender AN, Engel WK. Extrajunctional acetylcholine receptors. Alterations in human and experimental neuromuscular diseases. Arch Neurol 1976;33:751–758.
40. De Coster W, De Reuck J, Vander Eecken H. The target phenomenon in human muscle: a comparative light microscopic histochemical and electron microscopic study. Acta Neuropathol 1976;34:329–338.
41. Kovarsky J, Schochet SS Jr, McCormick WF. The significance of target fibers: a clinicopathologic review of 100 patients with neurogenic atrophy. Am J Clin Pathol 1973;59:790–797.

42. Dubowitz V. Pathology of experimentally re-innervated skeletal muscle. J Neurol Neurosurg Psychiatry 1967;30:99–110.

43. Jennekens FGI. Neurogenic Disorders of Muscle. In FL Mastaglia, JN Walton (eds), Skeletal Muscle Pathology. Edinburgh, UK: Churchill Livingstone, 1982;204–234.

44. Johnson MA, Polgar J, Weightman D, Appleton D. Data on the distribution of fiber types in thirty-six human muscles. an autopsy study. J Neurol Sci 1973;18:111–124.

45. Mahon M, Toman A, William PL, Bagnall KM. Variability of histochemical and morphometric data from needle biopsy specimens of human quadriceps femoris muscle. J Neurol Sci 1984; 63:85–100.

46. Gollnick PD, Armstrong RB, Saubert CW 4th, et al. Enzyme activity and fiber composition in skeletal muscle of untrained and trained men. J Appl Physiol 1972;33:312–319.

47. Sandstedt P, Nordell LE, Henriksson KG. Quantitative analysis of muscle biopsies from volunteers and patients with neuromuscular disorders. A comparison between estimation and measuring. Acta Neurol Scand 1982;66:130–144.

48. Lexell J, Downham D, Sjöström M. Morphological detection of neurogenic muscle disorders: how can statistical methods aid diagnosis? Acta Neuropathol 1987;75:109–115.

49. Lexell J, Downham D, Sjöström M. Distribution of different fiber types in human skeletal muscles. A statistical and computational study of the fiber type arrangement in the vastus lateralis of young healthy males. J Neurol Sci 1984;65:353–365.

50. Jennekens FGI, Tomlison BE, Walton JN. Data on the distribution of fiber types in five human limb muscles. An autopsy study. J Neurol Sci 1971;14:245–257.

51. Loughlin M. Morphometric Analysis of Muscle. In Muscle Biopsy. A Laboratory Investigation. Oxford: Butterworth–Heinemann,1993;194–228.

52. Gawel M, Butler R, Partridge TA, et al. Muscle Biopsy in Motor Neuron Diseases. In W Behan, F Clifford Rose (eds), Further Aspects in Progress in Neurological Research. Tunbridge Wells, UK: Pitman Medical, 1979;158–168.

53. Lester JM, Silbern DI, Cohen MH, et al. The co-dispersion index for the measurement of fiber type distribution patterns. Muscle Nerve 1983;6:581–587.

54. Bertorini T, Woodhouse C, Horner L. Muscle hypertrophy secondary to the tethered cord syndrome. Muscle Nerve 1994;17:331–335.

55. Rouques C, Jarnot N, Cathala HP, Castaigne P. Analyse de la distribution des fibres musculaires de differentes types au seign du muscle squellettique. Interest clinique resulat preliminares. Rev Neurol (Paris) 1973;129:300–303.

56. Hartlage PL, Soudmand R. Internalized capillaries in hypokalemic periodic paralysis [letter]. Arch Neurol 1981;38:602.

57. Polgar JS, Johnson MA, Weightman D, Appleton D. Data on fiber size in thirty-six human muscles. An autopsy study. J Neurol Sci 1973;19:307–318.

58. Brooke M, Engel WK. The histographic analysis of human muscle biopsies with regard to fiber type 1. Adult male and female. Neurology 1969;19:221–233.

59. Bell DG, Jacobs I. Muscle fiber area, fiber type, and capillarization in male and female body builders. Can J Sports Sci 1990;15:115–119.

60. Aherne W. A method of determining the cross-sectional area of muscle fibers. J Neurol Sci 1968;3:519–528.

61. Adams RC, Cöers C, Walton JN. Report of a subcommittee on the quantification of muscle biopsy findings. J Neurol Sci 1968;6:179–180.

62. Dubowitz V. Definitions of Changes Seen in Muscle Biopsies. In Muscle Biopsy. A Practical Approach (2nd ed). London: Bailliere Tindall, 1985;82–128.

63. Shy GM, Magee K. A new congenital nonprogressive myopathy. Brain 1956;7:610–621.

64. Bertorini TE. Myoglobinuria, malignant hyperthermia, neuroleptic malignant syndrome and serotonin syndrome. Neurol Clin 1997;15:649–671.

65. Frank JP, Harati Y, Butler IJ, et al. Central core disease and malignant hyperthermia syndrome. Ann Neurol 1980;7:11–17.

66. Neville HE, Brooke MH. Central Core Fibers: Structured and Unstructured. In BA Kakulas (ed), Basic Research in Myology. Amsterdam: Excerpta Medica, 1973;497–511.

67. Engel AG, Gomez MR, Groover RV. Multicore disease. A recently recognized congenital myopathy associated with multifocal degeneration of muscle fibers. Mayo Clin Proc 1971;46:666–681.

68. Koch B, Bertorini TE, Eng G, Boehm R. Severe multicore disease associated with reaction to anesthesia. Arch Neurol 1985;42:1204–1206.

69. Ferreiro A, Estoumet B, Chateau D, et al. Multi-minicore disease—searching for boundaries: phenotype analysis of 32 cases. Ann Neurol 2000;48:745–757.

70. Shy GM, Engel WK, Somers JE, Wanko T. Nemaline myopathy. A new congenital myopathy. Brain 1963;86:792–810.

71. Heffernan LP, Rewcastle NB, Humphrey JG. The spectrum of rod myopathies. Arch Neurol 1968;18:529–542.

72. Stuhlfauth I, Jennekens FG, Willemse J, Jockusch BM. Congenital nemaline myopathy. II. Quantitative changes in α-actinin and myosin in skeletal muscle. Muscle Nerve 1983;6:69–74.

73. Engel WK, Oberc MA. Abundant nuclear rods in adult-onset rod disease. J Neuropathol Exp Neurol 1975;34:119–132.

74. Brownell AK, Gilbert JJ, Shaw DT, et al. Adult onset nemaline myopathy. Neurology 1978;28: 1306–1309.

75. Spiro AJ, Shy GM, Gonatas NK. Myotubular myopathy. Persistence of fetal muscle in an adolescent boy. Arch Neurol 1966;14:1–14.

76. Sher JH, Rimalovski AB, Athanassiades TJ, Aronson SM. Familial myotubular myopathy: a clinical, pathological, histochemical, and ultrastructural study. Neuropathol Exp Neurol 1967;26:132–133.

77. Headington JT, McNamara JO, Brownell AK. Centronuclear myopathy: histochemistry and electron microscopy. Report of two cases. Arch Pathol 1975;99:16–24.

78. McLeod JG, Baker WD, Lethlean AK, Shorey CD. Centronuclear myopathy with autosomal dominant inheritance. J Neurol Sci 1972;15:375–387.

79. Engel WK, Gold GN, Karpati G. Type I fiber hypotrophy and central nuclei. A rare congenital muscle abnormality with a possible experimental model. Arch Neurol 1968;18:435–444.

80. Barth PG, van Wijngaarden GK, Bethlem J. X-linked myotubular myopathy with fatal neonatal asphyxia. Neurology 1975;25:531–536.

81. Laporate J, Hu LJ, Kretz C, et al. A gene mutation in X-linked myotubular myopathy defines a new putative tyrosine phosphatase family conserved in yeast. Nat Genet 1996;13:175–182.

82. Reske-Nielsen E, Hein-Soretisen O, Vorre P. Familial centronuclear myopathy: a clinical and pathological study. Acta Neurol Scand 1987;76:115–122.

83. Brooke MH. Congenital Fiber Type Disproportion. In BA Kakulas (ed), Clinical Studies in Myology, Part 2. Amsterdam: Excerpta Medica, 1973;147–159.

84. Lenard HG, Goebel HH. Unstructured congenital myopathies. Monatsschr Kinderheilkd 1977;125(5):496–498.

85. Clancy RR, Kelts KA, Oehlert JW. Clinical variability in congenital fiber type disproportion. J Neurol Sci 1980;46:257–266.

86. Goebel HH. Desmin-related neuromuscular disorders. Muscle Nerve 1995;18:1306–1320.

87. Engel AG, Angelini C, Gomez MR. Fingerprint body myopathy: a newly recognized congenital muscle disease. Mayo Clinic Proc 1972;47:377–388.

88. Jerusalem F, Engel AG, Gomez MR. Sarcotubular myopathy: a newly recognized, benign, congenital familial muscle disease. Neurology 1973;23:897–906.

89. Brooke MH, Neville HE. Reducing body myopathy. Neurology 1972;22:829–840.

90. Carpenter S, Karpati G, Holland D. New observations in reducing body myopathy. Neurology 1985;35:818–827.

91. Goebel HH, Schloon H, Lenard HG. Congenital myopathy with cytoplasmic bodies. Neuropadiatrie 1981;12:166–180.

92. Griggs RE, Mendell JR, Miller RS. Congenital Myopathies. In Evaluation and Treatment of Myopathies. Contemporary Neurology Series. Philadelphia: FA Davis, 1985;211–246.

93. Goebel HH, Muller J, Gillen HW, Merritt AD. Autosomal dominant "spheroid body myopathy." Muscle Nerve 1978;1:14–26.

94. Barohn RJ, Brumback RA, Mendell JR. Hyaline body myopathy. Neuromuscul Disord 1993; 4:257–262.

95. Reyes MG, Goldbarg H, Fresco K, Bouffard A. Zebra body myopathy. A second case of ultrastructurally distinct congenital myopathy. J Child Neurol 1987;2:307–318.

96. Ringel SP, Neville HE, Dusten MC, Carroll JE. A new congenital neuromuscular disease with trilaminar muscle fibers. Neurology 1978;28:282–289.

97. Rohkamm R, Boxler K, Ricker K, Jerusalem F. A dominantly inherited myopathy with extensive tubular aggregates. Neurology 1983;33:331–336.

98. De Groot JG, Arts WF. Familial myopathy with tubular aggregates. J Neurol 1982;227:35–41.

99. Brumback RA, Staton RD, Susag ME. Exercise-induced pain, stiffness, and tubular aggregates in skeletal muscle. J Neurol Neurosurg Psychiatry 1981;44:250–254.

100. Dick M, Bertorini TE, Igarashi M. Congenital muscular dystrophy presenting with respiratory failure. Dev Med Child Neurol 1992;34:264–265.

101. Pegoraro E, Marks H, Garcia CA, et al. Laminin alpha2 muscular dystrophy: genotype/phenotype studies of 22 patients. Neurology 1998;51:101–110.

102. Erb WH. Dystrophia muscularis progressiva—klinische und pathologischanatomische studien. Dtsch Z Nervenheilkd 1891;1:13–261.

103. Engel AG, Yamamoto M, Fischbeck KH. Muscular Dystrophies. In AG Engel, C Franzini-Armstrong (eds), Myology (2nd ed). New York: McGraw-Hill, 1994;1158–1162.

104. Arahata K, Engel AG. Monoclonal antibody analysis of mononuclear cells in myopathies: I. Quantitation of subsets according to diagnosis and sites of accumulation and demonstration and counts of muscle fibers invaded by T cells. Ann Neurol 1984;16:193–208.

105. Ten Houten R, De Visser M. Histopathological findings in Becker-type muscular dystrophy. Arch Neurol 1984;41:729–733.

106. Hopkins LC, Jackson JA, Elsas LJ. Emery-Dreifuss humeroperoneal muscular dystrophy: an X-linked myopathy with unusual contractures and bradycardia. Ann Neurol 1981;10:230–237.

107. Merlini J, Granata C, Dominici P, Bonfiglioli S. Emery-Dreifuss muscular dystrophy: report of 5 cases in a family and review of the literature. Muscle Nerve 1986;9:481–485.

108. Figarella-Branger D, El-Dassouki M, Saenz A, et al. Myopathy with lobulated muscle fibers: evidence for heterogeneous etiology and clinical presentation. Neuromuscul Disord 2002;12:4–12.

109. Vainzof M, Moreira ES, Canovas M, et al. Partial alpha-sarcoglycan deficiency with retention of the dystrophin-glycoprotein complex in a LGMD2D family. Muscle Nerve 2000;23:984–988.

110. Bethlem J, Van Wijngaarden GK, de Jong J. The incidence of lobulated fibers in the facioscapulohumeral type of muscular dystrophy and the limb-girdle syndrome. J Neurol Sci 1973;18:351–358.

111. Victor M, Hayes R, Adams RD. Oculopharyngeal muscular dystrophy. N Engl J Med 1962;267:1267–1272.

112. Tome FM, Fardeau M. Nuclear inclusions in oculopharyngeal dystrophy. Acta Neuropathol 1980;49:85–87.

113. Mastaglia FL, Laing NG. Distal myopathies. Clinical and molecular diagnosis and classification. J Neurol Neurosurg Psychiatry 1999;67:703–707.

114. Argov Z, Gardner-Medwin D, Johnson MA, Mastaglia FL. Congenital myotonic dystrophy: fibre type abnormalities in two cases. Arch Neurol 1980;37:693–696.

115. DiMauro S, Stern LZ, Mehler M, et al. Adult-onset acid maltase deficiency: a postmortem study. Muscle Nerve 1978;1:27–36.

116. Engel AG. Acid maltase deficiency in adults: studies in four cases of a syndrome which may mimic muscular dystrophy or other myopathies. Brain 1970;93:599–616.

117. Moufarrej NA, Bertorini TE. Respiratory insufficiency in adult-type acid maltase deficiency. South Med J 1993;86(5):560–567.

118. Hug G, Garancis JC, Schubert WK, Kaplan S. Glycogen storage disease, types II, III, VIII, and IX. A biochemical and electron microscopic analysis. Am J Dis Child 1966;111:457–474.

119. Swaiman KF, Kennedy WR, Sauls HS. Late infantile acid maltase deficiency. Arch Neurol 1968;18:642–648.

120. Baudhuin P, Hers HG, Loeb H. An electron microscopic and biochemical study of type II glycogenosis. Lab Invest 1964;13:1139–1152.

121. Cardiff RD. A histochemical and electron microscopic study of skeletal muscle in a case of Pompe's disease (glycogenosis II). Pediatrics 1966;37:249–259.

122. Dubowitz V. Muscle glycogenosis. Dev Med Child Neurol 1966b;8:432–436.

123. DiMauro S, Hartwig GB, Hays A, et al. Debrancher deficiency: neuromuscular disorder in five adults. Ann Neurol 1979;5:422–436.

124. Fernandes J, Huijing F. Branching enzyme-deficiency glycogenosis. Studies in therapy. Arch Dis Child 1968;43:347–352.

125. Bale P, Hammett JF, Neale FC. Histopathology of McArdle's disease in a family. J Pathol Bacteriol 1967;94:293–300.

126. Mitsumoto H. McArdle's disease: phosphorylase activity in regenerating muscle fibers. Neurology 1979;29:258–262.

127. Layzer RB, Rowland LP, Ranney HM. Muscle phosphofructokinase deficiency. Arch Neurol 1967;17:512–523.

128. DiMauro S, Dalakas M, Miranda AF. Phosphoglycerate kinase deficiency: another cause of recurrent myoglobinuria. Ann Neurol 1983;13:11–19.

129. DiMauro S, Miranda AF, Khan S, et al. Human muscle phosphoglycerate mutase deficiency. Newly discovered metabolic myopathy. Science 1981;212:1277–1279.

130. DiMauro S, Tsujino S. Nonlysosomal glycogenosis. In AG Engel, C Franzini-Armstrong (eds), Myology, Vol 2 (2nd ed). New York: McGraw-Hill, 1994;1554–1576.

131. DiMauro S, Lamperti C. Muscle glycogenoses. Muscle Nerve 2001;24:984–999.
132. Rebouche CJ, Engel AG. Carnitine metabolism and deficiency syndromes. Mayo Clin Proc 1983;58:533–540.
133. Karpati G, Carpenter S, Engel AG, et al. The syndrome of systemic carnitine deficiency—clinical, morphologic, histochemical, and pathophysiologic features. Neurology 1975;25:16–24.
134. DiMauro S, DiMauro PM. Muscle carnitine palmitoyl transferase deficiency and myoglobinuria. Science 1973;182:929–931.
135. Bertorini T, Yeh YY, Trevisan C, et al. Carnitine palmitoyl transferase deficiency: myoglobinuria and respiratory failure. Neurology 1980;30:263–271.
136. DiMauro S, Nicholson JF, Hays AP, et al. Benign infantile mitochondrial myopathy due to reversible cytochrome c oxidase deficiency. Ann Neurol 1983b;14:226–234.
137. Morgan-Hughes JA. Mitochondrial Myopathies. In FL Mastaglia, J Walton (eds), Skeletal Muscle Pathology. Edinburgh, UK: Churchill Livingstone, 1982;309.
138. Olson W, Engel WK, Walsh GO, Einaugler R. Oculocraniosomatic neuromuscular disease with 'ragged-red' fibers. Arch Neurol 1972;26:193–211.
139. DiMauro S. Exercise intolerance and the mitochondrial respiratory chain. Ital J Neurol Sci 1999;20:387–393.
140. Karpati G, Charuk J, Carpenter S, et al. Myopathy caused by a deficiency of Ca^{2+}-adenosine triphosphatase in sarcoplasmic reticulum (Brody's disease). Ann Neurol 1986;20:38–49.
141. Engel AG. Evolution and content of vacuoles in primary hypokalemic periodic paralysis. Mayo Clin Proc 1970c;45:774–814.
142. McFadzean AJ, Yeung R. Periodic paralysis complicating thyrotoxicosis in Chinese. BMJ 1967;1:451–455.
143. Howes EL, Price HM, Blumberg JM, Pearson CM. Hypokalemic periodic paralysis: electron microscopic changes in the sarcoplasm. Neurology 1966;16:242–256.
144. Tome FM. Periodic Paralysis and Electrolyte Disorders. In F Nesta, J Walton (eds), Skeletal Muscle Pathology. Edinburgh, UK: Churchill Livingstone, 1982;287–308.
145. Gamstorp I. Adynamia episodica hereditaria and myotonia. Acta Neurol Scand 1963;39:41–58.
146. Crews J, Kaiser KK, Brooke MH. Muscle pathology of myotonia congenita. J Neurol Sci 1976;28:449–457.
147. Bertorini TE. Histopathology of the Inflammatory Myopathies. In MC Dalakas (ed), Polymyositis and Dermatomyositis. Woburn, MA: Butterworths, 1988;157–194.
148. Carpenter S, Karpati G, Rothman S, Watters G. The childhood type of dermatomyositis. Neurology 1976;26:952–962.
149. Banker BQ, Victor M. Dermatomyositis (systemic angiopathy) of childhood. Medicine 1966;45:261–289.
150. Rose AL, Walton JN, Pearce GW. Polymyositis: an ultramicroscopic study of muscle biopsy material. J Neurol Sci 1967;5:457–472.
151. Hughes JT, Esiri M. Ultrastructural studies in human polymyositis. J Neurol Sci 1975;25:347–360.
152. Matsubara S, Mair WGP. Ultrastructural changes in polymyositis. Brain 1979;102:701–725.
153. Mintz G, Gonzalez-Angulo A, Fraga A, Zavala B. Ultrastructure of muscle in polymyositis. Am J Med 1968;44:216–224.
154. Bertorini TE. Inflammatory myopathies (polymyositis, dermatomyositis, inclusion body myositis). Comp Ther 1998;24:494–502.
155. Munsat T, Cancilla P. Polymyositis without inflammation. Bull Los Angeles Neurol Soc 1974;39:113–120.
156. Giorno R, Barden MT, Kohler PF, Ringel SP. Immunohistochemical characterization of the mononuclear cells infiltrating muscle of patients with inflammatory and noninflammatory myopathies. Clin Immunol Immunopathol 1984;30:405–412.
157. Bresnan M, Hauser SL, Weiner HZ, et al. Characterization of T cell subsets in peripheral blood and muscle in childhood dermatomyositis. Ann Neurol 1981;10:283.
158. Engel AG, Arahata K. Monoclonal antibody analysis of mononuclear cells in myopathies. II. Phenotypes of autoinvasive cells in polymyositis and inclusion body myositis. Ann Neurol 1984;16:209–215.
159. Magyar E, Talerman A, Mohacsy J, et al. Muscle changes in rheumatoid arthritis: a review of the literature with a study of 100 cases. Virchows Arch Pathol Anat Histol 1977;373:267–278.
160. Brooke MH, Kaplan H. Muscle pathology in rheumatoid arthritis, polymyalgia rheumatica, and polymyositis: a histochemical study. Arch Pathol 1972;94:101–118.
161. Ringel SP, Forstot JZ, Tan EM, et al. Sjögren syndrome and polymyositis or dermatomyositis. Arch Neurol 1982;39:157–163.

162. Tome FM, Fardeau M, Lebon P, Chevallay M. Inclusion body myositis. Acta Neuropathol Suppl (Berl) 1981;7:287–291.
163. Askanas V, Engel WK, Alvarez RB. Light and electron microscopic localization of beta-amyloid protein in muscle biopsies in patients with inclusion-body myositis. Am J Pathol 1992;141:31–36.
164. Mendell JR, Sahenk Z, Gales T, Paul C. Amyloid filaments in inclusion body myositis. Novel findings provide insight into nature of filaments. Arch Neurol 1991;48:1229–1234.
165. Askanas V, Engel WK, Mirabella M. Idiopathic inflammatory myopathies: inclusion-body myositis, polymyositis and dermatomyositis. Curr Opin Neurol 1994;7:448–456.
166. Schumacher HR. A scleroderma-like syndrome with fascitis, myositis and eosinophilia [Letter]. Ann Intern Med 1976;84:49–50.
167. Shulman LE. Diffuse fascitis with hypergammaglobulinemia and eosinophilia: a new syndrome? J Rheumatol 1984;11:569–570.
168. Simon DB, Ringel SP, Sufit RL. Clinical spectrum of fascial inflammation. Muscle Nerve 1982;5:525–537.
169. Myers GB, Gottlieb AM, Mattman PE, et al. Joint and skeletal muscle manifestations in sarcoidosis. Am J Med 1952;12:161–169.
170. Maurice PA. La participation de la musculature à la maladie de Bessier-Boeck-Schauman: étude anatomo-clinique portrant sur 13 cas. Helv Med Acta 1955;22:16–42.
171. Silverstein A, Siltzbach LE. Muscle involvement in sarcoidosis, asymptomatic myositis, and myopathy. Arch Neurol 1969;21:235–241.
172. Thompson WG. Trichinosis: a clinical study of fifty-two sporadic cases. Am J Med Sci 1910;140:157–166.
173. Jolly SS, Pallis C. Muscular psuedohypertrophy due to cysticercosis. J Neurol Sci 1971;12: 155–162.
174. Hendrick GF, Verhage J, Jennekens FG, Van Knapen F. Dermatomyositis and toxoplasmosis. Ann Neurol 1979;5:393–395.
175. Dalakas MC, Pezeshkpour GH, Gravell M, Sever JL. Polymyositis associated with AIDS retrovirus. JAMA 1986;256:2381–2383.
176. Dalakas MC, Pezeshkpour GH, Gravell M, et al. Polymyositis, viruses and immunodeficiency: a distinct syndrome. Ann Neurol 1986;20:142–143.
177. Khan R, Levin M, Bertorini TE, et al. Carnitine palmitoyl transferase (CPT) deficiency, rhabdomyolysis (RM), recurrent myositis, T-cell lymphoma, and human T-lymphophotrophic virus type 1 (HTLV1) in a single patient. J Clin Neuromuscul Dis 2001;2:231–232.
178. Zaidet O, Ruff R, Kaminski H. Endocrine and Toxic Myopathy. In A Shapira, RC Griggs (eds), Muscle Diseases. Boston: Butterworth–Heinemann, 1999;363–391.
179. Mastaglia F. Toxic Myopathies. In LD Rowland, S DiMauro (eds), Myopathies. New York: Churchill Livingstone, 1992;595–562.
180. Carella F, Riva E, Morandi L, et al. Myopathy during amiodarone treatment: a case report. Ital J Neurol Sci 1987;8:605–608.
181. Laconnis D, Giulani MJ, Vancott A. Acute myopathy of intensive care: clinical, electromyographic and pathologic aspects. Ann Neurol 1998;43:171–180.
182. Emser W, Schimrigk K. Myxedema myopathy: a case report. Eur Neurol 1977;16:286–291.
183. Mallette LE, Patten BM, Engel WK. Neuromuscular disease in secondary hyperparathyroidism. Ann Int Med 1975;82:474–483.
184. Bertorini TE. Histologic Studies in Muscle of Hyperparathyroidism. In SG Massry, T Fujita (eds), New Actions of Parathyroid Hormone. New York: Plenum Press, 1989;173–182.
185. Afifi AK, Bergman RA, Harvey JC. Steroid myopathy: clinical, histologic and cytologic observations. Johns Hopkins Med J 1968;123:158–174.
186. Muller R, Kugelberg E. Myopathy in Cushing's syndrome. J Neurol Neurosurg Psychiatry 1959; 22:314–319.
187. Mastaglia FL. Pathological changes in skeletal muscle in acromegaly. Acta Neuropathol (Berlin) 1973;24:273–286.
188. Dyck PJ, Lofgren EP. Method of fascicular biopsy of human peripheral nerve for electrophysiologic and histologic study. Mayo Clin Proc 1966;41:778–784.
189. King RHM. Biopsy Techniques. In Atlas of Peripheral Nerve Pathology. London: Arnold, 1999;21–24.
190. Dyck PJ, Lofgren EP. Nerve biopsy: choice of nerve, method, symptoms and usefulness. Med Clin North Am 1968;52:885–893.
191. Weller RO, Cervos-Navarro J. Techniques of Peripheral Nerve Biopsy and Histological Preparation. In Pathology of Peripheral Nerves. London: Butterworths, 1977;9–29.

192. Midroni G, Bilbao JM. Peripheral Neuropathy and the Role of Nerve Biopsy. In G Midroni, JM Bilbao, SM Cohen (eds), Biopsy Diagnosis of Peripheral Neuropathy. Boston: Butterworth–Heinemann, 1995;1–12.

193. Midroni G, Bilbao JM. Normal Anatomy of Peripheral (Sural) Nerve. In G Midroni, JM Bilbao, SM Cohen (eds), Biopsy Diagnosis of Peripheral Neuropathy. Boston: Butterworth–Heinemann, 1995;13–34.

194. Lorimier P, Mezin P, Labat Moleur F, et al. Ultrastructural localization of the major components of the extracellular matrix in normal rat nerve. J Histochem 1992;40:859–868.

195. Behse F. Morphometric studies on the human sural nerve. Acta Neurol Scand 1990;82(Suppl 132):1–38.

196. Behse F, Buchthal F, Carlsen F, Knappeis GG. Endoneurial space and its constituents in the sural nerve of patients with neuropathy. Brain 1974;97:773–784.

197. Honavar M, Tharakan JKJ, Hughes RAC, et al. A clinicopathological study of the Guillain-Barré syndrome. Nine cases and literature review. Brain 1991;114:1245–1269.

198. Jacobs JM, Love S. Qualitative and quantitative morphology of human sural nerve at different ages. Brain 1985;108:897–924.

199. Vital C, Valla TJM. Morphometric Features. In Ultrastructural Study of the Human Diseased Peripheral Nerve (2nd ed). New York: Elsevier, 1987;21–22.

200. Norton WT, Cammer W. Isolation and Characterization of Myelin. In P Morell (ed), Myelin (2nd ed). New York: Plenum Press, 1984;147–195.

201. Trapp BD. Myelin-associated glycoprotein. Location and potential functions. Ann N Y Acad Sci 1990;605:29–43.

202. Suter U, Welcher AA, Snipes GJ. Progress in the molecular understanding of hereditary peripheral neuropathies reveals new insights into the biopsy of the peripheral nervous system. Trends Neurosci 1993;16:50–56.

203. Ghabriel MN, Allt G. Incisures of Schmidt-Lanterman. Prog Neurobiol 1981;17:25–58.

204. Waller AV. Experiments on the section of the glossopharyngeal and hypoglossal nerves of the frog, and observations of the alterations produced thereby in the structures of their primitive fibers. Philos Trans R Soc Lond B 1850;140:423–429.

205. Donat JR, Wisniewski HM. The spatio-temporal pattern of Wallerian degeneration in mammalian peripheral nerves. Brain Res 1973;53:41–53.

206. Ghabriel MN, Allt G. The role of Schmidt-Lanterman incisures in Wallerian degeneration. 1. A quantitative teased fiber study. Acta Neuropathol 1979;48:83–93.

207. Dyck PJ, Hopkins AP. Electron microscopic observations on degeneration and regeneration of unmyelinated fibers. Brain 1972;95:223–224.

208. Midroni G, Bilbao JM. The Axon: Normal Structure and Pathological Alterations. In G Midroni, JM Bilbao, SM Cohen (eds), Biopsy Diagnosis of Peripheral Neuropathy. Boston: Butterworth–Heinemann, 1995;45–74.

209. Dyck PJ, Johnson WJ, Lambert EH, O'Brien PC. Segmental demyelination secondary to axonal degeneration in uremic neuropathy. Mayo Clin Proc 1971;46:400–431.

210. Spencer PS, Schaumburg HH. Central Peripheral Istal Axonopathy: The Pathology of Dying Back Polyneuropathies. In H Zimmerman (ed), Progress in Neuropathology. New York: Grune & Stratton, 1977;253–295.

211. Asbury AR, Johnson PC. Basic Pathologic Mechanisms. In AR Asbury, PC Johnson (eds), Pathology of Peripheral Nerve. Philadelphia: Saunders, 1978;50–71.

212. Vital C, Gherardi R, Vital A, et al. Uncompacted myelin lamellae in polyneuropathy, organomegaly, endocrinopathy, M-protein and skin changes syndrome. Ultrastructural study of peripheral nerve biopsy from 22 patients. Acta Neuropathol 1994;87:302–307.

213. Yoshikawa H, Dyck PJ. Uncompacted inner myelin lamellae in inherited tendency to pressure palsy. J Neuropathol Exp Neurol 1991;50:649–657.

214. Jacobs JM, Scadding JW. Morphological changes in IgM paraproteinaemic neuropathy. Acta Neuropathol 1990;80:77–84.

215. Quattrone D, Ganbarella A, Bono F, et al. Autosomal recessive hereditary motor and sensory neuropathy with focally folded myelin sheath. Clinical, electrophysiological and genetic aspects of a large family. Neurology 1996;46:1318–1324.

216. Dyck PJ, Chance P, Lebo R, Carney JA. Hereditary Motor and Sensory Neuropathies. In PJ Dyck, PK Thomas, et al. (eds), Peripheral Neuropathy (3rd ed). Philadelphia: Saunders, 1993; 1094–1136.

217. Lupski JR. Charcot-Marie-Tooth Polyneuropathy Syndrome: Molecular Biology and Neurobiology. In S Appel (ed), Current Neurology. Chicago: Mosby-Yearbook, 1993;13:41–58.

218. Hayasaka K, Himoro M, Sato W, et al. Charcot-Marie-Tooth neuropathy type 1B is associated with mutations of the myelin PO gene. Nat Genet 1993;5:31–34.

219. Warner LE, Mancias P, Butler IJ, et al. Mutations in the early growth response 2 (EGR2) gene are associated with hereditary myelopathies. Nat Genet 1998;18:382–384.

220. Bergoffen J, Scherer SS, Wang S, et al. Connexin mutations in X-linked Charcot-Marie-Tooth disease. Science 1993;262:2039–2042.

221. Behse F, Buchthal F. Peroneal muscular atrophy (PMA) and related disorders. II. Histological findings in sural nerves. Brain 1977;100:67–85.

222. Gherardi R, Bouche P, Escourolle R, et al. Peroneal muscular atrophy, part 2. Nerve biopsy studies. J Neurol Sci 1983;61:401–416.

223. Chance PF, Alderson MK, Leppig KA, et al. NA deletion associated with hereditary neuropathy with liability to pressure palsies. Cell 1993;72:143–151.

224. Mariman EC, Gabreels-Festen AAWM, van Beersum SEC, et al. Prevalence of the 1.5-Mb 17p deletion in families with hereditary neuropathy with liability to pressure palsies. Ann Neurol 1994;26:650–655.

225. Madrid R, Bradley WG. The pathology of neuropathies with focal thickening of the myelin sheath (tomaculous neuropathy): studies on the formation of the abnormal myelin sheath. J Neurol Sci 1975;25:415–448.

226. Behse F, Buchthal F, Carlsen F, et al. Hereditary neuropathy with liability to pressure palsies. Electrophysiological and histopathological aspects. Brain 1972;95:777–794.

227. Bouche P, Gherardi R, Cathala HP, et al. Peroneal muscular atrophy: part 1. Clinical and electrophysiological study. J Neurol Sci 1983;61:389–399.

228. Berciano J, Combarros O, Figols J, et al. Hereditary motor and sensory neuropathy type II. Clinicopathological study of a family. Brain 1986;109:897–914.

229. Guzzetta F, Ferriere G, Lyon G. Congenital hypomyelination polyneuropathy: pathological findings compared with polyneuropathies starting later in life. Brain 1982;105:395–416.

230. Harati Y, Butler IJ. Congenital hypomyelinating neuropathy. J Neurol Neurosurg Psychiatry 1985;48:1269–1276.

231. Dyck PJ. Neuronal Atrophy and Degeneration Predominantly Affecting Peripheral Sensory and Autonomic Neurons. In PJ Dyck, PK Thomas, JW Griffen, et al. (eds), Peripheral Neuropathy (3rd ed). Philadelphia: Saunders, 1993;1065–1093.

232. Thomas PK. Hereditary sensory neuropathies. Brain Pathol 1993;3;157–163.

233. Mandell J. Hereditary, Sensory and Autonomic Neuropathies. In J Mandell, JT Kissell, DR Cornblath (eds), Diagnosis and Management of Peripheral Nerve Disorders. Oxford, UK: Oxford University Press, 2001;460–476.

234. Maia M, Pires MM, Guimaraes A. Giant axonal disease: report of three cases and review of literature. Neuropediatrics 1988;19:10–15.

235. Tandan R, Little BW, Emery ES, et al. Childhood giant axonal neuropathy: case report and review of the literature. J Neurol Sci 1987;82:205–228.

236. Gambarelli D, Hassoun J, Pellisier JF, et al. Giant axonal neuropathy. Involvement of peripheral nerve, myenteric plexus and extra-neuronal area. Acta Neuropathol 1977;39:261–269.

237. Koch T, Schultz P, Williams R, et al. Giant axonal neuropathy: a childhood disorder of neurofilaments. Ann Neurol 1977;1:438–451.

238. Berard-Badier M, Gambarelli D, Pinsard N, et al. Infantile neuroaxonal dystrophy, or Seitelberger's disease. II. Peripheral nerve involvement: electron microscopic study in one case. Acta Neuropathol 1971;5(Suppl):30–39.

239. Caruso G, Santoro L, Perretti A, et al. Friedreich's ataxia: electrophysiological and histological findings. Acta Neurol Scand 1983;67:26–40.

240. Hughes JT, Brownell B, Hewer RL. The peripheral sensory pathway in Friedreich's ataxia: an examination by light and electron microscopy of the posterior nerve roots, posterior roots ganglia, and peripheral sensory nerves in cases of Friedreich's ataxia. Brain 1968;91:803–817.

241. Busard HL, Gabreels-Festen AA, Reiner WO, et al. Adult polyglucosan body disease: the diagnostic value of axilla skin biopsy. Ann Neurol 1991;29:448–451.

242. Plante-Bordeneuve V, Lalu T, Mirashi M, et al. Genotypic-phenotypic variations in series of 65 patients with familial amyloidotic polyneuropathy. Neurology 1998;57:708–714.

243. Mendell JR. Familial Amyloid Polyneuropathies. In JR Mendell, JT Kissel, DR Cornblath (eds), Diagnosis and Management of Peripheral Nerve Disorders. New York: Oxford University Press, 2001;477–491.

244. Nichols WC, Gregg RE, Brewer HB Jr, Benson MD. A mutation in apolipoprotein A-1 in the Iowa type o familial amyloidotic polyneuropathy. Genomics 1990;8:318–323.

245. Kiuru S. Familial amyloidosis of the Finnish type (FAF). A clinical study of 30 patients. Acta Neurol Scand 1992;86:346–353.

246. Darras BT, Adelman LS, Mora JS, et al. Familial amyloidosis with cranial neuropathy and corneal lattice dystrophy. Neurology 1986;36:432–435.

247. Kwiatkowski DJ, Westbrook CA, Bruns GAP, et al. Localization of gelsolin proximal to ABL on chromosome 9. Am J Hum Genet 1988;42:565–572.

248. Gross U, Sassa S, Jacob K, et al. 5-Aminolevulinic acid dehydratase deficient porphyria: a twenty-year clinical and biochemical follow-up. Clin Chem 1998;44:1892–1896.

249. Wang AL, Arrendondo-Vega FX, Giampietro PF, et al. Regional gene assignment of human porphobilinogen deaminase and esterase A4 to chromosome 11q23-11qter. Proc Natl Acad Sci U S A 1981;78:5734–5738.

250. Cacheau V, Martasek P, Fougerousse F, et al. Localization of the human coproporphyrinogen oxidase gene. Hum Genet 1994;94:557–559.

251. Taketani S, Inazawa J, Abe T, et al. The human protoporphyrinogen oxidase gene (PPOX): organization and localization to chromosome 1. Genomics 1995;29:698–703.

252. Potluri VR, Astrin KH, Wetmur JG, et al. Human δ-aminolevulinate dehydratase: chromosomal localization to 9p34 by in situ hybridization. Hum Genet 1987;76:236–239.

253. Cavanagh JB, Ridley AR. The nature of the neuropathy complicating acute intermittent porphyria. Lancet 1967;2:1023–1024.

254. Defanti CA, Sghirlanzoni A, Bottacchi E, Peluchetti D. Porphyric neuropathy: a clinical, neurophysiological and morphological study. Ital J Neurol Sci 1985;6:521–526.

255. Gibson JB, Goldberg A. The neuropathology of acute porphyria. Pathol Bacteriol 1956;71:495–509.

256. Anzil AP, Dozic S. Peripheral nerve changes in porphyric neuropathy: findings in sural nerve biopsy. Acta Neuropathol (Berl) 1978;42:121–126.

257. Di Trapani G, Casali C, Tonali P, Topi GC. Peripheral nerve findings in hereditary coproporphyria. Acta Neuropathol (Berl) 1984;63:96–107.

258. Kolodny EW, Fluharty A. Metachromatic Leukodystrophy and Multiple Sulfatase Deficiency: Sulfate Lipidosis. In CR Scriver, AL Beaudet, WS Sly, D Valle (eds), The Metabolic and Molecular Basis of Inherited Disease (7th ed). New York: McGraw-Hill, 1995;2693–2739.

259. Dayan AD. Peripheral neuropathy of metachromatic leukodystrophy: observations on segmental demyelination and remyelination and the intracellular distribution of sulphatide. J Neurol Neurosurg Psychiatry 1967;39:311–318.

260. Martin JJ, Ceuterick C, Mercelis R, Joris C. Pathology of peripheral nerves in metachromatic leukodystrophy: a comparative study of ten cases. J Neurol Sci 1982;53:95–112.

261. Dunn HG, Lake BD, Dolman DL, Wilson J. The neuropathy of Krabbe's infantile cerebral sclerosis (globoid cell leukodystrophy). Brain 1969;92;329–344.

262. Morgan SH, Rudge P, Smith JM, et al. The neurological complication of Anderson-Fabry disease (α-galactosidase A deficiency)—investigations of symptomatic and presymptomatic patients. QJM 1990;75:491–507.

263. Hashimoto K, Gross BG, Lever WF. Angiokeratoma corporis diffusum (Fabry): histochemical and electron microscopic studies of the skin. J Invest Dermatol 1965;44:119.

264. Tome FMS, Fardeau M. Lenoir G. Ultrastructural of muscle and sensory nerve in Fabry's disease. Acta Neuropathol 1977;38:187–194.

265. Toyoka K, Said G. Nerve biopsy findings in homozygous and heterozygous patients with Fabry's disease. J Neurol 1997;244:464–468.

266. Wichman A, Buchtal F, Pezeshkpour GH, Gregg RE. Peripheral neuropathy in abetalipoproteinemia. Neurology 1985;35:1279–1289.

267. Assmann G, von Ekardstein A, Brewer HB. Familial High Density Lipoprotein Deficiency: Tangier Disease. In R Scriber, AL Beaudet, WS Sly, D Valle (eds), The Metabolic and Molecular Basis of Inherited Disease, Vol 2 (7th ed). New York: McGraw-Hill, 1995;2053–2072.

268. Bale PM, Clifton-Bligh P, Benamin BH, Whyte HM. Pathology of Tangier disease. J Clin Pathol 1971;24:609–616.

269. Baxter JH. Absorption of chlorophyll phytol in normal man and in patients with Refsum's disease. J Lipid Res 1968;9:636–641.

270. Singh I, Pahan K, Singh AK, Barbosa E. Refsum disease: a defect in the α-oxidation of phytanic acid in peroxisomes. J Lipid Res 1993;34:1755–1764.

271. Refsum S. Heredopathia atactia polyneuritiformis: a familial syndrome not hitherto described. A contribution to the clinical study of the hereditary diseases of the nervous system. Acta Psychiatr Scand Suppl 1946;38:1–303.

272. Fardeau M, Engel WK. Ultrastructural study of peripheral nerve biopsy in Refsum's disease. J Neuropathol Exp Neurol 1969;28:278–294.

273. Moser HW. Adrenoleukodystrophy; phenotype, genetics, pathogenesis and therapy. Brain 1997; 120:1485–1508.

274. Moser HW, Moser AB, Naidu S, Bergin A. Clinical aspects of adrenoleukodystrophy and adrenomyeloneuropathy. Dev Neurosci 1991;13:254–261.

275. Schaumburg HH, Powers JM, Raine CS, et al. Adrenomyeloneuropathy: a probable variant of adrenoleukodystrophy. II. General pathology, neuropathology and biochemical aspects. Neurology 1977;27:1114–1119.

276. Asbury AKB, Arnason G, Adams RD. The inflammatory lesion in idiopathic polyneuritis. Its role in pathogenesis. Medicine 1969;48:173–215.

277. Arnason BGW, Soliven B. Acute Inflammatory Demyelinating Polyneuropathy. In PJ Dyck, PK Thomas (eds), Peripheral Neuropathy (3rd ed). Philadelphia: Saunders, 1993;1437–1497.

278. Ropper AH, Wijdicks EFM, Truax BT. Guillain-Barré Syndrome. Contemporary Neurology Series, Vol 34. Philadelphia: FA Davis, 1991;33–42.

279. Hart MN, Hanks DT, MacKay R. Ultrastructural observations in Guillain-Barré syndrome. Arch Pathol 1972;93:552–555.

280. Hafer-Mako CE, Sheikh KA, Li CY, et al. Immune attack on the Schwann cell surface in acute inflammatory demyelinating polyneuropathy. Ann Neurol 1996;39:625–635.

281. Feasby TE, Gilbert JJ, Brown WF, et al. An acute axonal form of Guillain-Barré polyneuropathy. Brain 1986;109:1115–1167.

282. Griffin JW, Li CY, Ho TW, et al. Pathology of the motor-sensory axonal Guillain-Barré syndrome. Ann Neurol 1996;39:17–28.

283. Griffin JW, Li CY, Ho TW, et al. Guillain-Barré syndrome in northern China. The spectrum of neuropathological changes in clinically defined cases. Brain 1995;118:577–595.

284. McKhann GM, Cornblath DR, Ho T, et al. Clinical and electrophysiological aspects of acute paralytic disease of children and young adults in northern China. Lancet 1991;338:593–597.

285. Kissel JT, Cornblath DR, Mendell JR. Guillain-Barré Syndrome. In JR Mendell, JT Kissell, DR Cornblath (eds), Diagnosis and Management of Peripheral Nerve Disorders. Oxford, UK: Oxford University Press, 2001;145–172.

286. Young RR, Asbury AK, Adams RD, Corbett JL. Pure pan-dysautonomia with recovery. Description and discussions of diagnostic criteria. Trans Am Neurol Assoc 1969;94:355–537.

287. Young RR, Asbury AK, Corbett JL, Adams RD. Pure pan-dysautonomia with recovery. Brain 1975;98:613–636.

288. Suarez GA, Fealey RD, Camilleri M. Idiopathic autonomic neuropathy: clinical neurophysiologic, and follow-up studies on 27 patients. Neurology 1994;44:1675–1682.

289. Watenberg R. Sensory Polyneuropathy. In R Watenberg (ed), Neuritis, Sensory Neurons, and Neuralgia. New York: Oxford University Press, 1958;160–162.

290. Oh S, LaGanke L, Clausen GC. Sensory Guillain-Barré syndrome. Neurology 2001;56:82–86.

291. Sterman AB, Schaumburg HH, Asbury AK. The acute sensory neuropathy syndrome: a distinct clinical entity. Ann Neurol 1987;7:354–358.

292. Danson M, Samuels MA, Morris J. Sensory form of acute polyneuritis. Neurology 1988;38: 728–731.

293. Dyck PJ, Lais AC, Ohta M, et al. Chronic inflammatory polyradiculoneuropathy. Mayo Clin Proc 1975;50:621–637.

294. Barohn RJ, Kissel JT, Warmolt JR, Mendell JR. Chronic inflammatory demyelinating polyradiculoneuropathy. Clinical characteristics, course, and recommendations for diagnostic criteria. Arch Neurol 1989;46:878–884.

295. Research criteria for diagnosis of chronic inflammatory demyelinating polyneuropathy (CIDP) from an Ad Hoc Subcommittee of the American Academy of Neurology (AIDS Task Force). Neurology 1991;41:617–668.

296. Oh SJ, Joy JL, Kuruoglu R. "Chronic sensory demyelinating neuropathy": chronic inflammatory demyelinating polyneuropathy presenting as a pure sensory neuropathy. J Neurol Neurosurg Psychiatry 1992;55:677–680.

297. Krendel DA, Parks HP, Anthony DC, et al. Sural nerve biopsy in chronic inflammatory demyelinating polyradiculoneuropathy. Muscle Nerve 1989;12:257–264.

298. Molenaar DS, Vermeulen M, de Haan R. Diagnostic value of sural nerve biopsy in chronic inflammatory demyelinating polyneuropathy. J Neurol Neurosurg Psychiatry 1998;64:84–89.

299. Julien J, Vital C, Lagueny A, et al. Chronic relapsing idiopathic polyneuropathy with primary axonal lesions. J Neurol Neurosurg Psychiatry 1989;52:871–875.

300. Stewart JD, McKelvy R, Duncan L, et al. Chronic inflammatory demyelinating polyneuropathy (CIDP) in diabetes. J Neurol Sci 1996;142:59–64.
301. Haaq RV, Friest TJ, Pendlebury WW, et al. Chronic inflammatory demyelinating polyneuropathy. A study of proposed electrodiagnostic and histologic criteria. Arch Neurol 2000;57:1745–1750.
302. Parry GJ, Clarke S. Multifocal acquired demyelinating neuropathy masquerading as motor neuron disease. Muscle Nerve 1988;11:103–107.
303. Pestronk A, Chaudhry V, Feldman EL, et al. Lower motor neuron syndromes defined by patterns of weakness, nerve conduction abnormalities and high titers of antiglycolipid antibodies. Ann Neurol 1990;27:316–326.
304. Lewis RA, Sumner AL, Brown MJ, et al. Multifocal demyelinating neuropathy with persistent conduction block. Neurology 1982;32:958–964.
305. Gibbels E, Behse F, Kentenich M, Haupt WF. Chronic multifocal neuropathy with persistent conduction block (Lewis-Sumner syndrome). A clinico-pathologic study of two further cases with review of the literature. Clin Neuropathol 1993;12:343–352.
306. Vital C, Aubertin J, Ragault JM, et al. Sarcoidosis of the peripheral nerve: a histological and ultrastructural study of two cases. Acta Neuropathol 1982;58:111–114.
307. Minahan RE. Sarcoid Peripheral Neuropathy. In J Mandell, JT Kissell, DR Cornblath (eds), Diagnosis and Management of Peripheral Nerve Disorders. Oxford, UK: Oxford University Press, 2001;256–271.
308. Oh SJ. Sarcoid polyneuropathy: a histologically proved case. Ann Neurol 1980;7:178–181.
309. Lovshin LL, Kernohan JW. Peripheral neuritis in periarteritis nodosa. A clinicopathologic study. Arch Intern Med 1948;82:321–338.
310. Claussen G, Thomas D, Goyne CH, et al. Diagnostic value of nerve and muscle biopsy in suspected vasculitis cases. J Clin Neuromuscul Disord 2000;1:117–123.
311. Midroni G, Bilbao JM, Cohen SM. Vasculitic Neuropathy. Biopsy Diagnosis of Peripheral Neuropathy. Boston: Butterworth–Heinemann, 1995;241–261.
312. Fujimura H, Lacroix C, Said G. Vulnerability of nerve fibres to ischaemia. A quantitative light and electron microscope study. Brain 1991;114:1929–1942.
313. Kissel JT, Slivka AP, Warmolts JR, Mendell JR. The clinical spectrum of necrotizing angiopathy of the peripheral nervous system. Ann Neurol 1985;18:251–257.
314. Dyck PJ, Benstead TJ, Conn DL, et al. Nonsystemic vasculitic neuropathy. Brain 1987;110:843–854.
315. Griffin JW, Cornblath DR, Alexander C, et al. Ataxic sensory neuropathy and dorsal root ganglionitis associated with Sjögren's syndrome. Ann Neurol 1990;27:304–305.
316. Dalmau JO, Posner JB. Paraneoplastic syndromes. Arch Neurol 1999;56:405–408.
317. Ropper AH, Gorson KC. Neuropathies associated with paraproteinemia. N Engl J Med 1998;338:1601–1607.
318. Kissel JT, Mendell JR. Neuropathies associated with monoclonal gammopathies. Neuromuscul Disord 1996;6:3–18.
319. Kyle R. "Benign" monoclonal gammopathy—after 20 to 35 years of follow-up. Mayo Clin Proc 1993;68:26–36.
320. Miescher GC, Latov N, Steck AJ. Dysglobulineic Neuropathies. In J Antel, G Birnbaum, P Hartung (eds), Neuroimmunology. Cambridge, UK: Blackwell Science, 1998;307–315.
321. Mendell JR, Sahenk Z, Whitaker JN, et al. Polyneuropathy and IgM monoclonal gammopathy: studies on the pathogenic role of anti-myelin-associated glycoprotein antibody. Ann Neurol 1985;17:243–254.
322. Ellie E, Vital E, Steck A, et al. Neuropathy associated with "benign" anti-myelin-associated glycoprotein IgM gammopathy: clinical, immunological, neurophysiological, pathological findings and response to treatment in 33 cases. J Neurol 1996;243:34–43.
323. Kyle RA, Dyck P. Neuropathy Associated with the Monoclonal Gammopathies. In PJ Dyck, PK Thomas (eds), Peripheral Neuropathy (3rd ed). Philadelphia: Saunders, 1993;1275–1287.
324. Reilly MM, Stuanton H. Peripheral nerve amyloidosis. Brain Pathol 1996;6:163–177.
325. Dellagi K, Dupouey P, Brouet JC, et al. Waldenström's macroglobulinemia and peripheral neuropathy: a clinical and immunologic study of 25 patients. Blood 1983;62:280–285.
326. Chad D, Pariser K, Bradley WG, et al. The pathogenesis of cryoglobulinemic neuropathy. Neurology 1982;32:725–729.
327. Nemni R, Corbo M, Fazio R, et al. Cryoglobulinaemic neuropathy. Brain 1988;111:541–552.
328. Adams D, Said G. Ultrastructural characterization of the M protein in nerve biopsy of patients with POEMS syndrome. J Neurol Neurosurg Psychiatry 1998;64:809–812.

329. Reulecke M, Dumas M, Meier C. Specific antibody activity against neuroendocrine tissue in a case of POEMS syndrome with IgG gammopathy. Neurology 1988;38:614–616.

330. Donaghy M, Hall P, Gawler J, et al. Peripheral neuropathy associated with Castleman's disease. J Neurol Sci 1989;89:253–267.

331. Simpson DM, Olney RK. Peripheral neuropathies associated with human immunodeficiency virus infection. Neurol Clin 1992;10:685–711.

332. Cornblath DR, McArthur JC, Pay GJ, Griffin JW. Peripheral Neuropathies in Human Immunodeficiency Virus Infection. In PJ Dyck, PK Thomas (eds), Peripheral Neuropathy. Philadelphia: Saunders, 1993;1343–1353.

333. De la Monte SM, Gabuda DH, Ho DD, et al. Peripheral neuropathy in the acquired immunodeficiency syndrome. Ann Neurol 1988;23:485–492.

334. Cornblath DR, McArthur JC, Kennedy PG, et al. Inflammatory demyelinating peripheral neuropathies associated with human T-cell lymphotrophic virus type III infection. Ann Neurol 1987;21:32–40.

335. Levy RM, Redesen DE, Rosenblum ML. Neurological manifestations of the acquired immunodeficiency syndrome (AIDS): experience at UCSF and review of the literature. J Neurosurg 1985;62:475–495.

336. Gherardi R, Lebargy F, Goulard P. Necrotizing vasculitis and the HIV replication in peripheral nerves [Letter]. N Engl J Med 1989;321:655–686.

337. Moulignier A, Authier FJ, Baurimont M, et al. Peripheral neuropathy in human immunodeficiency virus-infected patients with the diffuse infiltrative lymphocytosis syndrome. Ann Neurol 1997;41:438–445.

338. Bhigjee AI, Bill PLA, Wiley CA, et al. Peripheral nerve lesions in HTLV-1 associated myelopathy (HAM/TSP). Muscle Nerve 1993;116:21–26.

339. Ridley DS, Jopling WH. A classification of leprosy for research purposes. Lepr Rev 1962;33:119–128.

340. Job CK. Pathology of peripheral nerve lesions in lepromatous leprosy: a light and electron microscopic study. Int J Lepr Other Mycobact Dis 1971;39:251–268.

341. Job CK, Desikan KV. Pathologic changes and their distribution in peripheral nerves in lepromatous leprosy. Int J Lepr Other Mycobact Dis 1968;36:257–270.

342. Pearson JMH, Weddell AGM. Perineurial changes in leprosy. Lepr Rev 1975;46:51–62.

343. Shetty VP, Antia NH. Nerve damage in leprosy. Int J Lepr 1989;56:619–621.

344. McDonal WI, Kocen RS. Diphtheric neuropathy. In PJ Dyck, PK Thomas (eds), Peripheral Neuropathy (3rd ed). Philadelphia: Saunders, 1993;1412–1417.

345. Fisher CM, Adams RD. Diphtheric polyneuritis—a pathological study. J Neuropathol Exp Neurol 1956;15:243–268.

346. Reik L Jr. Peripheral Neuropathy in Lyme Disease. In PJ Dyck, PK Thomas (eds), Peripheral Neuropathy (3rd ed). Philadelphia: W.B. Saunders, 1993;1401–1411.

347. Halperin JJ, Little BW, Coyle PK, Dattwyler RJ. Lyme disease: cause of a treatable peripheral neuropathy. Neurology 1987;37:1700–1706.

348. Meier C, Grahmann F, Engelhardt A, Dumas M. Peripheral nerve disorders in Lyme-Borreliosis. Nerve biopsy studies from eight cases. Acta Neuropathol 1989;79:271–278.

349. Vinik A. Diabetic neuropathy: pathogenesis and therapy. Am J Med 1999;107:17S–26S.

350. Vinik AI, Park TS, Stansberry KB, Pittenger GL. Diabetic neuropathies. Diabetologia 2000;43:957–973.

351. Giannini C, Dyck PJ. Basement membrane reduplication and pericyte degeneration precede development of diabetic polyneuropathy and are associated with its severity. Ann Neurol 1995;37:498–504.

352. Thomas PK, Lacelles RG. The pathology of diabetic neuropathy. J Med 1966;35:489–509.

353. Vital C, Vallat JM, LeBlanc M, et al. Peripheral neuropathies caused by diabetes mellitus: ultrastructural study of 12 biopsied cases. J Neurol Sci 1973;18:381–398.

354. Dreyfus PM, Hakim S, Adams RD. Diabetic ophthalmoplegia: report of a case with postmortem study and comments on vascular supply of human oculomotor nerve. Arch Neurol Psychiatry 1957;77:337–349.

355. Raff MC, Sangalang V, Asbury A. Ischemic mononeuropathy multiplex associated with diabetes mellitus. Arch Neurol 1968;18:487–490.

356. Said G. Nerve biopsy findings in different patterns of proximal diabetic neuropathy. Ann Neurol 1994;35:559–569.

357. Krendal DA. Diabetic inflammatory vasculopathy. Muscle Nerve 1997;20:520–521.

358. Meier C, Bischoff A. Polyneuropathy in hypothyroidism. Clinical and nerve biopsy study of 4 cases. J Neurol 1977;215:103–114.

359. Low PA, McLeod JG, Turtle JR, et al. Peripheral neuropathy in acromegaly. Brain 1974;97: 139–152.

360. McCombe PA, McLeod JG. The peripheral neuropathy of vitamin B_{12} deficiency. J Neurol Sci 1984;66:117–126.

361. Sokol RJ, Kayden HJ, Bettis DB, et al. Isolated vitamin E deficiency in the absence of fat malabsorption: familial and sporadic cases: characterization and investigation of causes. J Lab Clin Med 1988;111:548–559.

362. Narayanaswami P, Bertorini TE, Frederick R. Gastric bypass neuropathy: clinical, electrophysiologic/histologic correlates (abstr). Muscle Nerve 1999;22(9):1332.

363. Jacobs JM, Costa-Jussa FR. The pathology of amiodarone neurotoxicity: II. Peripheral neuropathy in man. Brain 1985;108:753–769.

364. Tegner R, Tome FMS, Godeau P, et al. Morphological study of peripheral nerve changes induced by chloroquine treatment. Acta Neuropathol 1988;75:253–260.

365. Pilcher J, Chandrasekhar KP, Russell Rees J, et al. Long term assessment of perhexiline maleate in angina pectoris. Postgrad Med J 1973;49(Suppl 3):115–118.

366. Bradley WG, Lassman LP, Pearce GW, Walton J. The neuromyopathy of vincristine in man. Clinical, electrophysiological, and pathological studies. J Neurol Sci 1970;10:107–131.

367. Erdem S, Kissel JT, Mendell JR. Toxic Neuropathies: Drugs, Metals, and Alcohol. In JR Mendell, JT Kissel, DR Cornblath (eds), Diagnosis and Management of Peripheral Nerve Disorders. Oxford, UK: Oxford University Press, 2001;297–343.

368. Schaumburg H, Kaplan J, Windebank A, et al. Sensory neuropathy from pyridoxine abuse: a new megavitamin syndrome. N Engl J Med 1983;309:445–448.

369. Krinke G, Schaumburg HH, Spencer PS. Pyridoxine megavitaminosis produces degeneration of peripheral sensory neurons (sensory neuronopathy) in the dog. Neurotoxicology 1981;2:13–24.

370. Gutmann L, Martin JD, Welton W. Dapsone motor neuropathy—an axonal disease. Neurology 1976;26:514–516.

371. Bradley WG, Karlsson IJ, Rassol CG. Metronidazole neuropathy. BMJ 1977;2:610–611.

372. Yiannikas C, Pollard JD, McLeod JG. Nitrofurantoin neuropathy. Aust N Z J Med 1981;11: 400–405.

373. Tugwell P, James SL. Peripheral neuropathy with ethambutol. Postgrad Med J 1972;48:667–670.

374. Jones WA, Jones GP. Peripheral neuropathy due to isoniazid. Report of two cases. Lancet 1953;i:1073–1074.

375. Ochoa J. Isoniazid neuropathy in man: quantitative electron microscope study. Brain 1970;93: 831–850.

376. Ramirez JA, Mendell JR, Warmolts JR, Griggs RC. Phenytoin neuropathy: structural changes in the sural nerve. Ann Neurol 1986;19:162–167.

377. Kuncl RW, Duncan G, Watson D, et al. Colchicine myopathy and neuropathy. N Engl J Med 1987;316:1562–1568.

378. Erdem A, Freimer ML, O'Dorisio T, Mendell JR. Procainamide-induced chronic inflammatory demyelinating polyradiculoneuropathy. Neurology 1998;50:824–825.

379. Wilson JR, Conwit RA, Eidelman BH, et al. Sensorimotor neuropathy resembling CIDP in patients receiving FK506. Muscle Nerve 1994;17:528–532.

380. Victor M. Polyneuropathy Due to Nutritional Deficiency and Alcoholism. In PJ Dyck, PT Thomas, EH Lambert (eds), Peripheral Neuropathy. Philadelphia: Saunders, 1975;1050–1060.

381. D'Amour ML, Butterworth RF. Pathogenesis of alcoholic peripheral neuropathy: direct effect of ethanol or nutritional deficit? Metab Brain Dis 1994;9:133–142.

382. Walsh JC, McLeod JG. Alcoholic neuropathy. An electrophysiological and histological study. J Neurol Sci 1970;10:457–469.

383. Tredici G, Minazzi M. Alcoholic neuropathy. An electron-microscopic study. J Neurol Sci 1975;25:333–346.

384. Oh S. Lead neuropathy: case report. Arch Phys Med Rehabil 1975;56:312–317.

385. Lampert PW, Schochet SS Jr. Demyelination and remyelination in lead neuropathy: electron microscopic studies. J Neuropathol Exp Neurol 1968;27:527–545.

386. Donofrio PD, Wilbourn AJ, Albers JW, et al. Acute intoxication presenting as Guillain-Barré syndrome. Muscle Nerve 1987;10:114–120.

387. Dyck PJ, Gutrecht JA, Bastron JA, et al. Histologic and teased fiber measurements of sural nerve in disorders of lower motor and primary sensory neurons. Mayo Clin Proc 1968;43:81–123.

388. Bolton CF, Laverty DA, Brown JD, et al. Critically ill neuropathy: electrophysiological studies and demyelination from Guillain-Barré syndrome. J Neurol Neurosurg Psychiatry 1986;49:563–573.

389. Diaz-Arrastia R, Younger DS, Hair L, et al. Neurolymphomatosis: a clinicopathologic syndrome re-emerges. Neurology 1992;42:1136–1141.
390. Gherardi R, Gaulard P, Prost C, et al. T-cell lymphoma revealed by a peripheral neuropathy: a report of two cases with an immunohistologic study on lymph node and nerve biopsies. Cancer 1986;58:2710–2716.
391. Dyck PJ, Winkelman R, Bolton CF. Quantitation of Meissner corpuscles in hereditary neurological disorders. Neurology 1960;16:10–17.
392. Ridley A. Silver staining of nerve endings in human digital glabrous skin. J Anat 1973;115: 277–288.
393. Holland NR, Stokes A, Hauer P, et al. Intraepidermal nerve fiber density in patients with painful sensory neuropathy. Neurology 1997;48:708–711.
394. Hermann DN, Griffin JW, Hauer P, et al. Epidermal nerve fiber density and sural nerve morphometry in peripheral neuropathies. Neurology 1999;53:1634–1640.

20

Basic Medical Genetics and Molecular Diagnostics

J. Rafael Gorospe and Eric P. Hoffman

The impact of the new field of molecular genetics has nowhere been greater than in the practice of neurology. Today, neurologists (particularly those in the area of neuromuscular disorders) routinely use genetic tools to diagnose patients. As the field of molecular genetics matures and advances, so too do the important areas of pathophysiology delineation and its sister field of pathophysiology-based therapeutics. No doubt spurred by the completion of the Human Genome Project, researchers and practitioners have been so relentless in their pursuit of cutting-edge technologies that the diagnosis and treatment of patients can only be envisioned to get more sophisticated yet straightforward from here.

As with any changing field, however, advances in molecular genetics appear to have opened a "Pandora's box"—a thorny mix of ethical, legal, and political concerns—that threatens to complicate an already increasingly confusing picture. For instance, a hapless neurologist grappling with a difficult diagnostic case and scrambling to locate an appropriate laboratory has the added obligation to self-educate regarding the important ethical issues that come with testing. Issues concerning patient confidentiality, paternity, and insurability—to name only a few—may become as important and critical to physicians and their patients as what imaging modality to order or what treatment options to pursue. Fortunately, a number of Web-based resources have surfaced that can provide guidance in appropriate testing and keeping up to date with ethical, legal, and social implications of medical genetics.

In this chapter, basic concepts in medical genetics are first reviewed. In the second half of the chapter, an overview of molecular diagnostic methodologies is provided. In keeping with the basic thrust of the chapter, no attempt was made to discuss all of the molecular diagnostic tests that are currently available. Instead, only those methods considered "traditional" and in frequent use are emphasized. Finally, a number of exciting emerging technologies are introduced that are envisioned to transform molecular diagnostics as we currently know it.

WEB-BASED RESOURCES

Centralized reference sources, where continually updated information on genetics can be found, are now accessible through the Internet. The National Human Genome Research Institute of the National Institutes of Health maintains a Web site (http://www.nhgri.nih.gov/) containing important information and links to virtually any topic related to genetics (e.g., public policy, genomic and genetic resources, research). The educational resource section (http://www.nhgri.nih.gov/DIR/VIP/Glossary/) contains figures and explanations that are quite helpful, especially for those who wish to review basic genetic concepts.

Disease-specific information can be obtained from the following Web sites: On-Line Mendelian Inheritance in Man (OMIM), GeneTests, and GeneClinics. OMIM (http://www3.ncbi.nlm.nih.gov/Omim) contains clinical reviews on all known and suspected genetic disorders with each entry organized as a running synopsis of the accumulated literature. As such, it is extensively referenced and usually quite up to date. GeneTests (http://www.genetests.org) is a searchable database where one can locate laboratories offering specific molecular diagnostic tests. Information on the nature of the testing offered (e.g., clinical vs. research-based, gene vs. protein), the methods used (e.g., sequencing or mutation detection), and the contact person or laboratory to which patient samples can be sent are available on this Web site. GeneClinics (http://www.geneclinics.org) contains reviews of diagnostic categories focusing on genetic testing, genotype and phenotype correlations, and genetic counseling. Each review is written by an invited expert whose contribution is carefully screened by two or more expert peer reviewers and text-edited by the database curators to ensure consistency and completeness of the contributions. The expert guidance provided by the resource on the most appropriate and cost-effective genetic and biochemical tests can be particularly helpful to clinicians. This resource contains extensive bibliographies with direct links to abstracts via MedLine.

Finally, the journal *Neuromuscular Disorders* publishes in each edition a table that summarizes the most up-to-date information on genetic neuromuscular disorders. The table outlines the different diseases and their respective modes of inheritance, gene location, gene product (when available), OMIM reference number, and key references. It is anticipated that this information will soon be available as a Web-based resource. For the interested neurologist, another extensive outline in tabular form on the clinical and genetic classification of neurologic disorders can be found in Martin and Longo,[1] with information on mode of inheritance, phenotype, and disease mechanism.

BASIC CONCEPTS IN MEDICAL GENETICS

Genes

Human cells—and, by extension, whole human beings—grow, develop, and function in response to information contained in molecules of DNA found in each cell. A fragment of DNA that codes for a protein or ribonucleic acid (RNA) with a specific function is called a *gene*. The information in DNA must be stable, resistant to change, and faithfully replicated to ensure that mistakes (mutations) are not transmitted to daughter cells.

A gene has distinct components that are essential for the synthesis of the protein it codes for. The actual coding regions of a gene (*exons*) are not continuous but interspersed with noncoding sequences called *introns*. The exons of a gene form a mature transcript (mRNA) with the removal or splicing out of the introns; different yet related proteins can sometimes be encoded by the same gene through alternative splicing of different exons. Additionally, other sequences that can affect the synthesis of a protein are located upstream, within, or downstream a gene (e.g., promoters, splicing signals, regulatory elements).

DNA Structure

DNA molecules are made up of four types of nucleotides linked by phosphodiester bonds. Each nucleotide consists of a nitrogenous base, the sugar deoxyribose, and a phosphate group. The nitrogenous base could either be a purine (adenine [A] or guanine [G]) or a pyrimidine (cytosine [C] or thymine [T]). In forming the DNA chain, the 5' carbon of a deoxyribose of one nucleotide is covalently linked by phosphodiester bond to the 3' carbon of the deoxyribose of the next nucleotide in the chain.

DNA is usually found as a helical double-stranded structure coiled around a common axis with the individual strands running in opposite directions and the sugar and phosphate groups forming the backbone of the chain. The two strands are held together by highly predictable hydrogen bonds: A always pairs with T, and C always pairs with G. Because of this complementarity, the sequence of bases on one strand always determines the sequence on the other. The complementary nature of the strands also confers directionality in that one strand running in a 5' to 3' orientation is aligned to the opposite strand running 3' to 5'.

Reading Frame

The individual amino acids that make up a protein are each encoded by a sequence of three nucleotides called a *codon*. Thus, each RNA sequence transcribed from DNA can be translated in any one of three reading frames depending on where the decoding process begins. In almost every case, only one of these reading frames results in a functional protein. Alteration of the reading frame is one mechanism by which mutations (see Mutations) can exert their deleterious effect.

Mutations

A *mutation* can be broadly defined as any change in the nucleotide sequence of a gene that disables or alters the function of the protein or RNA for which it codes. A mutation may be lethal, but the majority are less deleterious—some are even thought to confer an evolutionary advantage. In general, if a mutation occurs in germ cells (the sperm or the egg), the mutation will be transmitted to all the cells of the offspring. Somatic mutations, on the other hand, will be confined to a clone of cells in a given tissue as exemplified by neoplasms.

Mutations versus Neutral Variations

Not all changes in the nucleotide sequence of a gene result in an abnormal protein or defective synthesis of the protein. Because the genetic code is thought to be degenerate (an amino acid can be coded for by more than one codon), single nucleotide changes in the coding region do not necessarily result in a different polypeptide product. These variations are called *polymorphisms*. Thus, it is imperative that any nucleotide change identified during genetic testing be absolutely confirmed as being the causative mutation and not merely a polymorphic variant of the normal sequence.

Nature of Mutations

It is estimated that 3–5% of diseases in the general population have a purely genetic basis,[2] although nearly all health problems have some genetic component. The nature of the mutations can range from global abnormalities involving whole genome sets (e.g., triploidy, tetraploidy) to abnormalities involving single genes (e.g., monogenic disorders). In between are disorders secondary to abnormalities of whole chromosomes or part of chromosomes (e.g., Down syndrome from trisomy of chromosome 21, cri du chat syndrome from deletion of the short arm of chromosome 5). For most monogenic disorders, the nature of the change in DNA sequence can take any of the following forms:

1. *Nucleotide substitution*. These are the most frequent mutations encountered, usually occurring during DNA replication. Roughly two-thirds are transitions (pyrimidine to pyrimidine or purine to purine), whereas one-third are transversions (pyrimidine to purine or vice versa). Substitutions that result in an amino acid change are called *missense mutations*. Those missense mutations that result in a stop codon are called *nonsense mutations*. Also included here are substitutions of nucleotides at splice site junctions (called *splice site mutations*) that may or may not alter the reading frame. See Figures 20.1 and 20.2 for examples.

2. *Deletions or insertions of a few nucleotides*. The majority of small deletions involve between one and five nucleotides, although deletions 20 bases long are not unusual. Small insertions are more rare, but both deletions and insertions frequently result in alteration of the reading frame (called *frame shift mutations*). See Figures 20.3 through 20.5 for examples.

3. *Large deletions*. Large deletion mutations usually result from the mispairing of homologous sequences with unequal recombination. The unequal crossover frequently can occur between repetitive elements in the sequence. Included in here are whole exon deletions in the extremely large dystrophin gene seen in many Duchenne's muscular dystrophy (DMD) patients (Figure 20.6). Nonhomologous or illegitimate recombination can also occur between two DNA sequences that share only minimal homology of a few base pairs.

4. *Large insertions*. The insertion of repetitive elements via retrotransposons (mobile genetic elements) is a common type of mutation in rodents but is an uncommon mechanism in humans. Insertions in introns may not be associated with any abnormality, but insertion in exons can result in alteration of the reading frame. Alternatively, large insertions can result from homologous recombination as in large deletions.

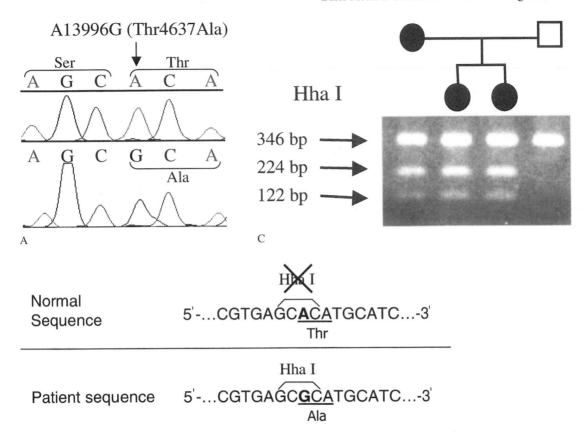

Hha I = GCGC

B

Figure 20.1 Restriction fragment length polymorphism detection of known gene mutations. Restriction enzyme digestion can be used as a molecular diagnostic test for genetic mutations. In this example, we show the analyses of patients with the same heterozygous point mutation for an autosomal dominant neuromuscular disorder. As shown in the automated sequence data **(A)**, the substitution of a guanine (G) nucleotide for an adenine (A) nucleotide (A13996G) changes a threonine amino acid residue to an alanine residue at amino acid position 4637 (Thr4637Ala). As shown in **(B)**, the A → G point mutation creates an Hha I restriction enzyme site not present in normal sequence in unaffected individuals. Shown in **(C)** is a polymerase chain reaction product from each of the pedigree members shown, digested with Hha I restriction enzyme. The unaffected father of the family shows a full-length polymerase chain reaction product with 346 base pairs (bp) that is not digested by Hha I; he has two normal copies of the gene (homozygous). His affected wife and two affected children show three bands after digestion with Hha I. They are each heterozygotes, with one normal gene and one abnormal gene. The normal gene shows the full-length undigested 346 bp polymerase chain reaction product, whereas the abnormal gene containing the Thr4637Ala change is cut into two bands by Hha I (224 bp and 122 bp, respectively). (C = cytosine; T = thymine.) (Reprinted with permission from Hoffman EP, Scacheri CA, Giron J. Genetic Testing. In R Pourmand [ed], Neuromuscular Diseases: Expert Clinicians' Views. Boston: Butterworth–Heinemann, 2001;51–65.)

5. *Inversions.* These are rare occurrences. The most common example is an inversion in the factor VIII gene found in patients with hemophilia A.

6. *Duplications.* The most frequent mechanism of duplications is homologous unequal crossover as described for deletions. Duplications may or may not be accompanied by a reciprocal deletion. A large and common duplication has been identified in most cases of Charcot-Marie-Tooth (CMT) disease type 1A.[3]

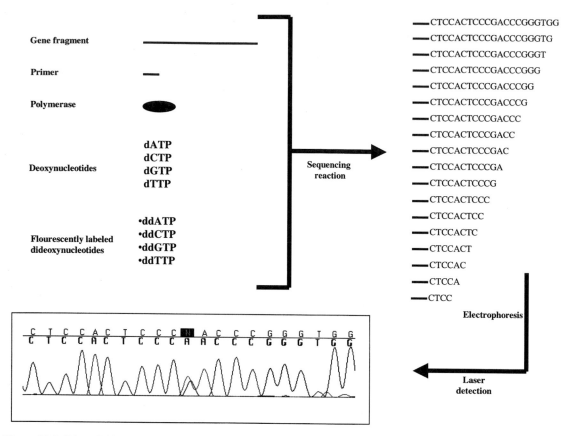

Figure 20.2 Direct DNA sequencing. DNA sequencing is the most detailed level of gene analysis. The reaction is a modification of the polymerase chain reaction in which a sequencing primer is used to bind to a template DNA (itself previously generated by polymerase chain reaction). The addition of dideoxynucleotides to the reaction leads to their incorporation in the 3' end of the newly synthesized strand. However, the polymerase is unable to add new bases from that point (chain termination). Electrophoresis of the reaction separates the elongation products detected by laser owing to the fluor attached to the dideoxynucleotides. The DNA sequence can then be downloaded and analyzed through a computer. Shown is an actual trace from a genetic test of a patient suspected of having Alexander's disease—an autosomal dominant white matter disorder. Exon 6 of the glial fibrillary acidic protein gene was polymerase chain reaction–amplified, sequenced, and analyzed using a capillary-based electrophoresis sequencing method. Analysis revealed heterozygosity at nucleotide position 1131 showing both guanine (G) (normal) and adenine (A) (mutant), indicating that one allele has undergone a G → A change. This changes an amino acid from glutamic acid to lysine, which is postulated to exert a toxic effect in astroglial cells. (C = cytosine; dATP = deoxyadenosine triphosphate; dCTP = deoxycytidine triphosphate; ddATP = dideoxyadenosine triphosphate; ddCTP = dideoxycytidine triphosphate; ddGTP = dideoxyguanosine triphosphate; ddTTP = dideoxythymidine triphosphate; dGTP = deoxyguanosine triphosphate; dTTP = deoxythymidine triphosphate; T = thymine.)

7. *Expansion of trinucleotide repeat sequences* (see the section Trinucleotide Expansion Disorders for a more detailed explanation). Expansion can occur either in the 5' untranslated region (e.g., fragile X syndrome), in the coding region (e.g., Huntington's disease), or in the 3' untranslated region (e.g., myotonic dystrophy) (Table 20.1). Expansion of the repeats results in disease when it eliminates the expression of a protein (gene silencing) or the expressed protein assumes an altered activity (dominant gain of function).

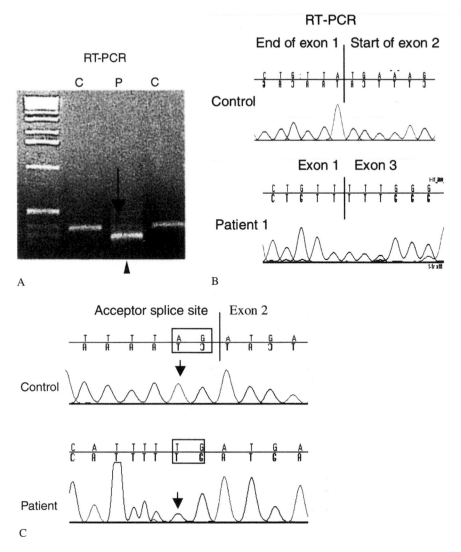

Figure 20.3 Splice site mutation causing exon skipping. Shown is an example of how sequencing, polymerase chain reaction (PCR), and electrophoresis can be used for mutation detection. The results of mutation studies reveal an A to T mutation in the acceptor splice site of intron 1 of the dystrophin gene. PCR of a reverse-transcribed messenger RNA (RT-PCR) reveals a smaller product (*arrowhead* in lane P flanked by two control samples [lane C] in **A**). Sequencing reveals that the PCR product lacks exon 2 in the transcript (**B**) but is clearly present in the genomic DNA of the patient (**C**, *arrow* shows the mutation). The loss of exon 2 leads to the use of a cryptic initiator methionine codon in exon 3, resulting in a dystrophin protein of abnormal smaller molecular weight. (A = adenine; C = cytosine; G = guanine; T = thymine.) (Courtesy of Drs. Sherifa Hamed and Eric Hoffman.)

Consequences of Mutations

Alterations in nucleotide sequence can result in quantitative and qualitative defects of protein synthesis. The physiologic activity of a protein may be reduced or completely eliminated or assume a different function such that critical pathways may be affected, resulting in a clinically observable phenotype. Different levels of gene reg-

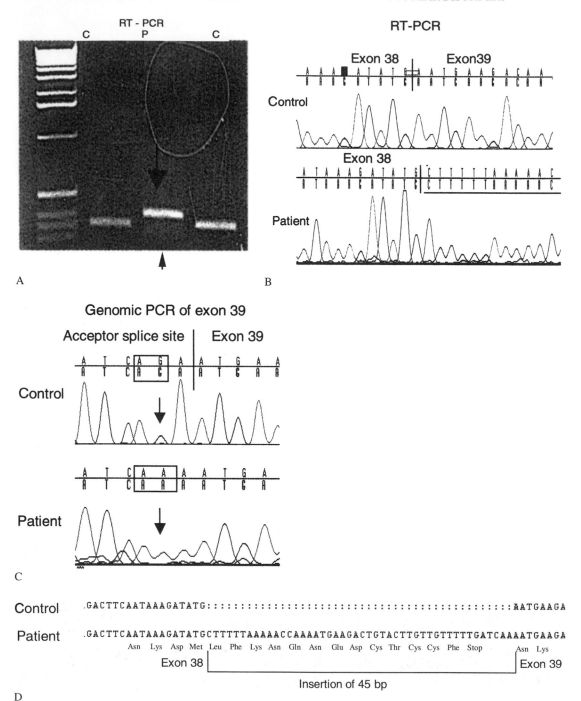

Figure 20.4 Splice-site mutation leading to a shift in the reading frame. A G to A mutation in the acceptor splice site in intron 38 of the dystrophin gene leads to the use of a cryptic splice site 45 base pairs (bp) upstream of the normal one in intron 38. Polymerase chain reaction of a reverse-transcribed messenger RNA (RT-PCR) reveals a larger product (*arrowhead* in lane P flanked by two control samples [lane C] in **A**). Sequencing reveals that the G to A change (*arrow* in **C**) causes an insertion of additional 45 nucleotides in the messenger RNA transcript (**B**). The disruption of the reading frame creates a premature stop codon (**D**). (A = adenine; Asn = asparagine; ASP = aspartic acid; C = cytosine; Cys = cysteine; G = guanine; Gln = glutamine; Glu = glutamic acid; Leu = leucine; Lys = lysine; Met = methionine; Phe = phenylalanine; T = thymine.) (Courtesy of Drs. Sherifa Hamed and Eric Hoffman.)

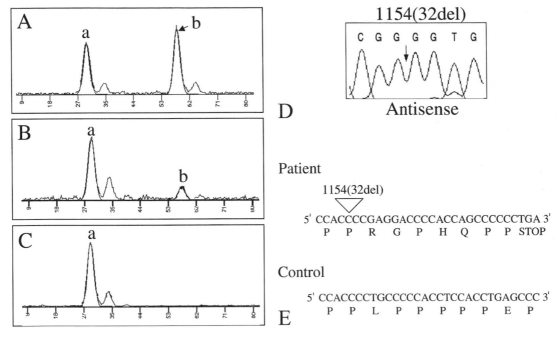

Figure 20.5 MeCP2 mutation in a hemizygous male infant with an Xq27-28 inversion and X-inactivation analysis of his nonmanifesting carrier mother. **D.** An electrophoregram of a 32–base pair C-terminal deletion [1154(del32)] in the MeCP2 gene of a hemizygous 16-month-old male infant with an Xq27-28 inversion and his mother who is a nonmanifesting carrier. The deletion resulted in frameshift in the reading frame of the MeCP2 protein and a stop codon eight amino acids downstream of the deletion, as shown in (**E**). Quantitative X-inactivation patterns in the mother are shown cut (**A**) and uncut (**B**). **A** and **C**, respectively, show results from polymerase chain reaction amplification of the alleles (peaks a, b) of the androgen receptor for the mother and her affected son. **B** shows the results for digestion of the active X chromosome (peak b) with the methylation sensitive enzyme (Hpa II) prior to polymerase chain reaction amplification (I-cut). The mother showed skewed X-inactivation (ratio, 86:14) with preferential inactivation of the allele (peak a) transmitted to her affected son, explaining her nonmanifesting status. Nucleotide sequence: A = adenine; C = cytosine; G = guanine; T = thymine. Protein sequence: E = glutamic acid; G = glycine; H = histidine; L = leucine; P = proline; Q = glutamine; R = arginine. (Courtesy of Dr. Kristen Hoffbuhr, Children's National Medical Center, Washington, DC.)

ulation may be affected, including transcription, RNA processing and maturation, translation, post-translation modification, and protein stability. Consequently, the identification of specific mutations can often assume added importance in detailing the functional map of a gene (i.e., transcription binding sites, receptor binding sites, catalytic sites).

Loss-of-function mutations functionally inactivate the gene and encoded protein. Deletions of one or more exons (or the entire gene) are common examples (e.g., DMD) (see Figure 20.6). Other causes include single-base deletions or insertions that shift the triplet codon reading frame for translation (frame-shift mutations) and single-base conversions that either introduce a new stop codon (nonsense mutations) or change splicing patterns (splice-site mutations) (see Figures 20.3 and 20.4). Likewise, missense mutations can also lead to loss-of-function recessive disorders if the amino acid change interferes with the function of the protein (e.g., active site in an enzyme) or if the amino acid change interferes with the processing of the protein (e.g., failure to transport the protein to the cell surface for correct function).

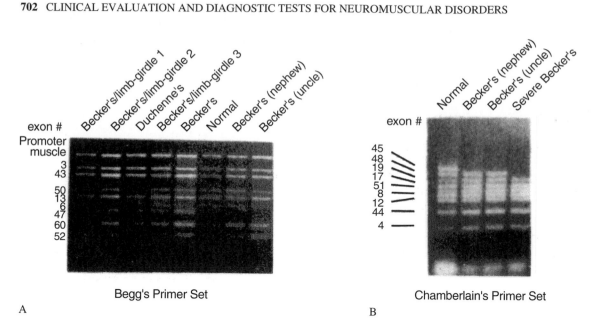

Figure 20.6 Direct DNA analysis of dystrophinopathy patients using multiplex polymerase chain reaction. Shown in **(A)** are three cases of Becker's muscular dystrophy with no missing polymerase chain reaction products (deletions). However, Becker's muscular dystrophy could not be ruled out, as 25% of Becker's muscular dystrophy patients have no detectable deletions. One Duchenne's muscular dystrophy patient had no detectable deletion, whereas one severe Becker's muscular dystrophy patient was found to have a deletion of exons 45–48 with the Chamberlain's primer set **(B)**. A nephew and uncle, both diagnosed with Becker's muscular dystrophy, were found to have an identical deletion of exons 45–47 using the Begg's and Chamberlain's primer sets.[90,91] All samples were compared to a normal control as shown. (Reprinted with permission from EP Hoffman, L Schwartz. Dystrophin and disease. Mol Aspects Med 1991; 12:175–194.)

Although loss-of-function mutations frequently form the basis for recessively inherited disorders, change- or gain-of-function mutations are characteristic of most dominantly inherited neurologic disorders in which the protein produced by the mutant gene exerts a toxic effect on the cell. The toxic product is usually the result of a subtle change in the gene that is still compatible with production of the protein (as opposed to the lack of protein production seen in loss-of-function mutations). The most common type of gain-of-function mutation is a missense mutation in which a single base pair change leads to an amino acid change in the encoded protein (see Figure 20.2). The toxic proteins can seriously disrupt cell and tissue function in a number of ways. Because of the amino acid change, the protein may exhibit altered solubility, causing it to precipitate into aggregates (i.e., inclusion bodies in astrocytes secondary to glial fibrillary acidic protein gene mutations in patients with Alexander's disease). Alternatively, the toxic protein can change its function, imposing a deleterious effect on the physiology of the cell. Illustrative examples are provided by a number of the sodium channels disorders: hyperkalemic periodic paralysis and myotonias,[4,5] long QT syndrome,[6] and generalized epilepsy with febrile seizures plus (GEFS+).[7] In these disorders, the toxic protein (abnormal sodium channel) exhibits failure of rapid inactivation, causing persistent inward sodium current; although half of the

Table 20.1 Examples of Repeat Expansion Disorders

Disorder	Gene	Repeat	Normal Repeat Number	Premutation	Full Mutation	Repeat Location	Reference
X-linked							
Fragile X syndrome	FMR1	CGG	6–52	60–200	230–1,000	5' UTR	76
Bulbospinal muscular atrophy	AR	CAG	11–33	—	38–66	Coding	59
Autosomal dominant							
Dentato-rubral-pallido-luysian atrophy	DRPLA	CAG	6–35	—	51–88	Coding	77
Huntington's disease	HD	CAG	6–39	—	36–121	Coding	78
Myotonic dystrophy	DMPK	CTG	5–37	—	50–3,000	3' UTR	63
Spinocerebellar ataxia 1	SCA1	CAG	6–39	—	41–81	Coding	79
Spinocerebellar ataxia 2	SCA2	CAG	14–31	—	35–64	Coding	80
Spinocerebellar ataxia 3	SCA3	CAG	12–41	—	40–84	Coding	81
Spinocerebellar ataxia 6	SCA6	CAG	4–19	—	21–27	Coding	82
Spinocerebellar ataxia 7	SCA7	CAG	7–17	—	38–130	Coding	83
Spinocerebellar ataxia 8	?	CTG	16–91	—	106–139	—	71
Autosomal recessive							
Friedreich's ataxia	FRDA1	GAA	6–34	80	112–1,700	Intron 1	74
Progressive myoclonus epilepsy 1	CSTB	CCCCGC-CCCGCG	2–3	—	35–50	5' flank-ing	84

sodium channels are abnormal (patients are heterozygous), the persistent inward sodium current has a dominant effect on the cell physiology.

MENDELIAN INHERITANCE

Inheritance often refers to the pattern by which observable traits are passed from generation to generation. Mendel made the first descriptions of inheritance in 1865 based on his experiments on the garden pea. In time, the term *mendelian inheritance* became synonymous with patterns of inheritance of characteristics and disorders that can be explained on the basis of single genes. From his experiments and the work of subsequent researchers, the following principles were drawn:

1. Genes come in pairs, one inherited from each parent.
2. *Principle of dominance and recessiveness.* Individual genes can have different alleles. Some alleles (dominant traits) exert their effects over others (recessive traits).
3. *Principle of segregation.* During meiosis, homologous alleles segregate such that each gamete receives only one allele.
4. *Principle of independent assortment.* Different pairs of alleles segregate (and combine) in an independent fashion.

For the most part, these principles are still valid and useful. This is especially true of genes in any of the 22 pairs of autosomes (chromosomes 1 through 22). However, we now know that genes on the X chromosomes of males have only one allele (not in pairs). Additionally, genes that are physically close to each other may not show independent assortment; this phenomenon has played a particularly important role in the mapping of genes through linkage analysis.

Autosomal Dominant Inheritance

Definition

In autosomal dominant disorders, a mutation in one of the homologous alleles on any of the 22 autosomes produces the clinical phenotype. Individuals who harbor both the wild type and the mutant alleles (heterozygotes) manifest the disorder. Autosomal dominant disorders exhibit the following necessary characteristics:

- Successive or multiple generations in a family are affected.
- Males and females are both affected.
- Either males or females can transmit the condition.
- At least one male-to-male transmission is seen.

Recurrence Risk

Because individuals are heterozygous, their gametes have a one in two (50%) chance of carrying either the normal or the mutant allele. With each pregnancy, therefore, the offspring of an affected individual will have a one in two chance (50%) of inheriting the disorder, assuming the partner of the affected individual is normal (Figure 20.7).

Other Important Features

The clinical manifestations of autosomal dominant disorders can vary among individuals who carry the mutant allele. The proportion of individuals with the allele concurrently showing any manifestations is an index of the *penetrance* of the disorder. If a large proportion of individuals deemed to be heterozygous by pedigree analysis or molecular investigation manifest any signs or symptoms of the disorder, the mutant allele is thought to be highly penetrant. As such, penetrance is a function of the thoroughness of the history taking, clinical examination, and the use of appropriate ancillary studies. For example, clinical examination of individuals suspected to have tuberous sclerosis or neurofibromatosis type II may not reveal any abnormalities. However, the appropriate neuroimaging study may reveal the phenotype. In some instances, penetrance is also dependent on the age of the individual (e.g., Huntington's disease).

The extent and variability that a sign or a symptom is manifested in an individual indicate the *expressivity* of the affected gene. Affected individuals carrying mutations of the same gene (even identical mutations) can vary considerably in the degree that they manifest the disorder. Neurofibromatosis patients in the same pedigree, for example, may not show the same structural and functional complica-

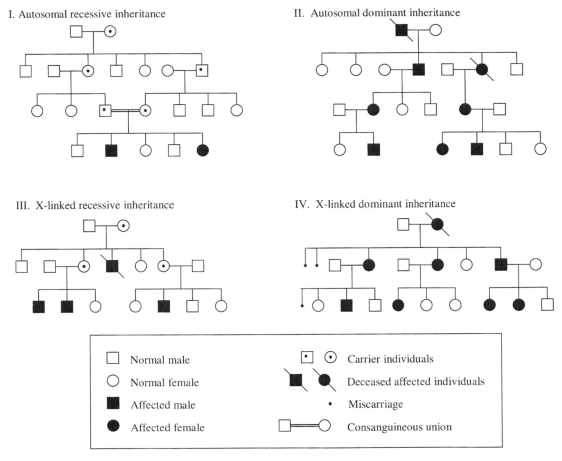

Figure 20.7 Representative pedigrees of different inheritance patterns. Shown are sample pedigrees of recessively inherited and dominantly inherited autosomal and X-linked disorders. Autosomal recessive disorders (**I**) are usually seen in a single sibship; the offspring may or may not result from consanguineous unions of parents who are both carriers of the mutated alleles. Autosomal dominant disorders (**II**) can be seen in multiple generations. X-linked recessive disorders (**III**) are primarily seen in boys whose mothers are obligate carriers; female carriers occasionally manifest the disorder when they have skewed inactivation of the normal X chromosome. X-linked dominant disorders (**IV**) are quite rare; an excess of female offspring is seen, and affected males transmit the disorder only to their daughters.

tions. On the other hand, *pleiotropism* refers to the phenomenon in which multiple, distinct, and seemingly unrelated phenotypic effects are produced by a single mutant gene. For instance, muscle weakness, cataracts, and insulin intolerance are pleiotropic manifestations of myotonic dystrophy. *Contiguous gene syndromes*, in which a number of unrelated manifestations are seen but multiple genes are involved, should not be confused with pleiotropy.

Dominant disorders typically involve a gene mutation that results in a toxic protein (change- or gain-of-function). Although they constitute the bulk of disorders seen in the adult neurology or neurogenetics clinic, they are generally refractory to protein testing owing to the fact that protein tests are not able to distinguish between normal and toxic proteins that may differ by as little as one amino acid (point mutation). Examples of autosomal dominant neuromuscular disorders include facioscapulohumeral dystrophy, myotonic dystrophy (DM) (myotonin-protein kinase), hyper- and hypokalemic periodic paralysis (sodium channel α subunit), spinocerebellar ataxia (SCA; ataxin), and CMT.

Autosomal Recessive Inheritance

Definition

In autosomal recessive disorders, both alleles of a homologous pair on any of the 22 autosomes are mutated, producing the clinical phenotype. Individuals who harbor both the wild-type and the mutant alleles (heterozygotes) are not affected and are called *carriers*. Autosomal recessive disorders exhibit the following necessary characteristics:

- Both males and females are affected.
- Affected individuals are usually seen in only one generation in a single sibship.
- Parents do not show phenotype.

Recurrence Risk

When a child is diagnosed as having an autosomal recessive disorder, both parents are assumed to be carriers. With each successive pregnancy, there is a one in two (50%) chance that either gamete carries the mutant allele. Thus, there are four possible combinations of these gametes. This results in a one in four (25%) chance that an offspring is homozygous affected, a two in four (50%) chance of being heterozygous unaffected, and a one in four (25%) chance of being homozygous unaffected (see Figure 20.7).

An affected individual only produces gametes with the mutant allele. This individual and a wild-type homozygous partner have offspring who are all unaffected heterozygous carriers. If the unaffected partner happens to be a heterozygous carrier, then each pregnancy has a one in two (50%) chance that the offspring is homozygous affected. In this instance, two generations are affected, and the pedigree is said to exhibit *pseudodominance*.

Recessive Mutations

Recessively inherited gene defects typically result in the loss-of-function of a single protein, and this loss of function is typically associated with the lack of detectable protein in patient tissues. In some instances, the protein deficiency is specific enough to be diagnostic, and in rarer instances, the detection of the protein deficiency can be more straightforward than detecting the guilty gene defect. Examples of autosomal recessive neuromuscular disorders include limbgirdle muscular dystrophies (LGMDs) secondary to *sarcoglycan* gene mutations, most metabolic myopathies, some forms of spinal muscular atrophies (Werdnig-Hoffman disease, Kugelberg-Welander disease), and Friedreich's ataxia (*frataxin*).

X-Linked Recessive Inheritance

Definition

Males have only one X chromosome and are therefore hemizygous for alleles on the X chromosome. Thus, a mutant allele is generally manifested in males and homozygous females but not in heterozygous females. Because homozygous females are rare, X-linked disorders usually affect only males. Important characteristics of X-linked recessive disorders include the following:

- Males are affected almost exclusively.
- Absence of male-to-male transmission.
- An unaffected (carrier) female transmits the disorder to her sons.
- Affected males may transmit the condition to grandsons through obligate carrier daughters.

Recurrence Risk

An affected male, if he survives to reproduce, will have daughters who are all obligate carriers and sons who are all unaffected. A carrier female, on the other hand, will have sons who have a one in two (50%) chance of being affected and daughters who have a one in two (50%) chance of being carriers (see Figure 20.7).

Manifesting Females

Occasionally, a female can be affected with an X-linked recessive disorder. The two most common situations when this arises are with (1) a female with a single X chromosome (as in Turner's syndrome), or (2) a female with nonrandom X-inactivation. The latter is the most common cause of symptoms in carriers for an inherited trait (as in manifesting carriers of DMD).

In females, one of the X chromosomes is inactivated early in embryonic development. X inactivation is a random process such that 50% of cells have a maternally derived active X, whereas the other 50% of cells have a paternally derived active X. A carrier female can become affected by skewed X-inactivation through the following mechanisms: (1) a chance occurrence, (2) preferential inactivation of a normal X because the other X is involved in an X-autosome translocation disrupting the causative gene, or (3) elimination of cells harboring one X that has lost a gene required for cell survival.

Examples

The most commonly encountered X-linked recessive disorder is DMD. In DMD, the causative gene has nearly 3 million base pairs, and all nonrelated patients have private or unique "personal" mutations. Although slightly more than half of patients have easily detectable genetic mutations in the dystrophin gene (deletions or insertions and duplications) (see Figure 20.6), detection of dystrophin deficiency in muscle biopsy is more sensitive in detecting all DMD patients and also in distinguishing the allelic disorders of DMD (complete absence of the protein) and Becker's muscular dystrophy (BMD) (expression of shorter or longer or less protein) (Figure 20.8). Other X-linked recessive disorders include

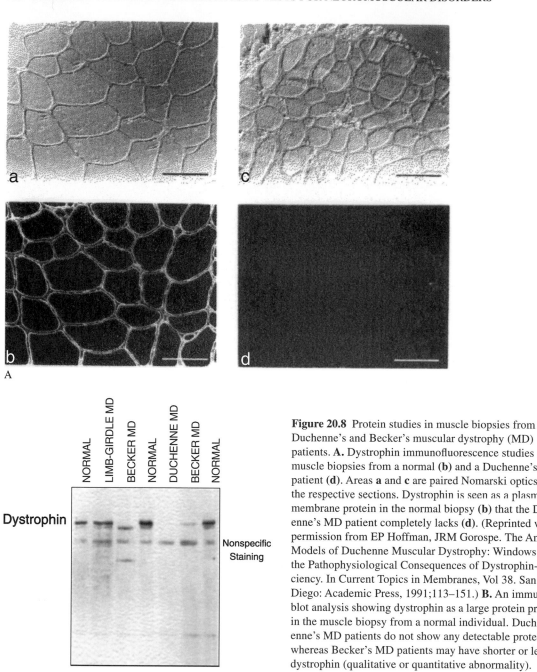

Figure 20.8 Protein studies in muscle biopsies from Duchenne's and Becker's muscular dystrophy (MD) patients. **A.** Dystrophin immunofluorescence studies on muscle biopsies from a normal (**b**) and a Duchenne's MD patient (**d**). Areas **a** and **c** are paired Nomarski optics of the respective sections. Dystrophin is seen as a plasma membrane protein in the normal biopsy (**b**) that the Duchenne's MD patient completely lacks (**d**). (Reprinted with permission from EP Hoffman, JRM Gorospe. The Animal Models of Duchenne Muscular Dystrophy: Windows on the Pathophysiological Consequences of Dystrophin-Deficiency. In Current Topics in Membranes, Vol 38. San Diego: Academic Press, 1991;113–151.) **B.** An immunoblot analysis showing dystrophin as a large protein present in the muscle biopsy from a normal individual. Duchenne's MD patients do not show any detectable protein, whereas Becker's MD patients may have shorter or less dystrophin (qualitative or quantitative abnormality). (Reprinted with author permission from RG Miller, EP Hoffman. Molecular diagnosis and modern management of Duchenne muscular dystrophy. Neurol Clin 1994;12:699–725.)

X-linked Emery-Dreifuss muscular dystrophy (*emerin*), myotubular myopathy (*myotubularin*), and Kennedy's syndrome (*androgen receptor*).

X-Linked Dominant Inheritance

Definition

Disorders of X-linked dominant inheritance are quite rare and are caused by dominant alleles on the X chromosome. Both males and females can be affected, but females tend to be less severely affected than hemizygous males unless the females are themselves homozygous for the mutant allele. The important characteristics of this group include the following:

- Affected males always transmit the disorder to their daughters.
- Affected males never transmit the disorder to their sons.
- Affected females can transmit the disorder to offspring of either gender.
- An excess of affected females is observed in the pedigrees.

Recurrence Risk

With each pregnancy, an affected female has a one in two (50%) chance of transmitting the disorder regardless of the gender of the offspring. On the other hand, only female offspring of affected males will be affected (see Figure 20.7).

Male Lethal Alleles

In some X-linked disorders, males with the disorder are rarely, if ever, seen. In these disorders, any hemizygous male conceptus is thought to be nonviable because the mutant allele adversely affects embryonic development. In the instance of an affected female, her offspring will have a female to male ratio of 2 to 1—none of the males is affected, half of the females inherits the disorder. Examples of this pattern are incontinentia pigmenti and Rett syndrome.

NONMENDELIAN INHERITANCE

Not all hereditary disorders follow the strict mendelian inheritance patterns described above. Although this fact has been known for many years, only recently has the molecular basis for some of these conditions been determined. A number of disorders included in this category are important neuromuscular diseases.

Mitochondrial Inheritance

Like nuclear chromosomes, mitochondria possess their own genome with their own semiautonomous replication, transcription, and translation systems. However, the inheritance pattern of mitochondrial DNA (mtDNA) is completely different in that mtDNA is strictly maternally inherited.[8,9] During fertilization, it has been shown that sperm mitochondria are selectively eliminated.[10] Thus, mitochondrial mutations can only be transmitted along maternal lines but affect both genders equally.

Recurrence Risk

All children of affected mothers are at risk of inheriting some mutated mitochondria. The number of mutant mitochondria in each offspring varies such that their phenotypes can, in turn, be extremely variable.

Heteroplasmy and Threshold Expression

Unlike nuclear DNA, which exists in only two copies per cell (with the exception of genes on the X chromosome of males), the mtDNA copy number can be variable. A single mitochondrion can contain up to 10 circular DNA molecules, and each cell may contain up to 100,000 mitochondria. A mutation in mtDNA results in a mixed population of normal and mutant molecules (*heteroplasmy*). During cell division, the mutant mtDNA is partitioned to daughter cells in a random process. Over time, different cell lineages can have pure mutant, pure normal (*homoplasmy*), or mixed mtDNA population.

The reliance on mitochondrial energy generation is different among tissues and organs. Indeed, the presence of mutant mtDNA can have a negative impact on energy production (i.e., the higher the number of mutant mtDNA, the less energy is available for cellular processes). It is thought that once energy production falls below a minimum level, normal tissue function is compromised, and clinical signs and symptoms begin to appear (threshold expression). Studies indicate that the expression thresholds for human organs are, in decreasing order, the central nervous system, heart and skeletal muscle, renal system, endocrine system, and liver.[11–14] Thus, it is no surprise that most mitochondrial disorders fall into the domain of neurologists.

Trinucleotide Expansion Disorders

Definition

Trinucleotide repeats are found throughout the human genome and are normally stable through generations of the same pedigree. The repeats are normally polymorphic in the general population; their number can vary among healthy individuals, and their function is largely unknown. Occasionally, an expansion occurs, which renders the DNA fragment unstable and susceptible to further expansion with additional cell divisions. Above a certain critical threshold, the number of repeats can be associated with disease (see Table 20.1).

Anticipation

The length of the expansion roughly correlates with age of onset and severity of the disease. Because the repeat length tends to increase with each transmission, the manifestations of the disease tend to occur at an earlier age with each successive generation. This phenomenon is called *anticipation*. This feature is particularly prominent in myotonic dystrophy and fragile X syndrome. In other disorders in this group, however, anticipation may be difficult to recognize and distinguish from random variations in age of onset (or even biased ascertainment of probands).

Premutations and Full Mutations

For most repeat sequences, there is no absolute cutoff between the normal range and repeat length associated with disease. In between are repeat lengths that may not be associated with disease but are unstable during transmission. Such expansions are deemed *premutations* and the individuals harboring them *carriers*. Expansions associated with disease state are termed *full mutations* (see Table 20.1). The exact mechanism by which expansion occurs is still poorly defined, as are the precise molecular mechanisms leading to the respective disorders in this group. Of note, however, is the observation that the repeat expansion can be influenced by the sex of the transmitting parent. For instance, myotonic dystrophy and fragile X syndrome expansions tend to be larger when transmitted by females.[15,16] Conversely, male transmission in Huntington's disease results in larger expansions and clinically earlier manifestations in offspring.[17]

Imprinting

Definition

Simply put, *imprinting* means parent-of-origin–dependent gene expression. An *imprinted gene* is one that is transcribed from only one parent's allele. An inactivated maternally derived allele is labeled as *maternally imprinted*, whereas an inactivated paternally derived allele is labeled as *paternally imprinted*. The exact nature of the epigenetic mark placed on imprinted genes as they pass through male or female gametogenesis is still unknown, but two common motifs that have been seen are differential methylation of CpG dinucleotides in DNA and differential chromatin structure in the imprinted region.[18] Imprinting is often suspected in the following cases:

- Pedigrees showing transmission of a disorder that is dependent on the sex of the transmitting parent
- Monozygotic twins who are discordant for a particular syndrome

Prader-Willi and Angelman Syndromes

To date, 19 genes are known to be imprinted in humans.[19] Clinical disorders secondary to imprinting effects can occur when there is lack of expression (i.e., deletion) or overexpression of a gene (i.e., duplication or loss of imprinting control). Two well-known neurobehavioral syndromes—Prader-Willi syndrome and Angelman syndrome—can be secondary to deletion of identical regions on the long arm of chromosome 15, but manifestations are dependent on the parent of origin of the affected chromosome.

Prader-Willi syndrome is characterized by hypotonia and failure to thrive early in life, but patients later exhibit obesity, developmental delay, and delayed puberty. The deletion is seen in the paternally derived chromosome 15.[20] On the other hand, Angelman syndrome is a disorder caused by deletion in the maternally derived chromosome 15 and is characterized by severe mental retardation, ataxia, seizures, and a happy disposition.[21,22] A specific test based on DNA methylation facilitates the identification of parental origin of the affected chromosome.

Uniparental Disomy

Imprinted genes can also manifest a clinical phenotype when both members of a chromosome pair are inherited from only one parent—a situation called *uniparental disomy*. In these cases, paternal duplication is attended by a concomitant maternal deficiency, whereas paternal deficiency is seen in maternal duplications. The primary mechanism for this phenomenon usually involves "trisomy rescue" after meiotic nondisjunction (Figure 20.9). Most trisomic conceptuses are lethal; most

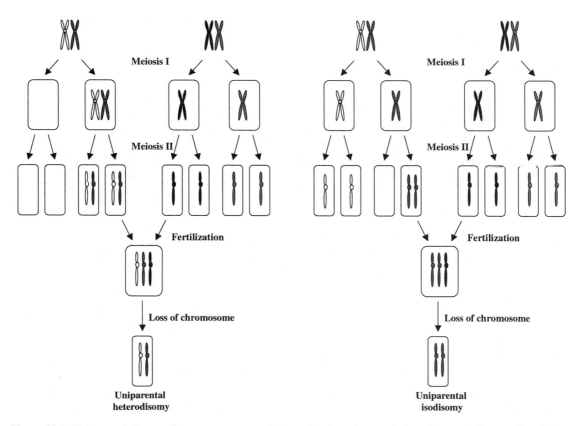

Figure 20.9 Uniparental disomy. Shown are two possible mechanisms that result in uniparental disomy. Nondisjunction can occur either in meiosis I or II, leading to the formation of a disomic gamete. Fertilization of a disomic gamete with a monosomic gamete results in a trisomic conceptus, most of which are aborted. Conceptions that survive are usually the result of loss of one of the trisomic chromosomes (trisomy rescue). (Adapted from RF Mueller, J Cook. Mendelian Inheritance. In DL Rimoin, JM Connor, RE Pyeritz [eds], Principles and Practice of Medical Genetics [3rd ed]. New York: Churchill Livingstone, 1997;87–102.)

conceptions that survive are the consequence of loss of one of the trisomic chromosomes. If the loss of a chromosome is a random event, uniparental disomy is expected in one-third of surviving cases.

MOLECULAR GENETIC TOOLS

Overview

The genetic test that one uses is frequently dictated by the nature of the suspected genetic defect. A physician confronted with a child showing a collection of seemingly unrelated symptoms or dysmorphology frequently starts by requesting a karyotype, which allows detection of gross chromosomal abnormalities. Barring any abnormal chromosomal report, additional diagnostic modalities are used to zero in on the diagnosis. The majority of genetic diseases are single-gene disorders whose molecular diagnosis ultimately rests on testing the specific gene or protein. Generally, a gene mutation is considered more specific than a protein abnormality given that quantitative abnormalities in protein may be primary or secondary to the actual genetic defect. In some instances, however, protein testing (by Western blot or immunofluorescence) may actually be as definitive as the genetic test. A good example is DMD, in which absence of dystrophin by immunoblot or immunofluorescence can be confirmatory when no deletion mutation is found from an initial multiplex polymerase chain reaction (PCR) screen (see Figure 20.8).

It stands to reason that a specific molecular test can be performed only when the gene responsible for a particular disease has been mapped or identified. If the sequence of a gene is known and mutations have been described, direct mutation analysis can be carried out. This is usually the method of choice because it offers direct confirmation of diagnosis. Alternatively, the sequence of interest can initially be screened for any changes that may warrant further testing with other molecular methods. If the gene has not been identified but its relative location in the genome is known based on DNA markers, linkage analysis can be done. The latter is thought to be less accurate than direct mutation analysis because it is dependent on statistical prediction. In either case, the strategy for mutation detection is determined by the nature of the specific mutation (i.e., point mutation, large deletion). In general, a molecular approach to analyzing a stretch of DNA (a gene or suspected disease locus) is possible only if sequence information or probes (for DNA markers) are available.

In the last couple of years, the development of molecular tools has proceeded with great speed and breadth such that the genetic bases for numerous disorders are unraveling at a frenetic pace. Similarly, a number of molecular tools that are simple yet sensitive and easy to automate have been developed by biotechnology companies as kits, complete with detailed instructions and relevant controls. In keeping with the basic thrust of this chapter, only the most commonly used molecular tools and the key concepts underlying each method are presented. For a more detailed discussion, the interested reader is directed elsewhere.[23–26] Additionally, we focus only on those methods of mutation detection that use a patient's genomic DNA sample (usually from a small peripheral blood sample). As genomic DNA contains all genes, it is not necessary for the gene to be expressed to detect the underlying gene mutation.

Cytogenetics

The first line of diagnostic test that a physician frequently uses when confronted with a likely genetic condition is direct visualization of the chromosomes. Chromosome or karyotype analysis offers a simple yet informative means of detecting large genetic abnormalities (numeric or structural defects). Clear examples of cytogenetic abnormalities are seen in patients with aneuploidies (too many or too few chromosomes), such as Down syndrome. Aneuploidies involve many scores of genes, and as a result, the abnormal "dosage" of so many genes typically results in multisystemic syndromes that may include neurologic symptoms. The resolution of detection is usually limited to changes larger than 10 million base pairs. Thus, even a "small" cytogenetic abnormality (10 million base pairs) can contain a hundred or more genes, given that a typical gene is only approximately 30,000 base pairs in size.

A cytogenetic technique that offers an additional level of resolution is *fluorescent in situ hybridization* (FISH). In this method, pieces of cloned and purified human genomic DNA are labeled with biotin using molecular genetic techniques, then hybridized to a cytogenetic spread of patient chromosomes. The biotinylated probe DNA hybridizes to the complementary sequence of the region of interest on each chromosome in each cell. The biotin is then detected using streptavidin linked to a fluorophore and visualized using fluorescence microscopy. This method can detect deletions (one chromosome will fluoresce instead of two) or rearrangements (incorrect chromosomes fluoresce) of chromosomes that are below the resolution of the light microscope (fewer than 10 million base pairs) (see Color Plate B54).

Polymerase Chain Reaction

One of the most innovative techniques developed to analyze DNA is PCR. With PCR, millions of copies of a specific DNA fragment can be synthesized in a few hours (Figure 20.10). The procedure consists of repeated cycles of the following steps:

1. Heat denaturation of double-stranded DNA
2. Primer annealing to DNA
3. Primer extension

During denaturation (94–98°C), the two strands of a target DNA are separated into single strands. In the next step, the temperature of the reaction is lowered (50–68°C) to allow annealing (complementary hybridization) of primers to the target sequence. The *primers* are synthetic oligonucleotides approximately 20–30 nucleotides long. They come in pairs of forward and reverse primers, each of which is complementary to opposite strands of the DNA segment of interest. As such, prior knowledge of at least part of the DNA sequence is required to make the necessary primers. Each primer then serves as a template used by a DNA polymerase (Taq polymerase isolated from a heat-resistant bacterium called *Thermus aquaticus*) to synthesize DNA from deoxynucleotide triphosphates (dNTPs) added to the reaction. This third step of primer extension occurs at a temperature of 72°C and ends when the next cycle commences. Given that DNA

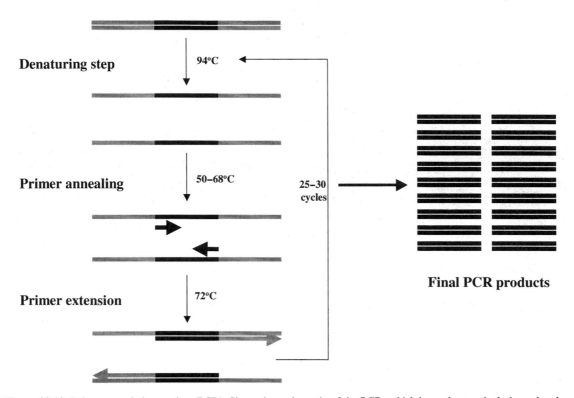

Denaturing step   94°C

Primer annealing   50–68°C

25–30
cycles

Final PCR products

Primer extension   72°C

Figure 20.10 Polymerase chain reaction (PCR). Shown is a schematic of the PCR, which is used extensively in molecular diagnostic laboratories today. In the presence of forward and reverse primers, deoxynucleotides, and Taq polymerase, a fragment of DNA can be amplified through repeated steps of denaturation, primer annealing, and primer extension. The PCR product can then be run on an agarose gel for visualization or processed further for sequencing or cloning experiments.

synthesis proceeds in a 5' to 3' direction, the end of the first cycle results in newly synthesized DNA strands whose 5' ends are fixed but whose 3' end varies in length. With repeated cycles, the lengths of the synthesized strands eventually become fixed with ends that are defined by opposite primers. The number of DNA molecules doubles at each cycle such that nearly a billion copies would have been synthesized after 30 sequential cycles. The PCR products can then be used for further molecular studies as detailed below.

Electrophoresis

Like PCR, electrophoresis is one of the most important techniques in molecular biology. Electrophoresis resolves DNA and RNA fragments according to size. At neutral pH, nucleic acid molecules are negatively charged and migrate toward the anode in an electric field. If the electrophoresis takes place within a polymer gel matrix, a mixture of DNA fragments will be separated and visualized as distinct bands with the smaller fragments migrating more rapidly than the larger fragments (see Figure 20.6). Two of the more commonly used matrices are agarose and poly-acrylamide. DNA fragments in the 0.1- to 20.0-kilobase (kb) range are usually resolved in agarose gels, whereas smaller DNA fragments (0.025- to 2.000-kb range) are separated in polyacrylamide gels. The addition of a denaturant (i.e., urea) to polyacrylamide gels allows resolutions down to single base differences—a method that is used to great advantage in sequencing reactions (see more detailed discussion in the section Direct DNA Sequencing) (see Figure 20.2).

A number of techniques are used for the visualization of DNA fragments after electrophoresis. Ethidium bromide is a chemical that intercalates in DNA and fluoresces under ultraviolet light. This DNA detection method is particularly useful for direct visualization of samples that are relatively abundant. Radioactive-based and newer fluorescence-based methods can also be used, especially for DNA samples whose amounts are too small for direct visualization.

Restriction Enzymes

Restriction enzymes or restriction endonucleases were the first widely used method for the discrimination of sequence variations. These endonucleases are naturally occurring bacterial enzymes that recognize specific DNA sequences such that any sequence change leads to either a gain or loss of cutting ability (see Figure 20.1). In simple terms, a DNA fragment incubated with a restriction enzyme in the appropriate buffer solution cuts the DNA into pieces of defined sizes.

Some restriction enzymes are also capable of distinguishing sites based on their methylation status such that enzymatic approaches can also be used for detection of X-inactivation and imprinting patterns. Maternal and paternal copies may be distinguished by using methylation sensitive isoschizomers (restriction enzymes that recognize the same sites). An example of such a pair is *MspI* and *HpaII*. Both recognize the site CCGG, but the latter cuts only unmethylated sites, whereas the former cuts irrespective of methylation.

Southern Blotting

Southern blotting is another tool available for studying and identifying DNA sequences that is dependent on nucleic acid hybridization. A segment of DNA containing the sequence of interest is digested with a restriction enzyme, resulting in DNA fragments of different sizes. When run on an agarose gel, distinct fragments may not be visible, and a smear is seen instead, with the smaller fragments moving faster in the gel. The DNA is then transferred from the gel to a nitrocellulose membrane filter, which is hybridized with a labeled nucleic acid probe to detect the target sequence. To detect where the probe binds, the filter is placed on an x-ray film. The film is consequently developed, and the presence of the target sequence is indicated by a darkening on the film, giving an estimate of its size when compared to the original gel and molecular weight standards. Although mostly used for physical mapping in the past, the use of southern blotting as a molecular diagnostic tool today lies in a variation called dot-blot or allele-specific oligonucleotide hybridization (see Allele-Specific Oligonucleotide Hybridization). In this method, the sequence of interest is simply spotted onto a nitrocellulose membrane, eliminating the need for electrophoresis. The sample is then probed and detected as above.

Table 20.2 Mutation Detection Methods

Analysis of Known Variants	Screening for Unknown Variants
Allele-specific oligonucleotide (ASO) hybridization[a]	DNA sequencing[a]
Restriction digestion[a]	Single-strand conformer polymorphism[a]
Microarray[a]	Heteroduplex analysis[a]
Amplification refractory mutation system (ARMS)[b]	Denaturing high-performance liquid chromatography[a]
Artificial creation of restriction site (ACRS)	Microarrays
Oligo-ligation assay (OLA)	Dideoxy fingerprinting
Molecular beacons	Denaturing gradient gel electrophoresis
	Chemical cleavage mismatch
	Protein translation truncation
	Differential sequencing with mass spectrometry

[a]Discussed in text.
[b]See Figure 20.17.

Screening Methods

In general, currently available methods to analyze nucleotide changes in the human genome fall in one of the following categories:

- Methods for detecting known mutations or polymorphisms
- Methods for detecting possible mutations

Table 20.2 lists the mutation detection strategies that fall under each class. Only the most commonly used methods are discussed. Interested readers are directed to consult the appropriate references.[23–26]

Screening for Known Mutations

As newer and more efficient methods for mutation detection are developed, it has become easier to identify disease-causing mutations. For many disorders, only a few common mutations may actually be responsible for most of the cases. Probably the most dramatic example is sickle-cell disease, in which a single mutation is responsible for all cases. In these cases, suspected patients can be screened for the common mutations, and a positive result negates the need for more extensive testing. The more common methods in this class are allele-specific oligonucleotide hybridization and restriction digestion. A promising new method involves the use of microarrays.

Allele-Specific Oligonucleotide Hybridization. In this method, also known as *dot blot*, PCR products of the region of interest are "dotted" in duplicate membranes. One membrane is hybridized (or probed) with a radioactively labeled oligonucleotide corresponding to the normal sequence. The other is hybridized with a probe that is complementary to the mutant sequence. After incubation in the appropriate buffer, the pattern is detected by autoradiography. Normal individuals show hybridization only to the normal probe, and heterozygotes hybridize to both probes, whereas individuals who are homozygous to the mutation show hybridization only to the mutant probe (Figure 20.11).

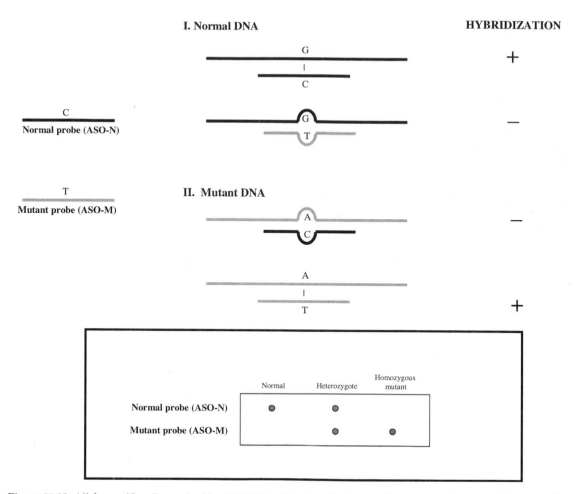

Figure 20.11 Allele-specific oligonucleotide (ASO) hybridization. To detect a known mutation, two oligonucleotides (probes) are synthesized—one to hybridize with the normal sequence (ASO-N), the other to hybridize with the mutation (ASO-M). Three control samples are spotted on a nitrocellulose filter along with the test sample. Hybridization of the mutant probe with the test sample indicates that the sample came from a patient carrying the mutant allele. (A = adenine; C = cytosine; G = guanine; T = thymine.)

Restriction Digest. Hundreds of restriction enzymes are commercially available today, and they provide a rapid and relatively cheap yet accurate method for detecting point mutations that have previously been identified. Cleavage by these enzymes is sequence-specific, so any deviation from the expected digestion pattern indicates a change in the sequence of the restriction site (see Figure 20.1).

Microarrays. Until recently, DNA microarrays (nucleotide sequences attached to a solid support) have largely been used in research and high-end clinical diagnostics. With newer manufacturing platforms, the production costs for the chips have lowered considerably so that it is now feasible and affordable to use DNA microarrays in detecting mutations. Although the process of fabricating and manufacturing the arrays may differ among platforms (capillary-based printing [Genometrix], electronic addressing [Nanogen], or photolithotripsy [Affymetrix]), the same basic principles in nucleic acid hybridization are exploited to assay the genotype of interest. Similarly, different assay methods have been developed and more are undoubtedly in the research and development pipeline; currently available methods for assaying hybridization use fluorescence, electronics, mass spectrometry, molecular beacons, or peptide nucleic acids. In general, a particular methodology usually involves the five basic steps:

1. The region of DNA to be tested is bound to a solid support (microarray production).
2. PCR amplification of test sample.
3. Hybridization.
4. Assay for presence or absence of hybridization.
5. Computer-assisted imaging and signal detection.

DNA microarray technology for the neonatal screening of the common mutations causing sickle-cell disease, α-1 antitrypsin deficiency, and factor V Leiden has been described.[27] Similarly, single nucleotide polymorphic discrimination by an electronic dot-blot assay on a semiconductor microchip has been reported.[28]

Screening for Possible Mutations

The methods discussed in this section exploit the properties of nucleic acids in the detection of sequence variations and do not require a prior knowledge of the mutation. These methods may depend on altered nucleic acid conformation, melting temperatures, or presence of mismatches. The length of the sequence that can be conveniently analyzed may differ, as may the sensitivity, among the different methods. As in the previous section, only the more commonly used methods are discussed.

The emerging field of microarray technology is again briefly mentioned here as imparting the potential advantages of speed, multiplexing, efficiency, and automation that current technologies do not. In the future, it will be possible for a patient whose clinical picture is consistent with leukodystrophy, for instance, to be tested simultaneously for multiple genes causing white matter disorder using a single "leukodystrophy chip." It is just as conceivable that a number of these tests will be transitioned from the lab to physician offices. These advances will be to the advantage of patients, as these will eliminate costly multiple testing and lengthy waiting times for obtaining results and initiating therapy.

Direct DNA Sequencing. The determination of the actual nucleotide sequence is the most direct method not only for screening the presence of mutations but also for detecting the exact nature of the mutation. Although several different techniques have been developed (capillary-based [Beckman], gel-based [LiCor]), most are variations of the dideoxy chain termination method originally developed by Sanger. The method involves an initial denaturation step in which the two strands of a DNA fragment are separated to allow hybridization with an oligonucleotide primer. In the presence of saturating quantities of dNTPs and small quantities of dideoxynucleotide triphosphates (ddNTPs), DNA polymerase copies the single-stranded DNA using the primer as template. During the elongation step, ddNTPs are incorporated in the 3' end of the newly synthesized strand, but no additional bases can be incorporated by the polymerase (chain termination). Thus, extension products of varying lengths are generated and can be separated by electrophoresis on polyacrylamide matrix (see Figure 20.2). Using fluorescently labeled ddNTPs, computer analysis of the sequence is possible.

Multiplex Polymerase Chain Reaction. Amplifying different fragments of DNA in one reaction mixture is a quick and easy method to detect large deletions or insertions. This approach is usually the first step in the molecular diagnosis of suspected DMD patients. In our laboratory, 18 dystrophin exons are examined in two amplification reaction mixes. The absence of a PCR product (positive result) is virtually diagnostic of a dystrophinopathy (see Figure 20.6). In contrast, a negative result (presence of all expected PCR products) does not completely rule out the diagnosis and requires additional testing if the diagnosis is highly suspected.

Single-Strand Conformation Polymorphism. *Single-strand conformation polymorphism* is a mutation detection method that is dependent on the three-dimensional shape of single-stranded molecules (Figure 20.12). The sequence of interest is first PCR-amplified, then the product is denatured by heating followed by rapid cooling. The single strands form sequence-specific secondary and tertiary structures that can be analyzed on a standard nondenaturing polyacrylamide gel. The two strands of DNA move separately, and when run with appropriate controls, an electrophoretic shift (conformer) indicates the presence of sequence variation. The identity of the exact sequence can then be confirmed by other methods. Although most labs still visualize the products by autoradiography, automation is now possible using fluorescently labeled fragments and automated capillary electrophoresis.[29]

Heteroduplex Formation and Denaturing High-Performance Liquid Chromatography. If the DNA from a patient carrying a point mutation in one allele (heterozygous) were PCR amplified, two populations of PCR products would be produced: normal and mutant. Heat denaturing of the PCR products separates the individual strands, which, when subsequently cooled, will reform, producing three products: normal/normal (homoduplexes), mutant/mutant (homoduplexes), or normal/mutant (heteroduplexes). These heteroduplexes form a nonhybridizing "bubble" at the location of the mutation, which can change the mobility characteristics of the gene fragment when subjected to electrophoresis.

Instead of using electrophoresis as a detection step, heteroduplexes can be analyzed by denaturing high-performance liquid chromatography (DHPLC) (Figure 20.13). Partially heat-denatured PCR products are run in a column of alkylated nonporous particles. The column retention time of the heteroduplexes relative to the homoduplexes (given a linear acetonitrile elution gradient) is dependent on internal sequence variation making separation and identification of polymorphic or mutant products possible. Automation of the method allows rapid analysis (approximately 5 minutes per sample). Additionally, large fragments of DNA, up to 1.5 kb, can be analyzed. Like single-strand conformation polymorphism, this method only says that something is different in the sequence; hence, DHPLC must be followed by DNA sequencing of heteroduplexes. A major advantage is that DHPLC does not require any labeling of the DNA under study. DNA fragments are detected simply through ultraviolet absorbance by the DHPLC machine.

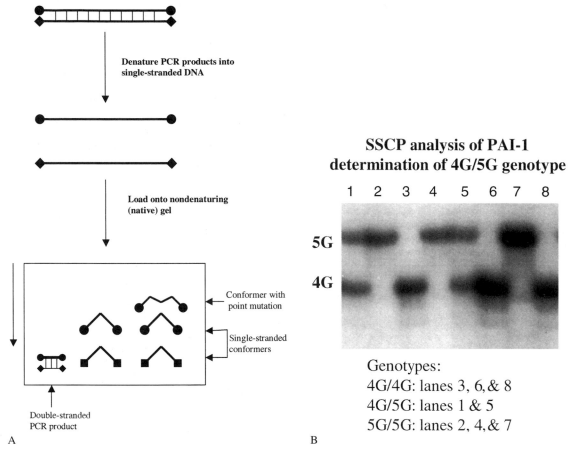

Figure 20.12 Single-stranded conformational polymorphism (SSCP) identification of changes in a polymerase chain reaction (PCR) product from a candidate gene. SSCP analysis requires amplification of the region of interest with the PCR. The double-stranded PCR product is heat denatured into single, separate strands, which fold onto themselves in a specific conformation or shape determined by the DNA sequence (**A**). Single nucleotide changes affect the conformation of each single stranded product, thereby altering the DNA migration on a native acrylamide gel (**A**, conformer with point mutation). This technique is often used to detect single nucleotide base changes and other small genetic mutations. (A = adenine; C = cytosine; G = guanine; T = thymine.) (Reprinted with permission from Hoffman EP, Scacheri CA, Giron J. Genetic Testing. In R Pourmand [ed], Neuromuscular Diseases: Expert Clinicians' Views. Boston: Butterworth–Heinemann, 2001;51–65.) **B.** An application of SSCP to detect changes in the plasminogen activator inhibitor (PAI-1). Here, the change in the PAI-1 gene is used to test its association with increased risk for myocardial infarction. This example demonstrates the SSCP technique used to distinguish the usual DNA sequence in the PAI-1 gene—five consecutive guanine residues—from a polymorphism that predisposes individuals with protein S deficiencies to myocardial infarction. The polymorphism has only four consecutive guanines and is a deletion of one nucleotide. (Courtesy of Dr. Peter Scacheri, National Human Genome Research Institute.)

Linkage Analysis

Occasionally, direct sequence analysis cannot be performed. This situation arises when (1) the disease gene has not been identified, or (2) no identifiable mutation in the highly suspected gene has been found. The latter is often the case in a number of DMD patients in whom point mutations may be difficult and laborious to identify given the enormous

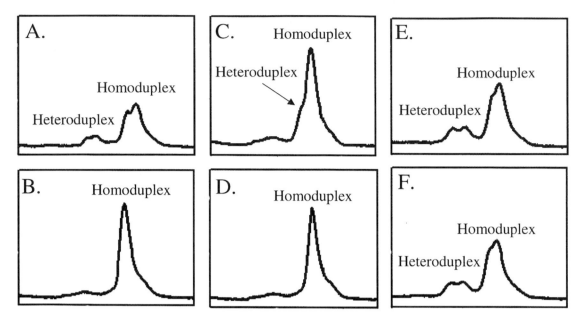

Figure 20.13 Denaturing high-pressure liquid chromatography for detection of genetic changes in Rett syndrome. Shown are a number of examples of denaturing high-pressure liquid chromatography analysis of polymerase chain reaction products corresponding to the MeCP2 gene in Rett syndrome patients (**A,C,E,F**) and controls (**B,D**). The polymerase chain reaction product is loaded onto the paired ion chromatography column and eluted at specific temperatures and denaturant concentrations. Heteroduplexes, which are double-stranded DNA containing both normal and mutant strands of DNA, come off the column at an earlier time, leading to extra leading peaks on the chromatogram. These heteroduplexes are then subjected to automated sequencing to identify the specific mutation. (Courtesy of Drs. Joseph Devaney and Kristen Hoffbuhr, Children's National Medical Center, Washington, DC.)

size of the dystrophin gene. In these instances, linkage analysis of a pedigree is possible provided that key family members are available and are willing to be tested.

Molecular diagnosis by linkage analysis is loosely based on the principle of *linkage disequilibrium*—determining whether two closely linked markers follow each other in a pedigree at a frequency greater than expected by chance. The frequency that the different markers are grouped in the same permutation as they are transmitted to the members of a given pedigree depends on the recombination between the genetic markers. The genetic markers that are used in diagnostic linkage analysis are sequences of DNA that are polymorphic and heterozygous in a random population. Restriction fragment length polymorphisms have been used for a number of years but have been replaced for the most part by the use of short tandem repeats. Tandem repeats are stretches of DNA composed entirely of repeating di-, tri-, or tetranucleotides. The precise number of repeats at any given locus varies, allowing their use for diagnostic linkage purposes. In our lab, CA repeats are used a great deal in combination with PCR for risk assessment, carrier status determination, and even for prenatal diagnosis.

Because linkage analysis is an indirect testing method, this requires that as many informative family members as possible are available to be tested. This is to ensure that the phase of the markers, particularly in an affected individual, can be established. Once the phase is established, this information can be applied in tracing the affected chromosome in other family members. Thus, linkage analysis permits tracking of the affected chromosome regardless of the precise mutation causing the disorder. Figure 20.14 details an example of linkage analysis in a pedigree of a dominantly inherited autosomal disorder.

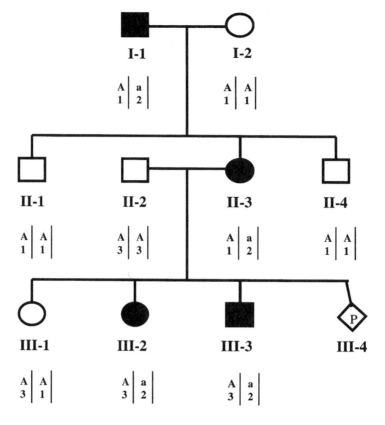

Figure 20.14 Linkage analysis in a dominantly inherited autosomal disorder. Linkage analysis is a method that can be used to determine whether two markers (the disease locus and a test marker) are on the same chromosome. This is dependent on knowing the phase of the two markers, which, in turn, requires that normal and affected individuals are available for analysis. In this pedigree, the grandfather (I-1) is affected with a dominantly inherited autosomal disorder and is heterozygous at the disease gene loci (A/a) and at the marker locus (1/2). He transmits the disorder to his daughter (II-3), who inherits allele 2 of the test marker from him and allele 1 from her mother. She (II-3) has three children herself, two of whom (III-2 and III-3) are affected, and both of whom inherited allele 2 from her; an unaffected child (III-3) inherited allele 1. Because allele 2 of the marker locus is linked to the disease locus, the unborn child (III-4) will have a 95% chance of being affected if he or she also inherits allele 2 of the marker locus from the mother (II-3).

GENE EXPRESSION PROFILING

When a gene is disabled and its corresponding protein is either losing or gaining function, a downstream pathophysiologic cascade is set into motion that ultimately results in some observable clinical phenotype. In some instances, the disorder may be manifested quite early (e.g., metabolic acidosis and seizures in organic acidurias). In some cases, it may take years before patients start experiencing symptoms (e.g., easy fatigability in juvenile cases of Alexander's disease). In still others, it is quite typical that the constellation of signs and symptoms becomes diagnostic of the disorder (e.g., the facial features, personality changes, myotonia, and distal weakness characteristic of myotonic dystrophy), so performing a genetic test would simply be confirmatory.

Frequently, however, the clinical outcome of a particular genetic defect is difficult to predict—a predicament that many researchers are hard at work to reverse. With the completion of the Human Genome Project and the identification of most genes, it has become possible to detect downstream changes in gene expression instigated by a primary genetic defect. Both generic responses and specific changes can be studied at the molecular level using microarrays or GeneChips (Affymetrix, Santa Clara, CA). The transcriptional profile of as many as 60,000 genes can be studied at the same time in a single experiment, providing a molecular fingerprint of a patient tissue that can be mined for insights on how and why the disease progresses (see reference 30 for illustration of the power of this technology). Already, this tool of molecular fingerprinting is gaining use in disease subcategorization (i.e., relapsers vs. nonrelapsers), prognostication (rapidly progressive vs. slowly progressive), and pharmacotherapeutics (responders vs. nonresponders).

SELECTED GENETIC NEUROMUSCULAR DISORDERS

Motor Neuron Diseases

Familial Spastic Paraparesis

Familial spastic paraparesis encompasses a group of genetically heterogeneous disorders characterized by progressive spasticity, mild sensory deficits, and upper motor neuron signs. The pathology in these disorders typically involves axonal degeneration of the pyramidal tracts and, to a lesser degree, the fasciculus gracilis and spinal cerebellar tracts. As with all the disorders discussed in this section, the molecular diagnosis of patients can be achieved by mutation screening of the gene (if known) or by linkage analysis.

Autosomal Dominant Forms. To date, five dominant loci have been mapped at the following regions: 14q11.2-q24.3, 2p21-p24, 15q11.1, 8q23-24, and 10q23.3-q24.2.[31–35] The gene and gene product for the 2p locus have been named *spastin*, an adenosine triphosphatase believed to be involved in the assembly or function of nuclear protein complexes.[36] The genes for the other forms have not been identified.

Autosomal Recessive Forms. Three loci for the recessive forms of familial spastic paraparesis have been mapped. The first was localized at 8q12-13 in four Tunisian families,[37] but the gene for this locus has not been identified. The second locus was identified at 16q24.3 from linkage analysis of a large consanguineous family from Italy.[38] The gene and protein were subsequently identified and named *paraplegin*,[39] a nuclear-encoded mitochondrial metalloprotease that has both proteolytic and chaperone-like activities at the inner mitochondrial membrane. A third recessive locus was mapped at 15q13-15, but the gene is still unknown.[40]

X-Linked Recessive Forms. Two distinct loci for X-linked recessive types have been identified: Xq28 (SPG1) and Xq21-q22 (SPG2). SPG1 is a complicated form of spastic paraparesis that is due to mutations in the neural cell adhesion molecule L1,[41] an axonal glycoprotein required for neuronal migration and differentiation.[42] SPG1 is allelic to two other disorders: X-linked hydrocephalus and

MASA syndrome (*m*ental retardation, *a*phasia, *s*pastic paraplegia, *a*dducted thumbs).[41]

SPG2 is a pure form of spastic paraparesis caused by mutations in the gene for proteolipid protein, one of the major myelin proteins.[43] It is allelic to Pelizaeus-Merzbacher disease.

Amyotrophic Lateral Sclerosis

Amyotrophic lateral sclerosis (ALS) is a lethal disease characterized histopathologically by loss of motor neurons. It clinically presents as progressive weakness with signs of both upper and lower motor neuron involvement and bulbar dysfunction. Most cases are sporadic, but approximately 10% are familial. Both autosomal dominant and recessive forms have been identified.

Autosomal Dominant Form. A dominant adult-onset locus, designated *ALS1*, was first demonstrated on 21q.[44] A gene in this region, Cu/Zn-binding superoxide dismutase 1 (*SOD1*) was later found mutated in ALS patients.[45] However, only 13% of dominant adult-onset cases appear to be due to mutations in SOD1.[46] Some pedigrees showing autosomal dominant adult-onset ALS did not link to this locus and have been designated *ALS3*. A dominant change in function of *SOD1* is postulated to induce oxidative stress leading to neuronal cell death.

In rare cases, mutations in the gene for neurofilament heavy polypeptide on 22q12 can be the primary cause for ALS.[47,48] When neurofilament heavy polypeptide is mutated, the transport of components required for axonal integrity is believed to be perturbed, causing axonal degeneration.[49]

A juvenile-onset autosomal dominant form of ALS has also been mapped to 9q34.[50] Designated *ALS4*, the locus has recently been narrowed to a 500-kb interval on 9q34, but the gene has not yet been identified.[51] Recently, another autosomal dominant locus for familial ALS has been mapped to 18q.[52]

Autosomal Recessive Forms. Two recessive forms of ALS with onset in the juvenile period have been mapped. One, designated *ALS2*, is localized to 2q33-35, whereas another one, designated *ALS5*, is on 15q12-21.[53,54] The genes for these forms of ALS have not yet been uncovered.

Anterior Horn Cell Disorders

Spinal Muscular Atrophy. Spinal muscular atrophies are a group of autosomal recessive disorders of variable onset characterized by degeneration of the lower motor neurons. Patients typically present with weakness, areflexia, fasciculations, and (in the more severe forms) prominent bulbar signs. Depending on severity and age of onset, the disease is subdivided into three forms (Table 20.3).[55] All three types were mapped by linkage analysis to 5q11.2-13.3, and subsequent studies indicate that a gene contained in this region is responsible for causing spinal muscular atrophies.[56,57] The gene has been designated *survival motor neuron* (SMN).

Kennedy's Syndrome (X-Linked Bulbospinal Muscular Atrophy). X-linked bulbospinal (or "spinal and bulbar") muscular atrophy is an adult-onset condition, which variably presents with a slowly progressive wasting and weakness of the muscles. The

Table 20.3 Classification of the Spinal Muscular Atrophies (SMAs)

Classification	Age of Onset	Course	Death
SMA type I	0–6 mos	Never sit	<2 yrs
SMA type II	<18 mos	Never stand	>2 yrs
SMA type III	>18 mos	Stands alone	Adult

proximal muscles of the shoulders and hips are initially affected. Later, bulbar muscles are affected as well, leading to swallowing and speech problems. Mild androgen insensitivity is not uncommon, resulting in gynecomastia and testicular atrophy.

Bulbospinal muscular atrophy is considered the prototype of genetic neurodegenerative disorders caused by expansion of trinucleotide repeats. Linkage to the proximal arm of the X chromosome was first reported in 1986,[58] and the gene was later identified as the androgen receptor.[59]

The genetic basis for the various motor neuron disorders is summarized in Table 20.4.

Hereditary Neuropathies

Charcot-Marie-Tooth Peripheral Neuropathies

CMT is a group of peripheral nerve disorders that shows genetic and clinical heterogeneity. Clinical features may include progressive muscle weakness, absent or diminished reflexes, gait disturbance (steppage gait), hammer toes, and cold intolerance. Two major types have been proposed, distinguished by measuring motor nerve conduction velocities (NCVs). Patients with CMT1 typically show slowed motor NCVs and onion bulb formation on histopathology. In contrast, CMT2 patients often have normal or near normal NCVs and histologic findings of axonal loss. The age onset of the CMT2 type is usually higher. Table 20.5 provides a summary of the genetic basis for the different CMT subtypes.

Hereditary Sensory Autonomic Neuropathies

Hereditary sensory autonomic neuropathies are a group of disorders typically manifested by sensory deficits and autonomic dysfunction. Patients can present with excessive or no sweating and problems with maintaining normal body temperature. Both autosomal dominant and recessive forms of the disorder are recognized, with the dominant form usually presenting much later in life with severe sensory deficits. The genetics of the various forms are summarized in Table 20.6.

Myopathies

Muscular Dystrophies

The muscular dystrophies are a heterogeneous group of degenerative disorders characterized by progressive muscle weakness and wasting. Although skeletal muscles are primarily involved, the heart could be variably affected. Over the last 5 years, the

Table 20.4 Hereditary Anterior Horn Cell Disorders

Disorder	Inheritance Pattern	MIM Number	Location/Gene	References
A. FSP	AD	182601	2p21-p-24/*spastin*	32
	AD	603563	8q23-24	34
	AD	601162	10q23.3	35
	AD	182600	14q	31
	AD	600363	15q11.1	33
	AR	270800	8q12	37
	AR	602783	16q24.3/*paraplegin*	38,39
	AR	604360	15q13-15	40
	X-linked	312900	Xq28/*L1CAM*	41
	X-linked	312920	Xq21-q22/*PLP*	43
B. ALS				
ALS1	AD	105400	21q/*SOD1*	44,45
	AD	105400	22q12/*NEFH*	47,48
ALS4	AD	602433	9q34	50
ALS6	AD	606640	18q	52
ALS2	AR	205100	2q33-35	53,54
C. Anterior horn disorders				
Spinal muscular atrophy	AR	600354	5q11.2/*SMN*	56,57
Kennedy's syndrome	X-linked	313200	Androgen receptor	58,59
Scapuloperoneal syndrome, myopathic type	AD	181430	12q13.3	87
Scapuloperoneal syndrome, neurogenic type	AD	181405	12q24.1	87
Distal spinal muscular atrophy	AD	600794	7p	88

AD = autosomal dominant; ALS = amyotrophic lateral sclerosis; AR = autosomal recessive; FSP = familial spastic paraparesis.

genetic basis has been elucidated for most forms (Table 20.7) and has given rise to a molecular classification of these disorders. Only selected disorders are presented here in some detail. Interested readers may find more information about specific disorders (and references) by following the respective OMIM entries.

Dystrophinopathies. Mutations in the dystrophin gene can result in either DMD, in which there is complete absence of the protein, or BMD, in which the abnormality of protein expression could be qualitative (higher or lower molecular weight) or quantitative (decreased synthesis). With few exceptions, the progression of the disease tends to be more benign in BMD compared to DMD patients. The diagnosis can be established by immunochemical methods (immunofluorescence or immunoblots) or by mutation studies. Females at risk for dystrophinopathy can be detected by elevation in serum creatine kinase, by analysis of the mutation present in an affected relative, or by linkage analysis. Prenatal diagnosis is provided by a number of laboratories and may be performed on either chorionic villus or muscle biopsy.

Table 20.5 Genetic Basis of the Different Charcot-Marie-Tooth (CMT) Subtypes[a]

Disorder	Inheritance Pattern	Location	Gene	Protein	MIM Number
A. *CMT1*					
CMT1A[b]	AD	17p12	PMP22	Peripheral myelin protein 22[c]	118220
CMT1B	AD	1q21	MPZ	Myelin protein zero (P_0)[c]	118200
CMT1C	AD	—	—	—	601098
CMT1X	X-linked	Xq13	Cx32	Connexin 32	304040
B. *CMT2*					
CMT2A	AD	1p36	KIF1B[d]	Kinesin family member 1B	118210
CMT2B	AD	3q13	—	—	600882
CMT2D	AD	7p14	—	—	601472
CMT2E	AD	8p21	NEFL	Neurofilament	162280
C. *CMT4*					
CMT4A	AR	8q12	—	—	214400
CMT4B	AR	11q23	—	—	601382
CMT4C	AR	5q23	MTMR2	Myotubularin-related protein	601596
HMSNL, CMT4D	AR	8q24	NDRG1	—	601455
CMT4E	AD	10q21	EGR2	Early growth response 2	129010
CMT4F, Dejerine- Sottas disease[e]	AD/AR	19q13	PRX	Periaxin	145900
		17p12	PMP22	Peripheral myelin protein 22[c]	145900
		1q22	MPZ	Myelin protein zero (P_0)[c]	145900

AD = autosomal dominant; AR = autosomal recessive; HMSNL = hereditary motor and sensory neuropathy, LOM type.

[a]Adapted from JR Lipski, CA Garcia. Charcot-Marie-Tooth Peripheral Neuropathies and Related Disorders. In CR Scriver, AL Beaudet, WS Sly, D Valle (eds), The Metabolic and Molecular Basis of Inherited Disease (8th ed). New York: McGraw-Hill, 2001;5759–5788.

[b]Allelic to hereditary neuropathy with liability to pressure palsy (HNPP).

[c]Allelic disorders.

[d]Adapted from C Zhao, J Takita, Y Tanaka, et al. Charcot-Marie-Tooth disease type 2a caused by mutation in a microtubule motor kif1bbeta. Cell 2001;105:587–597.

[e]CMT4F has also been seen classified separately from Dejerine-Sottas disease. The AD form of Dejerine-Sottas disease has also been classified as CMT3.

Table 20.6 Genetic Basis of the Hereditary Sensory Autonomic Neuropathies (HSAN)

Disorder	Inheritance Pattern	Location	Gene	MIM Number	Reference
HSAN I (hereditary sensory radicular neuropathy)	Autosomal dominant	9q22.1	Serine palmitoyl transferase, long-chain subunit 1	162400	85
HSAN II (neurogenic acroosteolysis)	AR	—	—	201300	—
HSAN III (Riley-Day syndrome; familial dysautonomia)	AR	9q31	I kappaB kinase complex-associated protein	223900	86,87
HSAN IV (congenital insensitivity to pain with anhidrosis)	AR	1q21	Neurotrophic tyrosine kinase receptor, type 1	256800	88,89

AR = autosomal recessive.

Table 20.7 Genetic Myopathies

Disorders	Inheritance Pattern	Location	Gene	MIM Number
A. Dystrophinopathies				
Duchenne's muscular dystrophy	X-linked	Xp21	Dystrophin	310200
Becker's muscular dystrophy	X-linked	Xp21	Dystrophin	310200
B. Limb-girdle muscular dystrophies (LGMDs)				
LGMD1A	Autosomal dominant (AD)	5q31	Myotilin	159000
LGMD1B	AD	1q11-21	Lamin A/C	159001
LGMD1C	AD	3p25	Caveolin-3	601253
LGMD1D	AD	6q23	—	602067
LGMD1E	AD	7q	—	603511
LGMD2A	Autosomal recessive (AR)	15q15.1-q21.1	Calpain 3	253600
LGMD2B	AR	2p13	Dysferlin	603009
LGMD2C	AR	13q12	γ-Sarcoglycan	253700
LGMD2D	AR	17q12-q21.33	α-Sarcoglycan	600119
LGMD2E	AR	4q12	β-Sarcoglycan	253700
LGMD2F	AR	5q33-q34	δ-Sarcoglycan	253700
LGMD2G	AR	17q11-q12	Telethonin	253700
LGMD2H	AR	9q31-q34.1	TRIM32	254110
LGMD2I	AR	19q13.3	FKRP*	—
C. Emery-Dreifuss muscular dystrophies (EDMDs)				
X-linked EDMD	X-linked	Xq28	Emerin	310300
Autosomal dominant EDMD	AD	1q11-q23	Lamin A/C	181350
D. Congenital muscular dystrophies (CMDs)				
Primary merosin deficiency (MDC1A)	AR	6q2	Merosin (lamin α2 chain)	156225
Primary integrin deficiency	AR	12q13	Integrin α7	600536
CMD (Fukuyama type)	AR	9q31-q33	Fukutin	253800
MDC1C	AR	19q13.3	FKRP	606596
CMD with rigid spine	AR	1p35-p36	—	602771
E. Other congenital myopathies				
Myotubular myopathy	X-linked	Xq28	Myotubularin	310400
Central core disease	AD	19q13.1	Ryanodine receptor	117000
Nemaline myopathy	AD	1q21-q23	α-Tropomyosin	161800
	AR	2q21.2-q22	Nebulin	256030
	AD	1q24.1	Skeletal muscle α-actin	101800
F. Other myopathies with known genetic defects				
Miyoshi myopathy	AR	2p12-p14	Dysferlin	254130
Bethlem myopathy	AD	21q22.3	Collagen type VI α-1 or α-2 subunit	158810
	AD	2q37	Collagen type VI α-3 subunit	158810
Oculopharyngeal muscular dystrophy	AD	14q11.2-q13	Poly(A) binding protein 2	164300
LGMD with epidermolysis bullosa	AR	8q24-qter	Plectin	226670
Desmin myopathy	AD	11q22	αβ-Crystallin	123590
	AD	2q35	Desmin	601419
Facioscapulohumeral muscular dystrophy	AD	4q35	—	158900

*Data from M Brockington, Y Yuva, P Prandini, et al. Mutations in the fukutin-related protein gene (FKRP) identify limb girdle muscular dystrophy 2I as a milder allelic variant of congenital muscular dystrophy MDC1C. Hum Mol Genet 2001;10:2851–2859.

Limb-Girdle Muscular Dystrophies. The LGMDs are a group of genetically heterogeneous disorders characterized by weakness of the shoulder and pelvic girdle muscles. Considerable clinical overlap with the dystrophinopathies is not infrequently observed. The age of onset and severity is variable, with the more severe forms usually labeled as *severe childhood autosomal recessive muscular dystrophies*. Autosomal dominant cases are designated *LGMD1*, of which five distinct genetic types are now recognized. Eight genetically distinct types are known to be inherited as autosomal recessive and are designated as *LGMD2*. Four of the latter involve genes that code for dystrophin-associated proteins (sarcoglycans). A summary of these disorders is presented in Table 20.7.

Emery-Dreifuss Muscular Dystrophy. Emery-Dreifuss muscular dystrophy is a primary myopathy characterized by slowly progressive muscle wasting and weakness akin to BMD, with early contractures of the elbows and Achilles' tendons. Life-threatening cardiomyopathy with conduction blocks is frequently observed in Emery-Dreifuss muscular dystrophy patients. The X-linked form of the disease is due to mutations of the emerin gene,[60] whereas the autosomal dominant form is caused by mutations in lamin A/C.[61]

Oculopharyngeal Muscular Dystrophy. Oculopharyngeal muscular dystrophy is a disorder characterized by progressive ptosis and dysphagia. Other manifestations could include proximal muscle weakness, facial muscle weakness, and tongue atrophy and weakness. Both autosomal dominant and recessive forms are recognized, but both forms involve the polyadenylation-binding protein 2 (PABP2) gene.[62] Molecular genetic diagnosis can be made with a demonstration of PABP2 trinucleotide repeat expansions by PCR analysis (Figure 20.15).

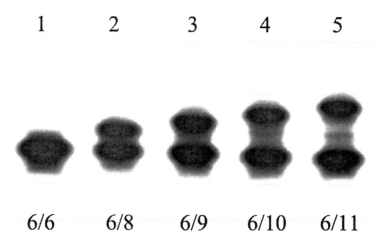

Figure 20.15 Molecular analysis of the poly (A) binding protein 2 (PABP2) gene trinucleotide repeat. Polymerase chain reaction analysis with primers flanking the (GCGn) repeat in five individuals referred for diagnostic testing for oculopharyngeal muscular dystrophy. Numbers denote GCG sizes. The patient in lane 1 is homozygous normal for two alleles carrying six GCG repeats. Patients in lanes 2–5 carry expanded alleles (GCG8–11) within the PABP2 gene. Alleles in this size range are associated with the clinical manifestations of oculopharyngeal muscular dystrophy. (Courtesy of Dr. Nicholas Potter, Department of Medical Genetics, University of Tennessee Medical Center, Knoxville.)

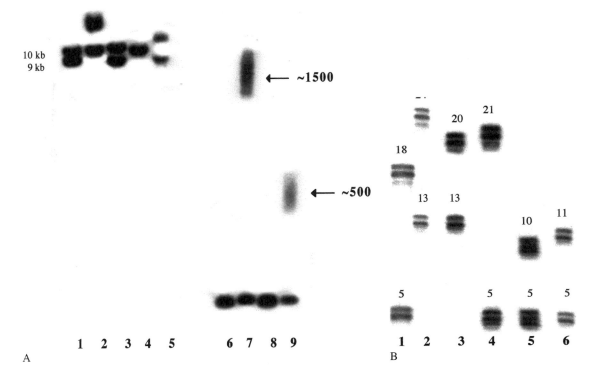

Figure 20.16 Molecular analysis of the myotonin protein kinase gene trinucleotide repeat. **A.** Southern blot analysis of patient genomic DNA digested with EcoR1 (lanes 1–5) and BamH1 (lanes 6–9) and probed with p5B1.4. Two restriction enzyme digests are used to aid the sizing of abnormal alleles containing CTG repeat expansions. A common 1-kb insertion/deletion polymorphism is detectable when using EcoR1 digests and gives rise to two fragments (9 kb and 10 kb) in some unaffected subjects having normal CTG repeats (lanes 1 and 3). Lanes 1 and 6: individual with no repeat expansion (alleles <35 as sized by polymerase chain reaction); lanes 2 and 7: patient with repeat expansion of approximately 1,500 (midpoint of smear) associated with congenital myotonic dystrophy; lanes 3 and 8: individual with repeats less than 35; lane 4: individual with repeats less than 35 and no insertion/deletion polymorphism; lanes 5 and 9: mother of patient in lanes 2 and 7 who has a repeat expansion of approximately 500 associated with adult onset myotonic dystrophy. **B.** Polymerase chain reaction sizing of stable alleles less than 35. Numbers denote estimated CTG repeat sizes. Large alleles beyond approximately 40–50 CTG repeats are difficult to amplify, and Southern blotting is needed to detect most pathologic alleles. (Courtesy of Dr. Jack Tarleton, Fullerton Genetic Center, Asheville, NC.)

Myotonic Dystrophy. DM is the most common adult-onset muscular dystrophy, characterized by muscle weakness and wasting and myotonia. DM is a multisystem disorder involving smooth and cardiac muscle, endocrine glands, the central nervous system, and the lens. Although DM follows an autosomal dominant pattern of inheritance, extreme variation in clinical presentation is seen despite the absence of genetic heterogeneity. As seen in a number of trinucleotide repeat expansion disorders, affected pedigrees show anticipation characterized by progressively younger age of onset and severity with successive generations. The parental origin of the mutation appears to influence presentation as well. The congenital and more severe forms are almost always maternally transmitted, whereas the first symptomatic and less severely affected generation is usually of paternal origin.

The molecular basis for DM was elucidated in 1992. The molecular defect is an unstable expansion of a trinucleotide (CTG) repeat at the 3' untranslated region of a gene encoding a protein kinase (DMPK) on 19q13 (Figure 20.16).[63–65] Patients with this genetic defect are now considered DM1, and a group of patients in which

Table 20.8 Spinocerebellar Ataxias (SCAs)

Disorder	Inheritance Pattern	Location	Gene/Gene Product	MIM Number
SCA1	AD	6p23	Ataxin-1	164400
SCA2	AD	12q24.1	Ataxin-2	183090
SCA3 (Machado-Joseph disease)	AD	14q24.3-q32	Ataxin-3	109150
SCA4	AD	16q24-qter	—	164400
SCA5	AD	11p11-q11	—	164400
SCA6	AD	19p13	Calcium channel	183086
SCA7	AD	3p12-p21.1	Ataxin-7	164500
SCA8	AD	13q21	SCA8	603680
SCA10	AD	22q13	SCA10	603516
SCA11	AD	15q14-q21.3	—	604432
SCA12	AD	5q31-q33	Protein phosphatase regulatory subunit B	604326
SCA13	AD	19q13	—	605259
SCA14	AD	19q13.4-qter	—	605361

AD = autosomal dominant.

the genetic defect is in chromosome 3q21 is now considered DM2. The defect in this group is a CCTG expansion located in intron 1 of the zinc finger protein 9 (ZNF9) gene.[66]

Proximal Myotonic Myopathy. Proximal myotonic myopathy is a recently recognized disease entity that resembles DM but has a somewhat slower progression. The inheritance pattern is also autosomal dominant but, unlike DM, does not seem to exhibit pronounced anticipation. Although a large kindred has recently been localized to 3q,[67] other studies have not shown a linkage to this locus, suggesting genetic heterogeneity for proximal myotonic myopathy.[68,69]

Spinocerebellar Disorders

Spinocerebellar Ataxias

The SCAs are dominantly inherited disorders characterized by degeneration of neurons in the cerebellum, spinocerebellar tract, and brain stem. Three major clinical categories have been proposed.[70] Autosomal dominant cerebellar ataxia (ADCA) type I is characterized by ataxia with other variable neurologic features (pyramidal signs, ophthalmoplegia, extrapyramidal signs, and dementia). ADCA type II disorders show ataxia with pigmentary maculopathy and striking anticipation, whereas those classified under ADCA type III are characterized by a relatively pure cerebellar syndrome. The genetic basis for the SCAs is summarized in Table 20.8. The precise molecular basis for eight of the SCAs has been elucidated, and the majority is due to expansion of CAG trinucleotide. SCA8 is due

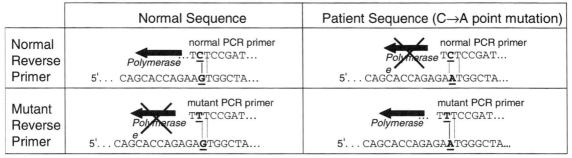

	Normal Sequence	Patient Sequence (C→A point mutation)
Normal Reverse Primer	normal PCR primer ...T**C**TCCGAT... *Polymerase* 5'... CAGCACCAGAA**G**TGGCTA...	normal PCR primer *Poly~~merase~~* T**C**TCCGAT... *e* 5'... CAGCACCAGAGA**A**TGGCTA...
Mutant Reverse Primer	mutant PCR primer T**T**TCCGAT... *Poly~~merase~~* *e* 5'... CAGCACCAGAGA**G**TGGCTA...	mutant PCR primer T**T**TCCGAT... *Polymerase* 5'... CAGCACCAGAGA**A**TGGGCTA...

A

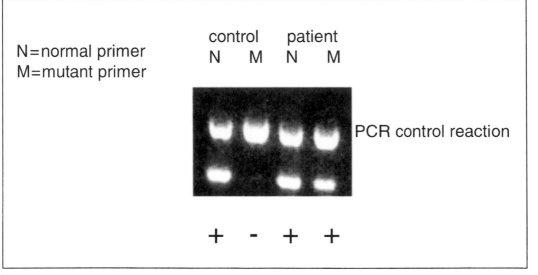

B

Figure 20.17 Amplification-refractory mutation system (ARMS) analysis of a mutation of the chloride channel gene. The ARMS technique is used to detect known single-base changes and exploits the premise that polymerase chain reaction (PCR) primers must be designed to very closely complement the sequence of interest; otherwise, they will fail to amplify the sequence under study. Two reactions must be run for each sample: one using a primer designed to amplify the normal sequence and one using a primer sequence designed to amplify the mutant sequence **(A)**. Intentional mismatches in the primer sequence determine which sequences will amplify with PCR, and a primer with more than one noncomplementary base to the DNA sample will not amplify that segment. Heterozygous positive controls must be run with each sample. An example of the use of ARMS is shown for the G230E mutation in the CLCN1 chloride channel gene causing myotonia congenita **(B)**. The "control" has two normal chloride channel genes, and thus amplifies only with the normal (N) primer set (in addition to an internal "PCR control reaction") and not with the mutation-specific primer set (M). The heterozygous myotonia congenita patient shows amplification with both N and M primer sets, proving that he has the G230E change in the chloride channel. Failure to detect this particular point mutation does not rule out other mutations in this gene. (A = adenine; C = cytosine; G = guanine; T = thymine.) (Reprinted with permission from Hoffman EP, Scacheri CA, Giron J. Genetic Testing. In R Pourmand [ed], Neuromuscular Diseases: Expert Clinicians' Views. Boston: Butterworth–Heinemann, 2001;51–65.)

Table 20.9 Channelopathies

Disorders	Inheritance Pattern	Location	Gene/Protein	MIM Number
A. Chloride channel				
Thomsen disease	AD	7q35	*CLC-1*/muscle chloride channel	160800
Becker's myotonia	AR	7q35	*CLC-1*/muscle chloride channel	255700
B. Sodium channel				
Hyperkalemic periodic paralysis	AD	17q23	*SCN4A*/sodium channel α subunit	170500
Paramyotonia congenita	AD	17q23	*SCN4A*/sodium channel α subunit	168300
C. Calcium channel				
Hypokalemic periodic paralysis	AD	1q31	*CACNL1A3*/calcium channel	170400
D. Potassium channel				
Episodic ataxia	AD	12p	*KCNA1*/voltage-gated potassium channel	160120

AD = autosomal dominant; AR = autosomal recessive.

to CTG expansion,[71] whereas one study involving SCA10 families revealed expansion of a pentanucleotide (ATTCT).[72] The SCA8 gene product is unusual in that it appears to be an antisense RNA to a brain-specific transcript encoding an actin-binding protein (KLHL1).[73]

Friedreich's Ataxia

Friedreich's ataxia is a progressive mixed cerebellar-sensory disorder of autosomal recessive inheritance. Age of onset is typically around puberty and can initially present as gait instability or generalized clumsiness. Later manifestations could include dysarthria, deep sensory loss, hearing loss, lower limb muscle weakness, cardiomyopathy, and impaired glucose tolerance.

The genetic basis for Friedreich's ataxia has been shown to be a massive expansion of a normally short GAA trinucleotide repeat region in intron 1 of the frataxin gene.[74] Disruption of the frataxin protein is believed to inactivate mitochondrial iron-sulfur proteins leading to accumulation of iron in the mitochondria.[75]

Channelopathies

Channelopathies are newly recognized episodic disorders of the nervous system secondary to defects in voltage- and ligand-gated ion channels. Alterations in ion channels perturb the regulation of membrane excitability and function of excitable cells, such as nerves and muscles. The prototypical disorders in this group are the periodic paralyses—autosomal dominant disorders characterized by episodic weakness or paralysis instigated by stress or fatigue and myotonia congenita caused by a defect of the muscle chloride channel gene (Figure 20.17). The major channelopathies involving muscles and nerves are summarized in Table 20.9.

CONCLUSIONS

With the evolution of newer and more sophisticated technology, it becomes imperative for a physician to become familiar with the basic concepts underlying each technology to fully realize its power and use. At the same time, physicians and the patient must become aware of the implications of genetic testing on confidentiality, insurance, and lifestyle even before a test is requested. Given the maze of ethical and legal concerns that accompany the communication of test results, the neurologist is enjoined either to become intimately familiar with relevant issues and what appropriate measures to take or to refer the genetic testing process to medical specialists (i.e., a genetic counselor or medical geneticist) who may be better informed on the same. As an initial resource, the University of Montreal has established a Web site (http://www.humgen.umontreal.ca/en/GenInfo.cfm) that can be consulted for current policies and regulations on genetics and patient care advocated by governments and professional organizations. The Web site has a searchable bibliography and links to Web pages of the appropriate organizations or government jurisdictions. For those neurologists who routinely convey gene test results to patients, it might be worthwhile to routinely access this resource.

REFERENCES

1. Martin JB, Longo FM. Molecular Neurobiology. In JL Jameson (ed), Principles of Molecular Medicine. Totowa, NJ: Humana Press Inc., 1998;871–890.
2. Koop P, Jameson JL. Transmission of Human Genetic Disease. In JL Jameson (ed), Principles of Molecular Medicine. Totowa, NJ: Humana Press Inc., 1998;43–63.
3. Pentao L, Wise CA, Chinault AC, et al. Charcot-Marie-Tooth type 1A duplication appears to arise from recombination at repeat sequences flanking the 1.5 Mb monomer unit. Nat Genet 1992;2:292–300.
4. Rudolph JA, Spier SJ, Byrns G, et al. Periodic paralysis in quarter horses: a sodium channel mutation disseminated by selective breeding. Nat Genet 1992;2:144–147.
5. Rojas CV, Wang JZ, Schwartz LS, et al. A Met-to-Val mutation in the skeletal muscle Na+ channel alpha-subunit in hyperkalaemic periodic paralysis. Nature 1991;354:387–389.
6. Zareba W, Moss AJ, Schwartz PJ, et al. Influence of genotype on the clinical course of the long-QT syndrome. International Long-QT Syndrome Registry Research Group. N Engl J Med 1998;339: 960–965.
7. Escayg A, MacDonald BT, Meisler MH, et al. Mutations of SCN1A, encoding a neuronal sodium channel, in two families with GEFS+2. Nat Genet 2000;24:343–345.
8. Giles RE, Blanc H, Cann HM, Wallace DC. Maternal inheritance of human mitochondrial DNA. Proc Natl Acad Sci U S A 1980;77:6715–6719.
9. Case JT, Wallace DC. Maternal inheritance of mitochondrial DNA polymorphisms in cultured human fibroblasts. Somatic Cell Genet 1981;7:103–108.

10. Kaneda H, Hayashi J, Takahama S, et al. Elimination of paternal mitochondrial DNA in intraspecific crosses during early mouse embryogenesis. Proc Natl Acad Sci U S A 1995;92: 4542–4546.

11. Shoffner JM, Lott MT, Lezza AM, et al. Myoclonic epilepsy and ragged-red fiber disease (MERRF) is associated with a mitochondrial DNA tRNALys mutation. Cell 1990;61:931–937.

12. Wallace DC. William Allan Award Address. Mitochondrial DNA variation in human evolution, degenerative disease, and aging. Am J Hum Genet 1995;57:201–223.

13. Wallace DC, Zheng X, Lott MT, et al. Familial mitochondrial encephalomyopathy (MERRF): genetic, pathophysiological, and biochemical characterization of a mitochondrial DNA disease. Cell 1988;55:601–610.

14. Wallace DC, Lott MT, Shoffner JM, Ballinger S. Mitochondrial DNA mutations in epilepsy and neurological disease. Epilepsia 1994;35(Suppl 1):S43–S50.

15. Mulley JC, Staples A, Donnelly A, et al. Explanation for exclusive maternal origin for congenital form of myotonic dystrophy. Lancet 1993;341:236–237.

16. Reyniers E, Vits L, De Boulle K, et al. The full mutation in the FMR-1 gene of male fragile X patients is absent in their sperm. Nat Genet 1993;4:143–146.

17. Andrew SE, Goldberg YP, Kremer B, et al. The relationship between trinucleotide (CAG) repeat length and clinical features of Huntington's disease. Nat Genet 1993;4:398–403.

18. Ohlsson R, Tycko B, Sapienza C. Monoallelic expression: "there can only be one." Trends Genet 1998;14:435–438.

19. Bartolomei MS, Tilghman SM. Genomic imprinting in mammals. Annu Rev Genet 1997;31: 493–525.

20. Robinson WP, Bottani A, Xie YG, et al. Molecular, cytogenetic, and clinical investigations of Prader-Willi syndrome patients. Am J Hum Genet 1991;49:1219–1234.

21. Vu TH, Hoffman AR. Imprinting of the Angelman syndrome gene, UBE3A, is restricted to brain. Nat Genet 1997;17:12–13.

22. Kishino T, Lalande M, Wagstaff J. UBE3A/E6-AP mutations cause Angelman syndrome. Nat Genet 1997;15:70–73.

23. Malcolm S. Molecular Methodology. In DL Rimoin, JM Connor, RE Pyeritz (eds), Principles and Practice of Medical Genetics (3rd ed). New York: Churchill Livingstone, 1996;67–85.

24. Grompe M, Johnson W, Jameson JL. Recombinant DNA and Genetic Techniques. In JL Jameson (ed), Principles of Molecular Medicine. Totowa, NJ: Humana Press Inc., 1998;9–24.

25. Hoffee P (ed). Medical Molecular Genetics. Madison, CT: Fence Creek Publishing, 1998.

26. Kristensen VN, Kelefiotis D, Kristensen T, Borresen-Dale AL. High-throughput methods for detection of genetic variation. Biotechniques 2001;30:318–332.

27. Dobrowolski SF, Banas RA, Naylor EW, et al. DNA microarray technology for neonatal screening. Acta Paediatr 1999;432(Suppl 88):61–64.

28. Gilles PN, Wu DJ, Foster CB, et al. Single nucleotide polymorphic discrimination by an electronic dot blot assay on semiconductor microchips. Nat Biotechnol 1999;17:365–370.

29. Larsen LA, Christiansen M, Vuust J, Andersen PS. High-throughput single-strand conformation polymorphism analysis by automated capillary electrophoresis: robust multiplex analysis and pattern-based identification of allelic variants. Hum Mutat 1999;13:318–327.

30. Chen YW, Zhao P, Borup R, Hoffman EP. Expression profiling in the muscular dystrophies: identification of novel aspects of molecular pathophysiology. J Cell Biol 2000;151:1321–1336.

31. Hazan J, Lamy C, Melki J, et al. Autosomal dominant familial spastic paraplegia is genetically heterogeneous and one locus maps to chromosome 14q. Nat Genet 1993;5:163–167.

32. Hazan J, Fontaine B, Bruyn RP, et al. Linkage of a new locus for autosomal dominant familial spastic paraplegia to chromosome 2p. Hum Mol Genet 1994;3:1569–1573.

33. Fink JK, Wu CT, Jones SM, et al. Autosomal dominant familial spastic paraplegia: tight linkage to chromosome 15q. Am J Hum Genet 1995;56:188–192.

34. Hedera P, Rainier S, Alvarado D, et al. Novel locus for autosomal dominant hereditary spastic paraplegia, on chromosome 8q. Am J Hum Genet 1999;64:563–569.

35. Lo Nigro C, Cusano R, Scaranari M, et al. A refined physical and transcriptional map of the SPG9 locus on 10q23.3-q24.2. Eur J Hum Genet 2000;8:777–782.

36. Hazan J, Fonknechten N, Mavel D, et al. Spastin, a new AAA protein, is altered in the most frequent form of autosomal dominant spastic paraplegia. Nat Genet 1999;23:296–303.

37. Hentati A, Pericak-Vance MA, Hung WY, et al. Linkage of "pure" autosomal recessive familial spastic paraplegia to chromosome 8 markers and evidence of genetic locus heterogeneity. Hum Mol Genet 1994;3:1263–1267.

38. De Michele G, De Fusco M, Cavalcanti F, et al. A new locus for autosomal recessive hereditary spastic paraplegia maps to chromosome 16q24.3. Am J Hum Genet 1998;63:135–139.

39. Casari G, De Fusco M, Ciarmatori S, et al. Spastic paraplegia and OXPHOS impairment caused by mutations in paraplegin, a nuclear-encoded mitochondrial metalloprotease. Cell 1998;93:973–983.

40. Martinez Murillo F, Kobayashi H, Pegoraro E, et al. Genetic localization of a new locus for recessive familial spastic paraparesis to 15q13-15. Neurology 1999;53:50–56.

41. Jouet M, Rosenthal A, Armstrong G, et al. X-linked spastic paraplegia (SPG1), MASA syndrome and X-linked hydrocephalus result from mutations in the L1 gene. Nat Genet 1994;7:402–407.

42. Joosten EA, Gribnau AA. Immunocytochemical localization of cell adhesion molecule L1 in developing rat pyramidal tract. Neurosci Lett 1989;100:94–98.

43. Saugier-Veber P, Munnich A, Bonneau D, et al. X-linked spastic paraplegia and Pelizaeus-Merzbacher disease are allelic disorders at the proteolipid protein locus. Nat Genet 1994;6:257–262.

44. Siddique T, Figlewicz DA, Pericak-Vance MA, et al. Linkage of a gene causing familial amyotrophic lateral sclerosis to chromosome 21 and evidence of genetic-locus heterogeneity. N Engl J Med 1991;324:1381–1384.

45. Rosen DR, Siddique T, Patterson D, et al. Mutations in Cu/Zn superoxide dismutase gene are associated with familial amyotrophic lateral sclerosis. Nature 1993;362:59–62.

46. Pramatarova A, Figlewicz DA, Krizus A, et al. Identification of new mutations in the Cu/Zn superoxide dismutase gene of patients with familial amyotrophic lateral sclerosis. Am J Hum Genet 1995;56:592–596.

47. Figlewicz DA, Krizus A, Martinoli MG, et al. Variants of the heavy neurofilament subunit are associated with the development of amyotrophic lateral sclerosis. Hum Mol Genet 1994;3:1757–1761.

48. Al-Chalabi A, Andersen PM, Nilsson P, et al. Deletions of the heavy neurofilament subunit tail in amyotrophic lateral sclerosis. Hum Mol Genet 1999;8:157–164.

49. Collard JF, Cote F, Julien JP. Defective axonal transport in a transgenic mouse model of amyotrophic lateral sclerosis. Nature 1995;375:61–64.

50. Chance PF, Rabin BA, Ryan SG, et al. Linkage of the gene for an autosomal dominant form of juvenile amyotrophic lateral sclerosis to chromosome 9q34. Am J Hum Genet 1998;62:633–640.

51. Blair IP, Bennett CL, Abel A, et al. A gene for autosomal dominant juvenile amyotrophic lateral sclerosis (ALS4) localizes to a 500-kb interval on chromosome 9q34. Neurogenetics 2000;3:1–6.

52. Hand CK, Khoris J, Salachas F, et al. A novel locus for familial amyotrophic lateral sclerosis, on chromosome 18q. Am J Hum Genet 2002;70:251–256.

53. Hentati A, Bejaoui K, Pericak-Vance MA, et al. Linkage of recessive familial amyotrophic lateral sclerosis to chromosome 2q33-q35. Nat Genet 1994;7:425–428.

54. Hentati A, Ouahchi K, Pericak-Vance MA, et al. Linkage of a commoner form of recessive amyotrophic lateral sclerosis to chromosome 15q15-q22 markers. Neurogenetics 1998;2:55–60.

55. Munsat TL. Workshop report: International SMA collaboration. Neuromuscul Disord 1991;1:81.

56. Brzustowicz LM, Lehner T, Castilla LH, et al. Genetic mapping of chronic childhood-onset spinal muscular atrophy to chromosome 5q11.2-13.3. Nature 1990;344:540–541.

57. Bussaglia E, Clermont O, Tizzano E, et al. A frame-shift deletion in the survival motor neuron gene in Spanish spinal muscular atrophy patients. Nat Genet 1995;11:335–337.

58. Fischbeck KH, Ionasescu V, Ritter AW, et al. Localization of the gene for X-linked spinal muscular atrophy. Neurology 1986;36:1595–1598.

59. La Spada AR, Wilson EM, Lubahn DB, et al. Androgen receptor gene mutations in X-linked spinal and bulbar muscular atrophy. Nature 1991;352:77–79.

60. Bione S, Maestrini E, Rivella S, et al. Identification of a novel X-linked gene responsible for Emery-Dreifuss muscular dystrophy. Nat Genet 1994;8:323–327.

61. Bonne G, Di Barletta MR, Varnous S, et al. Mutations in the gene encoding lamin A/C cause autosomal dominant Emery-Dreifuss muscular dystrophy. Nat Genet 1991;21:285–288.

62. Brais B, Bouchard JP, Xie YG, et al. Short GCG expansions in the PABP2 gene cause oculopharyngeal muscular dystrophy. Nat Genet 1998;18:164–167.

63. Brook JD, McCurrach ME, Harley HG, et al. Molecular basis of myotonic dystrophy: expansion of a trinucleotide (CTG) repeat at the 3' end of a transcript encoding a protein kinase family member. Cell 1992;68:799–808.

64. Fu YH, Pizzuti A, Fenwick RG Jr, et al. An unstable triplet repeat in a gene related to myotonic muscular dystrophy. Science 1992;255:1256–1258.

65. Mahadevan M, Tsilfidis C, Sabourin L, et al. Myotonic dystrophy mutation: an unstable CTG repeat in the 3' untranslated region of the gene. Science 1992;255:1253–1255.

66. Liquori CL, Ricker K, Moseley ML, et al. Myotonic dystrophy type 2 caused by a CCTG expansion in intron 1 of ZNF9. Science 2001;293(5531):864–867.

67. Ricker K, Grimm T, Koch MC, et al. Linkage of proximal myotonic myopathy to chromosome 3q. Neurology 1999;52:170–171.

68. Kress W, Mueller-Myhsok B, Ricker K, et al. Proof of genetic heterogeneity in the proximal myotonic myopathy syndrome (PROMM) and its relationship to myotonic dystrophy type 2 (DM2). Neuromuscul Disord 2000;10:478–480.

69. Wieser T, Bonsch D, Eger K, et al. A family with PROMM not linked to the recently mapped PROMM locus DM2. Neuromuscul Disord 2000;10:141–143.

70. Harding AE. Clinical features and classification of the inherited ataxias. Adv Neurol 1993; 61:1–14.

71. Koob MD, Moseley ML, Schut LJ, et al. An untranslated CTG expansion causes a novel form of spinocerebellar ataxia (SCA8). Nat Genet 1999;21:379–384.

72. Matsuura T, Yamagata T, Burgess DL, et al. Large expansion of the ATTCT pentanucleotide repeat in spinocerebellar ataxia type 10. Nat Genet 2000;26:191–194.

73. Nemes JP, Benzow KA, Moseley ML, et al. The SCA8 transcript is an antisense RNA to a brain-specific transcript encoding a novel actin-binding protein (KLHL1). Hum Mol Genet 2000;9:1543–1551.

74. Campuzano V, Montermini L, Molto MD, et al. Friedreich's ataxia: autosomal recessive disease caused by an intronic GAA triplet repeat expansion. Science 1996;271:1423–1427.

75. Rotig A, de Lonlay P, Chretien D, et al. Aconitase and mitochondrial iron-sulphur protein deficiency in Friedreich ataxia. Nat Genet 1997;17:215–217.

76. Fu YH, Kuhl DP, Pizzuti A, et al. Variation of the CGG repeat at the fragile X site results in genetic instability: resolution of the Sherman paradox. Cell 1991;67:1047–1058.

77. Koide R, Ikeuchi T, Onodera O, et al. Unstable expansion of CAG repeat in hereditary dentatorubral-pallidoluysian atrophy (DRPLA). Nat Genet 1994;6:9–13.

78. Huntington's Disease Collaborative Research Group. A novel gene containing a trinucleotide repeat that is expanded and unstable on Huntington's disease chromosomes. Cell 1993;72:971–983.

79. Orr HT, Chung MY, Banfi S, et al. Expansion of an unstable trinucleotide CAG repeat in spinocerebellar ataxia type 1. Nat Genet 1993;4:221–226.

80. Sanpei K, Takano H, Igarashi S, et al. Identification of the spinocerebellar ataxia type 2 gene using a direct identification of repeat expansion and cloning technique, DIRECT. Nat Genet 1996;14:277–284.

81. Kawaguchi Y, Okamoto T, Taniwaki M, et al. CAG expansions in a novel gene for Machado-Joseph disease at chromosome 14q32.1. Nat Genet 1994;8:221–228.

82. Zhuchenko O, Bailey J, Bonnen P, et al. Autosomal dominant cerebellar ataxia (SCA6) associated with small polyglutamine expansions in the alpha 1A-voltage-dependent calcium channel. Nat Genet 1997;15:62–69.

83. David G, Abbas N, Stevanin G, et al. Cloning of the SCA7 gene reveals a highly unstable CAG repeat expansion. Nat Genet 1997;17:65–70.

84. Lalioti MD, Scott HS, Buresi C, et al. Dodecamer repeat expansion in cystatin B gene in progressive myoclonus epilepsy. Nature 1997;386:847–851.

85. Dawkins JL, Hulme DJ, Brahmbhatt SB, et al. Mutations in SPTLC1, encoding serine palmitoyltransferase, long chain base subunit-1, cause hereditary sensory neuropathy type I. Nat Genet 2001;27:309–312.

86. Slaugenhaupt SA, Blumenfeld A, Gill SP, et al. Tissue-specific expression of a splicing mutation in the IKBKAP gene causes familial dysautonomia. Am J Hum Genet 2001;68:598–605.

87. Anderson SL, Coli R, Daly IW, et al. Familial dysautonomia is caused by mutations of the IKAP gene. Am J Hum Genet 2001;68:753–758.

88. Indo Y, Tsuruta M, Hayashida Y, et al. Mutations in the TRKA/NGF receptor gene in patients with congenital insensitivity to pain with anhidrosis. Nat Genet 1996;13:485–488.

89. Shatzky S, Moses S, Levy J, et al. Congenital insensitivity to pain with anhidrosis (CIPA) in Israeli-Bedouins: genetic heterogeneity, novel mutations in the TRKA/NGF receptor gene, clinical findings, and results of nerve conduction studies. Am J Med Genet 2000;92:353–360.

90. Chamberlain JS, Gibbs RA, Ranier JE, et al. Deletion screening of the Duchenne muscular dystrophy locus via multiplex DNA amplification. Nucleic Acids Res 1988;16:11141–11156.

91. Beggs AH, Koenig M, Boyce FM, Kunkel LM. Detection of 98% of DMD/BMD gene deletions by polymerase chain reaction. Hum Genet 1990;86:45–48.

Appendix 1

Diagnostic Pathways of Generalized Neuromuscular Disorders and Diagnostic Workup of Segmental or Focal Disorders

Tulio E. Bertorini, Pushpa Narayanaswami, and Kandasami Senthilkumar

This section provides, in a summarized way, our approach to patients with neuromuscular diseases—first, in a pathway form for generalized diseases, followed by a description of the diagnosis and workup for various segmental disorders (i.e., radiculopathy, mononeuropathy).

When using these pathways, it is obvious that decisions have to be made in the context of the patient's presentation and medical history. For example, a patient with generalized weakness who has relatives with the diagnosis of dystrophinopathy will be studied initially with measurements of creatine kinase or DNA analysis without having to go through other diagnostic tests outlined in the pathway (Figure A1.1A). Similarly, in a floppy infant with evidence of fasciculations, the clinician might wish to go directly to DNA testing, obviating the use of electromyography and particularly biopsy (see Figure A1.1B). An adult patient who presents with muscle weakness, atrophy, fasciculation, dysarthria, and positive Babinski signs would not need a repetitive stimulation test or an edrophonium test but a detailed electromyography.

In another example, if there is a clinical suspicion of myasthenia gravis, the first diagnostic test would be the edrophonium test, and, if negative, measurement of acetylcholine receptor antibody titers, followed by repetitive stimulation tests or single-fiber electromyography. The order of these will, however, change in a patient with a history of intermittent muscle weakness or diplopia that is not detected during the examination; as in this patient, the first diagnostic test would be a measurement of acetylcholine receptor antibody titers, followed by repetitive stimulation tests and single-fiber electromyography if necessary.

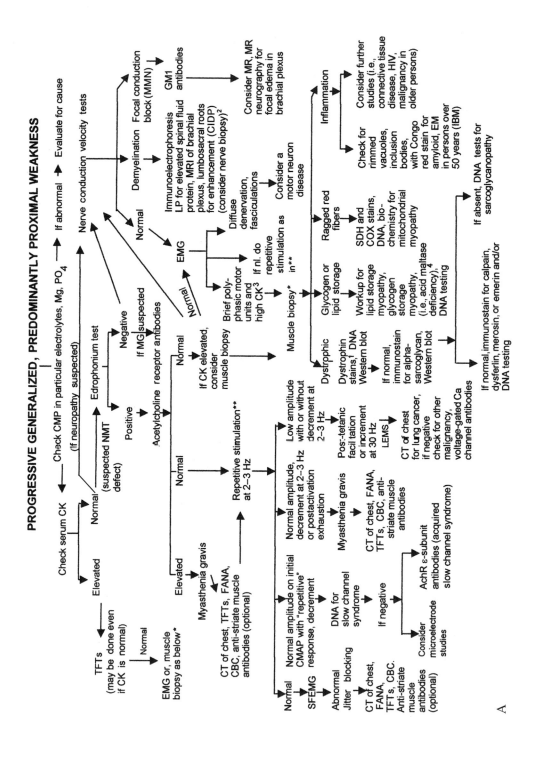

Figure A1.1 A. Progressive generalized predominantly proximal weakness. (1 = if phenotype of dystrophinopathy, can do DNA test prior to the biopsy [see (**B**)]; 2 = if uniformly slow and clinically suspected, check DNA for CMT [generalized weakness, however, is not a characteristic presentation]; 3 = if clinical and EMG myotonia, consider PROMM and do DNA testing; 4 = particularly if myotonia is seen on EMG but without symptoms of clinical myotonia.)

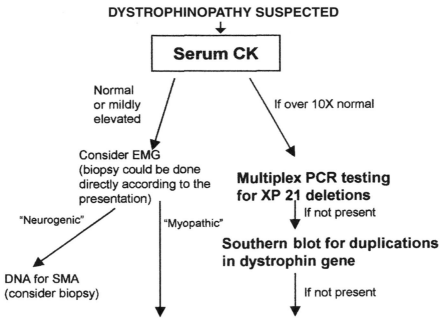

B. Workup of a patient suspected of dystrophinopathy.

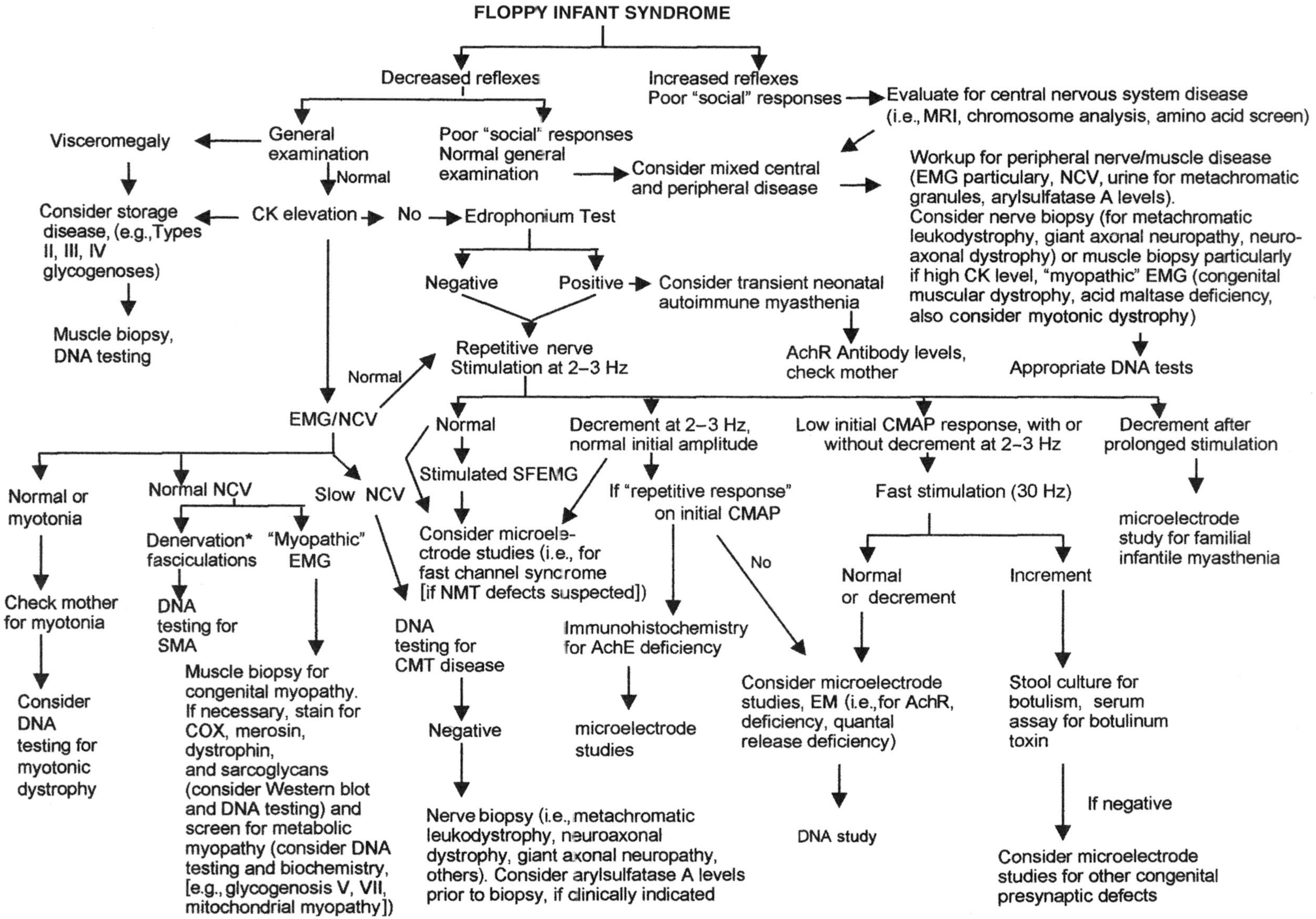

Figure A1.2 Floppy infant syndrome. (* = If negative, do histamine test for Riley-Day syndrome and consider a DNA test.)

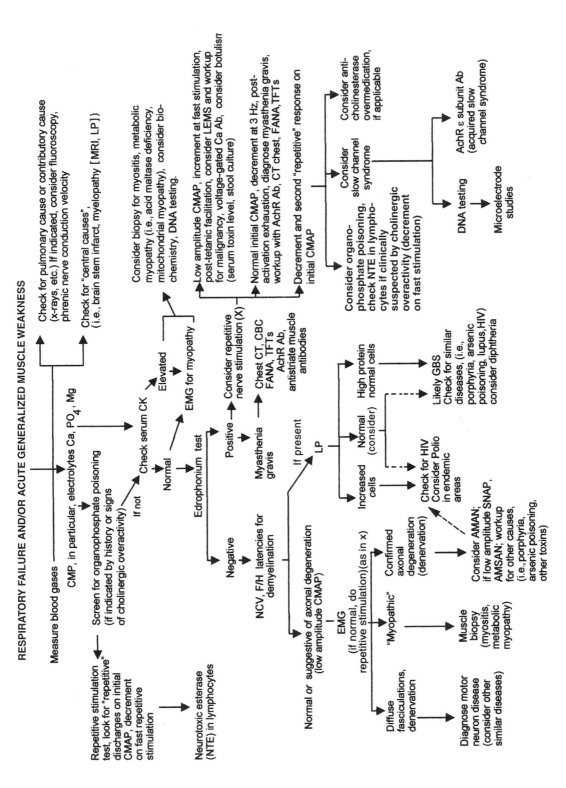

Figure A1.3 Respiratory failure and/or acute generalized muscle weakness.

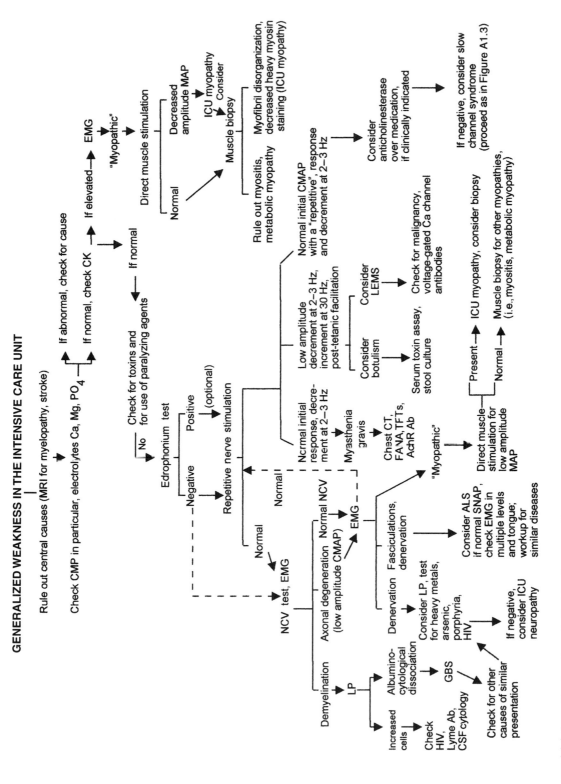

Figure A1.4 Generalized weakness in the intensive care unit.

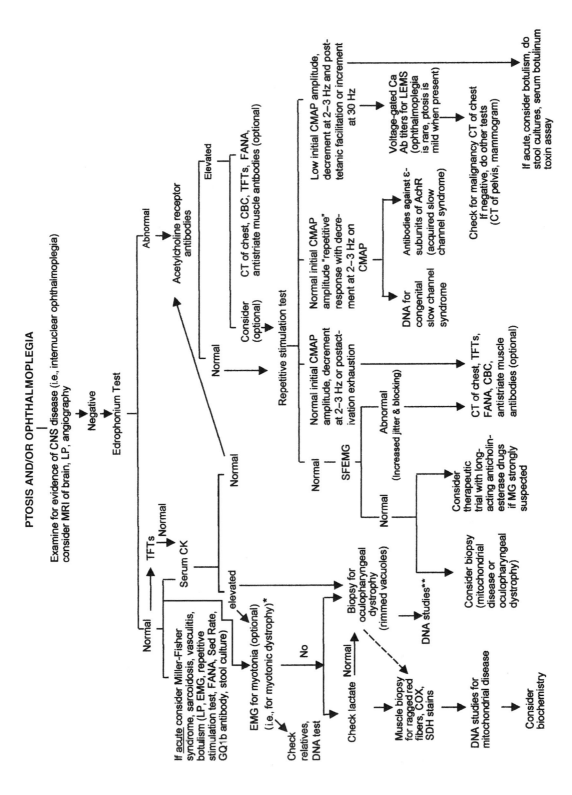

Figure A1.5 Ptosis and/or ophthalmoplegia. (* = If suspected even with normal CK; ** = may do prior to biopsy if clinical indication or positive family history.)

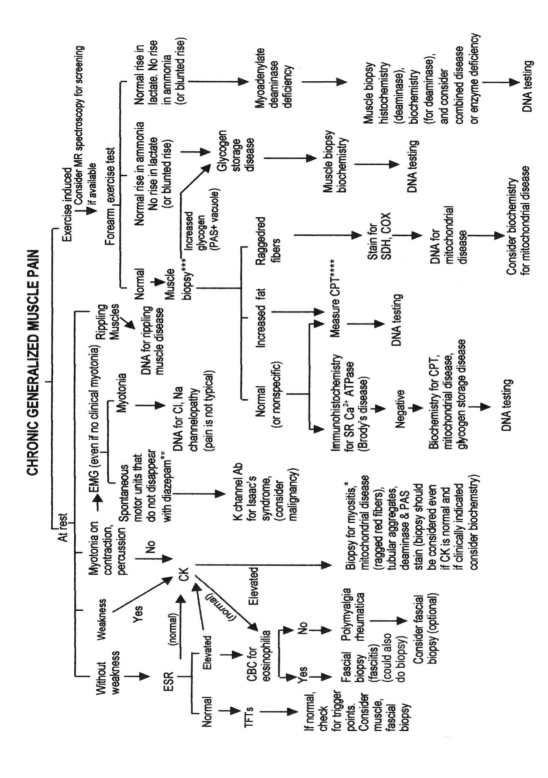

Figure A1.6 Chronic generalized muscle pain. (* = May do if indicated, even with normal CK. ** = If spontaneous motor units that disappear with diazepam, consider stiff-man syndrome, but both diseases present mainly with prominent muscle stiffness [see Figure A1.7]. *** = The biopsy should also be checked for tubular aggregates, deaminase, fat stains, glycogen enzymes, and PAS. **** = CPT deficiency causes pain mainly during myoglobinuric attack.)

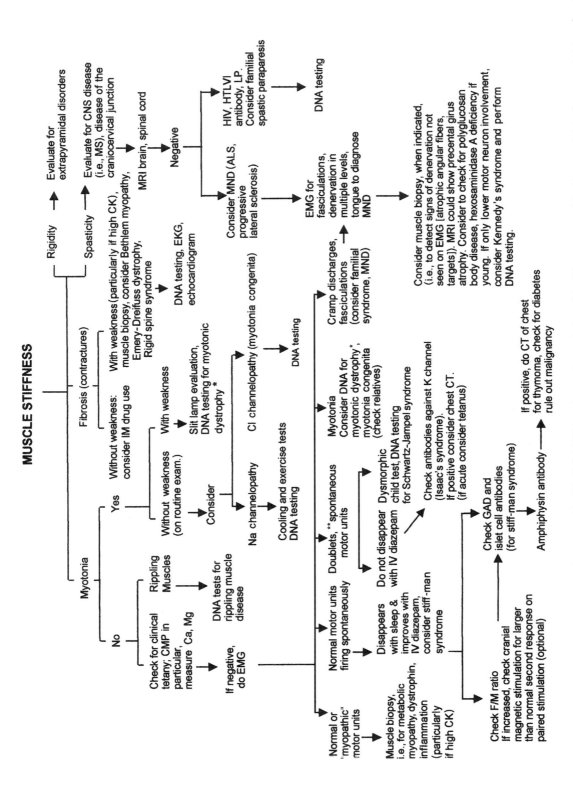

Figure A1.7 Muscle stiffness. (* = If proximal weakness, consider PROMM, DNA testing, and test relatives. ** = The presence of doublets or triplets also suggests tetany [need to check Ca, Mg, ionized Ca, and consider normocalcemic tetany].)

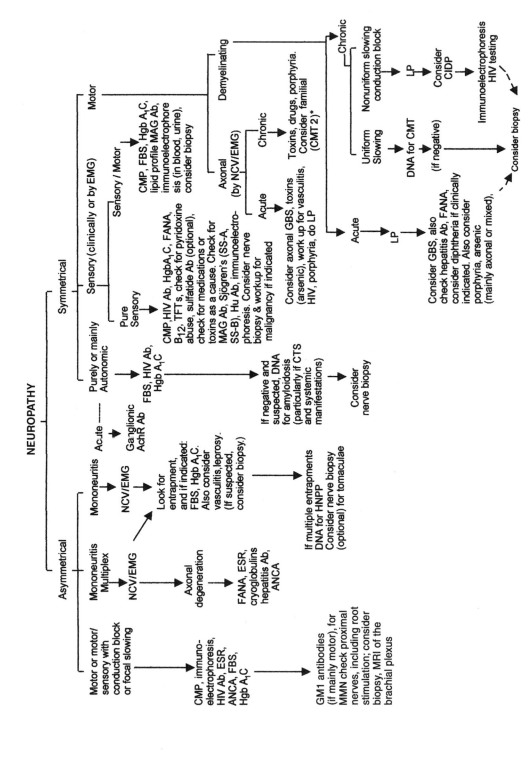

Figure A1.8 Signs and symptoms of neuropathy. In this, as in other pathways, a proper history should be considered along with the results of routine laboratory tests (i.e., familial diseases, history of alcoholism, diabetes, and medication or drug exposure). (* = Also consider distal myopathies in their initial clinical assessment, to be confirmed by EMG, CK levels, and biopsy.) (Modified from AK Asbury, PK Thomas. The Clinical Approach to Neuropathy. In AK Asbury, PK Thomas [eds], Peripheral Nerve Disorders. Boston: Butterworth, 1995;19.)

The following abbreviations are found in Figures A1.1 through A1.8: Ab = antibody; AChE = acetylcholinesterase; AChR = acetylcholine receptor; ALS = amyotrophic lateral sclerosis; AMAN = acute motor axonal neuropathy; AMSAN = acute motor and sensory axonal neuropathy; ANCA = antineutrophil cytoplasmic antibodies; ATP = adenosine triphosphate; BMD = Becker's muscular dystrophy; CMAP = compound muscle action potential; CK = creatine kinase; CBC = complete blood count; CIDP = chronic inflammatory demyelinating polyneuropathy; CMAP = compound muscle action potential; CMP = cardiomyopathy; CMT = Charcot-Marie-Tooth disease; CNS = central nervous system; COX = cytochrome oxidase; CPT = carnitine palmitoyl transferase; CSF = cerebrospinal fluid; CT = computed tomography; DMD = Duchenne's muscular dystrophy; DNA = deoxyribonucleic acid; EKG = electrocardiogram; EM = electron microscopy; EMG = electromyography; ESR = erythrocyte sedimentation rate; FANA = fluorescent antinuclear antibody; FBS = fasting blood sugar; F/H = F response/H reflex ratio; F/M = F wave/compound muscle action potential or H wave; GAD = glutamic acid dehydrogenase; GBS = Guillain-Barré syndrome; Hgb = hemoglobin; HIV = human immunodeficiency virus; HNPP = hereditary neuropathy with liability to pressure palsy; HTLVI = human T-cell lymphotrophic virus type I; IBM = inclusion body myositis; ICU = intensive care unit; LEMS = Lambert-Eaton myasthenic syndrome; LP = lumbar puncture; MAG = myelin-associated glycoprotein; MAP = muscle action potential; MMN = multifocal motor neuropathy; MND = motor neuron disease; MR = magnetic resonance; MRI = magnetic resonance imaging; MS = multiple sclerosis; NCV = nerve conduction velocity; NMT = neuromuscular transmission; NTE = neurotoxic esterase; PAS = periodic acid–Schiff; PCR = polymerase chain reaction; PROMM = proximal myotonic myopathy; SDH = succinate dehydrogenase; SF = single fiber; SFEMG = single-fiber electromyography; SMA = spinal muscular atrophy; SNAP = sensory nerve action potential; SS = Sjögren's syndrome; TFT = thyroid function test.

SUMMARY OF THE CLINICAL AND ELECTRODIAGNOSTIC APPROACHES TO FOCAL NEUROMUSCULAR CONDITION

C2 through C4 cervical roots/cervical plexus

Causes
Injuries of the high cervical roots can be caused by trauma or tumors involving the cervical spine, disk herniations, arthritic spurs, and herpetic lesions; lateral neck surgery, tumors, trauma, and radiation could damage the plexus.

Symptoms
Weakness of the trapezius and sternocleidomastoid muscles and/or unilateral diaphragmatic paralysis. There may be dermatomal sensory deficit in C2 through C4 dermatomes of the head and neck; in lesions involving the greater auricular nerve, there is decreased sensation behind and below the ear.

Clinical diagnosis
The diagnosis is made by the presence of weakness of the affected muscles and/or sensory loss in the cervical root dermatome.

Electrodiagnosis
Latency measurements of the accessory nerve to the upper trapezius and phrenic nerve to the diaphragm are useful in plexopathies. Denervation may be seen in affected muscles; denervation of paraspinal muscles helps to diagnosis radiculopathy. Electrophysiologic tests should rule out a diffuse condition (i.e., ALS).

Other tests
MRI of the spine or plexus. Plain chest x-rays or fluoroscopy to demonstrate diaphragmatic paralysis.

Spinal accessory nerve

Causes
Common causes of the spinal accessory nerve damage are surgery of the lateral neck, tumors, radiation, trauma, and jugular vein cannulation. Intracranially, the accessory nerve could be damaged by tumors also affecting the vagus and glossopharyngeal nerves (Vernet syndrome).

Symptoms
Atrophy and weakness of the upper trapezius, discomfort with variable pain in shoulder and upper scapular area; may also cause weak sternocleidomastoid muscle if the axons to this muscle are affected.

Clinical diagnosis
"Drop shoulder," weak and atrophic trapezius, sternocleidomastoid muscles; outward deviation and winging of the scapulae.

Electrodiagnosis
Denervation in the trapezius and sternocleidomastoid muscles, diminished CMAP amplitude with stimulation of the spinal accessory nerve and recording from the trapezius and stimulating the spinal accessory nerve, particularly when compared to the opposite side; otherwise, normal studies.

Phrenic nerve

Causes
Neck trauma, tumors, traction injuries, catheterization, thoracic surgery, fractures, tuberculosis, brachial neuritis, diabetes, and sarcoidosis.

Symptoms
Mild dyspnea; this could be severe in bilateral diaphragmatic paralysis.

Clinical diagnosis
May not be obvious clinically in unilateral lesions; in bilateral lesions, there could be paroxysmal abdominal movements during breathing and the use of accessory respiratory muscles.

Electrodiagnosis
Phrenic nerve conduction comparing with the opposite side; diaphragmatic EMG may show denervation. This should also be used to rule out other processes such as ALS, myopathies, and diffuse polyneuropathy.

Other tests
Chest x-rays, fluoroscopy, and MRI of the neck could be useful to rule out plexus lesion, if suspected.

Other cervical radiculopathies

Causes
These are not reviewed in detail. These are frequently caused by disk herniation and occasionally by tumors (e.g., neuromas) and osteophytes.

Symptoms
: Radicular pain, weakness, numbness.

Clinical diagnosis
: Diminished reflexes in the affected distribution, dermatomal sensory deficit, and weakness of the affected muscles.

Electrodiagnosis
: Electrophysiologic studies show normal nerve conduction velocities, although there could be prolongation of the F responses of the nerves with affected axons, and/or low amplitude of the CMAP in chronic cases. Absent H reflex in affected nerves such as flexor carpi radialis. Normal SNAP in the affected dermatome (i.e., normal radial, ulnar, and median nerve sensory studies). Electromyography may show reduced number of motor units and/or denervation in muscles innervated by the affected roots and in the paraspinal muscles. For example, involvement of C5 and C6 roots could cause a reduced number of motor units and denervation in biceps, brachioradialis, deltoids, and supra- and infraspinatus. The rhomboids are denervated only in C5 root lesions. C7 root lesions affect the triceps, extensor carpi radialis, extensor digitorum, pronator teres, and flexor carpi radialis. C8 and T1 root lesions involving the flexor digitorum, profundus (ulnar half) flexor carpi ulnaris, extensor indicis, and hand muscles *(for details about muscle innervation, see Table 2.14).*

  If paraspinal denervation is not present, denervation should include muscles innervated by different nerves but by the same roots. In C5 and C6 cervical radiculopathy, there is denervation in the serratus anterior, levator scapula, and the rhomboids, which nerves originate directly from the roots and not from the plexus. Thus, their denervation helps to diagnose radiculopathy and differentiate from focal brachial plexopathy. EMG should rule out a diffuse process such as ALS.

Other tests
: MRI of the neck, postmyelogram CT scan for diagnosis and to exclude other conditions (i.e., syringomyelic cavities produce muscle atrophy in involved segments).

Brachial plexus
Upper trunk

Causes
: Compression from the hypertrophic muscles, trauma, "burner's" or "stinger" syndrome from athletic trauma, stretching, rucksack paralysis, tumors, autoimmune brachial neuropathy, radiation, positioning from anesthesia, hereditary brachial neuropathy, Duchenne-Erb paralysis at birth.

Symptoms
: Weakness of the proximal muscles of the upper extremities, particularly the supra- and infraspinatus, deltoids, biceps, and brachioradialis.

Clinical diagnosis
: Weak affected muscles, diminished biceps, brachioradialis reflexes, and sensory deficit over the lateral aspect of the shoulder, lateral forearm, and first two digits.

Electrodiagnosis
: Electrodiagnostic studies may show prolonged motor latency to the involved muscles when stimulating at Erb's point or low-amplitude CMAP when compared to the opposite side. SNAP of the nerves supplying the affected territories (e.g., the first two digits of the hand or the lateral cutaneous nerve of the forearm) could be of low amplitude. EMG studies are used to differentiate from radiculopathy or a diffuse process. This could show denervation and myokymia in the affected muscles but not in the paraspinals, serratus, rhomboids, or other limb muscles, in which nerves do not pass through the upper trunk (in autoimmune brachial neuropathy, other limb muscles may be affected). If abnormalities are found, it may be necessary to perform nerve conduction tests and EMG in the opposite limb or a leg to exclude a more diffuse process. Somatosensory evoked responses and root stimulation may be useful.

Other tests
: MRI with contrast and MR neurography of the plexus.

Middle trunk

Causes
: Trauma, fracture of the clavicle, tumors, and radiation; these frequently also affect the upper trunk.

Symptoms	Weakness of wrist and finger extension, patchy arm numbness mainly in dorsum of forearm and hand. Affected muscles include the triceps, extensor carpi radialis, extensor digitorum, and normal strength in the brachioradialis, biceps, and hand muscles.
Clinical diagnosis	Diminished triceps reflex, normal brachioradialis and biceps reflexes, diminished sensation of dorsal forearm and hand.
Electrodiagnosis	Radial motor conduction may reveal low amplitude CMAP. SNAP of median nerve to the middle finger may be of low amplitude with normal SNAP to the index finger. Nerve conduction velocities should be measured on other nerves, such as the median motor and SNAPs to other digits. EMG could show denervation in the affected muscles listed above and in the latissimus dorsi, flexor digitorum, flexor carpi radialis pronator teres, flexor pollicis longus, and flexor digitorum and is normal in the brachioradialis, flexor carpi ulnaris, first dorsal interosseous, and, particularly, the paraspinal muscles. Myokymic discharges may be seen in affected muscles, particularly in radiation plexopathy.
Other tests	MRI with contrast of the plexus.

Lower trunk

Causes	Thoracic outlet syndrome from hypertrophic scalenus muscle, cervical rib. Upper lung cancer, other tumors (neuromas, lymphomas), aponeurotic bands, trauma, complication of thoracic surgery, and Klumpke's paralysis at birth.
Symptoms	Weakness of the ulnar and median innervated muscles of the hand, finger and thumb flexion and extension, pain and numbness of the last two digits.
Clinical diagnosis	Demonstration of weakness of affected muscles, sensory deficit in fifth finger, dorsum of hand, medial forearm; Horner's syndrome.
Electrodiagnosis	Nerve conduction velocities of the ulnar nerve to Erb's point may show proximal slowing, conduction block, or decreased amplitude CMAP compared to the opposite side. Prolonged F latency, the SNAP of the ulnar nerve to the fifth digit as well as its dorsal cutaneous branch, and the median cutaneous nerve of the forearm could be of low amplitude. EMG may show denervation in the lower trunk muscles such as the flexor and extensor carpi ulnaris, ulnar and median innervated muscles of the hand, flexor digitorum profundus (ulnar half), pronator quadratus, extensor pollicis longus, and extensor digitorum. EMG in other muscles such as the biceps, deltoid, flexor carpi radialis, pronator teres, brachioradialis, and paraspinals should be normal. Somatosensory evoked responses could be helpful to demonstrate slowing or absence of the Erb's potential.
Other tests	MRI with and without contrast, MR neurography, chest x-rays.

Brachial plexus cords

Causes	Similar to those affecting the trunks, including trauma, tumors, compressions, and radiation.
Symptoms	Weakness of muscles innervated by nerves whose axons pass through the affected cords and sensory loss in their dermatomes.

Lateral cord

Symptoms	Affects elbow flexion, supination, and pronation of the forearm and wrist flexion.
Clinical diagnosis	Involved muscles include the pectoralis major, biceps, flexor carpi radialis, and pronator teres with decreased sensation of the lateral forearm and thumb; absent biceps reflex.
Electrodiagnosis	Decreased SNAP amplitude of the medial nerve to the first and second digits and lateral antebrachial cutaneous nerve and denervation in the muscles listed above (Clinical diagnosis). Other shoulder and arm muscles as well as paraspinals should be normal

Posterior cord

Symptoms
Affects the elbow, wrist and finger extension, supination of the forearm, and shoulder abduction.

Clinical diagnosis
Weakness of affected muscles, including the deltoids, brachioradialis, triceps, extensor carpi radialis, extensor digitorum, and indicis proprius. There is decreased sensation in the dorsum of the forearm and hand, posterior aspect of the arm, and lateral aspect of the shoulder.

Electrodiagnosis
Decreased SNAP amplitude of the radial nerve to the base of the thumb. EMG could demonstrate denervation of the affected muscles described above and also teres and latissimus dorsi sparing the paraspinal muscles and muscles innervated by the lateral cord (see above) and medial cord (see below).

Medial cord

Symptoms
Weak wrist, finger, and thumb flexion and abduction; particularly weak hand muscles.

Clinical diagnosis
Decreased sensation in the medial forearm, medial palm, and fourth and fifth digits; absent finger flexion reflexes.

Electrodiagnosis
Decreased CMAP of median and ulnar nerves, decreased SNAP of ulnar nerve to the fifth digit, the dorsal cutaneous branch of the ulnar nerve, and the medial antebrachial cutaneous nerve. Denervation in hand muscles, flexor carpi ulnaris, flexor digitorum profundus, and pronator quadratus.

Long thoracic nerve

Causes
Stab wound, heavy shoulder bags, shoulder braces, thoracotomy, mastectomy, surgery for removal of the first ribs, vigorous athletic activities, and brachial neuritis.

Symptoms
Serratus anterior weakness, winging of the scapula pain.

Clinical diagnosis
Normal examination except for characteristic winging of weak serratus.

Electrodiagnosis
Motor latency testing the serratus, measure latency to other muscles of the shoulder girdle or opposite serratus to compare. EMG of serratus could show denervation; other shoulder muscles and paraspinal muscles should be normal. Tests should rule out radiculopathy, brachial neuropathy, or a diffuse process.

Dorsal scapular nerve

Causes
Stretching, trauma, and cervical masses.

Symptoms
Pain and weakness in the levator scapulae and rhomboids (causing difficulty raising the outstretched arm).

Clinical diagnosis
Weakness of the affected muscles (retraction of the scapulae) and winging of the scapula during wide abduction.

Electrodiagnosis
Could show denervation of levator scapulae and rhomboids but not in other shoulder girdle muscles or paraspinals. These are studied to rule out radiculopathy or a diffuse process.

Suprascapular neuropathy

Causes
Damage of the suprascapular nerve at the suprascapular notch by the ligament, other fibrous tissue, stretching the suprascapular nerve, trauma, brachial neuritis, compression at the spinoglenoid notch.

Symptoms
Pain in the scapular area with atrophy and/or weakness of the supra- and infraspinatus. Lesions at the spinoglenoid notch produce atrophy only in the infraspinatus.

Clinical diagnosis
Reproduction of pain on palpation and atrophy and weakness of the affected muscles. Clinical diagnosis should rule out brachial neuritis and C5 and C6 radiculopathy.

Electrodiagnosis — Prolonged latency or low-amplitude CMAP when recording the affected muscles with stimulation at Erb's point, when compared to the opposite side, other normal nerve conduction tests. Denervation of the affected muscles. EMG should rule out radiculopathy, high plexus lesion, brachial neuritis, and a diffuse process.

Axillary nerve

Causes — Brachial neuritis, fracture, and dislocation of the head of the humerus, intramuscular injections, intraoperative injury.

Symptoms — Pain, difficulty raising or abducting the arm, atrophy of the deltoids, and decreased sensation in the shoulder and arms.

Clinical diagnosis — Weakness and atrophy of the deltoid; decreased sensation in the axillary nerve territory in the shoulder.

Electrodiagnosis — Motor latency of the axillary nerve to deltoid, stimulating at Erb's point could be prolonged, and the CMAP may be of low amplitude when compared with the opposite side. Denervation is seen only in deltoid and teres minor and not in other shoulder girdle muscles or paraspinals. EMG should rule out C5 and C6 radiculopathy, upper trunk plexopathy, and a more diffuse process.

Other — Plain x-rays and MRI could be useful.

Musculocutaneous nerve

Causes — Fractures of the humerus, trauma, masses, excessive exercise, surgery, entrapment of the coracobrachialis muscle, brachial neuritis.

Symptoms — Weakness, atrophy of elbow flexion, and numbness in outer forearm.

Clinical diagnosis — Weak biceps, decreased or absent biceps reflex, and decreased sensation in the lateral aspect of the forearm.

Electrodiagnosis — Prolonged motor latency of the musculocutaneous nerve recording from the biceps, decreased CMAP amplitude, and decreased SNAP amplitude of lateral antebrachial cutaneous nerve. EMG shows denervation in the biceps, brachialis, and coracobrachialis. EMG should be normal in C5 and C6 and other upper extremity muscles or paraspinals (done to rule out radiculopathy). Should also rule out a more diffuse process.

Other tests — Plain x-rays, MRI.

Radial nerve

Compression at the spiral groove

Causes — Trauma, fracture of the humerus, pressure (Saturday night palsy), masses, tourniquets and compression during surgery, HNPP, multifocal motor neuropathy.

Symptoms — Radial sensory loss at the dorsum of the hand, wrist drop. Triceps muscle is spared (affected in higher lesions such as axilla, involving also the median and ulnar nerves in the triad syndrome [i.e., from crutches]).

Clinical diagnosis — Pain at the site of compression, weakness of the wrist and finger extensors, decreased sensation in the radial nerve territory, normal triceps reflex, and decreased brachioradialis reflex.

Electrodiagnosis — Radial nerve SNAP could be normal initially but is of low amplitude or absent later, particularly in severe lesions. Radial nerve CMAP could be of low amplitude in chronic cases, or there is evidence of conduction block at the level of the lesion. EMG shows denervation in radial innervated muscles except the triceps and anconeus (both affected in lesions of the radial nerve in the axilla). Electrodiagnostic tests should rule out C7 radiculopathy, plexopathies of the middle trunk or posterior cord, diffuse neuropathy, and other radial nerve lesions.

Other tests — Plain x-rays of the humerus, MRI.

"Radial tunnel syndrome"

Causes	Lesions of the whole radial nerve at different points at the elbow by fusion bands from the brachioradialis to the brachialis muscle, compression at the arcade of Frohse, and the extensor carpi radialis, tumors, trauma, and abnormal vessels such as the "leash of Henry," which are a group of vessels from the radial recurrent artery and veins.
Clinical diagnosis	Patients have very little sensory deficit, but they have pain, particularly in the lateral elbow when extending the middle finger with the elbow extended. In some, there is no weakness, just joint pain, but there could be finger and wrist extensor weakness. Some patients complain of nonspecific weakness in the arms.
Electrodiagnosis	Electrodiagnostic test could be normal or show chronic neurogenic changes or denervation in the radial innervated muscles of the forearm.
Other tests	MRI of the elbow.

Posterior interosseous syndrome

Causes	Compression of the posterior interosseous branch (motor) of the radial nerve. This occurs at the arcade of Frohse or at the supinator muscle itself due to repetitive pronation and supination of the hand, masses, vascular malformation, trauma, fractures, or dislocation of the radius.
Symptoms	Pain in the elbow, weakness of the finger extensors, and thumb abduction, and normal sensation in the radial nerve distribution.
Clinical diagnosis	Weakness of finger extension, thumb abduction; there could be a radial deviation of the wrist during wrist extension from a weak extensor carpi ulnaris muscle; normal sensation and otherwise normal examination.
Electrodiagnosis	Normal SNAP of the radial nerve. CMAP of the extensor indicis obtained with stimulation at the elbow could be of prolonged latency or low amplitude when compared to the opposite side. Denervation in muscles innervated by the posterior interosseous nerve (e.g., extensor digitorum communis, extensor indices propious, extensor carpi ulnaris, and abductor and extensor pollicis longus), sparing the triceps, the brachioradialis, supinator, and extensor carpi radialis. Electrophysiologic tests should rule out more proximal radial nerve lesions, plexopathy, and C7 radiculopathy.
Other tests	MRI of the elbow could be helpful.

Superficial radial nerve

Causes	Lesions between the brachioradialis and extensor carpi radialis longus and by hypertrophic fibrous bands. At the wrist, the nerve could be damaged by tight wristbands, handcuffs, intravenous needles, or surgery—all causing cheiralgia paresthetica.
Symptoms	Pain, numbness in radial territory in the dorsum of the hand.
Clinical diagnosis	Positive Tinel's sign; decreased sensation over the dorsum of the thumb; no weakness.
Electrodiagnosis	Absent or prolonged radial nerve SNAP latency with normal motor conduction and normal electromyography.

Median nerve

Elbow lesions

Causes	Compression of the median nerve at the ligament of Struthers by a fibrous band and hypertrophic pronator teres muscle (pronator syndrome), trauma, tumor, and vascular malformation. The nerve could also be damaged by masses or trauma in the arm and the axilla, where the ulnar and radial nerves could also be affected (triad syndrome).

Symptoms
Pain at the site of compression, weakness of median innervated muscles of the forearm or hand, numbness in median nerve territory in the hand dermatome, and pain during supination and pronation.

Clinical diagnosis
Pain at the site of compression, demonstration of weakness of the median innervated muscles, sensory deficit in the median nerve distribution, reproduction of pain on palpation and on pronation and supination (in the pronator syndrome).

Electrodiagnosis
Conduction velocity of the median nerve at or above the elbow to the wrist could be slow or could show evidence of conduction block. Motor latency of the flexor carpi radialis could be prolonged when compared to the opposite side. SNAP of the median nerve of low amplitude in chronic cases. EMG could show denervation or reduced motor unit recruitment in muscles innervated by the median nerve and anterior interosseous muscle in the forearm or hands. The pronator teres is frequently spared in the pronator syndrome.

Other tests
MR neurography and MRI could be helpful to detect the cause and site of the lesion.

Anterior interosseous syndrome

Causes
Compression of the anterior interosseous branch of the median nerve by fibrous tissue, anomalous muscles, tendinous origin of the ulnar head of the pronator teres, tumors, repeated supination or pronation, karate, venous access cut-downs, and catheterizations.

Symptoms
Pain in the forearm, weakness of flexion of the fingers and thumb.

Clinical diagnosis
Weakness of flexion of the distal phalanx of the thumb and second and third digits, normal thenar eminence muscle, normal sensation. Particularly important is the inability to produce the "O," "OK," or "pinch" sign.

Electrodiagnosis
Normal nerve conduction velocity of the median nerve. Prolongation of latency to the pronator quadratus (very difficult technically). Normal median SNAP latency and amplitude. EMG could show denervation or reduced motor unit recruitment only in muscles innervated by the anterior interosseous nerve, such as the flexor pollicis longus, flexor digitorum profundus, and pronator quadratus.

Other tests
MRI could detect masses or abnormal muscles. MR neurography could be useful.

Carpal tunnel syndrome

Causes
Compression of the median nerve at the wrist at the carpal tunnel could be caused by repetitive movements, such as typing, excessive computer use, and other causes such as rheumatoid arthritis, acromegaly, pregnancy, diabetes, HNPP, hypothyroidism, amyloids, masses, and cysts.

Symptoms
Pain in the hands, particularly at night, numbness in the first three digits and half of the fourth, and weakness of the thenar muscles.

Clinical diagnosis
Positive Phalen's test and Tinel's sign at the wrist and decreased sensation in the median nerve distribution in the hand. In chronic severe cases, there could be weakness and atrophy of the median thenar muscles.

Electrodiagnosis
Prolonged median nerve SNAP latency with stimulation at the median nerve digits and particularly palmar sensory responses. This should be compared to the ulnar, radial, and opposite median nerve. Prolonged distal median motor latency in chronic cases (less sensitive). EMG is usually normal early but could show decreased number of motor units in more severe chronic cases. EMG could be useful, when clinically indicated, to rule out other conditions that might also be present (i.e., radiculopathy) or to rule out more proximal lesions.

Other tests
MRI, MR neurography could be helpful to detect structural abnormalities. Other tests should be done to rule out a more diffuse process, such as polyneuropathy, and the patient should be worked up for predisposing causes (i.e., diabetes, hypothyroidism). If multiple entrapments are present, HNPP should be considered.

Digital nerve lesions

Causes
Median nerve digital branches could be entrapped by continuous pressure and in the intermetacarpal tunnels by inflammation and fractures.

Symptoms
Numbness in the involved digits, pain.

Clinical diagnosis
Should exclude carpal tunnel syndrome and should show evidence of abnormalities only in affected digits. The median innervated muscles are normal.

Electrodiagnosis
SNAP of the median nerve should be abnormal or low amplitude only in the affected digits. EMG is normal.

Ulnar nerve

Compression at the elbow

Causes
Bony abnormalities, rheumatoid arthritis, acute trauma, recurrent trauma, subluxation of the nerve at the elbow due to absence of the aponeurotic arcade, fibrous tissue, hypertrophic retinaculum, chronic compression, pressure during anesthesia. Predisposing factors such as diabetes or HNPP. (The nerve could also be damaged at the axilla by compression [i.e., crutches].)

Symptoms
Numbness in the fifth digit and half of the fourth digit, dorsum, ulnar area of the hand, atrophy and hand weakness, clumsy hand, poor grip. The patient could report that the fifth digit is caught when he or she places the hand in the pocket due to weak adduction.

Clinical diagnosis
Based on reproduction of symptoms, positive Tinel's sign, decreased sensation in the ulnar nerve distribution in the fifth digit and ulnar half of the fourth digit, dorsum, and ulnar palmar area of the hand, weakness and/or atrophy of the ulnar innervated muscles, and positive Froment's sign.

Electrodiagnosis
There may be a drop of motor nerve conduction velocity or conduction block across the elbow. Inching technique might be necessary to clearly localize this. The results need to be compared to the opposite side. Ulnar SNAP is of low amplitude in the fifth digit and the palm, as well as that of the dorsal cutaneous branch. EMG could show denervation and low recruitment of motor units in the ulnar-innervated muscles of the hand and the ulnar part of the flexor digitorum profundus. The flexor carpi ulnaris may be normal. Median nerve muscles and other C8 and T1 lower trunk innervated muscles are also normal. Electrodiagnosis should rule out C8-T1 radiculopathy, brachial plexus lesion at the lower trunk and medial cord, and distal ulnar entrapment, as well as a diffuse process such as polyneuropathy. ALS and multifocal motor neuropathy should also be ruled out by testing multiple segments, particularly if the deficit is purely motor.

Compression at the wrist and hand

Causes
Trauma, compression of the ulnar nerve at the canal of Guyon, or distal compression, such as at the hook of the hamate bone, or in the palm, neuromas, repetitive pressure, bicycling.

Symptoms
Pain, numbness (if the lesion is proximal to the sensory branch of the fifth digit), and atrophy or weakness of ulnar muscles according to the area of the compression. If the lesion is at or distal to the hamate, it spares the hypothenar muscles.

Clinical diagnosis
Positive Tinel's sign at the wrist, numbness in the ulnar distribution, and weakness in the affected muscles.

Electrodiagnosis
Low-amplitude or prolonged ulnar fifth digit SNAP if compression affects this branch at the Guyon's canal, normal dorsal cutaneous branch SNAP, prolonged latency to the first dorsal interosseous when compared to the abductor digiti minimi or when compared to the opposite side. EMG would determine if damage is distal and thus does not affect the hypothenar muscles and show denervation of the ulnar innervated hand muscles according to the location of the lesion. The tests should exclude other conditions, such as C8 and T1 radiculopathy, plexus lesions, and proximal ulnar entrapment.

Other tests
: MRI of the hand could be useful.

Lumbosacral radiculopathy

Lumbar radiculopathy

Causes
: Lumbar radiculopathy is caused by protruded intravertebral disks, bone spurs, and other intraspinal processes. (Cytomegalovirus infections affect the whole cauda equina.)

Symptoms
: Symptoms of the high lumbar roots produce pain, which may be radiated to the anterior thigh and the inguinal area. Numbness in the territory of affected root dermatome.

Clinical diagnosis
: Positive femoral stretch test, diminished sensation in the distribution of the affected root dermatome, weakness of the femoral and obturator innervated muscles, absent knee jerk, and adductor reflex. If L1 and L2 roots are affected, there could be a diminished cremasteric reflex.

Electrodiagnosis
: Normal motor conduction velocity, normal sensory evoked responses. There could be prolonged femoral nerve H reflex and femoral T reflex. EMG shows denervation and/or low motor unit recruitment in femoral and obturator innervated muscles and denervation in paraspinal muscles.

Other tests
: Lumbosacral MRI, CT scan, postmyelogram CT scan.

Lower lumbosacral radiculopathy

Causes
: Lower lumbosacral radiculopathy is most often caused by intervertebral disk protrusion and bone spurs and can also be caused by other intraspinal processes such as tumors and infections.

Symptoms
: Pain in the back, radiating to the posterior leg; numbness with weakness of muscles innervated by affected roots.

Clinical diagnosis
: Positive straight-leg raising test; ankle jerk could be absent in the S1 radiculopathy with evidence of sensory (see Figures 2.43 and 2.44) and/or motor deficit in areas of the affected roots. Motor deficit in affected muscles is discussed in Electrodiagnosis (see Table 2.14).

Electrodiagnosis
: Normal nerve conduction velocities; CMAP could have low amplitude in chronic cases when stimulating the peroneal nerve (L5) or tibial nerve (S1). Absent or prolonged latency of tibial H reflex in S1 radiculopathy. F responses could be prolonged in the peroneal nerve (L5) or tibial nerves (S1). Denervation in paraspinal and affected muscles (i.e., L4 through L5: tibialis anterior, extensor hallucis, tensor fascia lata, gluteus medius, sometimes in peroneus longus, short head of biceps and tibialis posterior; L5 and S1: hamstrings, gastrocnemius, soleus).

Lumbosacral plexus

Causes
: This involves lesions of the lumbar portion (lumbar plexus) or the lower portion (lumbosacral plexus). Retroperitoneal and pelvic neoplasms, intrapartum compression, diabetes and autoimmune plexopathy, radiation, surgery and abscess, severe trauma with hip fractures and hematoma.

Symptoms
: Pain in back and abdomen; weakness. Lumbar plexus lesions affect the femoral and obturator innervated muscles (hip flexion, knee extension, thigh adduction). The lower lumbosacral plexus lesions affect the sciatic innervated muscles tensor fascia latae and gluteus (hip abduction, extension, knee flexion, and foot flexion extension; adductors; abductors).

Clinical diagnosis
: In lumbar plexopathy, positive femoral stretch test. Weakness of iliopsoas, quadriceps, adductors of the thigh, absent knee jerk, decreased sensation (mainly in the inner thigh and anterior medial leg). In lower lumbosacral plexus lesions, there is weakness in the glutei, hamstrings, and tibial and peroneal innervated muscles; absent ankle reflexes, decreased sensation in posterior thigh, posterolateral lower leg, and foot.

Electrodiagnosis   Low-amplitude CMAP of affected muscles. Prolonged or absent F responses or H reflexes of affected nerves (i.e., femoral H in lumbar plexus; tibial H, F, and peroneal F in lumbosacral plexus). Low-amplitude SNAP saphenous, lateral femoral cutaneous in lumbar plexus lesions, low-amplitude sural, tibial nerve, SNAPs in lower lumbosacral plexus lesions. EMG could show decreased number of motor units, denervation of affected muscles or (as described in Clinical diagnosis and Table 2.14) sparing the paraspinals.

Other tests   MRI, CT scan of retroperitoneal area and pelvis; rule out coagulopathy and diabetes.

Ilioinguinal nerve

Causes   Surgery, trauma, dislocation of the hip joint, tumors, entrapment in abdominal muscles.

Symptoms   Pain in the inguinal area.

Clinical diagnosis   Pain on palpation of anterior-superior iliac spine radiating to inguinal area. Should rule out high lumbar disk, pelvic renal, abdominal and retroperitoneal masses.

Electrodiagnosis   Normal lower extremity and paraspinal muscles, possible denervation in the oblique internus and transversus abdominus muscles.

Genitofemoral nerve

Causes   Trauma, surgery, adhesions, compression, tumors.

Symptoms   Pain in inguinal area.

Clinical diagnosis   Absent cremasteric reflex, decreased sensation in femoral triangle.

Electrodiagnosis   Nerve conduction tests and EMG are normal.

Superior gluteal nerve

Causes   Trauma and compression by anterior-superior fibers of the piriformis muscle, complications of hip arthroplasty, intramuscular injections.

Symptoms   Pain in area above and lateral to sciatic notch.

Clinical diagnosis   Weak, atrophic gluteus medius, tensor fascia latae.

Electrodiagnosis   Denervation of gluteus medius, tensor fascia latae, and gluteus minimus; otherwise normal electromyography.

Other tests   MRI of hip area.

Inferior gluteal nerve

Causes   Trauma, intramuscular injections, colorectal cancer.

Symptoms   Pain in the buttocks, weak hip extension, atrophic gluteus maximus.

Electrodiagnosis   Denervation only of gluteus maximus; otherwise normal studies.

Other tests   MRI of hip area.

Femoral nerve

Causes   Compression at the inguinal ligament, trauma, hematomas, lesions during femoral catheterization, stretch injuries, surgery, childbirth, diabetes.

Symptoms   Pain, weakness of the knee extension, numbness of the thigh.

Clinical diagnosis   Pain on compression. Weakness of the knee extensors, normal adduction, absent knee jerk, decreased sensation in the anterior thigh and inner lower leg (saphenous nerve distribution).

Electrodiagnosis Prolonged distal latency, low amplitude of the femoral nerve CMAP, or slow conduction compared to the opposite side, absent or prolonged femoral H reflex, absent femoral T reflex, decreased number of motor units, denervation in the femoral innervated muscles; sparing the adductors and paraspinals as well as lower leg muscles.

Other test MRI of the inguinal, pelvic, and retroperitoneal areas should rule out other conditions such as diabetes and vasculitis.

Saphenous nerve

Causes Compression at the subsartorial Hunter's canal, trauma or stretching during removal of saphenous vein for cardiac bypass surgery, neuromas, fibrous bands.

Symptoms Pain in inner knee radiating to distal leg, worse with exercise.

Clinical diagnosis Pain on palpation, decreased sensation in saphenous nerve territory (inner leg).

Electrodiagnosis Low-amplitude saphenous SNAP, normal sural and superficial peroneal nerve, otherwise normal motor nerve conduction and EMG.

Lateral femoral cutaneous nerve

Causes Lesions of the lateral femoral cutaneous nerve at the anterior superior iliac spine and inguinal ligament, tight belts, corsets, carrying guns or keys in belt, surgery, retroperitoneal hematoma, tumors; predisposing factors, particularly obesity and diabetes.

Symptoms Burning paresthesias (meralgia paresthetica), numbness in the lateral femoral cutaneous distribution in the lateral thigh.

Clinical diagnosis Numbness in the lateral thigh, no weakness, positive Tinel's sign at the anterior superior iliac spine.

Electrodiagnosis Absent or low-amplitude lateral femoral cutaneous SNAP. This, however, is technically difficult, and one should check the response in the opposite side to compare. EMG of the lower extremity muscles to rule out radiculopathy, plexopathy, and femoral neuropathy is normal.

Other tests Blood sugar; consider MRI if a retroperitoneal lesion such as a hematoma is considered.

Obturator nerve

Causes The obturator nerve could be damaged by compression, hematomas, osteitis pubis, hernias, surgery at the adductor canal by the adductor membrane, or during labor.

Symptoms Pain in the inguinal area up to the inner aspect of the thigh and weakness of the thigh adductors.

Clinical diagnosis Weak adductor muscles of the hip, normal hip and knee extensors and flexors, and decreased sensation inner thigh. Normal knee reflexes and decreased or absent adductor reflex.

Electrodiagnosis Decreased number of motor units and denervation of the adductor muscles with normal quadriceps, glutei, hamstrings, and other leg muscles as well as paraspinals. Normal femoral nerve conduction and standard nerve conduction velocity tests of the leg.

Other tests MRI of obturator nerve area, particularly at the adductor canal.

Sciatic nerve

Causes Lesions of the sciatic nerve are caused by falls in the seated position, hip arthroplasty, tumors, fractures, intramuscular injections, fibrous bands, endometriosis and hypertrophy of the piriformis muscle.

Symptoms Pain at the sciatic notch, foot drop, weakness in sciatic muscles, numbness in sole of foot, posterior thigh, and posterior lateral leg.

Clinical diagnosis	Tenderness in the sciatic notch. Weakness in sciatic innervated muscles (e.g., hamstrings, gastrocnemius and soleus, tibialis posterior and tibialis anterior, peronei), absent ankle reflex, positive straight leg raise test. Tends to involve preferentially the peroneal division and thus may mimic peroneal palsy.
Electrodiagnosis	Could show absent or low-amplitude sural and superficial peroneal SNAP and prolonged or absent H reflex and F responses of the tibial and peroneal nerves. Normal nerve conductions in the tibial and peroneal nerves but could show low amplitude CMAP. EMG may show denervation of the tibial and peroneal innervated muscles and hamstrings, normal gluteus medius, tensor fascia latae, femoral innervated muscles, and paraspinal muscles. To diagnose involvement of the peroneal division of the sciatic nerve, the short head of the biceps may show denervation, which is not present in peroneal nerve lesions.
Other tests	MRI of the sciatic notch, hip, and upper thigh area.

Sural nerve

Causes	Cysts, tumors, and compression by thigh boots, surgery.
Symptoms	Pain, decreased sensation on outer aspect of foot and posterior lateral lower leg.
Clinical diagnosis	Decreased sensation in sural nerve distribution.
Electrodiagnosis	Low-amplitude prolonged sural nerve SNAP; otherwise normal tests.
Other tests	Not necessary.

Peroneal nerve

Causes	Compression, trauma, stretching at the fibular head, prolonged crossing of the legs, coma, arthroscopy, surgery of the popliteal fossa, knee surgery, compartment syndrome, prolonged general surgery.
Symptoms	Foot drop and numbness.
Clinical diagnosis	Weakness of the peroneal innervated muscles, sparing of the foot plantar flexors, and invertors, sensory deficits in the common peroneal distribution, deep peroneal or superficial peroneal distribution according to the site of the lesion.
Electrodiagnosis	Low amplitude of the superficial peroneal nerve SNAP compared to a normal sural nerve and compared to the opposite side. Conduction slowing or conduction block of the peroneal nerve across the knee. EMG may show denervation decreased number of motor units in the peroneal innervated muscles according the site of the lesion, sparing the short head of the biceps. The peroneus longus and brevis are affected in common peroneal and superficial peroneal nerve lesions but not in deep peroneal lesions. In deep peroneal (and common peroneal) nerve lesions, the tibialis anterior, extensor hallucis, and pollicis are affected. EMG should rule out a sciatic nerve lesion, plexopathy, and L5 radiculopathy. EMG studies should thus include tibial innervated muscles, hamstrings, tibialis posterior, tensor fascia latae, gluteus, and paraspinals. If a diffuse process is suspected, the other leg should be tested.
Other tests	Rule out predisposing causes, such as diabetes, vasculitis, HNPP, polyneuropathy, and other conditions that manifest by foot drop such as ALS.

"Anterior tarsal tunnel" syndrome

Causes	Stretching or compression of the deep peroneal nerve as it passes through the extensor retinaculum compressions, stretching.
Symptoms	Pain in dorsum of the foot and weakness of the extensor digitorum brevis muscle.

Clinical diagnosis — Pain on palpation, decreased sensation in the deep peroneal nerve territory, atrophic EDB muscle. Decreases in sensation in V-shaped area in between the first and second digits in the dorsum of the foot.

Electrodiagnosis — Normal electrophysiologic studies, except for low-amplitude CMAP at the EDB muscle when stimulating the peroneal nerve. EMG may show reduced number of units or denervation in the EDB but not in the tibialis anterior, extensor hallucis, or other leg muscles.

Tibial nerve

Proximal compression

Causes — Trauma, surgery in the knee, hematoma in the popliteal fossa, cysts, or aneurysms.

Symptoms — Pain, weakness of the foot flexion, inversion, numbness, and paresthesias in the sole of the foot.

Clinical diagnosis — Weak tibial innervated muscles including gastrocnemius, soleus and tibialis posterior, flexor digitorum, absent ankle jerks, and decreased sensation in sole of the foot.

Electrodiagnosis — Low-amplitude tibial nerve CMAP and plantar SNAPs, with normal sural superficial peroneal SNAPs. Tibial nerve conduction velocity could be slow from knee to foot. H reflex prolonged or absent.

Tarsal tunnel syndrome

Causes — Compression of the tibial nerve at the flexor retinaculum.

Symptoms — Burning and pain is produced mainly by stretching the foot.

Clinical diagnosis — Positive Tinel's sign, decreased sensation in the sole of the foot, and atrophy of the tibial foot muscles.

Electrodiagnosis — Prolonged distal motor latencies to the abductor hallucis and/or adductor digit quinti, low-amplitude or prolonged latency medial and/or lateral plantar SNAPs. Near nerve sensory conductions could detect slowing or temporal dispersion. EMG may show denervation of the foot muscles innervated by tibial nerve, sparing the EDB and leg muscles. Should rule out radiculopathy, plexopathy, sciatic nerve lesion, and proximal tibial nerve lesions.

Interdigital nerves

Causes — Exercise, hyperextension of metatarsal phalangeal joints, Morton's neuroma, compression at the transverse metatarsal ligaments, and arthritis.

Symptoms — Pain in the sole of the foot.

Clinical diagnosis — Tenderness on palpation relieved with local anesthetics. Decreased sensation in V-shaped ventral area of the foot between third and fourth toes.

Electrodiagnosis — EMG, when done to rule out other processes, is normal.

ALS = amyotrophic lateral sclerosis; CT = computed tomography; CMAP = compound muscle action potential; EDB = extensor digitorum brevis; EMG = electromyography; HNPP = hereditary neuropathy with liability to pressure palsies; MR = magnetic resonance; MRI = magnetic resonance imaging; SNAP = sensory nerve action potential.

Appendix 2

Important Neuromuscular Disorder Diagnostic Criteria

Tulio E. Bertorini, Pushpa Narayanaswami, and Kandasami Senthilkumar

Several diagnostic criteria that are useful in clinical practice and research trials have been published for various neuromuscular diseases. We include here those that have the most clinical value or are frequently used; in some, minor modifications have been made to incorporate more current diagnostic methods; in others, and for some diseases, more than one published criterion has been included if these have been widely used. For more specific details, the reader is referred to the original publication.

REVISED DIAGNOSTIC CRITERIA FOR AMYOTROPHIC LATERAL SCLEROSIS*

The diagnosis of amyotrophic lateral sclerosis (ALS) requires the presence of

- Evidence of lower motor neuron (LMN) degeneration by clinical, electrophysiologic, or neuropathologic examination,
- Evidence of upper motor neuron (UMN) degeneration by clinical examination, and
- Progressive spread of symptoms or signs within a region or to other regions, as determined by history or examination,

together with the absence of

- Electrophysiologic and pathologic evidence of other disease processes that might explain the signs of LMN and/or UMN degeneration, and
- Neuroimaging evidence of other disease processes that might explain the observed clinical and electrophysiologic signs.

---

*Adapted from BR Brooks, RG Miller, M Swash, TL Munsat. El Escorial revisited: revised criteria for the diagnosis of amyotrophic lateral sclerosis. Amyotroph Lateral Scler Other Motor Neuron Disord 2000;1(5):293–299.

DIAGNOSTIC CATEGORIES

Clinically definite ALS and *clinically probable ALS* are used to describe these categories of clinical diagnostic certainty on clinical criteria alone:

Clinically definite ALS is defined on clinical evidence alone by the presence of UMN, as well as LMN signs, in the bulbar region and at least two spinal regions, or the presence of UMN and LMN signs in three spinal regions.

Clinically probable ALS is defined on clinical evidence alone by UMN and LMN signs in at least two regions, with some UMN signs necessarily rostral to (above) the LMN signs.

The terms *clinically probable ALS–laboratory-supported* and *clinically possible ALS* are used to describe these categories of clinical certainty on clinical laboratory studies and criteria or only clinical criteria:

Clinically probable ALS–laboratory-supported is defined when clinical signs of UMN and LMN dysfunction are in only one region, or when UMN signs alone are present in one region and LMN signs defined by EMG criteria are present in at least two regions, with proper application of neuroimaging and clinical laboratory protocols to exclude other causes.

Clinically possible ALS is defined when clinical signs of UMN and LMN dysfunction are found together in only one region or UMN signs are found alone in two or more regions, or LMN signs are found alone in two or more regions; or LMN signs are found rostral to UMN signs and the diagnosis of clinically probable ALS–laboratory-supported cannot be proven by evidence on clinical grounds in conjunction with electrodiagnostic, neurophysiologic, neuroimaging, or clinical laboratory studies. Other diagnoses must have been excluded to accept a diagnosis of clinically possible ALS.

Clinically suspected ALS may be suspected in many settings in which the diagnosis of ALS could not be regarded as sufficiently certain to include the patient in a research study. Hence, this category is deleted from the revised *El Escorial Criteria for the Diagnosis of ALS.*

Electrophysiologic Studies Used in the Diagnosis of Amyotrophic Lateral Sclerosis

Electrophysiologic Features of Lower Motor Neuron Dysfunction

Conventional Electromyographic Studies. The features of LMN dysfunction in a particular muscle are defined by EMG concentric needle examination to provide evidence of active and chronic denervation, including fibrillations and fasciculations. Nerve conduction studies are also required to exclude motor neuropathy. Signs of *active denervation* consist of (1) fibrillation potentials and (2) positive sharp waves. Signs of *chronic denervation* consist of (1) large motor unit potentials of increased duration with an increased proportion of polyphasic potentials, often increased amplitude; (2) reduced interference pattern with firing rates higher than 10 Hz unless there is a significant UMN component, in which case the firing rate may be lower than 10 Hz; and (3) unstable motor unit potentials. The combination of active and chronic denervation findings is required, but the relative proportion may vary from muscle to muscle.

Fasciculation Potentials. Fasciculation potentials are characteristic clinical features of ALS. Their presence in EMG recordings is helpful in the diagnosis of ALS, particularly if they are of long duration and polyphasic and when they are present in muscles in which there is evidence of active or chronic partial denervation and reinnervation. Their distribution can vary. Their absence raises diagnostic doubts but does not preclude the diagnosis of ALS. Fasciculation potentials of normal morphology occur in healthy subjects (benign fasciculations), and fasciculation potentials of abnormal morphology occur in other denervations disorders (e.g., motor neuropathies).

Topography of Active and Chronic Denervation and Reinnervation

The electromyographic (EMG) signs of LMN dysfunction required to support a diagnosis of ALS should be found in at least two of the four central nervous system (CNS) regions: brainstem, (bulbar/cranial motor neurons), cervical, thoracic, or lumbosacral spinal cord (anterior horn motor neurons).

- For the brainstem region, it is sufficient to demonstrate EMG change in one muscle (e.g., tongue, facial muscles, jaw muscles).
- For the thoracic spinal cord region, it is sufficient to demonstrate EMG changes in the paraspinal muscles at or below the T6 level or in the abdominal muscles.
- For the cervical and lumbosacral spinal cord regions, at least two muscles innervated by different roots and peripheral nerves must show EMG changes.

Nerve Conduction Studies

Nerve conduction studies are required for the diagnosis principally to define and exclude other disorders of peripheral nerve, neuromuscular junction, and muscle that may mimic or confound the diagnosis of ALS. These studies should generally be normal or near normal. The motor conduction times should be normal unless the compound muscle potential is small. The sensory nerve conduction studies can be abnormal in the presence of entrapment syndromes and coexisting peripheral nerve disease.

Electrophysiologic features suggesting other disease processes include the following:

1. Evidence of motor conduction block.
2. Motor conduction velocities lower than 70% and distal motor latencies higher than 30% of the lower and upper limits of normal values, respectively.
3. Sensory nerve conduction studies that are abnormal. Entrapment syndromes, peripheral neuropathies, and advanced age may render sensory nerve action potentials difficult to elicit in the lower extremities.
4. F-wave or H-wave latencies more than 30% above established normal values.
5. Decrements greater than 20% on repetitive stimulation.
6. Somatosensory evoked response latency greater than 20% above established normal values.
7. Full interference pattern in a clinically weak muscle.
8. Significant abnormalities in autonomic function or electronystagmography.

Pathologic Studies in the Living Patient with Sporadic Amyotrophic Lateral Sclerosis

Indications for Biopsies

Biopsy of the skeletal muscle, peripheral nerve, and other tissues is not required for the diagnosis of ALS, unless the clinical, electrophysiologic, or laboratory studies have revealed changes that are atypical for ALS (e.g., inclusion body myositis [IBM]). In addition, the muscle biopsy may be used to demonstrate LMN involvement in a body region not shown to be involved by other techniques.

Muscle Biopsy

A feature required for the diagnosis is

- Evidence of chronic denervation/reinnervation in an affected muscle.

Features that are compatible with and do not exclude the diagnosis are

- Scattered hypertrophied muscle fibers
- No more than a moderate number of target or targetoid fibers
- Fiber-type grouping of no more than mild to moderate extent
- The presence of a small number of necrotic muscle fibers

Features that rule out the diagnosis or suggest the presence of additional disease are

- Significant monoclonal gammopathy, infiltration with lymphocytes and other mononuclear inflammatory cells
- Significant arteritis
- Significant numbers of muscle fibers involved with the following structural changes: necrosis, rimmed vacuoles, nemaline bodies, central cores, accumulation of mitochondria (ragged red fibers)
- Large fiber–type grouping
- Giant axonal swellings from accumulation of masses of neurofilaments, but not of periodic acid–Schiff–positive bodies, in intramuscular nerves.

DIAGNOSTIC CRITERIA AND CLASSIFICATION OF PROXIMAL SPINAL MUSCULAR ATROPHY*

Types According to Age at Onset

In spinal muscular atrophy (SMA) type 1 (severe form), onset ranges from the prenatal period to the age of 6 months.
In SMA type II (intermediate form), onset is usually before the age of 18 months.
In SMA type III (mild form), onset is usually after the age of 18 months

---

*Modified from K Zerres, KE Davies. 59th ENMC International Workshop: Spinal Muscular Atrophies: recent progress and revised diagnostic criteria 17–19 April 1998, Soestduinen, The Netherlands. Neuromuscul Disord 1999;9(4):272–278.

Throughout this Appendix, C = comment, E = exclusion, and I = inclusion.

Distribution of Muscle Weakness

I: Muscle weakness of the trunk and limbs (proximal more than distal; lower limbs weaker than upper).

I: Symmetric weakness.

E: Weakness of extraocular muscles, diaphragm, and myocardium, or marked facial weakness.

C: There are rare congenital-onset cases of SMA whose clinical picture also includes external ophthalmoplegia, facial diplegia, and early respiratory insufficiency.

C: Wasting is often not conspicuous in SMA type I.

Associated Features

I: Fasciculations of tongue and tremor of hands.

C: Tremor of the hands is frequently observed in SMA types II and III.

E: Sensory disturbances.

E: CNS dysfunction.

C: Arthrogryposis of the major joints is a rare finding in a severe form of SMA type I. In SMA type I, some mild limitation of abduction of the hips or extension of the knees or elbows is common.

E: Involvement of other neurologic systems or organs (e.g., hearing or vision).

Course/Life Expectancy

I: In SMA types I and II, there is an arrest of development of motor milestones. Children with SMA type I are never able to sit without support.
Children with SMA type II are unable to stand or walk without aid.
In SMA type III, the ability to walk will be achieved.

I: In SMA type I, the majority of patients have a life expectancy of less than 2 years.
In SMA type II, survival into adolescence or adulthood is common.
In SMA type III, life expectancy is most likely normal.

C: There will be certain patients who do not clearly fit any one category.

Electrophysiology

I: Abnormal spontaneous activity (e.g., fibrillations, positive sharp waves, and fasciculations by EMG).

I: Increased mean duration and amplitude of motor unit action potential by EMG.

E: In SMA types II and III, reduction of motor nerve conduction velocities (MNCVs) less than 70% of lower limit.

C: MNCVs may be markedly reduced in SMA type I.

E: Abnormal sensory nerve action potentials (SNAPs) in SMA types II and III.

C: There is a rare congenital-onset SMA with death within the first weeks of life, in which MNCVs are very low and SNAPs are absent.

Histopathology of Muscle

I: Groups of atrophic fibers of both types
  Hypertrophic fibers of type I
  Type grouping (chronic cases)
C: In early-onset cases of SMA type I, these characteristic features may not be present. Instead, there are small fibers of both types. In SMA type III there may be a concomitant "myopathic" pattern.

Laboratory Criteria

I: Creatine kinase (CK) is usually less than five times the upper limit of normal.

Molecular Genetics

I: The homozygous absence/mutation of the telomeric SMN (survival motor neuron) gene (SMN^T) in chromosome 5q in the presence of clinical symptoms is diagnostic.
C: In cases with absence/mutation of the telomeric SMN gene, further diagnostic procedures (e.g., EMG and muscle biopsy) are no longer needed.
C: The presence of both copies of SMN^T argues strongly against the diagnosis.

REVISED DIAGNOSTIC CRITERIA FOR GUILLAIN-BARRÉ SYNDROME*

I. Features required for diagnosis
  A. Progressive motor weakness of more than one limb. The degree ranges from minimal weakness of the legs, with or without mild ataxia, to total paralysis of the muscles of all four extremities and the trunk, bulbar and facial paralysis, and external ophthalmoplegia.
  B. Areflexia (loss of tendon jerks). Universal areflexia is the rule, although distal areflexia with definite hyporeflexia of the biceps and knee jerks suffices if other features are consistent.
II. Features strongly supportive of diagnosis
  A. Clinical features (ranked in order of importance):
    1. Progression. Symptoms and signs of motor weakness develop rapidly but cease to progress by 4 weeks into the illness. Approximately 50% reach the nadir by 2 weeks, 80% by 3 weeks, and more than 90% by 4 weeks.
    2. Relative symmetry. Symmetry is seldom absolute, but usually, if one limb is affected, the opposite is as well.
    3. Mild sensory symptoms or signs.
    4. Cranial nerve involvement. Facial weakness occurs in approximately 50% and is frequently bilateral. Other cranial nerves may be involved, particularly those innervating the tongue and muscles of deglutition, and sometimes the extraocular motor nerves. On occasion (less than 5%), the neuropathy may begin in the nerves to the extraocular muscles or other cranial nerves.

---

*Reprinted with permission from AK Asbury, DR Cornblath. Assessment of current diagnostic criteria for Guillain-Barré syndrome. Ann Neurol 1990;27(Suppl):S21–S24.

5. Recovery. It usually begins 2–4 weeks after progression stops. Recovery may be delayed for months. Most patients recover functionally.
6. Autonomic dysfunction. Tachycardia and other arrhythmias, postural hypotension, hypertension, and vasomotor symptoms, when present, support the diagnosis. These findings may fluctuate. Care must be exercised to exclude other bases for these symptoms, such as pulmonary embolism.
7. Absence of fever at the onset of neuritic symptoms.

Variants (not ranked)

1. Fever at onset of neuritic symptoms.
2. Severe sensory loss with pain.
3. Progression beyond 4 weeks. Occasionally, a patient's disease continues to progress for many weeks or the patient will have a minor relapse.
4. Cessation of progression without recovery, or with major permanent residual deficit remaining.
5. Sphincter function. Usually the sphincters are not affected, but transient bladder paralysis may occur during the evolution of symptoms.
6. CNS involvement. Ordinarily, Guillain-Barré syndrome (GBS) is thought of as a disease of the peripheral nervous system. Evidence of CNS involvement is controversial. In occasional patients, such findings as severe ataxia interpretable as cerebellar in origin, dysarthria, extensor plantar responses, and ill-defined sensory levels are demonstrable, and these need not exclude the diagnosis if other features are typical.

B. Cerebrospinal fluid (CSF) features strongly supportive of diagnosis
1. CSF protein. After the first week of symptoms, CSF protein is elevated or has been shown to rise on serial lumbar punctures.
2. CSF cells. Counts of 10 or fewer mononuclear leukocytes/mm^3 in CSF.

Variants

1. No CSF protein rise in the period of 1–10 weeks after at the onset of symptoms (rare).
2. Counts of 11–50 mononuclear leukocytes/mm^3 in CSF.

C. Electrodiagnostic features strongly supportive of diagnosis. Approximately 80% of affected individuals will have evidence of nerve conduction slowing or block at some point during the illness. Conduction velocity is usually less than 60% of normal, but the process is patchy and not all nerves are affected. Distal latencies may be increased to as much as three times normal. Use of F-wave responses often gives good indication of slowing over proximal portions of nerve trunks and roots. Up to 20% of patients have normal conduction studies. Conduction studies may not become abnormal until several weeks into the illness (criteria for demyelination used here include three of the four features listed in Research criteria for diagnosis of chronic inflammatory demyelinating polyneuropathy (CIDP). (Report from an Ad Hoc Subcommittee of the American Academy of Neurology AIDS Task Force. Neurology 1991;41[5]:617–618.)

Features casting doubt on diagnosis

1. Marked, persistent asymmetry of weakness
2. Persistent bladder or bowel dysfunction
3. Bladder or bowel dysfunction at onset
4. More than 50 mononuclear leukocytes/mm^3 in CSF
5. Presence of polymorphonuclear leukocytes in CSF
6. Sharp sensory level

Features that rule out the diagnosis

1. A current history of hexacarbon abuse (volatile solvents; n-hexane and methyl n-butyl ketone). This includes huffing of paint lacquer vapors and addictive glue sniffing.
2. Abnormal porphyrin metabolism indicating a diagnosis of acute intermittent porphyria. This manifests as increased excretion of porphobilinogen and δ-aminolevulinic acid in the urine.
3. A history or finding of recent diphtheritic infection, either faucial or wound, with or without myocarditis.
4. Features clinically consistent with lead neuropathy (e.g., upper limb weakness with prominent wrist drop; may be asymmetric) and evidence of lead intoxication.
5. The occurrence of a purely sensory syndrome.
6. A definite diagnosis of a condition such as poliomyelitis, botulism, hysterical paralysis, or toxic neuropathy, (e.g., from nitrofurantoin, dapsone, or organophosphorus compounds), which occasionally may be confused with GBS.

PROPOSED DIAGNOSTIC CRITERIA FOR GUILLAIN-BARRÉ SYNDROME*

The following criteria are for necessary for the clinical diagnosis of GBS (in combination, they are sufficient for the diagnosis).

1. Subacutely developing flaccid paralysis. (*Comment*: The nadir is reached within 2 weeks in more than 80% of the patients.)
2. Weakness starts from the onset at both sides of the body, and there is a strong tendency for symmetry. (*Comment*: Weakness usually starts in the legs, but onset in upper extremities or even cranial nerves also occurs.)
3. The myotatic reflexes decrease and usually disappear entirely.
4. Other causes for rapidly developing flaccid weakness should be highly unlikely based on history and, if necessary, additional tests.

---

*Adapted and modified from FG Van der Meche, PA Van Doom, J Meulstee, FG Jennekens. Diagnostic and classification criteria for the Guillain-Barré Syndrome. Eur Neurol 2001;45(3):133–139.

Other Elements Characteristic for Guillain-Barré Syndrome but with Limited Diagnostic Value That May Add to the Diagnosis If Criterion 4 Is Uncertain

- The total protein content in the CSF rises, and the cell count is either normal or only slightly raised. (*Comment:* As a rule, there are less than 3 cells/mm^3. In a series of 134 patients involved in a Dutch clinical trial, only 15 (11%) had more than 3 cells/mm^3 [author's unpublished observation].) (*Editor's note:* Conventionally, the normal number of cells is considered less than or equal to 5 cells/mm^3, and if there are higher cell counts, other causes should be considered.) (*Comment:* In 50% of patients, the protein is elevated during the first week; in 80% or patients, the protein is elevated during the second week.)
- The electrophysiologic investigation supports a polyneuropathy if, in at least two individual nerves, at least three of the following parameters are abnormal with respect to well-defined normal values:

   Distal motor latency.
   Nerve conduction velocity.
   F-wave latency (given a normal distal conduction velocity).
   Amplitude of the distal compound muscle action potential (CMAP).
   Abnormal increase in the duration of the CMAP with proximal stimulation versus distal stimulation.
   Amplitude of the compound sensory nerve potential.
   Recruitment pattern (either absent or "single pattern").
   Presence of spontaneous muscle fiber activity. (*Editor's note:* For the axonal variant, as this indicates axonal degeneration but does not appear until approximately after 3 weeks of onset, their presence early would suggest an alternative diagnosis.)

Subclassification of the Guillain-Barré Syndrome

Criteria 1–4 should be fulfilled for all subclassifications. The following criteria for subclassification should be added for either type.

Motor-Sensory Guillain-Barré Syndrome

Elements of motor-sensory GBS are

5. Sensory deficit is present at admission or during follow-up. The diagnosis is definitive if criteria 1–4 for GBS are fulfilled in addition to criterion 5.

Pure Motor Guillain-Barré Syndrome

Elements of pure motor GBS are

6. Sensory deficit is not present at admission or during follow-up. The diagnosis is definitive if criteria 1–4 for GBS are fulfilled in addition to criterion 6.

Miller-Fisher Variant of Guillain-Barré Syndrome

Elements of Miller-Fisher GBS are

7. Weakness starts in the external eye muscles.
8. Ataxia.
9. Immunoglobulin (Ig) G antibodies against ganglioside GQ1b.

The diagnosis of Miller Fisher syndrome (MFS) is definitive if criteria 1–4 for GBS are fulfilled in addition to criteria 7 and 8 or 7 and 9. The diagnosis is probable if criteria 1–4 and 7 are fulfilled.

Bulbar Variant of Guillain-Barré Syndrome

Elements of bulbar variant GBS are

10. The onset of weakness is in the facial muscles, the deglutition muscles, or the tongue muscles.

The diagnosis of the bulbar variant of GBS is definitive if criteria 1–4 are fulfilled in addition to criterion 10.

Demyelinating or Primary Axonal Forms of Guillain-Barré Syndrome

Elements of demyelination are

11. Physiologic criteria. One of the following has to be present in two or more nerves:
    a. Distal motor latency greater than 150% of upper limit of normal (ULN)
    b. Motor nerve conduction velocity less than 70% of lower limit of normal
    c. F-wave latency greater than 150% of ULN
    d. Abnormal compound muscle action potential (CMAP) amplitude decay more than the ULN
    e. Abnormal distal temporal dispersion: distal CMAP duration greater than 150% of ULN
    f. Abnormal temporal dispersion: distal to proximal CMAP duration ratio greater than 150% of ULN
12. Pathologic criterion. Evidence of demyelination in sural nerve biopsy or autopsy (if axonal changes are present, it remains uncertain if the process is primarily axonal or demyelinating).

Elements of axonal degeneration are

13. Electrophysiologic criteria for axonal degeneration in GBS:
    a. Decreased CMAP amplitude with distal stimulation (decreased distal CMAP could also be from demyelination-causing distal conduction block; therefore, the specificity is limited)
    b. The absence of any abnormality compared to normal in all parameters of conduction mentioned under criterion 11 in all nerves investigated with a minimum of three nerves; the only exception being decrease in conduction velocity at well-known places for compression neuropathy
    c. The absence of any of the six elements mentioned under criterion 11 for demyelination in all nerves investigated with a minimum of three nerves
14. Pathologic criteria for axonal degeneration: axonal degeneration found at autopsy over all segments, including roots, nerves, and endings in the absence of

demyelination (evidence of demyelination after 3–4 weeks of onset also indicates axonal degeneration).

PROPOSED DIAGNOSTIC CRITERIA FOR CHRONIC INFLAMMATORY DEMYELINATING POLYRADICULONEUROPATHY*

Mandatory Inclusion Criteria

All patients must have these features:

1. Progression of muscle weakness (steady, stepwise or relapsing) for 2 months
2. Symmetric proximal and distal weakness in upper or lower extremities
3. Areflexia or hyporeflexia

Mandatory Exclusion Criteria

Patients must be devoid of these features:

1. Clinical features, including pure sensory neuropathy, mutilation of hands or feet, retinitis pigmentosa, ichthyosis, orange tonsils, and history of exposure to drugs or toxins known to cause peripheral neuropathy.
2. Laboratory findings of low serum cholesterol levels, abnormal porphyrin metabolite values, fasting glucose levels of greater than or equal to 7.7 mmol/liter, low serum vitamin B_{12} levels, hypothyroidism, heavy metal intoxication, and CSF white blood cell count greater than $50/mm^2 \times 10^6/liter$.
3. Nerve biopsy specimen with features of vasculitis, neurofilamentous, swollen axons, intramyelinic blebs, amyloid deposits, Schwann cells with evidence of storage materials typical for Fabry's disease, adrenal leukodystrophy, metachromatic leukodystrophy, globoid cell leukodystrophy, or Refsum's disease.
4. Electrodiagnostic features of neuromuscular transmission defect, myopathy, or anterior horn cell disease.

Major Laboratory Criteria

1. Nerve biopsy specimens with predominant features of demyelination that include segmental demyelination, remyelination, loss of nerve fibers, onion-bulb formation, and perivascular inflammation.
2. Nerve conduction studies with features of demyelination, including slowing of conduction velocities in at least two motor nerves to less than 70% of lower limit or normal (two nerves required to avoid inclusion of patients with focal compression neuropathy).
3. CSF protein level greater than 0.45 g/liter.

---

*Reprinted with permission from RJ Barohn, JT Kissel, JR Warmolts, JR Mendell. Chronic inflammatory demyelinating polyradiculoneuropathy. Clinical characteristics, course, and recommendations for diagnostic criteria. Arch Neurol 1989;46(8):878–884. (*Editor's note*: Some of these authors have proposed new diagnostic criteria [see the section New Proposed Criteria for Chronic Inflammatory Demyelinating Polyneuropathy].)

Diagnostic Categories

Definite

1. Mandatory inclusion criteria
2. Mandatory exclusion criteria
3. All three major laboratory criteria

Probable

1. Mandatory inclusion criteria
2. Mandatory exclusion criteria
3. Two of three laboratory criteria

Possible

1. Mandatory inclusion criteria
2. Mandatory exclusion criteria
3. One of three laboratory criteria

Concurrent Illness

Patients in this group have an acquired demyelinating polyneuropathy accompanying another disorder; conditions described so far include thyrotoxicosis, HIV infection, monoclonal gammopathy, hereditary motor and sensory neuropathy, CNS demyelination, chronic active hepatitis, inflammatory bowel disease, and Hodgkin's disease.

RESEARCH DIAGNOSTIC CRITERIA FOR CHRONIC INFLAMMATORY DEMYELINATING POLYNEUROPATHY*

I. Clinical
  A. Mandatory
    1. Progressive or relapsing motor and sensory, rarely only motor or sensory, dysfunction of more than one limb of a peripheral nerve nature, developing over at least 2 months.
    2. Hypo- or areflexia. This will usually involve all four limbs.
  B. Supportive
    1. Large-fiber sensory loss predominates over small-fiber sensory loss.
  C. Exclusion
    1. Mutilation of hands or feet, retinitis pigmentosa, ichthyosis, appropriate history of drug or toxic exposure known to cause a similar peripheral neuropathy, or family history of a genetically based peripheral neuropathy.
    2. Sensory level.
    3. Unequivocal sphincter disturbance.
II. Physiologic studies

---

*Reprinted with permission from Research criteria for diagnosis of chronic inflammatory demyelinating polyneuropathy (CIDP). Report from an Ad Hoc Subcommittee of the American Academy of Neurology AIDS Task Force. Neurology 1991;41(5):617–618.

A. Mandatory—Nerve conduction studies including studies of proximal nerve segments in which the predominant process is demyelination. Must have three of four:
1. Reduction in conduction velocity (CV) in two or more motor nerves:
   a. <80% of LLN if amplitude >80% of LLN.
   b. <70% of LLN if amplitude <80% of LLN.
2. Partial conduction block or abnormal temporal dispersion in one or more motor nerves; either peroneal nerve between ankle and below fibular head, median nerve between wrist and elbow, or ulnar nerve between wrist and below elbow.
   a. Criteria suggestive of partial conduction block; less than 15% change in duration between proximal and distal sites and more than 20% drop in negative-peak (-p) area or peak-to-peak (p-p) amplitude between proximal and distal sites.
   b. Criteria for abnormal temporal dispersion and possible conduction block: more than 15% change in duration between proximal and distal sites and more than 20% drop in -p area or p-p amplitude between proximal and distal sites. These criteria are only suggestive of partial conduction block as they are derived from studies of normal individuals. Additional studies, such as stimulation across short segments or recording of individual motor unit potentials, are required for confirmation.
3. Prolonged distal latencies in two or more nerves:
   a. Greater than 125% of ULN if amplitude greater than 80% of LLN.
   b. Greater than 150% of ULN if amplitude less than 80% of LLN.
4. Absent F waves or prolonged minimum F-wave latencies (10–15 trials) in two or more motor nerves:
   a. Greater than 120% of ULN if amplitude greater than 80% of LLN.
   b. Greater than 150% of ULN if amplitude less than 80% of LLN.

B. Supportive
1. Reduction in sensory CV less than 80% of LLN.
2. Absent H reflexes.

III. Pathologic features
A. Mandatory—nerve biopsy showing unequivocal evidence of demyelination and remyelination.
1. Demyelination by either electron microscopy (more than five fibers) or teased fiber studies (>12% of 50 teased fibers, minimum of four internodes each, demonstrating demyelination/remyelination).

B. Supportive
1. Subperineurial or endoneurial edema.
2. Mononuclear cell infiltration.
3. Onion-bulb formation.
4. Prominent variation in the degree of demyelination between fascicles.

C. Exclusion
1. Vasculitis, neurofilamentous swollen axons, amyloid deposits, or intracytoplasmic inclusions in Schwann cells or macrophages indicating adrenoleukodystrophy, metachromatic leukodystrophy, globoid cell leukodystrophy, or other evidence of specific pathology.

IV. CSF studies
A. Mandatory

1. Cell count less than $10/mm^3$ if HIV seronegative, less than $50/mm^3$ if HIV seropositive.
2. Negative Venereal Disease Research Laboratory (VDRL) test.
   B. Supportive
   1. Elevated protein.

Diagnostic categories for research purposes:

Definite: Clinical A and C, Physiology A, Pathology A, and C, and CSF A
Probable: Clinical A and C, Physiology A, and CSF A
Possible: Clinical A and C, Physiology A

NEW PROPOSED CRITERIA FOR CHRONIC INFLAMMATORY DEMYELINATING POLYNEUROPATHY

	Proposed Criteria 2001
Mandatory clinical features	
Pattern of clinical involvement	Major: Symmetric, proximal + distal weakness loss
	Minor: exclusively distal weakness or sensory loss
Reflexes	Areflexia or hyporeflexia
Time course	At least 2 months
Laboratory features	
Electrodiagnostic studies	
Partial conduction block (definite, probable or possible) must be present in at least one motor nerve	At least two out of four criteria must be met (see American Association of Electrodiagnostic Medicine criteria in the next table for partial conduction block)
Conduction velocity (must be abnormal in at least two motor nerves)	Reduced <80% of LLN if CMAP amplitude >80% of LLN; reduced <70% of LLN if CMAP amplitude is reduced <80% of LLN
Distal latency (must be abnormal in at least two motor nerves)	Prolonged >125% of ULN if CMAP amplitude >80% of LLN; prolonged >150% of ULN if CMAP amplitude is <80% of LLN
F-wave latency (must be abnormal in at least two motor nerves)	Absent or prolonged >125% of ULN if CMAP amplitude >80% of LLN; prolonged >150% of ULN if CMAP amplitude is <80% of LLN
CSF studies	Mandatory: Protein >45 mg/dl
	Supportive[a]: Cell count <10/mm^3
Nerve biopsy features	Predominant features of demyelination[b]
	Inflammation (not required)
Requirements for diagnostic categories	
Definite	Clinical major, electrodiagnostic, and CSF (biopsy supportive but not mandatory)
Probable	Clinical major, electrodiagnostic or CSF, and biopsy
Possible	Clinical major and one out of three laboratory features or clinical minor and two of three laboratory features

[a]CSF cell count greater than 10 mm^3 (or >50/mm^3 if HIV seropositive) should prompt evaluation for HIV, Lyme disease, and lymphomatous or leukemic infiltration of nerve roots.
[b]To include segmental demyelination, remyelination, and onion-bulb formation.
Source: Reprinted with permission from DS Saperstein, JS Katz, AA Amato, RJ Barohn. Clinical spectrum of chronic acquired demyelinating polyneuropathies. Muscle Nerve 2001;24(3):311–324.

AMERICAN ACADEMY OF ELECTRODIAGNOSTIC MEDICINE PROPOSED CRITERIA FOR PARTIAL CONDUCTION BLOCK

Nerve Segment (Proximal/Distal)	Minimal Temporal Dispersion (Duration Increased by 30% or Less)				Moderate Temporal Dispersion (Duration Increased by 31–60%)	
	Definite Partial Conduction Block		Probable Partial Conduction Block		Probable Partial Conduction Block	
	Amplitude Reduction (%)	Area Reduction (%)	Amplitude Reduction (%)	Area Reduction (%)	Amplitude Reduction (%)	Area Reduction (%)
Median						
Forearm (E/W)	>50	>40	40–49	30–39	>50	>40
Arm (AX/E)	>50	>40	40–49	30–39	>50	>40
Proximal (EP/AX)	a	a	>40	>30	>50	>40
Ulnar						
Forearm (BE/W)	>50	>40	40–49	30–39	>50	>40
Across Elbow (AE/BE)	>50	>40	40–49	30–39	>50	>40
Arm (AX/AE)	>50	>40	40–49	30–39	>50	>40
Proximal (EP/AX)	a	a	>40	>30	>50	>40
Radial						
Forearm (E/DF)	b	b	>50	>40	>60	>50
Arm (AX/E)	b	b	>50	>40	>60	>50
Proximal (EP/AX)	b	b	>50	>40	>60	>50
Peroneal						
Leg (BF/ankle)	>60	>50	50–59	40–49	>60	>50
Across FH (AF/BF)	>50	>40	40–49	30–39	>50	>40
Thigh (SN/AF)	a	a	>50	>40	>60	>50
Tibial						
Leg (knee/ankle)	>60	>50	50–59	40–49	>60	>50
Thigh (SN/knee)	a	a	>50	>40	>60	>50

AE = above elbow; AF = above fibular head; AX = axilla; BE = below elbow; BF = below fibular head; DF = distal forearm; E = elbow; EP = Erb's point; FA = forearm; FH = fibular head; SN = sciatic notch; W = wrist.

[a]See technical consideration I.F.

[b]See technical consideration I.E.

Source: Reprinted with permission from RK Olney. Consensus criteria for the diagnosis of partial conduction block. Muscle Nerve 1999;22(Suppl 8):S225–S229.

I. Technical considerations used in these determinations
   A. All measurement of amplitude, area, and duration in these criteria refers to values for the negative peak of surface-recorded CMAPs. The *negative peak* is defined as that component aspect of the waveform from the first baseline crossing from negative to positive. CMAPs that have more than one negative peak are referred to as *multiphasic CMAPs*.
   B. These criteria are intended to apply only to nerves in which the negative-peak amplitude of the CMAP with distal stimulation is 20% or more of the lower limit of normal.
   C. The percent reduction in the table above is applicable to ulnar nerve in the forearm only if median-to-ulnar nerve crossover in the forearm (Martin-Gruber anastomosis) has been excluded by the recording of an initially positive hypothenar CMAP with stimulation of median nerve at the elbow. Furthermore, usage of excessive stimulation intensity at the wrist that activates both

median and ulnar nerves may result in the suggestion of partial conduction block in the forearm segment of the median nerve due to ulnar innervation of deep thenar muscles.

D. Although the specificity for determining partial conduction block is similar for median and ulnar nerves when stimulating at the axilla or Erb's point, the sensitivity is often lower with these proximal stimulation sites for the median nerve unless collision stimulation techniques are used. This is because of the common ulnar innervation of deep thenar muscles.

E. The criteria are more restrictive for the radial, peroneal, and tibial nerves than for the median and ulnar nerves. Even with surface recording of the CMAP, the vast majority of the expert panel agrees that reduction of amplitude and area of the radial motor response is considered sufficient only to support probable partial conduction block. A higher percentage of reduction in amplitude and area is required for the peroneal and tibial nerves than for the median and ulnar nerves. Furthermore, greater care is necessary to ensure that stimulation is supramaximal at the knee for the tibial nerve; special stimulation techniques may need to be used.

F. Stimulation at Erb's point and at the sciatic notch, with surface electrical or magnetic stimulator or stimulation at the sciatic notch with a needle, is not accepted by many of the panel as sufficiently reliable in producing supramaximal stimulation to be included in the criteria for definite partial conduction block. However, the expert panel accepts that the probability of achieving supramaximal stimulation is high if maximal amplitude and area of the CMAP are achieved with stimulus intensity at 70% or less of maximal stimulator output (i.e., the stimulator is able to deliver a supramaximal stimulus that is 30% more than maximal intensity).

G. With the commercial stimulators that are presently available in the United States, neither needle nor magnetic stimulation of nerve roots is accepted as sufficiently reliable in producing supramaximal stimulation of demyelinated nerve roots to be included in these criteria.

H. These criteria do not fully encompass all factors that experienced electrodiagnostic consultants consider before interpreting that partial conduction block is present. For example, certain anatomic variations such as body weight and limb edema are difficult to quantify. To ensure that supramaximal stimulation has been achieved, greater caution is required in obese rather than in thin individuals and in limbs with edema.

PROPOSAL FOR DIAGNOSTIC CHRONIC INFLAMMATORY DEMYELINATING POLYNEUROPATHY ASSOCIATED WITH MONOCLONAL GAMMOPATHY OF UNCERTAIN SIGNIFICANCE*

A causal relation between demyelinating polyneuropathy and monoclonal gammopathy of uncertain significance should be considered in a patient with

---

*Reprinted with permission from NC Notermans, H Franssen, M Eurelings, et al. Diagnostic criteria for demyelinating polyneuropathy associated with monoclonal gammopathy. Muscle Nerve 2000;23(1):73–79.

1. Demyelinating polyneuropathy according to the electrodiagnostic American Academy of Neurology criteria for idiopathic CIDP.*
2. Presence of an M protein (IgM, IgG, or IgA), without evidence of malignant plasma cell dyscrasias (e.g., multiple myeloma, lymphoma, Waldenström's macroglobulinemia, or amyloidosis).
3. Family history negative for neuropathy.
4. Age greater than 30 years.

The relation is *definitive* when IgM M proteins with anti–myelin-associated glycoprotein (MAG) antibodies are present.

The relation is *probable* when at least three of the following are present in a patient without anti-MAG antibodies:

1. Time to peak of the neuropathy greater than 2 years.
2. Chronic, slowly progressive course without relapsing or remitting periods.
3. Symmetric distal polyneuropathy.
4. Sensory symptoms and signs predominate over motor features.

A causal relation is unlikely when at least three of the following are present in a patient without anti-MAG antibodies:

1. Median time to peak of the neuropathy is within 1 year.
2. Clinical course is relapsing and remitting or monophasic.
3. Cranial nerves are involved.
4. Neuropathy is asymmetric.
5. Motor symptoms and signs predominate.
6. History of preceding infection.
7. Presence of abnormal median SNAP in combination with normal sural SNAP.

DIAGNOSTIC CRITERIA FOR MULTIFOCAL MOTOR NEUROPATHY†

Inclusion Criteria

Age of onset: 20–65 years

Asymmetric limb weakness at onset or motor involvement having a motor nerve distribution in at least two peripheral nerve distributions

Predominant upper limb involvement

Disabling weakness: Medical Research Council scale grade 4 or less in at least one muscle

Duration at least 6 months

Electrophysiologic evidence of one site with definite conduction block or one site with probable conduction block in the upper limb (see the section Electrophysiologic Criteria)

---

*See Research criteria for diagnosis of chronic inflammatory demyelinating polyneuropathy (CIDP). Report from an Ad Hoc Subcommittee of the American Academy of Neurology AIDS Task Force. Neurology 1991;41(5):617–618.

†Adapted from PR Hughes. 79(th) ENMC International Workshop: multifocal motor neuropathy. 14–15 April 2000, Hilversum, The Netherlands. Neuromuscul Disord 2001;11(3):309–314.

Exclusion Criteria

Clinical

Upper motor neuron signs
Bulbar or cranial signs or symptoms
Sensory signs
Associated systemic diseases that might cause neuropathy
Pregnancy, planned pregnancy, or unwillingness to practice contraception
Severe, concurrent medical conditions or previous neurologic deficit that would interfere with treatment or assessment.
Treatment with immunosuppressive agents during 6 months before randomization

Laboratory

CSF protein greater than 1 g/liter

Electrophysiologic Criteria

SNAP amplitude less than 80% of the lower limit of normal.

Electrophysiologic Criteria

Definite Conduction Block

Upper limb nerves, deep peroneal nerve: area reduction proximal/distal greater than or equal to 50%; duration prolongation proximal/distal less than 30%
Tibial nerve: area reduction proximal/distal greater than or equal to 60%; duration prolongation proximal/distal less than 30%

Probable Conduction Block

Upper limb nerves, deep peroneal nerve: area reduction proximal/distal greater than or equal to 50%; duration prolongation proximal/distal greater than 30%
Tibial nerve: area reduction proximal/distal greater than or equal to 60%; duration prolongation proximal/distal greater than 30%

Possible Conduction Block

Upper limb nerves, deep peroneal nerve: area reduction proximal/distal greater than or equal to 30%
Tibial nerve: area reduction proximal/distal greater than or equal to 50%

DIAGNOSTIC CRITERIA FOR CHARCOT-MARIE-TOOTH DISEASE (HEREDITARY MOTOR AND SENSORY NEUROPATHY TYPE I)*

A firm diagnosis of autosomal dominant hereditary motor and sensory neuropathy type I in a family to be used for linkage analysis requires the presence of all of the

---

*Modified from M De Visser. Hereditary motor and sensory neuropathy type Ia. Web site: European Neuromuscular Centre, 1998. http://www.enmc.org. Accessed April 30, 2002.

following clinical, electrophysiologic, and histopathologic and genetic criteria in the propositus within this family:

1. Slowly progressive symmetric muscle wasting and weakness, predominantly of the distal part of the lower limbs
2. Severely decreased motor conduction velocity (median nerve motor conduction velocity [MCV])
3. Pedigree consistent with autosomal dominant inheritance (ideally with evidence of male-to-male transmission)

Clinical Criteria—Muscle Wasting and Weakness

I: Muscle wasting and weakness of predominantly the distal part of the lower limbs.
I: Symmetric.
C: Later wasting and weakness of the intrinsic hand muscles and the distal part of the medial vastus muscle and other parts of the quadriceps muscle may develop.

Other associated features or diseases:

C: Impaired sensation is frequently observed but is not an obligatory feature.
E: Arthrogryposis with the exception of talipes or pes cavus.
C: Scoliosis and nerve hypertrophy are present in a proportion of patients.
E: CNS involvement.
C: The presence of brisk reflexes should mitigate against the diagnosis. Some patients may have extensor plantar responses. There may be tremor or slight limb ataxia.
E: Other major organ involvement (e.g., vision, hearing, cardiac).
C: There may be abnormalities of visual or auditory evoked responses but no overt clinical evidence of involvement of the optic or auditory nerves.
E: Impairment of oculomotor and bulbar function; marked facial weakness.
E: Myotonic dystrophy.
C: If an occasional patient shows one of the previously mentioned exclusion criteria, this does not necessarily exclude the whole family from linkage analysis.

Laboratory Criteria—Electrophysiology

I: Median nerve MCV: moderate to severe and uniformly (*Editor's addition*) slow motor nerve conduction velocity.
I: Sural nerve biopsy (usually sural nerve, although a fibular nerve may sometimes be sampled):
    An increase in total transverse fascicular area
    Marked reduction of density and total number of large and small myelinated fibers
    Onion bulbs
    Paranodal and segmental demyelination and remyelination
    Lack of prominent axonal degeneration (*Editor's addition*)

DNA Studies

Evidence of duplication on chromosome 17p11.2(IA)
Evidence of mutations in 1q22(IB)

CLASSIFICATION OF MYASTHENIA GRAVIS

I. Ocular myasthenia

II. A. Mild generalized myasthenia with slow progression; no crises; drug-responsive

   B. Moderately severe generalized myasthenia; severe skeletal and bulbar involvement but no crises; drug response less than satisfactory

III. Acute fulminating myasthenia; rapid progression of severe symptoms with respiratory crises and poor drug response; high incidence of thymoma; high mortality

IV. Late severe myasthenia, same as III but progression over 2 years from class I to class II (10%)

Source: Reprinted with permission from KE Osserman. Myasthenia Gravis and Related Disorders of Neuromuscular Transmission. In Myasthenia Gravis. New York: Grune & Stratton, 1958;79–80.

CLINICAL CLASSIFICATION OF MYASTHENIA GRAVIS FROM THE MYASTHENIA GRAVIS FOUNDATION OF AMERICA

Class	Symptoms
I	Any ocular muscle weakness.
	May have weakness of eye closure.
	All other muscle strength is normal.
II	Mild weakness affecting other than ocular muscles.
	May also have ocular muscle weakness of any severity.
IIa	Predominantly affecting limb, axial muscles, or both.
	May also have lesser involvement of oropharyngeal muscles.
IIb	Predominantly affecting oropharyngeal, respiratory muscles, or both.
III	Moderate weakness affecting other than ocular muscles.
	May also have ocular muscle weakness of any severity.
IIIa	Predominantly affecting limb, axial muscles, or both.
	May also have lesser involvement of oropharyngeal muscles.
IIIb	Predominantly affecting oropharyngeal, respiratory muscles, or both.
	May also have lesser or equal involvement of limb, axial muscles, or both.
IV	Severe weakness affecting other than ocular muscles.
	May also have ocular muscle weakness of any severity.
IVa	Predominantly affecting limb and/or axial muscles.
	May also have lesser involvement of oropharyngeal muscles.
IVb	Predominantly affecting oropharyngeal, respiratory muscles, or both.
	May also have lesser or equal involvement of limb, axial muscles, or both.
V	Defined by intubation, with or without mechanical ventilation, except when employed during routine postoperative management. The use of a feeding tube without intubation places the patient in class IVb.

Source: Reprinted with permission from A Jaretzki 3rd, RJ Barohn, RM Ernstoff, et al. Myasthenia gravis: recommendations for clinical research standards. Task Force of the Medical Scientific Advisory Board of the Myasthenia Gravis Foundation of America. Neurology 2000;55(1):16–23.

QUANTITATIVE MYASTHENIA GRAVIS SCORE FOR DISEASE SEVERITY

Test Item	None	Mild	Moderate	Severe	Score
Grade	0	1	2	3	
Double vision on lateral gaze right or left (circle one), secs	61	11–60	1–10	Spontaneous	
Ptosis (upward gaze), secs	61	11–60	1–10	Spontaneous	
Facial muscles	Normal lid closure	Complete, weak, some resistance	Complete, without resistance	Incomplete	
Swallowing 4 oz water ($\frac{1}{2}$ cup)	Normal	Minimal coughing or throat clearing	Severe coughing/ choking or nasal regurgitation	Cannot swallow (test not attempted)	
Speech after counting aloud from 1 to 50 (onset of dysarthria)	None at 50	Dysarthria at 30–40	Dysarthria at 10–29	Dysarthria at 9	
Right arm outstretched (90-degree setting), secs	240	90–239	10–89	0–9	
Left arm outstretched (90-degree setting), secs	240	90–239	10–89	0–9	
Vital capacity, % predicted	≥80	65–79	50–64	<50	
Right-hand grip, kg					
Men	≥45	15–44	5–14	0–4	
Women	≥30	10–29	5–9	0–4	
Left-hand grip, kg					
Men	≥35	15–34	5–14	0–4	
Women	≥25	10–24	5–9	0–4	
Head lifted (45 degrees, supine), secs	120	30–119	1–29	0	
Right leg outstretched (45 degrees, supine), secs	100	31–99	1–30	0	
Left leg outstretched (45 degrees, supine), secs	100	31–99	1–30	0	

Source: Reprinted with permission from RJ Barohn, D McIntire, L Herbelin, et al. Reliability testing of the quantitative myasthenia gravis score. Ann N Y Acad Sci 1998;841:769–772.

DIAGNOSTIC CRITERIA FOR DUCHENNE'S MUSCULAR DYSTROPHY*

Inclusion

1. Symptoms are present before the age of 5 years.
2. Clinical signs comprise progressive symmetric muscular weakness: proximal limb muscles more than distal muscles, initially only lower limb muscles. Calf hypertrophy is often present.
3. Exclusions: fasciculations, loss of sensory modalities.
4. Wheelchair dependency before the age of 13 years.
5. There is at least a 10-fold increase of serum CK activity (in relation to age and mobility).
6. Muscle biopsy: abnormal variation in diameter of the muscle fibers (atrophic and hypertrophic fibers), (foci of) necrotic and regenerative fibers, hyalin fibers, increase of endomysial connective and fat tissue.
7. Muscle biopsy: almost no dystrophin demonstrable, except for an occasional muscle fiber (less than 5% of fibers) (*Editor's note*: absent dystrophin by Western blot analysis).
8. DNA: Duchenne-type (frameshift) deletion, or other mutations such as duplication and point mutation within the dystrophin gene, with identical deletion or identical haplotype, involving closely linked markers, as in previous cases in the family.
9. Positive family history, compatible with X-linked recessive inheritance.

The diagnosis is definite when[†]
  A. First case in a family
    1. Age less than 5 years: (2), 3, 5, 6, 7, (8) all present
    2. Age 5–12 years: 1, 2, 3, 4, 5 (at least once), 6, 7, (8) all present
    3. Age greater than 12 years: (1), 2, 3, 4, 5 (at least once), 8, (or 6 and 7) all present
  B. Another case in the family (according to element 9) complies with the criteria under A[‡]
    1. Age less than 5 years: 5 and 9 present
    2. Age 5–12 years: 1, 2, 3, 5 (at least once) all present
    3. Age greater than 12 years: (1), 2, 3, 4, 5 (at least once) all present

---

*Modified from FG Jennekens, ten LP Kate, M de Visser, AR Wintzen. Diagnostic criteria for Duchenne and Becker muscular dystrophy and myotonic dystrophy. Neuromuscul Disord 1991;1(6):389–391. Also available at http://www.enmc.org. Accessed April 30, 2002.

[†]An element number is placed in parentheses when the information is desirable for diagnosis but not yet obtainable or reliable.

[‡]When family history is positive (according to element 9) and B is not valid, one should rule as specified under A.

DIAGNOSTIC CRITERIA FOR BECKER'S MUSCULAR DYSTROPHY*

1. Clinical signs comprise progressive symmetric muscular weakness and atrophy: proximal limb muscles more than distal muscles; initially only lower limb muscles. Calf hypertrophy is often present. Weakness of the quadriceps femoris may be the only manifestation for a long time. Some patients have cramps that are mostly induced by activity. Contractures of the elbow flexors occur late in the course of the disease.
2. Lack of fasciculations; loss of sensory modalities (exclusions).
3. No wheelchair dependency before sixteenth birthday.
4. There is a more than fivefold increase of serum CK activity (in relation to age and mobility).
5. Electromyography: short duration, low amplitude, polyphasic action potentials, fibrillations and positive waves; normal motor and sensory nerve conduction velocities.
6. Muscle biopsy: abnormal variation in diameter of the muscle fibers (disseminated or small groups of atrophic and hypertrophic fibers), (foci of) regenerative fibers, mostly disseminated necrotic fibers. Dependent on stage and course of the disease, there may be a minor degree of grouping of histochemical fiber types and increase of connective and fat tissue.
7. Dystrophin present but decreased or with nonuniform staining in muscle by immunohistochemistry, decreased by Western blot analysis (*Editor's note*).
8. DNA: Becker-type (in frame) deletion, or other mutations such as point mutation within the dystrophin gene, identical deletion or identical haplotype, involving closely linked markers, as in previous case(s) in the family.
9. Positive family history, compatible with X-linked recessive inheritance.

The diagnosis is definite when
  A. First case in a family: (1), 2, 3, 4, 5, and either 8 or 6 and 7 all present.
  B. Another case in the family (according to element 9) complies with the criteria under A.[†]
    1. The case is a first-degree relative: 4 (at least twice) present.
    2. In other situations: (1), 2, 3, 4, 5, and either 8 or 6 and 7 all present.

An element number is placed in parentheses when the information is desirable for diagnosis but not yet obtainable or reliable.

DIAGNOSTIC CRITERIA FOR FACIOSCAPULOHUMERAL MUSCULAR DYSTROPHY[‡]

There are four main criteria that define facioscapulohumeral muscular dystrophy (FSHD):

1. Onset of the disease in facial or shoulder girdle muscles; sparing of the extraocular, pharyngeal, and lingual muscles and the myocardium
2. Facial weakness in more than 50% of the affected family members

---

*Modified from FG Jennekens, LP ten Kate, M de Visser, AR Wintzen. Diagnostic criteria for Duchenne and Becker muscular dystrophy and myotonic dystrophy. Neuromuscul Disord 1991;1(6):389–391.
†When family history is positive (according to element 9) and B is not valid, one should rule as specified under A.
‡Modifed from GW Padberg, PW Lunt, M Koch, M Fardeau. Workshop report. Diagnostic criteria for facioscapulohumeral muscular dystrophy. Neuromuscul Disord 1991;1(4):231–234.

3. Autosomal dominant inheritance in familial cases
4. Evidence of myopathic disease in EMG and muscle biopsy in at least one affected family member without biopsy features specific to alternative diagnoses.

For a standard diagnosis, the following criteria are recommended:

Clinical Criteria

I: Onset of the disease is in facial or shoulder girdle muscles. Presenting symptoms usually relate to weakness or wasting of these muscles.

E: Onset in the pelvic girdle muscles suggests alternative diagnoses, although subsequent pelvic girdle involvement is common in FSHD.

C: Clinical recognizable age of onset is very variable; age at symptomatic onset is even more so. The mean age of recognizable onset (absent presymptomatic) is in the second decade. Onset before the age of 5 years is rare but does not exclude the diagnosis. Infantile or early childhood onset requires facial weakness to be present because the diagnosis cannot otherwise be made reliably.

Facial Involvement

I: Facial weakness affecting eye closure (orbicularis oculi) and peri-oral muscles (orbicularis oris) occurs in the vast majority of patients. In the absence of facial weakness, a diagnosis of FSHD can be accepted only if the majority of affected family members has facial weakness.

E: Extraocular, masticatory, pharyngeal, and lingual muscle weaknesses are not part of the disease. (*Editor's note*: Tongue weakness and atrophy can occur in FSHD, as reported in Yamanaka G, Goto K, Matsumura T, et al. Tongue atrophy in facio-scapulohumeral muscular dystrophy. Neurology 2001;57[4]:733–735; thus, this should not necessarily be an exclusion.)

C: Facial weakness may be very discrete and is sometimes noticeable by asymmetry of facial expression only.

Shoulders

C: The scapular fixators are the muscles most prominently involved. Also, the pectoralis major muscles become affected early in most cases. The deltoid muscles remain unaffected for a long period of time and often have a particular pattern of atrophy (i.e., partial and proximal).

Asymmetry

I: Asymmetry of involvement in the shoulder girdle muscles is the rule, usually affecting the right side first.

C: Symmetric weakness and atrophy at presentation are unusual and necessitate increased caution before accepting the diagnosis of FSHD. Asymmetric involvement of facial muscles occurs frequently.

C: Computed tomographic scan and magnetic resonance imaging (*Editor's addition*) may help to detect asymmetry of muscle atrophy. There appears to be no difference in mean age at death between patients and their nonaffected siblings.

Contractures

Contractures and pseudohypertrophy of muscles may be present.

E: Severe and diffuse contractures exclude the diagnosis of FSHD.

Cardiac Disease

E: Cardiomyopathy is not part of the disease. When present, it suggests an alternative diagnosis.

C: Hearing loss is part of the disease; it starts with high tone perceptive deafness and may progress to involve all frequencies. The severity of hearing loss varies between subjects at any age but tends to be progressive. It is recommended that the results of hearing assessments be documented for several affected members in each family.

C: A retinal vasculopathy with capillary telangiectasis, microaneurysms, and capillary closure has been reported in some members of some FSHD families. At present, it is unclear whether this is a specific association. It should not be used for diagnostic purposes.

C: A few cases have been reported with mental retardation. It is recommended that investigation of any such case should include chromosome analysis, concentrating on the distal long arm of chromosome 4.

Genetic Criteria

I: The pattern of inheritance is autosomal dominant (gene defect in 4q35).

C: Sporadic cases occur; their frequency is unknown, but they are not rare. Only if both parents have been examined can a case be accepted as "sporadic."

E: There is not substantial evidence for recessive inheritance.

Laboratory Criteria

C: CK levels can be normal but are often elevated, although they rarely exceed five times the upper limit of normal. Persistently high CK values above this level warrant exclusion of other neuromuscular diagnoses.

C: EMG often shows short-duration, low-amplitude polyphasic potentials. Some neurogenic features such as high-amplitude potentials and positive sharp waves are present occasionally, but do not characterize individual families. Motor and sensory nerve conduction velocities are normal.

E: Giant motor unit potentials.

C: Muscle biopsies may exhibit any of the standard myopathic criteria. In addition, small angular fibers are not uncommon, and moth-eaten fibers are frequently found. An occasional small group of atrophic fibers may be observed, in which case another biopsy in the same patient or in an affected sibling is desirable. Cellular infiltrates are not uncommon in FSHD and can be extensive. Their significance is unknown. In these cases, an autosomal dominant pattern of inheritance is required to establish the diagnosis of FSHD.

DIAGNOSTIC CRITERIA FOR LIMB-GIRDLE MUSCULAR DYSTROPHY*

Onset

I: Onset of the disease may be in the pelvic or shoulder girdle muscles, or both simultaneously; the initial symptoms usually relate to weakness in one of these muscle groups at any age. Early contractures are not usually a feature of recessive disease but may be seen in some dominantly inherited forms. Calf hypertrophy is a frequent but not invariable finding, and there may be considerable intrafamilial variability for this feature.

E: Onset of weakness in distal, facial, or extraocular muscles should suggest alternative diagnoses, although these muscle groups may be involved later in the course of the disease.

C: Onset of the disease may be at any age. In recessive families, onset beyond the early 20s is less common; in dominant cases, later onset can be seen.

Progression

C: Progression of the weakness is inevitable but ranges from very fast to very slow. Muscle involvement may show some asymmetry. Cardiac involvement has been reported in a minority of patients.

Mode of Inheritance

C: Limb-girdle muscular dystrophy (LGMD) may be inherited in an autosomal dominant or recessive fashion. In the absence of a family history there are, at present, no clear clinical indications to distinguish the two modes of inheritance.

Laboratory Criteria

I: Serum CK is always elevated in recessive cases (at least when the disease is active) and may be used as a presymptomatic test in families in which early elevation of serum CK has been documented.

Note: The diagnosis can be made by evidence of DNA mutation in patients or families associated with LGMD (e.g., sarcoglycans; calpain, dysferlin, or caveolin genes; or evidence of the lack of staining for the particular proteins, on immunohistochemistry of muscle biopsy specimens, if available).

I: Investigations such as EMG and muscle biopsy usually provide evidence of nonspecific myopathic or dystrophic changes. Muscle computed tomographic scanning may also provide evidence of hypodensity in the involved muscles. This

---

*Modified from KMD Bushby. Diagnostic criteria for the Limb Girdle muscular dystrophies. Report of the ENMC consortiums on Limb Girdle dystrophies. Neuromuscul Disord 1995;5(1):71–74. Also available at http://www.enmc.org. Accessed April 30, 2002.

may be useful in the differential diagnosis of LGMD and spinal muscular atrophy, as well as determining the exact pattern of muscle involvement.

E: The diagnosis of LGMD is excluded by the finding of abnormal dystrophin staining on muscle biopsy (providing there are adequate controls for membrane integrity) or the finding of a dystrophin gene abnormality.

In female patients presenting as the first case in their family, chromosome analysis should exclude the finding of an Xp; autosome translocation in association with Duchenne's muscular dystrophy.

In families with more than one affected boy in a sibship, examination with probes within the dystrophin gene can also be used to exclude X-linkage. The finding of muscle biopsy features diagnostic of a neuropathic process, inflammatory changes, and metabolic or mitochondrial abnormalities also excludes the diagnosis.

These exclusions are a vital part of the diagnosis of LGMD.

Note: Several genetic defects have been identified in various LGMDs, which can be recognized by DNA studies. In some, the protein defect can be identified by Western blot or immunohistochemistry (see Chapter 20, particularly Table 20.7, for details).

DIAGNOSTIC CRITERIA FOR MYOTONIC DYSTROPHY (STEINERT DISEASE)*

The clinical picture depends on the age of onset:
  A. Congenital (A1) and infantile myotonic dystrophy (A2), age less than 10 years
  B. Juvenile/adult myotonic dystrophy, age 10–50 years
  C. Late adult/senile myotonic dystrophy, age greater than 50 years

A1. Congenital myotonic dystrophy
   1. Stillbirth or generalized severe muscular weakness (including the face) and hypotonia with sucking, swallowing, and sometimes respiratory insufficiency; absence of tendon reflexes; club feet.
   2. Symptoms of myotonic dystrophy (see B, mentioned previously) in the mother.
   3. If mother is asymptomatic, immature fibers in the muscle biopsy.
   4. Same haplotype, involving closely linked markers, as affected first-degree relative (or evidence of increased number of CTG repeats in chromosome 19). (*Editor's note*: These patients with the defect in chromosome 19 are now considered DM1, and a group of patients with the genetic defect in chromosome 3q21 are now considered DM2.)
A2. Infantile myotonic dystrophy
   1. Mental retardation.
   2. Generalized weakness, especially of the face and distal limbs; myotonia starts usually between the ages of 5 and 10 years.
   3. EMG: Myotonic volleys in several muscles ("dive bomber") resemble repetitive denervation potentials with inconstant frequency of 20–120 Hz, dura-

---

*Adapted from FG Jennekens, LP ten Kate, M de Visser, AR Wintzen. Diagnostic criteria for Duchenne and Becker muscular dystrophy and myotonic dystrophy. Neuromuscul Disord 1991;1(6):389–391. http://www.enmc.org. Accessed April 30, 2002.

tion of at least 0.5 second. (Examination of orbicularis oris, masseter, thenar, and tibialis anterior muscles.)
   4. Symptoms of myotonic dystrophy in one of the parents.
   5. Same haplotype, involving closely linked markers, as affected first-degree relative (or evidence of increased number of CTG repeats in chromosome 19).
B. Juvenile/adult myotonic dystrophy
   1. Myotonia of grip and/or percussion myotonia of thenar.
   2. Weakness of one or more of the following: orbicularis oculi, pharyngeal, or distal limb muscles. Atrophy of masticatory muscles and/or distal limb muscles may be obvious.
   3. Cortical cataract* (slit-lamp examination mandatory).
   4. EMG: myotonic volleys in several muscles.
   5. Positive family history compatible with autosomal dominant inheritance.
   6. Same haplotype, involving closely linked markers, as affected first-degree relative (or evidence of increased number of CTG repeats in chromosome 19).
C. Late adult/senile myotonic dystrophy
   1. Cortical cataract*: mild or no neuromuscular symptoms.
   2. EMG: myotonic volleys in several muscles.
   3. Positive family history compatible with autosomal dominant inheritance.
   4. Same haplotype, involving closely linked markers, as affected first-degree relative (or evidence of increased number of CTG repeats in chromosome 19).

Asymptomatic heterozygotes occur, even in old age.[†]

Criteria for Definite Diagnosis

A. First case in the family	B.* There is a first-degree relative who complies with the criteria under A
A1—1, 2, (3) all present	1, 2, (3) all present
A2—(1), 2, (3), 4, (5) all present	(1), 2, (3), 4, (5) all present
B—1, 3, (5)	1, 2
or 2, 3, 4, (5)	2
or 1, 2, (5)	3
or 6 present	4
	or 6 present
C—more than 1 element	1
or 4 present	or 2
	or 4 present

Note: An element number is placed in parentheses when the information is desirable for diagnosis but not yet obtainable or reliable.
*When family history is positive and B is not valid, one should rule as under A.

---

*Cataract should be cortical, assessed by an experienced ophthalmologist with slit lamp, and should not be used as criterion if no first-degree family member is affected.
[†]Immature fiber: small in diameter. On cross-section, an increased percentage of the fibers have internal nuclei and lack of oxidative enzyme activity at the periphery of the fibers. Differentiation of fiber types on oxidative enzyme reaction is, in some cases, impossible.

DIAGNOSTIC CRITERIA FOR PROXIMAL MYOTONIC MYOPATHY*

Mandatory Inclusion Criteria

1. Weakness, predominantly proximal.
2. Myotonia on EMG.
3. Cataracts: Slit-lamp examination demonstrates posterior, subcapsular, lens opacities resembling the cataracts typically seen in myotonic dystrophy. Onset of cataracts is before 50 years of age. Exception to this is if cataracts have already been removed before 50 years of age.
4. Autosomal dominant inheritance: At least two generations; in large kindreds there must be male-to-male transmission.
5. Normal size of CTG repeat in the gene for myotonic dystrophy (*Note*: genetic defect in chromosome 3q21).

Supportive Findings

Muscle pain
Fluctuating weakness and fluctuating stiffness/myotonia
Calf hypertrophy
Painful muscle cramps
Intermittent muscle fasciculations
Deep tendon reflexes usually preserved
Intermittent episodes of chest pain
Cardiac conduction defects
CNS symptoms: cognitive impairment, hypersomnia, seizures
Deafness: sensorineural
Male hypogonadism: primary type hypogonadism
Insulin resistance/glucose intolerance/diabetes mellitus
Hypothyroidism
Gastrointestinal symptoms: dysphagia, constipation
Frontal baldness
Hyperhydrosis

Exclusion Criteria

Ophthalmoplegia
Predominant distal weakness or distal wasting at onset

Muscle Biopsy

Increased numbers of central nuclei: variation in fiber size; pyknotic clumps; a few small scattered angular fibers; occasional ring fibers; type I fiber predominance; no preferential type I fiber atrophy

---

*Reprinted with permission from RT Moxley 3rd. 54th ENMC International Workshop: PROMM (proximal myotonic myopathies) and other proximal myotonic syndromes. 10–12th October 1997, Naarden, The Netherlands. Neuromuscul Disord 1998;8(7):508–518.

The biopsy helps to exclude some other myopathic disorders:
 Mitochondrial disorders
 Progressive dystrophinopathic muscular dystrophies
 Autosomal recessive limb girdle muscular dystrophies (antibody screening for different membrane associated proteins)
 IBM
 Glycogen storage disease (e.g., acid maltase deficiency)

Laboratory Tests

CK: mildly elevated or normal
Liver function: gamma-glutamyl transferase—mildly elevated or normal
Electrocardiogram: increased frequency of cardiac conduction abnormality
Thyroid function: normal thyroid-stimulating hormone and T4
Glucose tolerance testing: may demonstrate increased insulin release after oral and intravenous glucose loading (findings typical for insulin resistance), and may show impaired glucose tolerance or, occasionally, diabetes mellitus
Gonadal function testing: may demonstrate increased follicle-stimulating hormone, increased luteinizing hormone, and decreased testosterone levels in males

Electromyography

Electrical myotonia; normal or borderline slowing of nerve conduction; normal repetitive stimulation. (Motor unit morphology may have myopathic or neuropathic features in different patients, and some patients have normal morphology of the motor unit potentials.)

DIAGNOSTIC CRITERIA FOR INFLAMMATORY MYOPATHIES*

Five major criteria may be used to define polymyositis (PM) and dermatomyositis (DM):

1. Symmetric weakness of the limb-girdle muscles and anterior neck flexors, progressing over weeks to months, with or without dysphagia or respiratory muscle involvement.
2. Muscle biopsy evidence of necrosis of type I and II fibers, phagocytosis, regeneration with basophilia, large vesicular sarcolemmal nuclei and prominent nucleoli, atrophy in a perifascicular distribution, variation in fiber size, and an inflammatory exudates, often perivascular.
3. Elevation in serum of skeletal-muscle enzymes, particularly creatine phosphokinase and often aldolase, serum glutamate oxaloacetate and pyruvate transaminases, and lactate dehydrogenase.
4. EMG triad of short, small, polyphasic motor units, fibrillations, positive sharp waves and insertional irritability, and bizarre, high-frequency repetitive discharges.

---

*Modified from A Bohan, JB Peter. Polymyositis and dermatomyositis (first of two parts). N Engl J Med 1975;292(7):344–347.

5. Dermatologic features, including a lilac discoloration of the eyelids (heliotrope) with periorbital edema; a scaly, erythematous dermatitis over the dorsum of the hands, especially the metacarpophalangeal and proximal interphalangeal joints (Gottron's sign); and involvement of the knees, elbows and medial malleoli, as well as the face, neck, and upper torso.

Diagnostic Criteria

Definite PM/DM—three or four criteria (plus the rash) for DM; four criteria (without the rash) for PM

Probable PM/DM—two criteria (plus the rash) for DM; three criteria (without the rash) for PM

Possible PM/DM—one criterion (plus the rash) for DM; two criteria (without the rash) for PM

Exclusion Criteria

1. Evidence of central or peripheral neurologic disease, including motor neuron disorders with fasciculations or long-tract signs, sensory changes, decreased nerve conduction times, and fiber-type atrophy and grouping on muscle biopsy.
2. Muscle weakness with a slowly progressive, unremitting course and a positive family history that suggests a muscular dystrophy.
3. Biopsy evidence of granulomatous myositis such as with sarcoidosis (*Editor's note*: vacuoles and inclusion bodies).
4. Infections, including trichinosis, schistosomiasis, trypanosomiasis, staphylococcosis and toxoplasmosis.
5. Recent use of various drugs and toxins, such as clofibrate and alcohol.
6. Rhabdomyolysis and metabolic disorders such as McArdle's syndrome.
7. Endocrinopathies such as thyrotoxicosis, myxedema, hyperparathyroidism, hypoparathyroidism, diabetes mellitus, or Cushing's syndrome.
8. Myasthenia gravis—the simultaneous occurrence of PM and myasthenia gravis has been noted, although some authorities dispute it.
9. Others—myositis after influenzal and rubella infections, vaccination for rubella, the use of penicillamine, multicentric reticulohistiocytosis, giant cell myositis, atheromatous microemboli, and carcinomatous thromboembolization with muscle necrosis.

DIAGNOSTIC CRITERIA FOR POLYMYOSITIS-DERMATOMYOSITIS*

1. Skin lesions
   a. Heliotrope rash (red-purple edematous erythema on the upper palpebra)

---

*Adapted from K Tanimoto, K Nakano, S Kano, et al. Classification criteria for polymyositis and dermatomyositis. J Rheumatol 1995;22(4):668–674.

b. Gottron's sign (red-purple keratotic, atrophic erythema, or macules on the extensor surface of finger joints)

c. Erythema on the extensor surface of extremity joints; slightly raised red-purple erythema over elbows or knees

2. Proximal muscle weakness (upper or lower extremity and trunk)
3. Elevated serum CK or aldolase level
4. Muscle pain on grasping or spontaneous pain
5. Myogenic changes on EMG (short-duration, polyphasic motor unit potentials with spontaneous fibrillation potentials)
6. Positive anti-Jo-1 (histidyl tRNA synthetase) antibody
7. Nondestructive arthritis or arthralgias
8. Systemic inflammatory signs (fever; more than 37°C at axilla, elevated serum c-reactive protein level or accelerated erythrocyte sedimentation rate of more than 20 mm/hour by the Westergren method)
9. Pathologic findings compatible with inflammatory myositis (Inflammatory infiltration of skeletal muscle with degeneration or necrosis of muscle fibers, active phagocytosis, central nuclei, or evidence of active regeneration may be seen.)

Criteria for Diagnosis

Diagnosis made with at least one item from 1 and at least four items from 2–9 = DM
Diagnosis made with at least four items from 2–9 = PM

DIAGNOSTIC CRITERIA FOR INCLUSION BODY MYOSITIS*

I. Characteristic features—inclusion criteria
  A. Clinical features
   1. Duration of illness greater than 6 months.
   2. Age of onset greater than 30 years old.
   3. Muscle weakness must affect proximal and distal muscles of arms and legs and patient must exhibit at least one of the following features:
     a. Finger flexor weakness
     b. Wrist flexor greater than wrist extensor weakness
     c. Quadriceps muscle weakness (≤grade 4 MRC [Medical Research Council])
  B. Laboratory features
   1. Serum CK less than 12 times normal.
   2. Muscle biopsy.
     a. Inflammatory myopathy characterized by mononuclear cell invasion of non-necrotic muscle fibers
     b. Vacuolated muscle fibers
     c. Either
       (1) Intracellular amyloid deposits
       (2) 15- to 18-nm tubulofilaments
     d. EMG must be consistent with features of inflammatory myopathy.

*Reprinted with permission from RC Griggs, V Askanas, S DiMauro, et al. Inclusion body myositis and myopathies. Ann Neurol 1995;38(5):705–713.

3. Family history. (Rarely, IBM may be observed in families. This condition is different from hereditary inclusion body myopathy without inflammation. The diagnosis of familial IBM requires specific documentation of the inflammatory component via muscle biopsy as well as the other laboratory features.)

II. Associated disorders. IBM occurs with a variety of other, especially immune-mediated, conditions. An associated condition does not preclude a diagnosis of IBM if the diagnostic criteria are fulfilled.

III. Diagnostic criteria for inclusion body myositis

A. Definite IBM: Patients must exhibit all muscle biopsy features, including invasion of non-necrotic fibers by mononuclear cells, vacuolated muscle fibers and intracellular amyloid deposits, or 15- to 18-nm tubulofilaments. (None of the other clinical or laboratory features is mandatory if the muscle biopsy features are diagnostic.)

B. Possible IBM: If the muscle shows only inflammation (invasion of non-necrotic muscle fibers by mononuclear cells) without other pathologic features of IBM, then a diagnosis of possible IBM can be given if the patient exhibits the characteristic clinical and laboratory features.

DIAGNOSTIC CRITERIA FOR CHRONIC FATIGUE SYNDROME*

Chronic, unexplained, persistent, or relapsing fatigue of new onset (i.e., not lifelong) that is

- Not alleviated by rest
- Not the result of ongoing exertion
- Severe enough to result in substantial reduction of activity

Four or more of the following present for at least 6 months and not predating the fatigue:

- Impairment of memory or concentration severe enough to interfere with activities
- Sore throat
- Tender cervical or axillary lymph nodes
- Muscle pain
- Pain in multiple joints without swelling or redness
- Headaches of new type, pattern, or severity
- Nonrestorative sleep
- Postexertional malaise lasting more than 24 hours

Major Criteria[†]

1. New onset of persistent or relapsing, debilitating fatigue in a person without a previous history of such symptoms that does not resolve with bed rest and is

---

*Reprinted with permission from K Fukuda, SE Straus, I Hickic, ct al. The chronic fatigue syndrome: a comprehensive approach to its definition and study. International Chronic Fatigue Syndrome Study Group. Ann Intern Med 1994;121(12):953–959.

†Adapted from GP Holmes, JE Kaplan, NM Gantz, et al. Chronic fatigue syndrome: a working case definition. Ann Intern Med 1988;108(3):387–389

severe enough to reduce or impair average daily activity to less than 50% of the patient's premorbid activity level for at least 6 months.
2. Fatigue that is not explained by the presence of other evident medical or psychiatric illness, based on history, physical examination and appropriate laboratory findings.

Minor Criteria

At least six symptoms, plus at least two signs, or at least eight symptoms from the following list.

Symptom Criteria

1. Mild fever or chills
2. Sore throat
3. Painful adenopathy (posterior or anterior, cervical or axillary)
4. Generalized muscle weakness
5. Muscle discomfort or myalgias
6. Prolonged (≥24 hours) generalized fatigue levels of physical activity that would have been easily tolerated in the patient's premorbid state
7. Generalized headaches (of a type, severity, or pattern that is different from headaches the patient may have had in the premorbid state)
8. Migratory arthralgia without swelling or redness
9. Neuropsychologic complaints (one or more of the following: photophobia, transient visual scotomata, forgetfulness, excessive irritability, confusion, difficulty thinking, inability to concentrate, depression)
10. Sleep disturbances (insomnia, hypersomnia)
11. Description of the main symptom complex as initially developing over a few hours to a few days (this is not considered as equivalent to the previously mentioned symptoms in meeting the requirements of the case definition)

Physical Criteria*

Low-grade fever (oral temperature between 37.6° and 36.0°C or rectal temperature between 37.8° and 38.8°C)
Nonexudative pharyngitis
Palpable or tender anterior or posterior, cervical or axillary lymph nodes (nodes >2 cm in diameter suggest other causes; further evaluation is warranted)

---

*To be documented by the physician on at least two occasions that are at least 2 months apart.

THE AMERICAN COLLEGE OF RHEUMATOLOGY 1990 CRITERIA FOR CLASSIFICATION OF FIBROMYALGIA*

1. History of widespread pain.

    Pain is considered widespread when all of the following are present: pain in the left side of the body, pain in the right side of the body, pain above the waist, and pain below the waist. In addition, axial skeletal pain (cervical spine, anterior chest, thoracic spine, or low back) must be present. In this definition, shoulder and buttock pain is considered as pain for each involved side. Low back pain is considered lower segment pain.

2. Pain at 11 of 18 specific tender point sites on digital palpation.

    Pain, on digital palpation, must be present in at least 11 of the following 18 tender point sites:

Occiput—Bilateral, at the suboccipital muscle insertions

Low cervical—Bilateral, at the anterior aspects of the intertransverse spaces at C5-7

Trapezius—Bilateral, at the midpoint of the upper border

Supraspinatus—Bilateral, at origins, above the scapula spine near the medial border

Second rib—Bilateral, at the second costochondral junctions, just lateral to the junctions on upper surfaces

Lateral epicondyle—Bilateral, 2 cm distal to the epicondyles

Gluteal—Bilateral, in upper outer quadrants of buttocks in anterior fold of muscle

Greater trochanter—Bilateral, posterior to the trochanteric prominence

Knee—Bilateral, at the medial fat pad proximal to the joint line

Digital palpation should be performed with an approximate force of 4 kg (when compared with the force to reach if 4 kg in a dolorimeter).

For a tender point to be considered "positive" the subject must state that the palpation was painful. "Tender" is not to be considered painful. (0 = no pain; 1 = mild; 2 = moderate; 3 = severe; 4 = unbearable.)

SUGGESTED PRELIMINARY CRITERIA FOR THE DIAGNOSIS OF PRIMARY FIBROMYALGIA SYNDROME†

Major Criteria

Presence of two or more of the following six historic variables:

- "Hurt all over"
- Pain at seven or more sites
- General fatigue

---

*For classification purposes, patients are said to have fibromyalgia if criteria 1 and 2 are satisfied. Widespread pain must have been present for at least 3 months. The presence of a second clinical disorder does not exclude the diagnosis of fibromyalgia. Data adapted from F Wolfe, HA Smythe, MB Yunus, et al. The American College of Rheumatology 1990 Criteria for the Classification of Fibromyalgia. Report of the Multicenter Criteria Committee. Arthritis Rheum 1990;33(2):160–172.

†Adapted from MB Yunus, AT Masi, JC Aldag. Preliminary criteria for primary fibromyalgia syndrome (PFS): multivariate analysis of a consecutive series of PFS, other pain patients, and normal subjects. Clin Exp Rheumatol 1989;7(1):63–69.

- Poor sleep
- Anxiety/tension
- Irritable bowel syndrome

Plus four or more of the following tender points (right or left for each):

- Upper mid-trapezius
- Sternomastoid muscle (lower)
- Lateral pectoral muscle
- Midsupraspinatus muscle
- Upper lateral gluteal region
- Greater trochanteric region
- Medial fat pad of the knee

Minor Criteria

Presence of three or more of the previously mentioned six historical variables, plus two or more tender points

Obligatory Criteria

1. Presence of pain or stiffness, or both, at four or more anatomic sites (counting unilateral or bilateral involvement as one site) for 3 months or longer
2. Exclusion of an underlying condition which may be responsible for the overall features of fibromyalgia

Diagnosis of Primary Fibromyalgia Syndrome

Requires major or minor criteria, plus the obligatory criteria

Appendix 3

Protocols of Evaluation and Neuromuscular Disorder Rating Scales

Tulio E. Bertorini, Pushpa Narayanaswami, and Kandasami Senthilkumar

This section summarizes published protocols that can be applied to various neuromuscular diseases during clinic follow-ups or research clinical trials. The first few pages include those that can be used in most neuromuscular diseases such as published clinical functional grading scale, grading muscle strength scales, and a pain grading system. The rest of the Appendix includes evaluation and rating scales to apply in selected specific neuromuscular diseases.

SCHWAB AND ENGLAND ACTIVITIES OF DAILY LIVING SCALE

100	Completely independent; able to do all activities without slowness, difficulty, or impairment; essentially normal; unaware of any difficulty
90	Completely independent; able to do all activities with some degree of slowness, difficulty, and impairment; might take twice as long; beginning to be aware of difficulty
80	Completely independent in most activities; takes twice as long; conscious of difficulty and slowness
70	Not completely independent; more difficulty with some activities; takes three to four times as long to perform some activities; must spend a large part of the day with activities
60	Some dependency; can perform most activities but exceedingly slowly and with much effort; errors; some impossible
50	More dependent; needs help with half of activities; is slower, etc.; has difficulty with everything
40	Very dependent; can assist in all activities but few alone
30	With effort, now and then does a few activities alone or begins alone; much help needed
20	Nothing alone; can be of slight help with some activities; severe invalid
10	Totally dependent, helpless; complete invalid; care impossible outside hospital setting
0	Basic bodily functions only; bedridden

MODIFIED RANKIN SCALE*

Grade	Description
0	No symptoms at all
1	No significant disability despite symptoms, able to carry out all usual duties and activities
2	Slight disability; unable to carry out all previous activities but able to look after own affairs without assistance
3	Moderate disability; requiring some help, but able to walk without assistance
4	Moderately severe disability; unable to walk without assistance and unable to attend to own bodily needs without assistance
5	Severe disability; bedridden, incontinent, and requiring constant nursing care and attention

*This is a disability scale used in stroke patients but that can be used in patients with neuromuscular disorders. Source: Adapted from J Rankin. Cerebral vascular accidents in patients over the age of 60: prognosis. Scott Med J 1957;2:200–215; and JC van Swieten, PJ Koudstaal, MC Visser, et al. Interobserver agreement for the assessment of handicap in stroke patients. Stroke 1988;19:604–607.

MUSCLE TONE: MODIFIED ASHWORTH SCALE

0	No increase in tone
1	Slight increase in muscle tone, manifested by a catch followed by minimal assistance throughout the remainder (less than half the range of motion)
2	More marked increase in tone through most of the range of motion by affected parts easily moved
3	Considerable increase in tone, passive movement difficult
4	Limb rigid in flexion or extension

Source: Reprinted with permission from R Bohannan, MD Smith. Reliability of a modified Ashworth scale of muscle spasticity. Phys Ther 1987;67:206–207.

MUSCLE FUNCTION PROTOCOL

Name _____

Age _____

Manual Muscle Test Scores

Muscle Strength	Date		Date		Date		Date	
	Right	Left	Right	Left	Right	Left	Right	Left
Neck								
Extension								
Flexion								
Shoulder								
Abduction								
Flexion								
Elbow								
Extension								
Flexion								
Wrist								
Extension								
Flexion								
Hand								
Finger extensor								
Finger flexor								
Abduction thumb								
Finger spread								
Hip								
Extension								
Flexion								
Abduction (gluteus medius)								
Knee								
Extension								
Flexion								
Ankle								
Flexion								
Dorsiflexion								
Eversion								
Inversion								
Total Score								
Mean Score								

Muscle Strength Scales

Standard Grading Scale	MRC Scale	MRC Modified Scale	Description
N	5	10	Normal strength
G+	4+	9	Barely detectable weakness
G	4	8	Holds test position against gravity and moderate resistance
F+	3+	6	Muscle moves joint fully against gravity—is capable of transient resistance but collapses abruptly
F	3	5	Muscle moves joint fully against gravity but cannot hold against resistance
F– & P+	3–	4	Muscle moves joint against gravity but not the full possible extent of mechanical range
P	2+	3	Muscle moves joint when gravity eliminated through full extent of mechanical range
P–	2	2	Muscle moves joint when gravity eliminated through partial extent of mechanical range
Tr	1	1	A flicker of contraction felt in muscles; no joint motion
0	0	0	No contraction felt in muscle

F = fair; G = gravity; MRC = Medical Research Council; N = normal; P = poor; Tr = trace.
Source: Reprinted with permission from TE Bertorini. Requirements for adequate clinical trials in Duchenne's muscular dystrophy. Muscle Nerve 1985;470–473.

Range of Motion Limitations from Contractures

	Date		Date		Date		Date	
	Right	Left	Right	Left	Right	Left	Right	Left
Pelvic flexion contracture								
Knee flexor contracture								
Hip flexor contracture								
Iliotibial band contracture								
Elbow flexor contracture								

*Functional Grade: Lower Extremity**

1. Walks and climbs stairs without assistance
2. Walks and climbs with aid of railing
3. Walks and climbs stairs slowly with aid of railing (longer than 12 seconds for four standard steps)
4. Walks unassisted and rises from chair but cannot climb stairs
5. Walks unassisted but cannot rise from chair or climb stairs

---

*Reprinted with permission from PJ Vignos. In Licht S (ed), Rehabilitation and Medicine. New Haven, CT: E. Licht, 1968;584–562.

6. Walks only with assistance or walks independently with long leg braces
7. Walks in long leg braces but requires assistance for balance
8. Stands in long leg braces but unable to walk even with assistance
9. Is in wheelchair
10. Confined to bed

*Functional Grade: Upper Extremity**

11. Starting with arms at sides, abducts the arms in full circle until they touch above the head; places a weight of 2 kg or more on a shelf above eye level
12. Raises arm above head as previously, but cannot place 2 kg of weight on a shelf
13. Raises arms above head only by flexing the elbow (i.e., shortening the circumference of the movement or using accessory muscles)
14. Cannot raise hands above head but raises 8-oz glass of water to mouth
15. Raises hands to mouth but cannot raise 8-oz glass of water to mouth
16. Cannot raise hands to mouth but can use hands to hold pen or pick up pennies from table
17. Cannot raise hands to mouth and has no useful function of hands

PAIN GRADING SCALE: VERBAL DESCRIPTOR SCALE OF PAIN SCORES

0	1	2	3	4	5	6	7	8	9	10	11	12	13	14	15	16	17	18	19	20
	S	L	I	G	H	T	M	O	D	E	R	A	T	E	S	E	V	E	R	E

No pain   Worst possible pain

_____

Patient's Name

_____

Date

_____

*Reprinted with permission from MH Brooke, RC Griggs, JR Mendell, et al. Clinical trial in Duchenne dystrophy. I. The design of the protocol. Muscle Nerve 1981;4(3):186–197.

GRADING SCALE FOR SENSORY DEFICIT: INFLAMMATORY NEUROPATHY COURSE AND TREATMENT SENSORY SUMSCORE (ISS)[a]

Pinprick Sensation, Sites of Examination and Corresponding Grades		Vibration Sensation, Sites of Examination and Corresponding Grades[b]		Two-Point Discrimination, Site of Examination and Corresponding Grades[c]
Arms	**Legs**	**Arms**	**Legs**	**Index finger (K)**
Normal sense	Normal sense	Normal sense	Normal sense	Normal sense
0 = at index finger (A)	0 = at hallux (F)	0 = at index finger (A)	0 = at hallux (F)	—
Abnormal sense	Abnormal sense	Abnormal sense	Abnormal sense	Abnormal sense
1 = at index finger (B)	1 = at hallux (G)	1 = at index finger (B)	1 = hallux (G)	1 = 5–9 mm
2 = at wrist (C)	2 = at ankle (H)	2 = at wrist (C)	2 = at ankle (H)	2 = 10–14 mm
3 = at elbow (D)	3 = at knee (I)	3 = elbow (D)	3 = at knee (I)	3 = 15–19 mm
4 = at shoulder (E)	4 = at groin (J)	4 = at shoulder (E)	4 = at groin (J)	4 = ≥20 mm

A, B = index finger (dorsum distal interphalangeal joint); C = ulnar styloid process; D = medial humerus epicondyle; E = acromioclavicular joint; F, G = hallux (dorsum interphalangeal joint); H = medial malleolus; I = patella; J = anterior superior iliac spine; K = index finger (ventral side of distal phalanx).

[a]ISS composition: pinprick arm grade (range, 0–4) and vibration arm grade (range, 0–4); pinprick leg grade (range, 0–4) and vibration leg grade (range, 0–4); and two-point discrimination grade (range, 0–4).

[b]Vibration was assessed using the Rydel-Seiffert graduated tuning fork, and the values obtained were compared with the published normative vibration threshold values. Pinprick and vibration sense examination took place distal to proximal, and only the highest extension of dysfunction of the most affected arm and leg was recorded separately for both qualities.

[c]ISS range: 0 (normal sensation) to 20 (most severe sensory deficit).

Source: Reprinted with permission from IS Merkies, PI Schmitz, FG van der Meche, PA van Doorn. Psychometric evaluation of a new sensory scale in immune-mediated polyneuropathies. Neurology 2000;54: 943–949.

NORRIS AMYOTROPHIC LATERAL SCLEROSIS SCORE

	Normal (3)	Impaired (2)	Trace (1)	No Use (0)
1. Hold up neck				
2. Chew food				
3. Swallow				
4. Speak				
5. Turn in bed				
6. Sit up				
7. Empty bowel and bladder				
8. Breathe				
9. Cough				
10. Write name				
11. Use buttons, zippers				
12. Feed self				
13. Grip-lift self				
14. Lift book or tray				
15. Lift fork, pencil				
16. Change arm position				
17. Climb stairs, one flight				
18. Walk one block				
19. Walk across room				
20. Walk with assistance				
21. Stand up				
22. Change leg position				
		Hyperactive/ hypoactive	**Absent**	**Clonic**
23. Stretch reflexes—arms				
24. Stretch reflexes—legs				
	Absent	**Present**	**Hyperactive**	**Clonic**
25. Jaw jerk				
	Flexor	**Mute**	**Equivocal**	**Extensor**
26. Plantar response—right				
27. Plantar response—left				
	None	**Slight**	**Moderate**	**Severe**
28. Fasciculation				
29. Wasting—face, tongue				
30. Wasting—arms, shoulders				
31. Wasting—legs, hips				
32. Labile emotions				
		None to mild		**Moderate to severe**
33. Fatigability				
34. Leg rigidity				

Source: Reprinted with permission from FH Norris Jr, PR Calanchini, RJ Fallat, et al. The administration of guanidine in amyotrophic lateral sclerosis. Neurology 1974;24:721–728.

QUANTITATIVE MOTOR ASSESSMENT IN AMYOTROPHIC LATERAL SCLEROSIS: TUFTS QUANTITATIVE NEUROMUSCULAR EXAMINATION PROTOCOL*

Pulmonary function. Two pulmonary function tests are conducted using a Collins Eagle II survey spirometer and microprocessor (Warren E. Collins, Inc., Braintree, MA). Forced vital capacity (best of two trials) and maximum voluntary ventilation are recorded, using standard techniques.

Oropharyngeal. This consists of measuring diadochokinetic syllable production. A stopwatch is used to measure the time required to repeat the sound "pa" 20 times and the sound "pata" 15 times (Table A3.1). The better of two trials is recorded.

Timed motor activities. Dexterity of each hand is tested by timing the speed of dialing a standard telephone number and placing standard pegs in a Purdue pegboard (Model 32020, JA Preston Corp, New York, NY) while subject is seated at a 64-cm-high table. The speed with which a patient walks 15 feet, with or without assistance or devices, is also measured (Table A3.1).

Maximal isometric strength. An electronic strain gauge tensiometer (Interface, Inc., Scottsdale, AZ) is used to measure the maximal isometric force of nine muscle groups bilaterally. Flexion and extension at the shoulder, elbow, hip, and knee and extension at the shoulder, elbow, hip, and knee and dorsiflexion at the ankle were tested in standard positions (Table A3.2). The subject is positioned on a standard examination table (180 cm long, 60 cm wide, and 75 cm high) with aluminum uprights and adjustable rings. The limb is attached to a leather strap connected to the strain gauge, which in turn is attached to a ring on the immobile upright. The height of the ring is adjusted to ensure that the strap and strain gauge are parallel with the table. Force is transduced electronically by the amount of distortion of a metal ring within the strain gauge, then amplified and recorded on a strip chart recorder. The better of two trials is used as the score for that test.

Bilateral grip strength is measured using a Jamar dynamometer (Asimow Engineering Co., Los Angeles, CA). The patient is seated with the elbow at 90 degrees and with the forearm not resting on the thigh. The examiner can support the forearm but is not to stabilize the wrist. The better of two attempts per hand is recorded.

Table A3.1 Timed Motor Activities

Test Item	Equipment Needed	Criteria for Test Completion
Speech rate "pa"	Stopwatch	20 repetitions
Speech rate "papa"	Stopwatch	15 repetitions
Phone dialing	Spring-loaded dial phone, stopwatch	Completing the seven-digit number 764-7172
Pegboard test	Purdue pegboard, stopwatch	Number of pegs placed in 30 secs
Timed 15-ft walk	Stopwatch	Crossing the 15 ft marker

*Source: Reprinted with permission from PL Andres, W Hedlund, L Finison, et al. Quantitative motor assessment in amyotrophic lateral sclerosis. Neurology 1986;36:937–941.

Table A3.2 Method of Isometric Strength Testing Using an Electronic Strain Gauge

Muscle Group	Position of Patient
Shoulder flexion	Supine
Shoulder extension	Supine
Elbow flexion	Supine
Hip extension	Trunk at 20 degrees, supported on pillows
Hip flexion	Trunk at 20 degrees, supported on pillows
Knee extension	Sitting upright, towel roll under distal thigh
Knee flexion	Sitting upright, towel roll under distal thigh
Dorsiflexion	Supine, towel roll under ankle

AMYOTROPHIC LATERAL SCLEROSIS RATING SCALE

Description	Points
Bulbar (6–30 points)	
Swallowing	
General diet	3
Soft diet (soft, cooked, eliminates popcorn, nuts, cornbread, etc.)	6
Mechanical soft diet (finely chopped or ground and thick liquids)	9
Pudding consistency diet (strained, pureed, blended, and thick liquids)	12
Tube feedings	15
Speech	
Clear	3
Slightly slurred on enunciation of "pa," "ta," "ka"	6
Slurred	9
Unintelligible	12
None	15
Respiratory (6–30 points)	
VC less than 500 cc from highest previous recording or within 500 cc of predicted value	6
Change in VC of more than 500 cc from highest previous recording or from predicted VC, or need for incentive spirometry, medication, or chest physiotherapy	12
Change in VC of more than 1,000 cc from highest previous recording or from predicted VC, or need for intermittent positive pressure breathing or suctioning	18
VC below 1,800 cc or only able to record tidal volume due to weakness	24
Endotracheal intubation or tracheostomy	30
Muscle strength (6–36 points) using Medical Research Council scores of 0–5	
Muscles of upper extremities (sum of R and L sides) (deltoids, biceps, triceps, wrist extensors, wrist flexors, finger extensors, finger flexors)	
70	2
62–69	4
54–61	6
46–53	8
32–45	10
18–31	12
≤17	14

Table A3.2. *Continued*

Description	Points
Muscles of lower extremities (sum of R and L sides) (iliopsoas, quadriceps, hamstrings, ankle dorsiflexion, plantar flexion, toe extension, toe flexion)	
70	2
62–69	4
54–61	6
46–53	8
32–45	10
18–31	12
≤17	14
Grip (lb R grip + lb L grip divided by 2) using a Jamar adjustable dynamometer	
≥60	1
46–59	2
20–45	3
<20	4
Lateral pinch (lb R pinch + lb L pinch divided by 2) using an Osco pinch gauge	
≥14	1
10–13	2
5–9	3
<5	4
Muscle function—lower extremities (6–35 points)	
Standing from chair (secs)	
0.0–1.0	1
1.5–3.0	2
3.5–5.0	3
>5	4
Unable	5
Standing from lying supine (secs)	
≤2	1
2.5–4.0	2
4.5–6.0	3
6.5–10.0	4
>10	5
Unable	6
Walking 20 ft (6 m) (secs)	
≤8	1
8.5–12.0	2
12.5–16.0	3
>16	4
Unable	5
Need for assistive devices	
None	1
AFO/cane/boots	2
Walker, crutches, and occasional wheelchair (for long trips, etc.), or a combination of these	3
Confined mostly or always to wheelchair	4
Confined to bed	5

Climbing and descending four standard steps (secs)

≤5	1
5.5–8.0	2
8.5–12.0	3
12.5–18.0	4
>18	5
Unable	6

Hips and legs

Walks and climbs stairs without assistance	1
Walks and climbs stairs with aid of railing	2
Cannot climb stairs but walks unassisted and rises from chair	3
Cannot climb stairs but walks unassisted with either AFO or cane	4
Cannot climb stairs but walks with minimal assistance or walks unassisted with crutches or walker	5
Cannot climb stairs but walks with crutches or walker with assistance or walks with total support	6
Confined to wheelchair	7
Confined to bed	8

Muscle function—upper extremities (6–33 points)

Dress and feed

Independent	1
Independent with aids (button hooks, zipper pull, padded utensils, plate holder; does not need assistance)	2
Minor assistance (needs assistance cutting meat, buttons, shifting clothing)	3
Major assistance (caretaker does most of dressing or feeding, or both)	4
Dependent	5

Propelling wheelchair 20 ft (6 m) (secs)

≤11	1
11.5–20.0	2
20.5–30.0	3
30.5–40.0	4
>40	5
Unable	6

Arms and shoulders (grade the most affected side)

Starting with arms at the sides, abducts the arms in a full circle until they touch above the head	1
Raises arms above the head only by flexing the elbow or using accessory muscles	2
Cannot raise hands above the head but raises glass of water to mouth	3
Raises hands to mouth but cannot raise glass of water to mouth	4
Cannot raise hands to mouth but can use hands to hold articles	5
Cannot raise hands to mouth and has no useful function of hands	6

Cutting Theraplast—dominant hand (secs)

≤5	1
5.5–10.0	2
10.5–15.0	3
15.5–20.0	4
>20.0	5
Unable	6

Table A3.2. *Continued*

Description	Points
Purdue peg board (60 secs): (No. of pegs R side + No. of pegs L side divided by 2)	
27–36	1
22–26	2
18–21	3
1–17	4
Unable	5
Blocks (60 secs): (No. of blocks R side + No. of blocks L side divided by 2)	
75–95	1
62–74	2
43–61	3
1–42	4
Unable	5

AFO = ankle-foot orthosis; L = left; R = right; VC = vital capacity.

Source: Reprinted with permission from V Appel, SS Stewart, G Smith, SH Appel. A rating scale for amyotrophic lateral sclerosis: description and preliminary experience. Ann Neurol 1987;22:328–333.

AMYOTROPHIC LATERAL SCLEROSIS FUNCTIONAL RATING SCALE

Speech

4   Normal speech processes
3   Detectable speech disturbance
2   Intelligible with repeating
1   Speech combined with nonvocal communication
0   Loss of useful speech

Salivation

4   Normal
3   Slight but definite excess of saliva in mouth, may have nighttime drooling
2   Moderately excessive saliva; may have minimal drooling
1   Marked excess of saliva with some drooling
0   Marked drooling; requires constant use of tissue or handkerchief

Swallowing

4   Normal eating habits
3   Early eating problems, occasional choking
2   Dietary consistency changes
1   Needs supplemental tube feeding
0   Nothing by mouth (exclusively parenteral or enteral feeding)

Handwriting

4   Normal
3   Slow or sloppy; all words are legible
2   Not all words are legible
1   Able to grip pen but unable to write
0   Unable to grip pen

Cutting food and handling utensils (without gastrostomy)

4   Normal
3   Somewhat slow and clumsy but no help needed

2   Can cut most foods, although clumsy and slow, no help needed

1   Food must be cut by someone but can still feed self slowly

0   Needs to be fed

Alternate scale for patients with gastrostomy

4   Normal

3   Clumsy but able to perform all manipulations independently

2   Some help needed with closures and fasteners

1   Provides minimal assistance to caregivers

0   Unable to perform any aspect of task

Dressing and hygiene

4   Normal function

3   Independent and complete self-care with effort or decreased efficiency

2   Intermittent assistance or substitute methods

1   Needs attendant for self-care

0   Total dependence

Turning in bed and adjusting bed clothes

4   Normal

3   Somewhat slow and clumsy, but no help needed

2   Can turn alone or adjust sheets, but with great difficulty

1   Can initiate but unable turn or adjust sheets alone

0   Helpless

Walking

4   Normal

3   Early ambulation difficulties

2   Walks with assistance (any assistive device including ankle-foot orthosis)

1   Nonambulatory functional movement only

0   No purposeful leg movement

Climbing stairs

4   Normal

3   Slow

2   Mild unsteadiness or fatigue

1   Needs assistance (including handrail)

0   Cannot do

Breathing

4   Normal

3   Shortness of breath with minimal exertion (e.g., walking, talking)

2   Shortness of breath at rest

1   Intermittent (e.g., nocturnal) ventilator dependence

0   Ventilator dependent

Source: Reprinted with permission from Amyotrophic Lateral Sclerosis Functional Rating Scale. Assessment of activities of daily living in patients with amyotrophic lateral sclerosis. The ALS CNTF Treatment Study (ACTS) Phase I–II Study Group. Arch Neurol 1996;53(2):141–147.

SICKNESS IMPACT PROFILE/AMYOTROPHIC LATERAL SCLEROSIS-19

Domain	Question	SIP Weight	% of SIP/ALS
Body care and management	I make difficult moves with help (e.g., getting in or out of cars, bathtubs).	0.84	4.5
	I do not move into or out of bed or chair by myself but am moved by person or mechanical aid.	1.21	6.5
	I am in a restricted position all the time.	1.25	6.7
	I do not bathe myself at all but am bathed by someone else.	1.15	6.2
	I use a bedpan with assistance.	1.14	6.1
	I get dressed only with someone's help.	0.88	4.7
Home management	I am doing less of the regular daily work around the house than I would usually do.	0.86	4.6
Mobility	I stay within one room.	1.06	5.7
	I stay home most of the time.	0.66	3.5
Social interaction	I am not going out to visit people at all.	1.01	5.4
Ambulation	I do not walk at all.	1.05	5.6
Communication	I am having trouble writing or typing.	0.7	3.7
	I communicate mostly by gestures (e.g., moving my head, pointing, sign language).	1.02	5.5
	My speech is understood only by a few people who know me well.	0.93	5.0
	I am understood with difficulty.	0.87	4.7
Recreation and pastime	I am not doing any of my usual physical recreation or activities.	0.77	4.1
Eating	I feed myself but only by using specially prepared food or utensils.	0.77	4.1
	I do not feed myself at all but must be fed.	1.17	6.3
	I am eating no food at all. Nutrition is taken through tubes or intravenous fluid.	1.33	7.1
Totals		**18.67**	**100.0**

ALS = amyotrophic lateral sclerosis, SIP = sickness impact profile.

Source: Reprinted with permission from D McGuire, L Garrison, C Armon, et al. A brief quality of life measure for ALS clinical trials based on a subset of items from the sickness impact profile. J Neurol Sci 1997;152:S18–S22.

NEUROPATHY SYMPTOM PROFILE SCREENING*

This questionnaire can be used to complement the history and staging severity of the disease, and to recognize patterns of involvement. The results can be analyzed visually or by computer. Patient to answer yes or no to each question.

1. Do you have muscle weakness?
   If yes, complete the following:
   a. Is your weakness in lower limbs only?
   b. Is your weakness in upper limbs only?
   c. Has your weakness taken another course?
   If yes, please describe.

2. Answer each of the questions:
   a. Do you sometimes feel full of energy?
   b. Do you feel tired much of the time?
   c. Are you unable to arise from a kneeling position without use of your arms?

3. Do you get muscle cramps or a "charley horse"?
   a. Are the cramps in muscles of both lower and upper limbs?
   b. Are the cramps of muscles of the lower limbs only?
   c. Have the cramps increased in frequency progressively since their onset?

4. Is your sensation (sense of feeling) abnormal?†
   If yes, complete the following:
   a. Is your abnormal sensation confined to both lower and upper limbs?
   b. Is your abnormal sensation confined to the lower limbs?
   c. Have you ever burned yourself without feeling pain?
   If yes, amplify or elaborate giving dates and events below.

5. Are you excessively unsteady (stumble) when walking?
   If yes, complete the following:
   a. Does the unsteadiness come only occasionally (only for a few seconds or minutes at a time)?
   b. Is the unsteadiness present most or all of the time?
   c. Has your unsteadiness taken another course?
   If yes, please explain.

6. Do you have a "prickly asleep-numbness" (i.e., when your hand goes asleep from lying on it) of the feet? (Do not include numbness as explained in item 4.)
   If yes, complete the following:
   a. Does the numbness come only occasionally (only for a few minutes at a time)?
   b. Is it present most or all of the time?
   c. Have areas of numbness appeared and persisted for more than a few hours in different parts of your body?

---

*Adapted from Dyck PJ, Karnes J, O'Brien PC, Swanson PJ. Neuropathy Symptom Profile in health, motor neuron disease, diabetic neuropathy, and amyloidosis. Neurology 1986;36(10):1300 1308.
†Do *not* include "prickling asleep-numbness" or "dead asleep-numbness" that develops from sitting too long in one position or from lying on a limb too long producing numbness for a few minutes only.

7. Do you have "prickly-sleep numbness" of hands? (Do not include numbness as explained in item 4.)
   a. Does the numbness come only occasionally (only for a few minutes at a time)?
   b. Is present most or all of the time?
   c. Has the numbness taken another course?
   If yes, please describe.

8. Do you have "dead-asleep numbness" "like Novocain" without prickling of the feet? (Do not include numbness as explained in item 4.)
   If yes, complete the following:
   a. Does the numbness come only occasionally (only for a few minutes at a time)?
   b. Is it present most or all of the time?
   c. Have areas the numbness appeared and persisted for more than a few hours in different parts of your body?
   If yes, please describe.

9. Do you have "dead-asleep numbness" "like Novocain" without prickling of the hands? (Do not include numbness explained in item 4.)
   If yes, complete the following:
   a. Does the numbness come only occasionally (only for a few minutes at a time)?
   b. Is it present most or all the time?
   c. Has the numbness taken another course?
   If yes, please describe.

10. Do you have "burning discomfort" of the hands?
    If yes, complete the following:
    a. Does this type of discomfort come only occasionally (only for a few minutes at a time)?
    b. Is it present most or all of the time?
    c. Has the discomfort taken another course?
    If yes, please describe.

11. Do you have "burning discomfort" of the feet?
    If yes, complete the following:
    a. Does this type of discomfort come only occasionally (only for a few minutes at a time)?
    b. Is present most or all of the time?
    c. Has the discomfort taken another course?
    If yes, please describe.

12. Do you have difficulty recognizing objects by feel with hands?
    If yes, complete the following:
    a. Is this difficulty in both hands?
    b. Is this difficulty in one hand only?
    c. Has the difficulty taken another course?
    If yes, please describe.

13. Are you unable to feel your feet when you walk?
    If yes, complete the following:
    a. Is this disability the same as it was 3 months ago?
    b. Is better than it was 3 months ago?
    c. Has the disability taken another course?
    If yes, please describe.

14. Are you unable to distinguish hot from cold water when you put your feet in the bath?
    If yes, complete the following:
    a. Is this disability the same as it was 3 months ago?
    b. Is it better than it was 3 months ago?
    c. Has the disability taken another course?
    If yes, please describe.

15. Are you unable to distinguish hot from cold water with your hands?
    If yes, complete the following:
    a. Is this disability the same as it was 3 months ago?
    b. Is better than it was 3 months ago?
    c. Has the disability taken another course?
    If yes, please describe.

16. Do you experience these symptoms in your hands?
    Answer for each symptom:
    a. Hurt with use
    b. Jabbing pain
    c. Deadness

17. Do you experience these symptoms in your feet?
    Answer for each symptom:
    a. Hurt with walking
    b. Jabbing pain
    c. Deadness

18. Do you experience any of these symptoms in your abdomen and/or chest?
    Answer for each symptom:
    a. Hurt with use
    b. Jabbing pain
    c. Deadness

19. Do you experience any of these symptoms in your face and/or mouth and/or throat?
    Answer for each symptom:
    a. Hurt with use
    b. Jabbing pain
    c. Deadness

20. Have you fainted more than once during the last year?
    If yes, complete the following:
    a. Usually while standing.

b. Usually while seated.
c. Do you faint more frequently now than 1 year ago?

21. Do you have blurring of vision?
    If yes, complete the following:
    a. Does it occur only with standing?
    b. Does it occur only with prolonged reading?
    c. Is it followed by a bad headache?

22. Do you have double vision?
    If yes, complete the following:
    a. Does it occur only with standing?
    b. Does it occur only for a second or two at one time?
    c. Does it occur in recurring episodes lasting at least several minutes?

23. Do you vomit (apart from during an infection like the flu)?
    If yes, complete the following:
    a. Does it include food from several meals?
    b. Does this occur occasionally (at least once per week)?
    c. Does this occur frequently (at least once per day)?

24. Do you have night diarrhea?
    If yes, complete the following:
    a. Does this occur occasionally (once per week)?
    b. Does this occur frequently (once per day)?

25. Do you have loss of control of normal bowel motions (not diarrhea) so that you soil yourself?
    If yes, complete the following:
    a. Do you have no control?
    b. Do you have occasional soiling?
    c. Do you have the loss of control due to urgency?

26. Do you have loss of control of bladder function?
    If yes, complete the following:
    a. Cannot void, so need catheterization?
    b. Incontinent, but no need for catheterization?
    c. In women: Occurs only with cough, sneeze, strain, or pushing?

27. In men: Can you have a penile erection?

28. In men: Can you ejaculate (emission of fluid with sexual climax)?

29. Do you overheat because you sweat insufficiently?

30. Are you unable to sweat on your hands?

31. Are you unable to sweat on your feet?

32. Do you have other symptoms you would like to report?
    If yes, please describe.

33. Do you smoke cigarettes?
    If yes, complete the following:
    a. Smoke more than one pack per day?
    b. Smoke less than one pack per day?

34. Do you drink alcohol?
    If yes, complete the following:
    a. Beer, ounces/week* _____
    b. Wine, ounces/week* _____
    c. Hard alcohol, kind* _____
       ounces/week* _____

---

*A can of beer is 12 oz, a cup is 8 oz, and an average "shot of whiskey" is approximately 1 oz.

NEUROPATHY SYMPTOM SCORE*

Neurologic Symptom Score[†]

Score 1 point for presence of a symptom.
  I. Symptoms of muscle weakness
     A. Bulbar
        1. Extraocular
        2. Facial
        3. Tongue
        4. Throat
     B. Limbs
        5. Shoulder girdle and upper arm
        6. Hand
        7. Glutei and thigh
        8. Legs
 II. Sensory
     A. Negative symptoms
        9. Difficulty identifying objects in mouth
        10. Difficulty identifying objects in hands
        11. Unsteadiness in walking
     B. Positive Symptoms
        12. "Numbness," "asleep feeling," "like Novocain," "prickling"—at any site
        13. Pain—burning, deep aching, tenderness—at any location
III. Autonomic symptoms
        14. Postural fainting
        15. Impotence in male
        16. Loss of urinary control
        17. Night diarrhea

---

*Reprinted with permission from PJ Dyck, WR Sherman, LM Hallcher, et al. Human diabetic endoneural sorbitol, fructose, and myoinositol relate to sural nerve morphometry. Ann Neurol 1980;8(6):590–596.

[†]This is a simplified grading system applicable not only during initial screening but also during follow-up; it is useful in research clinical trials.

NEUROLOGIC DISABILITY SCORE FOR PERIPHERAL NEUROPATHY ASSESSMENT*

Name _____ Evaluation # _____ Date _____

Scoring: Enter 0 for no deficit, 1 for mild deficit, 2 for moderate deficit, 3 for severe deficit, and 4 for complete absence of function or severest deficit.

Evaluation	Right	Left
Cranial nerves		
Papilledema		
EOM weakness, Cr III		
EOM weakness, Cr VI		
Face weakness		
Palate weakness		
Tongue weakness		
Muscle weakness		
Respiratory		
Shoulder abduction		
Biceps brachii		
Brachioradialis		
Extension at elbow		
Extension at wrist		
Flexion at wrist		
Extension of fingers		
Flexion of fingers		
Intrinsic hand		
Iliopsoas		
Glutei		
Quadriceps		
Hamstrings		
Dorsiflexors		
Plantar flexors		
Reflexes		
Biceps brachii		
Triceps brachii		

---

*This form is used to obtain the neurologic disability score. The right and left columns are summated and added together. These scores can be adapted to meet the needs of specific studies. Form adapted from PJ Dyck, WR Sherman, LM Hallcher, et al. Human diabetic endoneural sorbitol, fructose, and myo-inositol relate to sural nerve morphometry. Ann Neurol 1980;8(6):590–596.

Brachioradialis		
Quadriceps femoris		
Triceps surae		
Sensation		
Index finger (below base of nail)		
Touch pressure		
Pricking pain		
Vibration		
Joint position sense		
Great toe (below base of nail)		
Touch pressure		
Pricking pain		
Vibration		
Joint position sense		
Sum		
Total		

Cr = cranial nerve; EOM = extraocular muscle.

DETECTION AND STAGING OF DIABETIC NEUROPATHY*

Staging

The following methods are used to determine stages in diabetic neuropathy:

Nerve conduction tests (NC)
Neurologic examination (NE)
Quantitative motor examination (QME)
Quantitative sensory examination (QSE)
Quantitative autonomic examination (QAE)
Neuropathic symptoms (NS)
Abnormalities in nerve conduction: ($\geq$3SD) of one or more attributes in two or more nerves. Motor conduction velocity, amplitude or area of CMAP, distal latency of peroneal and median nerve amplitude, area or latency or conduction velocity of median sensory and sural nerves.

Abnormalities of neurologic examination (NE): Abnormality of one or more of muscle strength, tendon reflexes (normal = 0; reduced = 1, absent = 2).

Sensory deficit in great toe, foot or index finger of touch, pain, vibration sense, position sense (reduced = 1; absent = 2).

Lack of pupillary response to light, postural hypotension or anhydrosis.

Quantitative motor examination (QME): One or more abnormalities of quantitative strength (QME).

Quantitative sensory examination (QSE): One or more abnormalities in quantitative sensory testing (QME), which include vibratory detection threshold (VDT), cooling (CDT), or warming (WDT).

Quantitative autonomic examination (QAE): One or more abnormalities in autonomic sensory testing.

Neuropathic symptoms (NS): Occurrence of any of the following symptoms judged to be caused by diabetic neuropathy, if not disabling, are graded: not disabling, stage 2; disabling, stage 3; questionable degrees of symptoms, stage 0 or 1.

Symptomatic Neuropathy

Occurrence of any symptoms (among the 12 listed below) judged to be due to diabetic polyneuropathy but not disabling (see Stage 3 below) is sufficient to fulfill the criteria for stage 2. Patients with questionable degrees of symptoms are staged as 1 or 0.

Motor

- Symptoms of muscle weakness in acts of daily living

Sensory

- Any of the following symptoms:

---

*Modified from PJ Dyck. Detection, characterization and staging of polyneuropathy: assessed in diabetics. Muscle Nerve 1988;11(1):21–32.

1. Absence of feeling: reported deficiency of tactile, thermal, or nociceptive sensation encountered in acts of daily living.
2. Sensory ataxia: reported unsteadiness in walking.
3. Numbness or paresthesia ("dead asleep," "prickly asleep," "like novocaine," "like hand gone asleep," etc.): judged by its distribution, persistence, and duration to be due to neuropathy and not due to physiologic compression as occurs in acts of daily living or entrapment (e.g., carpal tunnel syndrome or to another condition).
4. Neuropathic pain: burning, aching, excessive discomfort of feet or hands with use, and lancinating pain.

Autonomic

- Any of the following symptoms attributed to diabetes mellitus and not due to medications, psychologic disturbance, intercurrent illness, disease of the organ, or previous injury or surgery:

1. Gastric atony
2. Urinary retention
3. Urinary incontinence
4. Rectal incontinence
5. Diarrhea
6. Impotence in men younger than 65 years of age
7. Postural hypotension, lightheadedness or fainting (with postural decrease of systolic blood pressure $\geq$30 mm Hg)

Disabling Neuropathy

Disabling neuropathy (stage 3) is considered the occurrence of one or more of the following:

Motor

- Symptoms of muscle weakness, confirmed by examination of sufficient severity that the patient is unable to walk independently.

Sensory

1. Symptoms of sensory loss of sufficient severity, confirmed by examination, that the patient cannot walk independently because of sensory ataxia.
2. Absence of feeling in hands so that the patient is disabled.
3. Symptoms of pain, having the characteristics of neuropathic pain, that is disabling. The following criteria (a, b, and c) have to be fulfilled:
   a. The patient has previously attended physicians for pain relief.
   b. Work and recreational activities have been curtailed by at least 25% because of pain.
   c. Medication for pain relief has been taken on a continuing ($\geq$50% of days) basis for at least 6 weeks.

Autonomic

1. Gastric atony, as demonstrated by gastric retention tests and by exclusion of other gastric or psychiatric causes of emesis, causing emesis of retained ($\geq$18 hours) food at least once weekly for at least 6 weeks
2. Urinary retention as demonstrated by manometer evidence of detrusor hypoactivity and not due to psychiatric disturbance or urinary bladder disease necessitating continuous use of a catheter for 6 weeks or longer
3. Urinary incontinence due to loss of sphincter function necessitating continuous ($\geq$50% of time) use of diapers or leg urinal for at least 6 weeks and not due to psychologic or bladder disease
4. Rectal incontinence due to loss of sphincter function of at least 6 weeks duration and not due to psychiatric or rectal disease
5. Diarrhea to the degree that it causes weight loss ($\geq$5 kg) and steatorrhea $\geq$10 mg per 24 hours and not due to psychiatric disturbance, laxative abuse, or other bowel disease
6. Symptomatic lightheadedness or fainting due to orthostatic hypotension ($\geq$30 mm Hg systolic) with concomitant blood pressure drop, present continuously (lightheadedness or fainting weekly) for at least 6 weeks

Grading

Notation of Staged Severity of Diabetic Neuropathy

For a given patient, a shorthand designation might be used. The first component (from left to right) of the notation reflects the overall stage of neuropathy (0–3). The second component of the notation (placed in parentheses) gives the severity of motor (M), sensory (S), or autonomic (A) symptoms and deficits using 0–3 staging criteria. The third component of the notation reflects which evaluations were abnormal.

First Component of Notation

The symptoms and deficits from motor (M), sensory (S), or autonomic (A) fiber dysfunction are staged separately using the general staging approach given previously. Attributes of nerve conduction and state of the tendon reflexes are not used in staging the second component.

Motor
M0 = No symptoms or findings of muscle weakness (NE or QME)
M1 = No symptoms of weakness, but muscle weakness is demonstrated (NE or QME)
M2 = Symptoms of muscle weakness as described in stage 2, and muscle weakness (NE or QME) but of lesser severity than M3
M3 = Symptoms of muscle weakness as described under Disabling Neuropathy (3), motor item 1 previously, and muscle weakness (on NE or QME)

Sensory
S0 = No sensory symptoms or loss (NE or QSE)
S1 = No sensory symptoms and sensory deficit (NE or QSE)

S2 = Symptoms of sensory involvement as described under Symptomatic Neuropathy (2), sensory items 1–4 but of lesser severity than in stage 3, and sensory loss (NE or QSE)

S3 = Symptom of sensory fiber involvement as described under Disabling Neuropathy (3); sensory items 1, 2, or 3; and sensory loss (on NE or QSE)

Autonomic

A0 = Autonomic symptoms and no autonomic abnormality (NE or QAE)

A1 = No autonomic symptoms and autonomic deficit (NE or QAE)

A2 = Autonomic symptoms as described under Symptomatic Neuropathy, autonomic items 1–6, and autonomic deficit (NE or QAE)

A3 = Autonomic symptoms as described under Disabling Neuropathy, autonomic items 1–6, and autonomic deficit (NE or QAE)

Note the (A) overall stage of neuropathy (0–3); (B) grade the severity of motor sensory (S), or autonomic (A) symptoms. Grade for 0–3 and another description which is an indication reflexes are abnormal (for details see PJ Dyck. Detection, characterization and staging of polyneuropathy: assessed in diabetics. Muscle Nerve 1988;11[1]:21–32).

Stage Definitions

Stage 0 (no neuropathy): Fewer than two abnormalities among (1) NC: (2) NE (e.g., neurologic examination or Neurologic Disability Score); (3) QME, QSE, or QAE, or (4) NS (e.g., neuropathic symptoms or Neuropathic Symptom Score [NSS]). See definitions below.

Stage 1 (asymptomatic neuropathy): Two or more abnormalities among (1) NC; (2) NE; or (3) QME, QSE, or QAE, but no abnormality of NS.

Stage 2 (symptomatic neuropathy): Two or more abnormalities among (1) NC; (2) NE; (3) QME, QSE, or QAE; or (4) NS. Neuropathic symptoms are present but are of lesser severity than stage 3.

Stage 3 (disabling neuropathy): Two or more abnormalities among (1) NC, (2) NE; (3) QME, QSE, or QAE; or (4) NS. Disabling neuropathic symptoms are present.

QUANTITATIVE MYASTHENIA GRAVIS SCORE FOR DISEASE SEVERITY

Test Item	None	Mild	Moderate	Severe	Score
Grade	0	1	2	3	
Double vision on lateral gaze right or left (circle one), secs	61	11–60	1–10	Spontaneous	
Ptosis (upward gaze), secs	61	11–60	1–10	Spontaneous	
Facial muscles	Normal lid closure	Complete, weak, some resistance	Complete, without resistance	Incomplete	
Swallowing 4 oz water (¹/₂ cup)	Normal	Minimal coughing or throat clearing	Severe coughing, choking, or both or nasal regurgitation	Cannot swallow (test not attempted)	
Speech after counting aloud from 1 to 50 (onset of dysarthria)	None at 50	Dysarthria at 30–49	Dysarthria at 10–29	Dysarthria at 9	
Right arm outstretched (90-degree setting), secs	240	90–239	10–89	0–9	
Left arm outstretched (90-degree setting), secs	240	90–239	10–89	0–9	
Vital capacity, % predicted	≥80	65–79	50–64	<50	
Right-hand grip, kg					
Men	≥45	15–44	5–14	0–4	
Women	≥30	10–29	5–9	0–4	
Left-hand grip, kg					
Men	≥35	15–34	5–14	0–4	
Women	≥25	10–24	5–9	0–4	
Head lifted (45 degrees supine), secs	120	30–119	1–29	0	
Right leg outstretched (45 degrees supine), secs	100	31–99	1–30	0	
Left leg outstretched (45 degrees supine), secs	100	31–99	1–30	0	

Source: Reprinted with permission from RJ Barohn, D McIntire, L Herbelin, et al. Reliability testing of the quantitative myasthenia. Ann N Y Acad Sci 1998;841:769–772; and RJ Barohn. How to Administer Quantitative Myasthenic Tests [video]. Chicago: Myasthenia Gravis Foundation of America, 1996.

MYOTONIC DYSTROPHY: MUSCULAR IMPAIRMENT RATING SCALE

Grade	Description
1	No muscular impairment
2	Minimal signs—myotonia, jaw and temporal wasting, facial weakness, neck flexor weakness, ptosis, nasal speech, no distal weakness except isolated digit flexor weakness
3	Distal weakness—no proximal weakness except isolated elbow extensor weakness
4	Mild to moderate proximal weakness
5	Severe (Modified Medical Research Council scale, ≤ –3/5) proximal weakness

Source: Reprinted with permission from J Mathieu. Assessment of a disease-specific muscular impairment rating scale in myotonic dystrophy. Neurology 2001;56:336–340.

Appendix 4
Important Neuromuscular Web Sites

Tulio E. Bertorini, Pushpa Narayanaswami,
and Kandasami Senthilkumar

This list has useful addresses and Web sites, but as Web site addresses change
frequently, these addresses can be accessed by using search engines such as
Netscape, Yahoo!, or Google to find particular groups.

AMYOTROPHIC LATERAL SCLEROSIS AND OTHER MOTOR NEURON DISEASES

The ALS Association
National Office
27001 Agoura Rd
Suite 150
Calabasas Hills, CA 91301-5104
Information and referral service:
　(800) 782-4747
All other calls: (818) 880-9007
http://www.alsa.org

The ALS Association of Canada
265 Yorkland Blvd
Suite 300
Toronto, Ontario M2J 1S5
Canada
Phone: (800) 267-4257
http://www.als.ca

The ALS C.A.R.E Program-Center for
　Outcomes Research
University of Massachusetts School of
　Medicine
Supported by an unrestricted grant from
　Aventis Pharmaceuticals
http://www.umassmed.edu

World Federation of Neurology,
　Amyotrophic Lateral Sclerosis
http://www.wfnals.org

ALS Survival Guide
http://www.lougehrigsdisease.net
http://www.alssurvivalguide.com

Hope for ALS
http://www.hopeforals.com/index.html

International Alliance of MND/ALS
　Associations
http://www.alsmndalliance.org

The Motor Neurone Disease (MND)
   Association
PO Box 246
Northampton NN1 2PR
United Kingdom
Phone: +44 01604 250505
Fax: +44 01604 638289/624726
Help line: +44 08457 626262
E-mail: enquiries@mndassociation.org
http://www.mndassociation.org

Families of Spinal Muscular Atrophy
PO Box 196
Libertyville, IL 60048-0196
Phone: (800) 886-1762
http://www.fsma.org

Spinal Muscular Atrophy.net
http://www.affari.com/smanet

ATAXIA

National Ataxia Foundation
2600 Fernbrook Ln
Suite 119
Minneapolis, MN 55447
Phone: (763) 553-0020
Fax: (763) 553-0167
E-mail: naf@ataxia.org
http://www.ataxia.org

A-T Children's Project
668 S. Military Trail
Deerfield Beach, FL 33442
Phone: (800) 5-HELP-A-T
E-mail: info@atcp.org
http://www.atcp.org

Friedreich's Ataxia Parents Group
http://www.fortnet.org/fapg

Friedreich's Ataxia Research Alliance
2001 Jefferson Davis Hwy
Suite 209
Arlington, VA 22202
Phone: (703) 413-4468
Fax: (703) 413-4467
E-mail: fara@frda.org
http://www.members.home.net/frda

International Network of Ataxia Friends
E-mail: internaf-owner
   @yahoogroups.com
http://www.internaf.org

CLINICAL TRIALS

CenterWatch Clinical Trials Listing
   Service
CenterWatch
22 Thomson Pl, 36T1
Boston, MA 02210-1212
Phone: (617) 856-5900
Fax: (617) 856-5901
http://www.centerwatch.com

ELECTROMYOGRAPHY AND NERVE CONDUCTION

EMG and Nerve Conductions
   Homepage
A site featuring nerve and muscle
   disease testing, doctor/patient
   discussion groups, anatomical charts,
   and technical descriptions of
   electromyography and nerve
   conduction studies.
http://www.teleemg.com

Nerve Conduction Studies
http://madison-tate.virtualave.net/
   nerve_conduction_studies.html

EMG Teaching Cases—University of
   Texas Health Science Center at San
   Antonio
Daniel Dumitru, M.D., Professor and
   Deputy Chairman
Department of Rehabilitation Medicine
http://www.daffodil.uthscsa.edu/faculty/
   dumitru/emgs/Default.htm

American Academy of Physical
   Medicine and Rehabilitation
AAPM&R EMG Cases
http://www.aapmr.org/cme/emg.htm

Disabled Peoples' International
http://www.dpi.org/links.html

Clinical Neurophysiology
Department of Neuroscience
University Hospital Uppsala
SE-751 85 Uppsala
Sweden
Phone: +46 18 611 34 35
Fax: +46 18 55 61 06

FIBROMYALGIA

Fibromyalgia Network
PO Box 31750
Tucson, AZ 85751
Phone: (800) 853-2929
http://www.fmnetnews.com

American Fibromyalgia Syndrome
    Association, Inc.
6380 E. Tanque Verde
Suite D
Tucson, AZ 85715
Phone: (520) 733-1570
http://www.afsafund.org

GENETICS

OMIM
Online Mendelian Inheritance in Man
http://www3.ncbi.nlm.nih.gov/Omim

GeneClinics
Funded by the NIH
Developed at the University of
    Washington, Seattle
http://www.geneclinics.org

GeneTests
Funded by the National Library of
    Medicine of the NIH and Maternal
    Child Health Bureau of HRSA
http://www.genetests.org

Glossary of Genetic Terms
http://www.nhgri.nih.gov/DIR/VIP/
    Glossary

Genetic Information
http://www.humgen.umontreal.ca/en/
    GenInfo.cfm

MITOMAP
A Human Mitochondrial Genome Data-
    base
Center for Molecular Medicine
Emory University
Atlanta, GA
http://www.gen.emory.edu/mitomap.html

University of Montreal Information
    Center for Policies and Registration
    for Genetic Testing
http://www.humgen.umontreal.ca/en/
    GenInfo.cfm

MALIGNANT HYPERTHERMIA

Malignant Hyperthermia Association of
    the United States
39 E. State St
PO Box 1069
Sherburne, NY 13460
Phone: (607) 674-7901
Fax: (607) 674-7910
E-mail: Jo@mhaus.org
http://www.mhaus.org

MEDLINE

PubMed, a service of the National
    Library of Medicine
http://www4.ncbi.nlm.nih.gov/entrez/
    query.fcgi

MedExplorer: Neurology
http://www.medexplorer.com/
    subcategory.dbm

MUSCULAR DYSTROPHY

Muscular Dystrophy Association-USA
National Headquarters
3300 E. Sunrise Dr
Tucson, AZ 85718
Phone: (800) 572-1717
http://www.mdausa.org

Muscular Dystrophy Association of
  Canada
National Office
2345 Yonge St
Suite 900
Toronto, ON M4P 2E5
Canada
Phone: (416) 488-0030
  (800) 567-2873
Fax: (416) 488-7523
E-mail: info@mdac.ca
http://www.mdac.ca

Muscular Dystrophy Association-
  Australia
GPO Box 9932
Melbourne 3001
Australia
Phone: +61 3 9370 0477
Free call: 1 800 656 MDA
Fax: +61 3 9370 0393
E-mail: bms@mda.org.au
http://www.mda.org.au

Parent Project Muscular
  Dystrophy
Headquarters
1012 N. University Ave
Middletown, OH 45044
Phone: (513) 424-0696
  (800) 714-KIDS
Fax: (513) 425-9907
E-mail: patfurlong@aol.com
http://www.parentdmd.org

The Muscular Dystrophy Family
  Foundation, Inc.
2330 N. Meridian St
Indianapolis, IN 46208-5730
Phone: (800) 544-1213
E-mail: mdff@prodigy.net
http://www.mdff.org

Duchenne Muscular Dystrophy
  Research Center (DMDRC)
  International
http://www.dmdrc.org/dmdrc.html

The Cooperative International
  Neuromuscular Research Group
Children's Research Institute
Children's National Medical Center
111 Michigan Ave, NW
Washington, DC 20010
Phone: (202) 884-3813
Fax: (202) 884-6014
http://63.75.201.101/cinrg

Duchenne Muscular Dystrophy
  Research Center
University of California
5833 Life Science Bldg
University of California
Los Angeles, CA 90095
E-mail: dmdrc@physci.ucla.edu
http://www.physci.ucla.edu/DMD

FacioScapuloHumeral Muscular
  Dystrophy Society
3 Westwood Rd
Lexington, MA 02420
Phone: (781) 860-0501
Fax: (781) 860-0599
E-mail: carol.perez@fshsociety.org
http://www.fshsociety.org

The Muscular Dystrophy
  Campaign
Nattrass House
7-11 Prescott Pl
London SW4 6BS
United Kingdom
Phone: +44 020 7720 8055
Fax: +44 020 7498 0670
E-mail: info@muscular-dystrophy.org
http:// www.muscular-dystrophy.org

Muscular Dystrophy—Ireland
Carmichael Centre
Coleraine House
Coleraine Street
Dublin 7
Ireland
Phone: +353 01-8721501 / 8723826
E-mail: info@mdi.ie
http://www.mdi.ie

European Alliance of Muscular
Dystrophy Associations (EAMDA)
EAMDA Secretariat
7-11 Prescott Pl
London, SW4 6BS
United Kingdom
Phone: +44 71 720805
Fax: +44 71 4980670
E-mail: mail@eamda.sonnet.co.uk
http://www.sonnet.co.uk/eamda

The World Alliance of Neuromuscular Dis-
order Associations (WANDA) c/o The
Muscular Dystrophy Association, Inc.
GPO Box 414
Adelaide SA 5001
Australia
Phone: +61 8 82345266
Fax: +61 8 82345866
E-mail: info@mdasa.org.au
http://www.w-a-n-d-a.org

Patient Resources: Neuromuscular
Diseases
http://www.neuro.wustl.edu/
neuromuscular/over/resource.htm

Emery-Dreifuss Muscular Dystrophy
Mutation Database
Dr. John Yates
Cambridge University
Department of Medical Genetics
Box 134 Addenbrookes Hospital
Cambridge CB2 2QQ
United Kingdom
E-mail: jyates@hgmp.mrc.ac.uk
http://www.path.cam.ac.uk/emd

Muscular Dystrophy Association of
New Zealand
National Office
7A Taylors Rd
Morningside, Auckland
PO Box 16-238
Sandringham, Auckland 1030
New Zealand
Phone: +64 9 815 0247
Fax: +64 9 815 7260
Free phone: 0800-800-337
E-mail: director@mda.org.nz
http://www.mda.org.nz

Leiden Muscular Dystrophy pages
Department of Human and Clinical
Genetics,
Leiden University Medical Center
http://www.dmd.nl

International Myotonic Dystrophy
Organization
764 Old Westbury Rd
Crystal Lake, IL 60012
Phone: (815) 477-0047
http://www.myotonicdystrophy.com

MYASTHENIA GRAVIS

Myasthenia Gravis Foundation of
America
5841 Cedar Lake Rd
Suite 204
Minneapolis, MN 55416
Phone: (952) 545-9438
    (800) 541-5454
Fax: (952) 545-6073
http://www.myasthenia.org

MYOPATHY

Myositis Association of America
755 Cantrell Ave
Suite C
Harrisonburg, VA 22801
Fax: (540) 432-0206
E-mail: maa@myositis.org
http://www.myositis.org

United Mitochondrial Disease
Foundation
http://www.umdf.org

Advancement of Research in
Myopathies
Non-profit foundation with the primary
goal of speeding up the research on
HIBM
PO Box 261926
Encino, CA 91426
Phone: (800) ARM-2000 (1-800-276-
2000)
http://www.hibm.org

Association Française contre les
   Myopathies
http://www.afm-france.org

CARMEN
Concerted Action for Research into
   Myopathies due to Enzyme
   Deficiencies
http://carmen.bi.umist.ac.uk

NEUROFIBROMATOSIS

National NF Foundation
95 Pine St, 16th Floor
New York, NY 10005
Phone: (212) 344-6633
   (800) 323-7938
Fax: (212) 747-0004
E-mail: NNFF@nf.org or
   NNFF@aol.com
http://www.nf.org

Neurofibromatosis, Inc.
8855 Annapolis Rd
Suite 110
Lanham, MD 20706-2924
Phone: (301) 577-8984
   (800) 942-6825.
Fax: (301) 577-0016
http://www.nfinc.org

NEUROMUSCULAR CENTERS

Neuromuscular Disease Center
Washington University School of
   Medicine, St. Louis, Missouri
http://www.neuro.wustl.edu/
   neuromuscular

European Neuromuscular Centre
Information on the diagnosis and epidemiology of neuromuscular diseases.
http://www.enmc.org

European Neuromuscular Centre:
   Diagnostic Criteria for
   Neuromuscular Disorders
http://www.enmc.org

MuscleNET
http://www.telethon.bio.unipd.it

The World Muscle Society (WMS)
http://www.ior.it/wms

New York Online Access to Health
   (NOAH)
Ask NOAH about: Neurological
   Problems
http://www.noah-health.org/english/
   illness/neuro/neuropg.html

Information on Human Neurological
   Diseases
http://www.neuroguide.com/
   neurodis.html

Neuroland-Neuromuscular Disease Info
   Center
http://www.neuroland.com/nm

Karolinska Institutet: Nervous System
   Diseases (Sweden)
http://www.mic.ki.se/Diseases/c10.html

Enfermedades Neuromusculares
   (Argentina)
http://www.neuromuscular.com.ar

NEUROPATHOLOGY

Neuropathology of the Internet
A searchable and browsable directory
   compiled for medical students,
   residents, and other health
   professionals.
http://www.neuropat.dote.hu

NEUROPATHY

Guillain-Barré Syndrome Foundation
   International
PO Box 262
Wynnewood, PA 19096
Phone: (610) 667-0131
Fax: (610) 667-7036
E-mail: gbint@ix.netcom.com
http://www.guillain-barre.com

Guillain-Barré Syndrome Support
Group
http://www.gbs.org.uk

Guillain-Barré Syndrome Support
Group: Chronic Inflammatory
Demyelinating
Polyradiculoneuropathy
http://www.gbs.org.uk/cidp.html

The Neuropathy Association
60 E. 42nd Street
Suite 942
New York, NY 10165
Phone: (212) 692-0662
E-mail: info@neuropathy.org
http://www.neuropathy.org

The Charcot-Marie-Tooth Association
2700 Chestnut St
Chester, PA 19013-4867
Phone: (610) 499-9264
    (610) 499-9265
    (800) 606-2682
Fax: (610) 499-9267
http://www.charcot-marie-tooth.org

The Charcot-Marie-Tooth International
1 Springbank Dr
St. Catharine's
Ontario, L2S 2K1
Canada
Phone: (905) 687-3630
Fax: (905) 687-8753
E-mail: cmtint@vaxxine.com
http://www.passy-muir.com/
    resource.htm

Charcot-Marie-Tooth International of
the United Kingdom
121 Lavernock Rd
Penarth
CF64 3QG
United Kingdom
Phone: +44 02920 709537
http://www.cmt.org.uk

CMTnet
http://www.ultranet.com/~smith/
    CMTneto.html

The Peripheral Neuropathy Italian
Association
http://www.neuropatia.it

ORGANIZATIONS

American Academy of Neurology
1080 Montreal Ave
St. Paul, MN 55116
Phone: (651) 695-1940
Fax: (651) 695-2791
http://www.aan.com

American Neurological
Association
5841 Cedar Lake Rd
Suite 204
Minneapolis, MN 55416
Phone: (952) 545-6284
Fax: (952) 545-6073
http://www.aneuroa.org

Myasthenia Gravis
Association
http://www.mgauk.org

American Association of
Electrodiagnostic Medicine
(AAEM)
421 First Avenue SW
Suite 300 East
Rochester, MN 55902
Phone: (507) 288-0100
Fax: (507) 288-1225
E-mail: aaem@aaem.net
http://www.aaem.net

Child Neurology Society
1000 W. County Rd E
Suite 126
St. Paul, MN 55126
Phone: (651) 486-9447
Fax: (651) 486-9436
E-mail: nationaloffice@
    childneurologysociety.org
http://www.childneurologysociety.org

Child Neurology Society
http://www.cparent.com/rcsourccs/
    associations/cns.htm

The Centers for Disease Control and
Prevention (CDC)
http://www.cdc.gov/default.htm

National Institute of Arthritis and
Musculoskeletal and Skin Diseases
http://www.nih.gov/niams

National Institute of Neurological
Disorders and Stroke
http://www.ninds.nih.gov

National Organization for Rare
Disorders, Inc.
PO Box 892
New Fairfield, CT 06812-8923
http://www.rarediseases.org/cgi-bin/
nord

Office of Rare Diseases
National Institutes of Health
31 Center Dr, MSC 2084
Bldg 31, Room 1B-19
Bethesda, MD 20892-2084
Phone: (301) 402-4336
Fax: (301) 480-9655
E-mail: hh70f@nih.gov
http://www.rarediseases.info.nih.gov/
ord/index.html

National Institute of Neurological
Disorders and Stroke
For inquiries regarding NINDS
Extramural Programs:
NINDS-Neuroscience Center
Division of Extramural Research
6001 Executive Blvd
Suite 3309
Bethesda, MD 20892-9531
For health or medical questions and
general information:
NIH Neurological Institute
PO Box 5801
Bethesda, MD 20824
Phone: (800) 352-9424
http://www.ninds.nih.gov

Capítulo Argentino de Lucha contra las
Enfermedades de la Motoneurona
Tucuman 950 Piso 4 Dto 23
1049-Buenos Aires
Argentina
Phone/Fax: +54 11 4393 6753
http://www.calmo.org.ar

Child Neurology Home Page
http://www.waisman.wisc.edu/child-
neuro/index.html

American Association of Neuroscience
Nurses
4700 W. Lake Ave
Glenview, IL 60025
Phone: (888) 557-2266 (inside of the
United States only)
Phone: (847) 375-4733
http://www.aann.org

The National Association For Home Care
228 Seventh St SE
Washington, DC 20003
Phone: (202) 547-7424
Fax: (202) 547-3540
http://www.nahc.org

American Physical Therapy Association
1111 N. Fairfax St
Alexandria, VA 22314-1488
http://www.apta.org

American Occupational Therapy
Association
4720 Montgomery Ln
PO Box 31220
Bethesda, MD 20824-1220
Phone: (301) 652-2682
Fax: (301) 652-7711
http://www.aota.org

American Speech-Language-Hearing
Association, Inc.
10801 Rockville Pike
Rockville, MD 20852
Phone: (800) 638-8255
http://www.asha.org

Case Management Association of America
8201 Cantrell Rd
Suite 230
Little Rock, AR 72227
Phone: (501) 225-2229
Fax: (501) 221-9068
http://www.cmsa.org

PHYSIOLOGY

Muscle Physiology Home Page
University of California, San Diego
The Muscle Physiology
    Laboratory
VA Medical Center (mail code 151)
3350 La Jolla Village Dr
San Diego, CA 92161
Phone: (858) 552-8585 ext. 7016
Fax: (858) 552-4381
http://www-neuromus.ucsd.edu

Index

Note: Page numbers followed by *f* indicate figures; numbers followed by *t* indicate tables.